ARCHIVES OF DISEASE IN CHILDHOOD

VOLUME XXXIII, 1958

LONDON
BRITISH MEDICAL ASSOCIATION
TAVISTOCK SQUARE, W.C.1

CONTENTS

No. 167. *FEBRUARY 1958*

	PAGE
Some Physical Measurements in the First Three Years of Life. FRANK FALKNER	1
Growth and Development in a Group of Children of Very Low Birth Weight. CECIL M. DRILLIEN	10
The Prognosis of Bronchiectasis in Childhood. ALFRED WHITE FRANKLIN	19
A Consideration of Colostrum and Milk as Sources of Antibodies which may be Transferred to the Newborn Baby. KATHLEEN E. BOORMAN, BARBARA E. DODD and MAVIS GUNTHER	24
The Serum Proteins at 6 Months of Age in Infants Fed on Human or Cow's Milk or on Both. FATMA HASSAN and MAVIS GUNTHER	30
The Dietary Treatment of Phenylketonuria. L. I. WOOLF, RUTH GRIFFITHS, ALAN MONCRIEFF, STEPHEN COATES and F. DILLISTONE	31
Parathyroid Adenoma in a Child Presenting as Rickets. B. S. B. WOOD, W. H. GEORGE and A. W. ROBINSON	46
Acromegaly in a Girl of 8 Years. R. MCLAREN TODD	49
Malignant Non-chromaffin Paraganglioma of the Thigh. A. MACFARLANE and A. R. MACGREGOR	55
Gumma of the Liver in Congenital Syphilis. D. WHITEHOUSE and W. V. MACFARLANE	58
Paper Electrophoresis of Serum Proteins in Children. W. W. PAYNE and CONSTANCE C. FORSYTH	61
A Clinical and Haemodynamic Study of Ventricular Septal Defect in Infants. GEORGE M. MAXWELL, GEORGE G. ROWE and CHARLES W. CRUMPTON	67
Sweat Analysis in Fibrocystic Disease, Chronic Pulmonary Disease and Controls. MARY M. WEEKS and G. A. BROWN	74
The Gastro-oesophageal Region in Infants. G. S. MULLER BOTHA	78
Paediatric Societies in the British Isles	95
Book Reviews	96

No. 168. *APRIL 1958*

Regional Obstructive Emphysema in Infancy. JAMES THOMSON and JOHN O. FORFAR	97
An Inborn Error of Metabolism with the Urinary Excretion of α-Hydroxy-Butyric Acid and Phenyl-pyruvic Acid. ALAN J. SMITH and LEONARD B. STRANG	109
A Case of Hartnup Disease. WALTER HENDERSON	114
Dissociation as a Guide to Developmental Assessment. R. S. ILLINGWORTH	118
Dysmaturity. S. SJÖSTEDT, G. ENGLESON and G. ROOTH	123
Congenital Interruption of the Aortic Arch. BRIDGET V. FOLEY	131
Normal Diameter of the Heart in Radiographs of Pre-School Children. DAVID HEWITT	134
The Changing Aetiology of Erythema Nodosum in Children. JOHN LORBER	137
Clinical and Biochemical Changes During Exchange Transfusion. JAMES W. FARQUHAR and HYLTON SMITH	142
Treatment of Persistent Enuresis with the Electric Buzzer. IAN G. WICKES	160
Recurrent Abdominal Pains: A Field Survey of 1,000 School Children. JOHN APLEY and NORA NAISH	165
Salmonella Meningitis. KENNETH C. WATSON	171
Calcified Mesenteric Lymphangioma. R. L. BISHTON, C. P. SAMES and HUGH R. E. WALLIS	176
Sweat Test for the Diagnosis of Fibrocystic Disease of the Pancreas. K. A. MISCH and H. M. HOLDEN	179
Paediatric Pathology Club	181
Book Reviews	183

No. 169. *JUNE 1958*

PAGE

ABO Incompatibility and Haemolytic Disease of the Newborn. G. H. VALENTINE 185

The Disappearance of Foetal Haemoglobin in Congenital Cyanotic Heart Disease. M. K. COGHLAN and M. C. JOSEPH 191

Basophilic Leucocytes in Children in Health and Disease. ROSS G. MITCHELL 193

Intraperitoneal Blood Transfusion in Children in Accra with Special Reference to the Treatment of Kwashiorkor. SUSAN B. G. OFORI ATTA 202

Traumatic Subperiosteal Haematoma of the Femur in the Newborn. ROSS G. MITCHELL and K. RHANEY 205

Subglottic Haemangioma: Two Infants with Laryngeal Stridor. C. A. HOLBOROW 210

Intraspinal Neuroblastoma in a Newborn Baby. E. ELEFANT, V. VOJTA and V. BENEŠ .. 212

Some Unusual Findings in a Family with Friedreich's Ataxia. PETER E. SYLVESTER 217

A Case of Intracranial Dermoid Cyst Associated with the Klippel-Feil Deformity and Recurrent Meningitis. A. PETER ROBERTS 222

Sirenomelia: Sympus Dipus ('Mermaid'). HUGH JOLLY and EDITH M. LAMONT 226

Gargoylism: Clinical, Radiological and Haematological Features in Two Siblings. S. B. GRIFFITHS and M. FINDLAY 229

Hydranencephaly (Hydrencephaly). L. CROME and PETER E. SYLVESTER 235

The Wenckebach Phenomenon and Auricular-ventricular Dissociation in Children. M. H. SHNIER 246

A Salt Wasting Syndrome in Infancy. DONALD B. CHEEK and JOHN W. PERRY 252

Anorexia and Severe Inanition Associated with a Tumour Involving the Hypothalamus. HELEN KAGAN 257

Acute Spinal Epidural Abscess: A Case in an Infant with Recovery. R. G. RUSHWORTH and P. B. MARTIN 261

Cow's Milk Allergy in Infancy. W. DAVIES 265

Frank Beriberi in a 4-month-old Infant. TADEUSZ GIZA and JERZY ARMATA 269

William Heberden's Cases of Anaphylactoid Purpura. ARTHUR ROOK 271

Book Reviews 272

No. 170. *AUGUST 1958*

Paediatrics in Western Nigeria. MALCOLM MACGREGOR 277

Phlyctenular Conjunctivitis in African Children. HARRY STEIN and IDA FREIMAN 292

Hormone Excretion in Precocious Puberty in Girls. R. D. BULBROOK, F. C. GREENWOOD and A. H. SNAITH 295

Urinary Excretion of 17-Ketosteroids in Children. MARGARET PROUT and A. H. SNAITH .. 301

The Urinary Excretion of 17-Hydroxysteroids in Children. R. GARDNER and A. H. SNAITH .. 305

The Prognosis in Juvenile Obesity. A. G. MULLINS 307

Diabetes Insipidus following Tuberculous Meningitis. JOHN LORBER 315

Diabetes Mellitus in a Child showing Features of Refsum's Syndrome. J. B. HEYCOCK and J. WILSON 320

The Post-Natal Weight Loss of Babies Born to Diabetic and Non-diabetic Women. JAMES W. FARQUHAR and STANLEY A. SKLAROFF 323

Jaundice and Infantile Diarrhoea. R. G. F. PARKER 330

Congenital Spherocytosis in Infancy. DAVID BURMAN 335

Congenital Heart Disease in One of Identical Twins. H. EVERLEY JONES 342

The Electrocardiographic Recognition of Ventricular Hypertrophy in Congenital Cardiovascular Disease during the First Year of Life. J. S. OLDHAM 346

The Differential Diagnosis of Rheumatic Fever. K. A. HALLIDIE-SMITH and E. G. L. BYWATERS 350

PAGE

A Small Outbreak of Neonatal Meningitis in a Maternity Unit. ERIC McKAY and JOHN SMITH 358
Neonatal Perforation of the Colon. LEONARD HAAS 362
Bilateral Pulmonary Agenesis. ALBERT E. CLAIREAUX and H. P. FERREIRA 364
Atresia of the Oesophagus with Common Tracheo-Oesophageal Tube. R. G. WELCH and O. A. N. HUSAIN 367
Psychogenic Megacolon in Children: The Implications of Bowel Negativism. PHILIP PINKERTON 371
British Paediatric Association: Proceedings of the Twenty-ninth Annual General Meeting .. 381
Book Reviews 384

NO. 171. *OCTOBER 1958*

Severe Infantile Hypercalcaemia with Special Reference to the Facies. M. C. JOSEPH and D. PARROTT 385
Congenital Absence of the Intrahepatic Bile Ducts. LEONARD HAAS and RICHARD H. DOBBS .. 396
Replacement Transfusion as a Means of Preventing Kernikterus of Prematurity. V. MARY CROSSE, PATRICIA G. WALLIS and ANNA M. WALSH 403
Serum Transaminase Variations in Childhood. PAOLO TOLENTINO and MARCELLA ROSSI .. 409
A Test for Coeliac Disease. W. W. PAYNE and V. JENKINSON 413
A Longitudinal Study of the Growth and Development of Prematurely and Maturely Born Children.
Part I. Introduction. CECIL MARY DRILLIEN 417
Part II. Physical Development. CECIL MARY DRILLIEN 423
Pancreatitis in Young Children. J. COLLINS 432
Herpes Zoster Ophthalmicus in Children. S. M. TUCKER 437
Observations on the Bromide Partition Test in the Diagnosis of Non-purulent Meningitis. V. S. NICOL and H. T. FAWNS 440
Pneumatosis Intestinalis in Chinese Children. C. S. MUIR 445
Physical Development of Schoolgirls in Upper Burma. C. V. FOLL 452
The Prevalence of Dental Caries in Relation to Maturity. J. N. MANSBRIDGE 455
Familial Dysautonomia. T. McKENDRICK 465
Autopsy Findings in a Case of Pituitary Dwarfism. A. T. SANDISON 469
Insufficient Glucuronide Formation in the Newborn and its Relationship to the Pathogenesis of Icterus Neonatorum. M. VEST 473
The First Arch Syndrome. J. McKENZIE 477
Book Reviews 487

NO. 172. *DECEMBER 1958*

The Fluid Shift from the Vascular Compartment Immediately After Birth. DOUGLAS GAIRDNER, JOHN MARKS, JANET D. ROSCOE and R. O. BRETTELL 489
The Plasma Amino Acids in Malnutrition: Preliminary Observations. ROLAND G. WESTALL, ÉLLEN ROITMAN, CARMEN DE LA PEÑA, HOWARD RASMUSSEN, JOAQUIN CRAVIOTO, FEDERICO GÓMEZ and L. EMMETT HOLT, JR. 499
Hypocalcaemic Tetany Developing within 36 Hours of Birth. W. S. CRAIG and M. F. G. BUCHANAN 505
Cellular Immunity at Birth: The Mechanism and Nature of the Phagocytic Response. M. S. EDWARDS, L. L. GRIFFITHS and P. N. SWIFT 512
Thrombotic Microangiopathic Haemolytic Anaemia. M. J. ROBINSON, N. P. ORCHARD and A. R. EDEN 520

PAGE

Acute Acquired Haemolytic Anaemia Associated with Herpes Simplex Infection. R. McLaren Todd and N. V. O'Donohoe 524

Haemolytic Anaemia in a Child Receiving Nitrofurantoin. David Levy and Alice Porgess .. 527

Erythrocyte Sedimentation Rate, C-Reactive Protein Determination, Serum Protein Fractions, Fibrinogen Level and Antistreptolysin Reaction in 52 Rheumatic Children. N. Popov and S. Stanisheva 529

The Prognosis of Idiopathic Renal Acidosis in Infancy with Observations on Urine Acidification and Ammonia Production in Children. Elizabeth U. Buchanan and G. M. Komrower .. 532

Diastematomyelia. C. C. Michael James and L. P. Lassman 536

A Case of Cushing's Syndrome in an Infant. E. Goldblatt and A. H. Snaith 540

Epidemics of Gastro-enteritis Associated with *Esch. coli* O119 Infection. K. Hugh-Jones and G. I. M. Ross 543

Book Reviews 552

Index to Volume 33 553

SOME PHYSICAL MEASUREMENTS IN THE FIRST THREE YEARS OF LIFE

BY

FRANK FALKNER*

From the Child Study Centre, Institutes of Child Health and Education, University of London

(RECEIVED FOR PUBLICATION JULY 1, 1957)

There are few standards of physical measurements available for pre-school children in the British Isles. Gore and Palmer (1949) published cross-sectional data of the pre-school period based on measurements taken in 1947. Within each age-group sample there were differences of weeks or months between ages of individual children. The most recent publication of cross-sectional data in this age period was from the Oxford Child Health Survey in 1955 (Acheson, Kemp and Parfit, 1955) and gives standards of height and weight for children born between 1944 and 1948. This was a longitudinal study, but no incremental data were given. The late Professor Low's (1952) raw data have been published on several measurements for a group of children followed for the first five years of life and who were born between 1923 and 1927. So far as is known these are the only longitudinal data in this age period in the United Kingdom published up till now.

The following standards of children born between 1952 and 1954 are presented. For details of the sample, method of recruitment and investigations carried out, etc., reference may be made to Moore, Hindley and Falkner (1954). Briefly, the sample consists of 'healthy' unselected children, and these same children are followed regularly from birth. They are drawn from an area in London. The children are seen at the ages of 4 weeks (± 2 days), 13, 26, 39 weeks, 1 year, 18 months (± 7 days), 2 years and thence yearly (± 14 days). The majority of children are seen very close to the correct date and never outside these stated limits.

It may be remarked that at 3 years the number of children forming the sample drops considerably. At the time of analysis not all the original children had reached 3 years of age—a common happening in running analyses of longitudinal studies.

Measurements

All the measurements were taken by one of four measurers, the majority being taken by one person, and the rest divided equally between the other three. All were trained. When a new measurer joined the team he or she was taught by a trained member, and checks of individual errors and variations were made from time to time. Lincoln (1930) has shown the very great improvement in accuracy after such training whereby important large errors are reduced to minimal ones.

Increments

Known gains in specific measurements are a valuable indication of rate of growth and progress. Krogman (1956) has said: 'It is a source of great weakness that this aspect of growth analysis is so consistently neglected.' Increments may be calculated only from children followed longitudinally and not from cross-sectional data. Increments presented in this paper are means calculated on children seen at the beginning and end of an incremental period. (Not all the children are able to present themselves for their appointed examinations every time.) 'Adjusted mean increments' will be given and the term needs explanation. It was clearly convenient to use 13 weeks as the standard comparative incremental period. Not all the intervals are 13 weeks; for example, 4 to 13 weeks is 9 weeks. These intervals were therefore 'adjusted' to bring them to a comparable 13-week period. This may not be entirely permissible, for it presumes that the rate of growth of the particular measurement is rectilinear at that time which may not, in fact, be so; but the periods between examinations are felt to be short enough to justify this where it has been necessary.

In presenting the increments of the children it might be argued that those children who were able to be included by virtue of being seen at the beginning and end of each incremental period, and

* Present address: University of Louisville Medical School, Louisville, Kentucky.

TABLE 1

MEAN RECUMBENT-LENGTH OF CHILD STUDY CENTRE CHILDREN AT 4 WEEKS TO 3 YEARS
(In inches to nearest 0·1 inch, and cm. to nearest mm. 1 S.D. of mean given)

Ages	Boys					Girls				
	No.	Inches		Cm.		No.	Inches		Cm.	
		Mean	S.D.	Mean	S.D.		Mean	S.D.	Mean	S.D.
4 wks.	82	21·2	0·9	53·9	2·3	77	20·7	0·7	52·5	1·8
13 wks.	96	23·7	0·9	60·2	2·4	85	22·9	0·6	58·2	1·6
26 wks.	94	26·3	0·9	66·7	2·4	81	25·5	0·8	64·8	2·6
39 wks.	84	28·1	1·0	71·3	2·6	78	27·3	1·0	69·3	2·6
1 yr.	80	29·5	1·1	75·0	2·7	78	28·9	1·0	73·3	2·6
18 mos.	77	32·0	1·2	81·2	3·2	66	31·4	0·9	79·7	2·4
2 yrs.	55	34·0	1·5	86·5	3·7	54	33·3	1·2	84·5	3·1
3 yrs.	28	37·1	1·9	94·1	4·8	21	37·0	1·4	94·1	3·4

thus more regularly, were not necessarily representative of the whole group. With this in mind, this possibility was examined and there was found to be no significant difference between the different groups, at the different ages, in size of recumbent-length, weight, crown–rump measurement or head circumference.

Length and Weight Measurements

Length. There is a difference in an individual's recumbent-length and standing height. Boyd (1929), on children aged 2–5 years, found differences of 1·0 to 1·5 cm., and with older children differences up to 3·0 cm. occur. Since children who can actually stand are not necessarily able to be stood erect in the correct position (Krogman, 1950), it is felt that measurement of standing height before the age of 3 years and possibly 4 is probably unreliable. All measurements of length in this series of children were taken with the child nude lying on a horizontal measuring table. Such tables have been developed by Todd at Western Reserve University, Thompson at Yale, Schultz at Johns Hopkins University and by Knott (1941), Hindley (1953), Thomson (1956) and Falkner (1957). The technique used is well summarized by Krogman (1950). The estimated maximum error was $\pm 0{\cdot}5\%$. Children were measured either in the morning or in the afternoon. Time of day is important in measuring height, for children can 'lose' 2 cm. in a day and 1 cm. can be lost in the first hour. This can be 'put back' again after a rest (Palmer, 1930; Redfield and Meredith, 1938; Boyd, 1929). This source of error is lessened in measuring recumbent-length, but at the same time the children were stretched (not severely) just before actual measurement.

Weight. All children were weighed in the nude to the nearest ounce on either a basket-scale or a platform beam balance (both periodically checked) according to age. Percentiles are given in the weight tables rather than standard deviations, for weight is not normally distributed (it is positively skewed), whereas recumbent-length is nearly so.

Figs. 1 and 2 show graphically* the data from Tables 1, 2, 3 and 4.

* In a study such as this there are several ways of plotting the data (Tanner, 1951), for not all the children are seen every time. Those that are at the beginning and the end of each incremental period only may be used to plot the velocity curve. Hence the distance curve can be plotted by using the maximum number of children seen at each age—in other words, using the longitudinal study cross-sectionally—or by plotting it from the velocity curve, having started with a mean size at birth or 4 weeks of age. (These are not the only ways (see Tanner, 1951), but the most simple, practical and least complicated.) All the distance curves plotted in this paper are from means at each age, but in each case curves were also plotted from the velocity data. On this sample of children both methods produced almost identical curves.

TABLE 2

MEAN 'ADJUSTED' INCREMENTS OF RECUMBENT-LENGTH OVER 13-WEEK PERIODS OF CHILD STUDY CENTRE CHILDREN FROM 4 WEEKS TO 3 YEARS
(In inches to nearest 0·1 inch, and cm. to nearest mm. 1 S.D. of mean given)

Ages	Boys					Girls				
	No.	Inches		Cm.		No.	Inches		Cm.	
		Mean	S.D.	Mean	S.D.		Mean	S.D.	Mean	S.D.
4–13 wks.	77	3·6	0·8	9·1	2·1	66	3·4	0·6	8·6	1·6
13–26 wks.	87	2·5	0·5	6·4	1·3	74	2·6	0·6	6·7	1·5
26–39 wks.	80	1·9	0·6	4·8	1·4	69	1·9	0·5	4·7	1·3
39 wks.–1 yr.	71	1·5	0·5	3·7	1·3	69	1·5	0·6	3·8	1·5
1 yr.–18 mos.	63	1·2	0·3	3·1	0·8	58	1·3	0·4	3·2	0·9
18 mos.–2 yrs.	51	1·0	0·3	2·6	0·7	45	1·0	0·2	2·6	0·6
2–3 yrs.	23	0·8	0·1	2·1	0·3	20	0·8	0·1	2·2	0·3

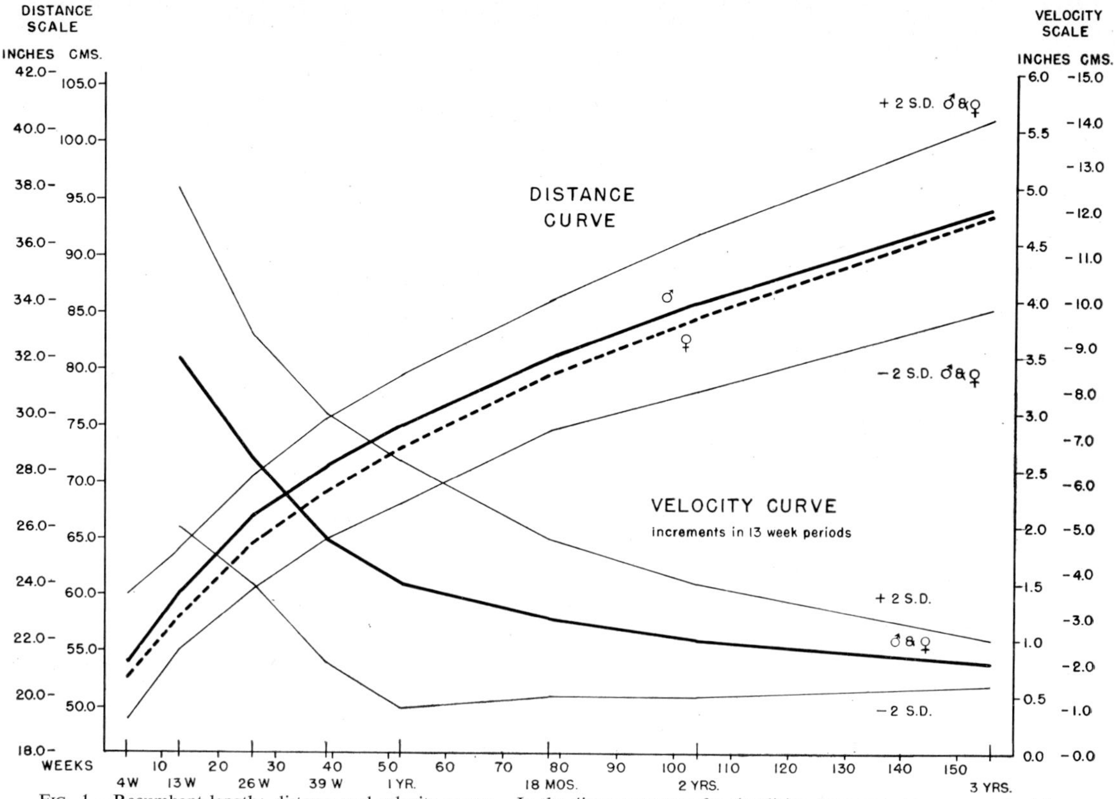

FIG. 1.—Recumbent-length: distance and velocity curves. In the distance curves, for simplicity, boys and girls are combined for ±2 S.D. curves. Boys and girls are combined to give the velocity curves, since their increments are so very similar.

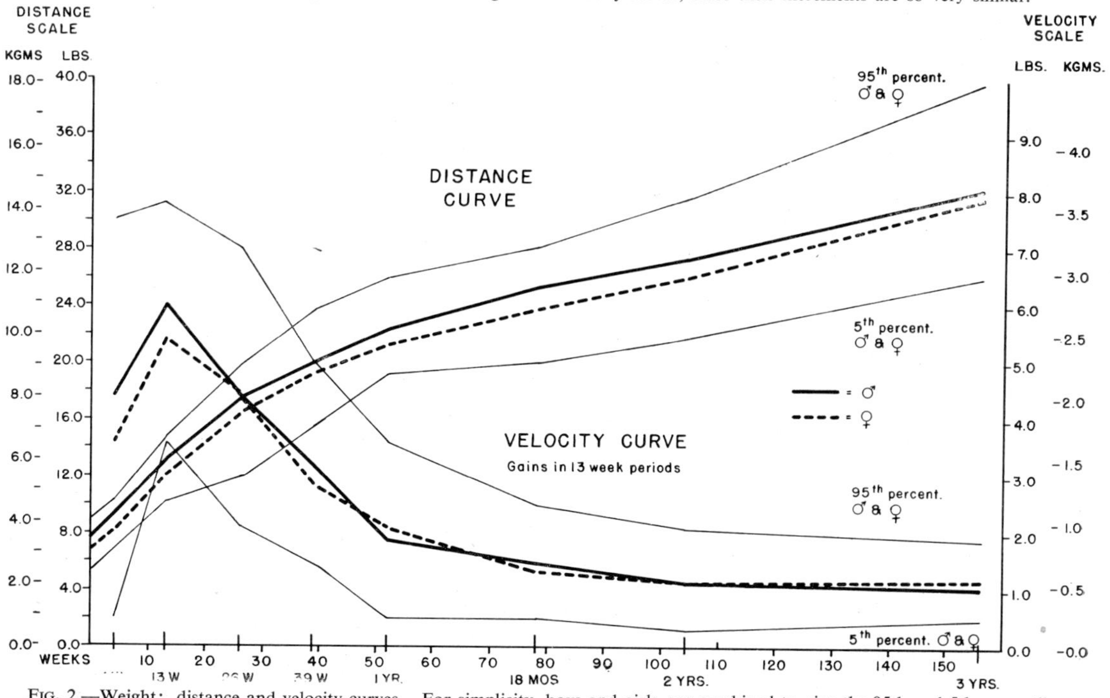

FIG. 2.—Weight: distance and velocity curves. For simplicity, boys and girls are combined to give the 95th and 5th percentiles.

TABLE 3

MEAN WEIGHT OF CHILD STUDY CENTRE CHILDREN AT BIRTH TO 3 YEARS

(In lb. to nearest 0·1 lb., and kg. to nearest 10 g.)

Boys

Ages	No. of Subjects	Percentiles							Mean Weight	
		1	5	20	50	80	95	99		
		Weight (lb.)							Lb.	Kg.
At birth	96	5·6	5·9	6·7	7·7	8·4	9·5	11·2	7·6	3·46
4 wks.	82	6·4	7·0	7·9	9·1	9·9	10·8	12·2	8·9	4·05
13 wks.	96	7·8	10·8	11·6	12·9	14·6	15·7	16·9	13·1	5·91
26 wks.	94	10·9	14·6	16·0	17·6	19·0	19·9	21·9	17·4	7·91
39 wks.	84	13·0	16·3	18·6	20·9	22·4	24·1	26·6	20·4	9·25
1 yr.	81	14·6	17·0	20·3	23·0	24·5	26·3	27·0	22·4	10·15
18 mos.	74	18·9	20·1	22·8	25·9	27·7	28·5	30·4	25·4	11·50
2 yrs.	57	21·7	22·0	25·3	27·6	30·1	31·9	32·6	27·5	12·48
3 yrs.	33	25·0	25·1	27·7	32·6	35·4	39·5	50·2	32·2	14·60

Girls

Ages	No. of Subjects	Percentiles							Mean Weight	
		1	5	20	50	80	95	99		
		Weight (lb.)							Lb.	Kg.
At birth	93	4·6	5·1	6·2	7·2	8·0	8·8	9·4	7·1	3·23
4 wks.	77	6·2	6·5	7·4	8·2	9·1	9·7	10·7	8·2	3·73
13 wks.	84	8·4	9·5	10·9	12·2	13·0	13·7	14·7	11·9	5·39
26 wks.	81	12·6	13·1	14·7	16·5	17·9	19·7	21·0	16·4	7·43
39 wks.	78	14·0	14·8	17·1	19·3	21·2	23·6	25·7	19·2	8·69
1 yr.	78	15·8	17·4	19·2	21·0	23·1	25·9	26·9	21·3	9·64
18 mos.	67	18·6	19·8	21·9	23·9	26·2	28·0	31·3	23·9	10·85
2 yrs.	57	20·8	21·5	23·6	25·8	28·3	31·3	32·6	26·1	11·81
3 yrs.	22	24·1	27·2	28·8	30·9	34·3	40·3	43·3	31·8	14·43

TABLE 4

'ADJUSTED' MEAN INCREMENTS OF WEIGHT GAIN OVER 13-WEEK PERIODS OF CHILD STUDY CENTRE CHILDREN FROM BIRTH TO 3 YEARS

(In lb. to nearest 0·1 lb., and kg. to nearest 10 g.)

Boys

Ages	No. of Subjects	Percentiles							Mean Increments	
		1	5	20	50	80	95	99		
		Increments (lb.)							Lb.	Kg.
Birth–4 wks. ..	73	−2·2	0·3	2·8	4·5	5·9	8·2	9·7	4·4	2·00
4–13 wks.	77	3·0	4·1	4·8	5·7	7·4	8·4	12·2	6·1	2·74
13–26 wks.	87	1·3	2·1	3·4	4·4	5·4	6·8	7·5	4·4	2·01
26–39 wks.	80	0·7	1·5	2·4	3·1	4·1	4·9	7·2	3·2	1·45
39–52 wks.	72	−1·3	0·2	1·2	2·0	2·4	3·8	4·3	1·9	0·86
1 yr.–18 mos. ..	60	−0·05	0·6	0·9	1·4	2·0	2·4	2·6	1·5	0·66
18 mos.–2 yrs. ..	51	0·2	0·5	0·7	1·2	1·5	2·1	2·4	1·2	0·53
2–3 yrs.	29	0·3	0·5	0·8	1·1	1·3	1·7	2·4	1·1	0·49

Girls

Ages	No. of Subjects	Percentiles							Mean Increments	
		1	5	20	50	80	95	99		
		Increments (lb.)							Lb.	Kg.
Birth–4 wks. ..	72	−1·2	0·7	2·1	3·5	5·0	6·8	7·8	3·6	1·64
4–13 wks.	65	2·5	3·2	4·3	5·1	6·7	7·2	8·4	5·3	2·42
13–26 wks.	73	1·1	2·1	3·3	4·4	5·8	7·2	7·6	4·5	2·05
26–39 wks.	69	0·2	1·3	2·0	2·6	3·9	5·4	6·0	2·9	1·30
38–52 wks.	69	0·1	0·9	1·4	2·0	2·7	3·4	4·4	2·1	0·93
1 yr.–18 mos. ..	59	−0·2	0·3	0·9	1·3	1·9	4·6	3·0	1·4	0·62
18 mos.–2 yrs. ..	48	−0·4	0·2	0·7	1·2	1·7	2·1	2·4	1·2	0·53
2–3 yrs.	21	0·5	0·6	0·7	1·0	1·4	2·2	2·7	1·2	0·52

Discussion. While it is well known that boys are taller and heavier than girls, it is interesting to see how closely similar they are in increments (rate of growth) of recumbent-length and weight in this age period, except in the case of weight gain between birth and 3 months. Their birth weight and early recumbent-length differences are maintained.

From other studies (example: Simmons, 1944) it appeared that the size of the newborn baby is not related strongly to his size at, say, 2 years, and Tanner, Healy, Lockhart, MacKenzie and Whitehouse (1956) have shown that birth size is only very slightly related to adult size. It would seem that the genetically determined factor in the growth pattern of the child does not start to become evident until after 1 year of age and is quite apparent at 2 years, presumably the prenatal environmental influences having now been mainly eliminated. Tanner found a high relationship between adult size and size at 3 years.

The London data were examined to verify this hypothesis. Since weight is subject so much to the vicissitudes of life in this period, recumbent-length only was examined.

To check the possible effect of illness on these assumptions the groups were subdivided into children who had been (*a*) ill and not hospitalized, (*b*) hospitalized and (*c*) not ill at all. The correlations remained almost identically the same. Table 5 shows there is little relationship between recumbent-length at 4 weeks and 1 year, but a close relationship between 1 year and 2 years.

TABLE 5

CORRELATIONS BETWEEN RECUMBENT-LENGTHS OF CHILD STUDY CENTRE CHILDREN AT 4 WEEKS AND 1 YEAR AND AT 1 YEAR AND 2 YEARS

	4 Weeks and 1 Year		1 Year and 2 Years	
	No.	r	No.	r
Boys and girls	124	0·30	120	0·83
Boys	60	0·19	51	0·84
Girls	64	0·54	69	0·80

Regarding rate of growth, increments of recumbent-length between 4–13 weeks and 1 year–18 months were examined for relationships. Table 6 shows there is a very low relationship and confirms Tanner's (1956) observation that rate and size seem practically independent.

The Oxford, Aberdeen and another London set of

TABLE 6

CORRELATIONS OF RECUMBENT-LENGTH INCREMENTS OF CHILD STUDY CENTRE CHILDREN BETWEEN 4–13 WEEKS AND 1 YEAR–18 MONTHS

	No.	r
Boys and girls	124	0·08
Boys	54	0·07
Girls	50	0·23

TABLE 7

MEAN COMPARATIVE LENGTHS

(In inches to nearest 0·1 inch)

Ages	London, 1926 (Myers, 1926)		Aberdeen (Low, 1952)		Oxford (Acheson *et al.*, 1955)		London, 1952 (Child Study Centre)	
	Boys	Girls	Boys	Girls	Boys	Girls	Boys	Girls
Birth	—	—	19·6	19·5	—	—	—	—
4 wks.	21·0	20·9	—	—	—	—	21·2	20·7
13 wks.	23·0	22·7	—	—	—	—	23·7	22·9
26 wks.	25·0	25·3	—	—	—	—	26·3	25·5
39 wks.	26·2	26·8	—	—	—	—	28·1	27·3
1 yr.	27·9	27·5	28·9	28·6	—	—	29·5	28·9
18 mos.	31·0	30·6	—	—	31·9*	31·1*	32·0	31·4
2 yrs.	32·4	32·1	32·9	32·9	34·0*	33·2*	34·0	33·3
2½ yrs.	34·0	33·4	—	—	35·6*	35·1*	—	—
3 yrs.	36·1	35·4	36·2	36·4	37·3*	36·7*	37·1	37·0

* Standing height.

TABLE 8

MEAN COMPARATIVE INCREMENTS IN LENGTH

(In inches to nearest 0·1 inch)

Ages	Boys			Girls		
	Aberdeen	Oxford	London, 1952	Aberdeen	Oxford	London, 1952
1 yr.–2 yrs.	1·0	—	1·1	1·1	—	1·1
18 mos.–2 yrs.	—	1·0*	1·0	—	1·0*	1·0
2–3 yrs. ..	0·8	0·8*	0·8	0·9	0·9*	0·9

* Standing height.

TABLE 9

MEAN COMPARATIVE WEIGHTS

(In lb. to nearest 0·1 lb.)

Ages	London, 1926 (Myers, 1926)		Aberdeen (Low, 1952)		London, 1947 (Gore and Palmer, 1949)		Oxford (Acheson *et al.*, 1955)		London, 1952 (Child Study Centre)	
	Boys	Girls	Boys	Girls	Boys	Girls	Boys	Girls	Boys	Girls
Birth	—	—	7·0	6·9	—	—	7·6	7·3	7·6	7·1
4 wks.	8·3	8·2	—	—	8·6	8·5	—	—	8·9	8·2
13 wks.	11·5	10·7	—	—	13·1	12·2	—	—	13·1	11·9
26 wks.	15·4	15·8	—	—	17·5	16·4	17·5	16·1	17·4	16·4
39 wks.	18·1	18·1	—	—	20·5	19·3	—	—	20·4	19·2
1 yr.	20·5	19·5	20·6	19·9	22·6	21·0	22·7	21·1	22·4	21·3
18 mos.	22·7	22·1	—	—	25·5	24·1	25·4	23·9	25·4	23·9
2 yrs.	26·5	25·0	25·2	24·6	28·3	26·9	27·8	26·1	27·5	26·1
2½ yrs.	28·2	24·7	—	—	30·8	29·5	29·9	28·6	—	—
3 yrs.	30·2	29·3	28·7	29·4	32·8	31·6	32·2	31·0	32·2	31·8

TABLE 10

COMPARATIVE MEAN INCREMENTS OF WEIGHT

(In lb. to nearest 0·1 lb.)

Ages	Aberdeen (Low, 1952)		London, 1947 (Gore and Palmer, 1949)		Oxford (Acheson *et al.*, 1955)		London, 1952 (Child Study Centre)	
	Boys	Girls	Boys	Girls	Boys	Girls	Boys	Girls
Birth–4 wks.	—	—	—	—	—	—	4·4	3·6
4–13 wks.	—	—	6·5	5·3	—	—	6·1	5·3
13–26 wks.	—	—	4·4	4·2	—	—	4·4	4·5
26–39 wks.	—	—	3·0	2·9	—	—	3·2	2·9
39 wks.–1 yr.	—	—	2·1	1·7	—	—	1·9	2·1
1 yr.–18 mos.	—	—	1·5	1·5	1·4	1·4	1·5	1·4
1 yr.–2 yrs.	1·2	1·2	1·4	1·5	1·3	1·2	1·3	1·2
18 mos.–2 yrs.	—	—	1·2	1·4	1·2	1·1	1·2	1·2
2–3 yrs.	0·9	1·2	1·1	1·2	1·1	1·1	1·1	1·2

children are compared in means in Tables 7 and 8. The Aberdeen and London data in Table 8 are true mean increments. The Oxford increments have been obtained by subtracting mean heights at the ages stated; they are thus an approximation only.

Comparative weights are given in Tables 9 and 10. Because of the arrangement of age groups in Table 10 the London 1926 data did not permit increments to be obtained. The London 1947 and Oxford 1948 increments in this table have been obtained by subtracting the means at the ages stated and are thus approximations; the Aberdeen and London 1952 increments are true increments.

Tables 7, 8, 9 and 10 show that, although the samples are not strictly comparable, the trend of children to become taller and heavier as time goes on is apparently maintained (Annotation in *Lancet*, 1955; Tanner, 1955). This is apparently due to the consistent biological fact that children are reaching physical maturity earlier and earlier. Skeletal maturity assessments upon the early samples of children would be most interesting had they been

TABLE 11

MEAN CROWN–RUMP MEASUREMENTS OF CHILD STUDY CENTRE CHILDREN AGED 4 WEEKS TO 3 YEARS

(In inches to nearest 0·1 inch, and cm. to nearest mm. S.D. = 1 standard deviation of mean)

Ages	Boys					Girls				
	No.	Inches		Cm.		No.	Inches		Cm.	
		Mean	S.D.	Mean	S.D.		Mean	S.D.	Mean	S.D.
4 wks.	82	13·8	0·7	35·0	1·7	77	13·7	0·5	34·3	1·3
13 wks.	95	15·4	0·7	39·2	1·7	84	14·9	0·5	37·9	1·2
26 wks.	94	17·0	0·6	43·3	1·6	81	16·6	0·5	42·1	1·3
39 wks.	84	18·0	0·7	45·8	1·8	77	17·5	0·6	44·5	1·5
1 yr.	79	18·7	0·6	47·5	1·6	77	18·2	0·8	46·2	2·0
18 mos.	85	19·8	0·7	50·2	1·8	75	19·4	0·7	49·3	1·9
2 yrs.	55	20·7	0·9	52·6	2·4	53	20·3	0·7	51·6	1·7
3 yrs.	31	22·2	1·1	56·3	2·7	26	21·6	1·1	54·9	2·7

available. The Oxford 1948 and London 1952 data are very similar. It is also apparent how very similar are all the incremental figures irrespective of the date of the study. Again, rate of growth and size have been suggested to be independent.

Other Measurements

Upper Segment (or Crown–Rump Length) and Lower Segment (or Lower-stem Length). The crown–rump measurement was obtained on the same measuring-board as for recumbent-length. The child's legs are raised vertically, the measurement representing the distance between the crown of the head and the rump over a line connecting the ischial tuberosities. (See Bean, 1922; Knott, 1941; Falkner, 1957, etc.) Results are given in Tables 11 and 12.

Lower-segment length is obtained by simple subtraction of crown–rump length from total recumbent-length. The ratio of upper to lower segment is a useful index of growth and is commonly expressed as the percentage of the total length that is made up by the upper segment. It is known as the stem-stature index, and is expressed as:

$$\frac{\text{Stem-length (crown–rump length)} \times 100}{\text{Recumbent-length (or height)}}$$

The maximum standard deviation of the mean at any age in the Aberdeen or London children (where the raw data were available) was $\pm 1 \cdot 6$.

The index varies remarkably little between some widely different samples and decreases with age, as the lower limbs grow more rapidly than the upper segment. It reaches its final adult stable figure at approximately 12 years in the female and 16 years in the male. At the third month of foetal life it is of the order of 80·0 (Schultz, 1926), and at birth indexes from different racial groups vary little between 66·0 and 67·5 (examples: Japanese—Ito,

TABLE 12

MEAN 'ADJUSTED' INCREMENTS OF CROWN–RUMP MEASUREMENT IN 13-WEEK PERIODS OF CHILD STUDY CENTRE CHILDREN AGED 4 WEEKS TO 3 YEARS

(In inches to nearest 0·1 inch, and cm. to nearest mm.)

Ages	Boys			Girls		
	No.	'Adjusted' Mean Increment		No.	'Adjusted' Mean Increment	
		Inches	Cm.		Inches	Cm.
4–13 wks.	76	2·4	6·1	65	2·2	5·5
13–26 wks.	86	1·6	4·0	73	1·7	4·2
26–39 wks.	80	1·0	2·6	68	0·9	2·4
39 wks.–1 yr.	70	0·7	1·7	66	0·7	1·8
1 yr.–18 mos.	70	0·5	1·4	66	0·6	1·6
18 mos.–2 yrs.	50	0·5	1·2	44	0·5	1·2
2–3 yrs.	25	0·4	1·1	24	0·3	0·8

TABLE 13

MEAN STEM-STATURE INDEX OF CHILD STUDY CENTRE CHILDREN COMPARED WITH OTHER CHILDREN

Ages	London, 1952		Aberdeen (Lowe, 1952)		Detroit (Hejinian and Hatt, 1929)		New York (Wallis, 1931)	
	Boys	Girls	Boys	Girls	Boys	Girls	Boys	Girls
Birth	—	—	67·8	68·1	—	—	—	—
4 wks.	65·0	65·2	—	—	—	—	—	—
13 wks.	65·0	65·1	—	—	—	—	—	—
26 wks.	64·8	64·9	—	—	—	—	—	—
39 wks.	64·1	64·0	—	—	—	—	—	—
1 yr.	63·3	63·0	63·1	63·3	—	—	63·6	62·8
18 mos.	61·7	61·7	—	—	—	—	—	—
2 yrs.	60·8	61·0	61·4	61·1	61·2	60·8	60·8	60·2
3 yrs.	59·7	58·3	59·9	59·2	59·3	59·2	58·8	58·4

TABLE 14

MEAN HEAD CIRCUMFERENCES OF CHILD STUDY CENTRE CHILDREN AGED 4 WEEKS TO 3 YEARS

(In inches to nearest 0·1 inch, and cm. to nearest mm.)

Ages	Boys					Girls				
	No.	Inches		Cm.		No.	Inches		Cm.	
		Mean	S.D.	Mean	S.D.		Mean	S.D.	Mean	S.D.
4 wks.	82	14·7	0·4	37·4	1·1	77	14·4	0·4	36·5	1·0
13 wks.	96	16·0	0·4	40·7	1·1	84	15·6	0·5	39·7	1·2
26 wks.	94	17·3	0·5	43·8	1·2	81	16·8	0·4	42·7	1·1
39 wks.	83	18·0	0·5	45·7	1·3	78	17·6	0·5	44·6	1·2
1 yr.	79	18·4	0·5	46·8	1·3	75	18·0	0·5	45·7	1·2
18 mos.	83	19·0	0·5	48·3	1·3	74	18·5	0·4	47·0	1·1
2 yrs.	58	19·4	0·6	49·3	1·4	57	18·8	0·4	47·9	1·1
3 yrs.	35	19·8	0·5	50·4	1·3	32	19·5	0·4	49·5	1·1

1936; American—Bakwin and Bakwin, 1934; Italian—Tatafiore, 1935). At 8 years it approximates 54·5 (Wallis, 1931). By puberty it is of the order of 51·5 to 52·0 in both sexes, and thereafter remains at this minimum amount. The index is influenced by age, sex, race and constitutional type. There are two areas of very low upper-segment length—Central Africa and Native Australasia; and two 'high' areas—Central Africa (Pygmies) and the Arctic (Bean, 1922); but otherwise the index appears remarkably stable and comparable in distribution.

Bean (1922) stated that in different samples the female index was generally larger than the male, regardless of constitutional type and stature. The present sample of children does not indicate that such differences appear in the first three years of life at least.

In certain diseases the index is altered and may give a useful additional diagnostic indication. As an example, in cretinism the dwarfism includes retardation of growth of the lower limbs, and this manifests itself in the index. Five cretins recently seen had the following indices: two aged 4 weeks—mean of 69·0; two aged 3 months—mean of 68·1; and one aged 6 months—66·9. By comparison with Table 13 it will be seen that these indices are high.

Head Circumference. This is taken with a flexible, narrow-width steel tape and represents the maximum circumference, with the tape passing round the occipital and frontal areas and held perpendicular to the mid-sagittal plane.

TABLE 15

'ADJUSTED' MEAN INCREMENTS OF HEAD CIRCUMFERENCE IN 13-WEEK PERIODS OF CHILD STUDY CENTRE CHILDREN AGED 4 WEEKS TO 3 YEARS

(In inches to nearest 0·1 inch, and cm. to nearest mm.)

Ages	Boys			Girls		
	No.	'Adjusted' Mean Increment		No.	'Adjusted' Mean Increment	
		Inches	Cm.		Inches	Cm.
4–13 wks.	77	1·9	4·8	65	1·9	4·8
13–26 wks.	87	1·2	3·1	73	1·2	3·1
26–39 wks.	79	0·8	2·0	69	0·7	1·9
39 wks.–1 yr.	69	0·5	1·2	67	0·4	1·1
1 yr.–18 mos.	67	0·3	0·7	62	0·3	0·7
18 mos.–2 yrs.	49	0·2	0·5	26	0·2	0·5
2–3 yrs.	33	0·1	0·3	28	0·1	0·4

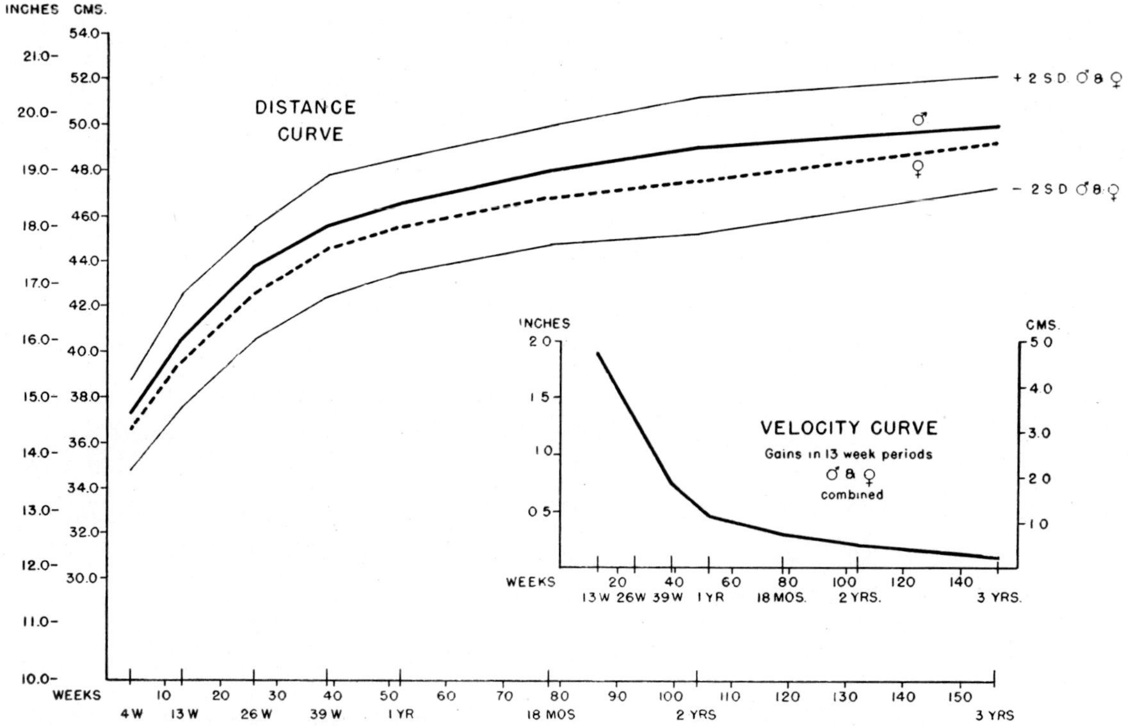

FIG. 3.—Head circumferences: distance and velocity curves. In the distance curves, for simplicity, boys and girls are combined to give the 2 S.D. curves. Boys and girls are combined to give the velocity curves, since their increments are almost identical.

Head circumference is a useful measurement clinically in early childhood, particularly when hydrocephalus, subdural haematoma or neoplasms are in question. Correlations between head measurement, cranial capacity and intelligence are, however, uniformly low and of the order of 0·12 (Broom, 1932; Paterson, 1930). Incremental data may be of most use. Although the boys' mean head circumferences are consistently larger than the girls', the mean increments are practically identical.

Fig. 3 shows graphically* the data from Tables 14 and 15. The incremental curve is of boys and girls combined.

Summary

Means and mean increments of recumbent-length, weight, crown–rump length and head circumference are given for children from a longitudinal developmental study in London. The children were born in 1952–4. Standard deviations and percentiles are given. Comparative lengths and weights, and increments of both, are given for samples of children born from 1923 to 1954. The secular trend for children to become larger continues. The relationship between early, late and adult life is discussed. There is very little relationship between size at 4 weeks and 1 year, but a good relationship between 1 year and 2 years. Size appears independent of rate of growth, which shows little relationship from any age to any age. Stem-stature indices are given and comparisons with other samples made. Their usefulness is discussed.

I am much indebted and grateful to Professor Alan Moncrieff for constant encouragement and guidance; to Dr. W. M. Krogman, who read and criticized this paper; and to Miss Coral Tibbetts, Mr. Richard Westland and Mrs. Nancy Singleton for computational and secretarial assistance.

REFERENCES

Acheson, R. M., Kemp, F. H. and Parfit, J. (1955). *Lancet*, **1**, 691.
Annotation (1955). *Ibid.*, **2**, 1327.
Bakwin, H. and Bakwin, R. M. (1934). *Hum. Biol.*, **6**, 612.
Bean, R. B. (1922). *Amer. J. phys. Anthrop.*, **5**, 349.
Boyd, E. (1929). *Ibid.*, **13**, 389.
Broom, M. E. (1932). *School and Society*, **36**, 703.
Falkner, F. (1957). Ed. Internationally Cooperative Research in Child Development. Centre Int. de l'Enfance, Paris.
Gore, A. T. and Palmer, W. T. (1949). *Lancet*, **1**, 385.
Gray, H. and Ayres, J. G. (1931). *Growth in Private School Children.* University of Chicago Press.
Hindley, C. B. (1953). *Lancet*, **2**, 142.
Ito, P. K. (1936). *Amer. J. Dis. Child.*, **52**, 321.
Hejinian, L. and Hatt, E. (1929). *Amer. J. phys. Anthrop.*, **13**, 287.
Knott, V. B. (1941). *Univ. Iowa Studies in Child Welfare*, **18**, No. 3. [1948].
Krogman, W. M. (1950). *Monogr. Soc. Res. Child Dev.*, **13**, No. 3.
—— (1956). *Ibid.*, **20**, No. 1. [1955].
Lincoln, E. A. (1930). *J. genet. Psychol.*, **38**, 445.
Low, A. (1952). *Growth of Children.* Univ. of Aberdeen.
Moore, T., Hindley, C. B. and Falkner, F. (1954). *Brit. med. J.*, **2**, 1132.
Myers, B. (1926). *Brit. J. Child. Dis.*, **23**, 87.
Palmer, C. E. (1930). *Anat. Rec.*, **45**, 234.
Paterson, D. G. (1930). *Physique and Intellect.* New York.
Redfield, J. E. and Meredith, H. V. (1938). *Child Developm.*, **9**, 293.
Schultz, A. H. (1926). *Quart. Rev. Biol.*, **1**, 465.
Simmons, K. (1944). *Monogr. Soc. Res. Child Dev.*, **9**, No. 1.
Tanner, J. M. (1951). *Hum. Biol.*, **23**, 93.
—— (1955). *Growth at Adolescence.* Oxford.
—— Healy, M. J. R., Lockhart, R. D., MacKenzie, J. D., and Whitehouse, R. H., (1956). *Arch. Dis. Childh.*, **31**, 372.
Tatafiore, E. (1935). *Pediatria (Napoli)*, **43**, 422.
Thomson, J. (1956). *Arch. Dis. Childh.*, **31**, 382.
Wallis, R. S. (1931). Univ. Iowa. *Studies in Child Welfare*, Vol. **5**, No. 1.

* See footnote on page 2.

GROWTH AND DEVELOPMENT IN A GROUP OF CHILDREN OF VERY LOW BIRTH WEIGHT

BY

CECIL M. DRILLIEN

From the Department of Child Life and Health, University of Edinburgh

(RECEIVED FOR PUBLICATION JULY 22, 1957)

In recent years improved techniques in premature baby care have resulted in a greatly improved expectation of life for the very small, premature baby. Table 1 gives the survival rates from one large Edinburgh maternity hospital for six premature weight groups in the years 1945 and 1954. It will be seen that the most striking improvement is found in the lowest weight groups. This raises the important question of what happens to these very small babies in later life. Although there is an extensive literature on the growth and development of premature babies, the majority of investigators have considered premature babies as a whole, *i.e.*, all those with a birth weight of 5½ lb. (2,500 g.) or less, the samples studied being heavily weighted by the larger premature infants. A recent survey of all premature births in Edinburgh, in the years 1952 to 1953 (Drillien and Richmond, 1956), showed that 57% of all births registered as being premature by weight were between 4 lb. 9 oz. and 5 lb. 8 oz. at birth. In another investigation (Drillien, 1957), it was shown that amongst primiparae 49% of babies considered premature on a weight basis were reported as having a gestation time of 38 weeks or longer; the comparable figure amongst higher parities was 37%. The majority of these small, full-time babies weighed between 5 and 5½ lb. at birth, and practically all of them were over 4½ lb. (2,041 g.).

TABLE 1

SURVIVAL RATES FOR BABIES OF 5½ LB. AND UNDER AT BIRTH IN ONE EDINBURGH MATERNITY HOSPITAL

Weight in lb.	Percentage Survival	
	1945	1954
5 to 5½ ..	91·6	96·3
4½ to 5 ..	83·3	84·6
4 to 4½ ..	81·6	82·4
3½ to 4 ..	51·8	71·4
3 to 3½ ..	35·0	73·0
Under 3 ..	4·5	28·2

It appears, therefore, that the effect of prematurity on later growth and development may be seriously underestimated if the sample studied contains an undue proportion of small but mature infants.

Hess and Lundeen (1949) in their book, 'The Premature Infant', describe briefly a follow-up investigation of 259 infants born between 1922 and 1947 whose birth weights varied from 735 to 1,260 g. (1 lb. 10 oz. to 2 lb. 8 oz.). Two hundred and twelve (82%) were traced and examined. These cases were graded as to physical and mental development: 48% were considered to be of average physical development and 59% of average mental development. Unfortunately no details are given of the criteria of normality used.

Howard and Worrell (1952) quote a personal communication from Hess regarding the progress of 317 children who were then 8 years or older, of birth weight between 605 and 1,260 g. (1 lb. 5 oz. to 2 lb. 8 oz.). Of these, 51% were considered to be of normal physical status and 64% of average mental development, figures closely paralleled by the previous investigation.

Kunstadter and Bartelme (1934) describe in detail the findings in 17 children surviving a birth weight of less than 1,000 g. (2 lb. 3 oz.). Of these, five died after discharge from hospital and before the age of 2 years. Developmental testing was carried out on 10 of the children: five were considered to be of normal or superior intelligence, and five definitely retarded. Out of eight cases, in which reports were given as to emotional stability, four were regarded as having marked behaviour problems, two as having minor behaviour problems and two were said to be stable and emotionally mature. Nine children over the age of 1 year were weighed and measured: eight were found to be underweight, most of them considerably so. These eight children were also retarded in height, but not to the same extent as in weight.

Knobloch, Rider, Harper and Pasamanick (1956) describe the findings in 57 infants at 9 months of age, whose birth weight was 1,500 g. (3 lb. 4 oz.) or less, this being a part of a wider study of premature infants of different birth weights. They considered that in this low birth weight group 44% of the infants had an abnormal condition of sufficient magnitude to cause serious concern about the prognosis for future development. The comparable incidence for the rest of the premature infants was 8·6% and for full-term infants 2·6%.

Method of Investigation

A long-term study of the growth and development of premature and mature infants, born in Edinburgh hospitals between the years 1953 and 1955, yielded 20 children whose weight was 3 lb. or less at birth. In view of the small number it was decided to continue to follow up all cases in this low birth weight group born after 1955, and also to go back over a period of years in order to collect a larger number of these children. In all a total of 75 names was obtained. In every case the family has been traced, and in all but one where the family had moved out of the district, the mother has been interviewed and living children examined.

Table 2 gives the numbers of children by age of

TABLE 2
COMPOSITION OF THE SAMPLE

Age	Total	Boys	Girls
6 months	5	1	4
1 year	4	1	3
1½ years	5	1	4
2 years	12	4	8
2½ years	1	–	1
3 years	10	6	4
4 to 5 years . .	12	5	7
5 to 6 years . .	5	1	4
6 to 7 years . .	7	2	5
7 to 8 years . .	3	–	3
8 to 9 years . .	5	2	3
Total	69	23	46

the last examination. It will be noticed that there are nearly twice as many girls as boys in this sample, due no doubt to their slightly longer gestation time for any given birth weight, associated with the fact that girls withstand the hazards of birth better than boys of like weight. All cases of 3 years and under are included in the larger survey and are seen at regular six-monthly intervals. Over this age the children have been seen on one or two occasions only. Five children died before the age of 2 years.

In one case the child died at 18 months, the cause of death being bronchopneumonia. In the other four cases, in which death occurred at 6 months or earlier, the cause of death was not known. In two cases the child was found dead in the cot, having been apparently quite well a few hours earlier. In the other two cases, the child appeared fretful and refused feeds in the evening and died the following morning before medical aid was summoned.

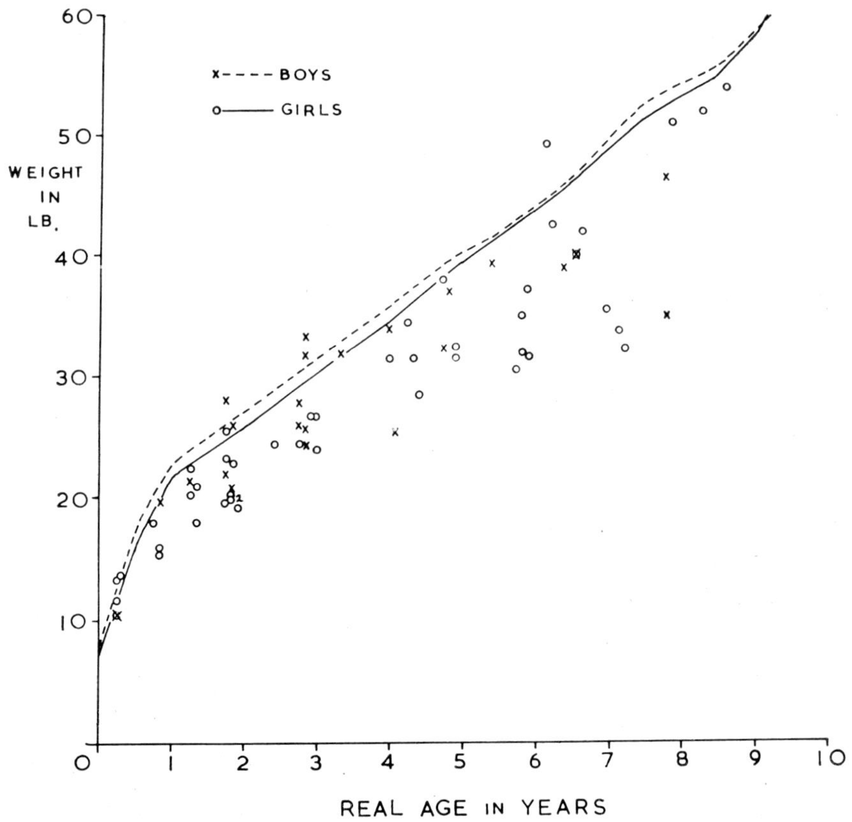

FIG. 1.– Weights of prematurely born children compared with mean weights of normal children.

Physical Development

The children were weighed in light, indoor clothes without shoes, and an appropriate deduction was made for the amount of clothing still worn. All children of 2 years and over were measured recumbent, without shoes, on a portable measuring board.

Normal weight and length curves were constructed from means for Edinburgh infants, pre-school and school children (1951 to 1956) given in 'Disease in Infancy and Childhood' Ellis (1956).

In the accompanying figures the weeks of prematurity have been deducted from the chronological age to give the real age.

Fig. 1 gives the weights of 69 children, 46 girls and 23 boys, at the time of their last examination. Except in the first six months of life almost all are underweight, many considerably so, even when allowance is made for the degree of prematurity.

Fig. 2 shows the lengths of 54 children, 35 girls and 19 boys. The retardation in length is not so marked as for weight. This is demonstrated in Fig. 3, where curves have been constructed from the figures used previously for normal weight and length, giving the expected ratio of weight to length. It will be seen that many of the premature children are markedly underweight for their height, as well as being generally small for their age.

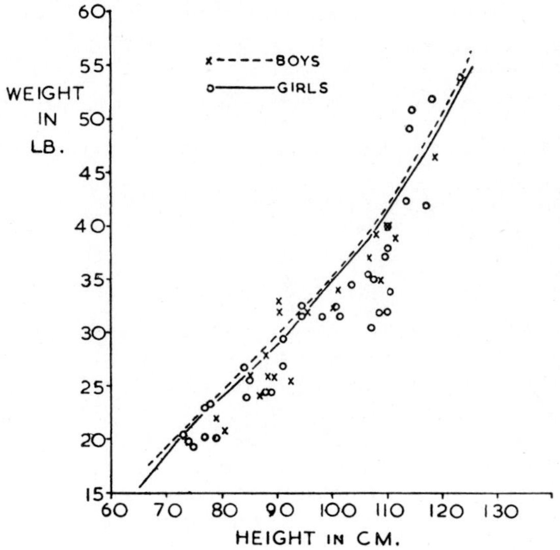

FIG. 3.—Height/weight ratios in prematurely born children compared with those for normal children.

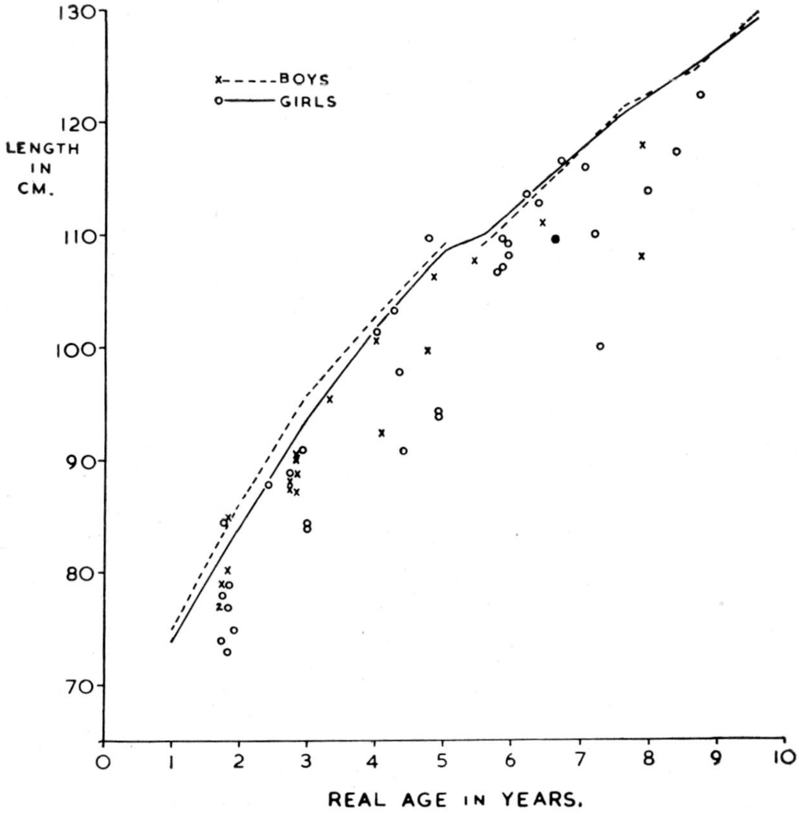

FIG. 2.—Lengths of prematurely born children compared with mean lengths of normal children.

Figs. 4 and 5 present the same data in a different way. For every case, excepting those of 6 months and younger, the ratio is given, expressed as a percentage, of the 'weight age' to the real age of the child, the 'weight age' being the age at which a 'normal' child would have the weight of the child in question. For children of 2 years and over, a similar ratio has been calculated of 'length age' to real age. Again allowance has been made for degree of prematurity. The data are summarized in Table 3. The figures show that there is no apparent tendency for physique to improve with age, the proportion of undersized children remaining steady throughout the age period under review.

Mental Development

All children of 3 years and under were given developmental tests based on those described by Gesell (1941, 1950). It was not possible to carry out the complete battery of tests in every case, but in the majority information has been obtained as to ability in locomotor activities, hand manipulation, language and social adjustment. These cases are included in the larger survey and have been tested at regular six-monthly intervals. For each case the developmental quotient (D.Q.) has been calculated.

The D.Q. is the relationship between 'maturity age' and actual age, expressed as a percentage value.

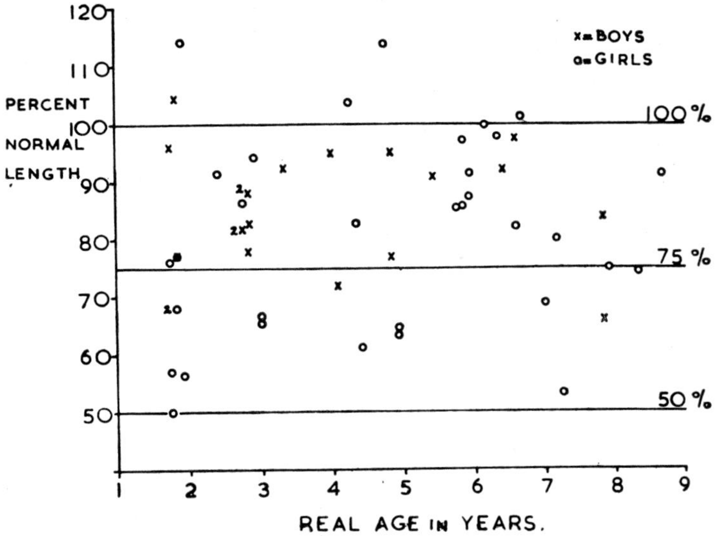

FIG. 5.—Ratios of 'length age' to real age in prematurely born children.

$$\text{D.Q.} = \frac{\text{Maturity age}}{\text{Chronological age} - \text{weeks of prematurity}} \times 100$$

Children over the age of 3 years were tested on the Terman Merrill L. test. In those cases where the child was markedly retarded, Gesell tests were used up to the 3-year level, and Terman Merrill tests also used if the child showed an average result, at the 3-year level, on the Gesell tests.

TABLE 3

RATIO OF WEIGHT AND LENGTH AGES TO REAL AGE IN PREMATURE GROUP

Ratio of Weight and Length Ages to Real Age (%)	Weight	Length
100 or over	5 (7·8%)	6 (11·3%)
76 to 100	19 (29·7%)	32 (60·4%)
51 to 75	32 (50·0%)	15 (28·3%)
50 or less	8 (12·5%)	—
Total	64 (100 %)	53 (100 %)

In assessing the mental development of the school age group much assistance has been given by the school medical officers, who either obtained a report from the child's class teacher, or arranged for the child to be given an I.Q. test. Five children in this group are attending the Royal Blind School, Edinburgh, and an assessment of intelligence was supplied by the Headmaster.

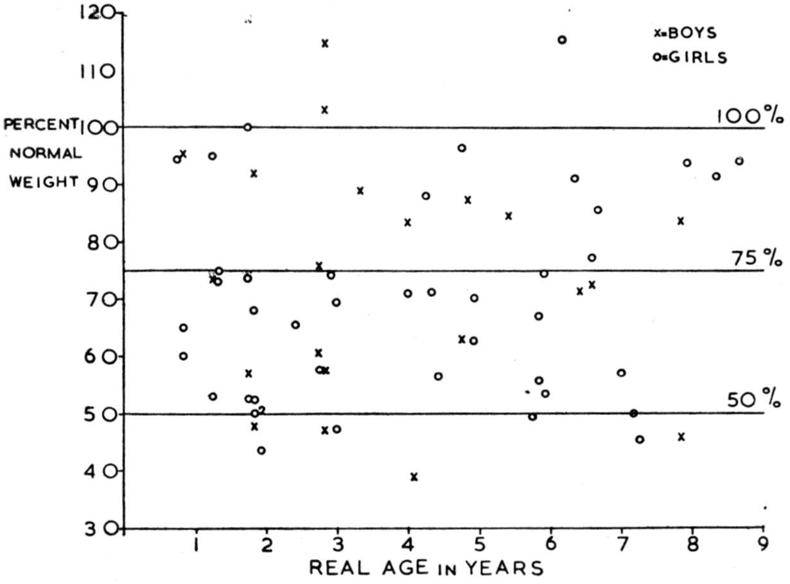

FIG. 4.—Ratios of 'weight age' to real age in prematurely born children.

Mental Development in the Pre-School Period

Fig. 6 gives the D.Q. for 38 children, 22 girls and 16 boys, between the ages of 1 and 5 years. Only 14 children (37%) have a D.Q. of 90 or over. These

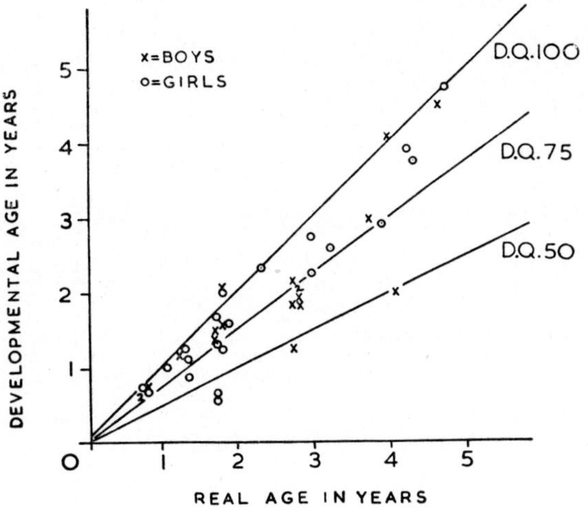

FIG. 6.—Developmental quotients for 38 pre-school prematurely born children.

can be considered normal, or superior in mental ability. Thirteen children (34%) have a D.Q. between 75 and 89, and are definitely dull; seven (18%) between 50 and 74 may be considered high-grade defectives; and four (11%) below 50 as grossly defective.

The children of 3 years and under, who are included in the larger survey, have been compared with other children in the survey of different birth weights. In each case the child included in this study has been matched with others of like age and sex selected at random from the main survey. Allowance has been made for the degree of prematurity in each of the three premature groups. Table 4 gives the average D.Q. for children in four birth weight groups, the difference in D.Q. compared with children mature at birth, and tests of significance for this difference. It will be seen that the average D.Q. rises steadily with increasing birth weight, and in each case the difference is significant. However, it is only in the smallest weight group that a substantial difference in D.Q. is found. The prematurely born children, as a whole, tend to come from an inferior socio-economic level than those in the mature group, and there is no doubt that the intelligence of the parents in the latter group tends to be higher and the home environment more favourable. This, by itself, may account for the

TABLE 4

AVERAGE D.Q. LEVELS IN PREMATURE AND MATURE CHILDREN

	Birth Weight (lb. oz.)			
	5·9 and Over	4·9 to 5·8	3·1 to 4·8	3 and Under
Average D.Q.	106	99	95	81
Difference from mature group		7	11	2·5
t		2·36	2·98	7·84
p		0·025	0·01	0·001

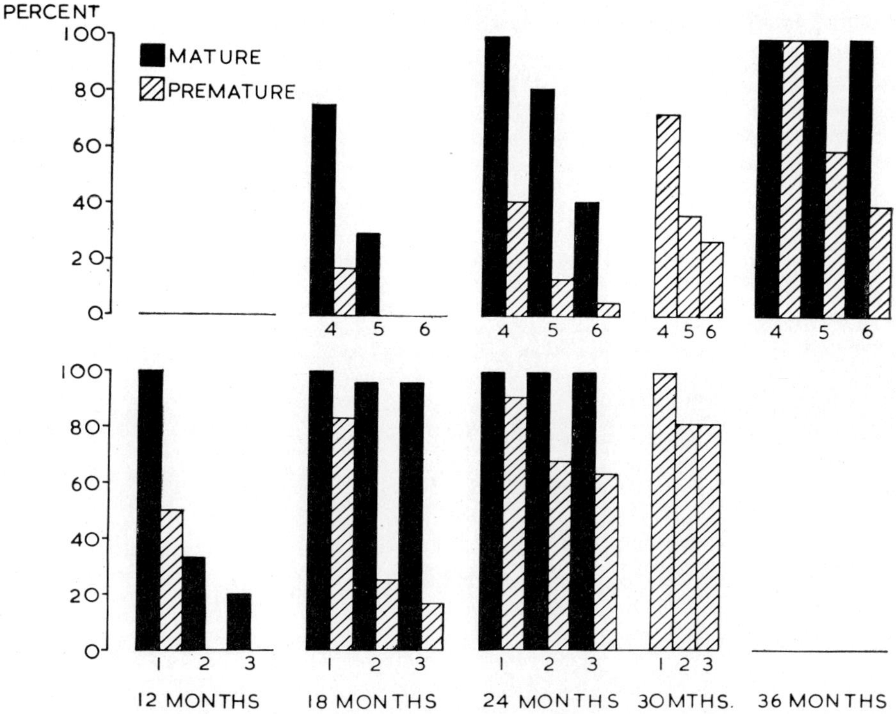

FIG. 7.—Milestones of development in premature and mature children: (1) sitting, (2) standing, (3) walking, (4) single words, (5) phrases, (6) sentences.

small differences found in D.Q. level between the larger premature children and the mature children. However, in the smallest weight group the difference is so great that it seems probable that the low D.Q. scores are directly connected with the low birth weight.

The ages at which certain milestones were passed in locomotion and speech development in the first three years have been compared in those who were 3 lb. or under at birth and those over 5½ lb. and the results are shown in Fig. 7.

The lower section of the figure shows the number of children, expressed as a percentage, at any given age who were able to (1) sit unsupported for 10 minutes or longer; (2) stand unsupported for 30 seconds or longer; (3) walk alone across a room.

The upper section shows the percentage who (4) had five or six definite words, apart from Mamma and Dadda; (5) had many single words and several two- or three-word phrases; (6) were speaking in broken sentences.

The maturely born children were not examined at 30 months. It will be seen that for locomotor activities the premature group had nearly reached the 18-month mature level by the age of 30 months, and, in speech, at 3 years they were still rather behind the mature 2-year-old level.

It is not possible to say at this stage whether there is likely to be any substantial improvement as the children get older. Out of 21 children under 3 years of age seen at regular intervals, 13 have remained at approximately the same D.Q. level (a change up or down of 8 points or less), six have definitely improved and two have deteriorated.

An attempt has been made to correlate conditions at birth and during the first few weeks of life with later mental development. In 59 cases, full records were available. In 15 cases, the baby's condition at birth was very poor, respiration was established with difficulty and cyanotic or cerebral attacks occurred during the next two weeks. Ten of these babies later showed definite mental retardation. In 36 cases, the babies caused little anxiety either at the birth or during their stay in hospital. Of these, 15 later appeared to be definitely retarded. In general one may say that it appears very difficult to judge from immediate post-natal findings what the ultimate prognosis will be.

Mental Development in School Age Children

Five school age children are attending the Royal Blind School, Edinburgh. In supplying an estimate of intelligence, the Headmaster stressed the difficulty of obtaining accurate I.Q. scores in the presence of emotional difficulties.

Age		I.Q.
Yr.	Mth.	
5	10	80 approximately
6	2	80 to 95
6	11	80 approximately
6	2	Testing impossible owing to considerable degree of emotional disturbance, but both appear retarded
6	9	

Thirteen children attending the ordinary primary schools were given intelligence tests. Terman and Merrill L or M scale tests were used except in the case of one Polish boy with a poor grasp of the English language, who was also given the Wechsler intelligence scale for children.

The estimated I.Q.s of these children and assessments of educational attainments are as follows:

Age		I.Q.	Educational Attainment
Yr.	Mth.		
5	5	109	Satisfactory start with formal work
6	1	77	Not ready for formal work
6	5	84	Below average, especially in number work
6	6	87	Below average, especially in number work. To be kept back one year. Twin (3 lb. 6 oz.) is in class for age
6	10	Wechsler Verbal 81 Performance 101	Successfully overcoming handicaps of poor health (spastic) and language difficulties
6	11	82	Severely retarded but has defective vision and hearing
7	4	89	In class for age
7	6	80	Severely retarded. Has been kept back one year
8	3	91	Is in class for age
8	3	83	Is in class for age
8	3	85	Severely retarded especially in number work. Has been kept back one year
9	2	84	Is in class for age

Three children have not been given intelligence tests. Class teachers' reports are given below:

Age		Educational Attainment
Yr.	Mth.	
6	4	Below average but making progress
7	0	Below average. Has been kept back one year. Twin (3 lb. 7 oz.) is in class for age
8	8	Below average in all subjects

Of a total of 21 children, therefore, only three are considered to be of average intelligence and the majority are very dull. However, they all entered school at the usual age and at present are considered to be of sufficient intelligence to benefit from normal primary schooling. In the pre-school group of 38 children, at least seven appear to be so grossly retarded that it seems unlikely that they will be able to begin school at 5 years, or attend normal school.

In general the school age children appear to show

less mental damage than those born in the past three years. This may be due to the fact that there is steady improvement with increasing age, but it seems more likely that with improved techniques in premature baby care damaged children are now surviving who would not have done so some years ago. This supposition is strengthened by the fact that of a total of six children with cerebral diplegia, only one is of school age, the other five being 3 years old or younger.

Illness in Early Life

The amount of illness suffered in the early years of life by the very small premature babies has been compared with that reported during the same age period for an equal number of mature babies of like sex and age.

Table 5 gives the number of children in each

TABLE 5

MORBIDITY IN FIRST THREE YEARS IN PREMATURE AND MATURE CHILDREN

Age	No.	No Illnesses		Percentage	
		Premature	Mature	Premature	Mature
Birth to 6 months	36	20	29	56	81
6 to 12 months ..	31	12	24	39	78
12 to 18 months ..	26	14	16	54	62
18 to 24 months ..	20	11	16	55	80
24 to 36 months ..	9	3	3	33	33

group who were reported as having had no illnesses, apart from head colds and minor digestive disturbances, during the previous six months. Eleven hospital admissions, for medical illness, were reported, 10 of them in the premature group. In each case, except one where the baby was admitted to hospital for failure to thrive, the diagnosis was bronchitis or pneumonia. The premature babies appeared to be particularly susceptible to lower respiratory infections. Twenty-four episodes of bronchitis or pneumonia were reported in this group compared with seven in the mature group. Frequent chesty colds during the previous six months (the mother stating that 'the doctor is never away from the door') were reported on 24 occasions in the premature group compared with six in the mature group. The figures for other illnesses are approximately equal in the two groups, except for specific infections which were more common amongst mature babies, particularly between 2 and 3 years, no doubt due to the fact that fewer of these children were firstborn, and also that in general they were allowed out to play and mixed with other children at an earlier age.

In the premature group there were two cases of spastic diplegia, one of spastic paraplegia and two of spastic hemiplegia. One child had a considerable degree of deafness, and one suffered from epilepsy. Out of a total of 12 boys, three had unilateral or bilateral inguinal hernia.

Out of a total of 29 children between the ages of 3 and 9 years, about whom a reliable history could be obtained, 12 were reported as having had frequent chesty colds, bronchitis and pneumonia. One boy, aged 5 years, improved as he grew older, but in the other 11 cases the predisposition to lower respiratory infections had persisted since infancy. One school age boy suffered from spastic diplegia.

Visual Defects

A high proportion of the very small, premature babies were later found to have a visual defect. Out of 43 children between the ages of $2\frac{1}{2}$ years and 9 years, 21 (49%) were found to have some visual defect, as shown in Table 6. Twenty of the total

TABLE 6

VISUAL DEFECTS IN 43 CHILDREN AGED $2\frac{1}{2}$ TO 9 YEARS

Retrolental fibroplasia			5
Multiple congenital abnormalities			1
Myopia			11
Low myopia		2	
Moderate myopia		3	
High myopia		6	
Associated squint	7		
No associated squint	4		
Hypermetropia with squint			1
Convergent squint with negligible refractive error			3
Total			21

were of school age and all of them had been seen by the school ophthalmologist. Twenty-three were under school age and had not been seen by an ophthalmologist, except in cases of obvious defect. In the school age group, 13 were found to have some abnormality, *i.e.*, 65%. In the pre-school group, 35% had an obvious defect. It therefore seems probable that some of the pre-school children may be found to have some minor defect of vision when they go up for routine examination on entry into school.

The commonest disorder found was myopia of varying degree. Eleven children were found with this condition, six of them with a considerable degree involving fundal changes. Five children had retrolental fibroplasia with very little useful vision. Of the school age group, five were attending the Royal Blind School.

Emotional Disorders

All the mothers were questioned as to the behaviour of the child: how he reacted to other children and adults, whether there had been any particular problems associated with toilet training, sleeping or feeding habits, and in particular whether the child had been more difficult to handle than his siblings.

Children under the age of 3 years are not included in these results as minor behaviour problems are so common between the ages of 18 months and 3 years as to be considered a part of normal development.

Out of a total of 42 children between the ages of 3 and 9 years, 14 mothers stated that the child had been easy to handle and that there had not been any but minor problems of behaviour. In 28 cases (66·7%), there were, or had been, problems of sufficient degree to be considered abnormal in the particular age group concerned. In 14 cases (33·3%), the emotional disorders could be considered of quite a severe degree. In 17 cases, the child was described as being excessively timid and shy and very dependent on the mother. Characteristically the mother would state that the child was reluctant to go out to play, could never be left with a neighbour, refused to attend Sunday school with older brothers and sisters, and, in the case of school-age children, took a long time to settle down at school. One boy, who lived close to his school, ran away home at play time every day during his first two years at school. Developmental testing with these children was very difficult, cooperation was poor, the child clinging to mother and crying, or remaining obstinately silent. Physical examination and measuring were often resisted vigorously.

Eleven children were described as being highly strung, excitable and nervous, with many fears. Toilet problems and persistent bedwetting after the age of 5 years were reported in six cases. One boy, who attended the ordinary public school, was totally incontinent until the age of 7. Nine children were said to indulge in wild temper tantrums. Head banging, induced vomiting and breath holding were reported in the 3-5 age-group. Two school-age children would throw themselves on the floor, kicking and screaming when thwarted. Sleeping problems and night terrors were described in six cases. One boy of 6 years wakes nearly every night screaming and has to be taken into the parents' bed. This had been going on for several years.

The Headmaster of the Royal Blind School stated that the cases of retrolental fibroplasia attending the school were generally more difficult to handle, and less mature emotionally than other blind children of normal birth weight.

Thirty of the children examined had older or younger siblings. In 11 cases the mother stated that the premature baby had been no more difficult to handle than her other children. In 19 cases (63%) the child has always been more difficult than siblings of normal birth weight.

In four cases the child was one of twins, the other child being over 3 lb. at birth.

Case 1. These twins are aged 7 (twin I, birth weight, 2 lb. 14 oz., twin II, birth weight, 3 lb. 7 oz.), and both children have always been easy to handle. Neither has exhibited any marked behaviour problems. However, the mother says that the smaller twin has always been 'mothered' and protected by the larger and is very dependent on her.

Case 2. These twins are 3 years old. (twin I, birth weight, 2 lb. 12 oz., twin II, birth weight, 5 lb. 2 oz.). The mother has little control over either child. They both exhibit marked temper tantrums and are generally difficult to handle. However, the larger twin is much more independent. The smaller twin is said to be more excitable and highly strung and very dependent on the mother.

Case 3. These twins are 3½ years old (twin I, birth weight, 2 lb. 15 oz., twin II, birth weight, 4 lb. 2 oz.). The larger twin was friendly and cooperative and had always been much easier to handle. The smaller twin showed marked sleeping and feeding problems, was much more dependent on the mother, and was excessively timid and shy. She still indulged in temper tantrums 12 months after her brother had grown out of this phase.

Case 4. The twins are 7 years old (twin I, birth weight, 2 lb. 15 oz., twin II, birth weight, 3 lb. 6 oz.). The mother described the smaller twin as having always been highly strung, nervous and very excitable, in contrast to the larger twin who had never given any anxiety.

It is difficult to know whether the emotional immaturity of many of these children is a direct consequence of their low birth weight or whether it results from over-protection by the parents, and a transference of maternal anxiety to the child. It is possible that the deprivation of normal maternal care during the first few months of life may have some bearing on this problem. Bowlby (1953) suggests that the bad effects of separation from the mother may be evident from the age of a few weeks.

It seems likely that in at least one-third of these cases the emotional instability and immaturity may be as great a handicap to the child in later life as physical inferiority and mental slowness.

Discussion

A study of the growth and development of these 69 children with a very low birth weight suggests that the prognosis for the very small, premature infant is considerably worse than that reported by other workers. American writers suggest that at least 50% will be physically normal and rather more will be average in mentality. Corner (1952) reports on 70 surviving babies weighing less than 3 lb. 4 oz. at birth and states that 53 (76%) were absolutely normal physically and mentally. However, in few of these investigations are details given of physical measurements, mental testing, or any indication as to what standards of normality are employed. It is possible that more detailed examination would have led to different conclusions.

When each case in this study was considered separately, it was found that at least two-thirds of the total were definitely handicapped as a result of their small birth weight. Moreover, if cases of retrolental fibroplasia are excluded, it was found that as many children in the 1-3-year-old group were severely handicapped as those in the school age group. It appears likely that as the survival rate in this low birth weight group improves an increasing number of damaged children will survive.

Summary

The results can be summarized as follows:

Physical Growth. The majority were considerably below average in both weight and height. Out of 64 children, only five had reached the expected weight for their age, and six out of 53 had reached the expected height. The retardation in weight was the most marked, the children being underweight for their height as well as generally small.

Mental Development. In a group of 38 pre-school children, only 14 were considered to have a development quotient of 90 or over. In the school age group of 21 children, three were considered to be of average intelligence.

Morbidity. Children in this low birth weight group appeared to be particularly susceptible to lower respiratory infections. In children of 3 years and under, the incidence was four times as high as that in a matched control group of maturely born children.

Physical Handicaps. Out of 31 children between the ages of 1 and 3 years, five were found to suffer from cerebral diplegia. One further case was found in the school-age group.

One-half of the children had a visual defect, and in one-third this could be considered a definite handicap.

Emotional Disorders. Behaviour problems were reported in two-thirds of the cases, and in one third the emotional disorder could be considered of quite a severe degree.

At least two-thirds of infants in the low birth weight group sustained physical, mental or emotional handicap in later infancy and childhood. This figure is considerably in excess of previous estimates and, moreover, about twice as many under-3-year-old children were severely handicapped as in those of school age. It is suggested that as the survival rate of very small premature infants improves an increasing proportion of damaged infants will survive.

I am indebted to the following, who supplied the data for the section on mental development in the school age group: Dr. W. N. Boog Watson, Chief Executive School Medical Officer, Edinburgh; Miss A. T. Paterson, Principal Educational Psychologist, Edinburgh; Dr. J. Riddell, Medical Officer of Health, Midlothian and Peeblesshire; Dr. C. B. Ross, County Medical Officer of Health, West Lothian; Dr. H. D. Wilson, County Medical Officer, East Lothian; Dr. A. Allan, Medical Officer of Health, Berwickshire; Mr. C. H. W. G. Anderson, Headmaster of the Royal Blind School, Edinburgh, and Dr. G. S. Dhillon, School Ophthalmologist, who provided ophthalmic reports on school age children. I would also like to thank Professor R. W. B. Ellis for his assistance and encouragement throughout.

This research programme has been supported by a grant from the Scottish Hospital Endowments Research Trust.

References

Bowlby, J. (1953). *Child Care and the Growth of Love*, ed. M. Fry. London.
Corner, B. (1952). *Bristol med.-chir. J.*, **69**, 117.
Drillien, C. M. (1957). *J. Obstet. Gynaec. Brit. Emp.*, **64**, 161.
—— and Richmond, F. (1956). *Arch. Dis. Childh.*, **31**, 390.
Ellis, R. W. B. (1956). *Disease in Infancy and Childhood*, 2nd ed. Edinburgh.
Hess, J. H. and Lundeen, E. C. (1949). *The Premature Infant*, 2nd ed. Philadelphia.
Howard, P. J. and Worrell, C. H. (1952). *Pediatrics*, **9**, 577.
Knobloch, H., Rider, R., Harper, P. and Pasamanick, B. (1956). *J. Amer. Med. Ass.*, **161**, 581
Kunstadter, R. H. and Bartelme, P. F. (1934). In Hess, J. H., Mohr, G. J. and Bartelme, P. F. *The Physical and Mental Growth of Prematurely Born Children*, p. 221. Chicago.

THE PROGNOSIS OF BRONCHIECTASIS IN CHILDHOOD*

BY

ALFRED WHITE FRANKLIN

From the Children's Department, St. Bartholomew's Hospital, London

(RECEIVED FOR PUBLICATION JULY 5, 1957)

In England Ogilvie (1941), Field (1949) and Conway (1952) have collected cases of childhood bronchiectasis over the long term and on the large scale needed for worthwhile information. The gloomy prognostication, based on old clinical and necropsy studies, that the bronchiectatic child will not grow up or will be a burden to himself and his neighbours, is not generally true. Since 1926—that is, during 20 to 30 years of active bronchography—the diagnosis has depended on an x-ray appearance of dilatation in more or less of the bronchial tree. On this basis it seems now established that : (1) dilatation once present always persists, except where tubular widening is confined to lobes or segments temporarily collapsed (atelectatic reversible bronchiectasis); (2) under natural conditions the distribution of the affected areas does not alter; and (3) the clinical picture changes little and the tendency is for any change to be for the better even without surgery and without chemotherapy.

In 1944, I (Franklin, 1944) reviewed 24 personal cases of bronchiectasis, observed for periods of four and a half to 13 years, and found 15 of them completely well and free from symptoms, while four were assessed as invalids, and five were classed as delicate according to criteria described below. The x-ray evidence of bronchiectasis had remained constant in distribution throughout the period of observation in all but one of the cases. This boy had the severest form of bronchiectasis clinically, with the added complications of steatorrhoea, an anaemia of pernicious type, and for a short period signs of subacute combined degeneration of the cord. Despite all this and the fact that the bronchiectatic areas spread he is, at the age of 23, well grown, normal and healthy and has been free from respiratory symptoms for six years. With a further follow-up it is possible to take from this whole group 19 cases with an interval from the onset of symptoms of between 13 and 26 years, and one with an interval of 34 years. In all but two the period of observation exceeds 10 years. Of the 20 patients (Table 1), one died aged 20 years of cerebral abscess (before 1944) and three are invalids with severe cough and much purulent sputum. Three, despite large amounts of sputum, are usually well and in light employment. Two are well except for occasional attacks of pneumonia. The remaining 11 patients are completely well and free from symptoms. Of those graded well in 1944, in only one case has there been deterioration, with the copious production of sputum, following an A1 assessment and entry into the British Army. In all the others any change has been for the better.

In 1945 the Meath School of Recovery (for the care of bronchiectatic children aged 5 to 8 years) was opened by the Invalid Children's Aid Association of London through the stimulus of Dr. Elaine Field. I had to assess cases for admission and to see them over their six to 18 months' stay, and have recently reviewed them all or seen clinical reports or x-ray series from their own paediatricians or chest surgeons. Out of 191 admissions between January, 1946, and December, 1952, eight were non-proven cases, 12 were inadequately followed up and the remaining 171 are included in the survey. Children were admitted because too ill to attend day school from home; for convalescence and schooling before, between and sometimes after lung resection; for social reasons, for example, to allow an unmarried mother to work; or when home conditions were considered too bad for a child with chronic respiratory disease.

As the school provided physiotherapy and postural drainage the amount of sputum and cough was stressed at first, but it soon became evident that some ill and undernourished children had little sputum or cough, while others with a great deal of both were extremely well and full of energy. The cases were then grouped (Table 2) as invalid (38 cases), delicate (70 cases) and well (63 cases). The label *invalid* is applied where sputum is of inexhaustible amount or there is failure to

* A paper presented to the combined meeting of the American Pediatric Society, British Paediatric Association, Society for Pediatric Research and Canadian Paediatric Society, Quebec, June, 1955.

TABLE 1

LONG-TERM ASSESSMENT OF 20 PREVIOUSLY REPORTED CASES OF BRONCHIECTASIS (FRANKLIN, 1944)

Assessment in 1944 and Case No.		Age at Follow-up (years)	Observation Period (years)	Age at Onset (years)	Duration of Symptoms (years)	Final Assessment
Invalid ..	3	20	10	4	16	Died aged 20 years
	4	20	12	9/12	19	Delicate (1944)
	6	18	12	4	14	Invalid (1944)
	7	25	19	3/12	25	Well
	11	19	15	2	17	Invalid
Delicate ..	6	18	6	1	17	Delicate (1944)
	12	23	16	Birth	23	Invalid. (Left lower lobectomy at age 19)
	19	25	21	6/12	25	Age 23: empyema. Age 25: light employment. (Gross sputum)
	21	25	22	2	23	Delicate. Light employment. (Gross sputum)
Absolutely well	1	34	22	3/52	34	Well
	2	18	9	8/12	18	Well (1944)
	5	27	17	6/12	26	Well
	9	23	12	4	19	Well
	10	23	20	Birth	23	Well, but treated for duodenal ulcer
	13	20	14	4	16	Well
	15	26	19	6	20	Well
	17	22	10	8	14	Well
	18	15	11	2	13	Well
	20	22	15	4	18	Well
	24	22	19	3	19	Well. (A1 in Army. Gross sputum)

thrive or crippling bronchitis or asthma; a child is labelled *well* not only in the absence of symptoms but also, if growth and energy are normal, when there are minimal amounts of sputum easily cleared, or periodic bronchitis, asthma or fever. The middle group, called *delicate*, have sputum that can be cleared though with difficulty, are capable of some exertion, but tire easily and cannot be described as well. The dividing lines, though not exact, are drawn by one observer.

At the final assessment with the same grouping standards, 15 are invalid, 23 delicate, three have died and 130 out of 171 are well, the follow-up time (not the duration of disease) being three to 10 years. Those classed as well are well grown and lead a full, normal life at school or in employment; 91 are completely free from symptoms, but 39 have traces of sputum, occasional cough, bronchitis or febrile attacks, without notable interference with the conduct of life. Table 2 shows that of 38 originally classed as invalid 14 are well, while of 63 originally well three have become invalid. All three have been operated on, none with complete removal of all affected areas. Three patients have died, one from chloramphenicol treatment, one from cor pulmonale at 16 years after a temporary improvement following partial surgery. The third died as the result of anaesthesia for bronchography, and a fourth might have joined her but for a timely tracheotomy. In these deaths treatment or diagnosis is deeply involved. This might at least discourage the routine annual stocktaking bronchogram.

TABLE 2

FINAL ASSESSMENT OF CASES GROUPED ACCORDING TO ORIGINAL ASSESSMENT

Assessment at Entry to Meath School	Total Cases	Final Assessment			
		Invalid	Delicate	Dead	Well
Invalid	38	10	12	2	14
Delicate ..	70	2	6	1	61
Well	63	3	5	0	55
Total ..	171	15	23	3	130

Tradition demands a statement about finger-clubbing, which in this series was a measure of the degree and activity of infection, disappearing with symptomatic improvement or recovery. The more lobes involved—'lobes' meaning lobe or segment of a lobe—(Table 3) the worse the condition, and much purulent sputum is more likely with saccular than with tubular dilatation. Collapse is commonly reported in radiographs of bronchiectasis, but except in the 'well' group there is usually dilatation of

TABLE 3

NUMBER OF LOBES AND TYPE OF DILATATION IN EACH GROUP

No. of Lobes	Assessment at Entry			Total (171 cases)
	Invalid (38 cases)	Delicate (70 cases)	Well (63 cases)	
1	3	19	18	40
2	6	17	13	36
3	10	18	20	48
4	15	14	11	40
5	4	2	1	7
Saccular ..	22	18	8	48
Fusiform ..	2	3	2	7
Tubular ..	14	49	53	116

bronchi outside the collapsed area and a permanent airless shadow may well be cast by a shrunken fibrous lobe.

Evidence of upper respiratory tract disease was present in all but 30 of the cases (Table 4). In another 46 cases there was either a history of removal of tonsils and adenoids or a simple nasal discharge, or both. In at least half of the invalid and the delicate cases upper respiratory symptoms contributed to the clinical picture. The relation between upper respiratory infection in general, and sinus disease in particular, and bronchiectasis is open to dispute, and the problem of which causes which may be solved by regarding bronchiectasis as sometimes part of a disease of the entire respiratory tract, improvement in one part leading to improvement in the other, but improvement in both being needed for the relief of symptoms. Lobectomy alone has accomplished little in the presence of chronic bronchitis and sinusitis, but if sinus or aural disease can be cleared up the lung condition usually improves.

TABLE 4

UPPER RESPIRATORY INFECTION

	Assessment at Entry		
	Invalid (38 cases)	Delicate (70 cases)	Well (63 cases)
Nasal discharge	19	28	23
Sinus infection	19	28	23
Sinus operation ..	13	21	17
Aural discharge	6	9	13
Aural operation	1	3	3
Removal of tonsils and adenoids	16	45	41
Nasal discharge or removal of tonsils and adenoids alone or in combination ..	8	25	13
No upper respiratory disease	12	10	8

The early onset of symptoms is striking, these starting before the age of 2 years in 99 of 171 cases (Table 5). Some prognostic importance for this is suggested by the fact that this onset of symptoms before the age of 2 years occurred in 13 of 15 judged invalid at the final assessment, in five of the seven cases where all five lobes are involved in 19 of the 20 with severe nutritional disturbance and in 20 of the 22 cases of saccular dilatation in those classed as invalid at entry. That this cannot be blamed on the character of the onset of symptoms is shown in Table 6, which compares the mode of onset in all cases and those beginning under the age of 2 years. There is no appreciable difference in the percentage distribution. Could the greater severity of the disease when the onset is early be due to infection of the lung at a particular stage of its growth?

TABLE 5

AGE AT ONSET OF RESPIRATORY SYMPTOMS

Age at Onset (years)	No. of Cases	Age at Onset (years)	No. of Cases
Under 1 ..	61 } 99	5–6	7 } 15
1–2 ..	38 }	6–7	2
2–3 ..	30	7–8	2
3–4 ..	18 57	8–9	3
4–5 ..	9	Uncertain	1

TABLE 6

CHARACTER OF ONSET

Type of Onset	Total (171 cases)	Per cent. of All Cases (100)	Onset Under 2 Years (99 cases)
From birth	6*	3·5	6
No acute illness ..	56	32·8	35
Pneumonia	51	29·8	31
Whooping-cough ..	32	18·6	16
Measles	19	11·1	9
Other	7	4·2	2

* Plus one case of neonatal pneumonia.

NOTE: Only one case presented as tuberculosis, but four more were probably cases of primary infection, and tuberculosis was present in at least 12 cases, all arising after the age of 2 years.

Although elaborate classifications of bronchiectasis have been suggested in the past, we are inclined now to think and speak of and to treat bronchiectasis as an entity. Accuracy in prognosis might be helped by classifying cases into aetiological groups and clinical types. Certainly the progressive and serious lung lesions in cases of pancreatic fibrosis should be excluded. At the other end of the scale atelectatic unilobar disease should also be excluded unless time proves that the changes persist following expansion of the lung. Empyema complicating pneumonia at onset was found in seven cases, and all these benefited from surgery. The role of tuberculosis is more difficult to determine. The tuberculin state is known only in 50 cases, and was positive in 15 and negative in 35. Only one case presented as tuberculosis, but review suggests that it was important in 11 others, four with primary lesions and seven with collapse or bronchostenosis secondary to enlarged lymph nodes. The particularly suggestive clinical features are an onset after the age of 2 years, involvement localized to one lobe or one lung, temporary finger-clubbing (in two only while there was cough and sputum), a high incidence of 'collapse' and a low one of upper respiratory disease. All cases but one are now in the 'perfectly well' group. Surgery is usually unnecessary for the relief of cough and sputum, and its use depends on the general policy adopted for the surgical treatment of childhood intrathoracic tuberculosis.

Prognosis has been considered in relation to the major clinical types of the disease. In the classical case there is much purulent sputum, often abnormal physical signs in the chest and finger-clubbing. The patient at rest punctuates time with the typical cough, a deep and effortless rattle, while exertion, emotion or changes of posture cause periodic productive paroxysms. There is a small group with some clinical symptoms and signs suggesting the disease, but with bronchitis and asthma as the prominent features, and a still smaller group with recurrent fever and occasional respiratory signs and symptoms. Haemoptysis as the sole evidence of bronchiectasis must be rare in children. Table 7 correlates the assessment at entry with these clinical types, and shows the high incidence of classical cases in the invalid group in contrast with the low incidence of invalids in either bronchitic or febrile cases. The large number of patients, 40, who are classed as well in the group labelled classical needs comment. These children had a classical history and many had the clinical evidence of bronchiectasis at the preliminary examination and even on arrival at the home. The picture though clear was always mild and was short-lived, so that within a few days or weeks of arrival neither cough nor expectoration could be induced by exercise, tipping or tapping.

TABLE 7

ASSESSMENT AT ENTRY AND TYPE OF CLINICAL PICTURE

Assessment at Entry	Total Cases	Classical: Cough and Purulent Sputum	Bronchitic and Asthmatic	Recurrent Febrile Attacks
Invalid ..	38	36	2	0
Delicate ..	70	52	14	4
Well ..	63	41	11	11*
Total ..	171	129	27	15

* Including one case of inhaled foreign body and one of tuberculosis.

This review covers the most active period in the surgical attack on children with bronchiectasis. A total of 71 cases were operated on, including 60 of the 129 classical cases, 26 of which had complete excision of all affected areas and 34 excision of part only. Some of these operations, as judged by the clinical rather than the radiological picture, seem to have been cosmetic, and some to have been carried out to allay the unjustified fear of spread of disease or of deterioration of health. Where there was complete resection of all areas known to be affected 17 of 26 patients are well, but nine retain symptoms of cough and sputum. Of the 34 with partial surgical treatment, 12 are well despite the continued presence of bronchiectatic areas. In one-half of the non-surgical classical cases the patients are well. This group contains milder cases, but also 14 patients with large amounts of sputum who escaped surgery because of the wide-spread disease. Of the 28 bronchitic cases, seven had complete, three partial and 18 no operation. Few if any would have been treated surgically now. One case of recurrent fever out of 15 had complete surgery with improvement. The presentation of figures is difficult and may be misleading, since numbers are small and anything approaching matched controls is impossible. The series lacks consistency because many physicians and surgeons using different criteria were in charge of the cases. The results may at least be claimed to show that surgery is not the complete therapeutic answer. The risk of post-operative pulmonary collapse and consequent spread of bronchiectasis is less than was feared at first, but extensive surgery may increase dyspnoea on exertion and diminish mixing efficiency in the lungs.

The prognosis of any chronic or disabling disease cannot be made on a purely anatomical basis. Sixteen patients (almost one in 10) were of sufficiently low intelligence to require special educational methods, and such cases do badly. The doctor's advice, as well as his methods of diagnosis and treatment, may affect the situation in unintended ways. The only unmanageable boy had been away from home continuously from the age of 10 months to 5 years because of respiratory illness. Twenty-nine other patients were separated from home in early life for long periods on medical advice, though only four of these were led by behaviour disturbance to the Child Guidance Clinic. In six cases great fear of the disease had been induced in parents and children by the doctor's terrible prognosis or by his arguments in favour of surgery. Repeated bronchograms, radiographs and surgical operations take a toll of morale. The record is held by one boy who had 56 *x*-ray exposures in two years. Thirty-five homes were judged physically unsatisfactory, and 10 children from slums undoubtedly improved after rehousing in a new area. Although in three cases operative treatment was considered wisest because of relapse on return to bad housing conditions, in the whole series the physical environment affected the results surprisingly little.

To sketch briefly the course of the commonest, the classical case, the onset is early in life following pneumonia, perhaps complicating whooping-cough or measles or both in succession. The cough, the sputum, with clubbing, cyanosis, abnormal physical signs in the chest and chest deformities, are severe from the outset and continue for five or six years punctuated by recurrent pneumonia. In the lucky case the symptoms gradually improve and at 12 or 13 years of age the child is in comparatively good health except for some productive cough, increasing with any respiratory infection. Later in adolescence the symptoms disappear. In the unlucky case with severe and extensive bilateral saccular disease, chronic pneumonitis leads to permanent invalidism, possibly with cor pulmonale. Such cases are usually too extensive for surgery, while the use of antibiotics, despite a reduction in sputum and a disappearance of bacterial infection, leaves the secretion of copious mucus and the abnormal physical and radiological signs and causes little improvement in the patient's symptoms. By contrast, the mild case dries up with a course of the appropriate antibiotic and may remain free from symptoms for many months or years.

The results in the series reviewed seem quite good. The bad cases, the 15 who remain invalids, are bad indeed, and to prevent such cases seems the only solution. May I suggest that the prognosis is worst with an onset under 2 years of age, that the respiratory tract is often involved as a whole, the bronchial dilatation being only a part of what is wrong; that the extent of the disease is unlikely to change, so that repeated bronchography with its slight though definite risk is unnecessary; that selection of cases for operation requires prolonged observation and deep knowledge of the individual case; and that in assessing prognosis before deciding on treatment the natural history of bronchiectasis be remembered and the whole child and his environment be considered, so that treatment is avoided that might be more harmful than the disease itself.

I acknowledge gratefully the help of Miss Gosling, the Matron at the Meath Home at the relevant period, the staff of the Invalid Children's Aid Association, and the many colleagues in the fields of paediatrics, thoracic surgery and radiology, who have so unselfishly produced clinical records and radiographs and have sanctioned the follow-up visits of their patients. I would also thank the children and their parents for their cooperation, including much travelling.

REFERENCES

Conway, D. J. (1952). M.D. Thesis, Cambridge University.
Field, C. E. (1949). *Pediatrics*, **4**, 21, 231, 355.
Franklin, A. W. (1944). *Proc. roy. Soc. Med.*, **37**, 576.
Ogilvie, A. G. (1941). *Arch. intern. Med.*, **68**, 395.

A CONSIDERATION OF COLOSTRUM AND MILK AS SOURCES OF ANTIBODIES WHICH MAY BE TRANSFERRED TO THE NEWBORN BABY

BY

KATHLEEN E. BOORMAN, BARBARA E. DODD and MAVIS GUNTHER

From the South London Transfusion Centre, the Department of Forensic Medicine, London Hospital Medical College, and the Obstetric Hospital, University College Hospital, London

(RECEIVED FOR PUBLICATION JULY 19, 1957)

The fact that antibodies can be conveyed to a newborn animal by colostrum was first shown by Ehrlich (1892). In his experiments artificial antibodies to abrin and ricin were induced in mice; after exchange of litters of immunized and non-immunized animals, the litters suckled from immunized mothers had acquired some measure of protection to abrin and ricin. Although the antibodies of colostrum are known to be absorbed unaltered by the newborn calf and lamb (Mason, Dalling and Gordon, 1930), there has been no clear evidence that such absorption occurs in human beings. If it does occur it is of less significance and is harder to detect because the baby, unlike a calf or lamb, is endowed before birth with maternal antibodies which it receives transplacentally. Thus the maternal serum, and therefore the infant's serum, will contain antibodies of the same specificity as the colostrum. When the baby is fed by its mother, absorption from the colostrum can be recognized only by an increase of the antibodies already in the baby's serum.

The question of absorption, even in small quantities, of unaltered antibodies is of importance, although the effects of depriving the child of colostrum or breast milk are not dramatic as in ungulates. We need to know what qualities or substances in breast milk contribute to the baby's defences and make the incidence of infection lower than among the bottle-fed. The lower incidence of gastro-enteritis among breast-fed babies (Douglas, 1950) could be explained by postulating less exposure to infection, but Douglas also found a significant protection against measles conferred by suckling. This protection showed a correlation with the length of lactation and lasted longer. The finding suggested that over a long period of breast feeding small amounts of globulin or antibody are absorbed or derived from the milk, or alternatively that breast milk influences the baby's hormonal or other control of its own antibodies. The widespread belief in the benefit of breast milk for premature babies conforms with the idea of antibody transfer, since the serum globulin is low in premature infants (Rimington and Bickford, 1946). If the protection which milk confers depends on the absorption of unaltered antibodies, heat treatment of breast milk should be avoided so far as is possible. If, on the other hand, the globulins of colostrum and milk are broken down in digestion and yet contribute to the baby's specific immunity, they do so presumably by providing the material for the rebuilt globulins, and heat treatment might be expected to have little or no effect. The possibility of absorption of unaltered antibodies is also of more direct and obvious importance in deciding whether an Rh-negative mother with Rh antibodies in her serum, colostrum and milk should feed her Rh-positive infant from the breast, or whether this would increase the severity of the haemolytic disease of the newborn from which it was already suffering.

In the investigation described here the anti-A and anti-B content of maternal serum, colostrum and milk, and of infant's serum taken at birth and at 3 and 10 days post partum, was determined. This was done in order to find the range of titration values and whether there was any correlation between them, for instance, whether a high titre of agglutinins in the maternal serum is associated with a high titre of the same agglutinins in the colostrum and milk, and whether the agglutinins of colostrum and milk pass unaltered through the digestive tract of the infant and appear in its serum. It was hoped in this way to measure the contribution of maternal antibodies which might be expected in completely normal physiological circumstances when any other effects such as the antitryptic effect of colostrum would be in full play. The question also arose whether the agglutinins might cause or prolong haemolytic disease of the newborn.

In the second part of the study a number of Rh-negative babies were bottle-fed with fluids containing anti-D antibodies and their sera examined at intervals for the appearance of these antibodies.

Serological Methods

The ABO grouping and Rh typing of maternal and cord samples was by the standard tube technique. The ABO grouping included tests on the cells and serum of each individual.

Titration of Antibodies. The anti-A and anti-B agglutinins were titrated in the maternal serum taken at the time of delivery, in the colostrum on the third day and in the milk on the tenth day. In the infant the anti-A and anti-B agglutinins of the cord serum were titrated, also those of serum obtained by heel prick on the third and tenth days after birth.

The method used for titration of antibodies in serum was essentially as described by Taylor and Ikin (1939). Doubling dilutions of test serum were made in saline with a Pasteur pipette graduated to deliver a constant volume (about 0·03 ml.). To each of the dilutions an equal volume of a 2% suspension of appropriate red cells was added, the cells being always from the same donors and freshly drawn each day. The titrations were made in duplicate and allowed to stand at room temperature for two to three hours, after which the contents of the tubes were examined for agglutination both macroscopically and microscopically. The presence of evenly distributed clumps of three or more cells was accepted as evidence of agglutination. The titre of a serum sample was expressed as the reciprocal of the highest dilution of serum causing agglutination.

The maternal colostrum and milk were titrated in exactly the same way as the serum. It was, however, found necessary to centrifuge these fluids rapidly for five minutes so that the cream could be removed from the surface and discarded. Colostrum and milk also agglutinated Group O cells but the titration value was low; however, a titration against Group O cells was included for each sample (see also Hirszfeld and Lille-Szyszkowicz, 1949).

Complete or saline-agglutinating Rh antibodies were titrated in a similar way, but were incubated at 37° C. instead of at room temperature. Owing to the fragile nature of the agglutinates, great care was taken in handling the contents of each tube when reading the tests. The standard red cells used were of the genotypes R_1R_1 (CDeCDe) and R_2r (cDEcde), together with rr (cdecde) as a negative control.

For the titration of incomplete or albumin-agglutinating Rh antibodies a slightly modified technique was used. The serial dilutions of the serum being tested were made in AB serum instead of saline and an equal volume of a 2% suspension of standard red cells in bovine albumin was added to each tube. The same precautions were taken in reading the tests.

Detection of Rh Antibodies. Four techniques were employed for the detection of anti-Rh (anti-D) antibodies in the baby's serum.

(*a*) Saline Technique. Equal volumes of the serum to be tested and a 2% suspension of standard cells were incubated for two hours and then the red cells were examined microscopically for agglutination, the Rh genotypes of the cells used being the same as those for the titration of saline agglutinins.

(*b*) Albumin Technique. Equal volumes of serum and a 2% suspension of red cells made in 30% bovine albumin were incubated for two hours and the tests read in the same manner as for the saline technique. For this test the standard cells used were of genotypes R_1R_2 (CDecDE) and rr (cdecde).

(*c*) Indirect Coombs Technique. Equal volumes of serum to be tested and a 5% suspension of standard red cells were incubated for two hours at 37° C. The red cells were then carefully washed three times in saline and a drop of anti-human-globulin serum was mixed with them on a slide. The slide was then gently rocked and the smear examined for agglutination, if necessary microscopically. The results were not recorded as negative until the slides had been under observation for five minutes. The anti-globulin reagent was controlled against known sensitized cells with each batch of tests. Each serum examined was tested against three D-positive and two D-negative samples of standard cells.

(*d*) Trypsin Technique. A stock solution was made by dissolving 0·1 g. of crystalline trypsin (Armour) in 10 ml. $\frac{N}{20}$ HCl. Each day before use the trypsin solution was diluted 1 in 10 with 0·1 M phosphate buffer at *p*H 7·7. This buffered enzyme was added to twice-washed cells of the appropriated Rh type in the proportion of four parts of solution to one part of packed red cells. (The red cells used for trypsin testing are freshly bled into 3·7% sodium citrate solution, separated by centrifugation and washed twice with 0·85% saline.) After adding buffered trypsin solution the red cells were incubated at 37° C. for 30 minutes, then washed twice in warm saline at 37° C. Before adding the trypsin-treated cells to the test sera a 2-4% suspension of the cells was made in warm saline. Equal volumes of test serum and trypsinized red cells were incubated for approximately one hour at 37° C. and the tests read for agglutination. In the case of trypsin tests it is not advisable to handle the cell sediments too gently or false positive results may be obtained. The same standard cells were used for the test as for the indirect Coombs test.

Part I: Titres of Anti-A and Anti-B Isoagglutinins in Colostrum and Milk and Infants' Sera

Samples were taken from 97 mothers and their babies. Of the mothers, 52 belonged to Group O, 39 to Group A, four to Group B and two to Group AB. The anti-A and anti-B agglutinins were titrated in the maternal serum taken at the time of delivery, in the colostrum on the third day post partum and in the milk on the tenth day. The baby's serum was tested for the presence of anti-A and anti-B agglutinins in the cord blood at birth and at the third and tenth days of life. Cases in which the baby was small were not included, nor were those in which breast feeding was unsuccessful.

Results. The titres of anti-A and anti-B agglutinins in the maternal serum ranged from 16 to 1,000; in the milk, from 1 to 1,000; and in the colostrum, from 2 to 64,000. In most cases the concentration of agglutinins was higher in colostrum than in milk.

The titres of anti-A and anti-B agglutinins in the infant's serum were low, ranging from 0 to 16, and the majority of them were less than 8. The relationship between titres of agglutinins in colostrum and in milk and those in maternal serum and colostrum, and the change of titre in the infant's serum and colostrum, are shown in Figs. 1-3. (In these diagrams the titre is expressed in units of the number of serial dilutions and not in the actual dilution.) These relationships are all in respect of the anti-B agglutinin, because owing to the distribution of ABO blood groups there are many more cases in which the anti-B agglutinin is compatible with the infant's red cells.

A true picture of the state of affairs with regard to agglutinins that are incompatible with the infant's red cells cannot be obtained owing to absorption of these agglutinins by the infant's tissues and body fluids.

Discussion. Figs. 1 and 2 show that there is some correlation between titres of agglutinins in colostrum and milk and between those of maternal serum and colostrum, the tendency being for women with high serum titres to possess the highest colostrum titres, and also, as might be expected, high colostrum titres were followed by higher titres of antibody in the milk.

Evidence of an effect of colostrum titre on that of the infant's serum was sought by plotting the colostrum titre against the change in titre in the infant's serum between birth and the tenth day (Fig. 3). No significant correlation was found, nor was there any correlation when the titres of milk were similarly plotted.

The range of titre of the agglutinin in colostrum in this group of cases was between 2 and 8,000. Assuming that the effect of dilution would be similar if it were absorbed unchanged, it was thought that some difference in titre in the sera of babies after the ingestion of colostrum with this range of titre variation might be detectable. With complete absorption the dilution in the baby's intravascular fluids would be of the order of one in six for each ounce taken. By the tenth day a baby fully fed from the breast may have received between one-half and two-thirds of its birth weight in colostrum and milk. Even if most of the secretion were milk a substantial absorption of agglutinins might reasonably be expected to be reflected in the infant's serum. The

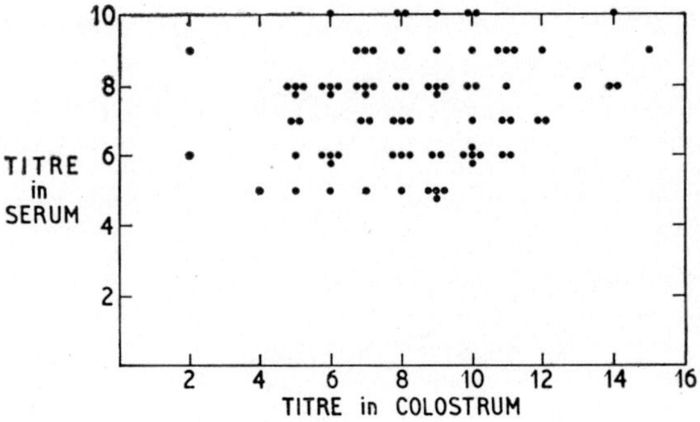

FIG. 2.—Relationship between titres of agglutinins in maternal serum and colostrum.

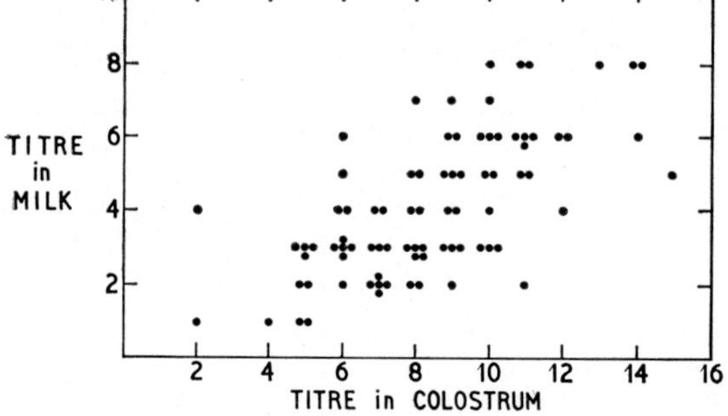

FIG. 1.—Relationship between titres of agglutinins in colostrum and milk.

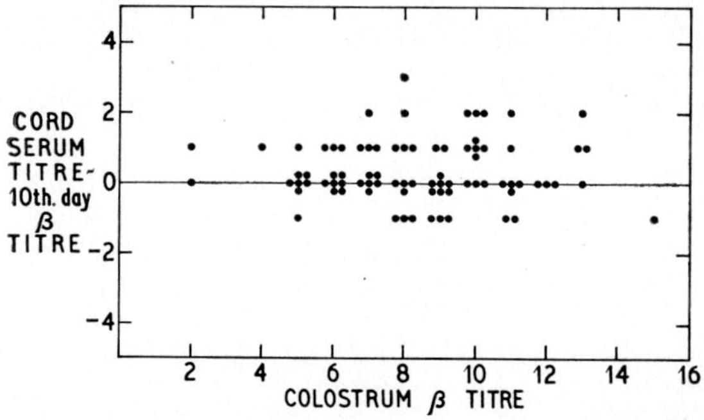

FIG. 3.—Showing effect of colostrum titre on that of infant's serum.

range of titre in the colostrum and milk was so great that it is unlikely that variations in the amount taken would have obscured evidence of absorption if it had occurred in more than trace amounts.

It is of interest to note that in the cases in which the infant was taking large quantities of incompatible agglutinin with the colostrum and milk, for example, Group A babies of Group O mothers in some of whom the colostrum titres were 512-4,000, no sign of jaundice or anaemia was observed in the baby.

The fact that a few infants' sera showed agglutinin titres above 8 seems to indicate that occasionally saline agglutinins as opposed to incomplete antibodies are able to cross the placental barrier and enter the foetal circulation. In the opinion of some workers only incomplete antibodies are capable of this.

The above study of anti-A and anti-B content of maternal serum, milk and colostrum are an early one and a measure of incomplete antibodies was made. Very recently some evidence in a few cases had been obtained for the transfer of incomplete anti-A from mother to milk and from milk to infant (Munk-Anderson, Aagaard and Dyggve, 1957).

Part II: Inhibition of Rh Antibodies by Newborn Babies

Method. Either milk or serum containing Rh antibodies of high titre was given by mouth to normal babies. The Rh type was determined from the cord blood at birth, and feeding of the material was started as soon as possible afterwards. The antibody containing material had been collected from suitable donors and stored at −18° C. until required. It was gently warmed to a suitable temperature for the baby, and the residue from each feed was saved and titrated to confirm that the heat had not altered the titration value. The infant's serum was obtained by heel puncture and in every case samples were taken during feeding and approximately daily for two or three days afterwards.

In all, 21 babies were fed with either serum or milk containing Rh antibodies. The first 11 of these were investigated before the introduction of the very sensitive trypsin technique for the detection of incomplete antibodies, and the last 10 cases were investigated with this technique as well as the indirect Coombs technique.

With one exception Rh-negative babies were selected to avoid possible injury to the baby and also to eliminate the risk of antibodies becoming attached specifically to tissue cells and thus not being detectable in the circulation.

Milk containing Rh antibodies was given to one Rh-negative and one Rh-positive baby, and serum containing Rh-antibodies of both complete and incomplete types was fed to the remaining 19. High-titre fluids were deliberately selected in order to obtain the maximum chance of detecting antibody in the infant's circulation if present. The first dose of the material was given as early as possible in life; two babies even received it within two hours of birth. This timing was chosen to test the possibility that absorption in human beings resembles that in ungulates: absorption is almost quantitative in calves and lambs during the first 24 hours, but virtually ceases after 48 hours. The serum was either fed

TABLE

Case No.	Rhesus Group	Age of Baby when Antibody Received	Material Taken and Volume (ml.)	Titre and Type of Antibody	Maximum Effective Volume (litres)	Birth Weight (kg.)	Fraction of Dose Estimated Detectable in Intravascular Plasma
1	Rh+	4–9 days	Milk 278	64	26	3·71	1 in 40
2	Rh−	12 hrs.–5 days	Serum 340	64	16	3·97	1 in 80
3	Rh−	12 hrs.–2 days	Serum 119	16	2	2·79	1 in 13
4	Rh−	12 hrs.–3 days	Serum 153	32	6	3·09	1 in 40
5	Rh−	2–5 days	Serum 26	1,000	27	3·69	1 in 140
6	Rh−	18 hrs.–4 days	Milk 810	8	3	3·00	1 in 20
7	Rh−	11–19 hrs.	Serum 17	1,000; saline	17	4·17	1 in 82
8	Rh−	12–24 hrs.	Serum 25	1,000; saline	25	3·32	1 in 150
9	Rh−	12–24 hrs.	Serum 25	1,000; saline	25	3·00	1 in 166
10	Rh−	2–10 hrs.	Serum 17	2,000; saline	34	4·03	1 in 170
11	Rh−	2–4 hrs.	Serum 18	2,000; saline	36	3·74	1 in 194
12	Rh−	13–38 hrs.	Serum 47	1,000; saline	47	3·44	1 in 273
13	Rh−	15–35 hrs.	Serum 18	1,000; albumin	18	3·64	1 in 100
14	Rh−	17–36 hrs.	Serum 22	512; albumin	10	3·34	1 in 61
15	Rh−	15–36 hrs.	Serum 22	1,000; albumin	22	3·05	1 in 44
16	Rh−	10–29 hrs.	Serum 20	512; albumin	8	3·05	1 in 52
17	Rh−	27–50 hrs.	Serum 17	512; albumin	8	3·76	1 in 43
18	Rh−	53–85 hrs.	Serum 21	256; saline	5	3·10	1 in 32
19	Rh−	36–41 hrs.	Serum 12	512; albumin	6	3·08	1 in 39
20	Rh−	3–40 hrs.	Serum 23	256; saline	5	3·60	1 in 28
21	Rh−	8–33 hrs.	Serum 16	512; albumin	8	3·40	1 in 47

Cases 12–21 received the serum together with colostrum.

mixed with measured amounts of fresh colostrum, or given immediately after the feed from the breast in eight cases in order that the antitryptic effect of colostrum or any other unsuspected factor which might assist in antibody absorption might play its physiological rôle.

Results. The accompanying Table gives the volume and titre of the material and the time it was given, together with the birth weight of the baby. Some measure is needed to show what proportion of the antibody would have to be absorbed in order to be detected, although an estimation of this kind can be only approximate. From this it will be assumed that the material, if absorbed unaltered, dispersed round the body, and when obtained in serum from a heel prick would agglutinate cells at a final dilution corresponding to that in the original serum. This leaves no allowance for any 'carry-over' effect in the original titration. If the number of millilitres of each dose of material is multiplied by the highest dilution at which agglutination is obtained, the sum of all the products for all the doses given to one baby amounts to a volume to which the entire dose might be diluted and still be detectable. If this hypothetical effective volume is compared with the baby's intravascular fluid volume a proportion is obtained which shows very roughly how much of the dose would have to be absorbed to be detectable. These findings are also summarized in the Table, which gives the hypothetical effective volume and its relation to the baby's intravascular fluid. In no case were Rh antibodies detected in the serum after the infant had been fed with milk or serum containing these antibodies in high titre. In the first 11 cases tests were made by saline and indirect Coombs techniques, using red cells from individuals homozygous for antigen D as well as Rh-negative cells as a negative control. In the last 10 cases tests by the trypsin technique were also included, since in some instances it has been shown that this technique will reveal the presence of antibodies when other techniques fail.

Discussion. The volume of milk or serum fed to the babies was necessarily less than the amount of milk a baby obtains by suckling, but the titre of the material was very much higher than the titres commonly found in the breast secretion of women with antibodies. In the course of the search for colostrum and milk with Rh antibodies of high titre many samples were examined. The milk eventually obtained and used for feeding was of exceptionally high titre.

If one may assume that antibodies of high titre, when diluted, are comparable to weak ones, the amounts of antibodies received by the babies were within the range of doses commonly transferred by suckling in the first days of life. It is, however, possible that the absorption of antibodies from colostrum might be different from absorption from serum since, for instance, colostrum contains trypsin inhibitors (Laskowski and Laskowski, 1951).

Antibodies, if absorbed, would be detectable only if the rate of their destruction or removal were relatively slow. The rate of disappearance of other passive immune bodies has been found to extend over weeks rather than days (Barr, Glenny and Randall, 1949). This slow rate was confirmed in the present investigation by studying the fall in titre in babies' sera. Two babies, the unaffected children of mothers with Rh antibodies from previous sensitization, received Rh antibodies transplacentally. These remained detectable for two weeks. Two were given antibody intravenously and the rate of disappearance of the antibody in these two cases is given in Fig. 4. It is concluded that the negative

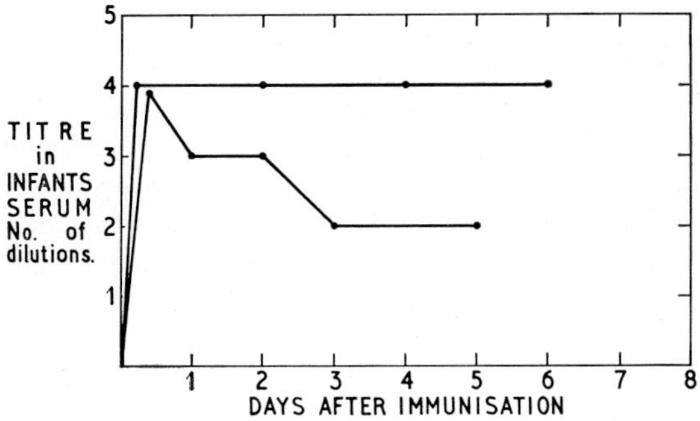

FIG. 4.—Showing rate of disappearance of antibody given intravenously to two babies.

result of the tests for absorbed agglutinins was not attributable to quick removal of the antibody or to ill timing of the sampling of the infant's serum.

Cathie (1947) also found no evidence of absorption of unaltered antibodies. His material was given to Rh-positive individuals, one man and several children, the youngest apparently being 1 week old. He concluded that there was no justification for weaning infants with haemolytic disease on account of the presence of Rh antibodies in the breast milk. Since his subjects were Rh positive there was a likelihood that if partial absorption occurred, the antibodies might become attached to tissues without becoming detectable in the serum. The dosage given in the present investigation and the fact that the subjects were Rh negative are believed to have ensured that if even only a small proportion of the antibody given were absorbed it would have been detected. The fact that no absorbed antibody was found in the infant's serum is not regarded as conclusive evidence that Rh-positive babies of mothers with Rh antibodies may be fed from the breast during the first days of life. It seems undesirable to give a baby, whether mildly or severely affected with haemolytic disease, more of the one substance from which it is suffering. The mechanism, whether it is intestinal juice, gut wall or liver, which prevents free absorption is unknown; nor is it known whether the mechanism is injured in affected babies. Since affected babies are nearly always the offspring of multiparae, the maintenance of lactation without putting the baby to the breast is usually practicable for the seven or eight days until the agglutinin titre of the milk has fallen. During this time expressed milk may be boiled and given to the baby, and direct feeding started on the eighth day.

The slow elimination of passive immune bodies and the range of dosage used in this investigation still leave a possibility that a baby could slowly accumulate rather than lose antibodies although no absorption has been detected. The protection afforded by breast milk against measles (Douglas) already mentioned hints that this is so. It is therefore recommended that a baby born with cells sensitized by Rh agglutinins should be fed from the breast after eight days and fed with heated expressed breast milk until then. Moreover, since we have not been able to demonstrate the transfer of antibodies from milk and colostrum to the infant, there is no reason to suppose that by heating the breast milk the baby is being deprived of other kinds of antibody which are beneficial.

Summary

Part I. Samples of serum, colostrum and milk from 97 mothers and their infants were tested for their anti-A and anti-B content.

The titres of anti-A and anti-B agglutinins in the maternal serum ranged from 16 to 1,000, in the milk from 1 to 1,000, in the colostrum from 2 to 64,000 and in the infant's serum from 0 to 16. Some correlation was noted between titres of agglutinins in colostrum and milk and between those of maternal serum and colostrum. No correlation was established between titres of colostrum or milk and the infants' serum.

Part II. Serum and milk containing Rh antibodies were given to one Rh-positive and 20 Rh-negative infants in the first days of life.

The infants' sera were tested for Rh antibodies by saline and indirect Coombs techniques in the first 11 cases, and by saline, indirect Coombs and trypsin techniques in the last 10 cases. No Rh antibodies were detected.

The material given would have been detectable after dilution in the baby's intravascular fluid if approximately one in 150 parts was absorbed unaltered.

The material was given to some babies within 24 hours of birth. Absorption comparable to that which occurs in ungulates immediately after birth was not found.

The sensitivity of the methods used does not preclude absorption of traces of unaltered antibodies by babies already affected by Rh antibodies. Expression and heat treatment of breast milk during the first eight days is recommended where the baby's cells are sensitized.

Our thanks are due to Dr. J. F. Loutit, Dr. R. A. Zeitlin and Miss Doreen Daley for their help and cooperation in this work, most of which was carried out while we were employed by the Medical Research Council.

References

Barr, M., Glenny, A. T. and Randall, K. J. (1949). *Lancet*, **2**, 324.
Cathie, I. A. B. (1947). *Brit. med. J.*, **2**, 650.
Douglas, J. W. B. (1950). *J. Obstet. Gynaec. Brit. Emp.*, **57**, 335.
Ehrlich, P. (1892). *Z. Hyg. Infekt.-Kr.*, **12**, 183.
Hirszfeld, L. and Lille-Szyszkowicz, J. (1949). *Rev. Immunol. (Paris)*, **13**, 265.
Laskowski, M., Jr., Laskowski, M. (1951). *J. biol. Chem.*, **190**, 563.
Mason, J. H., Dalling, T. and Gordon, W. S. (1930). *J. Path. Bact.*, **33**, 783.
Munk-Anderson, G., Aagaard, K. and Dyggve, H. (1957). VI Congress of the European Society of Haematology Abstracts, p. 153.
Rimington, C. and Bickford, J. A. (1946). *Biochem. J.*, **40**, xxvi.
Taylor, G. L. and Ikin, E. W. (1939). *Brit. med. J.*, **1**, 1027.

THE SERUM PROTEINS AT 6 MONTHS OF AGE IN INFANTS FED ON HUMAN OR COW'S MILK OR ON BOTH

BY

FATMA HASSAN and MAVIS GUNTHER
From the Department of Child Welfare, University College Hospital, London

(RECEIVED FOR PUBLICATION JULY 19, 1957)

The finding by Douglas (1950) that breast-fed babies possess an immunity to measles which bottle-fed babies do not, and the fact that the administration of γ globulin can protect a baby from the infection, suggested that babies receiving human milk might have a greater serum γ globulin content than those giving cow's milk from a bottle. In a serological investigation of neonatal antibodies Boorman, Dodd and Gunther (1958) could detect no increase in the baby's circulating Rh antibodies as a result of feeding high-titre serum; nor could they find any effect on serum isoagglutinins from the consumption of colostrum and milk of varying titres of anti-A and anti-B agglutinins which the babies received from their mothers. It seemed possible, however, that γ globulins were more readily absorbed or rebuilt, even though they might lose their particular immunological specificity, from human rather than bovine globulins taken by mouth. The absorption of serum proteins of the animal's own species and not of others has been suggested by Dent and Schilling (1948) from their work on dogs. Although the total quantity of γ globulin needed to alter a baby's susceptibility to measles is small, it seemed worth while to see whether a detectable difference in the serum proteins was produced over a period of months by different methods of feeding.

Present Investigation

In the investigation here reported comparison was made of the serum from babies who were known to have received only one kind of milk, human or bovine, from birth or a mixture of both. By 6 months of age they had, however, all received other foods in small quantities. The total protein in the serum at 6 months of age was estimated by the density method of Linderstrøm-Lang and Lanz (1938) as modified by Lowry and Hunter (1945). The serum was subjected to electrophoresis on a paper strip (Flynn and de Mayo, 1951) and the components were estimated by a scanner and direct transmission of light (Crook, Harris and Warren, 1952).

Results

The sera from the three groups of infants, receiving (*a*) breast milk, (*b*) cow's milk or (*c*) a mixture of human and cow's milk, showed no significant differences in their content of total protein and none in the content of the components of albumin and of α_1, α_2, β and γ globulin (see Table).

It is concluded that no differences in the serum protein levels resulting from feeding the infants with human or cow's milk could be detected in the samples by micro-electrophoretic analysis.

Our best thanks go to Professor F. L. Warren and to Dr. N. R. Butler for their help.

REFERENCES

Boorman, K. E., Dodd, B. E. and Gunther, M. (1958). *Arch. Dis. Childh.*, **33**, 24.
Crook, E. M., Harris, H. and Warren, F. L. (1952). *Biochem. J.*, **51**, xxvi.
Dent, C. E. and Schilling, J. A. (1948). *Ibid.*, **42**, xxix.
Douglas, J. W. B. (1950). *J. Obstet. Gynaec. Brit. Emp.*, **57**, 335.
Flynn, F. V. and de Mayo, P. (1951). *Lancet*, **2**, 235.
Linderstrøm-Lang, K. and Lanz, H. (1938). C.R. Lab. Carlsberg (Ser. chim.), **21**, 315. (No. 24).
Lowry, O. H. and Hunter, T. H. (1945). *J. biol. Chem.*, **159**, 465.

TABLE

SERUM PROTEINS OF BABIES AT 6 MONTHS FED WITH HUMAN OR COW'S MILK OR A MIXTURE OF BOTH

Feeding	No. of Cases	Mean Birth Weight (g.)	Total Protein (g./100 ml.)		Albumin %		α_1 Globulin %		α_2 Globulin %		β Globulin %		γ Globulin %	
					Rel.	Absol.	Rel.	Absol.	Rel.	Absol.	Rel.	Absol.	Rel.	Absol.
Breast	11	3,400	Mean	6·42	64·56	4·16	4·61	0·293	10·12	0·64	12·87	0·82	7·64	0·48
			S.D.	0·55	3·69	0·55	0·95	0·048	2·43	0·14	1·89	0·13	2·59	0·127
Bottle	6	3,515	Mean	6·37	65·1	4·15	5·42	0·41	10·01	0·64	11·75	0·72	7·74	0·49
			S.D.	0·57	2·38	0·34	0·69	0·073	1·28	0·097	2·24	0·09	2·52	0·19
Mixed	11	3,285	Mean	6·16	62·5	3·79	5·58	0·34	10·91	0·67	13·25	0·81	7·80	0·48
			S.D.	0·47	4·24	0·91	1·32	0·073	1·66	0·117	1·64	0·085	1·92	0·12

THE DIETARY TREATMENT OF PHENYLKETONURIA

BY

L. I. WOOLF, RUTH GRIFFITHS, ALAN MONCRIEFF, STEPHEN COATES and F. DILLISTONE

From the Institute of Child Health and The Hospital for Sick Children, Great Ormond Street, London

(RECEIVED FOR PUBLICATION JULY 10, 1957)

Phenylketonuria is an inborn error of the metabolism of phenylalanine associated almost invariably with grave mental deficiency, and often with epilepsy resembling petit mal. It was suggested that the mental deficiency was due to an intoxication by phenylalanine or one of its metabolites and might be relieved by feeding a diet low in phenylalanine (Woolf and Vulliamy, 1951). An economically practicable form of such a diet, based on a charcoal-treated casein acid hydrolysate, was devised by one of us (L.I.W.) and first fed to a phenylketonuric child by Bickel, Gerrard and Hickmans (1953).* They reported a dramatic improvement in mentality in their patient and Woolf, Griffiths and Moncrieff (1955), using objective psychometric methods, found a marked improvement in three other cases. Since then there have been a number of reports of the successful application of the dietary treatment of phenylketonuria (*e.g.*, Armstrong and Tyler, 1955; Braude, 1956; Horner and Streamer, 1956; Blainey and Gulliford, 1956), and it is evidently being widely adopted. We are reporting here our experiences both with the original three patients (now followed for a further 32 months) and with a further seven phenylketonuric children who have been treated on the diet for periods varying from 11 to 34 months. One of these has been treated from the age of a few weeks for over two years, and has remained in the normal range of intelligence. Another, treated from the age of 4 months, has not shown the further deterioration in intelligence which would be expected if untreated. The rest have all improved in intelligence rating; in two of the four cases with fits these ceased soon after the children were placed on the diet, and the E.E.G. became nearly normal (*cf.* Wolf, 1956).

Of the children who have been or are being treated with the diet at this hospital, all but eight are reported here. Of these eight, one lives at a considerable distance, while the other seven have been treated for too short a time to enable any conclusions to be drawn.

Clinical Summaries

Case 1. This child, a sibling of Case 9, was born in February, 1955, weighing 6 lb. 3 oz. (her twin sister, born first, weighed 7 lb. 10 oz. at birth). Urine obtained on the seventeenth day of life contained phenylpyruvic acid and both twins were admitted at the age of 3 weeks. Phenylpyruvic acid could not be detected in the urine of the twin sister and paper chromatography showed that her urinary phenylalanine concentration was normal. Dr. Cedric Carter kindly saw them and tests showed conclusively that they are dizygous. The blood group of Case 1 was O, NN, CD (probable genotype R_1R_1) and of the normal twin O, NN, CDc (probable genotype R_1r). Both children appeared normal physically, and clinically about identical in behaviour. Intelligence tests were carried out on both twins and will be discussed later. The affected twin was weaned from the breast and a special synthetic 'milk', low in phenylalanine was started (see page 39), and she was quickly worked up to an intake of 50 calories per lb. per day. She lost a little weight and the intake was increased at first to 60 calories per lb. and then to 70 calories as she appeared to be hungry. The weight increased rather slowly and the amount of cow's milk added to the diet was several times increased, each increase accelerating the weight gain. She became anaemic in appearance, the haemoglobin fell and a blood transfusion was given. Clinically, she did not appear quite as bright as her twin sister but intelligence testing gave a very satisfactory result, showing her to be average at the age of 15 weeks, with a 'general quotient'* (G.Q.) of 99. She was re-admitted with a bad 'cold' at the age of 5 months having continued on her special 'milk' as an out-patient. At the age of 6 months, she weighed 14 lb. 10 oz. and was doing very well physically and mentally. The urine remained free from phenylpyruvic acid. She became difficult over feeds and was re-admitted for weaning on to a more solid diet but this proved an impossible task, and weaning was delayed for a further few months. She was successfully weaned on to solids at 15 months and is now getting a mixed diet like that of her older sister (Case 9). Her mother did not think

* It was Dr. Bickel who undertook the laborious task of preparing the charcoal-treated casein hydrolysate, now commercially available, and who courageously first gave it to a phenylketonuric patient.

* The G.Q. is derived from a scale (Griffiths, 1954) suitable for testing very young children of low mental age (see page 34).

her progress quite so good as her twin sister's but intelligence tests were satisfactory, the child's G.Q. having reached a 'plateau' of about 88. An E.E.G. was performed on June 13, 1956, and was within normal limits as far as could be ascertained on a short record with the eyes open.

For several months she had very little hair on her head. When it finally grew it was golden, exactly the same colour as her normal twin sister's and unlike the grey-blonde characteristic of phenylketonuria. (The family was fair-haired, see Case 9.)

Case 2. This girl, born on October 9, 1951, was under the care of Dr. P. R. Evans. She originally attended at the age of just over 1 year for muscular weakness and failure to thrive. There had been a few attacks which were possibly 'fits'. The urine was not examined for phenylpyruvic acid at this time. Her retardation was not great and progress continued. She walked at just under 2 years. At this time phenylketonuria was diagnosed but no treatment was instituted. A year later in view of success with the diet in other cases she was admitted, and a phenylalanine-free diet was started in September, 1954. She was at this time a blue-eyed blonde with an I.Q. of 71. There have been no fits since the age of 2 years (on no medicaments). An E.E.G. in 1954, before the condition was first treated, was normal. Her physical development is normal. She had been a contact with a patient with active pulmonary tuberculosis, and her Mantoux reaction became positive in November, 1954, but the child has shown no evidence of the disease. The phenylalanine-free diet has been maintained since the autumn of 1954, though with occasional mild lapses. In the autumn of 1956, her I.Q. having reached the level of 92, she started school, being nearly 5 years old. Her teacher has said, 'She is a normal child, no different from the others.'

Case 3. This child was born on February 17, 1951, and the following is a summary of the previous clinical account (Woolf *et al.*, 1955).

One older brother is a proved phenylketonuric. Case 3 was late in sitting up, standing and walking. She had no illnesses and no fits. Phenylketonuria was discovered at the age of 2 years 7 months and dietary treatment was begun in October, 1953. An E.E.G. was normal and her G.Q. was 42. Her very pale hair became dark under treatment.

Continuation of History. She was re-admitted for assessment in January, 1954, and appeared to be progressing. She was more active than before. Phenylpyruvic acid was absent from the urine. Similar results were found when admitted in April, 1954, and again in July, 1954. She was admitted to Tadworth Branch Hospital in September, 1954, for three weeks while her parents had a holiday. Her urine remained free from phenylpyruvic acid. She had a slight gastro-intestinal upset in October, 1954. The clinical impression was one of continuing improvement. In April, 1956, it was noted that her parents were inclined to be careless and phenylpyruvic acid was found in the urine on one occasion. Her I.Q., which had been rising steadily, levelled off at 57, and then slipped back to 52 at this time. The dietary errors were corrected and her I.Q. has risen to 65 (January, 1957). She is now aged 6 years, and has lessons several times a week from a visiting Surrey County Council teacher.

Case 4. This boy was born on February 20, 1951. The following is a summary of a previous clinical account (Woolf *et al.*, 1955).

The milestones were passed late. Fits occurred at 6 months of age. Phenylketonuria was discovered at the age of 2 years and 8 months. An E.E.G. in October, 1953, was abnormal, and diagnostic of epilepsy. The special diet was started in October, 1953. By January, 1954, an E.E.G. showed none of the previously reported abnormal features. A subsequent E.E.G. showed no specific epileptic activity. His ash-blonde hair became darker. Difficulties over the diet at home caused him to be admitted to the branch hospital at Tadworth. During the period September, 1953, to October, 1954, his G.Q. rose from 20 to 31 while he was on the diet.

Continuation of History. He was admitted to The Hospital for Sick Children and its country branch from July 28, 1954, to August 3, 1955, mainly because of home difficulties. He had acute appendicitis in January, 1955, but made an uneventful post-operative recovery. Walking improved and he had no fits. The general impression of his last few months at Tadworth in 1955 was that there was no noticeable improvement in physical and mental achievements. He was seen in the Out-patient Department in September, 1955, at the age of 4½ years. He weighed 17·8 kg. He could walk unaided, though unsteadily, but could not talk and was still doubly incontinent. He had had no fits. After careful consideration of his physical state and the results of intelligence testing, it was decided to discontinue the special diet, especially in view of recurrent difficulties at home. An E.E.G. in June, 1955, showed in a sleep record evidence of some epileptic activity, with high-voltage spikes and slow components, but it was not strictly comparable with previous records which were taken with the eyes open. Only slight 'fits' have recurred, confined to his waking on occasional mornings three times or so each week. Another E.E.G. in June, 1956, did not show any epileptic outbursts but there were frequent artefacts which makes the record unreliable. Clinically he was still having occasional fits when wakening out of sleep but these were not so severe as previously. He is on no sedative drugs or any special diet now (June, 1956). His mother thinks he is continuing to improve slowly in all he does and is not going back. He actually continues at a low level of G.Q. 20, the same as before treatment was started.

Case 5. This child born on December 13, 1948, was described by Woolf *et al.*, 1955, and the following is a summary:

An older brother is a proved phenylketonuric ament, and there is one normal sister. At the age of 3 months it was thought that she did not recognize her parents.

She could sit by 1 year. At the age of 15 months she began to have fits. An E.E.G. showed spike-and-wave discharges. Her I.Q. was estimated to be about 40 at the age of 20 months. Phenylpyruvic acid was found in the urine. Fits, resembling petit mal, continued but ceased abruptly in December, 1953, on aloxidone and amphetamine sulphate. She could stand with support at 3 years. An E.E.G. in April, 1954, showed slow spike-and-wave complexes during sleep. Dietary treatment began at the age of 5 years 4 months in May, 1954. There was a curious attack of major epilepsy after 25 days of diet with unconsciousness and cardiac failure. Her hair darkened very markedly during treatment.

CONTINUATION OF HISTORY. She was admitted to Tadworth Branch Hospital to give her parents a holiday. The cardiac failure had completely resolved. No fits occurred (she was still on sedatives), but she was still very retarded. She was seen in the Out-patient Department from time to time and also admitted for re-assessment in September, 1954. An E.E.G. in September, 1954, showed very frequent bursts of irregular spike-and-wave complexes in the sleeping record, but no epileptic activity when awake. Later she developed some severe fits. She began to crawl about the end of the year. It was eventually decided to stop the special diet gradually, starting on April 21, 1955, as very little progress was being made. Several severe fits occurred and she was admitted in 'status epilepticus' on May 8, 1955. The fits were controlled with intramuscular paraldehyde followed by aloxidone, and she remained free from fits up to November, 1956, when last seen, continuing treatment by aloxidone. On that date she was still unable to walk alone or to swallow solids. Her mother thinks she has deteriorated and is losing skills she once possessed.

Case 6. This child, born on March 10, 1955, is the second of two children. He was brought to hospital under the care of Dr. P. R. Evans at the age of 16 months with an older backward brother who was found to have phenylketonuria. This child's urine was therefore tested and he was found to have phenylketonuria. He had been thought to be normal up to 8 months of age although he did not hold up his head until 6 months. When first seen he could not crawl or walk and had only been sitting up for two months. He was a fair-haired, blue-eyed child. There was no history of fits but a doubtful episode resembling petit mal occurred while he was an in-patient. The E.E.G. was not abnormal except for tracings from the pre-frontal region which were perhaps abnormally flat. The G.Q. was 57 on the Griffiths scale. A low phenylalanine diet was started. He has attended the Out-patient Department regularly with clinical improvement and only minor difficulties over diet. A second E.E.G. three months after the diet was begun was normal. Clinically he was thought to show some slow improvement but speech was delayed. In January, 1957, his I.Q. was 76 (Merrill-Palmer); on the Griffiths scale his G.Q. was 68 but this was an incomplete test, since he scored the maximum on several items.

Case 7. This child, born on January 6, 1951, was brought to the Out-patient Department at the age of 2½ years because she was not walking. The patient had been slightly backward with her other milestones. Phenylpyruvic acid was discovered in the urine. The parents were uncooperative from the start, refusing to accept that the child was severely retarded. A brief attempt to start a low-phenylalanine diet was abandoned because the child was removed by the parents. The E.E.G. was within normal limits. The G.Q. on the Griffiths scale was 49 (on July 2, 1953, aged 2 years 6½ months) and, on a repeat test, again 49 (August 5). The parents came back to the Out-patient Department some months later but it was decided that lack of cooperation would preclude use of a special diet. Frequent respiratory tract infections led to a further admission at the age of 4½ years when her tonsils were removed. The G.Q. at this time on the Griffiths scale was 35. She continued to attend erratically and physically made reasonable progress. The G.Q. in May, 1956, was 37, and she was being considered for an occupation centre despite her mother's continued opposition to acceptance of the diagnosis. The child never had any fits.

Case 8. This child, born on August 10, 1955, is a sister of a known phenylketonuric boy. When his condition was diagnosed her urine was examined, and she was found also to be passing phenylpyruvic acid. She was then 4 months of age and had been thought by her parents to be normal in her mental development, but clinically she seemed a little retarded. Her G.Q. (Griffith's scale) was 57. She was put on a low phenylalanine diet and proved difficult to feed on this diet. As with Case 1, phenylalanine tended to vanish completely from her blood and so cow's milk was given and increased several times in an effort to restore the blood phenylalanine level to normal. The serum proteins dropped to 4·56 g. per 100 ml., and the blood urea level rose to 67 mg./100 ml., but both returned to normal when phenylalanine reappeared in the blood in response to an increase in intake of cow's milk. After being stationary for over three weeks, her weight began to rise and she was eventually discharged. Her G.Q. at the age of 6 months was 64. Progress at home continued but seemed to slow up. At the age of 11 months she could sit only with assistance. An E.E.G. was normal. This child emigrated at the age of 14 months, preventing further testing, but the mother reports (January 3, 1957) that, at 16 months, the child stands alone and says a few words.

Case 9. This child is the sister of Case 1. She was born on March 9, 1953, and first attended The Hospital for Sick Children in April, 1954, at the age of 11 months for backwardness. She held up her head at 6 months, and sat alone at 1 year. Minor 'fits' began at about 20 months in which she dropped forward. At this time phenylpyruvic acid was found in the urine and she was admitted for further investigation. She was a typical blonde, backward child with a general intelligence quotient of 24 (Griffiths scale). An E.E.G. was severely abnormal with very high voltage, slow delta activity associated with 'sharp' components. A low phenylalanine diet was started. Some initial loss of weight occurred with the diet as usual, but was later made good. Her hair, which had been almost albino, changed to a medium brown colour with a sharp line of demarcation between white and brown. She had no fits while she was in hospital, but no obvious improvement occurred in her mental state. She was discharged home to continue on the diet but re-admitted a few weeks later with an acute respiratory tract infection which yielded to routine treatment. The mother was pleased with progress and the child was crawling. In February, 1956, she was reported to be saying single words and had begun to walk. Aloxidone was being used but the 'fits' were not entirely controlled. Further intelligence testing in May, 1956, gave a G.Q. of 31, an improvement of four points since October, 1955, and of seven points over the lowest score of 24 in March and June, 1955. An E.E.G. on March 14, 1957, showed only doubtful or slight improvement over the one before treatment started, and was still severely abnormal with large irregular sharp waves, spikes, and slow waves, but with an unstable alpha rhythm. It is probable that except for a special feature in this case the special diet might well have been abandoned after about a year's trial but when it was started the mother was again pregnant and gave birth to twins. One of these was affected, with phenylpyruvic acid in the urine, and one was not. This very important pair of twins from the point of view of study merited great care for all the family.

Case 10. This boy (under the care of Dr. P. R. Evans) was born on December 23, 1952, and is an only child. He was said to be normal up to 3 months of age. Minor fits began at 5 months and he has been retarded ever since. The urine was found to contain phenylpyruvic acid at the age of 18 months. The G.Q. was 20 on the Griffiths scale. An E.E.G. showed diffuse epileptic changes. Major epilepsy developed about a month later. A low phenylalanine diet was started in July, 1954. Slight clinical improvement was noted. He was admitted for re-assessment about five months later. The E.E.G. was reported as erratically normal. (He was on phenobarbitone and the improvement could be due to this.) Fits were continuing but less frequently. He was re-admitted six months later. He was now aged 2½ years and for two months he had been standing and walking. There had been no fits for three months (phenobarbitone ½ grain at night). He had some difficulty over solid food. An E.E.G. was reported as 'mildly abnormal'. He has continued to attend as an out-patient. He had no more fits. The G.Q. in August, 1955, was 27 and in May, 1956, it was 34, indicating a very definite intellectual improvement. He has continued throughout on his low phenylalanine diet, but with numerous serious lapses, his mother being apparently unable to keep forbidden foods from him.

Case 11. This child was born on February 7, 1955, and was first seen (under the care of Dr. P. R. Evans) in March, 1956, at the age of 13 months, because his mother thought he ought to be doing more. Phenylpyruvic acid was found in the urine. There were no fits at any time. The G.Q. (Griffiths scale) was 21 in April, 1956. An E.E.G. showed diffuse abnormal bursts of sharp spike-and-wave activity, such as are often associated with the condition of phenylketonuria. A phenylalanine-free diet was begun but, through a manufacturer's error, *N*-acetyl-DL-tryptophan was fed instead of DL-tryptophan for the first eight weeks. His weight dropped over six days from 11·3 kg. to 11 kg., rose to 11·7 kg. soon after cow's milk was added to the diet, and then dropped steadily to 10·7 kg. During this time the blood phenylalanine level remained high, though phenylpyruvic acid did not reappear in the urine. When tryptophan was added to his diet, his weight began to increase at once, the blood phenylalanine level dropped to normal, and he obviously became much more cheerful. His hair remained the grey-blond colour characteristic of phenylketonuria throughout the period when he was unintentionally deprived of tryptophan; three days after adding tryptophan to his diet the new growth at the base of the hair was almost black, making a striking contrast with the rest of the hair.

His G.Q. (Griffiths scale) on November 8, 1956, was 23, and on April 18, 1957, it was 32. An E.E.G, on April 16, 1957, still showed a generalized abnormality with large amplitude, irregular sharp waves, spikes and slow waves, but there was an improvement over the E.E.G. of April 19, 1956, though the records are not strictly comparable.

Psychological Examinations

Careful psychometry was necessary if we were not to rely on subjective impressions of any improvement on dietary treatment. The test used had to be suitable for children of low mental age. A recently devised test (Griffiths, 1954), which had been standardized by one of us (R.G.) on about 600 children between the ages of 2 weeks and 2 years has been used throughout. The nature of this test provides for very detailed information by virtue of items divided into five sub-scales, each measuring a significant aspect of mental growth and development. This makes it possible to observe from time to time the progress in, *e.g.*, eye-hand coordination, or alertness to sounds. After the second year the scale merges into the Terman-Merrill which was the test used for children of mental age over 2 years, except in Case 6 where the Merrill-Palmer scale was used. The youngest infants were tested every six weeks, the intervals being gradually lengthened to three months during the second year.

The results are best shown in graphs of mental age plotted against chronological age (Figs. 1-4).

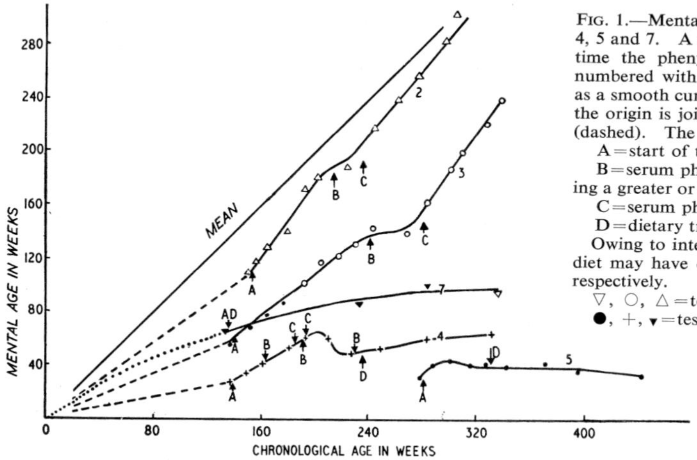

FIG. 1.—Mental age plotted against chronological age for Cases 2, 3, 4, 5 and 7. A smoothed curve is drawn through the points from the time the phenylalanine-restricted diet was started (each curve is numbered with the case no.); in Case 7 this line is continued back as a smooth curve (dotted) through the origin and in Cases 2, 3 and 4 the origin is joined to the first point in each curve by a straight line (dashed). The mean for the whole population is also shown.

A = start of the diet low in phenylalanine

B = serum phenylalanine concentration found to be raised, indicating a greater or lesser departure from the diet

C = serum phenylalanine level found to have returned to normal

D = dietary treatment terminated.

Owing to intermittent testing, the departure from or return to the diet may have occurred a little earlier than is indicated by B or C respectively.

▽, ○, △ = test results obtained on the Terman-Merrill scale.

●, +, ▾ = test results obtained on the Griffiths scale.

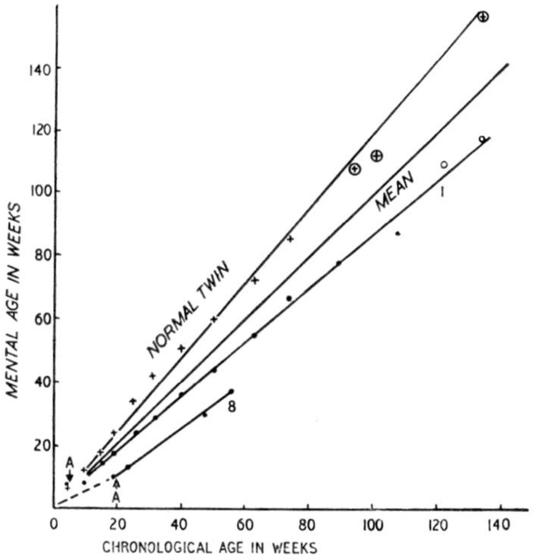

FIG. 2.—Mental age plotted against chronological age for Cases 1, 8 and the normal twin of Case 1. A as in Fig. 1.

○, ⊗ = test results obtained on the Terman -Merrill scale.

●, + = test results obtained on the Griffiths scale.

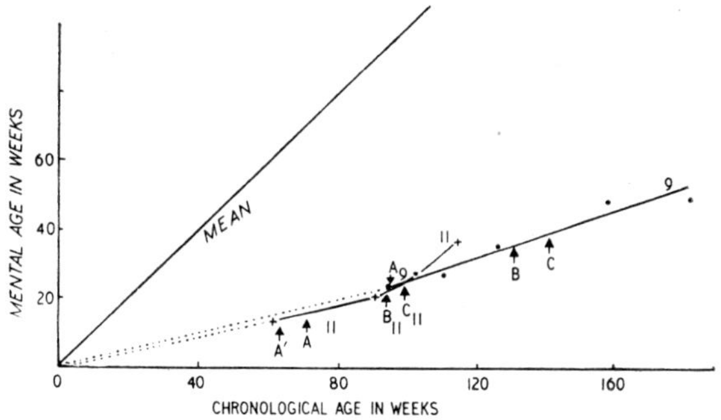

FIG. 4.—Mental age plotted against chronological age for Cases 9 and 11.

●, + = test results (Griffiths scale).

A′ = phenylalanine and tryptophan-restricted diet started.

A, B and C as in Fig. 1; where confusion might arise, the case no. is added to A, B or C as a subscript.

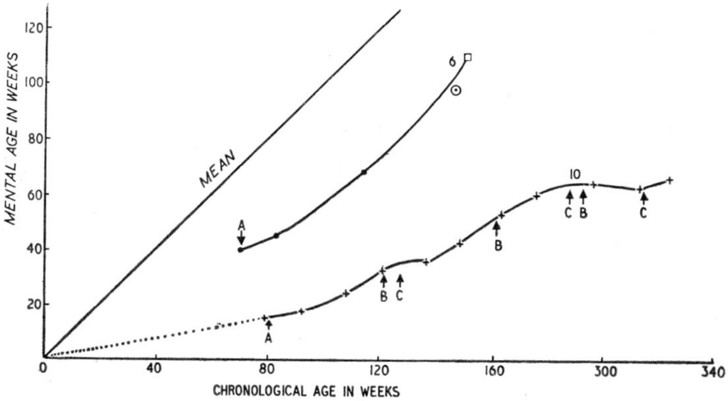

FIG. 3.—Mental age plotted against chronological age for Cases 6 and 10. A, B and C as in Fig. 1.

●, + = test results obtained on the Griffiths scale.

⊙ = result of an incomplete test on the Griffiths scale.

□ = test result on the Merrill-Palmer scale.

Fig. 5 shows the changing general intelligence quotients as time passes.*

Case 1. When first tested, at the age of 4 weeks, she was more active than her normal twin; in fact she displayed a certain hyperactivity. For example, when placed in the prone position she suddenly lifted head and shoulders well up, turned her head first to the left, then to the right, and then placed her cheek against the pillow again. Apart from this unusual physical activity, her test results were in general and in detail very like her twin sister's, and the two children actually passed and failed exactly the same test items in scales C, D and E. In subsequent tests the healthy twin continued to do well. After one very good test result (119) the G.Q. of Case 1 dropped to a fairly steady level of between 88 and 92. This has been maintained.

Case 2. Even before she went on to the diet, this child had a G.Q. of 71. She was already able to do a few tests of the Terman-Merrill scale, and this test was used for all subsequent psychological examinations. The child has made steady and quite rapid progress ever since (Fig. 1). Her speech was at first indistinct and largely babble, but this stage has long ago been left behind and her speech is now clear and fluent and developing rapidly.

Case 3. This child has been followed since October, 1953, when her G.Q. was 42. Her intelligence has improved almost continuously. At one stage (see Fig. 1, point B) there was a pause in progress; she did not do so well on tests and much of the restlessness noticed earlier had returned. It was found that the blood phenylalanine level was raised (both in this case and all the others, the blood and urinary phenylalanine levels were not known till after the intelligence testing). The diet has since then been strictly adhered to and the child has not only regained her former position but has advanced still further. When tested in November, 1956, she had reached a new level of 62.

It is highly probable that this child will prove to be educable, at least at an educationally subnormal level, but she will be continually under observation and in another year or so may be found capable of accepting education in a normal school.

Case 4. This child was described in a previous paper as Case 1 (Woolf *et al.*, 1955) as improving quite rapidly

* The raw quotients and mental ages have been given in Figs. 1-5, Differences in the standard deviations make the quotients slightly different in meaning as one passes from one type of test to another, but these do not obscure the improvement. Dr. J. A. Fraser Roberts advised us that, owing to the doubtful accuracy of the standard deviations for children of such low I.Q., it would be misleading to give the results for most of these children in terms of standard scores at the different ages.

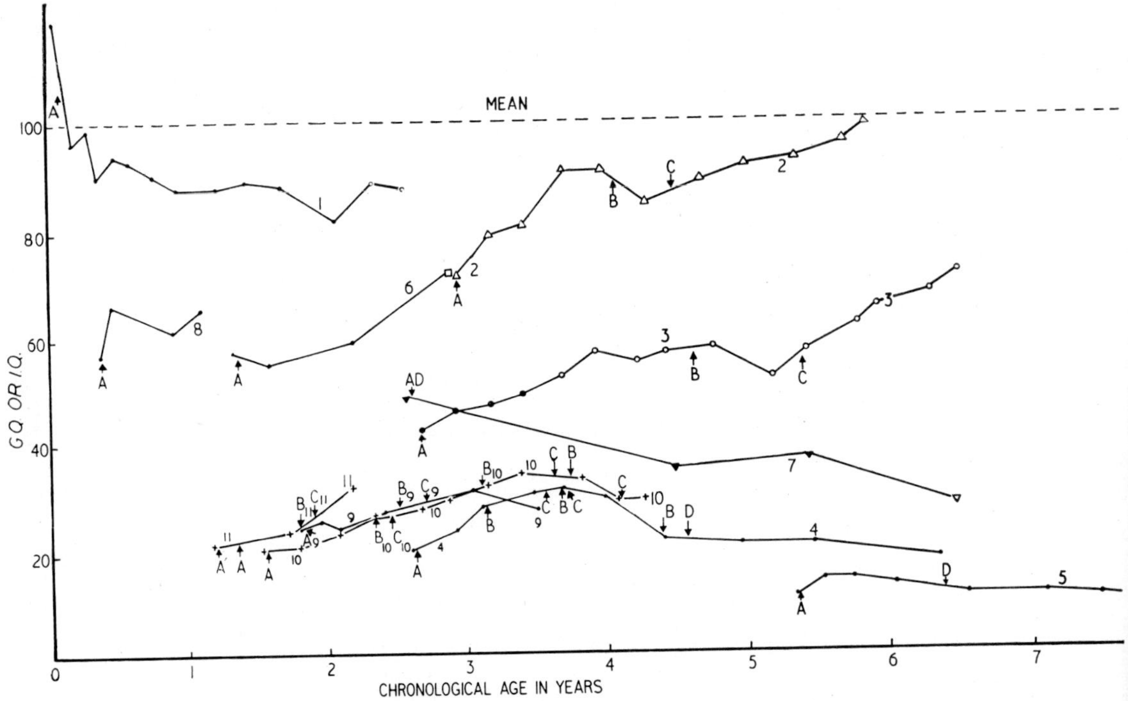

FIG. 5.—Intelligence quotient plotted against chronological age for all 11 cases, A′ A, B, C and D as in Figs. 1 to 4. ●, +, ▾=test results obtained on the Griffiths scale. ▽, ○, △=test results obtained on the Terman-Merrill scale. □=test result obtained on the Merrill-Palmer scale.

in all directions, but particularly in regard to speech. On the diet his G.Q. rose from 20 to 30 in 10 months and his speech from Q.C.8 to Q.C.32 during the same period.

Soon after this encouraging progress, however, it was found that the child was not being kept strictly on the diet at home and phenylpyruvic acid was again found in the urine.

The results of a test on March 2, 1955, were surprising, for not only did his mental age remain exactly the same as on the last test, but every item in the test was passed or failed exactly as before. This naturally produced a drop in the G.Q. from 31 to 29. He was content to do various tests, but appeared not to recognize the examiner. He was unsteady on his feet, produced very few sounds, and the nurses reported no speech. He did not laugh or smile. He did not always fixate objects shown to him, and manipulation was vague and momentary, objects being immediately relinquished after handling. He deliberately bumped his head on the floor twice.

On June 29, 1955, he had made no progress in learning; he had in fact deteriorated, failing a few items he could previously do. He walked unsteadily, without direction, round and round in circles, and did not go after toys. He appeared not to make contact with people. Speech had regressed seriously; he had ceased to masticate, and was being fed with a spoon.

It was felt at that time that the child was suffering from a degree of emotional deprivation in this long period (10 months) away from home, sufficient to produce some signs suggestive of an early psychosis and to cause intellectual regression. As the youngest child in the home, he had previously had a good deal of attention and devoted care from his mother. The separation was working against the success of the diet. The child was apparently sent home, but the parents made little attempt to keep to the diet and he was taken off it. He has maintained his level at about G.Q. 21 to 22. He is happy, smiling and laughing, vocalizing and quite different in appearance since he was seen in the summer at Tadworth. He has re-learnt to walk upstairs, holding his mother's hand, can seat himself at table, is less vague, going towards people and after toys on the floor. He produces several clear sounds, *e.g.*, 'me-me, Babby, Dada'. His use of his hands, too, is slightly better.

Case 5. The progress of this child on the diet was slight, her G.Q. rising in the course of 12 months from 11 to 14. No further progress could be obtained. Subsequently she was taken off the diet.

Since the child came off the diet her mental age has actually dropped from 42 weeks in September, 1954, to 38 weeks in June, 1956. This negative progress rate indicates continuing deterioration and her G.Q. has dropped sharply to 10. At 7½ years of age she is intellectually and in all developmental respects like a baby of 8 months.

Case 6. This case is of interest since there was no sharp inflexion at the start of the diet, but the progress rate increased steadily (Fig. 3). During the first 10 months of treatment the G.Q. did not change significantly, but during the next eight months it rose by 17 points on the Merrill-Palmer scale. The Griffiths scale test was not completed, but even in its partial form already showed a rise of eight points. The diet was strictly adhered to throughout.

Case 9. The test results on this child demonstrate the irreversibility of some effects of the phenylketonuria if the child is too old when treatment starts. This girl was 21 months old and her G.Q. was 24; after 20 months o treatment it has only risen to 27, although it did reach a peak of 31.

For the past six months, this child has been showing behaviour which increasingly qualifies to be called psychotic. She does not make any progress in relating to people, and does not look at people. Her increasing motor skill makes more evident the poverty of the content of her thought; she staggers about aimlessly, hurting herself, biting the furniture, completely withdrawn, though her mental age is now about 12 months.

Case 10. The rise in the actual quotient of 13 points, from 20 to 33, is not in itself dramatic, but a slow and steady rise of the quotient by a few points each time is definitely significant. To know this boy, however, is to be aware of a continuous improvement, for, where he previously lay in his cot, contented enough but unable to sit or speak or play, he is now, two years later, walking and trotting about and climbing. He has a small vocabulary of words and can throw a ball and manipulate toys and bricks a little.

When seen on January 30, 1957, he was very restless and miserable and his G.Q. had dropped to 29. His urine and blood, obtained immediately after the intelligence test, contained quite a high concentration of phenylalanine, and his mother was again warned not to depart from the diet. A similar G.Q. was found on April 3, but he was much more cheerful and cooperative; his blood and urinary phenylalanine concentrations were normal.

Case 11. This child went on the diet when he was 1 year and 2 months old. Six months later the quotient had only risen two points, but the diet had not been kept strictly; six months later it had risen 11 points. This child has a persistently unhappy disposition; whenever seen in hospital, he cries continually and inconsolably; no attention his mother gives him is of any help and all activities seem equally distasteful to him. Twice the test had to be abandoned. This crying is very like that seen in a child with cerebral damage, but, on the other hand, the mother says he is not like this at home. She agrees that the home circumstances, necessitating a day nursery, are by no means ideal and may be the cause of the abnormal behaviour.

It is of interest to note that, as these children begin to progress on the diet, improvement in different kinds of activities is not uniform but tends to accentuate what may be a characteristic profile. The first and most striking observation, patent to everybody concerned, is the increased physical activity with the accompanying progress in locomotor development. In a few weeks or months, the child may learn to sit, creep, stand and walk. He also shows improved social alertness, enjoying the contact with other people and losing some of the apathy and general mental dullness previously observed. Progress in speech and also in hand-eye coordination is frequently much slower, and manual skill may be delayed for some time. The number of cases studied in this way so far is too few for any statistical evaluation of a characteristic profile to be valid, but it appears that the child, still limited in general mental capacity, tends to concentrate on one type of activity at a time, locomotor improvement being at first most strikingly present in the majority of cases.

Feeding more protein than allowed seems, in some cases, to cause restlessness and hyperactivity. The child seems unable to concentrate on the test or to cooperate with the examiner. He seems miserable. On a number of occasions when this type of behaviour was noted, blood obtained immediately after the psychological examination was found to have a raised phenylalanine concentration. Return to the diet (as shown by subsequent chemical investigation) produced a happier, calmer and more cooperative mood.

Chemical Investigations

The diet was controlled, in each case, by repeated chemical investigation of the blood and urine. In the first three cases treated, the daily phenylalanine intake, as milk protein, was at first reduced till phenylpyruvic acid was no longer detectable in the urine, using the direct ferric chloride reaction and the more sensitive method of Berry and Woolf (1952). It was found that the concentration of phenylalanine in the blood and urine, though reduced to about one-third of its former value, was still considerably above normal when phenylpyruvic acid vanished from the urine. The amount of cow's milk fed daily was therefore controlled by keeping the phenylalanine concentration in the blood and urine at the same level as in normal children. This resulted in the milk intake being roughly halved for the first three cases (3, 4 and 5).

Paper chromatography (Woolf, 1951) was used to follow the blood and urinary amino-acids; this enabled the phenylalanine concentration to be compared with the concentrations of the other amino-acids and this balance, particularly for the blood, is more nearly related to the body's needs than is a simple determination of phenylalanine. One advantage of using this method was that any drop to below normal in blood phenylalanine level could be detected and corrected by increasing the intake of cow's milk, usually by 15 or 30 ml. per day. After each such increase or reduction, the blood phenylalanine concentration took about a fortnight to reach a new steady level.

In Case 1, the daily phenylalanine requirements rose steadily between the ages of 5 weeks and 9 months. The blood phenylalanine level was found on several occasions to be very low and there was necessarily a time lag between the subsequent increases in intake of cow's milk and retesting. The infant's growth rate was unsatisfactory at times, probably as a result of this, and on one occasion the blood urea concentration rose to 60 mg. per 100 ml., reflecting the catabolism of the unbalanced amino-acid mixture being fed. Case 8 showed similar effects of too low a phenylalanine intake.

Case 11 ceased to gain weight when placed on the diet and his blood and urinary phenylalanine concentrations remained raised, though below the point at which phenylpyruvic acid is excreted. This continued for five weeks, in spite of progressively decreasing his intake of cow's milk. His hair remained very fair and did not show the darkening at the roots that appeared so dramatically in most other phenylketonurics when placed on the diet. It was noticed that he was excreting very little tryptophan, and the various components of the diet were examined. It was found that, through an error of the manufacturer, he was being fed acetyl-DL-tryptophan instead of DL-tryptophan. When this was corrected there was a dramatic rise in his weight, his blood and urinary phenylalanine concentrations dropped sharply, and his hair turned dark at the roots within three days.

In every case, the diet did not affect the post-absorptive blood concentrations of any amino-acids except phenylalanine, methionine and α-amino-butyric acid. The blood levels of methionine and α-aminobutyric acid rose slightly when 1 g. of DL-methionine was fed daily. The urinary concentrations of methionine and tryptophan were very high; presumably the D form of both amino-acids was not appreciably reabsorbed by the kidney tubules and accounted for their high excretion. The urinary excretion of tyrosine, leucine, valine, serine and lysine was also somewhat higher than the average, though far below the levels met in diseases such as cystinosis. Probably feeding the bulk of the dietary nitrogen as a mixture of amino-acids resulted in a higher rate of absorption from the gut than when protein is fed; this would lead to an unusually high blood amino-acid level and hence to a greater 'overflow' of amino-acids into the urine. The daily intake of casein hydrolysate was kept on the high side to correct for inefficient utilization, and a fairly high calorie intake was maintained by feeding extra carbohydrate, since dietary carbohydrate is known to affect the utilization of amino-acids (Harris and Harris, 1947; Munro and Thomson, 1953).

In every case, within a few days of starting the diet, the previously normal urinary taurine concentration fell to an extremely low level and taurine sometimes vanished from the urine. It was thought that sulphur-containing amino-acids might be deficient in the diet and so DL-methionine was added (1 g. per day for children over 1 year). This raised the urinary taurine excretion very slightly in a few cases, but had no effect at all in most, even though the urinary cystine excretion rose markedly in all cases. L-cystine was fed to Case 1 to see whether the slow absorption of this amino-acid from the gut was necessary for the production of taurine (*cf.* the anomalous effect of feeding cystine to cystinurics), but no extra taurine was excreted. Pyridoxine may be necessary for converting cystine to taurine (Blaschko, Datta and Harris, 1953) and 25 mg. extra pyridoxine was fed daily to Case 1 for three days, but there was no increase in taurine excretion. Acid hydrolysis of urine showed that taurine was not present in conjugated form except in traces; the quantity of conjugated taurine adsorbed by the acid resin, Zeo-Karb 225, was normal (*cf.* Woolf and Norman, 1957). The concentration of taurine in the blood was normal, or even above normal when the urinary concentration rose slightly; taurine in the blood was identified as in Woolf and Norman's (1957) analysis. The only conclusion is that in some unexplained way the diet increases the renal tubular reabsorption of taurine.

In Case 1 the urinary excretion of hydroxyproline, previously marked (*cf.* Woolf and Norman, 1957), fell almost to zero as soon as the diet was started. The excretion of proline and of all other amino-acids was unaffected except as discussed above.

Indolyllactic acid was present in all the specimens of urine examined before the children were placed on the diet, and indolylacetic acid could be detected in about half of them (*cf.* Armstrong and Robinson, 1954). Within a few days of starting the diet neither acid could be detected in the urine, in spite of the large amount of DL-tryptophan being given. Phenyllactic acid and the unidentified reducing keto-acid (Berry and Woolf, 1952) also vanished from the urine shortly after starting treatment, while the concentrations of phenolic acids and phenylacetylglutamine dropped to normal values.

The Diet

Basically the diet has differed very little from that described by Woolf *et al.* (1955). The major differences have been: (*a*) The reduction in the intake of cow's milk when the blood phenylalanine level, rather than urinary phenylpyruvic acid, was made the criterion (the amount of casein hydrolysate fed was raised to compensate for the diminished protein intake); (*b*) the adaptation of the diet for a very young infant; (*c*) modifications as the patients got older; (*d*) the addition of methionine.

The daily intake of cow's milk was between 60 and 120 ml. per day, providing an estimated 100 to 200 mg. of phenylalanine daily for children over 18 months of age. The daily requirements were higher during the first 18 months. Afterwards changes in phenylalanine requirement were slow for any given child, but there was some variation between one child and another. Potatoes were given to the older children in strictly controlled amounts, 2 oz. mashed potato being taken as equivalent to 1 oz. cow's milk in phenylalanine content.

Cases 1 and 8 presented a special problem as they were only 17 days old and 4 months old respectively when treatment was decided on. The soup, vegetables, bread, etc., of the older children had to be replaced by a thin liquid which had to contain, as far as possible, all the nutrients of human milk, except phenylalanine, in their correct concentrations. The greatest difficulty was in incorporating the fat; experiments with coconut oil and glyceryl monostearate were unsuccessful, the emulsion invariably breaking when the mixture with amino-acids, sugar, salts, etc. was sterilized. Eventually the fat was added as double cream and this was completely successful. The composition of the 'milk' is shown in Table 1 (Appendix).

The thick cream supplied a proportion of the protein required (for phenylalanine) and the rest was supplied by the cow's milk. A diet completely free from phenylalanine was never given to these very young infants, in contrast to the older phenylketonurics who were given a phenylalanine-free diet for a few days to bring the blood phenylalanine level down quickly before adding cow's milk. The amount of cow's milk fed to the young infants had to be increased frequently as it was repeatedly found insufficient to keep the blood phenylalanine level up to normal. At its maximum, when Case 8 was 7 months old and weighed 7·4 kg., the daily intake of cow's milk was 120 ml. in addition to 90 ml. of double cream, and slightly less for Case 1. Another case, not reported here in detail, at 11 months required 200 ml. of cow's milk and 100 ml. of double cream daily to keep the blood phenylalanine level normal. After the eleventh month the phenylalanine requirements began to drop. Inositol and choline were given in such large amounts because they are present in milk (Robinson, 1951) though of unknown function. The salts were also added to give a mixture resembling the inorganic constituents of human milk and of the same *p*H, though the calcium phosphate had to be in suspension. Vitamin B_{12} was added as 'cytagon' oral syrup in preference to crude liver extract, and folic acid was added to the vitamin tablets (*cf.* Collins, Harper, Schreiber and Elvehjem, 1951).

As the children got older and could take a more solid diet than the original soup, some variety was introduced. The cow's milk was omitted from the soup, and was given with a cereal at breakfast. The 'soup' was made thicker, flavoured with tomato and given at the mid-day meal only, sometimes poured over potatoes, swedes, cabbage, etc., but more often as a separate course. Vegetables (except potatoes and pulses) were allowed freely. Stewed fruit, or a pudding (made from cornflour or sago with sugar, flavouring and colouring) followed; the parents were given a number of recipes. Bread, made from gluten-free wheat starch, with margarine and honey or jam was given at teatime and at other meals as required. Biscuits made from wheat starch, fat, sugar and flavouring were allowed freely, as were oranges and apples and sugar confectionery.

It is difficult to get much variety into the menu since all forms of protein are almost wholly barred. In spite of all efforts it is impossible to disguise completely the taste of the casein hydrolysate. It is remarkable that the children have taken the diet so well; there has been very little difficulty in getting any child to accept the diet in the first place, and they mostly continue to take it without any trouble—even the older children of fairly high I.Q. Some difficulty has sometimes arisen where a normal child in the same family awakens the phenylketonuric to the fact that her food differs from the normal sibling's, but this has always been smoothed over by the exercise of a little tact. A number of commercial firms have become interested in supplying a casein hydrolysate of better flavour, or in providing a ready mixed 'soup' powder, containing all the ingredients of the diet, to which the mother need only add hot water and flavouring.

DL-methionine was added to the children's diets when it was suspected that they were getting insufficient sulphur-containing amino-acids. Although this was shown to be a misinterpretation of the facts, DL-methionine is still added to the diet, a child over 1 year of age getting 1 g. daily. Casein is not very rich in sulphur-containing amino-acids, and hydrolysis and charcoal treatment removes the cystine; it seemed logical to provide an additional source of sulphur. Methionine was chosen in preference to cystine because methionine can replace cystine in the diet but not *vice versa*.

After the first few weeks the patients were all treated at home. The parents showed varying degrees of ability to cope with the special diet. Of the 11 patients, the parents of eight were fully cooperative. The parents of Case 7 refused to cooperate. In Case 4 there was very little attempt to keep to the diet. In Case 10 the child was quite obviously given forbidden foods on many occasions; a talk with the mother would result in a temporary drop in the urinary phenylalanine concentration, but sooner or later she lapsed. Case 2 also had an occasional lapse, shown by a temporary rise in urinary phenylalanine excretion; the child may have been taking food from the larder herself. Case 3 showed at one time a moderate rise in phenylalanine excretion that persisted and even increased in spite of cutting down her daily allowance of cow's milk and potatoes. Eventually phenylpyruvic acid appeared in the urine and her I.Q. remained stationary for six months, *i.e.*, progress, previously marked, ceased. It was only after close questioning that the parents, who were intelligent and cooperative, mentioned that the child was very fond of tea, drinking several cups a day. Each cup contained perhaps 60 ml. of milk. As soon as this beverage was omitted, phenylalanine excretion fell to normal and her I.Q. started to rise. In the other seven cases the parents seemed well able to make up the diet and repeated checks showed it was being adhered to. Thus in only two out of 10 cases did the parents seriously fail to keep to the diet.

Discussion

When Fölling (1934) first described phenylketonuria it was immediately apparent that this condition was an inborn error of metabolism closely analogous to those described by Garrod (1908, 1923). It has since been shown by Jervis (1953) that the enzyme phenylalanine hydroxylase, which converts phenylalanine to tyrosine in the normal liver, is absent from the liver of phenylketonurics. The simplest hypothesis is that in phenylketonurics the gene normally responsible for an essential stage in the synthesis of phenylalanine hydroxylase is replaced by a mutant gene incapable of this synthesis. Thus the inheritance of phenylketonuria as a recessive character is explicable if the patient is assumed to be homozygous for the mutant gene. Probably all the abnormal biochemistry of phenylketonuria results from the absence of phenylalanine hydroxylase.

The almost invariable association of severe mental defect with phenylketonuria, and its frequent association with epilepsy, have been explained as being due to either a pleiotropic effect of the same recessive gene, or an intoxication by phenylalanine or one of its metabolites, or a deficiency of tyrosine due to its not having been formed from phenylalanine. All three theories have been put forward at various times and, to some extent, investigated, *e.g.*, by Jervis (1937, 1950), Borek, Brecher, Jervis and Waelsch (1950), Woolf *et al.* (1955), Cowie (1951a) and Woolf and Vulliamy (1951).

If the mental deficiency is due to an intoxication, whether by phenylalanine or by one of its abnormal metabolites formed as a result of a high concentration of phenylalanine in the cells, it might be reversible by giving a diet low in phenylalanine unless permanent mental damage has occurred. The success attending the giving of such a diet is reported above and confirms and extends previous reports of success (Woolf *et al.*, 1955; Bickel *et al.*, 1953; Armstrong and Tyler, 1955; Braude, 1956; Blainey and Gulliford, 1956; Horner and Streamer, 1956). This improvement in the mental state is evidence of the correctness of the intoxication hypothesis.

The clearest evidence of a mental effect of the diet is given by the curves of mental age plotted against chronological age (Figs. 1-4). The slope of this line at any given point is the progress rate of the child at that time (Woolf *et al.*, 1955). In most cases there was a sharp inflexion upwards as soon as the low-phenylalanine diet was started. This improvement has been maintained while the child stayed on the diet, *i.e.*, the curve did not return to its original slope, although often the slope has remained well below the mean for the population as a whole. This finding can be explained only as an effect of restricting the phenylalanine intake.

There is no evidence of a spontaneous increase in progress rate or intelligence quotient in untreated phenylketonuria; in fact all the evidence is that there is a steady decline in both, rapid at first and gradual later (*e.g.*, Cases 5 and 7). These children are normal at birth and signs of mental deficiency are usually first noted at an age of 6 months or later. By about 1 year the child is usually an idiot, and mental deterioration seems to continue thereafter at a reduced rate. It is estimated that the majority of all older untreated phenylketonurics have intelligence quotients below 30 and fewer than 1% have intelligence quotients over 70 (Penrose, 1951). The probability of finding a phenylketonuric of average intelligence is very low indeed. Apart from the cases reported above and others treated elsewhere, only two cases have come to our notice, one of a boy aged 6 with an I.Q. of 103, who will be reported elsewhere (Coates, Norman and Woolf, 1957), and one of a 6-year-old boy who scored 94 on some intelligence tests (Cowie, 1951b). It is unlikely that any considerable number of phenylketonurics of normal intelligence are not being detected because: (*a*) the ferric chloride test has been so widely used for urinary 'acetone bodies', it is unlikely that a strong green coloration would be overlooked or not reported, and (*b*) the shape of the distribution curve of intelligence quotient among phenylketonurics, with its mode at 10, indicates (unless it is bimodal) that very few indeed would come within the normal range (*cf.*, Larson, 1956). Thus there is only a very low probability that in Cases 1 or 2 the intelligence would be at its present level if untreated.

In addition to the effect on the intelligence, with all that this implies, the electroencephalogram has become more nearly normal in two cases after the child was placed on the diet and epileptic fits have ceased (Cases 4 and 10). The epilepsy, often closely resembling petit mal, which occurs in a proportion of phenylketonurics is unusually resistant to drug therapy and the success of the low-phenylalanine diet in controlling it is all the more striking. However, in Case 9 the diet did not control the fits and the E.E.G. showed little improvement. In Case 5, starting the phenylalanine-restricted diet seemed to cause major epilepsy leading to status epilepticus, and the return to a normal diet seemed to have the same effect, in each case two to four weeks after the change in the diet. Both these cases showed evidence of mental deterioration even while they were on the diet; the continuing epilepsy may well be partly or wholly responsible for this. Epilepsy is more common in phenylketonurics of low I.Q. than in high-grade ones, and the intellectual defect may be partly due to the epilepsy in these cases or both may be the expression of more severe intoxication. As in other causes of epilepsy, once the condition is well established it appears to be not always controlled by removal of the precipitating agent.

Among minor effects of the diet, the eczema-like skin condition frequently found in phenylketonurics clears up rapidly. The dramatic darkening of the hair is one of the most striking effects of the diet. The relative deficiency of melanin in hair, skin and eyes in phenylketonuria is well known (*cf.*, Cowie and Penrose, 1951), and it has recently been shown that this is probably due to competitive inhibition of tyrosine oxidase by phenylalanine (Dancis and Balis, 1955). The inhibition is reversible *in vivo* by giving massive doses of tyrosine (Snyderman, Norton and Holt, 1955). It is not unexpected that the inhibition should also be reversible by reducing the phenylalanine concentration in the body by dietary means; the amounts of tyrosine given by us were insufficient of themselves to account for the hair darkening.

It is tempting to try to link this inhibition by phenylalanine of the formation of dihydroxyphenylalanine with the effects on the central nervous system, adrenaline and noradrenaline being synaptic transmission agents chemically related to dihydroxyphenylalanine. In fact, Weil-Malherbe (1955) has found that the concentrations of adrenaline and noradrenaline in the blood are unusually low in phenylketonuria. However, Pare, Sandler and Stacey (1957) have found that the serum concentration of 5-hydroxytryptamine, a neurohumoral agent chemically unrelated to dihydroxyphenylalanine, is also low in phenylketonuria and rises when a low phenylalanine diet is fed (Sandler and Stacey, 1957, private communication). It may be that the low blood concentrations of adrenaline, noradrenaline and 5-hydroxytryptamine are merely a reflection of a lowered level of activity of the central nervous system, and not due to a direct chemical inhibition of their formation.

In phenylketonuria the effects of the intoxication are not completely reversible. In almost every case the progress rate, although accelerated once the child was put on a low-phenylalanine diet, has been less than 100, suggesting that there is an irreversible component, as well as a reversible one, in the mental deterioration. Nor is this unexpected: from the age of a very few days the child has been subjected to the continuous action of a depressant substance—the period when the normal child is acquiring its first knowledge of the outer world, its first mastery of itself and its environment, is spent in a 'drugged' state. However completely the intoxicant is later removed, the effects of this time lost at a vital period will show in later years.

The brain is undergoing continuous structural development in the early months of life. (It is noteworthy that no consistent morphological changes in the brain have been reported to be associated with phenylketonuria.) It has been suggested (Hebb, 1949) that the neural mechanisms necessary for the earlier steps in learning may be altered by normal growth and development in such a way that they are not so readily available to an older child. This may explain why, in most of the cases considered here, although the brain has been restored to physiological normality by removal of an intoxicant, there is some impairment of the ability to learn. The lowering of the intelligence quotient in phenylketonuria is due to two factors: this irreversible component, and the immediate effect of the intoxication.

In Figs. 1-4 it can be seen that the slope of the curve of mental age plotted against chronological age is less than the average normal even after treatment has started. This reflects the permanent element of the mental deterioration. The time lag when treatment is started, *i.e.*, the difference between chronological and mental ages, is due to both temporary and permanent factors; it represents a gap between normal and phenylketonuric that may never be closed. From Fig. 1, curves 2 and 3, a temporary departure from the diet appears to result in a temporary flattening of the curve, but the slope returns to its previous value on resumption of the diet. We may tentatively conclude that a fairly short period of intoxication at the age of 4 or 5 years causes a reversible mental deterioration; nonetheless the time lag has been increased and the I.Q. consequently may always be lower than it would otherwise have been. Earlier in life, a period of intoxication increases the degree of permanent mental damage as is shown by the slope of the curve.

Cases 4 and 9 raise two interesting and perhaps related problems. Both children showed behaviour which could be called psychotic. In Case 4 this withdrawal most probably was the result of the 10 months in hospital, since on his return home he became more normal in his play and relationships. This withdrawal coincided with, and perhaps produced, a period when the mental age remained stationary though the diet was being kept to. The return to more normal behaviour at home led to a renewed but slow rise in mental age even though the diet was abandoned. Periods in hospital are known in general to depress the mental development of children (*e.g.*, Spitz, 1955). The deterioration in Case 9's emotional relationship seems to have a different origin. There have been no prolonged periods of separation from the mother, though the birth of twins has absorbed the mother's attention to some extent. The quality of the behaviour is more like that of a child with psychotic behaviour of organic origin. This observation can, perhaps, be correlated with the fact that the E.E.G. in Case 9 has remained abnormal, though in Case 4 it returned to normal on the diet. It seems possible that Case 4 may have suffered from a temporary psychosis of psychological origin, and Case 9 may have a permanent psychotic condition, additional to the lowering of the intelligence, following brain damage which is observable also on the E.E.G. Case 11 is the only other case with an E.E.G. which has remained abnormal, though there have been no fits, and it is interesting that he has always cried and been very actively miserable on every visit to the hospital.

The mental deterioration in untreated phenylketonurics follows an approximately exponential curve; it is most rapid during the first few months of life, *e.g.*, Case 8, I.Q. 57 at 4 months, higher than the great majority of older phenylketonurics; after the second year it proceeds more slowly, but still measurably, *e.g.*, Case 7. Even in Case 1, where the diet low in phenylalanine was started by the fifth week, some slight degree of mental deterioration had already occurred and appears to have been arrested but not reversed. In Case 8 the diet, started at 4 months, appears to have prevented further deterioration though there is as yet no significant rise in the G.Q. As one would expect, the younger the child and the less the degree of mental damage (as measured by the I.Q.), the greater the effect of the diet. This indicates the necessity for diagnosing phenylketonuria and instituting treatment as early in life as possible. The test for phenylpyruvic acid in the urine is extremely simple,* and the implications of a positive result are most important.

We advocate that every child's urine should be tested at the age of 21 days. In the light of further experience it may be possible to shorten this period between birth and testing. The urine of a sib of a known case of phenylketonuria should be examined daily, as far as possible, from birth up to at least 3 weeks of age (perhaps using paper chromatography as well as the ferric chloride test) both for his own sake and to help to close a gap in our knowledge, since there is a one in four chance that he will be affected, and we know neither the age at which the blood phenylalanine level begins to rise nor the age at which phenylpyruvic acid first appears in the urine in affected cases.

If this scheme is followed, all future cases of phenylketonuria will be detected and treatment begun before the fifth week of life. We estimate that from 20 to 40 new cases are born every year in Great Britain, basing this on Munro's (1947) figure of two to six cases of phenylketonuria per 100,000 population, and the 600,000 live births every year. It is probable that the incidence is rather higher than Munro estimated, because his figures are based on the population of institutions for low-grade mental defectives and their relatives, and there is a small but appreciable number of phenylketonurics of too high a grade to be admitted to institutions (*e.g.*, Case 2; *cf.* Coates *et al.*, 1957). The local health authorities should work out the necessary administrative measures to see that health visitors collect and test the urine of every baby. A coloured card with instructions as to testing is being prepared.† Already one large local authority has asked one of us to talk on the subject to health visitors and midwives in the area.

Even in older children a worthwhile improvement often results from dietary treatment. It is obviously a gain even if a child's mental rating is raised only from idiot to imbecile level. As a rough guide we consider treatment worth initiating if the child is 2 years old or under and the G.Q. not less than 20, or 3 years old with a G.Q. of 30 or over, or 4 years old with a G.Q. of 40 or over. In any border-line cases it is probably wise to try six months' treatment with careful psychological testing at the beginning, at 3 months and at the end of this period. A decision would then be reached in the light of any improvement effected. It is also important to rule out any other form of brain disease. For example, in the presence of spasticity or any suggestion of birth trauma in the widest sense, investigations such as air studies should be undertaken to eliminate the possibility of structural brain damage of a gross type.

We do not know for how long the diet must be strictly adhered to. It may be impossible to relax it throughout life. On the other hand, once development of the brain has reached a stage where permanent mental damage is unlikely, a certain degree of intoxication resulting from some relaxation of the diet may be tolerable. However, from Case 3, it appears that 5 years is too early an age for this.

The effects of giving a normal diet, after the child had been on a low-phenylalanine intake, have been reported by Bickel *et al.* (1953) and by Armstrong and Tyler (1955). They both noted reversal of the previous improvement. In Case 5 above, the mental age actually started to decline, causing a marked decrease in I.Q., when her diet was changed from one low in phenylalanine to a normal one; previously her I.Q. had been maintained at a steady though very low level. Somewhat similar findings were noted in Case 4, but here

* To a fresh specimen of urine is added a little 5% ferric chloride solution. A green coloration, reaching a maximum within five minutes and fading only slowly, constitutes a positive result. Acidification is unnecessary and can invalidate the test. The ferric chloride can be spotted on to a wet napkin but this is much less reliable than the test-tube method.

† This may be obtained from the Secretary, The Hospital for Sick Children, Great Ormond Street, London, W.C.1, price 6d.

the results are complicated by other psychological factors.

None of the children considered here has been given any psychological treatment or tuition likely to affect the score in intelligence tests. All, except Case 4, have been treated at home and received the ordinary attention a child receives from parents who have not been instructed in any special teaching or training. Only one child, Case 3, has received part-time tuition from a trained teacher, and this for a limited period. Thus we can eliminate disturbing factors in evaluating the effect of the diet on mentality.

These children have special educational problems. As the child emerges from his semi-intoxicated state and begins to function more normally in the intellectual sphere, his capacity to learn is accelerated. Learning takes time, and his climb to a state nearer to his innate level will take several years and may involve some strain. Thus the child of imbecile level with a rising I.Q. may eventually need, not an occupation centre, but a school for educationally subnormal children, and even here full justice may require an open mind, for the child may be capable of travelling still further, in fact to the normal school. Each case should therefore be considered individually and sympathetically by education authorities, and re-assessed frequently so that suitable adjustments can be made in the type of education available to him.

A further question is whether definite psychological help, other than periodic testing of intelligence, should not be seriously considered. These children, while improving rapidly, need sympathetic handling. Some of them tend to be nervous and, having much to catch up educationally, and socially may need individual tuition, or remedial education, or even psychotherapy. It is possible that even more rapid progress might be obtained through attendance at a child guidance clinic or other centre for individual or group play therapy.

Summary

The results of treating 10 phenylketonurics with a diet low in phenylalanine are described.

In almost every case there was a sharp and significant rise in I.Q. The I.Q. continued to rise, the mental age plotted against chronological age showing a point of inflexion at the time the diet was started.

An infant treated from the age of 5 weeks has remained at I.Q. 88 for nearly two years, indicating that relatively slight deterioration had occurred during the five weeks before treatment. Mental deterioration (dementia) proceeds most rapidly in untreated cases during the first weeks of life, then gradually slows down, but is still continuing appreciably at 2 years of age.

As it seems likely that mental deterioration in this condition can be prevented by early treatment, we suggest that every infant's urine be tested with ferric chloride at the age of 21 days (though this age may have to be modified), and treatment instituted immediately if a positive reaction is obtained.

It is important to keep the blood phenylalanine concentration at the normal level. If it is too high the child's progress slows down measurably, if too low, the child ceases to grow or thrive. The diet must supply all essential nutrients.

The success attending the use of this diet confirms the theory that the mental deficiency in phenylketonuria is the result of intoxication by phenylalanine or one of its abnormal metabolites.

We wish to thank Drs. P. R. Evans and A. P. Norman for permission to quote their cases; Drs. D. A. Pond, C. C. Evans and G. Pamplgione for the E.E.G. reports; the nursing staff for their intelligent cooperation; and the Research Committee of The Hospital for Sick Children for financial support.

References

Armstrong, M. D. and Robinson, R. S. (1954). *Arch. Biochem. Biophys.*, **52**, 287.
—— and Tyler, F. H. (1955). *J. clin. Invest.*, **34**, 565.
Berry, J. P. and Woolf, L. I. (1952). *Nature (Lond.)*, **169**, 202.
Bickel, H., Gerrard, J. and Hickmans, E. M. (1953). *Lancet*, **2**, 812.
Blainey, J. D. and Gulliford, R. (1956). *Arch. Dis. Childh.*, **31**, 452.
Blaschko, H., Datta, S. P. and Harris, H. (1953). *Brit. J. Nutr.*, **7**, 364.
Borek, E., Brecher, A., Jervis, G. A. and Waelsch, H. (1950). *Proc. Soc. exp. Biol. (N.Y.)*, **75**, 86.
Braude, H. (1956). *S. Afr. med. J.*, **30**, 83.
Coates, S., Norman, A. P. and Woolf, L. I. (1958). *Arch. Dis. Childh.*, **32**, 313.
Collins, R. A., Harper. A. E., Schreiber, M. and Elvehjem, C. A. (1951). *J. Nutr.*, **43**, 313.
Cowie, V. (1951a). *J. ment. Sci.*, **97**, 505.
—— (1951b). *Lancet*, **1**, 272.
—— and Penrose, L. S. (1951). *Ann. Eugen. (Camb.)*, **15**, 297.
Dancis, J. and Balis, M. E. (1955). *Pediatrics*, **15**, 63.
Fölling, A. (1934). *Hoppe-Seyl. Z. physiol. Chem.*, **227**, 169.
Garrod, A. E. (1908). *Lancet*, **2**, 1, 73, 142, 214.
—— (1923). *Inborn Errors of Metabolism*, 2nd ed. London.
Griffiths, R. (1954). *The Abilities of Babies*. London.
Harris, M. M. and Harris, R. S. (1947). *Proc. Soc. exp. Biol. (N.Y.)*, **64**, 471.
Hebb, D. O. (1949). *The Organization of Behaviour*. New York.
Horner, F. A. and Streamer, C. W. (1956). *J. Amer. med. Ass.*, **161**, 1628.
Jervis, G. A. (1937). *Arch. Neurol. Psychiat. (Chicago)*, **38**, 944.
—— (1950). *Proc. Soc. exp. Biol. (N.Y.)*, **75**, 83.
—— (1953). *Ibid.*, **82**, 514
Larson, C. A. (1956). Gedda's *Novant'anni delle Legge Mendeliane*, Rome.
Munro, H. N. and Thomson, W. S. T. (1953). *Metabolism*, **2**, 354.
Munro, T. A. (1947). *Ann. Eugen (Camb.)*, **14**, 60.
Pare, C. M. B., Sandler, M. and Stacey, R. S. (1957). *Lancet*, **1**, 551.
Penrose, L. S. (1951). *Ann. Eugen.* (Camb.) **16**, 134.
Robinson, F. A. (1951). *The Vitamin B Complex*. London.
Sandler, M. and Stacey, R. S. (1957). Personal communication.
Snyderman, S. E., Norton, P. and Holt, L. E. Jr. (1955). *Fed. Proc.*, **14**, 450.
Spitz, R. (1955). In *Mental Health and Infant Development*, ed. K. Soddy, Vol. 1. London.
Weil-Malherbe, H. (1955). In *Biochemistry of the Developing Nervous System*: Proc. 1st int. Neurochemical Symposium, Oxford, 1954, ed. H. Waelsch. New York.
Wolf, H. (1956). *Medizinische*, 883.
Woolf, L. I. (1951). *Gt Ormond Str. J.*, **1**, 61.
—— and Norman, A. P. (1957). *J. Pediat.*, **50**, 271.
—— and Vulliamy, D. G. (1951). *Arch. Dis. Childh.*, **26**, 487.
——, Griffiths, R. and Moncrieff, A. (1955). *Brit. med. J.*, **1**, 57

Addendum

In November, 1957, Case 9 had an attack of tonsillitis and refused all food for five days. At the end of this period her urine was found to contain phenylpyruvic acid in a concentration approaching that found in untreated cases of phenylketonuria, and her blood phenylalanine level was also very high.

The most likely explanation is that phenylalanine was released in the proportion relative to the other amino-acids in which it occurs in the tissue proteins which are spontaneously breaking down. This would be, of course, the ideally balanced amino-acid mixture for a normal person (and is approached by ordinary dietary proteins), but the phenylketonuric, owing to the absence of the enzyme phenylalanine hydroxylase, cannot catabolize the phenylalanine released from the tissues and therefore, in the fasting state, it accumulates in the blood and tissues. The low phenylalanine diet provides the other amino-acids in proportions giving a balanced mixture for a phenylketonuric, permitting all the phenylalanine released by tissue breakdown to be used in the synthesis of new tissue protein, and allowing for growth and for the small loss of phenylalanine in the urine and by reactions not involving phenylalanine hydroxylase.

APPENDIX

The following items of the diet can be provided by the National Health Service: Casein hydrolysate, tyrosine, tryptophan, methionine, calcium hydrogen phosphate, the items listed in Table 2, a mixture of salts in solution, namely, potassium chloride, sodium chloride,* magnesium sulphate, potassium iodide,* sodium citrate,* citric acid.*

* Only in the case of infants under 1 year old.

The parents have to buy sucrose, cow's milk, gluten-free wheat starch, kosher margarine, double cream, iodized salt, tomato juice, fruit, cornflour, sago, flavourings, vegetables, breakfast cereal, honey, jam and sweets.

TABLE 1

COMPOSITION OF 'MILK' GIVEN TO CASES 1 AND 8

Ingredient	Daily Intake
Casein hydrolysate*	24 g.
L-Tyrosine	2 g.
DL-Tryptophan	1 g.
DL-Methionine	1 g.
Sucrose	90 g.
Cow's milk	0 to 200 ml.
Double cream†	85 ml.
Calcium hydrogen phosphate	0·71 g.
Potassium chloride	0·65 g.
Sodium chloride	0·016 g.
Magnesium sulphate	0·165 g.
Sodium citrate	0·177 g.
Potassium iodide	0·00013 g.
Citric acid	0·08 g.
Water	to 850 ml.

* Acid hydrolysed casein passed through charcoal to remove phenylalanine and tyrosine.
† 48% fat, 1·7% protein.

TABLE 2

DAILY INTAKE OF SUPPLEMENTS TO ABOVE 'MILK'

Ingredient	Daily Intake
Choline chloride	100 mg.
Inositol	216 mg.
Vitamin B_{12}	4 µg.
Aneurine hydrochloride	0·5 mg.
Riboflavine	0·5 mg.
Pyridoxine	0·33 mg.
Nicotinamide	3·33 mg.
Ascorbic acid	40 mg.
α-Tocopherol	0·33 mg.
Acetomenaphthone	0·5 mg.
Biotin	0·17 mg.
Folic acid	0·25 mg.
Vitamin A	3,000 I.U.
Vitamin D	500 I.U.
Ferrous sulphate	0·15 g.
Manganous sulphate	0·0008 g.
Zinc sulphate	0·0014 g.
Cupric sulphate	0·003 g.

PARATHYROID ADENOMA IN A CHILD PRESENTING AS RICKETS

BY

B. S. B. WOOD, W. H. GEORGE and A. W. ROBINSON

From Dudley Road Hospital, Birmingham

(RECEIVED FOR PUBLICATION JULY 4, 1957)

Primary hyperparathyroidism in childhood is rare. Anspach and Clifton found only 12 cases up to 1939 and since then a few cases in children have been reported by Pugh (1946), Tsumori, Jensen, Hunnicutt, Foreman and Kinsell (1955), Crawford, Stefanelli and Alvarez (1956); these have in general, shown the changes typical of the adult.

The case described here is thought worthy of notice, not only in view of the age, but also because the degree of renal involvement and the radiological features were misleading at the time; in addition, as Dent and Hodson (1954) have stated, primary parathyroid disease in childhood may help to elucidate further the mode of action of parathyroid hormone.

Case Report

John W., aged 12, was first seen in March, 1956, with a five months' history of lethargy, vomiting, anorexia, thirst and polyuria, following a fracture to the left radius and ulna. This fracture resulted from a fall while wrestling with another boy and no obvious radiological abnormality was seen in the bone. No definite clinical abnormality was detected at this time. His blood pressure was 100/60 mm. Hg and his urine was normal apart from 4 white blood cells per high-power field.

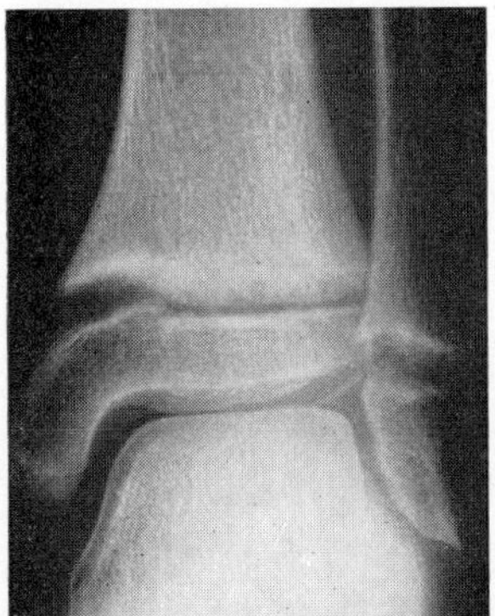

FIGS. 1.—Radiographs showing changes of late rickets.

His symptoms continued and a few months later he complained of pain in the left ankle, which on radiographs showed changes of late rickets (Figs. 1 and 2). He was therefore admitted for further study 17 months after the onset of symptoms. The muscles were flabby, the skin slightly pigmented and his blood pressure had risen to 130/100 mm. Hg.

Investigations gave the following results:

There was no albumin in the urine, but 4-6 white blood cells per high-power field. The specific gravity after a 12-hour fluid fast was 1010. Other results were as follows:

Blood	March 11, 1957	March 20, 1957	April 3, 1957
Calcium ..	14 mg. %	16 mg. %	17·5 mg. %
Phosphorus	3·8 mg. %	2·1 mg. %	4·7 mg. %
Urea ..	46 mg. %	40 mg. %	28 mg. %
CO_2 ..	40 vol. %	52 vol. %	48 vol. %

(Soon after admission he developed acute appendicitis; this was treated by appendicectomy and at this time his blood urea rose to 80 mg. % and his alkali reserve fell to 20 vol. %.)

Excretion pyelography showed poor concentration of the dye but normal calyces were seen.

Urine excretion studies on a low-calcium diet (less than 100 mg. calcium per day) gave 0·41 g. calcium per day and 1·23 g. phosphorus per day.

The calcium content of C.S.F. was 5·5 mg. %. According to Howard, Carey, Rubin and Levine (1949) a level below 6·0 mg. % in the presence of hypercalcaemia suggests primary hyperparathyroidism.

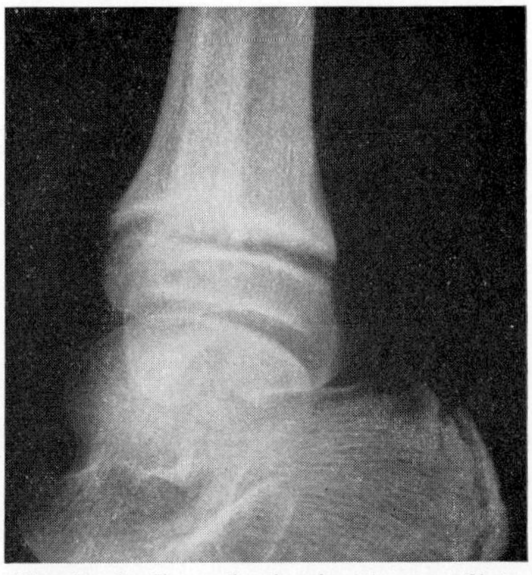

FIG. 2.—Radiographs showing changes of late rickets.

The principal features radiologically were generalized osteoporosis and subperiosteal erosions, particularly in the phalanges and the upper medial and lower posterior margins of the tibiae (see Fig. 2). The confusing element was the rachitic changes at the lower radial, ulnar, tibial

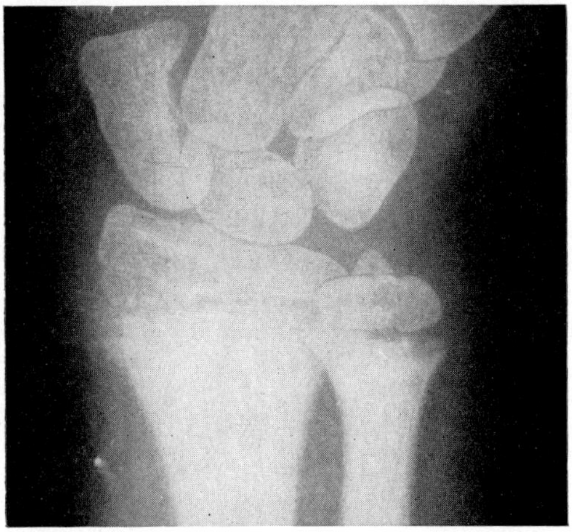

FIG. 3.—Radiographs showing changes of late rickets.

and fibular metaphyses on both sides (see Figs. 1, 2 and 3). A dental radiograph was also taken and showed intact lamina dura (as also did Tsumori and his colleagues' (1955) child of 10 with primary hyperparathyroid disease), a feature pointing against parathyroid hyperactivity of any duration.

The differential diagnosis between primary and secondary hyperparathyroidism has been summarized by Dent and Hodson (1954); this boy's biochemical findings fell neatly into the primary group, while the radiological features were equally typical of secondary or renal osteodystrophy, the impaired kidney function also tending to support the latter diagnosis. It was, however, clear that if a parathyroid tumour were suspected, the neck must be explored.

At operation an oblong tumour, 1 in. by ¾ in., was removed from behind the left lower pole of the thyroid, which on histology was found to be an adenoma of the wasserhelle cells (Figs. 4 and 5). Both sides of the neck were explored without any further abnormality being encountered.

The post-operative course was uneventful, the serum calcium level falling to 8·9 mg. % by the end of a week and the urinary calcium on a high calcium intake falling to below 0·05 g. per day.

When last seen two months after operation he was in good health with a blood pressure of 130/80 mm. Hg and normal calcium and phosphorus levels in the serum.

Discussion

A review of the literature makes it clear that quite severe renal impairment can occur as the result of primary hyperparathyroidism, atypical cases presenting as diabetes insipidus (Albright and Reifenstein, 1948) or hypertension (Race, 1952).

We should not therefore have been much influenced by the failure of this boy's kidneys to concentrate. We were, however, considerably disturbed by the radiological appearances of rickets, as Dent and Hodson (1954) imply that the essential difference between primary hyperparathyroidism and the secondary form due to renal disease is that in the former there is no sign of rachitic change. This is instanced by the 8-year-old boy reported by Pugh (1946) and similar statements are made by Albright and Reifenstein (1948) and Snapper (1949). However, Caffey (1950) states that in pre-adolescent primary hyperparathyroidism 'rachitic-like changes in the metaphyses have been described', presumably referring to the cases of Duken (1928) and Anspach

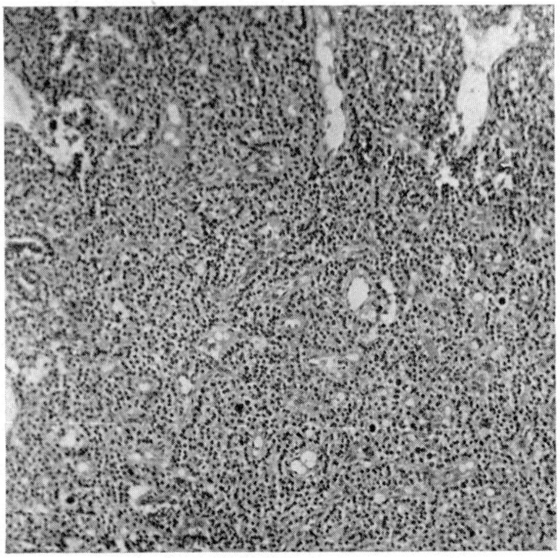

Fig. 4.—×90.

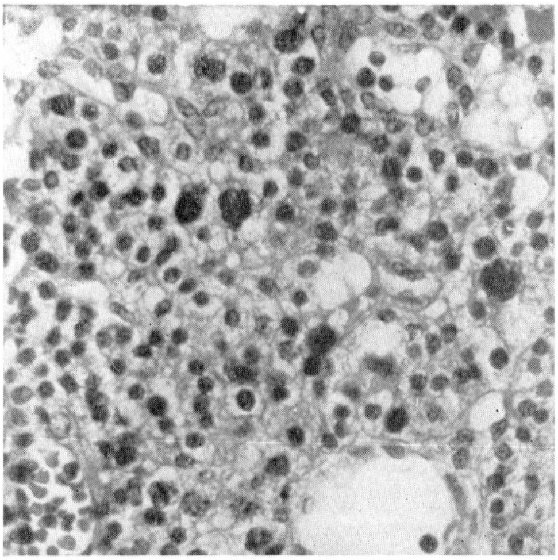

Fig. 5.—×375.

FIGS. 4 and 5.—Photomicrographs of the adenoma. Haematoxylin and eosin.

and Clifton (1939). Brailsford (1953) too states that in hyperparathyroidism before adolescence the radiographic appearance may be similar to type B renal rickets and he illustrates a case of primary hyperparathyroidism with rachitic changes in the lower ends of the radius and ulna.

Hunter and Turnbull (1931) differentiated the bone histology resulting from primary hyperparathyroidism, in which there is osteoporosis and no increase in osteoid tissue, from that of osteomalacia and rickets where osteoid is increased. They explained that in Schmorl's (1926) cases, where osteomalacia co-existed with hyperparathyroidism, the dietary state in Germany at that time led to the widespread occurrence of both osteomalacia and rickets in the general population. Such is unlikely to be the explanation in our case, as since infancy he regularly imbibed 2 to 3 pints of milk daily and took one teaspoonful of cod-liver oil throughout the winter months. The fact that he developed rickets on such a diet suggests perhaps that the phosphate diuretic effect of the parathyroid hormone predominated over its osteoclastic effect upon the bone. He had been growing 3 in. a year up to the time of his illness and any tendency towards a negative calcium or phosphorus balance might be expected to precipitate a rachitic change at the epiphyses. It does not seem possible to invoke an acidosis as the cause in view of the high serum calcium levels and the normal alkali reserve.

Summary

A boy of 12 presenting with radiological rickets was found to have the biochemical findings of primary hyperparathyroidism. This was confirmed by removal of a parathyroid adenoma at operation. It appears that radiological rickets can occur in primary hyperparathyroidism without primary renal disease or acidosis.

We are indebted to Dr. A. Booth for permission to reproduce the early radiographs, to Dr. W. H. Caldwell for the histological report on the tumour, to Mr. S. Smith for the biochemical investigations and to Mr. A. J. Higgs for the photomicrographs.

References

Albright, F. and Reifenstein, E. C. (1948). *The Parathyroid Glands and Metabolic Bone Disease*, p. 59. Baltimore.
Anspach, W. E. and Clifton, W. M. (1939). *Amer. J. Dis. Child.*, **58**, 540.
Brailsford, J. F. (1953) *The Radiology of Bones and Joints*, 5th ed. p. 108. London.
Caffey, J. (1950). *Pediatric X-ray Diagnosis*, 2nd ed., p. 782. Chicago.
Crawford, D. J. M., Stefanelli, J. and Alvarez, A. F. (1956). *Brit. J. Surg.*, **44**, 193.
Dent, C. E. and Hodson, C. J. (1954). *Brit. J. Radiol.*, **27**, 605.
Duken, J. (1928). *Z. Kinderheilk.*, **46**, 114.
Howard, J. E., Carey, R. A., Rubin, P. S. and Levine, M. D. (1949). *Trans. Ass. Amer. Phys.*, **62**, 264.
Hunter, D. and Turnbull, H. M. (1931). *Brit. J. Surg.*, **19**, 203.
Pugh, R. J. (1946). *Proc. roy. Soc. Med.*, **39**, 694.
Race, G. J. (1952). *N.C. med. J.*, **13**, 659.
Schmorl, G. (1926). *Klin. Wschr.*, **5**, 496.
Snapper, I. (1949). *Medical Clinics on Bone Diseases*, 2nd ed., p. 104. New York.
Tsumori, H., Jensen, E., Hunnicutt, A., Foreman, N. and Kinsell, L. W. (1955). *J. clin. Endocr.*, **15**, 1141.

ACROMEGALY IN A GIRL OF 8 YEARS

BY

R. McLAREN TODD

From the Department of Child Health, University of Liverpool

(RECEIVED FOR PUBLICATION JUNE 21, 1957)

Pierre Marie in 1886 first suggested the name acromegaly for a clinical condition associated with enlargement of the extremities (ἀκρα) which he had observed in two women aged 37 and 54 years. Marie reviewed the literature and found records of five male patients (two of whom were brothers) with similar features; the earliest of these descriptions concerned a man of 39 years reported by Saucerotte (1772). Marie also discussed the differential diagnosis of acromegaly from myxoedema, Paget's disease of bone (osteitis deformans) and leontiasis ossea of Virchow.

Although Saucerotte's account is probably the earliest medical description of acromegaly, the condition was well known to ancient writers. For example, the height of Goliath of Gath (1 Samuel 17. 4) was 6 cubits and a span (9½ ft.) and the record suggests that he may have suffered from a pituitary tumour which caused bitemporal hemianopia and so he was unable to see the stone slung at him by David. It is also of interest that Goliath's son was a man of great stature (2 Samuel 22. 20) and that he had polydactyly (six fingers on each hand and six toes on each foot); Goliath's brother was also a giant and the staff of his spear was like a weaver's beam (2 Samuel 22. 19).

The first paper suggesting a relationship between acromegaly and the pituitary gland was that of Verga (1864) of Milan. He reported the necropsy findings of a woman of 59 years who began to develop evidence of acromegaly at the age of 35 years; the post-mortem examination revealed a tumour extending from the sella turcica and compressing the optic nerves.

Acromegaly is exceedingly rare and is especially uncommon in childhood. Atkinson (1931) reviewed the world literature from 1890 to 1929 and found 15 boys and 10 girls under the age of 15 years suffering from acromegaly; during the past 25 years a few cases have been reported (Schlesinger, 1931; Behrens and Barr, 1932; Seale, 1934 and 1935; Hurxthal, 1943). The only previous case recorded in the *Archives of Disease in Childhood* since this journal was first published in 1926 concerns a boy of 6 years who lived in Brno (Traub, 1939) and showed acromegalic gigantism associated with bony changes in the right hip, tarsal scaphoids, metatarsals and vertebral bodies.

Case Report

G.O. was born on August 23, 1947, after a normal pregnancy and delivery. She weighed 7½ lb. at birth and developed normally until the age of 5 years when she had a mild attack of whooping cough. After this illness her mother noticed that she tired easily and that she was putting on weight excessively. It was not until two years later that the symptoms became more obvious. She consulted her family doctor (Dr. W. Jones Morris) in July, 1954, when she was 6 years 11 months old because of persistent nasal catarrh and he observed the acromegalic features. Her height at this time was 54½ inches. Her general health was good, her appetite was rather excessive, but she did not complain of visual disturbances (she had worn glasses from the age of 3 years), headaches or vomiting. A study of family photographs suggests that acromegaly had been present for some years. A photograph of the patient with her elder sister and younger brother taken when she was 3 years old did not show the features of acromegaly (Fig. 1) but a photograph taken when her brother was 4 years old and she was 5½ years old shows the enlarged hands and abnormal facial appearance of acromegaly (Fig. 2).

She was admitted to Alder Hey Children's Hospital, Liverpool, in February, 1956, for further investigation.

On admission (aged 8½ years) she weighed 116 lb., her height was 60 inches (height-age of 12½ years) and head circumference was 22 in. She was a heavily-built, coarse-featured child, with black hair, bushy eyebrows and the typical features of acromegaly. There was slight but definite generalized pigmentation of the skin, and pigmentation was especially marked in the axillae, groins, areolae and umbilical area. There was no axillary hair and no breast enlargement, but a small amount of pubic hair. There were no abnormal signs in the heart or lungs, blood pressure was 125/75 mm. Hg, and the abdomen was enlarged due to deposition of subcutaneous fat. Examination of the central nervous system, including optic fundi, was negative.

Table 1 records the measurements made of the patient, and of a girl one year older who was in the ward at the same time for investigation of 'dizzy spells'.

Further comparison is afforded by photographs of the hands (Fig. 3) and feet (Fig. 4), and by a full-length

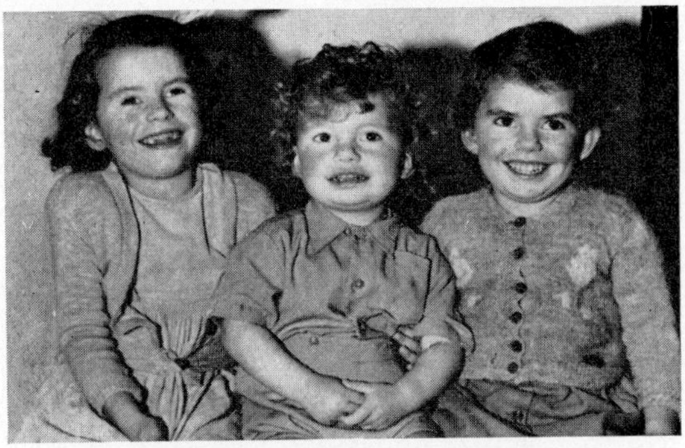

FIG. 1.

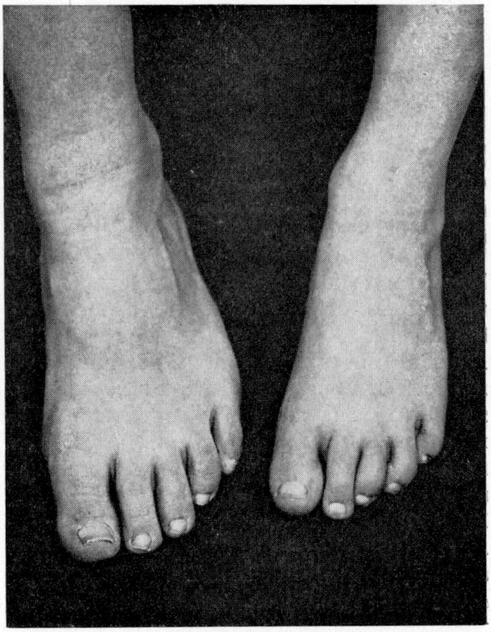

FIG. 4.

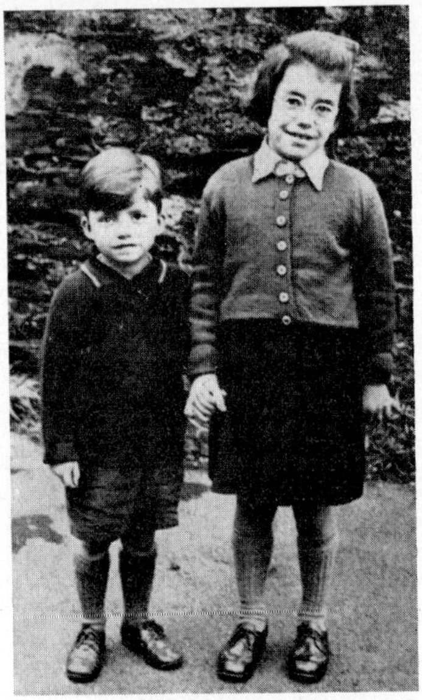

FIG. 2.

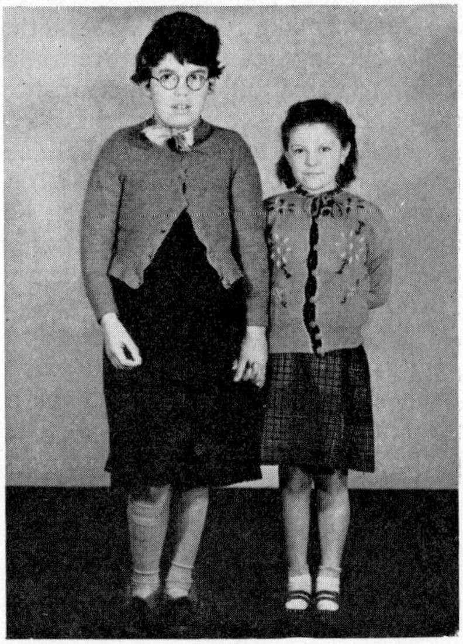

FIG. 5.

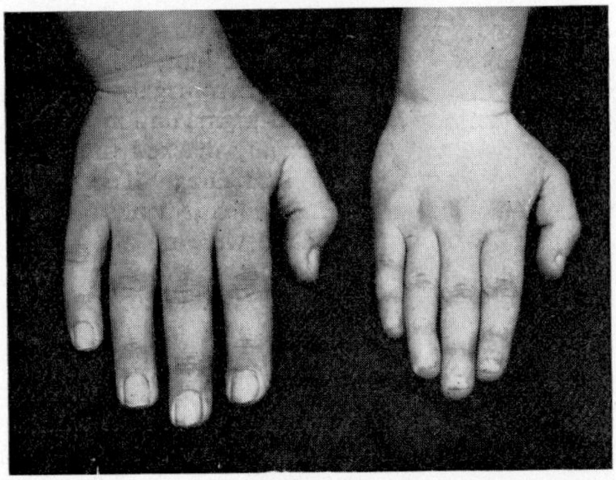

FIG. 3.

FIG. 1.—Patient (extreme right) at age of 3 years with brother and sister.

FIG. 2.—Patient at age of 5½ years with brother.

FIG. 3.—Right hand of patient and control.

FIG. 4.—Left foot of patient and control.

FIG. 5.—Full-length photograph of patient and control.

TABLE 1

MEASUREMENTS COMPARED WITH THOSE OF A CONTROL

	Control	Patient
Date of birth . .	23.6.46	28.8.47
Age (March, 1956) . .	9 years 9 months	8 years 7 months
Weight	67 lb. 4 oz. (50th percentile)	116 lb. 2 oz.
Height	51½ in. (50th percentile)	60 in. (height age 12½ yr.)
Upper measurement	26 in. (normal)	31½ in. (normal 26)
Lower measurement	25½ in. (normal)	28½ in. (normal 25)
Ratio upper/lower . .	1 to 1	1·1/1
Span	50½ in. (normal 52)	59 in. (normal 50)
Head circumference	21 in. (normal)	22 in. (normal 21)
Bone age	Same as chronological age	Same as chronological age

TABLE 2

MEASUREMENTS OF PATIENT'S FAMILY

	Height	Weight
Father	5 ft. 8 in.	160 lb.
Mother	5 ft. 3 in.	98 lb. 6 oz.
Sister (aged 10 yr.)	4 ft. 7 in.	67 lb. 8 oz.
Brother (aged 7 yr.)	4 ft. 1 in.	58 lb. 12 oz.

photograph (Fig. 5). The height and weight of other members of the patient's family are recorded in Table 2.

Investigations. Urine was of *p*H 5·5 and specific gravity 1020. No albumin, no reducing substances and nothing abnormal was seen in a centrifuged deposit.

Blood urea was 27 mg. %.

A blood count gave Hb 78% (11·5 g. %), leucocytes 9,000 per c.mm. (normal differential count).

Serum protein was 6·8 g. %, serum calcium 5·0 mEq/l., serum phosphorus 6·8 mg. %, serum alkaline phosphatase 14 K-A units %, serum potassium 4 mEq/l., serum cholesterol 190 mg. %, alkali reserve 19 mEq/l.

A glucose tolerance test gave the fasting blood sugar 100 mg. %, and half an hour after 35 g. glucose 130 mg. %, one hour 130 mg. %, two hours 140 mg. % and three hours 160 mg. %.

An insulin tolerance test gave the fasting blood sugar 107 mg., 20 minutes after 6 units of insulin 85 mg. %, 30 minutes 85 mg. %, 45 minutes 112 mg. %, one hour 95 mg. %, two hours 110 mg. %.

The total 17-ketosteroid content of a 24-hourly collection of urine was 2·8 mg. (average 0·3 to 1·99 mg.). The total 17 ketogenic steroids (corticosteroids) content of a 24-hourly collection of urine was 4·22 mg. (average 0·3 to 1·99 mg.).

An eosinophil test before intramuscular injection of A.C.T.H. gave 238 eosinophils per c.mm., after one hour 241, two hours 155, three hours 113, four hours 113.

Radiographs of the wrists and elbows show a bone

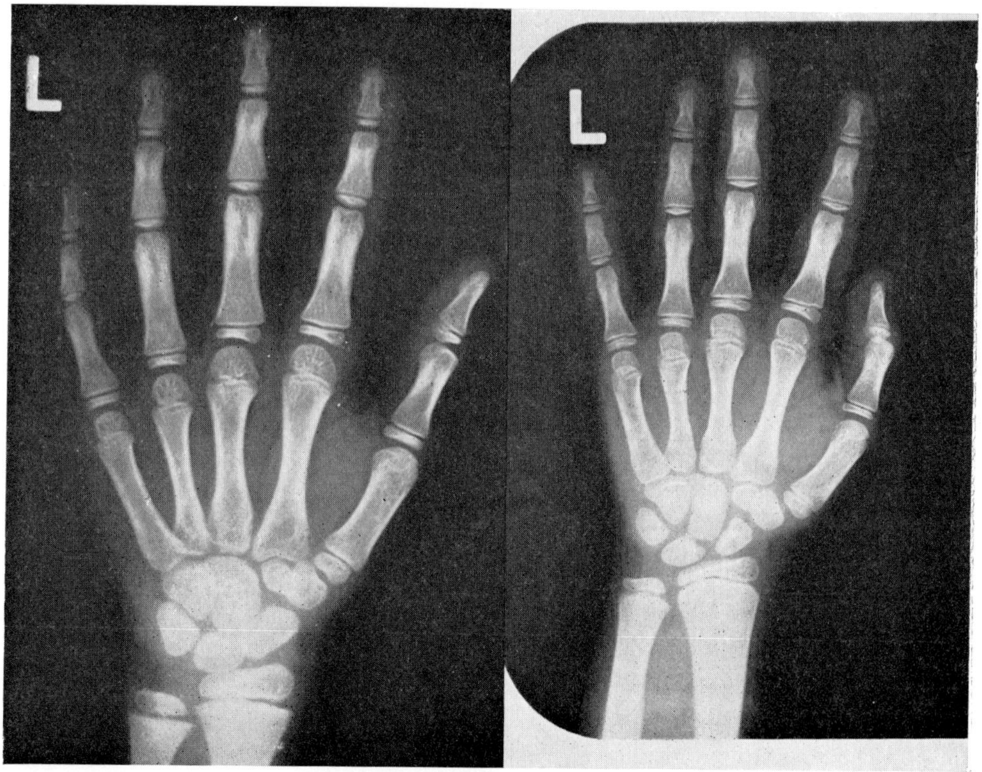

FIG. 6.—Radiograph of left wrist of patient and control.

age of 8 to 9 years (Fig. 6). The sella turcica was larger and deeper than that of the control (Fig. 7). No destructive changes were shown and there was no evidence of intracranial calcification.

An intravenous pyelogram was normal.

At rest an E.E.G. (Fig. 8) showed an irregular 9 per second alpha rhythm, and a considerable amount of slow activity within theta and delta ranges. There was no significant change on hyperventilation or on photic stimulation. The slow activity was very prominent and the delta activity was outside the limits of normal for a child of this age (report by Dr. R. R. Hughes).

A urinary nitrogen excretion test was carried out over a period of two weeks. The patient excreted 4·5 g. N_2 daily in urine, whereas a control excreted 7·2 g. per day.

The visual fields were entirely normal, and central colours also normal.

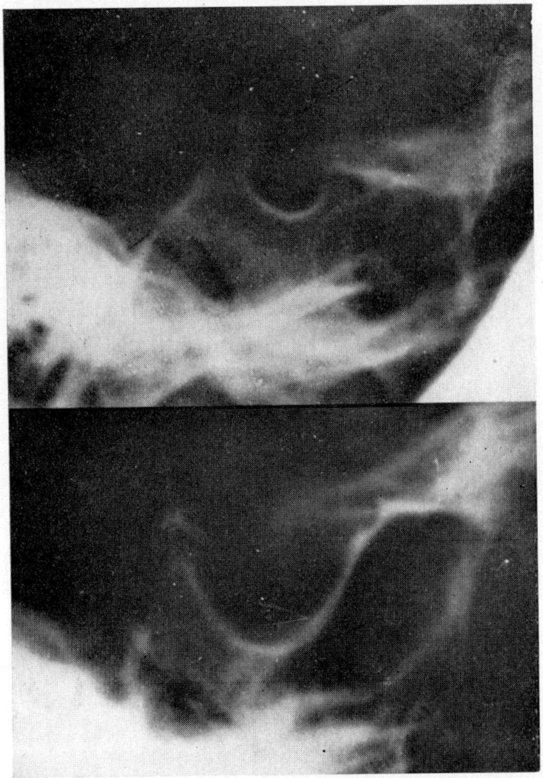

FIG. 7.—Radiographs of pituitary fossa of patient and control.

The patient was under observation in hospital for 11 weeks and during this period her height increased from 60 to 60½ in. and weight increased from 116 lb. 2 oz. to 125 lb. 4 oz. During this time the optic fundi remained normal, and she did not suffer from headache, vomiting or visual disturbance. She was seen, as an out-patient, by a radiotherapist (Dr. D. M. Fraser) who reported: 'I agree with you that acromegalic gigantism is the most probable diagnosis but I do not think that we should be justified in giving radiotherapy to the pituitary without more positive evidence of the presence of a tumour.'

In view of her continued growth and the embarrassment it caused her, particularly at school, it was decided to give oestrogens in an effort to promote epiphyseal fusion and thus prevent further excessive

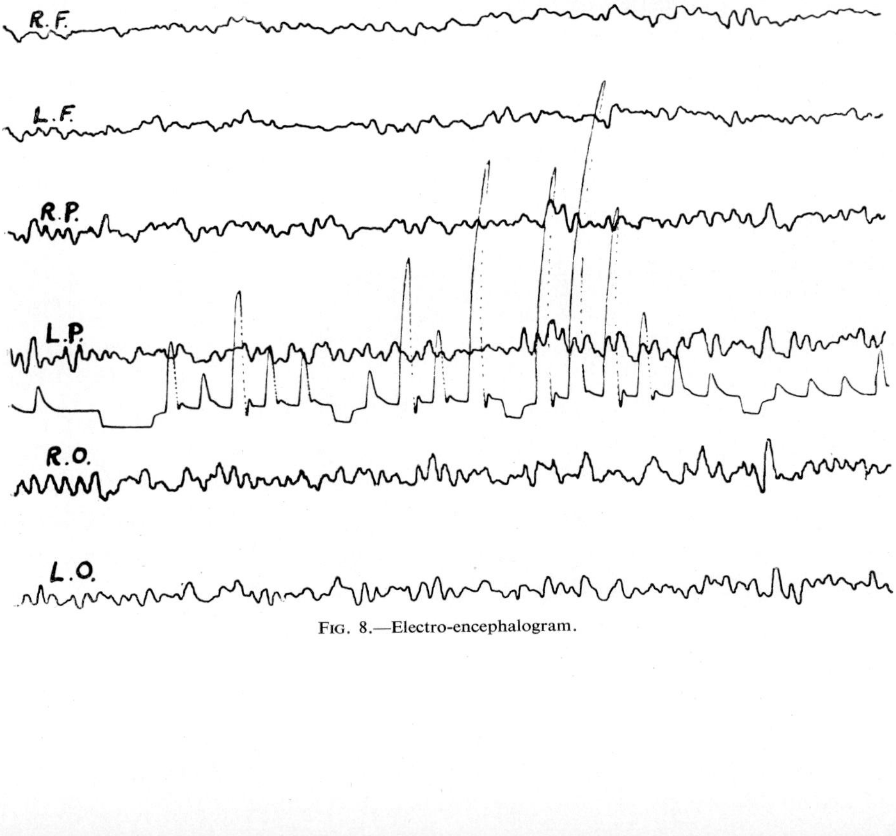

FIG. 8.—Electro-encephalogram.

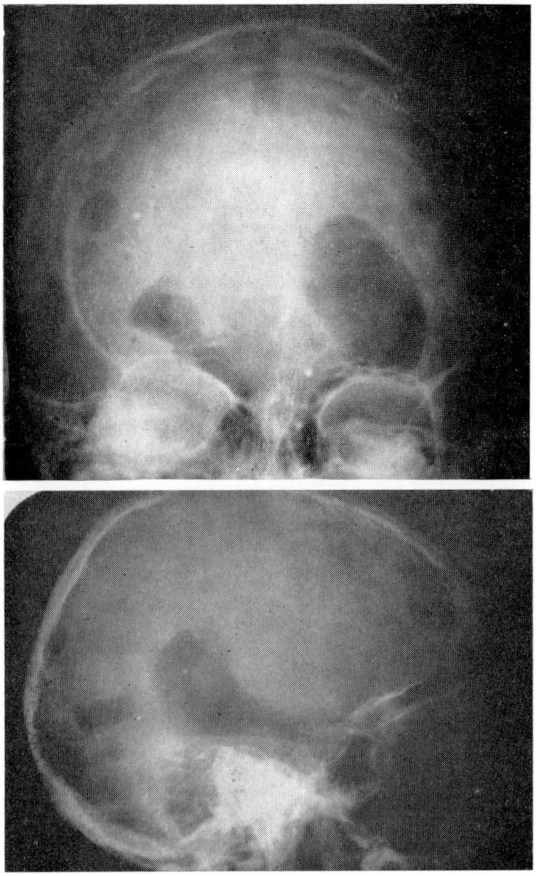

FIGS. 9A and 9B.—Ventriculogram.

growth of the long bones. She received stilboestrol, 1 mg. daily, for three weeks, and then 1 mg. twice daily for three weeks. It was discontinued because of vomiting and severe headaches. Menstrual bleeding started one week after stilboestrol was stopped and bleeding continued for four days. She was readmitted to hospital on September 24, 1956, because of increasingly severe headaches in the frontal and occipital regions, and vomiting several times daily.

The fundi were examined and bilateral papilloedema of about 3 dioptres swelling was observed. She was seen by Mr. Hannah (neurosurgeon) who agreed to relieve the raised intracranial tension surgically. A ventriculogram (Fig. 9A and 9B) showed evidence of a large suprasellar lesion which was partially blocking the ventricles. It was felt that a direct approach to the tumour was fraught with danger and it was decided to perform a Torkildsen's operation, making a short circuit between the lateral ventricle and the cisterna magna. The symptoms were relieved after operation and she was then given *x*-ray therapy over a period of four weeks to a tumour dose of 3,000 roentgen units. At a follow-up examination on February 18, 1957, her general condition was satisfactory, she had not suffered from headaches, the visual fields were normal, and the papilloedema had completely subsided. The acromegalic features were not more marked.

Discussion

The diagnosis of pituitary gigantism is founded upon the clinical and radiological manifestations Talbot, Sobel, McArthur and Crawford (1952) have described the main clinical features as follows: (*a*) Rapid growth of the skeleton and supporting mesenchymal structures; (*b*) no acceleration of skeletal maturation; (*c*) usually no gross evidence of hyperthyroidism, hyperadrenocorticism or hypergonadism; (*d*) occasionally signs of an expanding lesion in the region of the pituitary.

(*a*) The patient reported in this paper shows these clinical features. Growth has been rapid from about 5 years of age, and her height was $54\frac{1}{2}$ in. at the age of 7 years (height age of $10\frac{1}{2}$ years) and 60 in. at $8\frac{1}{2}$ years (height age of $12\frac{1}{2}$ years). (*b*) The excessive growth is due to excessive production of pituitary growth hormone and this hormone does not cause early skeletal maturation or closure of epiphyses. The bone age of this patient was the same as her chronological age. (*c*) There was no clinical evidence of overactivity of the thyroid, adrenal or sex glands and the following investigations support the clinical findings: serum cholesterol normal, excretion of 17 ketosteroids only slightly above the average normal, response to A.C.T.H. normal, blood electrolytes normal. (*d*) The patient also showed clinical evidence of an expanding intracranial lesion (headache, vomiting, papilloedema) and this was confirmed by encephalography.

In addition to these main clinical features, the diagnosis is supported by haematological and radiological abnormalities. The glucose tolerance curve was of the diabetic type and the patient showed insulin resistance. There was also evidence from balance studies of retention of nitrogen (pituitary growth hormone increases the utilization of amino-acids for synthesis of tissue proteins, causing thereby retention of nitrogen). Wilkins (1950) states that the finding of a high serum phosphorus level of the order of 5 to 6 mg. % may be valuable in confirming the diagnosis of hyperpituitarism and in this patient the serum phosphorus level was 6·8 mg.%. Patients with pituitary gigantism sometimes show radiological changes of the terminal phalanges, cancellous tufts develop, and small spaces of bone may be observed. This patient showed cancellous tufting of some of the terminal phalanges. Seale (1935) reported an eosinophilia

(12 to 16%) in an acromegalic boy of 12 years but could find no reports of similar blood changes; the blood count of our patient showed no increase of eosinophil cells.

The treatment recommended for pituitary gigantism will vary with the severity of the disease but involves either surgery, irradiation or hormones.

Surgical removal of an eosinophil tumour of the pituitary gland is a difficult procedure and the mortality rate is high. Surgical treatment is usually restricted, as in this patient, to relief of intracranial tension by a short circuit operation, especially when vision is threatened. Irradiation of the sella turcica is the most usual form of therapy and is often carried out (as in this patient) after relief of intracranial tension by surgical means. There is a risk of damage to other pituitary cells, and after radiotherapy symptoms of diabetes insipidus may be observed.

The use of hormones to hasten bone maturation and epiphyseal fusion seems a rational form of therapy. Testosterone or stilboestrol hasten epiphyseal fusion and also inhibit the secretion of pituitary hormones. This patient received stilboestrol for a short period only but there was some radiological evidence to suggest that bone maturation was hastened even by such a short course of therapy. Other hormones, e.g., posterior pituitary extract, may also be required to control the symptoms of diabetes insipidus which may develop either because of the pressure of a rapidly growing eosinophil tumour on the posterior pituitary gland, or after irradiation of the sella turcica.

Summary

The clinical features and results of investigations of a girl of 8 years suffering from acromegaly are recorded.

The diagnosis and treatment of this endocrine disorder are discussed.

References

Atkinson, F. R. B. (1931). *Brit. J. Child. Dis.*, **28**, 121.
Behrens, L. H. and Barr, D. P. (1932). *Endocrinology*, **16**, 120.
Hurxthal, L. M. (1943). *J. clin. Endocr.*, 3, 12.
Marie, P. (1886). *Rev. Medecine*, **6**, 297.
Saucerotte, (1772). See Weinberg, S. J. (1931). *Ann. med. Hist.*, n.s., 3, 650.
Schlesinger, B. (1931). *Proc. roy. Soc. Med.*, **24**, 1352.
Seale, E. A. (1934). *S. Afr. med. J.*, **8**, 371.
—— (1935). *Ibid.*, **9**, 295.
Talbot, N. B., Sobel, E. H., McArthur, J. W. and Crawford, J. D. (1952). *Functional Endocrinology from Birth through Adolescence*. Cambridge, Mass.
Traub, E. (1939). *Arch. Dis. Childh.*, **14**, 203.
Verga, A. (1864). See Weinberg, S. J. (1931). *Ann. med. Hist.*, n.s., 3, 650.
Wilkins, L. (1950). *The Diagnosis and Treatment of Endocrine Disorders in Childhood and Adolescence*, Springfield, Illinois.

MALIGNANT NON-CHROMAFFIN PARAGANGLIOMA OF THE THIGH

BY

A. MACFARLANE and A. R. MACGREGOR

From the Pathology Department, Royal Hospital for Sick Children, Edinburgh

(RECEIVED FOR PUBLICATION JULY 16, 1957)

Within recent years it has become recognized that some tumours arising in skeletal muscle have a close resemblance histologically to tumours of non-chromaffin paraganglia such as the carotid body and glomus jugulare (Smetana and Scott, 1951). Such tumours are rare and have previously been designated granular cell myoblastomata or, more recently, alveolar soft-part sarcomas (Christopherson, Foote and Stewart, 1952). They occur mainly in children and young adults and are often malignant.

The case recorded here is that of a boy who developed a tumour of the left rectus femoris muscle, which recurred after local excision and subsequently gave rise to widespread metastases from which he died a year later.

Case Report

J.T., a boy aged 6 years, attended the Royal Hospital for Sick Children, Edinburgh, in June, 1950, with the complaint of a swelling in the front of the left thigh for three weeks. It had been gradually increasing in size but had given rise to no symptoms.

The swelling was excised locally. He remained well for eight months but then complained of frontal headaches and vomiting. He was found to have bilateral papilloedema and raised intracranial pressure due to a space-occupying lesion in the posterior part of the left cerebral hemisphere. Left occipital craniotomy and decompression were performed. He gradually deteriorated, with herniation of the brain through the craniotomy and paraplegia as a result of spinal metastases. The tumour recurred in the front of the left thigh and there was lymphatic spread to the left inguinal nodes.

Morbid Anatomy

The primary tumour in the left rectus femoris muscle measured $7 \times 3 \times 3$ cm. It was oval, fleshy and generally white with several pale pink areas (Fig. 1). It was embedded in muscle and its margin was well defined except in one region where it appeared to be infiltrating.

At necropsy a year later, the tumour had recurred locally and formed a large, fleshy mass, $15 \times 5 \times 4$ cm., adherent to the femoral periosteum. The left inguinal lymph nodes were enlarged and replaced by tumour. Secondary deposits were present in the liver, lungs, vertebral column and spinal cord, brain (Fig. 2), skull, palate and the medulla of the right adrenal gland. In all these situations except the brain the metastatic deposits were similar macroscopically to the original tumour in the thigh. The large neoplastic mass in the brain differed in that

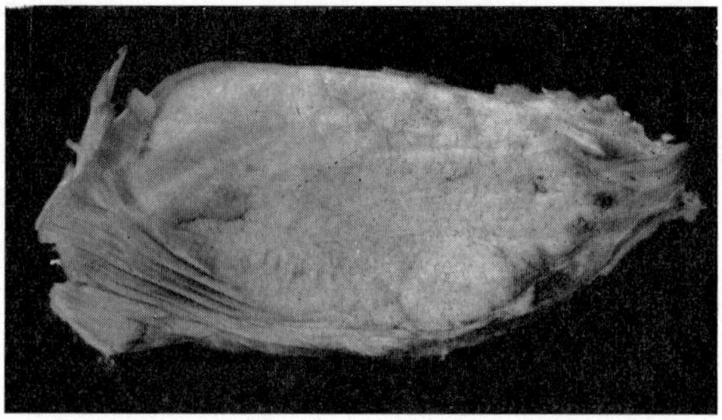

FIG. 1.—The primary tumour in the left rectus femoris muscle. About actual size.

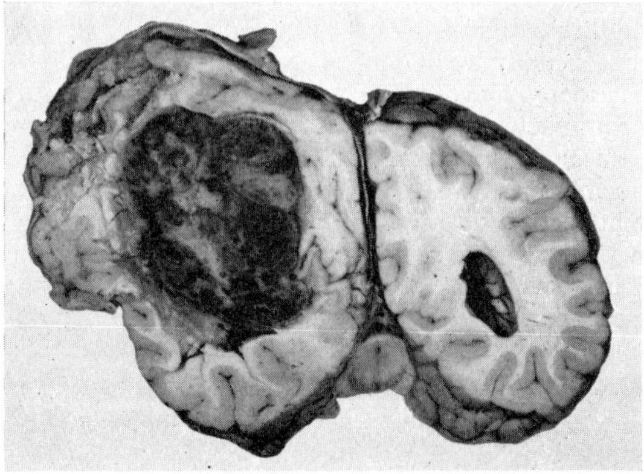

FIG. 2.—Large secondary deposit in posterior parieto-temporal region of left cerebral hemisphere. Note the extensive haemorrhage.

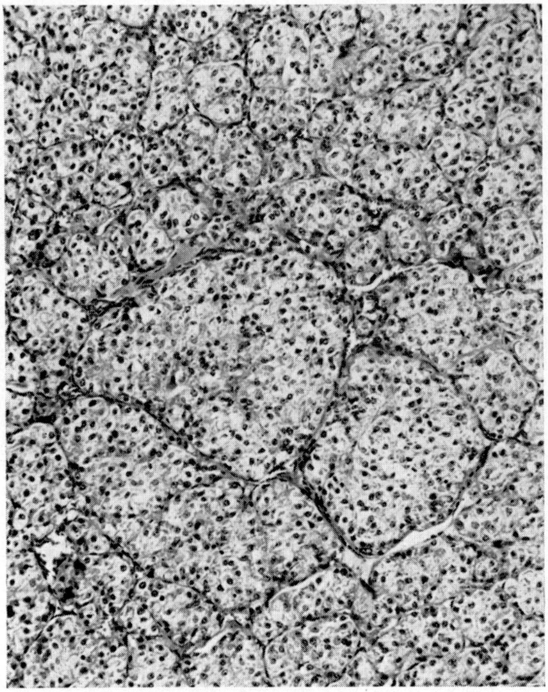

FIG. 3.—Primary tumour composed of discrete groups of granular cells. Note the vascular channels in several areas. H. & E. × 120.

widespread necrosis and haemorrhage had occurred. All epithelial tissues were examined with particular care to exclude a possible primary growth other than that in the thigh muscle.

Histology

Both primary and secondary tumours showed an identical histological pattern which is very characteristic and striking. The tumour cells were arranged in discrete groups which were enclosed by delicate, but usually well defined collagen fibres (Fig. 3). In many areas, these cell groups were separated from each other by vascular channels the walls of which were formed by the limiting collagenous membranes with an inner layer of extremely flattened endothelial cells (Figs. 4 and 5). These vascular spaces sometimes contained blood (Fig. 4), but were more often empty (Fig. 5). In the secondary deposit in the brain they were very large and engorged with blood. This delicate layer of endothelium was sometimes extremely thin and in places deficient (Fig. 5) so that tumour cells bulged into the lumina.

The neoplastic cells were large and polyhedral with indistinct cell boundaries and coarsely granular eosinophilic cytoplasm. The nuclei were large, variable in position and usually vesicular. Many contained prominent nucleoli. Mitotic figures were scanty. A striking feature in several areas was the production of a pseudo-acinar structure by degeneration of the central cells in the tumour masses (Fig. 6). Invasion of veins was observed in the primary tumour (Fig. 6).

Discussion

Tumours of this type have usually been classified as granular cell myoblastomata because of their relationship to skeletal muscle and granularity of the cytoplasm of the neoplastic cells. They can be readily identified by their distinctive histological pattern in the illustrations of several cases reported as granular cell myoblastomata, *e.g.*, Case 6 of Klemperer (1934), Case 4 of Horn and Stout (1943) and the case of Schwidde, Meyers and Sweeney (1951). Horn and Stout noted the striking pseudo alveolar structure of this group and used the term 'organoid' granular cell myoblastoma to describe them. Christopherson *et al.* (1952) reported 12

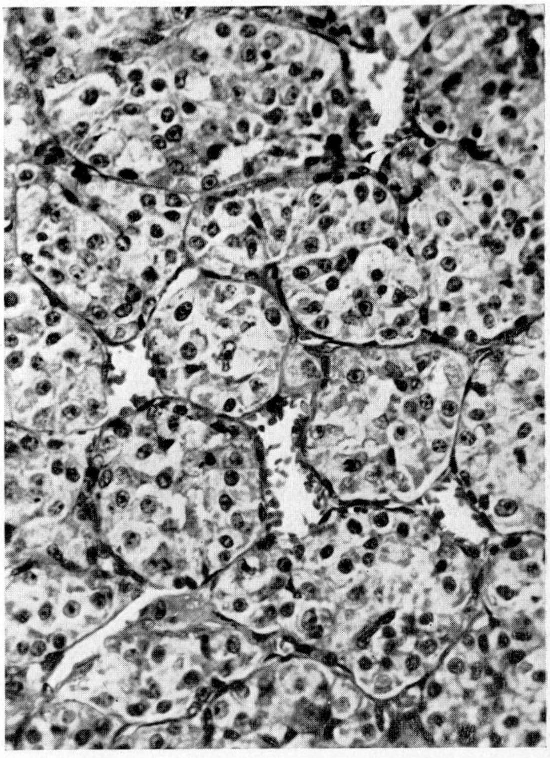

FIG. 4.—Delicate membranes of connective tissue enclose the groups of tumour cells. Several vascular channels containing red blood cells also present. H. & E. × 300.

tumours of this type, mainly in young adults and arising in skeletal muscle; 50% of them metastasized. They drew attention to their resemblance to paragangliomata but knew of no identification of any paraganglionic tissue in the extremities. They termed them alveolar soft-part sarcomas.

Smetana and Scott (1951) collected 14 examples of this tumour and showed that there was a close similarity to tumours of the carotid body and glomus jugulare. They considered they were paragangliomata and to support this view provided illustrations in their paper of structures removed from the vicinity of the large femoral vessels in Hunter's canal which they interpreted as normal paraganglionic tissue. Since then further examples have been described (Randall and Walter, 1954; Hicks and Leitch, 1955). Willis (1953) reported that he had seen five such tumours and was of the opinion that they were paragangliomata.

We agree with Smetana and Scott that these tumours are most probably non-chromaffin paragangliomata because of their striking resemblance to tumours of undoubted paraganglia, but conclusive proof of their origin must await confirmation of the presence of normal paraganglia in the limbs. We have attempted, without success so far, to identify such structures in the lower limbs of children and adults at necropsy.

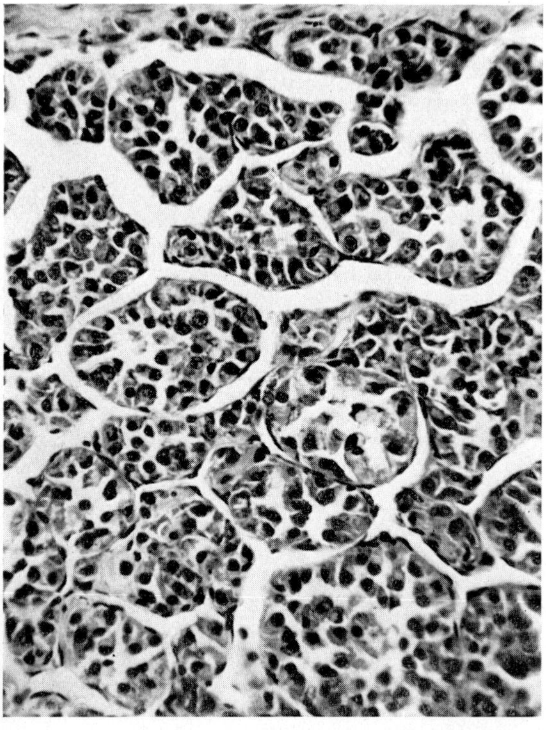

FIG. 5.—The endothelial lining of the vascular channels is extremely thin and deficient in places. H. & E. × 270.

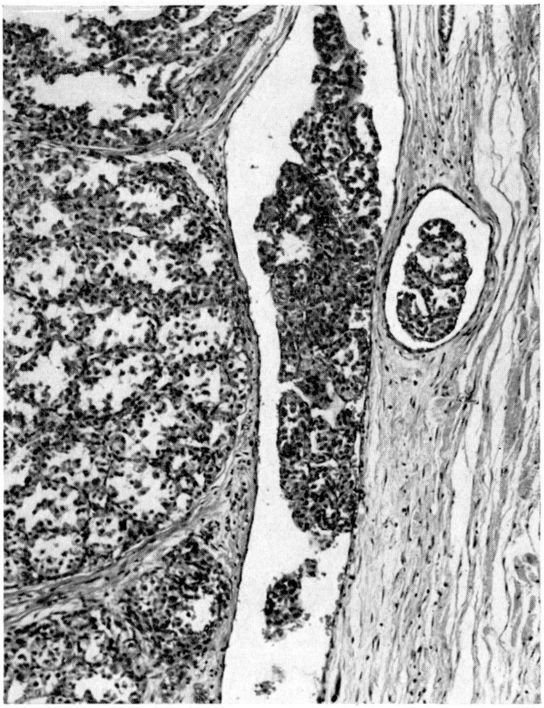

FIG. 6.—Venous invasion at periphery of primary tumour. Note pseudo-acinar structure in the left half of the field due to degeneration of central tumour cells. H. & E. × 85.

There seems little doubt, however, that this tumour is an entity whatever its tissue of origin. The histological pattern has been reproduced fairly uniformly in all the examples so far published. It appears to arise within or in close proximity to skeletal muscle, usually of the limbs, and affects mainly young adults or children. Many metastasize though they may appear histologically benign. Invasion of veins in the primary growth, as was demonstrated in this case, may indicate the future behaviour of these tumours.

Summary

A malignant tumour arising in the rectus femoris muscle of a young boy is described. It is considered to be a non-chromaffin paraganglioma.

We wish to thank the Photomicrography Department, University of Edinburgh, for the illustrations.

REFERENCES

Christopherson, W. M., Foote, F. W. and Stewart, F. W. (1952). *Cancer*, **5**, 100.
Hicks, N. D. and Leitch, O. W. (1955). *Med. J. Aust.*, **1**, 395.
Horn, R. C. and Stout, A. P. (1943). *Surg. Gynec. Obstet.*, **76**, 315.
Klemperer, P. (1934). *Amer. J. Cancer*, **20**, 324.
Randall, K. J. and Walter, J. B. (1954). *J. Path. Bact.*, **67**, 69.
Schwidde, J. T., Meyers, R. and Sweeney, D. B. (1951). *J. Neuropath*, **10**, 30.
Smetana, H. F. and Scott, W. F. (1951). *Milit. Surg.*, **109**, 330.
Willis, R. A. (1953). *Pathology of Tumours*, 2nd ed., p. 744. London.

GUMMA OF THE LIVER IN CONGENITAL SYPHILIS

BY

D. WHITEHOUSE and W. V. MACFARLANE

From the Departments of Child Health and Venereology, Newcastle General Hospital, Newcastle upon Tyne

(RECEIVED FOR PUBLICATION MARCH 5, 1957)

Modern methods of serological testing for syphilis in pregnancy combined with highly efficient anti-syphilitic therapy should now be making congenital syphilis a relatively rare disease. In addition, past reports have frequently emphasized the ease with which gummata of the liver, and, indeed, elsewhere, may be misdiagnosed. In these circumstances unusual manifestations of this condition are more than ever likely to be missed, and for this reason we feel our recent experience with gumma of the liver should be described.

Case Report

W.G., a boy of 6 years, the only son of parents both aged 40 years living in a small market town, was sent to the Out-patient Department with the suggested diagnosis of leukaemia. His history was of vague ill-health for one year, beginning with an episode called by his parents 'the blues', consisting of a period of extreme sensitivity to cold, with shivering and a blue-black appearance of the face and legs during the winter weather. This was followed by episodes of loss of appetite, pallor and pain in the left side of the abdomen lasting three or four weeks, but apparently without fever and without vomiting.

On examination he was pale, lethargic and febrile. The main physical sign consisted of a striking enlargement of the liver, especially the left lobe. The edge was well defined, reaching half-way to the umbilicus, and its surface was nodular. There was no generalized lymphadenopathy and the spleen was not palpable. The provisional diagnosis was secondary neoplasm, involving the liver.

During his first few days in hospital he showed a sustained fever averaging 100° F. and had a persistently high E.S.R. to 100 mm. in one hour. The blood picture was as follows: Hb 73%, P.C.V. 35%, M.C.H.C. 31%, W.B.C. 7,000/c.mm. (polymorphs 47%, eosinophils 2%, lymphocytes 42%, abnormally large lymphocytes 5% and monocytes 7%).

Liver function was tested by zinc sulphate, thymol turbidity, thymol flocculation and cephalin cholesterol tests, which were all normal. The alkaline phosphatase was 27·5 units (Jenner and Kay) and the serum bilirubin was 0·3 mg./100 ml.

Mantoux testing (10 international units) was negative and *x*-ray examination of the chest, abdomen and long bones showed no abnormality.

At laparotomy the liver was found to be studded throughout with round greyish nodules with a large mass coalescing in the left lobe to cause the enlargement which constituted the presenting physical sign. Careful search of the abdomen did not reveal any primary neoplasm, but the findings were thought to bear out the original diagnosis.

Histology. The report, by Dr. J. Hart-Mercer, was as follows :

'There is no sign of neoplasm. The nodular lesion is essentially a necrotizing chronic granuloma with almost complete obliteration of the local parenchyma. Included in the specimen are surviving areas of liver tissue but these are also being invaded by the granulomatous process which is spreading here mainly by the lymphoreticular tissue of the larger portal tracts. With a picture of necrotic foci rather resembling caseation associated with epithelioid reaction and Langhans giant cells, tubercle has to be considered.'

Serological Tests. As the Mantoux test was again negative a Wassermann reaction was performed and found to be positive. Blood Wassermann tests were repeatedly strongly positive, but examination of the cerebrospinal fluid revealed no evidence of syphilis. The parents were then investigated and the mother was found to have latent spyhilis. She had a strongly positive blood Wassermann reaction but normal cerebrospinal fluid with a negative Wassermann reaction. There was no clinical evidence of syphilis. The father was entirely negative. Detailed review of the child revealed no other sighs of congenital syphilis, and, in particular, re-examination of radiographs of the long bones showed no evidence of osteoperiostitic changes.

Treatment. Treatment was initially with potassium iodide, starting with 1 grain daily and increasing rapidly up to 10 grains three times daily. To this was added bismuth metal suspension ('chlorostab' brand) beginning with 50 mg. weekly and increasing gradually until the patient was receiving 150 mg. per injection, which was given deeply intramuscularly in the upper outer quadrant of alternate buttocks.

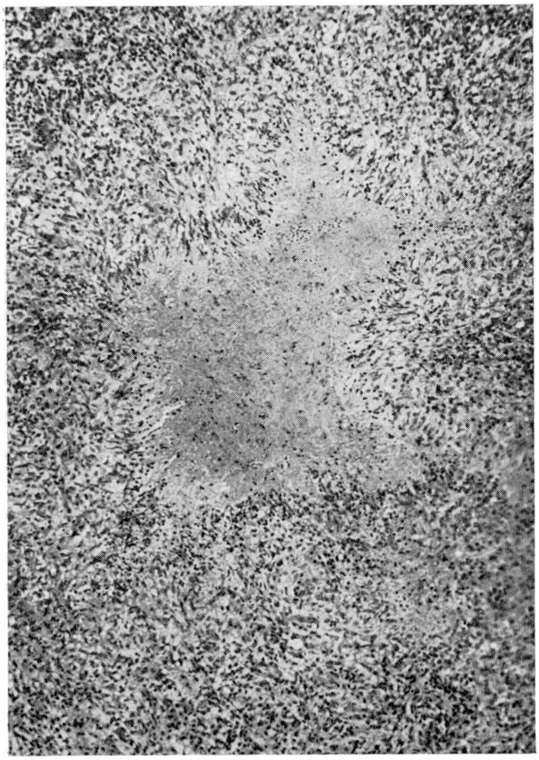

FIG. 1.—A small gummatous nodule in the liver. (× 90)

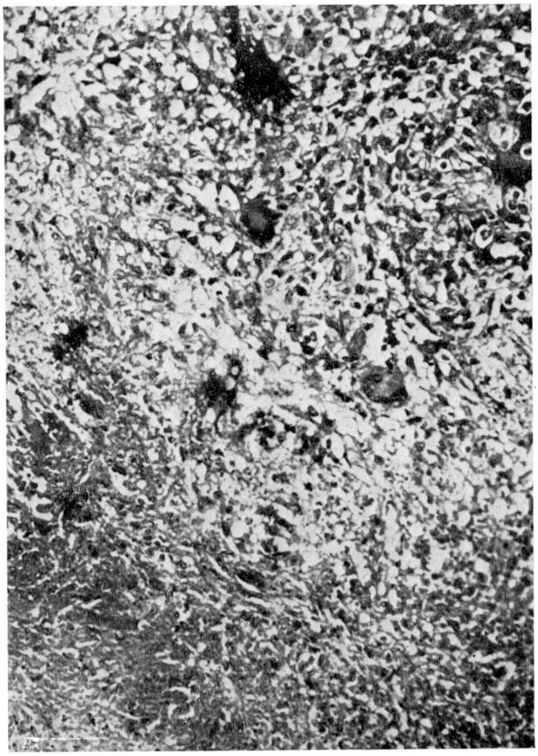

FIG. 2.—High-power view of liver showing multinucleate giant cells. (× 190)

An aqueous crystalline penicillin preparation was started on the tenth day after commencing treatment, beginning with 5,000 units six hourly and increasing to 50,000 units per injection in a further 10 days. After two weeks a delayed absorption product ('prolopen', Messrs. Glaxo Laboratories) was given once daily until a total of 6·3 mega units of penicillin had been administered.

After nearly three months, out-patient treatment was begun, consisting of 0·2 ml. bismuth weekly for 10-week periods alternating with 900,000 units penicillin per week for seven-week periods. A total of six courses of bismuth and 39 mega units of penicillin has been given to date.

Even the short pre-penicillin course produced a dramatic decrease in the size of the liver, and by the time penicillin was begun it had receded to only half an inch below the costal margin.

Liver function tests on discharge from hospital and repeated one year later were normal and the boy has now attained a negative serology for syphilis.

Comment

Nabarro (1954), with his very extensive experience of congenital syphilis, states that hepatic gummata are of great rarity in this variety of the disease. He says that the usual histological picture in the liver consists of a diffuse small cell infiltration occurring *in utero* and in the first months of life, succeeded later in some cases by fibrosis or cirrhosis varying from a microscopic lesion to complete destruction of the liver architecture. He quotes only two cases of gumma of the liver, described by Carpenter (1901) and Hutinel (1926), the former in an infant aged 8 months and the latter in a newborn infant, and says that he personally has not seen one.

McCrae and Caven (1926) reviewed 100 cases of tertiary syphilis of the liver, including five patients diagnosed as having congenital syphilis, aged 3, 13, 16, 18 and 19 years respectively. In the latter the liver was diffusely enlarged but the exact histology was unrecorded. Hahn (1943) examined 66 tertiary syphilic livers at necropsy in adults, and pointed out that in only nine was the true diagnosis made in life. Shapiro and Weiner (1951) described a further 79 necropsies, all in adults, and made the observation that 'the visceral manifestations of late syphilis through their rarity have been neglected'.

Flegel (1951) gave very detailed accounts of the livers in 22 children examined at necropsy at ages ranging from a stillborn infant to one aged $2\frac{1}{2}$ years of age. All had syphilitic changes, but in very few had the liver architecture been replaced by granulation tissue, and in none was there a striking picture of naked-eye gummata, the liver being always enlarged but usually smooth. His account of the histology accords closely with that of Nabarro.

Jeans (1957) states that 'gummata may occur in almost any part of the body but they are rare in the liver, spleen and lungs'. He refers to one case he had seen which probably had gummata of the liver, but without any details.

Only one other reference to gumma of the liver, in an infant, was found in an article by Gerlóczy (1939), but this article could not be obtained. Isolated gummata of the pancreas (Raeburn, 1951), and the stomach (Willeford, Childers and Hepner, 1952) have also been recorded.

A recent report by Macfarlane, Johns and Schofield (1955) has emphasized these points. Their survey covered 200 patients with congenital syphilis of whom 172 (86%) were found to have late syphilis. Of these, 105 had ocular lesions, including interstitial keratitis, optic atrophy choroiditis and iridocyclitis. Twenty-five had evidence of neurosyphilis, including juvenile and general paresis, tabes dorsalis, eighth nerve deafness, epilepsy and mental changes. Bone changes were found in 11 patients and joint changes in 16.

Only two patients had gummata, a girl of 9 years with a gumma of the larynx, and a man aged 28 years with a gumma of the testis, which had been removed as a malignant tumour.

These reports serve to emphasize the rarity of gumma in the viscera, and particularly in the liver, in childhood, and also the difficulty which may arise in diagnosis at any age. The striking features in this child are that such a condition can develop so early and with no other signs of the disease, presenting, as in many adults with tertiary syphilis, signs imitating malignant disease.

Summary

The case is reported of a child aged 6 years presenting with an isolated picture of gummata of the liver.

Allowing for the rarity of gummatous hepatitis in children, the remarkable ability of this disease to masquerade as other conditions serves as a reminder that a serological test for syphilis before operation in similar cases is worthy of consideration.

Bibliography

Carpenter, G. (1901). *The Syphilis of Children in Every-day Practice*, p. 51. London.
Flegel, H. (1951). *Zbl. allg. Path. path. Anat.*, **87**, 302.
Gerlóczy, F. (1939). *Budapesti orvosi ujság.*, **37**, 317.
Hahn, R. D. (1943) *Amer. J. Syph.*, **27**, 529.
Hutinel, V. (1926). *Bull. Soc. Pédiat. Paris*, **24**, 37.
Jeans, P. C. (1957). Brenneman's *Practice of Paediatrics*, Vol. 2, Ch. 26, pp. 9 and 33. Hagerstown, Maryland.
McCrae, T. and Caven, W. R. (1926). *Amer. J. med. Sci.*, **172**, 781.
Macfarlane, W. V., Johns, H. M. and Schofield, C. B. S. (1955). *The Background of Congenital Syphilis.* (Dept. of Venereology, Newcastle upon Tyne General Hospital.)
Nabarro, D. (1954). *Congenital Syphilis.* London.
Raeburn, C. (1951). *J. Path. Bact.*, **63**, 158.
Shapiro, E. and Weiner, H. (1951). *Amer. J. med. Sci.*, **222**, 494.
Willeford, G., Childers, J. H. and Hepner, W. R. (1952). *Pediatrics*, **10**, 162.

PAPER ELECTROPHORESIS OF SERUM PROTEINS IN CHILDREN

BY

W. W. PAYNE and CONSTANCE C. FORSYTH

From The Hospital for Sick Children, Great Ormond Street, London, and the Department of Child Health, University of St. Andrews, Queen's College, Dundee

(RECEIVED FOR PUBLICATION JULY 29, 1957)

Since the description of paper electrophoresis in 1950 by Cremer and Tiselius and by Durrum among others, considerable interest has been shown in this cheap and relatively quick method of separating the various protein fractions. The serum proteins move through the fine cellulose mesh of the paper under the influence of an electric current, the separation of the various fractions being brought about by differences in their electrophoretic mobility at a selected *p*H. The bands are then shown up by staining with a protein dye. Usually five separate fractions are seen: albumin and four globulin fractions, designated α_1, α_2, β and γ (Fig. 1). The albumin fraction is more or less homogeneous, but the various globulin fractions are heterogeneous and can be further subdivided by the use of other physical methods or biological techniques. The protein fractions obtained by paper electrophoresis approximate closely to those obtained by the original Tiselius method of electrophoresis in free solution. It is technically difficult, however, to estimate the various proteins quantitatively by the paper method (Wolstenholme and Millar, 1956).

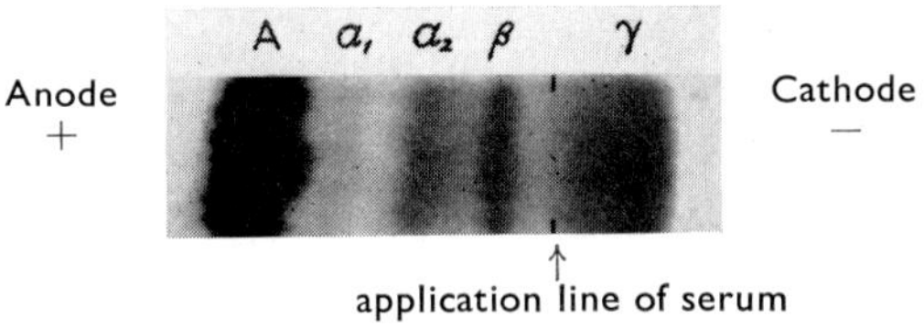

FIG. 1.—Paper electrophoresis slip showing the five serum protein fractions. Protein molecules are negatively charged at *p*H 8·6 and move towards the anode.

As we wished to study protein changes in large numbers of children we decided not to attempt elution or scanning of the strips and to accept a visual comparison with normal controls as adequate for our purpose. The technique described by Flynn and de Mayo (1951) was used with a few minor modifications. A slightly larger quantity of serum —namely, 0·02 ml.—than those authors used was applied to the paper from an accurately calibrated siliconed pipette, and we chose azocarmine B as the protein dye. When collecting blood samples by finger-prick care was taken to avoid haemolysing the specimen, because if free haemoglobin was present it appeared as a dense band in the $\alpha_2\beta$ region

The aim of the investigation was to study the value of the method in paediatric hospital practice. Several reports on electrophoretic pattern changes in adults have been published, including those of Flynn (1954) and Penman (1956), but only one dealing specifically with sick children has come to our notice, that of Corbeel (1954), and his results were not very detailed.

Normal Patterns

To establish the normal pattern from birth to 12 years of age 130 paper strips were prepared from children without physical disease who attended the out-patient department. Average strips and those representing the extreme limits of normal for each year of age were mounted on cards and used as controls in the study of diseases. Bands which were outside the range of normal for the relevant age were interpreted as showing an increased or decreased intensity. The variations with age proved to be more or less identical with those described by Knapp and Routh (1949) using the classical Tiselius method. The most striking change is in the γ globulin, which at birth is at the adult level, but falls rapidly in the next three or four months until it almost disappears, only a faint stain being visible on the strip. Thereafter it gradually increases, but is still low at 1 year. By 2 years it has increased considerably, and between 6 and 10 years the adult level is again reached. The α_2 globulin band is well marked in the infant and gradually decreases to the adult level by about 12 years of age

The albumin and α_1 and β globulin bands do not alter significantly with age (Fig. 2).

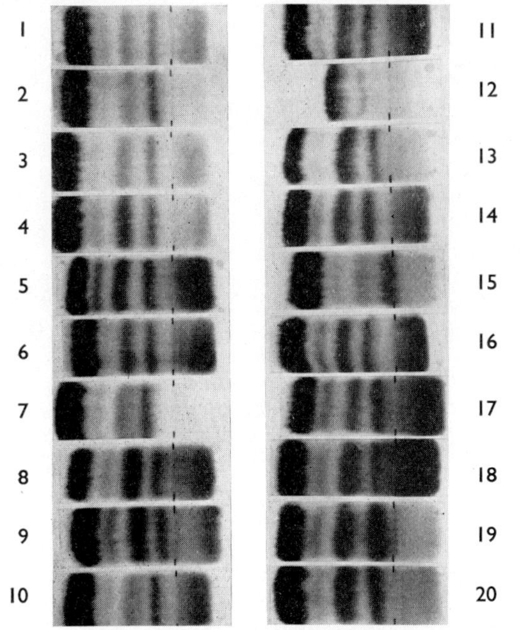

FIG. 2.—Normal serum protein electrophoretic patterns (Nos. 1-3) and those of various diseases (Nos. 4-20). Details are given in the table below.

abnormal. Early in the course of the disease the α_1 and α_2 globulin bands were increased, and later on the γ globulin became increased unless the infection had been very rapidly overcome. Out of 23 examples of acute infection, such as streptococcal tonsillitis, lobar pneumonia or bronchopneumonia, gastro-enteritis and staphylococcal osteomyelitis, there were only two normal strips; 11 showed α_1 and α_2 globulin increases, and 10 a γ globulin increase as well. This type of response was seen also in eight out of nine infants under 1 year with acute infections. The γ globulin, normally low in this period, was capable of increasing in response to infection. Once the infection was overcome the protein patterns reverted to normal.

In subacute infections it was usual to find an increase in α_2 and γ globulins—for example, in active bronchiectasis or in fibrocystic disease of the pancreas or ulcerative colitis. Of 22 cases of fibrocystic disease, nine showed α_2 and γ globulin increases and seven showed γ globulin increases only; five were normal and one had a low γ globulin. Of eight cases of ulcerative colitis, five showed α_2 and γ globulin increases and three showed γ globulin increases only. Two early cases showed α_1 and α_2 globulin increases only. In three cases of Caffey's disease (infantile cortical hyperostosis) α_2 and and γ globulin increases occurred which after several months returned to normal. This suggests that there is an inflammatory basis to Caffey's disease.

KEY TO SERUM PAPER ELECTROPHORETIC PATTERNS IN FIG. 2

Number	Sex	Age	Disease	Pattern Changes				
				A	α_1	α_2	β	γ
1	M	1 day	Normal					
2	M	4 mos.	Normal					
3	F	20 mos.	Normal					
4	M	7 yrs.	Acute tonsillitis		+	+		
5	F	5 yrs.	Fibrocystic disease		+	+		+
6	F	3 yrs.	Chronic pulmonary tuberculosis					+
7	M	2 yrs.	Agammaglobulinaemia					−
8	F	10 yrs.	Acute rheumatic fever		+	+		+
9	M	2 yrs.	Still's disease		+	+		+
10	M	12 yrs.	Rheumatoid arthritis					+
11	M	4 yrs.	Acute nephritis			+		+
12	M	4 yrs.	Nephrotic syndrome	−		+	+	−
13	M	4 yrs.	Nephrotic syndrome during treatment			+		−
14	M	7 yrs.	Infective hepatitis			+		+
15	M	2 mos.	Neonatal hepatitis			−		
16	F	10 mos.	Congenital obliteration of bile ducts		+			+
17	M	10 yrs.	Cirrhosis					+
18	F	8 yrs.	Haemosiderosis					γ_1+ γ_2+
19	F	16 mos.	Liver disease with hypercholesterolaemia			+	+	
20	F	8 mos.	Idiopathic hypercalcaemia of infants			+	+	

Abnormal Patterns

Infections. No change in electrophoretic pattern was detected in mild infections such as colds, bronchitis or low-grade urinary infections. However, where fever, leucocytosis and constitutional disturbance were present the proteins were usually

In chronic infections the γ globulin only was raised, for example, in six cases of chronic tuberculosis.

The serum of seven out of 14 children with a history of constantly recurring infections showed

TABLE 1

COMPARISON OF SERUM PROTEIN ELECTROPHORESIS FINDINGS IN RHEUMATIC FEVER, STILL'S DISEASE, RHEUMATOID ARTHRITIS AND ACUTE NEPHRITIS

Condition	Total Number of Cases	α_1, α_2 and γ Globulin Raised	α_2 and γ Globulin Raised	γ Globulin Raised	Normal Pattern
Rheumatic fever	20	5	4	7	4
Still's disease	8	6	1	1	0
Rheumatoid arthritis	7	0	2	2	2
Average E.S.R. (mm./1 hr.)	—	51	44	35	13
Range of E.S.R. (mm./1 hr.)	—	11–80	12–112	6–95	6–24
Acute nephritis*	32	0	12	3	12

* In three cases γ globulin was low; in two α_2 globulin only was raised.

normal protein patterns, while in three cases there were α_2 and γ globulin increases of the order already noted in acute and chronic infections. Two showed a low γ globulin, a condition one might term 'hypogammaglobulinaemia'; in the remaining two no γ globulin at all was visible on the strip. In these cases the diagnosis of 'agammaglobulinaemia' was confirmed by the classical Tiselius technique, as the γ globulin concentration was less than 0·1 g. per 100 ml. It is of considerable interest that in a third case of agammaglobulinaemia there was no history of recurrent infections and the child was examined by us because he had rheumatoid arthritis (a condition which we were studying at the time) with typical bilateral involvement of knees and ankles. The association of rheumatoid arthritis with agammaglobulinaemia is unexpected in view of the hypogenesis of reticulo-endothelial tissue associated with the latter condition.

Very high γ globulin levels were found in three children with severe chronic staphylococcal infections, two with empyema and one with enteritis. Janeway, Craig, Davidson, Downey, Gitlin and Sullivan (1954) described this condition in a group of infants, calling it 'hypergammaglobulinaemia' as the γ globulin level was higher than that seen in the usual chronic infection. The titre of antibodies was high in their cases, so that the failure to overcome the infection speedily lay elsewhere than in the immunity mechanism.

Rheumatic Fever, Still's Disease and Rheumatoid Arthritis. The rheumatic diseases were selected for study because a rise in total globulin commonly occurs in these conditions, but it soon became apparent that the globulin patterns were in no sense diagnostic and resembled closely those seen in subacute and chronic infections. When tests were made within a day or two of the onset of rheumatic symptoms the γ globulin level was always raised, a finding which was helpful on one occasion in differentiating acute osteomyelitis from rheumatic fever, as the γ globulin level is not raised in the early stages of acute osteomyelitis. Twenty children with rheumatic fever were studied, eight with Still's disease (joint swellings, adenopathy and splenomegaly, with or without rash or pericarditis) and seven with rheumatoid arthritis (arthritis being the only clinical manifestation of disease). The results obtained when the children were first seen are shown in Table 1. A rise of α_1, α_2 and γ globulins occurred in the most acute cases of rheumatic fever, three of which had pericarditis, and in children with the widespread tissue involvement of Still's disease. Changes in α_2 and γ globulins, or γ globulin increases alone, were found in the less acute cases of rheumatoid arthritis and in the later stages of rheumatic fever and Still's disease. With clinical improvement the α_2 globulin fell to normal before the γ globulin. Children showing normal patterns were, without exception, very mildly affected or had passed the acute phase of illness before coming to hospital.

As with simple infections, the more acute cases tended to have higher erythrocyte sedimentation rates (E.S.R.). Great variation, however, occurred and, although the average E.S.R., as seen in the table, worked out in descending order as the cases decreased in acuteness, the range of E.S.R. was almost the same in each group with abnormal globulins. In assessing the stage and severity of rheumatic fever, Still's disease and rheumatoid arthritis, therefore, it may be an advantage to take the electrophoretic findings as well as the E.S.R. into consideration. This may be particularly useful in cases with cardiac failure.

When followed throughout the course of these disorders the E.S.R. and electrophoretic pattern did not run parallel (Table 2). The tests were performed weekly on the same blood sample. Out of nine cases of rheumatic fever thus followed, four showed abnormal electrophoretic patterns for weeks or even months after the return of the E.S.R. to 10 mm. in one hour or less. In two cases, on the other hand,

TABLE 2

RELATION BETWEEN RETURN TO NORMAL OF SERUM PROTEIN ELECTROPHORESIS PATTERN (S.P.E.) AND E.S.R.

Conditions	Total Number of Cases	S.P.E. and E.S.R. Normal Together	S.P.E. Normal before E.S.R.	E.S.R. Normal before S.P.E.
Rheumatic fever ..	9	3	2	4
Still's disease and rheumatoid arthritis	6	5	1	0
Acute nephritis ..	10	4	6	0

the electrophoretic pattern became normal before the E.S.R., and in three the tests corresponded exactly. So few cases of rheumatoid arthritis had returned to normal at the time of assessment that the numbers are too small to be of much value.

To summarize, the changes in serum protein electrophoretic pattern which may be found in rheumatic fever, Still's disease and rheumatoid arthritis are of no help diagnostically and closely resemble those seen in simple infections. Electrophoresis may, however, be a useful adjunct to determination of the E.S.R. in assessing the stage and severity of the disorder and in deciding how long to continue treatment, whether by cortisone, salicylates or bed rest.

Acute Nephritis. In view of the aetiological similarity between acute nephritis and the rheumatic conditions, it was of interest to find how closely the patterns resembled each other in the two groups. The study covered 32 children with acute nephritis (see Table 1). None showed the α_1, α_2 and γ globulin increases seen in the most acute rheumatic conditions; 12 showed an α_2 and γ globulin rise, two an α_2 globulin rise only, while in three there was a slight increase and in three a slight decrease in γ globulin. Twelve showed a normal pattern, but nine of these children had passed the most acute phase when first seen. Consecutive studies (Table 2) showed that in four out of 10 cases the E.S.R. and serum protein electrophoretic pattern returned to normal together, while in six cases the electrophoretic pattern returned to normal first. Usually, but not invariably, the albumin disappeared from the urine before the results of blood tests became normal.

Of five cases of chronic nephritis of long standing with uraemia, four showed a slight reduction of γ globulin.

Nephrotic Syndrome. Changes in serum proteins in the nephrotic syndrome are dramatic and well recognized, the fall in γ globulin being in contrast to the rise seen in the acute stage of nephritis. The electrophoretic pattern is diagnostic with a low albumin, an $\alpha_2\beta$ complex, the two bands having been replaced by one broad deeply staining band, and a low γ globulin; the latter disappears in the most severe cases to give an acquired agammaglobulinaemia. In milder cases a pattern which might be termed 'partially nephrotic' occurs: the albumin is slightly reduced, the α_2 band is broader and more densely stained than normal, and the γ globulin is reduced. This partial pattern, which we first recognized in nephrotic patients improving under hormone therapy, was of value in assessing the cause of symptomless albuminuria in three cases. These children gave no history of oedema and had no urinary infection, their albuminuria being discovered on routine testing. In two the serum cholesterol was raised. None showed a reversal of albumin:globulin ratio, as the rise in α_2 globulin was offset by the fall in γ globulin. In each case the blood urea and an intravenous pyelogram were normal. One progressed to classical nephrosis, but in the other two the electrophoretic patterns returned to normal with disappearance of the albuminuria without treatment, and these children might be considered to have suffered *formes frustes* of the nephrotic syndrome. When stains for lipid or cholesterol are used, increased amounts of both fat and cholesterol are seen in the $\alpha_2\beta$ region.

In 25 cases of nephrosis a serial study of the pattern changes during hormone therapy was made. At the time of the disappearance of albuminuria the pattern began to alter. The $\alpha_2\beta$ complex separated into α_2 and β bands; later on the albumin re-formed, and finally after several weeks the γ globulin returned to normal. The serum cholesterol level fell to normal at about the same time as the γ globulin regenerated. The final return of the γ globulin to normal was used in determining the duration of full hormone therapy; the periods of treatment required to achieve it varied from case to case and did not always correspond with the apparent initial severity. With other forms of treatment, such as with resins, urea or mercurial diuretics, resulting in loss of oedema, but not to disappearance of albuminuria, no improvement in the nephrotic pattern was seen. When relapse occurred the first abnormality noted was the reappearance of albuminuria, and only after a week or so did the serum protein picture alter. This is consistent with present concepts of serum protein synthesis and storage.

Liver Disease. Alteration in serum proteins is the basis of the turbidity tests—for example, the thymol turbidity, Takata-Ara and Kunkel tests, the last being largely dependent on an increase in

TABLE 3

SERUM PROTEIN ELECTROPHORESIS CHANGES IN CERTAIN LIVER DISEASES

Disease	Total Number of Cases	α_1 Globulin		α_2 Globulin		β Globulin		γ Globulin		Normal Pattern
		−	+	−	+	−	+	−	+	
Infective hepatitis	21	0	0	2	3	1	1	0	3	14
Neonatal hepatitis	7	0	0	2	0	2	0	0	0	4
Congenital obliteration of bile ducts	8	0	4	0	0	0	0	0	3	3
Cirrhosis	15	0	0	5	0	0	0	0	11	2

γ globulin. In infancy these tests are notoriously unreliable, and this may be because of the difference in globulin pattern normally seen at this age, particularly the low γ globulin. By comparing the electrophoretic patterns of jaundiced babies with those of normal infants it was hoped that more valuable information might be obtained than from the turbidity tests alone. However, the results, although useful in some cases, were by no means uniform.

Of 21 cases of infective hepatitis in childhood (Table 3), 14 showed normal strips, three a rise in α_2 and β globulins, two a reduction in α_2 globulin, one a raised β globulin and one a lowered β globulin. From seven cases of neonatal hepatitis, four strips were normal, one showed a low $\alpha_2\beta$, one a low α_2 and one a low β globulin. Of eight cases of congenital obliteration of the bile ducts, proved at operation or necropsy, three showed normal strips, three an increase in α_1 and γ globulins, and one an increase in α_1 globulin only; the other showed variable changes in α_2 and β globulins. In 15 cases of cirrhosis only two strips were normal, and 11 showed a rise in γ globulin. Of these, two cases of haemosiderosis showed a dense band filling in the space between the β and γ globulins, an increase in the so-called γ_1 globulin. In four cases the α_2 globulin was low in association with a raised γ globulin, and in one the α_2 globulin was low with a normal γ globulin. Of 16 cases diagnosed incompletely as 'hepatosplenomegaly', 12 were normal. In three the α_2 globulin was low and the γ globulin raised, a pattern seen in cirrhosis of the liver. In one interesting case of galactosaemia in an infant the depression of α_2 and β globulins seen on the strip reverted to normal a week after the introduction of a lactose-free diet. In two cases of hepatic coma the α_2 and β globulins were low and the γ globulin high. Two rather unusual cases with jaundice and hypercholesterolaemia in which no liver biopsy was performed showed marked α_2 and β globulin increases.

In reviewing the changes in liver disease certain general patterns were apparent. The α_1 globulin was increased only in congenital obliteration of the bile ducts, and the α_2 globulin only in infective hepatitis. A decrease in α_2 globulin was a fairly common finding and was seen in other cases of infective hepatitis, in neonatal hepatitis and in cirrhosis. Changes in β globulin were rare and variable. A rise in γ globulin was almost the rule in cirrhosis, and occurred occasionally in infective hepatitis and in congenital obliteration of the bile ducts.

Idiopathic Hypercalcaemia of Infants. A study was made of 18 infants with idiopathic hypercalcaemia, but 10 of them had already passed the acute phase. In eight the serum calcium level was still raised, and in four of these there was a very definite increase in α_2 and β globulins, similar to the pattern seen in the two cases of liver disease with hypercholesterolaemia mentioned above. Two strips were also stained for fat and showed a rise in β lipoprotein concentration. One infant showed a rise in α_2 and γ globulins, and one a rise of γ globulin only. The other two infants with an increased blood calcium had a normal pattern. Two of the 10 infants with a normal serum calcium level by the time of examination showed abnormalities in the α_2 and β band persisting beyond the hypercalcaemic phase—a finding of some interest.

Miscellaneous Conditions. Strips were prepared from nearly 200 children in hospital, but no changes of diagnostic value were found. Conditions investigated included, among many others, the following: malignant tumours, leukaemia, Hodgkin's disease, haemolytic anaemia, histiocytosis, Gaucher's disease, thyrotoxicosis, cretinism, coeliac disease and pink disease.

Discussion

Five serum protein bands have been studied by paper electrophoresis. The albumin band is homogeneous or nearly so, but the other bands are mixtures of several proteins (Table 4). It will be seen that many specific proteins have been isolated from these fractions, although the α_2 globulin band is still largely unidentified. Some proteins are

TABLE 4

PROTEIN COMPONENTS OF PLASMA (ADAPTED FROM HUGHES, 1954)

Electrophoretic Band	Known Components	Concentration in Plasma (g./100 ml.)
Albumin	Crystalline albumins	4·30
α_1 Globulin ..		0·30
	α_1 Mucoprotein	0·05
	α_1 Lipoprotein	0·20
α_2 Globulin ..		0·70
	Ceruloplasmin	0·03
	α_2 Lipoprotein	0·02
	Complement	—
β Globulin		1·10
	Transferrin	0·25
	β Lipoprotein	0·40
γ_1 Globulin		0·50
	Fibrinogen	0·30
	Antihaemophilic globulin	—
	Isohaemagglutinins	—
γ Globulin or γ_2 Globulin		0·90
	Diphtheria antitoxin	0·001
Total plasma protein	.. .. ..	7·80

present in such low concentration that they are not likely to contribute much to the fairly gross quantitative levels required for visual appreciation; for example, it would appear that the increase in γ globulin found in chronic infections is greater than could be accounted for by a rise in specific antibodies, as they form such an infinitesimal part of the γ globulin total. The function of the apparently inert proteins in the various fractions is unknown, and their presence may be masking changes of specific active proteins occurring in disease. With the further identification of serum proteins diagnostic changes may be discovered which are not revealed by the present rather crude methods. To date only nephrosis, agammaglobulinaemia and multiple myeloma have pathognomonic patterns. The changes in infections, rheumatic conditions and liver disease may occasionally be of help in diagnosis, but, on the whole, their chief value lies in following the return to normal during the course of treatment.

The disorders which may be associated with an increase or decrease in the various globulin bands are shown in Table 5. Consideration of these may help to clarify the interpretation of the protein changes found in disease in childhood.

TABLE 5

DISEASES WHICH MAY BE ASSOCIATED WITH GLOBULIN CHANGES

Globulin	Decreased	Increased
α_1	None	Acute infections Rheumatic fever Still's disease Congenital obliteration of bile ducts
α_2	Infective hepatitis Neonatal hepatitis Cirrhosis Galactosaemia	Acute infections Subacute infections Rheumatic fever Still's disease Rheumatoid arthritis Acute nephritis Nephrotic syndrome Infective hepatitis Liver disease with hypercholesterolaemia Idiopathic hypercalcaemia of infants
β	Infective hepatitis Neonatal hepatitis Galactosaemia Hepatic coma	Nephrotic syndrome Infective hepatitis Liver disease with hypercholesterolaemia Idiopathic hypercalcaemia of infants
γ	Hypogammaglobulinaemia Agammaglobulinaemia Chronic nephritis with uraemia Nephrotic syndrome	Subacute infections Chronic infections Rheumatic fever Still's disease Rheumatoid arthritis Acute nephritis Infective hepatitis Congenital obliteration of bile ducts Cirrhosis Hepatic coma

Summary

The normal serum protein patterns obtained by paper electrophoresis in childhood have been described. Assessment of abnormal paper strips by visual comparison with the range of normal for the age was considered adequate for clinical purposes.

Changes occurring in a variety of conditions, including simple infections, rheumatic affections, acute nephritis, nephrosis, liver disease, and idiopathic hypercalcaemia, have been discussed.

The method of paper electrophoresis has only limited diagnostic value, but it may provide a useful additional guide to progress in the rheumatic conditions, nephrosis and diseases of the liver in particular.

We wish to thank the physicians at The Hospital for Sick Children, Great Ormond Street, and Professor J. L. Henderson, Dundee, for access to their cases. The work was begun with the aid of a grant from the Research Fund at Great Ormond Street. We are grateful to Mr. R. Fawkes, A.I.M.L.T., Dundee, for the photographs.

REFERENCES

Cremer, H. D. and Tiselius, A. (1950). *Biochem. Z.*, **320**, 273.
Corbeel, L. (1954). *Acta paediat. belg.*, **8**, 101.
Durrum, E. L. (1950). *J. Amer. chem. Soc.*, **72**, 2943.
Flynn, F. V. (1954). *Proc. roy. Soc. Med.*, **47**, 827.
—— and de Mayo, P. (1951). *Lancet*, **2**, 235.
Hughes, W. L. (1954). In *The Proteins*, ed. Neurath, H. and Bailey, K., Vol. 2, Part B, p. 740. New York.
Janeway, C. A., Craig, J., Davidson, M., Downey, W., Gitlin, D. and Sullivan, J. C. (1954). *Amer. J. Dis. Child.*, **88**, 388.
Knapp, E. L. and Routh, J. I. (1949). *Pediatrics*, **4**, 508.
Penman, H. G. (1956). *Practitioner*, **177**, 295.
Wolstenholme, G. E. W. and Millar, E. C. P. (1956). Ciba Foundation Symposium on Paper Electrophoresis, London.

A CLINICAL AND HAEMODYNAMIC STUDY OF VENTRICULAR SEPTAL DEFECT IN INFANTS

BY

GEORGE M. MAXWELL, GEORGE G. ROWE and CHARLES W. CRUMPTON

From the Department of Pediatrics and the Cardiovascular Laboratory, University of Wisconsin, Madison 6, Wisconsin, U.S.A.

(RECEIVED FOR PUBLICATION JULY 5, 1957)

The concept of ventricular septal defect as a disease of little severity (Roger, 1879; Brown, 1950), has been upset by the observations of Marquis (1950) and Engle (1954). The median age at death in Abbott's (1951) cases was 14½ years; however, in common with others, we have observed severe disability and death in many younger children.

The advent of surgical therapy for this defect (Lillehei, Cohen, Warden, Ziegler and Varco, 1955), and the desirability of correction at an early age make it worth while to review the clinical features in the earliest age group. The haemodynamic findings will be given in some detail.

Material and Methods

Sixteen cases of ventricular septal defect occurring in infants aged 1 year or less were studied in 1955. Table 1 shows the age at onset of symptoms and examination. Special studies were undertaken because of significant disease, and a large percentage thus observed was less than 6 months of age. Cardiac catheterization was done in the usual fashion using the Waters-Conley cuvette oximeter for oxygen saturation assessment. Its accuracy was checked by two or more Van Slyke specimens. Expired air was collected in a Tissot spirometer and analysed for oxygen and carbon dioxide content by the Scholander method. Calculations of shunts and resistances were by the usual formulae.

The catheter was normally placed in the femoral vein after the infant had received light basal (barbiturate) anaesthesia. Procaine (1%) was used as a local supplement. Two patients who had suffered congestive failure received oxygen throughout the catheterization, as it was felt that arrhythmias were less frequent in this circumstance. Difficulty was found in recording adequate pulmonary capillary pressures. We have found this also in adults with a large left-to-right shunt where more advantageous circumstances exist. The femoral vein was routinely ligated. No death or complication attributable to catheterization occurred.

Clinical Features

The Symptoms. These (Table 2) are surprisingly constant, and compare well with those found in other severe left-to-right shunts. They consist principally in failure of growth, refusal to feed. frequent respiratory infections and a 'murmur',

TABLE 2

CLINICAL HISTORY IN 16 CASES

	Number	Percentage
Presenting Complaints		
Cough and respiratory infections ..	10	62
Failure of growth	9	56
Dyspnoea	3	19
'Murmur'	3	19
Easy fatiguability	2	12·5
Cyanosis	1	6
Rapid heart	1	6
All Complaints		
Cough and respiratory infections ..	13	81
'Murmur'	13	81
Feeding difficulties	9	56
Failure of growth	9	56
Excessive sweating	7	44
Dyspnoea	5	31
'Rapid heart'	2	12·5
Easy fatiguability....	2	12·5
Cyanosis	2	12·5
Slow motor progress	1	6
Pallor	1	6
Hoarseness	1	6

TABLE 1

DISTRIBUTION OF PATIENTS ACCORDING TO ONSET OF SYMPTOMS AND AGE AT CATHETERIZATION

	Birth to 1 Month	2–3 Months	4–5 Months	5–7 Months	8–9 Months	10–12 Months
Age at onset of symptoms	4	5	4	–	3	–
Age seen and catheterized	2*	1	2	2	4	4

* Not catheterized until 2 months of age.

This latter was only rarely noted by the parents themselves. The early onset (Table 1) is noteworthy in some of the cases. Cyanosis—a rare feature in most adult series—occurred in some children. Excessive sweating in the absence of overt infections was not unusual. This has, however, been observed by us in other types of congenital heart disease. Lassitude—so commonly noted by the paediatrician —was seldom remarked upon by the parents. In a few cases the thrill was obvious to the family. Epistaxes, though common in older children with this defect, were absent in the patients studied.

The Signs. The most remarkable sign (Table 3) is growth failure; it occurs in most infants whose parents seek medical advice. Table 4 expresses this phenomenon in terms of growth percentile. It is seen that weight deficit is greater than height deficit though this latter is considerable. Head and chest size also tend to fall in the lower percentiles.

TABLE 3

PRINCIPAL SIGNS

	Number	Percentage
Systolic murmur	16	100
Systolic thrill	13	81
Chest deformity	13	81
Cardiomegaly (clinical)	13	81
Right ventricular apex type	11	69
Anaemia (excluding physiological) ..	7	44
Dyspnoea (exertional)	7	44
Associated defects (3 herniae, 2 telangiectases)	5	31
Dyspnoea (at rest)	4	25
Triple rhythm	4	25
Congestive failure	3	19
Cyanosis {At rest	2	12·5
Cyanosis {Exertional		
Split pulmonic second sound	2	12·5
Pulmonary thrust	1	6
Recurrent laryngeal palsy	1	6

Further inspection often reveals Harrison's grooves (Fig. 1); these seem to be associated with dyspnoea or frequent respiratory infections. Breathlessness at rest is variable; this symptom occurs more often on exercise—usually crying and defaecation. Two cases showed cyanosis. Minor associated defects were found in five infants. The severe nature of the lesion is illustrated by the onset of congestive cardiac failure in three children. In two this responded adequately to therapy. Cough was by far the commonest sign in some of the infants; usually unassociated with cardiac failure, it may be subsequent to a change in the pulmonary blood flow.

Cardiovascular examination gave a constant picture. Enlargement of the heart was usual, as this was one of the criteria for further study. The apical impulse was frequently of the right ventricular type. A gallop rhythm was occasionally palpated inside the displaced apex. A systolic thrill was felt over the lower left interspaces. It was coarse and widespread, corresponding well to Roger's original description. The thrill, however, may not appear for several months after birth. We have had the opportunity to observe two patients from birth, in whom no thrill could be felt until 3 and 4 months of age respectively. Similar findings have been observed in some cases of Fallot's tetralogy (Maxwell, 1954).

The character of the second sound at the pulmonary area is of some interest. It has been observed by Leatham (1952) that a widely split second sound is common in left-to-right shunts, usually in association with electrocardiographic evidence of right bundle branch block. Wood (1950) noted this sign in older patients with ventricular septal defect. This elegant clue was seldom found in the infant group studied here. Generally auscultation reveals a single sound, as in normal infants. Again, pathological intensity of this sound has not been observed, an expected finding in view of the wide range in normals of this age.

Apical diastolic murmurs were not heard in this group, which contrasts with Wood's (1950) findings for older patients with the same defect.

Anaemia is not uncommon. An attempt was made to exclude the 'physiological' anaemia of infancy in assessing the figures, and there is some

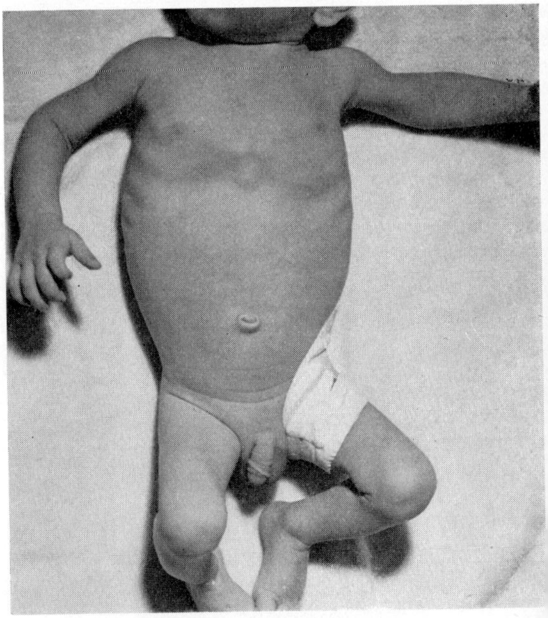

FIG. 1.—Note the Harrison's grooves.

evidence that a true iron-deficiency state exists. Certainly difficulty is found in introducing a mixed, iron-containing diet to these infants, and a staple diet of cow's milk is usually deficient in this element. The frequent infections introduce another need for iron (Wintrobe, 1951) and aggravate the condition.

These infants are lethargic and inactive. Muscular hypotonia is not unusual and this combination results in failure to pass the milestones of motor development at the proper time. Thus the ages of rolling over, sitting up and crawling may be delayed. Observation of other older cases suggests that those who live may catch up in the second and third years.

The single case of laryngeal palsy is not very unusual, though it is perhaps more common in cases of atrial septal defect.

Discussion of Clinical Features

The history is that of any severe left-to-right shunt, resembling most closely that of a 'malignant' patent ductus. Like the latter, the symptoms may exist from the perinatal period and are characterized by feeding problems, failure of growth, respiratory infections and a murmur. This latter corresponds with the description given for older children and adults. The thrill, however, may not appear until some months have elapsed. The murmur and thrill may be confused with that of aortic or subaortic stenosis; we have encountered four such cases in the period of this study. In these the murmur and thrill were not distinguishable from those of ventricular septal defect. However, good growth and lack of cardiomegaly and pulmonary plethora were useful differential points. They are more difficult to tell from cases of ventricular septal defects without pulmonary hypertension. A similar difficulty was reported by Taussig (1955). Brachial arterial tracing may be a useful distinguishing point.

Radiology

As a result of selection, enlargement of the heart was usual. Biventricular increase was common, and differentiation of the major chamber enlargement was difficult in these circumstances. The pulmonary arc was prominent, and the lung fields engorged: relative peripheral hypovascularity was seen in several patients, reflecting perhaps the situation reported by Hultgren, Selzer, Purdy, Holman and Gerbode (1953), in cases of patent ductus with pulmonary hypertension. The linear markings of Kerley (1951) were not seen. This was not unexpected, as this sign is related to the level of the pulmonary capillary pressure and not to the pulmonary arterial tension (Bruwer, Ellis, and Kirklin, 1955).

A corollary to increased pulmonary blood-flow is increased left atrial size. This has been said (Keats and Steinbach, 1955) to be characteristic of patent ductus. However, the left atrium may be prominent in any condition with pulmonary plethora and intact atrial septum. Brostoff and Rodbard (1956) have demonstrated the hydrodynamic cause in simulated ventricular septal defect.

Common radiological findings are illustrated in Figs. 2, 3, 4 and 5.

It will be seen that the findings in severe ventricular septal defect are very similar to those reported in 'malignant' patent ductus by Adams, LaBree and Stauffer (1950); it is probable that many cases are radiologically indistinguishable by ordinary techniques. While hypervascularity and right ventricular enlargement will occur in some cases of atrial septal defect, we have not noted left atrial enlargement in this condition. This is perhaps a useful differential point.

Routine angiocardiography has been of little value in delineating this lesion, and has only occasionally been employed by us. The size of the right ventricle and pulmonary arteries may sometimes be shown by this method, and the left ventricular dimension assessed by difference.

Electrocardiography

Most cases showed a right bundle branch block, often of the complicated type associated with increase in the right ventricular work (Wasserburger, 1956). Some cases may also show evidence of delay in activation time over the left ventricle in addition to the previous finding.

However, the electrocardiogram of ventricular septal defect is by no means unique; similar patterns may be found in patent ductus, again with signs of right and left ventricular overloading. The haemodynamic coincidence of these two lesions render this a reasonable finding. A common E.C.G. pattern is seen in Fig. 6.

Cardiac Catheterization

A. Diagnosis. The primary reason for the studies was confirmation and quantitation of the clinical diagnosis, and this was readily done in most cases. The increase in oxygen content from atrium to ventricle averaged 2·5 vol. in those studied while breathing room air. One case (No. 3 in Table 4) required 100% oxygen before the level of shunt was apparent. This was because of the extraordinayr degree of unsaturation present. Table 5 illustrates this point comparatively. In no case did we require to give adrenalin to show the level of shunt as has been suggested by Condorelli (Turchetti, 1954).

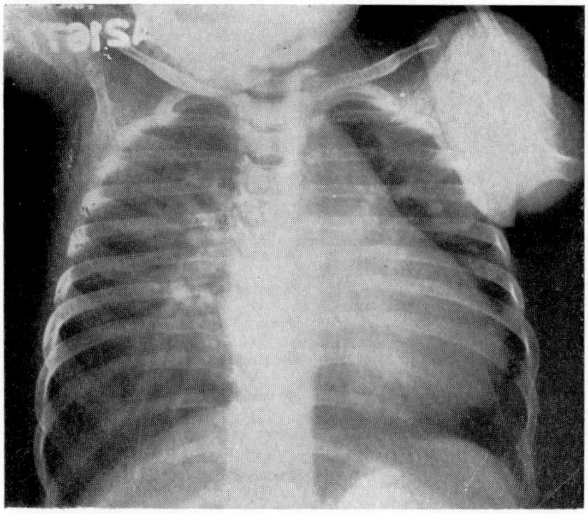

FIG. 2.—In this postero-anterior view there is cardiac enlargement, pulmonary plethora and prominence of the pulmonary arc.

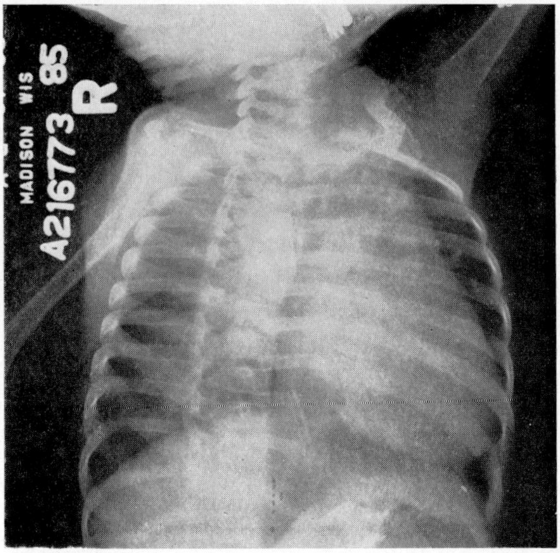

FIG. 3.—This R.A.O. view shows the right ventricular enlargement.

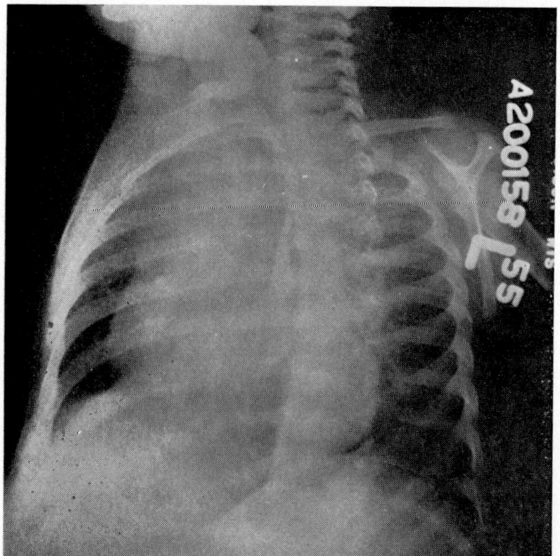

FIG. 4.—Note the enlarged left ventricle in this L.A.O. view.

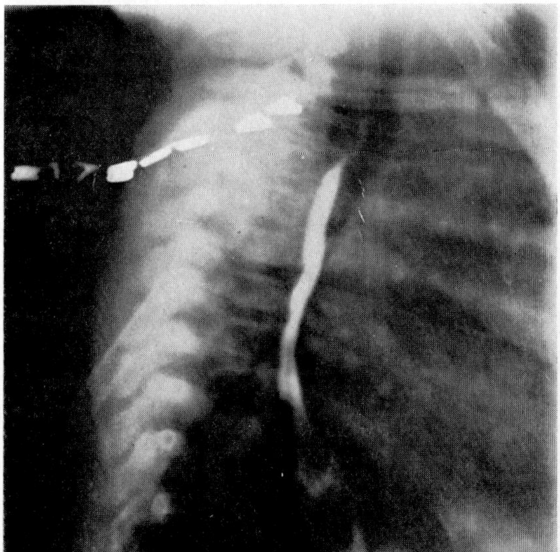

FIG. 5.—The left atrium has displaced the oesophagus in this right oblique view.

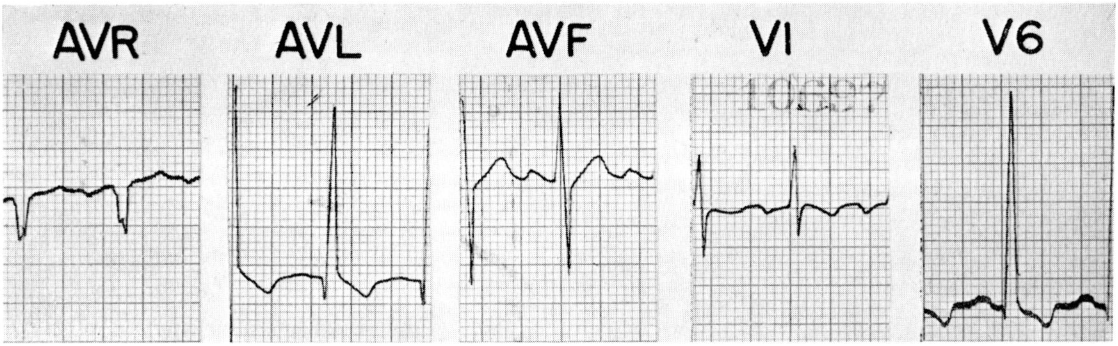

FIG. 6.—The E.C.G. of a case of ventricular septal defect aged 7 months. There is a delay in ventricular activation time over the left ventricle, *i.e.*, V.A.T. = 0·035-0·040 sec.

In some cases the left atrium was entered by way of a foramen ovale; that this was not a functioning defect was suggested by the lack of arterialization of the right atrium, and full saturation of the left atrium as compared with the pulmonary veins. The left ventricle was occasionally explored by this route also. In this age group, the technical problem of moving the catheter within the pulmonary circuit makes the exclusion of a patent ductus difficult*

* In one case since operated upon, a functioning patent ductus was found.

TABLE 5

SATURATION LEVELS IN CASE 3 BREATHING AIR AND OXYGEN

Site	O_2 Saturation %	
	Air	100% Oxygen
Superior vena cava	22	72
Mid right atrium	23	77
Low right ventricle	23	90
Main pulmonary artery	23	97
Left pulmonary artery	24	96
Femoral artery	52	97

TABLE 4

VENTRICULAR SEPTAL DEFECT

Nutrition in 16 Cases

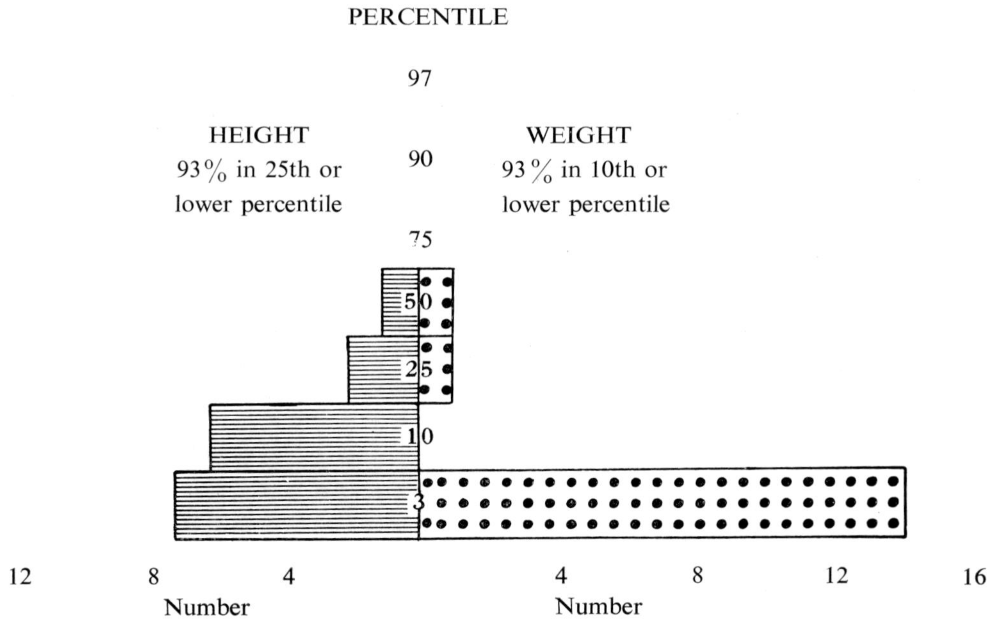

The percentile table shows that the majority of patients were severely malnourished.

TABLE 6

HAEMODYNAMICS OF VENTRICULAR SEPTAL DEFECT

Case No.	Age	Cardiac Output (l./min.)	Cardiac Index (l./M²)	Shunt L——R (l./min.)	L——R Shunt as % of C.O.	Pulmonary Arterial Mean (mm. Hg)	Femoral Arterial Mean (mm. Hg)	Pulmonary Arterial Mean as % Femoral Arterial Mean	Arterial Saturation (%)	Pulmonary Arterial Resistance	Peripheral Resistance	Right Ventricular Work	Right Ventricular Work Index	Left Ventricular Work	Left Ventricular Work Index	Total Work Index	Cardio-thoracic Ratio	Weight (%)
1	2/12	1·0	4·3	0·76	76	58	53	109	58	2,636	4,227	0·8	3·5	1·3	5·7	9·2	61	−3
2	7/12	2·4	8·1	0·83	34	77	71	108	85	2,522	2,326	2·5	8·3	2·4	8·0	16·3	66	−3
3	3/12	See Table 5																3
4	4/12	1·5	5·4	4·5	300	42	70	60	92	618	3,813	0·8	3·0	4·0	14·3	17·3	59	3
5	9/12	1·1	3·2	2·0	182	67	77	87	89	2,279	5,432	0·7	2·0	2·5	7·0	9·0	63	3
6	3/12	1·0	4·1	0·5	50	50	71	70	93	2,724	5,802	0·6	2·8	1·2	5·2	8·0	62	3
7	2/12	1·1	3·7	0·9	82	26	73	35	93	1,057	5,313	0·4	1·3	1·1	3·7	5·1	56	−3
8	6/12	1·7	5·6	3·6	211	54	79	68	93	737	3,751	1·1	3·7	4·2	14·2	17·9	69	−3
9	8/12	1·6	5·0	6·3	343	33	69	47	87	340	3,457	0·7	3·3	7·4	23·0	26·3	58	−3
10	9/12	1·4	4·4	4·2	300	57	66	86	95	795	3,684	1·1	3·4	4·6	14·4	17·8	58	−3
11	8/12	2·6	8·6	3·0	115	30	65	46	90	466	1,950	1·4	4·4	3·1	10·0	14·4	60	−3
12	4/12	1·5	6·3	1·9	126	50	73	68	95	1,163	4,051	1·0	4·3	3·3	14·4	18·7	60	−3
13	11/12	2·8	7·5	1·3	46	56	68	82	85	1,338	1,905	2·0	3·2	3·1	5·0	8·2	61	−3
14	12/12	4·0	7·7	1·7	42	55	59	93	92	715	1,192	2·6	5·0	3·9	7·9	12·9	62	25
15	12/12	1·7	3·8	4·4	258	26	60	41	90	346	5,511	0·5	1·0	5·0	11·0	12·0	53	−3
16	12/12	3·7	7·8	3·1	84	18	74	24	96	209	1,610	0·4	2·0	6·9	14·6	16·6	46	50

since no faith can be put in the failure to traverse the ductus. An associated defect of this type therefore cannot be readily excluded in this age group by catheterization alone.

B. The Haemodynamics. These are summarized in Table 6.

1. THE PRESSURES. Except in infants with congestive failure at the time of study, the levels in the great veins and right atrium were normal by comparison with adult standards.

Right ventricular hypertension was found in all but one case (16) of the series; this was carried forward into the pulmonary circuit essentially unchanged. No case was found to have the 'relative' pulmonary stenosis occasionally found in older persons with large left-to-right shunts. Its absence is probably related to the severe clinical condition and elevated total pulmonary resistance found in these infants.

Normal pressure levels for this age group have not been published, but sporadic observations in this unit in infants with compensated aortic stenosis suggest that adult standards hold good at least as early as 6 months of age. Case 16 would be normal by these criteria. Comparison of the pulmonary arterial mean pressures with the mean in the femoral artery showed that the former was 68% or more of the latter in 10 of the 16 cases. The implication of this is that these 10 children would be considered as poor surgical risks by the criteria of Lillehei *et al.* (1955). This pressure relationship if abnormal does not appear to be associated with the clinically assessed severity of these cases, *e.g.*, by nutrition, presence of dyspnoea or cardio-thoracic ratio. A normal relationship, as seen in Case 16, was in a child who had the highest growth percentile and a normal (46%) cardio-thoracic ratio. As expected, there is a suggestive relationship between a high mean pulmonary femoral pressure and the presence of arterial desaturation. However, as in Case 14, full saturation may be present even if the pulmonary arterial pressure mean is 93% of that in the femoral vessel.

Perusal of the peripheral saturation values, however, does show that significant oxygen unsaturation was present in seven of the 16 cases. This is again a contraindication to surgery in the views of Lillehei and his colleagues.

The pulmonary wedge pressures, where obtainable, were commonly within normal limits for the adult range.

2. CARDIAC OUTPUT AND SHUNTS. In the absence of control values for this age group, these figures are presented without comment. The high cardiac index in several of these children has been observed by us in older infants and children found to have no abnormality at cardiac catheterization. An index may be an unreliable concept in these small patients whose surface area is disproportionately greater per unit volume than in the adult. Additionally, the effect of the anaesthetic must be considered in the assessment of these results. The volume of shunt was three times or more the cardiac output in five of the patients and less than the cardiac output in six. As compared with older children studied in our laboratory, the left-to-right shunt is less in this group

which had a higher incidence of right ventricular hypertension. Conversely, right-to-left shunts were more common, and caused the high incidence of arterial unsaturation which has already been commented upon.

The resistances echo the phenomena already described; a high total pulmonary resistance was usual. This is in contradistinction to the normal or lower resistances found in many older children with a more benign lesion. Our only exception was Case 16, a patient who is perhaps more typical in this respect. The pulmonary arteriolar resistance (where calculable) contributes somewhat to this increase. The total peripheral resistances are in many cases high by adult standards, but this again may not be pathological for this group as it has been sporadically observed in normals of the same age studied in this department.

3. Cardiac Work. The right ventricular work was calculated on the assumption that the shunt occurs in systole and that this chamber does not contract upon the shunted blood. The results show that the amount of work done by the right ventricle is greatly increased by adult standards when expressed as a work index $\frac{\text{(R.V. work)}}{\text{(Surface area)}}$. This is, of course, a function of the raised pulmonary pressure. The left ventricular work is similarly increased by index values because of the left-to-right shunt.

Summation of the left and right ventricular work indices gives an estimate of the total work done by the heart in this condition. It is very likely, however, that values for normals in this age group are higher than for adults in this respect, because of the high peripheral resistance already mentioned, and the exaggerating tendency of a low surface area.

Discussion

This group illustrates the severe clinical and haemodynamic change in a series of infants with ventricular septal defect. It is seen that the problem in this age group is not of the shunt, but of the resultant or coincident pulmonary hypertension. This may occur very early in life. It was proven to exist as early as 2 months of age in Case 1. Clinically in this and in Case 3, the condition may have been present in the first two weeks of life. The resultant rise in ventricular and total work indices is very marked in the majority, and explains the high incidence of right-sided failure in this and other series (Engle, 1954). Growth failure is severe, but cannot be statistically related to the pulmonary arterial pressure if this is abnormal; nor in the absence of normal values to the cardiac output. If pulmonary pressure and arterial desaturation is considered in relation to operability, over half of these infants might not be aided by surgery. This trend might be reversed if these children are studied very early in life, though again cases occurred as early as 2 months in which surgery could not be advised. During the period of follow-up one child (Case 14) died of congestive cardiac failure; three others died suddenly at the beginning of a respiratory infection before surgery could be carried out.

Summary

The clinical and radiological features of a series of infants with ventricular septal defects are presented. The resultant effects on the haemodynamics are noted and discussed.

This study was supported in part by the Wisconsin Alumni Research Foundation and the Wisconsin Heart Association.

References

Abbot, M. E. (1951). In *Disorders of the Heart and Circulation*, ed. R. L. Levy. New York.
Adams, F. H., LaBree, J. and Stauffer, H. M. (1950). *Pediatrics*, **5**, 390.
Brostoff, P. and Rodbard, S. (1956). *Amer. Heart J.*, **51**, 325.
Brown, J. W. (1950). *Congenital Heart Disease*, 2nd ed. London.
Bruwer, A. J., Ellis, F. H., Jr. and Kirklin, J. W. (1955). *Circulation*, **12**, 807.
Engle, M. A. (1954). *Pediatrics*, **14**, 16.
Hultgren, H., Selzer, A., Purdy, A., Holman, E. and Gerbode, F. (1953). *Circulation*, **8**, 15.
Keats, T. E. and Steinbach, H. L. (1955). *Radiology*, **64**, 528.
Kerley, P. (1951). In *A Textbook of X-ray Diagnosis*, 2nd ed., ed. Shanks, S. C. and Kerley, P. Vol. 2. London.
Leatham, A. (1952). *Brit. med. Bull.*, **8**, 333.
Lillehei, C. W., Cohen, M., Warden, H. E., Ziegler, N. R. and Varco, R. L. (1955). *Surg. Gynec. Obstet.*, **101**, 446.
Marquis, R. M. (1950). *Brit. Heart J.*, **12**, 265.
Maxwell, G. M. (1954). Congenital Heart Disease in the Paediatric Age and Group. M.D. Thesis. University of Edinburgh.
Roger, H. (1879). *Bull. Acad. Méd. (Paris)*, ser. 2, **8**, 1074, 1189.
Taussig, H. B. (1955). Proc. Ann. Meet. Amer. Heart. Ass. New Orleans.
Turchetti, A. (1954). Proc. 2nd World Cong. of Cardiology, Washington, 1954. Abstract in *Acta cardiol. (Brux.)*, **9**, 592.
Wasserburger, R. W. (1956). Proc. Ann. Meet. Wisc. Heart Ass. To be published.
Wintrobe, M. M. (1951). *Clinical Hematology*, 3rd ed., p. 540. Philadelphia.
Wood, P. (1950). *Brit. med. J.*, **2**, 639.

SWEAT ANALYSIS IN FIBROCYSTIC DISEASE, CHRONIC PULMONARY DISEASE AND CONTROLS

BY

MARY M. WEEKS and G. A. BROWN

From the Department of Paediatrics and Child Health, the University of Birmingham, and Birmingham Children's Hospital

(RECEIVED FOR PUBLICATION AUGUST 1, 1957)

Recent findings of abnormalities of sweat composition in patients with fibrocystic disease of the pancreas have stimulated broader interest in this disease and provided a new laboratory diagnostic procedure. A simplified method for collecting samples of sweat is presented, together with analytical results for sodium, chloride and urea concentrations in patients with fibrocystic disease and in patients with chronic pulmonary disease.

Previously described methods of sweat collection have required either special heating apparatus or controlled environmental humidity. Webb, Flute and Smith (1957) describe a method using enveloping polythene bags to encourage sweating and filter paper instead of pads of gauze to absorb the sweat.

The present method allows children to carry on with their normal activities during the collection. The small amounts of sweat obtained are adequate for analysis as the methods are the same as those used by Webb *et al.* with corresponding results. Gauze was found to be an advantage as the absorbed sweat and water did not require filtering before analysis.

The method described here, together with the analytical procedures, require no apparatus other than that available in any biochemical laboratory. In many centres the chloride content only of sweat is being estimated as this is considered diagnostic.

Patients Studied

Twenty children with proven fibrocystic disease of the pancreas, six children with chronic pulmonary disease unassociated with fibrocystic disease and six apparently healthy siblings of five of the fibrocystic patients were studied. Forty in-patients in whom there was no reason to suspect a sweat abnormality were selected as controls.

Method

The materials used were washed cotton gauze, transparent plastic sheeting and 1-in. wide waterproof adhesive strapping.

Ordinarily gauze contains small amounts of sodium chloride. All the 3-in. gauze squares used in the investigation were, therefore, prepared by first leaving them to soak in distilled water for two hours, and then completing the extraction of salt by passing approximately two gallons of distilled water through each 100 squares. They were dried at 70° C.

A dry 50-ml.-flask containing a gauze square and closed by a ground-glass stopper was weighed. This piece of gauze was placed over the lumbar region of the patient, the site having been washed with distilled water and dried. It was covered with a larger square of plastic sheeting the edges of which were fixed to the skin with adhesive strapping to make an airtight seal.

The gauze was left in position for two to six hours, depending on the temperature of the external environment. It was then returned to the flask and reweighed, the weight of sweat thus being determined. At least 0·1 g. of normal sweat is required for accurate analysis, although 0·06 g. is sufficient in cases of fibrocystic disease of the pancreas.

Five millilitres distilled water were added to the flask which was restoppered and left for 12 hours.

The solution obtained by compressing the soaked gauze with a glass rod and decanting was used for estimating the chloride by mercurimetric titration, the sodium by flame photometry and the urea by urease and nesslerization. With very small amounts of sweat, extraction was performed by centrifuging the gauze in a tube containing a 1 cm. length of narrow bore polythene

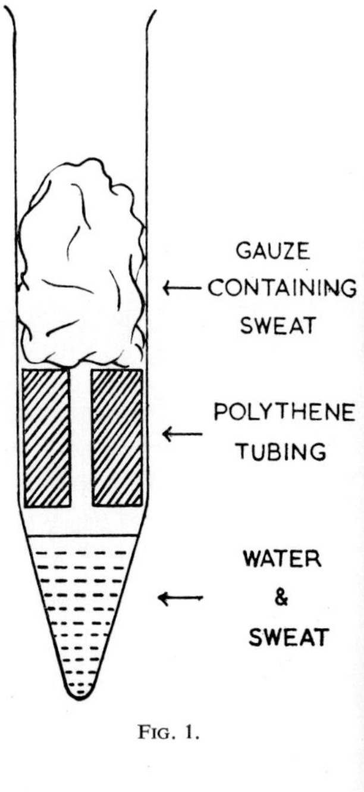

FIG. 1.

TABLE 1

MEAN VALUES AND RANGES OF SODIUM AND CHLORIDES

Group	Number of Cases	Range		Mean Values	
		Sodium (mEq/1.)	Chloride (mEq/1.)	Sodium (mEq/1.)	Chloride (mEq/1.)
Controls	40	6·6– 37·6	6·0– 38·4	21·2	21·8
Fibrocystic disease	20	36·4–189·4	49·6–196·1	104·0	111·5
Children with chronic pulmonary disease	6	48·1– 69·4	20·6– 40·5	58·2	31·5

tubing fixed in a conical centrifuge tube (Fig. 1). On centrifuging, the sweat and water passed through the polythene tubing into the small chamber below, from which it was removed with the aid of a Pasteur pipette.

Results

Sodium and Chloride Concentrations. Mean values and ranges are summarized in Table 1, and the correspondence between sodium and chloride concentrations in individual specimens is shown in Fig. 2. It is evident from the graph that the concentrations of sodium and chloride are much greater in the children with fibrocystic disease than in the controls.

Sweat from six children with chronic pulmonary disease showed high sodium but normal chloride levels. This may be an important finding but its significance is not apparent at the moment.

Six siblings of children with fibrocystic disease were investigated. All were healthy with no clinical evidence of disease. Two of these children were from one family, one having normal and one abnormal sweat. The remaining four were unrelated and of these three had abnormal, and one normal, sweat.

Urea Concentration. Sweat samples from 24 children were also analysed for urea, the results being summarized in Table 2.

There was a similar wide range of urea concentrations in both normal and fibrocystic groups, with an average concentration in the controls of 181 mg./

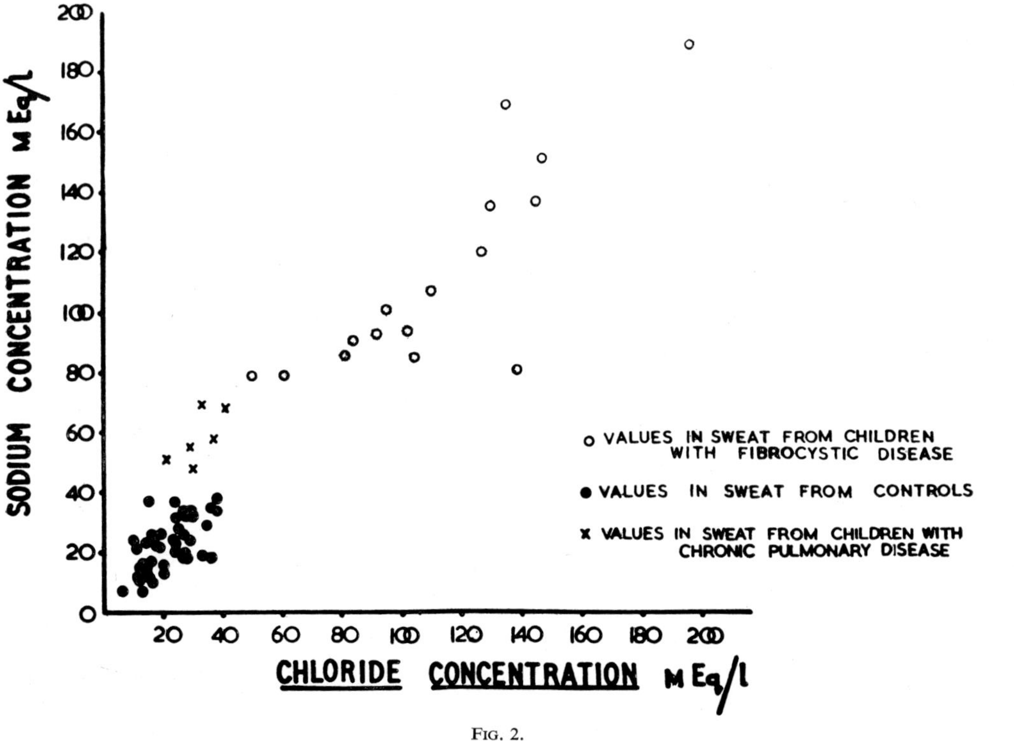

FIG. 2.

TABLE 2

RESULTS OF UREA ANALYSIS

Group	Number of Cases	Urea Range (mg./l.)	Urea Mean (mg./l.)
Controls ..	13	63–339	181
Fibrocystic disease	11	47–370	191

100 ml. and 191 mg./100 ml. in the group of fibrocystic children. Repeat estimations were performed on several children. The results were often far removed from those obtained originally, thus confirming that sweat urea concentrations vary in the individual though tending to exceed blood levels, *e.g.*, in one child with a raised blood urea (78 mg./100 ml.) the sweat urea was 755 mg./100 ml.

Amino-acid Concentration. The amino-acid pattern of the sweat estimated by paper chromatography was similar in both normal and fibrocystic groups and corresponded with the pattern shown by Dent and Walshe (1954).

Discussion

Since the occurrence in 1948 of heat prostration in 10 children of whom five had fibrocystic disease (Kessler and Andersen, 1951) many papers on abnormal sweat have been published.

The results of di Sant' Agnese, Darling, Perera and Shea (1953), who presented a series of 43 patients and 50 controls, and those of Schwachmann (1956), who investigated 200 patients and 800 controls, show that the concentrations of sweat sodium and chloride in fibrocystic disease are two to four times higher than normal. A similar difference has been obtained in the present series although the range of normality is lower than in previously published papers. This may be due to different methods and conditions of collection. Therefore it would appear that each investigator should establish his own standard according to his method.

The way in which the sweat becomes abnormal in patients with fibrocystic disease and in some of their relatives is unknown. Di Sant' Agnese *et al.* (1953) demonstrated by metabolic studies that disturbance in neither renal nor adrenal function was responsible, and no change could be seen in the sweat gland when examined microscopically.

Gochberg and Cooke (1956) came to the conclusion that the increased concentration of sodium chloride in sweat from fibrocystic children was due to an increase of sodium chloride in the precursor solution and suggested that there might be an absence of an enzyme, co-enzyme or substrate in secretory cells altering the release of energy producing the abnormal secretion. In this paper he reported sweat urea concentrations in nine children with fibrocystic disease, finding an average of 58 mg./100 ml. in controls and 55 mg./100 ml. in fibrocystics with little variation.

Examination of the sweat is becoming one of the most useful and reliable diagnostic tests for fibrocystic disease as illustrated by the two cases described.

Case Reports

Case 1. For three weeks before admission a girl aged 13 months had an exacerbation of the cough present since birth. There was no history of abnormal stools. She was cyanosed and febrile with crepitations heard over both lung fields. Radiographical changes were those of bronchopneumonia.

Analysis of the sweat on two separate occasions gave values typical of those in fibrocystic disease, viz.:

Sodium 92·5 mEq/l.	Chloride 170·0 mEq/l.
Sodium 142·0 mEq/l.	Chloride 86·2 mEq/l.

A three-day fat balance showed normal fat absorption, there was no excess fat in the faeces on microscopic examination, and the 'lipiodol' test (Silverman and Shirkey, 1955) was not indicative of fibrocystic disease.

Treatment was of no avail and the patient died three months after admission. At necropsy the findings in the pancreas and lungs were typical of fibrocystic disease.

This case resembles one reported by di Sant' Agnese (1955).

Case 2. A boy aged 9 weeks was admitted with suspected fibrocystic disease of the pancreas. He had passed pale, fatty and offensive motions and had failed to thrive. Radiological examination of the lungs revealed bilateral basal consolidation, fat globules were seen in the faeces on microscopical examination, and analysis of the fasting duodenal contents showed no trypsin and a very low activity of lipase.

Despite these findings repeated analyses of the sweat at monthly intervals gave normal results:

Sodium 12·9 mEq/l	Chloride 6·8 mEq/l.
Sodium 13·3 mEq/l.	Chloride 15·9 mEq/l.
Sodium 36·4 mEq/l.	Chloride 31·2 mEq/l.
Sodium 18·5 mEq/l.	Chloride 23·3 mEq/l.

His general condition improved slowly and his motions became normal without treatment. Subsequent analyses of the duodenal fluid revealed first low, and finally normal, activity of lipase and trypsin. It appeared, therefore, that the pancreatic dysfunction had been temporary.

Two other cases, brothers, attended this hospital during recent years. The elder boy had a splenectomy in 1953 when a diagnosis of portal hypertension with oesophageal varices was made. Subsequently he developed a severe pulmonary infection and in 1956 his sweat was found to contain high concentrations of sodium and chloride. His brother, who was thought to have coeliac disease in 1951, was readmitted in 1953 with faecal impaction which necessitated laparotomy. He has since been found to have fibrocystic disease of the pancreas with abnormal sweat. A third child in the family died when 12 days old.

Summary

A simple method of sweat collection is outlined.

Two cases are described in which investigation of the sweat was helpful diagnostically.

The results fall into three groups: sweat from children with fibrocystic disease containing salt in concentrations two to four times that of the concentration in the control group, and children with chronic pulmonary disease having a normal chloride concentration in the sweat but a high sodium value.

There is no difference between the amino-acid and urea concentrations in controls and children with fibrocystic disease.

We would like to express our gratitude to Professor J. M. Smellie, Mr. H. B. Salt and Dr. O. H. Wolff for their encouragement and helpful criticism; to Mr A. E. Marston, Chief Pharmacist, for providing the salt-free gauze; to Mr. J. G. Williamson for the photographs; and to the consultant staff of the Children's Hospital, Birmingham, for permitting us to investigate their patients.

References

Dent, C. E. and Walshe, J. M. (1954). *Brit. med. Bull.*, **10**, 247.
di Sant' Agnese, P. A. (1955). *Pediatrics*, **15**, 683.
——, Darling, R. C., Perera, G. A. and Shea, E. (1953). *Ibid.*, **12**, 549.
Gochberg, S. H. and Cooke, R. E. (1956). *Ibid.*, **18**, 701.
Kessler, W. R. and Andersen, D. H. (1951). *Ibid.*, **8**, 648.
Silverman, F. N. and Shirkey, H. C. (1955). *Ibid.*, **15**, 143.
Schwachmann, H. (1956). Personal Communication.
Webb, B. W., Flute, P. T. and Smith, M. J. H. (1957). *Arch. D Childh.*, **32**, 82.

THE GASTRO-OESOPHAGEAL REGION IN INFANTS

OBSERVATIONS ON THE ANATOMY, WITH SPECIAL REFERENCE TO THE CLOSING MECHANISM AND PARTIAL THORACIC STOMACH

BY

G. S. MULLER BOTHA

From the University of Birmingham Medical School

(RECEIVED FOR PUBLICATION MAY 24, 1957)

The nature of the closing mechanism between the oesophagus and the stomach has attracted considerable anatomical study in the past 300 years. Main interest has centred on the adult; the anatomy of the infant, which does not necessarily correspond, has not received the same attention. The present investigation is therefore concerned with infants. It was undertaken with two objects: first, from the anatomical study, both macroscopic and microscopic, to assess the importance of the various components of the normal closing mechanism; secondly, to consider the abnormal infant, in whom this mechanism is incompetent, in the light of clinical experience and radiological observation.

Material

The diaphragm, lower oesophagus, upper stomach, aorta and surrounding tissue were removed *en bloc* from 115 human subjects and fixed in 10% formol saline. Every specimen was carefully dissected and drawings were made of the essential features in all. Histological confirmation was obtained in doubtful cases. In age, the patients varied from a 32-week foetus to 8 years. In the great majority the ages ranged from a few hours to 1 month (average weight of 5½ lb.). One foetus of 1 lb. 2 oz. and one girl of 13 years were also studied. The sexes were about equally represented. In addition to the dissected specimens, numerous studies were carried out in the necropsy room where the organs were examined *in situ*. The following observations were made.

Diaphragm

Anatomy textbooks describe, and interesting pictures convincingly show, decussation of the crural fibres dorsal to the oesophagus. This is rare. Only a few specimens were found where the overlap of muscle fibres at their origin from the median arcuate ligament in the standard type could possibly be mistaken for decussation. Low (1907) and Collis, Kelly and Wiley (1954) found no decussation in a series of 25 and 50 diaphragms respectively. Considerable normal variation occurs, the functional significance of which has not been fully appreciated.

The Standard Pattern. The aorta, a midline structure, divides the crura into a right and left crus (Fig. 1a, 1b, 4). The right crus is better developed, more fleshy and wider than the left one. It arises from the bodies and discs of the upper three or four lumbar vertebrae (sometimes five); it passes cranially and divides into a large right and a smaller left limb which embrace the gullet and join again anteriorly. The fibres of the right limb arise from the vertebral column and right border of the median arcuate ligament and run straight upwards to insert into the central tendon. The right limb is always anterior. The spinal fibres of the left limb run upwards behind the right limb, arch obliquely over the aorta and then ascend immediately to the left of the gullet to insert into the central tendon. The lateral fibres of the left limb are short and arise from the central portion of the median arcuate ligament. The medial fibres sometimes curve acutely to the right, caudal to the oesophagus to gain origin from aponeurotic fibres to the right of the hiatus. The right limb is therefore visualized from the ventral aspect whereas the left limb can only be displayed fully from the back (Fig. 1b, 4). This arrangement results in a perfect overlap. The twisted figure of eight which is so well depicted in most drawings was not seen in a single instance; one must therefore conclude that it is not an anatomical fact. On the contrary, the 'straight' arrangement of the fibres is usually conspicuous.

The left crus is small and almost separate from the lateral fibres of the left limb; it takes no part in the formation of the hiatus. Decussation of muscle

(a) The standard pattern seen from the abdomen.

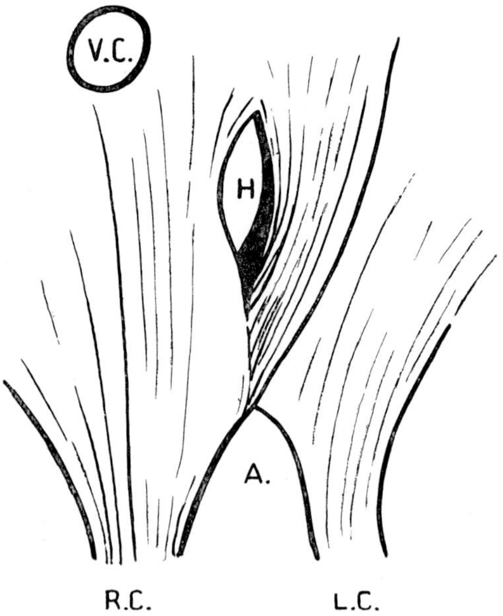

(b) The standard pattern seen from the chest.

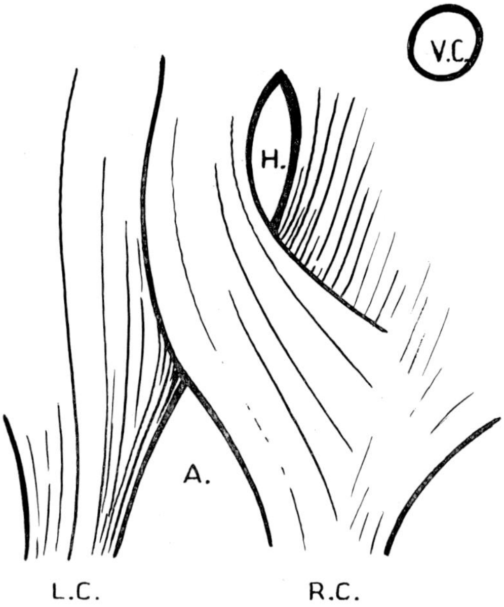

(e) Stage 1 shift to the left.

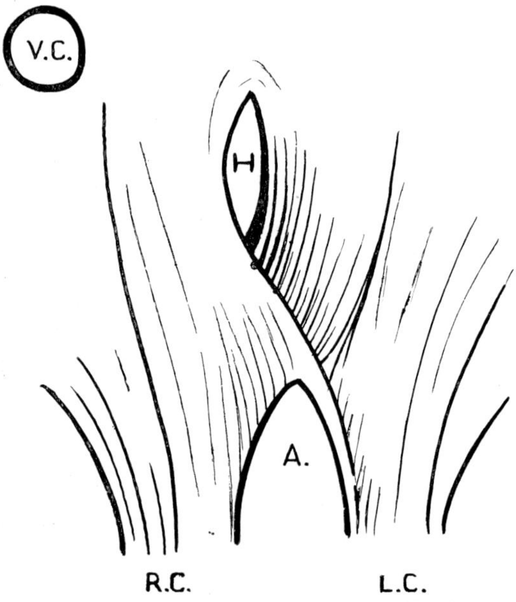

(f) The broad dorsal band consists of almost half the fibres of the left crus.

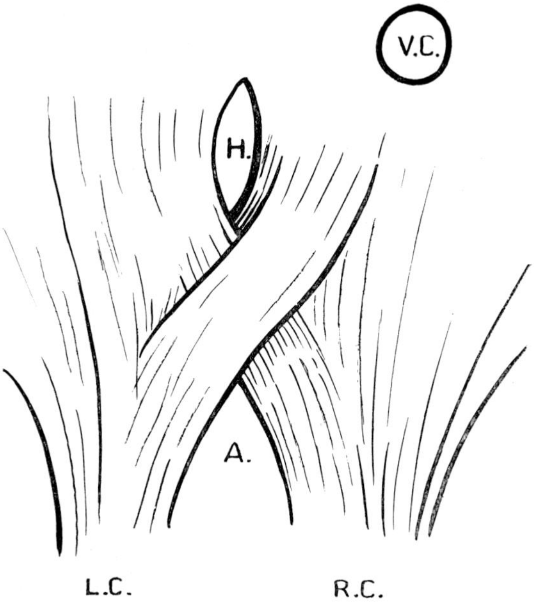

FIG. 1.—Variations in crural anatomy

R.C.=right crus L.C.=left crus A.=aortic opening H.=hiatus V.C.=vena cava

(c) Shift to the right.

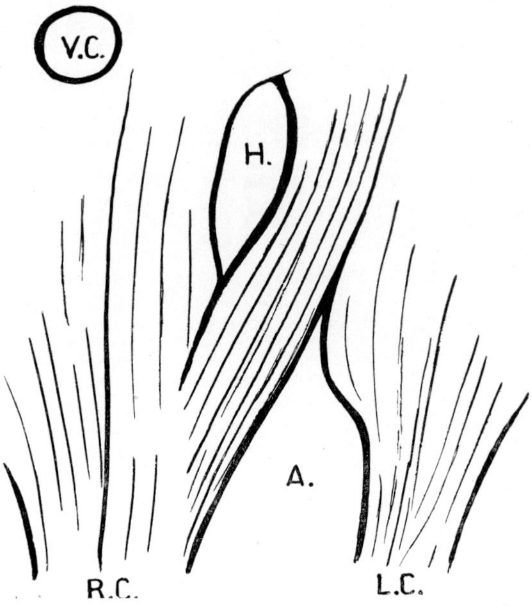

(d) A large hiatus approximates the aortic opening.

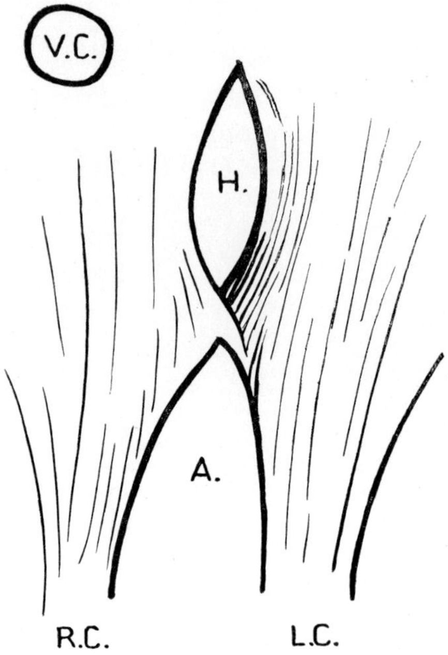

(g) A narrow dorsal band.

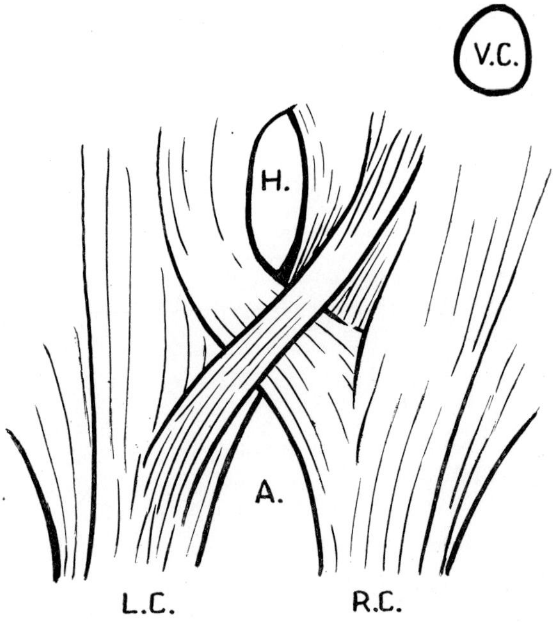

(h) A transverse band.

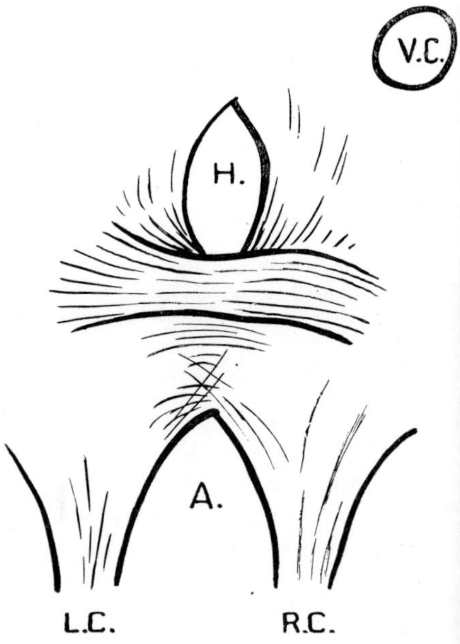

fibres does not occur dorsal to the hiatus, but is often present where the fibres arise from the median arcuate ligament.

Deviations from the standard pattern are very common.

Shift to the Right. In this variation, instead of the ventral and dorsal 'waistcoat effect' of the standard pattern, the right crus merely splits into two limbs so that a pyriform hiatal opening is formed (Fig. 1c). There is little or no overlap. The left limb does not arise from the median arcuate ligament, which is non-existent, but itself forms the right border of the aortic opening. The left crus is small and takes no part in the hiatus.

Shift to the Left: Stage 1. The medial fibres of the right crus sometimes transgress the midline to gain origin from the left border of the arcuate ligament (Fig. 1e). This encroachment on the left side may be slight or so complete as to extend down to the tendinous origin of the left crus, but essentially it remains part of the right crus. The left crus still does not partake in the formation of the hiatus.

The Scissors Overlap: Stage 2. The right and left crura may be equally well developed, but commonly the right one is still bigger. The left crus, which is for the first time taking part in the formation of the hiatus, forms a perfect overlap by criss-crossing with the right crus. The most common variation is a broad band from the left crus which crosses anteriorly to form the right hiatal margin, supplemented by a posterior band from the right crus which forms the left hiatal margin. These bands constitute the 'scissors'. They are easily separated and run antero-medially on each side of the aorta as the right and left borders of the median arcuate ligament which, as such, is non-existent. The treble or quadruple overlap when three or more bands criss-cross, is more uncommon (Fig. 2). The relative size and origin of the bands vary tremendously and no two are quite alike.

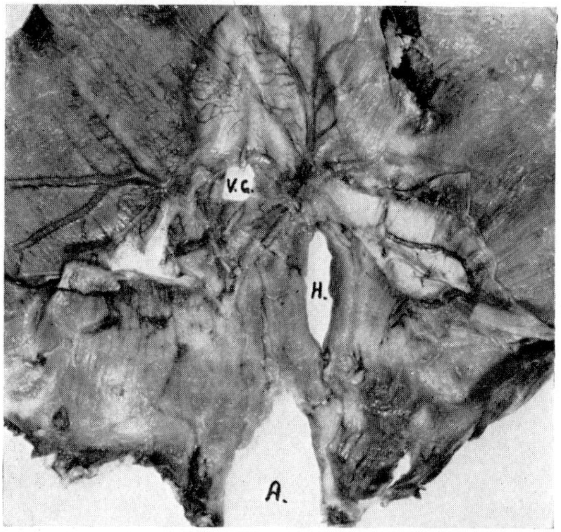

FIG. 3.—Stage 3 to the left. Diaphragm seen from the abdomen.

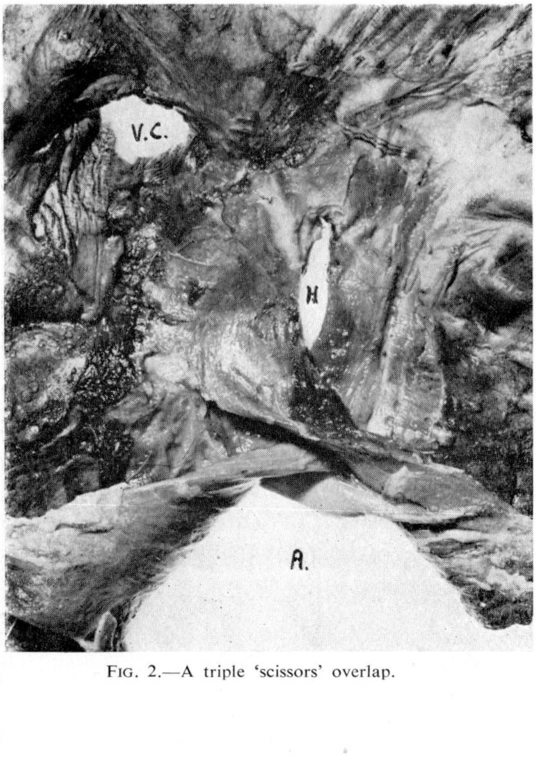

FIG. 2.—A triple 'scissors' overlap.

The Hiatus Formed Completely by Left Crus: Stage 3. This variation must be relatively uncommon. It was encountered in only one specimen and no previous descriptions of it have been seen. The left crus formed the entire hiatus and presented a mirror image of the 'shift to the right' (Fig. 3). There was no overlap in this case.

Accessory Bands. Low (1907) first described an accessory muscle band, 4 mm. wide, that extends from the superior aspect of the left crus, in front of the aorta and within the fibres of the right crus, to the caval orifice. He found four of these bands in 25 specimens. In an excellent paper Collis and his colleagues (1954) described a variant of Low's band as well as a transverse inter-tendinous bundle which they displayed in dissections of 50 diaphragms. Examples of all three types were found in this study, as well as other variants (Figs. 1f, 1g, 1h). The Low bands varied from a few muscle strands to a

TABLE 1

NORMAL VARIATIONS IN THE PATTERN OF THE CRURA

Crural Pattern	Standard Type	Shift to the Right	Shift to the Left: Stage 1	Shift to the Left: Stage 2	Shift to the Left: Stage 3	Accessory Bands	
						Small	Large
Total 115	67	12	28	7	1	20	19
Percentage ..	58·6	10·3	24·2	6	0·9	34	

bundle as thick as the left limb of the right crus and then formed a powerful 'scissors overlap'. The fibres either passed to the right, superficial to the right crus (the great majority), or through the substance of the left limb or lay in front of it. The obliquity varied from almost vertical to almost transverse. Some bands were long, thin and insignificant; other bundles were short, flat and powerful. Whereas most of the small bands are of academic interest only, there can be little doubt that on contraction they tend to decrease the size of the hiatal opening. When well developed, they may become an important factor in, first, enhancing the supportive function of the crura to maintain gastro-oesophageal competence and secondly, to reinforce the posterior weak spot in the hiatus.

The postero-medial branches of the phrenic nerves are the sole motor supply to the crura of the diaphragm (Botha, 1957a). Each nerve innervates the muscle on the ipsilateral side of the hiatus irrespective of its origin.

Table 1 indicates the wide variation that exists in crural pattern.

The Median Arcuate Ligament. In the standard type it is tendinous, well developed and gives origin to crural fibres from both sides. It does not always form the arching 'ligament' so well figured in text-books. It is weakest in the 'scissors' type (Fig. 2) or when the hiatus has shifted to the right and may sometimes be completely absent. In a few dissections the tendinous crural fibres joined in the midline, posterior to the aorta, and thus formed a fibrous ring for the passage of this big vessel.

Overlap. This is one of the most characteristic features of crural architecture and is by far most marked in the standard type. It obviously serves three purposes:

(1) TO STRENGTHEN A POTENTIALLY WEAK AREA. Anteriorly the crura are inserted into the central tendon by short, decussating, musculo-tendinous fibres. Clinical weakness never occurs at this site and therefore no anatomical overlap is indicated. Posteriorly, however, there is little stability and the criss-cross fibres might be easily separated by a force that acts on the hiatus. This is only too well demonstrated by the frequent occurrence of hiatus hernia in late adult life. Overlap is still Nature's best way of providing the greatest protection for the weakest area with the minimum available tissue.

(2) RIGHT LIMB ALWAYS OVERLAPS ANTERIORLY. This creates an oblique hiatus which is essential to accommodate the lower oesophagus with its marked deviation to the left. Overlap is not the cause of the obliquity of the gullet, as this is present if there is poor or no overlap (as found in some types), but it maintains its position more firmly and embraces the oesophagus more snugly during diaphragmatic or swallowing movements. A secure fixation decreases the chances of herniation.

(3) OVERLAP CHANGES ALIGNMENT OF MUSCLE FIBRES. This is specially noticeable in the 'scissors' type where not only the longitudinal, but also the transverse diameter of the hiatus is decreased when the diaphragm contracts. In the standard type, the right limb mainly pulls caudally, but the left limb pulls down and to the right, thus narrowing the hiatus from side to side. This tendency to constrict the hiatus is least marked in stage 3 and 'shift to the right', which on theoretical grounds should therefore be inferior functionally.

The Hiatus. Unlike the adult, the hiatus in the infant is of very uniform size. In all the above dissections, it was small, so small that the narrowest portion of the oesophagus could just pass through (Fig. 4). The oesophagus was gripped firmly.

The presence of a hiatal tunnel in the adult is doubtful. In the infant it is a fact. The crural muscle is round and 'heaped up' at the hiatal margins especially on the right side. In the 7 cm embryo the length of the right hiatal wall is twic the diameter of the oesophageal opening (Botha 1958). This length gradually decreases as th foetus develops, but it is still well marked at birth The length of the canal depends on the degree o obliquity. Where no overlap is present, the hiatu consists of a straight hole through the diaphragn (Fig. 3). The obliquity can easily be seen when th diaphragm is looked at from the front. The hiatu appears as a small, ovoid slit, which sometime almost disappears (Fig. 4). When viewed obliquel

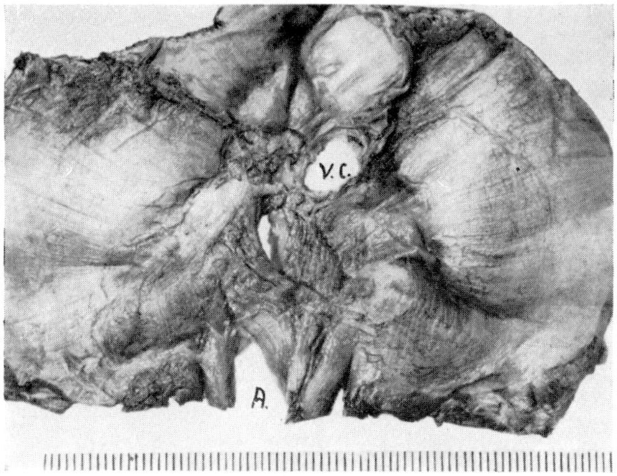

FIG. 4.—The hiatus in the standard pattern is slit-like when seen directly from above.

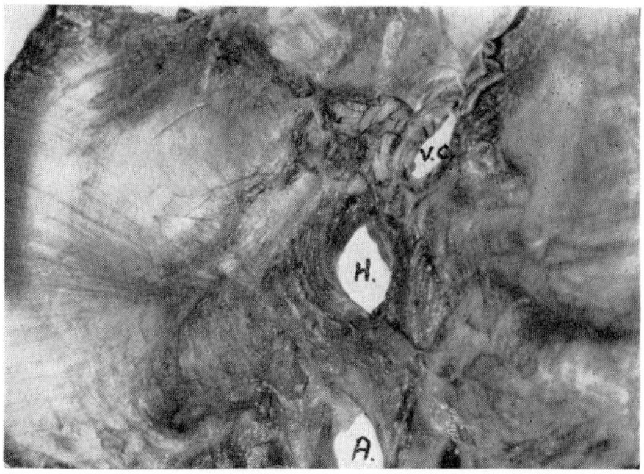

FIG. 5.—The hiatus in Fig. 4 appears large and ovoid or round when viewed obliquely.

in the line of the tunnel, the true size becomes apparent (Fig. 5). As in the adult, but less marked, the anterior wall of the canal is much shorter than the posterior one. This is primarily due to the wide overlap behind and the oblique upward slope of the diaphragm. In the older subjects in this series the canal was relatively shorter, wider and the oesophagus less securely fixed. In infants it was mostly from 3 to 8 mm. long, and proportionately much longer and firmer than in the adult.

The relative distance from the aorta to the caudal margin of the hiatus is also much greater in the infant than in the adult, suggesting that with age the oesophagus gradually approximates to the aorta. This is most certainly due to opening of the overlap and attenuation of the muscle fibres. In one specimen the median arcuate ligament and the inferior hiatal margin were very close together (which is most unusual in infants) and no overlap was present. In addition, the hiatus was relatively big (Fig. 1d). Although the oesophagus was firmly attached in the crural tunnel, this type of diaphragm with short fibres, lack of overlap and a wide hiatus may in future, when the necessary strain is present, give way to herniation.

Phreno-oesophageal Membrane. Any doubt as to the existence of this structure would be quickly dispelled by an examination of the infant diaphragm. There is no basic difference in its formation, position and attachments from that in the adult. It is, however, a much more definite structure that could be seen in every specimen as a thick, closely woven, creamy-white layer that bridged the potential gap between diaphragm and oesophagus. The main component is formed by the well-developed subdiaphragmatic fascia that divides at the level of the hiatus into a short, stout inferior limb and a thinner, long superior limb. The lower portion is usually stronger and is easily seen after removal of the fat and peritoneum as it splays out to a broad insertion into the cardia and adjacent stomach. The superior limb passes upwards through the hiatus and is joined above by the supra-diaphragmatic fascia which is a very definite layer but less well developed than its counterpart below. This strengthened limb then ascends in a circular fashion to insert into the terminal 5-10 mm. of thoracic oesophagus. The insertion of the membrane is never abrupt but in successive concentric layers of elastic strands with small areolar spaces in between. Individual strands are tough and can withstand considerable pressure. Some appear to be attached to the outer connective adventitia of the oesophagus, fascia propria, whereas others penetrate the external lomgitudinal muscle coat and can be traced down to the submucosa. The greatest concentration of fibres is inserted immediately above the diaphragm. Fat is absent in this structure.

The importance of this structure, which has been called a figment of the imagination, cannot be overestimated. It is the sole fixation of the oesophagus in the diaphragmatic hiatus, as the supportive value of the serosal layers above and below is negligible. The stomach and oesophagus were soundly secured in every specimen that I dissected, yet sufficient resiliency was present to allow adequate physiological movement. Fixation was much more firm in infants and movement was less than in children, and even more noticeable when compared with the adult. This difference is essentially due to the anchoring ability of an unattenuated phreno-oesophageal membrane and secondly, to a narrow, tight-fitting hiatus.

This structure is not a ligament. It is a fibro-elastic layer which is specially adapted to stand the strain of incessant movement at the hiatus during diaphragmatic contraction for 70 or 80 years. The histological appearance of the elastic fibres as well as their ratio to collagen is the same as that of a normal adult. Commonly 40-60% of elastic fibres occur but the proportion varies from 10 to 90%. The fibres vary in size, shape and form. Short, stout, blunt-ended strands appear next to thin, long filamentous fibrils. They vary from place to place and are mostly single. Branching does occur but is not marked. Resiliency and strength are obtained by wavy intertwining of the strands. As the fibres run in lamellae or bundles, different layers may be recognized on cross section.

Lower Oesophagus

Anatomically the lower oesophagus can be divided into a supra-diaphragmatic portion, a narrowed hiatal area and the abdominal oesophagus (Fig. 6).

The Supra-diaphragmatic Portion. This part of the oesophagus was generally wide and in the majority the diameter gradually decreased towards the diaphragm. In the older children it appeared wide right up to the hiatus. In only one specimen (a stillborn female of 9 lb.) was there a definite saccular dilatation above the diaphragm. As in the adult, the 'phrenic ampulla' is not an anatomical entity. It must be regarded as a radiological concept for a physiological phenomenon.

The Area of Constriction. In almost all the specimens a constricted area on the oesophagus coincided with the diaphragmatic hiatus which is always terminal in infants. The crura fit tightly around the oesophagus immediately above the cardia so that the abdominal part of this organ is very short. As the infant grows, the abdominal oesophagus increases in length so that the area of constriction shifts proximally. A narrowing was also observed in specimens where the oesophagus was removed from the diaphragm before fixation in formalin, but it was never so pronounced as when the specimen was fixed with the organs *in situ*. This clearly suggests that the diaphragm is mainly responsible for the localized area of constriction, but that another factor is present as well. This factor is the inferior oesophageal sphincter. Evidence of an anatomical sphincter was found in a small proportion of these subjects (Fig. 7). The fibres are thick, coarse and more irregular. Inter-lacing and cross bundles are common. The width depended on the age, but it was mostly 5 mm. wide in infants, and could only be inspected properly if the mucosa was removed. It was more difficult to see this in small specimens, but in the older age groups it became more evident. Sometimes it began at the oblique fibres, but in most cases it was above and separate from this bundle. In one specimen, a definite ring-like muscle band of 3 mm. wide was found a few millimetres above the cardia.

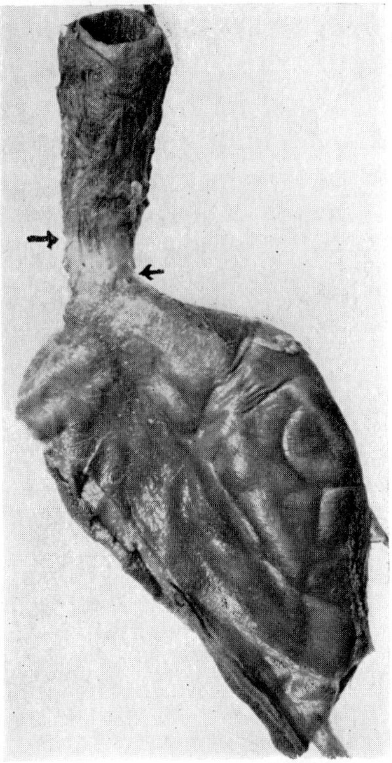

FIG. 6.—The lower oesophagus: the arrows indicate the crural tunnel.

The Abdominal Oesophagus. In the 18 mm. embryo the abdominal oesophagus is half as wide as the stomach and almost as long as the lesser curve of this organ (Botha, 1958a). When the embryo is 9·5 cm. long, it is still very well marked. Gradually the abdominal oesophagus gets shorter. At birth it is so short as to be almost non-existent in some cases. After a few months it is usually a few millimetres long and within a few years it measures from 5 to 15 mm.

The left wall is short or non-existent. The right wall is long and curves towards the left in a characteristic fashion to join the lesser curve at the cardia. The distal widening before the oesophagus joins the stomach is slight in the infant, but becomes more apparent in the first five to 10 years.

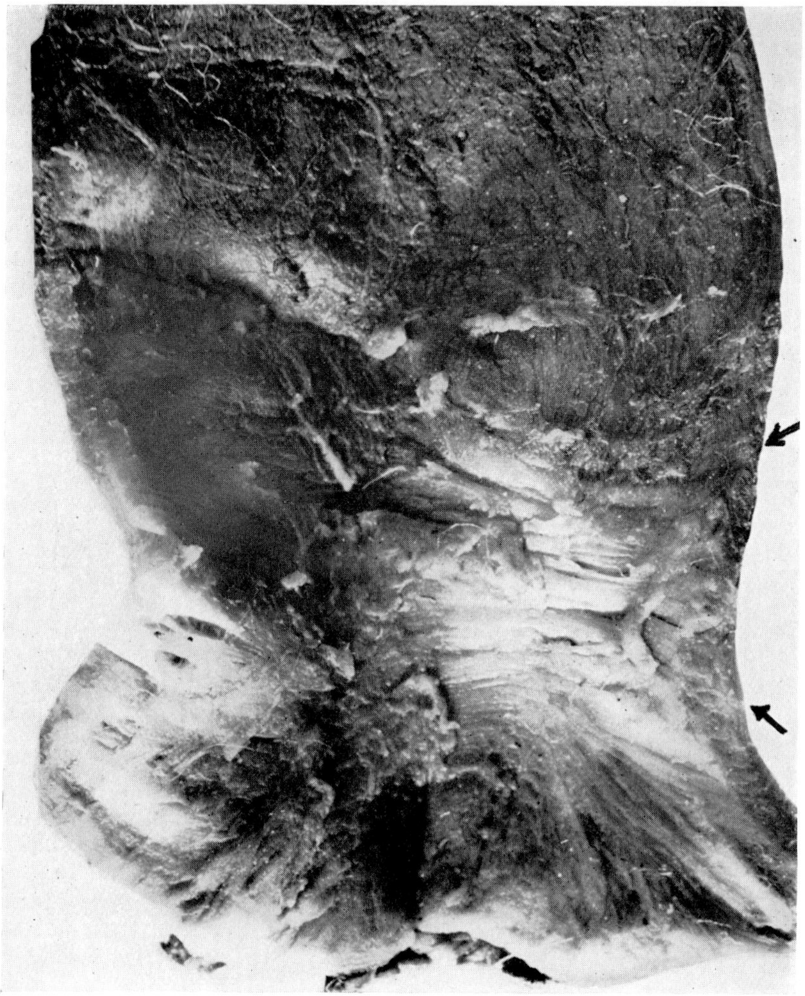

FIG. 7.—The inferior oesophageal sphincter after removal of the mucous membrane.

Cardia

The site where the oesophagus joins the stomach is called the cardia, and in infants it is always well defined. It is narrow in the infant but wider in older children. Internally, the sling fibres are the only guide as to the level of the cardia. They were present in every specimen, but better developed in some. These fibres are already macroscopically evident in the 8 cm. foetus, and form a much sharper ridge in the infant than in the adult.

Cardiac Angle

Several angles are formed by the foregut in the region of the diaphragm. The most widely discussed of these is the gastro-oesophageal angle (cardiac angle or incisura of His, 1903) which is formed on the left side between the abdominal oesophagus and the gastric fundus. Unfortunately this is often confused with the lower oesophageal angle which is formed at the hiatus as the abdominal oesophagus deviates to the left. The other angle is formed by the almost vertical oesophagus entering the stomach which lies at an oblique, horizontal plane.

The first angle is very variable. Its acuteness mainly depends on the fullness of the stomach. In the empty organ it is mostly more than 90°. In the full stomach, especially when a large gastric air bubble is present, the fundus rises higher and bulges medially so that this angle becomes more acute; but even in a full stomach it may still be a blunt angle.

Serosa

The peritoneal reflections in the infant are similar to those in the adult.

Fat Pads. Subperitoneal fatty deposits around the cardia are commonly present in the adult and especially large and lobular in obese individuals with a lax hiatus. These fat pads are either very small or absent in children and infants.

Gastro-phrenic Band. This was present, at least to some extent, in all the specimens. It is formed by a double fold of peritoneum that extends to the left from the abdominal oesophagus and fixes the superior border of the fundus to the under surface of the diaphragm. Sometimes this fold is narrow and almost non-existent. Commonly it forms an appreciable layer and may even extend as far laterally as the spleen. Loose, areolar connective tissue and elastic fibres are present, especially near the hiatus. Histologically the structure resembles closely the phreno-oesophageal membrane, except that elastic fibres are not nearly so abundant.

Infracardiac Bursa. Persistence above the diaphragm of the pneumato-enteric recess on the right side is common (Fig. 8). In this series 16 mesothelial-lined cavities were found of which seven were quite big. Histological sections proved the serosal lining. In two of these the cavity extended downwards on the right of the oesophagus, through the hiatus into the lesser omentum, where it ended blindly. In none of the present series was any freely communicative sac with the peritoneal cavity found, but this was demonstrated in adult dissections. These serosal pockets or bursae are uncommon in adults, which indicates that most are obliterated after birth.

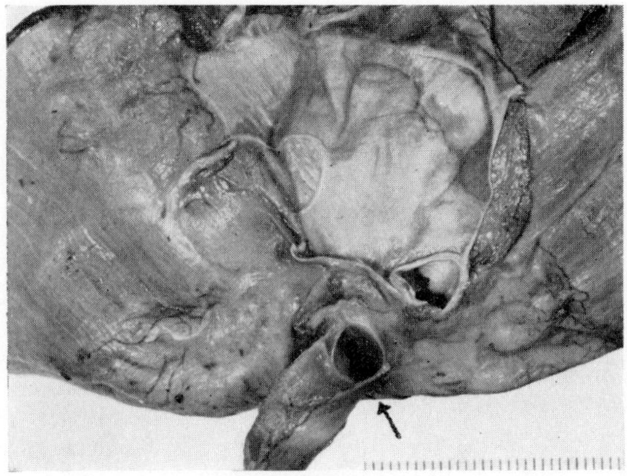

FIG. 8.—Infracardiac bursa on the right of the oesophagus seen from above.

Mucosa

Great variation occurred in the level at which the squamous epithelium changed to gastric mucous membrane. In the great majority the change took place near the gastro-oesophageal junction. In 63% the change took place at the cardia. Although the squamous epithelium was never found to extend well down into the stomach (as in the horse, rat or pig), it did in some cases descend below the cardia for a few millimetres. In 33% the change was above the cardia and in 4% it was well above the cardia. In 69% it occurred below the diaphragm, in 27% at and in 5% above.

The junction was usually clearly visible as a serrated, irregular line where the smooth, pale, stratified squamous epithelium changed to the darker, more granular, glandular mucosa. In some cases, however, it was almost impossible to define the junction on macroscopic examination. The junction lies obliquely in the line of the cardia and is therefore always more distal on the right side.

Longitudinal oesophageal folds are tightly pressed together and no change occurs up to the cardia. There the folds terminate in small irregular triangular pads that radiate away from the cardiac orifice. The gastric folds begin separately at this level, and sometimes appear puckered and bunched up at the level of the hiatus. The folds bear no relation to the level of mucosal change. Even in those cases where this level does appear above the cardia, no alteration can be seen in the longitudinal arrangement of the oesophageal folds. It is quite certain that the site of mucosal change (as distinct from the cardia) cannot be located by *x*-ray examination.

Discussion

The Closing Mechanism. The exact role of the diaphragm, as a factor in preventing abnormal reflux of gastric contents in the adult, is still a matter of dispute. From the present dissections, however, there is little personal doubt as to the important function of the diaphragm in assisting the gastro-oesophageal closing mechanism of the infant. The crural muscle fibres are long, thick and well developed. The excellent overlap provides a small hiatus which is very oblique and relatively long. This, together with a tough, unstrained phreno-oeosophageal membrane ensures firm fixation. The short, almost non-existent abdominal oesophagus minimizes movement and rests snugly in the crural canal. The diaphragm thus forms a most important accessory mechanism which acts during all phases of respiration, although the marked overlap and criss-cross of the broad, stout bundles must result in a maximum constriction when it contracts. Compared with the adult, this special adaptation appears very necessary at the beginning of life. The infant is almost always supine. The stomach is relatively small, and filled every three or four hours with fluid and excess gas. Furthermore, the closing mechanism is frequently subjected to sudden bouts of raised intra-abdominal pressure during crying, hiccoughing or defaecation. Despite this, competence is excellent. In fact, competence is so remarkable that even the conventional posture and traditional tap on the back might sometimes fail to dislodge the gas bubble for five or 10 minutes after a feed. When the gas bubble eventually escapes, it does so with a characteristic burst which is easily perceptible by the flat of the hand on the abdomen; and deflation is as rapid as pricking a balloon. Practically speaking, cardiac incompetence in the normal infant is very uncommon. Thomsen (1955) examined 145 children (7 months to 7 years) radiologically, who were admitted to hospital for diseases other than gastro-intestinal. Despite steep Trendelenburg and manual compression of the abdomen, reflux was never demonstrated. However, cardiac incompetence in infants with partial thoracic stomach (where support of the diaphragm is lost) is much worse than in adults with hiatus hernia. The excellent competence in infancy is therefore not primarily due to a superior closing mechanism, but to the more efficient function of a less attenuated hiatus.

The existence of a physiological inferior oesophageal sphincter is now well accepted (Lyons, Ellis and Olsen, 1956). In a combined cine-radiographic and manometric study of the gastro-oesophageal junction, Botha, Astley and Carré (1957) proved that this sphincter extends over a considerable segment of the lower oesophagus: it is not confined to the cardia alone. The present study supports these views. In a few specimens, definite macroscopical thickening was present in the circular muscle coat, but this was never confined only to the cardia. These anatomical sphincters should not be compared with the pyloric sphincter as a standard. It is furthermore essential to remove the mucous membrane carefully before inspection of the muscle. Lerche (1950), who conducted a similar investigation in adults, concluded that anatomical sphincters do exist. Histology is notoriously unhelpful in the localization of anatomical sphincters and their presence cannot be refuted on microscopy alone.

The cardiac mucosal folds in the infant appeared without exception to be of a rosette pattern. Minor variations were frequent but no special folds, as seen in the adult, occurred. There were no 'curtains' on the greater curve side and no evidence to suggest a valve mechanism. The cardiac orifice was mostly round: the centre of symmetrically radiating mucosal folds. These folds are bunched together by the inferior sphincter so that a watertight seal is formed at the cardia. Together, these two factors act in perfect harmony and constitute the normal closing mechanism between stomach and oesophagus (Botha, 1958b).

Partial Thoracic Stomach

It has been shown that cardiac competence and oesophageal fixation are proportionately much better in infancy than in the adult. A partial thoracic stomach which causes vomiting immediately after birth is therefore not merely a 'slight herniation', but a major derangement.

The occurrence of part of the stomach in the posterior mediastinum was before considered to be rare in children. Thomsen (1949), who reviewed 70 reported cases up to 1947, published 58 cases of his own in 1955. Carré, Astley and Smellie (1952) found reference to just over 100 cases, yet they found an annual incidence of 18 infants with a partial thoracic stomach at the Children's Hospital in Birmingham. As there is no reason to suspect any recent alteration in the incidence of the condition, it is reasonable to assume that most cases have remained undiagnosed in the past. There are several reasons for this; sliding hiatal hernia has only become a recognized clinical entity over the last 20 or 30 years, and then mainly in adults. Many centres have lacked diagnostic facilities as well as experienced radiologists in this field. Recent advances in thoracic surgery have made this region readily accessible, when once the disorder is diagnosed. Another important reason for improved understanding of this condition is that a widespread interest in the oesophagus and closing mechanism has developed in the last decade, referred to in the American literature as 'esophagology'.

A considerable difference of opinion exists as to the aetiology of this abnormality. The mechanism of sliding hiatal hernia in adults has been admirably described by Allison and other workers in numerous publications. Partial thoracic stomach in infants has subsequently been regarded, without reservation, as a similar condition that developed in the same way. Husfeldt, Thomsen and Wamberg pointed out in 1951 that this explanation does not directly apply to children. The findings now recorded strongly support their view. The present confusion is considerable, partly because the evolution of the disorder is not fully appreciated. It is essential, therefore, first to point out why the mechanism of partial thoracic stomach in infants and that of sliding hiatal hernia in adults is not the same.

Evolution of Sliding Hiatal Hernia. The outstanding feature of the above anatomical observation, is the small, powerful hiatus with secure oesophageal fixation in marked contrast to the findings in the elderly. It is therefore not justified to discuss 'hiatal hernia' in infancy by referring to adult anatomy (Thomsen, 1955). It cannot be accepted that a normally developed and situated stomach with normal attachments would herniate through a normal hiatus, either shortly before or after birth, as a result of extrinsic forces that might act on the viscus.

Within the first few years of life, however, certain changes become manifest in the anatomical relationships of the cardiac region. The hiatus enlarges and the tunnel becomes shorter and less oblique. The abdominal oesophagus lengthens and becomes less securely fixed so that freer movement takes place.

These changes are even more exaggerated in the adult, due to the continuous strain on one of the potentially weak spots of the abdominal wall. The crural muscle becomes thin, stretched and weak. The force acting on the hiatus continually tends to enlarge the opening, separate the crural limbs and diminish the posterior overlap. The hiatal tunnel looses its obliquity, becomes shorter and wider until ultimately it constitutes a direct hole through the diaphragm. The phreno-oesophageal membrane stretches to a thin, attenuated layer, located only with difficulty. The elastic fibres are fragmented, dissociated and less wavy. This encourages greater mobility, so that on straining the cardia is forced into the hiatus and the aperture is further stretched, thus setting up a vicious circle. Small additional strains in the form of obesity, posture, constipation, bronchitis, corsets, etc., are sufficient to force the cardia progressively through the weakened hiatus until it lies in the posterior mediastinum. A benign situation then rapidly becomes significant. Displaced into an abnormal position, deprived of the important support of the diaphragm, the closing mechanism acts at a functional disadvantage; and when subjected to a sudden, forceful jet of gastric contents, it must give way in one direction only—into the oesophagus. As the sphincter weakens, reflux occurs more readily, until the sensitive squamous epithelium is continuously exposed to the relentless activity of gastric juice.

Oesophagitis follows. The acute inflammatory reaction is gradually followed by chronic fibrosis. The hernia increases in size, partly due to pressure from below and partly due to pull from above (the negative pressure, suction force and the remarkable longitudinal retraction of the outer muscle coat). As the cardia ascends the oesophagus maintains its straight contour, but gradually the lower portion is fixed in this position by ulceration and scarring; thus the patient ultimately ends up with a short oesophagus complicated by a stricture. The many variations on this theme need no elaboration.

In the vast majority of adults, sliding hiatal hernia is an acquired condition that usually develops in the later decades of life without any obvious congenital abnormality. It signifies a degenerative change in a normal hiatal region which is closely analogous to certain types of herniation of the anterior abdominal wall or pelvic floor and subject to the same predisposing causes.

Partial thoracic stomach in infants, I believe, is a congenital abnormality in the great majority of cases. The following facts substantiate this view.

Age Incidence. In the vast majority of infants with partial thoracic stomach (proved radiologically), symptoms date from birth or the early neonatal period: this in itself is highly suggestive of a congenital origin. In a series of 58 children with 'hiatus hernia', Thomsen (1955) found only three cases which presented after the age of 7 years. Two of these had para-oesophageal herniae (14 and 15 years) and therefore fall into a separate group and in the other child symptoms were present from birth. More than half of the infants in this series were admitted to hospital within the first year of life.

On the other hand, the incidence of sliding hiatal hernia in the 10-20 year age group without any previous symptoms is extremely small. If partial thoracic stomach is the result of simple herniation as in the adult, the incidence must increase, or at least some cases must present during this time, as the hiatus gets weaker with advancing age; the condition should not become rare.

Sex Incidence. Although Astley (1956) gives the sex incidence as equal, Thomsen (1955), Greenwald and Steiner (1929) and Truesdale (1935) found a much higher incidence amongst boys. In adult herniae, females predominate.

Familial Incidence. 'Enough familial instances occur to indicate a hereditary factor; in 10% there are one or more other cases in the family' (Astley, 1956). There may be as many as three infants in one family. The condition also occurs in twins (Wamberg, 1947) and in mother and daughter (Myles, 1939). No familial tendency has been noted in adults with herniation.

Radiology. The hiatus is sometimes unexpectedly small in adult sliding herniae. Where the hiatus is wide, a large portion of the stomach usually lies in the chest. As small herniae get bigger, reflux occurs more easily and stricture may develop.

The hiatus in infants with partial thoracic stomach is on the whole surprisingly wide; it is out of proportion to that in the adult. This lax, wide, and at times conical or tented hiatus contrasts very sharply with the normal crural pattern. With this wide gap, it is reasonable to expect further deterioration and increase in the size of the hernia as the infant gets older, if in fact, thoracic stomach is due to simple herniation. Instead, the supradiaphragmatic loculus remains small and insignificant in the majority of cases; it may even get smaller—or disappear completely. Regurgitation, however, is very free and competence relatively poor; the mechanism at the cardia is disturbed out of proportion to its radiological appearance. The fact that this wide hiatus later assists cardiac control with greater efficiency suggests that a congenitally deranged or maldeveloped diaphragm might with advancing age become more normal either by further development or by accommodation.

Clinical Course. In adults symptoms often have no relation to the radiological appearance of hiatus hernia; the tendency, however, is to deteriorate. Just the opposite happens in infants. The great majority follow a benign course and become completely asymptomatic by the age of 5 years with no subsequent relapse in childhood. The incidence of stricture varies in different centres. Untreated it is less than 10%; with adequate medical treatment it should be much less (Carré *et al.*, 1952).

Symptomatic cure does not necessarily imply restoration to normal anatomical relationships. Astley (1956) found that symptoms usually disappeared at the time of weaning to solids, although often gastro-oesophageal incompetence could still be demonstrated. At first reflux might occur from the abdominal to the thoracic portion of the stomach, although little barium passed back into the oesophagus. Later reflux ceased at the level of the diaphragm. This suggested to him an initial improvement in the sphincteric power of the oesophagus, followed later by improvement in the 'pinchcock' mechanism.

Surgery. The outcome of surgical treatment in partial thoracic stomach in infants is not nearly so good as in adults. This is the opposite to what might be expected. In at least a proportion of infants it means that either the oesophagus is congenitally short so that the tendency for the stomach to herniate is too great; or that the diaphragmatic crura are abnormal and therefore unable to maintain the stomach in its normal position after surgical repair.

Associated Abnormalities. The simultaneous occurrence of partial thoracic stomach and other malformations have been reported (Williams, 1945; Radloff and King, 1947; Thomsen, 1955; Astley, 1956; Kohler, 1957). The significance of this association is doubtful but it has been suggested as corroborative evidence in favour of a congenital origin of thoracic stomach. There is no indication that infectious diseases during pregnancy, complicated labours or prematurity have any relation to this condition. The interesting association of hypertrophic pyloric stenosis and partial thoracic stomach is too common to be disregarded. Roviralta (1952) described this combination as the 'phreno-pyloric syndrome'. Astley and Carré (1954) found five infants with pyloric stenosis as well as three other children with 'infantile pylorospasm' in a series of 115 cases with thoracic stomach. Forshall (1955) reported a series of 93 cases of 'cardio-oesophageal syndrome' in childhood in which eight infants were subjected to Rammstedt's operation. Four were irrefutable cases of pyloric stenosis. It has been suggested that herniation follows as a result of the stenosis. However, this is not true in most cases: vomiting is often present from birth; the hiatus is normal in cases of pyloric stenosis alone; and symptoms as well as the radiological appearance persist after division of the pyloric sphincter.

It is reasonable to conclude that sliding hiatal hernia in the adult is an acquired, degenerative condition that affects a normal hiatal region. Partial thoracic stomach in the infant is either due to a congenital short oesophagus or to herniation of the stomach through a congenitally malformed or undeveloped diaphragm. The relative frequency of each type is unknown. Despite statements to the contrary, it is impossible in the great majority of these cases to identify, beyond doubt, the 'congenital short oesophagus' or the 'hiatal hernia'; therefore the non-committal term 'partial thoracic stomach' is preferred.

Congenital Short Oesophagus

Tonndorf in 1923 postulated that thoracic stomach is the result of incomplete descent of the gastric organ due to failure of the oesophagus to elongate. During the fourth to seventh weeks of embryonic life, the oesophagus lengthens rapidly to keep up with the extension of the pharynx and the development of the lung buds (Botha, 1958a). If this elongation fails, the oesophagus will be partly or completely shortened. The stomach will lie somewhere in the posterior mediastinum, not because it has herniated to that position but because it has never descended into the abdomen, and it may therefore occur anywhere from the pharynx to the diaphragm. A case of extreme short oesophagus is to be published elsewhere (1958c) where the entire oesophagus consisted of a constriction of 2 or 3 mm. (Figs. 9 and 10). The stomach was in the neck, covered by peritoneum that stretched upwards like a funnel. The cardiac angle was obliterated. The poorly developed membranous diaphragm was tented up over the stomach and spleen. In the place of the hiatus was a huge, wide defect. Iniencephaly and cleft palate were also present. This maldevelopment of the diaphragm is secondary to insufficient lengthening of the oesophagus. This extreme degree of shortening, of which a previous description has not been found, must be relatively rare. More commonly the

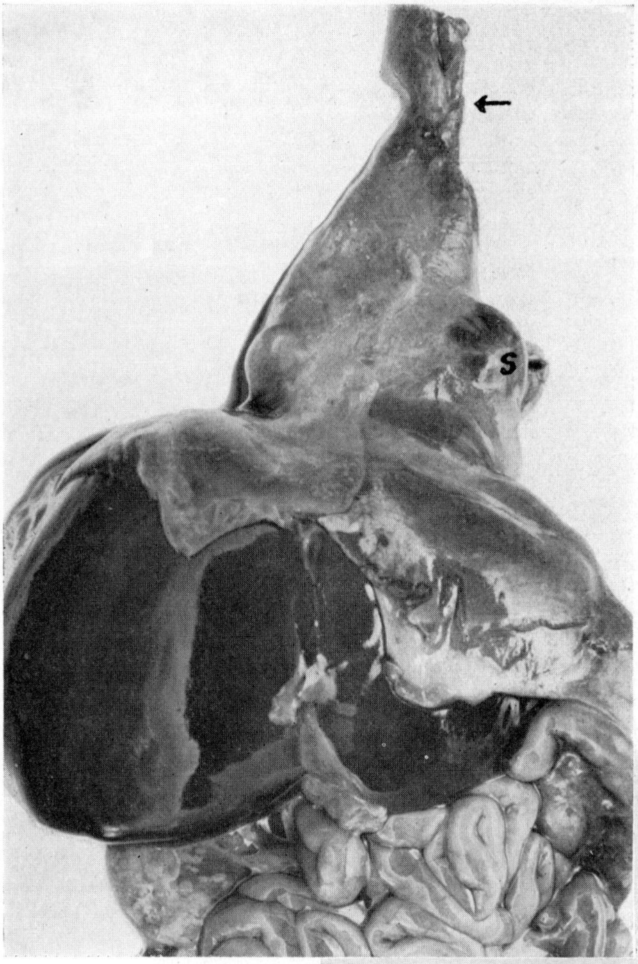

FIG. 9.—The mediastinal organs and abdominal viscera of an iniencephaly which shows complete failure of the oesophagus to elongate. The spleen (S) lies in the chest enveloped by a thin serosal membrane.

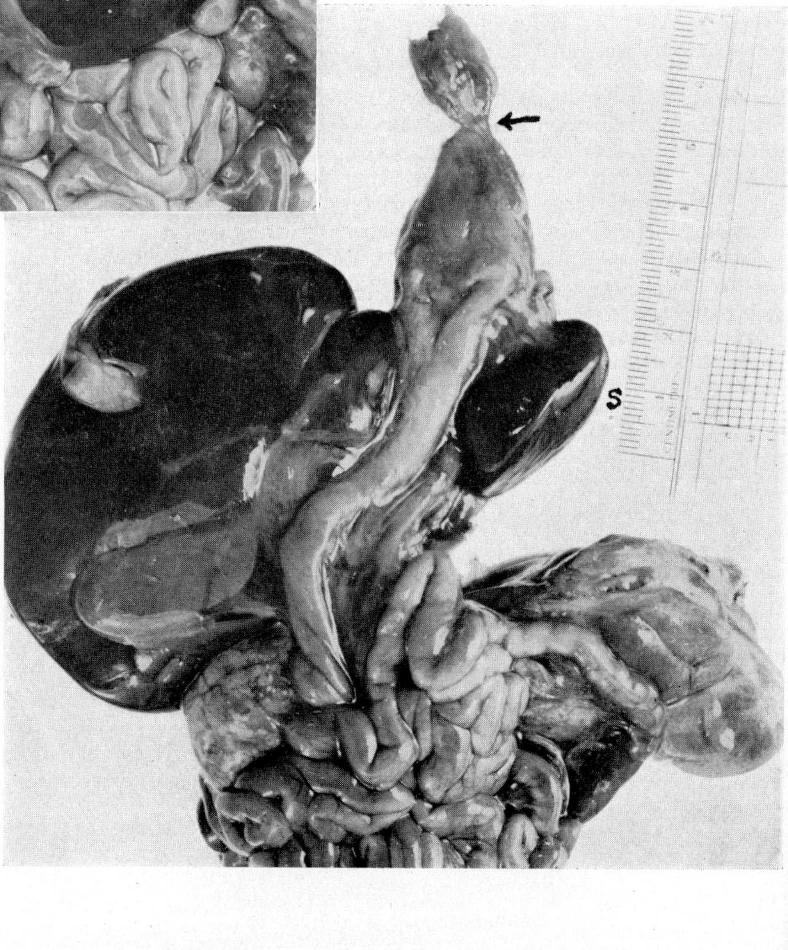

FIG. 10.—The serosal membrane in the specimen in Fig. 9 is removed. The arrow indicates the oesophagus, a mere constriction between stomach and pharynx.

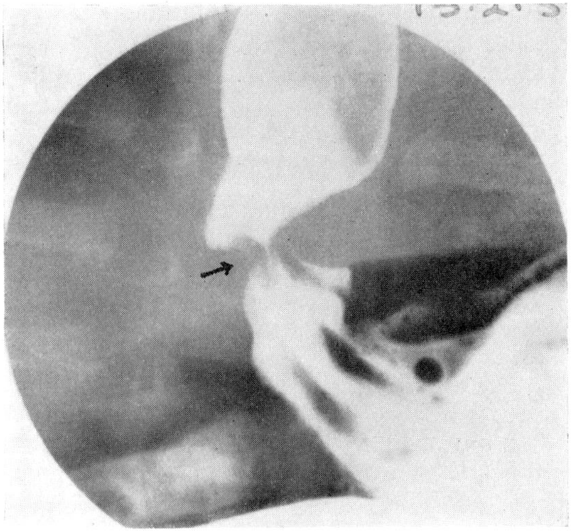

FIG. 11.—Partial thoracic stomach in an infant. The arrow indicates the 'empty segment', which is due to the contraction of the inferior oesophageal sphincter.

oesophagus extends to or below the level of tracheal bifurcation.

The oesophagus has remarkable powers of retraction. The organ may therefore shorten, after herniation of the stomach (as in a simple hiatus hernia), without any signs which might indicate its true length. It may become secondarily fixed in this position due to inflammatory changes which follow oesophagitis and ulceration; the shortening may be further aggravated by chronic fibrosis and scar contraction. Gastric mucosa is then present above the hiatus and the supradiaphragmatic loculus of stomach may in the course of years elongate to resemble the lower third of the oesophagus very closely. This well known clinical entity, which is not uncommon, is truly called 'short oesophagus' although it is not a 'congenital short oesophagus', a confusion of identity which has led to considerable misunderstanding. For this reason Tonndorf's conception fell into disrepute, especially after the papers of Johnstone (1943), Allison (1948) and others, so that later authors regarded congenital short oesophagus as a rare anomaly (Belsey, 1954; Thomsen, 1955 and Forshall, 1955). Certainly, many of the cases reported as congenital short oesophagus were really due to acquired shortening with associated hiatus hernia—described at a stage when the mechanism of hiatal herniation was imperfectly understood; but the diagnosis of congenital short oesophagus cannot be ruled out in the infant who vomits from birth and shows the following radiological features (Fig. 11): (1) A small, tubular, gastric loculus above the diaphragm; (2) a relatively fixed cardia above the diaphragm as evidenced by the distal border of the 'empty segment'. (This is due to the constriction of the inferior oesophageal sphincter and has been wrongly attributed to 'spasm' or 'stricture'). (3) A straight oesophagus; (4) obliteration of the cardiac angle; (5) a very wide, lax hiatus which may be tented.

The complete absence of oesophagitis in many infants with partial thoracic stomach entirely excludes any retraction or fixation due to chronic inflammatory scarring. Because oesophageal changes developed after one or two years in 'sliding hernia' where the gullet was normal before, Thomsen (1955) concluded that 'as is the case in adults, the shortening is due to reflux oesophagitis'. However, congenital short oesophagus necessarily implies that part of the stomach lies above the hiatus. As this deranged, insecurely fixed viscus is subject to all the forces that normally predispose to herniation, the loculus of stomach above the diaphragm may slowly increase in size. The normal closing mechanism is further disturbed, displaced and deprived of the important support of the crura. The reflux that follows leads to oesophagitis, fibrosis and more shortening. Thus 'congenital short oesophagus' and 'sliding hiatal hernia' may produce an indistinguishable end-result, and may co-exist.

Sliding Hiatal Hernia Due to a Malformed Hiatus

Instead of ascribing a primary inhibition of growth in the lower oesophagus (Tonndorf, 1923; Kelly, 1936; Lelong, 1947) as a cause for thoracic stomach, Bund (1918), Bailey (1919) and Åkerlund (1926) blamed the lack of fixation of the cardia on a persistence of the pneumato-enteric canal. This is considered unlikely because a relatively big thoracic stomach is sometimes seen at birth and even the biggest bursa should not allow this degree of mobility. Furthermore, little evidence of this peritoneal recess has been found at operation and the hiatus, which should be normally developed if the peritoneal sac is the only factor, is often abnormal. Harrington's (1940) theory that descent of the stomach is disturbed, with poor subsequent fixation to a wide hiatus, cannot be substantiated embryologically (Botha, 1958a). Shanks (1948) felt that the hiatus was congenitally enlarged, but the crural muscle was normal. Dunhill (1935 and 1948) described hiatal hernia with congenital absence of the left crus—the aorta bowed far to the left. Although this type of anomaly occurs it must be rare, and, relatively speaking, not an aetiological factor of clinical importance.

Bremer (1943) stated that hernia in the region of the tendinous antrum on the left side near the oesophagus is less common than herniation through the trigonum lumbocostale. He thought it 'due to failure of the last step in the closure of the pleural passage, the growth above the descending stomach of the thin strip of liver and septal extension to join the mediastinum. Except for the large opening the diaphragm in this type is normal'. This writer's view on the development of the diaphragm cannot be accepted (Botha, 1958a) and no clinical or experimental evidence has been found to support his theory.

Numerous vague references to 'hiatal insufficiency' appear in the literature (Allison, 1948; Johnstone, 1943), but no satisfactory explanation has been advanced as to the cause of herniation in children. Forshall (1955) found at operation in 30 cases of partial thoracic stomach that the right crus invariably appeared poorly developed, especially the left limb and the posterior fibres. The diaphragm as a whole was often unduly thin, almost flaccid to the touch. She thought that a poorly developed hiatus is the congenital element of this sliding hernia in which the cardia is drawn through the hiatus by the difference in intra-thoracic and intra-abdominal pressures. Her operative findings, supported by the findings at operation of other workers, contrast so sharply with the normal anatomy of the crura that one must accept some congenital maldevelopment at the hiatus.

The nature of this abnormality is not yet known, but the following suggestions may be considered:

(1) Congenital absence of one or both crura is rare.

(2) Failure of muscularization of hiatal muscle so that a membrane forms at the site of the crura which envelops the cranial portion of the stomach (Christiansen, 1941). However, muscularization of the diaphragm begins in the 12 mm. embryo (Botha, 1957b), when the oesophagus has already become fully elongated and the stomach has reached its normal position. There is, furthermore, no selective failure of the muscle cells to invade the septum transversum so that the rest of the diaphragm must show signs of such an anomaly if it does occur. In any case, muscle fibres are easily demonstrated in the hiatal margins in cases of partial thoracic stomach at operation and necropsy.

(3) The wide hiatus, with no muscular defect. *X*-ray appearances certainly confirm the wide hiatus. It is difficult to understand though, why infants should be born with such a wide opening in the diaphragm and the rest of the anatomy normal. A study of the embryology and development definitely points against this theory. If the oesophagus is of normal length and such a big hole exists, one would expect a progressive, large, freely movable hernia; partial thoracic stomach is small and fixed. It is also unlikely that such a primary defective lax hiatus should later resume a normal function. Thomsen (1955) stated that 'hernia' in infants is not present at birth but only develops afterwards as a consequence of the change in pressure in the thorax and abdomen, and is due to a 'lacking or abnormal fixation of the cardiac region'. From what has been said before, this statement cannot be accepted.

Very large, mobile herniae are sometimes found where the oesophagus appears of normal length and they are quite unlike the usual case of partial thoracic stomach. Although it may only be a difference of degree, it is thought that these herniae are true sliders, probably in part due to either a poorly formed hiatus or atypical arrangement of the crura (Fig. 3 and 1d).

(4) Malformed hiatus secondary to congenital short oesophagus. When the oesophagus fails to elongate, the cardia is retained in the chest. The serosa is drawn out to this level and may form a membranous sac around the upper stomach. Crural development has been interfered with; the fibres are attenuated and underdeveloped; the crura are thin and the wide hiatus is tented upwards. In the very short oesophagus (Figs. 9 and 10; Christiansen, 1941, and many others) the phreno-oesophageal elastic and serosal attachment to the high cardia has attenuated the crura to an insignificant membrane-like covering. When the abnormality is minimal, a wide hiatus and poorly developed crura, as found at operation by Forshall, may be the only anatomical signs of abnormality.

Smithers (1945) found it 'difficult to believe that short oesophagus has nearly always been overlooked at post-mortem'. However, after spending some time in the necropsy room examining hiatuses of normal subjects as well as others with hiatus hernia, I fully sympathize and agree with Anders and Bahrmann (1932) and other authors on this subject; the degree of herniation is difficult if not impossible to assess after death.

It has been said that reduction of a partial thoracic stomach at operation refutes the diagnosis of a congenital short oesophagus. This is not necessarily true. The gullet not only possesses amazing qualities of retraction but also of extension. The hiatus in the adult may move as much as two and a half vertebral bodies during respiration (Botha, 1957b). At operation, with the patient in the supine position, the oesophagus is mobilized to 'above the aortic arch level' and pulled down while the diaphragm is completely paralysed by relaxants. The cardia, after reduction, is maintained in the sub-diaphragmatic position by approximating the crura and fixing the oesophagus to the hiatal margin. This procedure might be impossible on inspiration or in the erect posture !

In conclusion, partial thoracic stomach is a relatively common disorder in infancy that might be due to congenital short oesophagus or a sliding hernia (or a combination of these conditions).

The two abnormalities cannot be distinguished in the majority of patients either by radiography or by endoscopy. I believe that a large proportion of instances of partial thoracic stomach are due to a congenital short oesophagus—a far greater percentage than has hitherto been recognized.

Para-oesophageal Hernia

Para-oesophageal herniae are uncommon. A portion of the stomach, usually the fundus, herniates through a relatively wide but otherwise normal hiatus while the cardia maintains its normal position. Cases in which the gastro-oesophageal junction has been displaced upwards, whether primary or secondary, cannot be regarded as true para-oesophageal types, but of a mixed variety. Para-oesophageal herniae are seldom present in infancy but usually occur later in childhood, adolescence or in the adult. They are always on the right side: left-sided ones are either of the mixed type or diaphragmatic. As the closing mechanism is acting in its normal position with optimum function, reflux and oesophagitis are unusual. However, this type of distortion frequently leads to ulceration, haemorrhage and even perforation.

The peritoneal sac which is commonly found is undoubtedly derived from the right pneumato-enteric recess (Åkerlund, 1926; Barrett, 1954; Botha, 1958a). Examples of these small empty sacs have been found on the right side as well as posteriorly, without any sign of herniation or any other abnormality around the hiatus. A large sac clearly invites early herniation, whereas the small ones remain as potential spaces which might later give way under strain. It then leads to a para-oesophageal hernia, a mixed hernia or it might weaken the attachment sufficiently to predispose to an ordinary sliding hernia with a sac. Harrington (1940, 1948) and Olsen and Harrington's (1948) views that these herniae, as with the sliding varieties, are due to congenital dilatation of the hiatus have not been verified.

Oesophagus Lined with Glandular Epithelium

Barrett (1950) first aroused interest in a condition which he called 'oesophagus lined by gastric mucous membrane'. Unfortunately this has been confused with congenital short oesophagus.

I have already indicated that some variation exists as to the level at which the squamous epithelium changes to glandular mucosa. In the adult, this variation is more marked and the level may occur anywhere from just below the cardia to the cricoid (Barrett, 1954). The epithelium is, however, not gastric epithelium, but glandular epithelium that closely resembles the 'zone of cardiac glands' in animals and man (Botha, 1958d). The tubules are short and tortuous; mucus-secreting alveoli are in abundance and oxyntic cells are either absent or very scanty. It is suggested that these glands represent a more primitive epithelial cell type, which, for one or other reason, has not fully differentiated into squamous epithelium (Botha, 1958d). There is evidence that these aberrations might predispose to oesophagitis and ulceration (Allison and Johnstone, 1953). Normally this condition has no relation whatsoever to short oesophagus or hiatus hernia. It might, however, be present in the lower oesophagus of a patient who later develops a hernia or it might line the lower portion of an oesophagus that is congenitally short, but it is then unusual and purely coincidental. Some of the cases reported as of gastric-lined oesophagi are actually cases of hiatal hernia or congenital short oesophagus where the cardia lies well above the diaphragm. One of the main reasons for this misconception is the view held by some workers that the squamo-glandular junction is the dividing line between stomach and oesophagus. If this is used as a standard, some animals will either possess an oesophagus and no stomach or others will only have a stomach without a gullet (Botha, 1958d). The site at which squamous and glandular epithelium meet cannot be regarded as the dividing line between stomach and oesophagus in man; it so happens that in the vast majority of people it takes place at or near the cardia.

Cardio-oesophageal Relaxation or 'Chalasia'

Neuhauser and Berenberg in 1947 reported 12 infants with 'persistent vomiting evidently due to relaxation or dysfunction of the hiatus portion of the esophagus with failure of the normal "sphincter" action of the cardia'. They called this 'cardio-esophageal relaxation or chalasia'. With conservative treatment symptoms disappeared after a few months and the infants showed no physical or fluoroscopic abnormalities. It was thought to be a temporary neuromuscular dysfunction of the hiatus portion of the oesophagus and diaphragm (Berenberg and Neuhauser, 1950). Forshall (1955) preferred the term 'lax oesophagus', because 'it is not only the cardia which is relaxed but also the whole lower two-thirds of the oesophagus'. However, it has been shown that the lower oesophagus in normal infants is characteristically wide, readily distensible and even sac-like on occasions, with irregular contractions and contours (Lelong and Aimé, 1934; Bakwin, Galenson and Le Vine, 1944; Thomsen, 1955; Henderson, 1942; Malenchini, Roca and Banzas, 1948).

There are other reasons why this condition is not likely to be a neuromuscular imbalance: the hiatus is usually wide and lax though there is no obvious autonomic connexion with the phrenic nerves or the diaphragmatic crura (Botha, 1957a). The cardiac angle is lost (Forshall) and the cardia itself appears on a higher level than normal, as if it has been ' drawn up ' into the hiatus. Drugs have no effect on this condition but recovery is remarkable in the great majority by nursing in the sitting posture. In adults, the level of the diaphragm as seen radiologically does not necessarily correspond to the level of the hiatus (Botha, 1957b). This is probably true in children, to a lesser degree, which makes it impossible to say with certainty that the cardia is below, at, or above the hiatus. One knows that in at least some of these cases, partial thoracic stomach later develops (and not necessarily associated with oesophagitis). Post-mortem and operative findings cannot be regarded as reliable. The radiological appearances are often extremely difficult to interpret and one may still be uncertain as to the diagnosis even after several examinations (Astley and Carré, 1954).

I believe that patients with 'chalasia' really suffer from mild degrees of partial thoracic stomach, but instead of the cardia being clearly in the chest, it is lying in or just above the hiatus. This slight distortion is sufficient to render the normal closing mechanism incompetent. Some deteriorate into sliding herniae. The great majority are treated medically in the sitting posture with permanent cure. Gravity assists the descent of the cardia to its normal position and thus normal competence is re-established.

Summary

The anatomy of the gastro-oesophageal region in more than 115 infants and children has been studied. The outstanding features were: a small powerful hiatus with marked overlap and an oblique lengthy tunnel; a formidable phreno-oesophageal membrane and secure fixation of a narrow terminal oesophagus. These features were considered to be mainly responsible for the superior gastro-oesophageal competence in infancy. In contrast, hiatus hernia in the elderly is a terminal degenerative manifestation in the evolution of the cardiac region.

Differences in age, sex and familial incidence, clinical course, radiological features, associated abnormalities and in the outcome of surgery support the view that the mechanism of partial thoracic stomach in infancy and hiatus hernia in adults are not identical conditions. The noncommittal term 'partial thoracic stomach' is preferred as it is impossible in the great majority of cases to distinguish between sliding hiatal hernia and congenital short eosophagus.

Evidence suggests that a large proportion of cases of partial thoracic stomach are due to congenital short oesophagus.

I am indebted to Professor F. A. R. Stammers for his interest in this work and to the Endowment Fund for a grant. I wish to thank Dr. Roy Astley for valuable advice and criticism in the preparation of this manuscript and for the radiograph: Dr. H. S. Baar, pathologist to the Children's Hospital, Birmingham, and Dr. H. G. Kohler, pathologist to the Maternity Hospital, Birmingham, for most of the anatomical material and Mr. T. F. Dee for the photographs.

References

Åkerlund, Å. (1926). *Acta radiol.* (*Stockh.*), **6**, 3.
Allison, P. R. (1948). *Thorax*, **3**, 20.
—— and Johnstone, A. S. (1953). *Ibid.*, **8**, 87.
Anders, H. E. and Bahrmann, E. (1932). *Z. klin. Med.* **122**, 736.
Astley, R. (1956). *Radiology of the Alimentary Tract in Infancy.* London.
—— and Carré, I. J. (1954). *Radiology*, **62**, 351.
Bailey, P. (1919). *Anat. Rec.*, **17**, 107.
Bakwin, H. Galenson, E. and Le Vine, B. E. (1944). *Amer. J. Dis. Child.*, **68**, 243.
Barrett, N. R. (1950). *Brit. J. Surg.*, **38**, 175.
—— (1954). *Ibid.*, **42**, 231.
Belsey, R. (1954). *Ann. roy. Coll. Surg. Engl.*, **14**, 303.
Berenberg, W. and Neuhauser, E. B. D. (1950). *Pediatrics*, **5**, 414.
Botha, G. S. Muller (1957a). *Thorax*, **12**, 50.
—— (1957b). *Lancet*, **1**, 662.
—— (1958a). *Anat. Rec.* In the press.
—— (1958b). *Brit, J. Surg.* In the press.
—— (1958c). To be published.
—— (1958d). *Acta Anat.* (*Basel*, In the press.
——, Astley, R. and Carré, I. J. (1957). *Lancet*, **1**, 659.
Bremer, J. L. (1943). *Arch. Path.* (*Chicago*), **36**, 539.
Bund, R. (1918). *Frank. z. Path.*, **21**, 243.
Carré, I. J., Astley, R. and Smellie, J. M. (1952). *Lancet*, **2**, 1150.
Christiansen, H. (1941). *Acta radiol.* (*Stockh.*), **22**, 360.
Collis, J. L., Kelly, T. D. and Wiley, A. M. (1954). *Thorax*, **9**, 175.
Dunhill, T. (1935). *Brit. J. Surg.*, **22**, 475.
—— (1948). In *British Surgical Practice*, ed. E. Rock Carling and J. Paterson Ross, Vol. 4, p. 451. London.
Forshall, I. (1955). *Arch. Dis. Childh.*, **30**, 46.
Greenwald, H. M. and Steiner, M. (1929). *Amer. J. Dis. Child.*, **38**, 361.
Harrington, S. W. (1940). *Amer. J. Surg.*, **50**, 381.
—— (1948). *Surg. Gynec. Obstet.*, **86**, 735.
Henderson, S. G. (1942). *Amer. J. Roentgenol.*, **48**, 302.
His, W. (1903). *Arch. Anat. Physiol.* [*Anat. Abt.*] (Lpz.), p. 345.
Husfeldt, E., Thomsen, G. and Wamberg, E. (1951). *Thorax*, **6**, 56
Johnstone, A. S. (1943). *Brit. J. Radiol.*, **16**, 357.
Kelly, A. B. (1936). *J. Laryng.*, **51**, 78.
Kohler, H. G. (1957). Personal communication.
Lelong, M. (1947). *Paediat. danub.*, **2**, 65.
—— and Aimé, P. (1934). *Arch. Mal. Appar. dig.*, **24**, 305.
Lerche, W. (1950). *The Esophagus and Pharynx in Action.* Springfield, Illinois.
Low, A. (1907). *J. Anat.* (*Lond.*), **42**, 93.
Lyons, W. S., Ellis, F. H. and Olsen, A. M. (1956). *Proc. Mayo Clin.*, **31**, 605.
Malenchini, M., Roca, J. and Banzas, T. (1948). *Pren. méd. argent.*, **35**, 1698.
Myles, R. B. (1939). *Brit. J. Radiol.*, **12**, 645.
Neuhauser, E. B. D. and Berenberg, W. (1947). *Radiology*, **48**, 480.
Olsen, A. M. and Harrington, S. W. (1948). *J. thorac. Surg.*, **17**, 189.
Radloff, F. F. and King, R. L. (1947). *Gastroenterology*, **9**, 249.
Roviralta, E. (1952). *Les Vomissements du Nourrisson.* Paris.
Shanks, S. C. (1948). *Brit. J. Radiol.*, **21**, 55.
Smithers, D. W. (1945). *Ibid.*, **18**, 199.
Thomsen, G. (1949). *Acta radiol.* (*Stockh.*), **32**, 193.
—— (1955). *Ibid.*, Suppl. 129.
Tonndorf, W. (1923). *Dtsch. Z. Chir.*, **179**, 259.
Truesdale, P. E. (1935), *New Engl. J. Med.*, **213**, 1159.
Wamberg, E. (1947). *Acta paediat.* (*Uppsala*), **34**, 293.
Williams, E. R. (1945). *Brit. J. Radiol.*, **18**, 323.

PAEDIATRIC SOCIETIES IN THE BRITISH ISLES

The following is a list of paediatric societies and their principal officers at the time of compilation. Alterations when they occur, information on new societies or any omissions from this list should be passed to the Secretary of the British Paediatric Association.

I: National

British Paediatric Association
President: Dr. K. H. Tallerman
Secretary: Dr. P. R. Evans
Institute of Child Health,
The Hospital for Sick Children
Great Ormond Street,
London, W.C.1.

The Royal Society of Medicine, Section of Paediatrics
President: Dr. A. Doyne Bell
Secretaries: Dr. Trevor P. Mann
H. H. Nixon, F.R.C.S.
The Royal Society of Medicine,
1, Wimpole Street,
London, W.1.

The British Association of Paediatric Surgeons
President: Miss Isabella Forshall, F.R.C.S. (Ed.)
Secretary: R. B. Zachary, Esq., F.R.C.S.
Children's Hospital,
Sheffield.

The Scottish Paediatric Society
President: Professor John Craig
Secretary: Dr. R. G. Mitchell,
Department of Child Health,
Medical School,
Dundee.

Scottish Surgical Paediatric Club
President: Matthew White, Esq., F.R.C.S (Ed.), F.R.F.P.S.G.
Secretary: Wallace M. Dennison, Esq., M.D., F.R.C.S.(Ed.), F.R.F.P.S.G.
Department of Paediatric Surgery,
Royal Hospital for Sick Children,
Glasgow, C.3.

Paediatric Pathology Club
Secretary: Dr. J. L. Emery,
Children's Hospital,
Sheffield.

Ulster Paediatric Society
President: Dr. R. W. M. Strain
Secretary: Dr. W. A. B. Campbell
19, Adelaide Park,
Belfast.

Irish Paediatric Association
President: K. M. Maughan, Esq., M.B., B.Ch.
Secretary: Dr. Raymond Rees
18, Fitzwilliam Square,
Dublin.

Welsh Paediatric Club
Secretary: c/o Professor A. G. Watkins
Department of Child Health
Llandough Hospital,
Penarth, Glam.

II: Regional

South West Paediatric Club
President: Professor A. V. Neale
Secretary: Dr. John Apley
Children's Hospital,
St. Michael's Hill,
Bristol, 2.

The Liverpool Paediatric Club
Chairman: Dr. F. P. Hudson
Secretary: Dr. R. McL. Todd,
Department of Child Health,
Alder Hey Children's Hospital,
Eaton Road,
Liverpool, 12.

Paediatric Society of the South-East Metropolitan Region
Chairman: Dr. R. C. Mac Keith
Secretary: Dr. David Morris
16 Ferncroft Avenue,
London, N.W.3.

The Aberdeen Child Health Society
President: Professor John Craig
Secretary: Dr. Norman S. Clark
374, Great Western Road
Aberdeen.

Caernarvonshire and Anglesey Paediatric Club
President: Dr. Gwyn Griffith,
Secretary: Dr. Margaret Slater
Bryniau,
Belmont Road,
Bangor, N. Wales.

Kent Paediatric and Child Health Society
President: Dr. Kenneth Cameron
Secretary: Dr. E. L. Huppert
12, Montpelier Row,
Blackheath, London, S.E.3.
Chairman: R. H. Percival, Esq., F.R.C.S.

The Leeds Regional Paediatric Club
President: Dr. W. P. Sweetnam,
Secretary: Dr. M. W. Arthurton,
The Children's Hospital,
St. Mary's Road,
Bradford, Yorks.

Leicester Paediatric Club
President: Dr. J. Vernon Braithwaite
Secretary: Dr. Leo Hahn
71, Knighton Drive,
Leicester.

Manchester Paediatric Club
President: Dr. W. H. Patterson
Secretary: Professor Wilfrid Gaisford
Department of Child Health,
St. Mary's Hospital,
Manchester, 13.

Midland Regional Paediatric Society
President: Dr. Jean M. Mackintosh
Secretaries: Dr. W. H. P. Cant and Dr. B. S. B. Wood
The Children's Hospital,
Ladywood Road,
Edgbaston,
Birmingham, 16.

Sheffield Regional Paediatric Society
President: Dr. A. P. M. Page,
Secretary: Dr. R. R. Gordon
58, Nether Edge Road,
Sheffield, 7.

The North of England Paediatric Society
President: Professor S. D. M. Court
Secretary: Dr. J. N. Stansfeld
"Hillcrest",
Farnley Hey Road,
Durham.

BOOK REVIEWS

Congenital Anomalies of the Viscera. By J. L. BREMER. (Pp. ix+202; 98 figures. 40s.) Harvard University Press (London: Oxford University Press). 1957.

The author is breaking new ground in attempting to give in book form a reasoned explanation, based on the embryology of the parts, of congenital visceral anomalies. His intention is to supplement the knowledge of human development usually gained by a medical student, and to show how slight variations in the timing of events, or changes in the relative positions of structures, lead up to many of the congenital malformations found in paediatric practice. The author gives a clear, succinct, and, at times, a very revealing account of the normal events, although some of the generalizations necessary in such a summary will not be unequivocally accepted by all embryologists as valid for human development. The normal development of each organ or system is first reviewed before the anomalies of that part are discussed. In this way the reader can readily follow the significance of variations from normal developmental sequences. Anomalies of the brain and spinal cord are omitted, except in so far as they are associated with anomalies of other viscera, as forming too vast a subject for a book of this compass. The face, the respiratory and the alimentary systems are dealt with in the first five chapters; the urinary system and suprarenals, and the male and female genital apparatus in the next two; while the heart and great vessels are considered in the four remaining chapters. The only serious omission of a common anomaly noted is that in which the apex of the developing lung is split by the right common cardinal vein, to give rise to the 'lobe of the azygos vein' in the fully formed state. It is surprising to find the statement (p. 55) that Hirschsprung's disease 'is due to no intrinsic maldevelopment or disease of the colon itself, but to a malfunctioning or stenosis' of the bowel below the dilated portion. Bodian, Stephens and Ward (1949) clearly demonstrated that a congenital absence of ganglion cells from the intramural plexuses of the narrowed distal colon is the underlying cause of the malfunctioning of the bowel in this condition.

The emphasis on alimentary and cardiovascular anomalies produces a certain imbalance in the book. The work of Barr and subsequent investigators on the sex chromatin of the female cell nucleus, and the fascinating problems of intersexuality have not been discussed. In view of the present very great interest in anomalies of the sex organs, and of the associated hormonal and chromosomal derangements, this is greatly to be regretted. These remarks are not intended in any way to detract from the many and brilliant explanations of visceral abnormality based on the logical follow-up of slight variations in the normal mechanics of development. Rather it is a matter of regret that an author, so well equipped to deal with the variations of human development, has failed in some degree to give an adequate lead in suggesting possible fundamental causal mechanisms for structural defects, or to integrate the newer knowledge of biochemical and hormonal factors which influence growth mechanisms, into the fabric of the book.

The book as a whole is beautifully set out and a pleasure to read, so that misprints, when they occur, are all the more noticeable. 'Sphincter', for example, is misspelt twice (pp. 121, 123), and 'patten' becomes 'pattern' (Fig. 12). It is inferred (Fig. 89) that rats remain in the embryonic condition for seven weeks, although the gestation period for these animals is only three weeks. Apart from such relatively unimportant faults as these, the book is to be highly commended to all seeking a clear account of the embryological basis of congenital visceral anomalies.

Bodian, M., Stephens, F. D. and Ward, B. C. H. (1949). *Lancet*, **1**, 6.

The Mentally Ill Child: A Guide for Parents. By STEVEN B. GETZ and ELIZABETH LODGE REES. (Pp. xiv+88. 25s.) Oxford: Blackwell Scientific Publications; Springfield, Illinois: Charles C. Thomas. 1957.

A book of this kind was certainly needed, for the problem of the mentally ill or psychotic child is still very imperfectly understood. It is important that those in administrative charge of children, school medical officers, doctors in infant welfare clinics, and so on, should be able to distinguish psychosis from mental defect.

This book, however, is written for parents, and for American parents at that. For the English parent inevitably much of the information about certification and placement is inappropriate to this country. A worse fault is that the book contrives to leave a confused effect; the description of the child could have given some explanation of his needs, rather than describing them in a catalogue, and the very difficult problem of relationships within the family containing a mentally ill child is discussed at a quite superficial level.

The bibliography, of 10½ pages, is a full one (with a few rather surprising omissions), but is mainly a bibliography for the professional reader. It would certainly startle a conscientious parent who embarked on it.

It is to be hoped that the success of the parents' association for children of this kind, which has been formed in America, may lead to something similar in this country. For these are children for whom administrative provisions are woefully inadequate, and who are often too sick to remain at home, too disturbed for the child guidance clinic and who tend to be relegated to occupation centres and hospitals for the mentally defective because no other provision is possible.

REGIONAL OBSTRUCTIVE EMPHYSEMA IN INFANCY

BY

JAMES THOMSON and JOHN O. FORFAR

From the Royal Infirmary, Dundee, and the Western General Hospital, Edinburgh, and from the Departments of Child Health, University of St. Andrews and University of Edinburgh

(RECEIVED FOR PUBLICATION JULY 31, 1957)

Over a quarter of a century ago Chevalier Jackson (1930) showed that the bronchi could act as valves in such a way that with respiration a lung or a lobe of a lung could become over-inflated. This valvular action would appear to be dependent on two physiological facts, first that the bronchi dilate on inspiration and contract on expiration (Reinberg, 1925; Heinbecker, 1927; Jackson, 1930), and that inspiration is predominantly an active muscular movement and is consequently more powerful than expiration which is largely a passive recoil. Thus on progressive reduction of the bronchial lumen by any obstruction a point will be reached at which the lumen is closed on expiration but allows air to enter on inspiration due to the greater power of this action and the slight bronchial dilatation which accompanies it. In the adult a functional disorder of this nature appears to be rare; in the infant, possibly due to the narrower bronchial lumen and greater elasticity of the bronchial wall, it can occur much more readily.

In generalized as opposed to regional obstructive emphysema the whole of the lung and both lungs are equally involved in the emphysematous process. Such may be seen in asthma or in acute bronchiolitis of infancy. In regional obstructive emphysema the emphysema is focal in distribution. It is more commonly unilateral but can be bilateral.

Valvular obstruction of the main lobar bronchus produces obstructive lobar emphysema in virtue of the fact that a lung lobe is a sealed self-contained unit (Fig. 1). Obstruction of smaller bronchi and bronchioles will not produce lobular emphysema provided the interalveolar pores (pores of Kohn) remain patent (Van Allen and Soo, 1933). In any segment of a lung less than a lobe these interalveolar pores allow escape of air from the alveoli in the affected segment to alveoli in the unaffected segment and thus prevent over-inflation in the affected segment. If, however, sticky secretions or other material or inflammatory swelling of the interalveolar septa cause obstruction of the interalveolar pores lobular emphysema may occur (Fig. 1). If, too, all the lobular bronchi are equally involved in the obstructive process so that no escape route for air remains, generalized lobular emphysema will result.

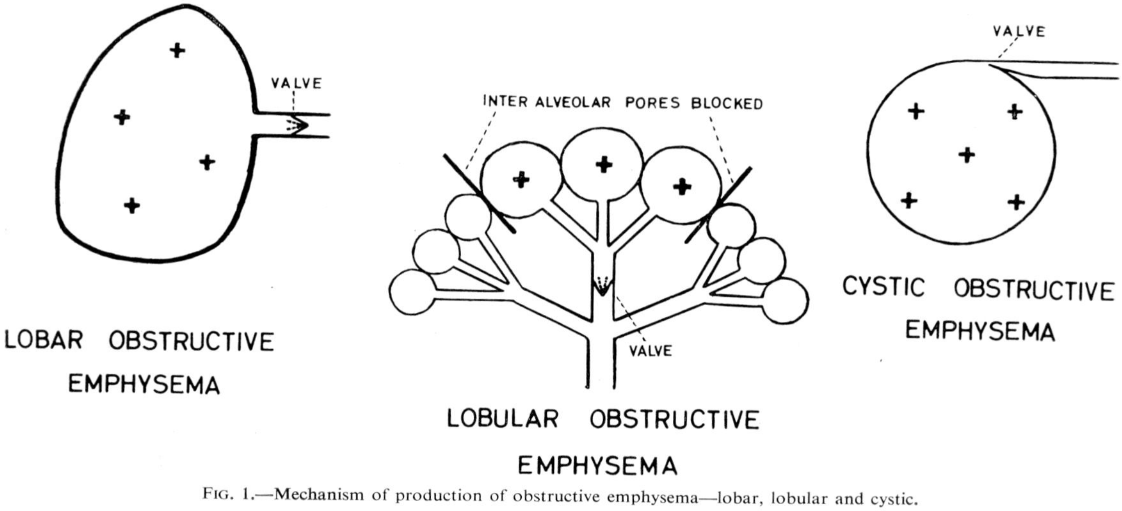

FIG. 1.—Mechanism of production of obstructive emphysema—lobar, lobular and cystic.

We report here a number of cases in which regional obstructive emphysema occurred in infants due to a variety of causes, and we classify the emphysema into three main anatomical types—lobar, lobular and cystic—with subsidiary groupings dependent on the pathogenesis of the condition.

LOBAR OBSTRUCTIVE EMPHYSEMA

Congenital Lobar Emphysema: Presumed Bronchial Obstruction

Case 1. This male infant, born at full term, was admitted to hospital on March 22, 1945, when 10 days old with the history that from the third day he had been having frequent breathless attacks. During these attacks he became cyanosed. Between attacks his breathing appeared normal. His birth had been normal.

On admission to hospital he was noted to be cyanosed and the respiration rate was rapid (60-70 per minute). The respirations were laboured. He had a cough, producing thin mucoid material. The percussion note over the left lung was hyper-resonant and over the right was impaired. On auscultation air entry was much diminished in all areas. The heart sounds were most distinctly heard on the right side of the chest.

Radiological examination revealed gross tension emphysema of the left lung, probably the left upper lobe with secondary collapse of the left lower lobe. The left side of the diaphragm was depressed, the left intercostal spaces widened and the mediastinum was displaced to the right (Fig. 2).

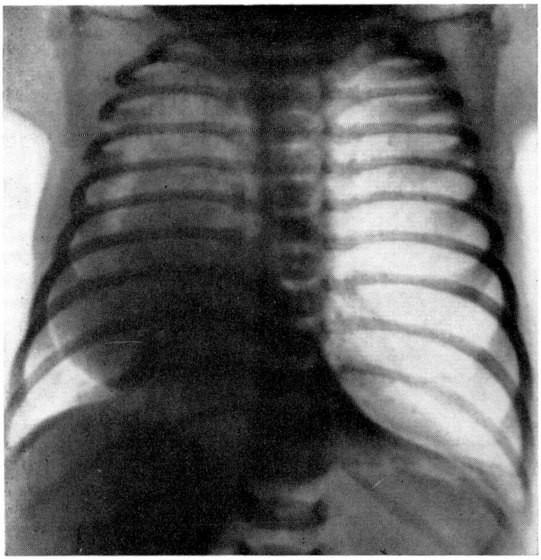

FIG. 2.—Case 1: Congenital lobar emphysema of the left upper lobe.

His condition deteriorated rapidly and he died a few hours after admission. No post-mortem examination was carried out.

Congenital Lobar Emphysema: Presumed Bronchial Obstruction

Case 2. A boy aged 4 weeks was admitted to hospital on September 26, 1955. He was the fourth child, born at full term after an uncomplicated labour lasting four hours. His birth weight was 9 lb. 5 oz. (4,198 g.).

Throughout his stay in a maternity unit his cry had been weak and his respirations noted to be somewhat laboured with accentuated respiratory movements. He was breast fed but required frequent rests during his feeds. He was discharged home on the tenth day.

On the fifteenth day of life he developed a sudden attack of cyanosis in which his lips were described as 'inky'. He held his head back and rolled it continuously from side to side. He did not lose consciousness and after one hour his colour gradually improved.

During the next two weeks he had several similar attacks of 10 to 60 minutes' duration. These bore no relation to feeding. For a week before admission he had a cough.

On admission he was a well-nourished baby with a weak cry. The temperature and pulse rate were normal. The respiration rate was 50 per minute. He had a slight cough and the alae nasi were moving. The chest remained fully expanded in all phases of respiration and the apex beat could not be detected. There was marked indrawing of the lower intercostal spaces and upper abdomen associated with vigorous respiratory efforts. Over the right lung the percussion note was hyper-resonant and over the left it was relatively diminished. The breath sounds were much reduced on the right side and to a lesser extent on the left. Radiological examination showed well-marked obstructive emphysema of the right lung with displacement of the mediastinum to the the left (Fig. 3). The right lower and probably right

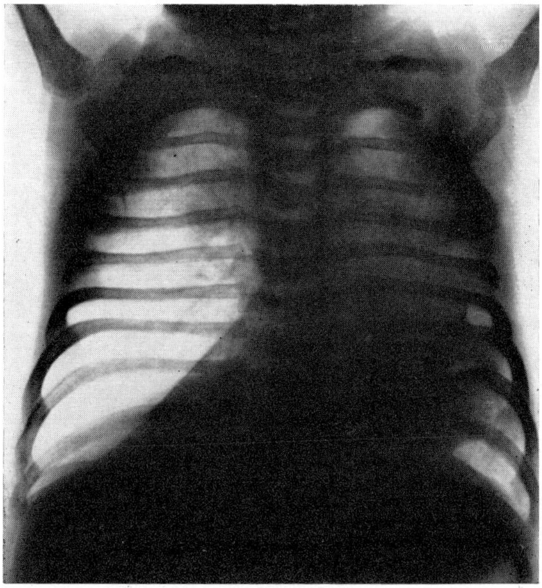

FIG. 3.—Case 2: Congenital lobar emphysema of the middle lobe of the right lung.

upper lobes were subject to pressure collapse, suggesting that it was the middle lobe which was emphysematous. The intradermal tuberculin test was negative up to a strength of 1/1,000.

On the second day after admission he had two brief cyanotic attacks accompanied by marked respiratory embarrassment and a severe degree of cyanosis not immediately relieved by oxygen.

Two days later bronchoscopy (Mr. M. Fallon) was carried out. During induction of anaesthesia and during the operation there was considerable respiratory difficulty. The left bronchus appeared normal. The right showed no evidence of a foreign body, but a bleb of pus was present in it and appeared to be coming from the right upper lobe bronchus.

On the following day he suddenly developed glottic oedema and required an emergency tracheotomy. Frequent suction was maintained through the tracheotomy tube and during this time there was no respiratory embarrassment. Thereafter the tracheotomy wound was allowed to close. When it did so episodic respiratory difficulty returned.

Radiologically right-sided emphysema persisted ; paradoxical movement of the mediastinum was not observed but absence of movement of the right side of the diaphragm was evident on screening.

Operative removal of the affected lobe was decided on, and was carried out at the age of 7 weeks. The operation was preceded by paracentesis through the chest wall, and the intrapulmonary pressure within the emphysematous lobe was found to be greater than the 35 cm. of water which was the highest pressure which our manometer could record. The normal pressure at this age is said to be less than 5 cm. of water. Deflation of the emphysematous lung facilitated anaesthesia. At operation the right middle lobe was seen to be grossly distended even in spite of decompression. It was resected. The adjacent lobes re-expanded immediately.

Post-operatively the child made a satisfactory recovery although he subsequently suffered an attack of pneumonia. Apart from that he has remained well over the past 18 months and radiologically the lung fields have remained normal.

Pathological examination of the excised middle lobe (Dr. K. Rhaney) showed that the whole of the right middle lobe was grossly over-inflated. Injected fluid passed freely in and out of the main bronchus. Cartilage in the walls of the bronchus appeared deficient but this may have been due to overdistension, giving a false appearance of disproportion. No mucous membrane folds or aberrant blood vessels likely to cause obstruction were found. Thus no convincing pathological cause for the obstruction could be demonstrated.

The possibility remains that deficiency of cartilage or some obstruction of the portion of the main bronchus not removed at operation was the responsible factor. It is possible also that functional distortion of the bronchus not evident in the excised lobe was present in life and contributed to the valvular obstruction.

Congenital Lobar Emphysema : Presumed Bronchial Obstruction

Case 3. This boy was born on September 3, 1956, some three weeks prematurely by spontaneous vertex delivery, birth weight 6 lb. 2 oz. (2,778 g.). He cried lustily after birth but the hands, feet, and face were cyanosed. A good deal of liquor was aspirated. Oxygen lessened but did not abolish the cyanosis. Some five hours after birth the respirations had become shallow and rapid (approximately 100 per minute). A few hours later there was marked costal margin recession and intercostal indrawing. It was noted that he was less distressed when lying on the right side. At that stage there was some diminution of air entry over the left lung. Radiologically the left lung was only slightly aerated, aeration of the right lower lobe was diminished and it was apparently normal in the right upper lobe. Despite this a lateral view showed anterior bowing of the sternum, suggesting emphysema, and well-marked aeration of the retrosternal space.

Three days later the respiration rate fell suddenly to 50-60 per minute, most of the symptoms disappeared and a chest film showed normal aeration of both lungs. Thereafter over a period of a month there were several episodes of sudden tachypnoea and slight cyanosis, not usually of longer than 15 minutes' duration. Periodic radiological examination showed varying degrees of collapse of the right middle and lower lobes. There was evidence of increased pressure within the right upper lobe with increased density of air, widening of the intercostal spaces and horizontal positioning of the ribs (Fig. 4). On screening the right upper lobe remained inflated on expiration and herniated across the mediastinum (Fig. 5).

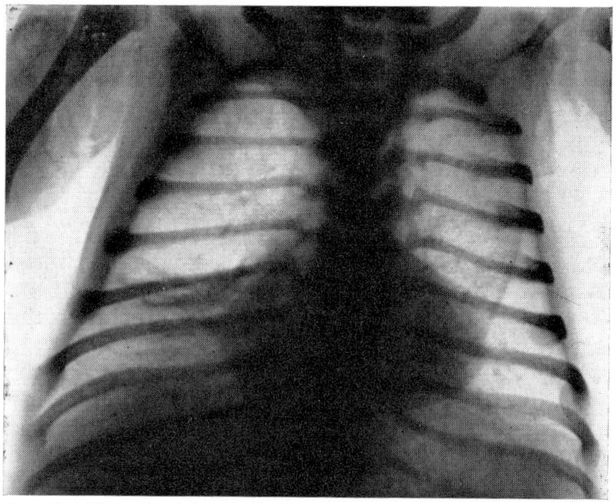

FIG. 4.—Case 3: Obstructive emphysema of the right upper lobe, showing horizontal position of ribs, widened intercostal spaces, and partial collapse of right middle and lower lobes.

At the age of 2 months a bronchogram was carried out. Lipiodol freely entered the collapsed right lower and middle lobes showing no evidence of bronchial obstruction. The right upper lobe bronchus was filled much less satisfactorily despite attempts to accomplish

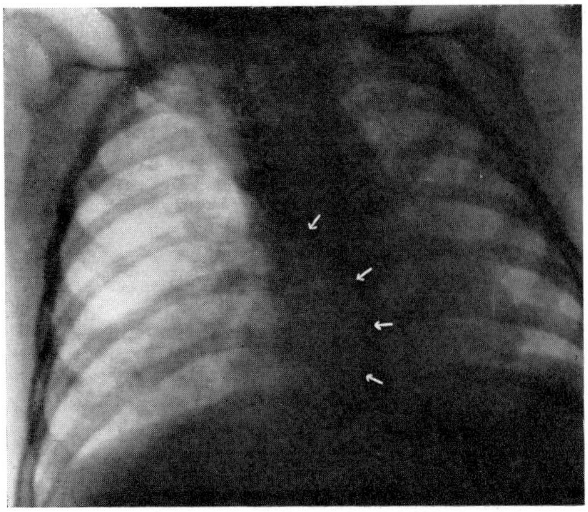

FIG. 5.—Case 3: Obstructive emphysema of the right upper lobe and mediastinal pleural herniation on expiration.

this. At this stage the air entry over the right upper lobe was markedly diminished.

This infant was considered to be suffering from congenital lobar emphysema of the right upper lobe. In the first few days of life this had prevented adequate expansion of the left lung and right lower lobe, presumably due to pressure on them, and latterly had caused pressure collapse of the right lower lobe.

After the age of 1 month his symptoms became less severe and he began to feed well and to gain weight satisfactorily. By the age of a year he was relatively symptom free, although he became severely distressed during an intercurrent respiratory infection. Radiologically there was little change in the lung.

Lobar Obstructive Emphysema: Extrabronchial Compression by an Enlarged Heart

Case 4. This girl had been born at term, birth weight 6 lb. (2,722 g.). Her progress appeared to be satisfactory until she was 9 months old, when she developed cough, anorexia and fretfulness. Five days after the onset of these signs she was admitted to hospital.

At the time of admission, on November 8, 1948, she was relatively symptom free but radiological examination of the chest showed cardiac enlargement with some emphysema of the lower lobe of the right lung. There were no cardiac murmurs. Two days after admission there occurred a sudden incident of respiratory embarrassment when her respiration rate rose to 80 per minute, and the percussion note over the right lung became hyper-resonant as compared with the left. These signs disappeared after a few hours. For 10 days she remained well then developed, quite suddenly, a further episode of tachypnoea with respiratory distress. Clinically the heart was displaced to the left and there was intercostal indrawing. Radiological examination after the worst of her symptoms had passed off showed tension emphysema of the right middle and lower lobes (Fig. 6). A lateral film showed the trachea displaced backwards by the enlarged heart (Fig. 7).

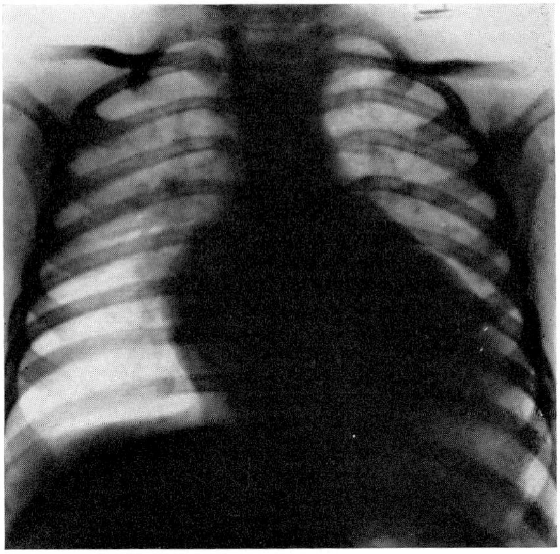

FIG. 6.—Case 4: Enlarged heart and obstructive emphysema of the right lower lobe.

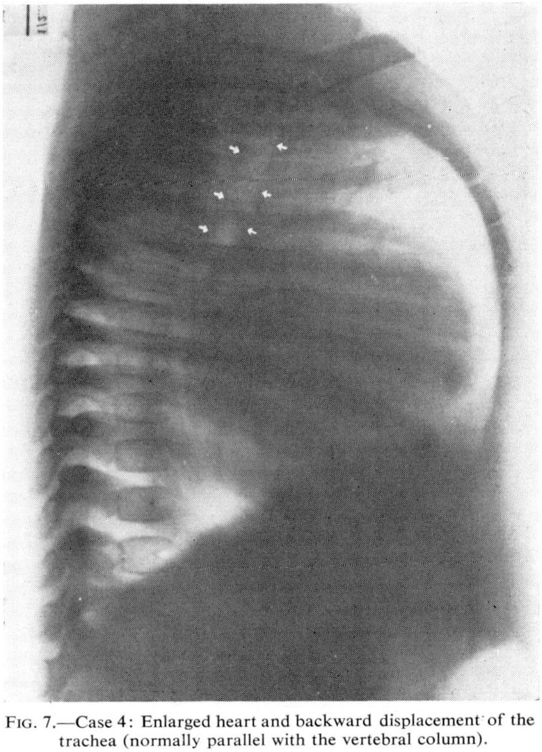

FIG. 7.—Case 4: Enlarged heart and backward displacement of the trachea (normally parallel with the vertebral column).

Over the next few weeks a minor degree of emphysema of the right middle and lower lobes persisted. Finally the left lung collapsed suddenly and completely causing gross respiratory distress and she died 24 hours later.

At post-mortem examination the heart was enlarged 75% above the normal weight for this age. There were no valvular or septal defects. Unfortunately the heart was not examined histologically. The left lung was collapsed due to the pressure of the large heart on the left bronchus. The right lower lobe bronchus appeared liable to pressure from the same cause. There was emphysema of the right middle and lower lobes with partial collapse of the right upper lobe. Histological examination of the lungs confirmed the macroscopic findings.

Thus external pressure on the right lower lobe bronchus appeared to be the mechanism producing tension emphysema in this case.

Lobar Obstructive Emphysema : Extrabronchial Compression by Enlarged Glands and Bronchial Obstruction by Mucopus

Case 5. This boy, whose birth weight was 6½ lb. (2,948 g.), was a first child of a British mother and an Indian father. There was no family history of tuberculosis. At the age of 4½ months he was admitted urgently to hospital. For 11 days he had had a cough and wheezy respiration, and a few hours before admission to hospital he had become remarkably breathless and restless.

On admission on September 6, 1948, he showed well-marked respiratory distress with intercostal indrawing and a respiration rate ranging from 40 to 60 per minute. The chest remained in the position of full inspiration. After a few hours his symptoms passed off but returned on the following day when there was diminished air entry over the lower lobe of the right lung with fullness of the right side of the chest. The percussion note over the right lung was resonant.

Radiological examination showed marked tension emphysema of the middle and lower lobes of the right lung, cardiac displacement to the left, depression of the right diaphragm, increase in the width of the intercostal spaces, upward displacement of the interlobar fissure and a mediastinal pleural hernia (Fig. 8). Radiological examination three days later when his acute symptoms had abated showed that the tension emphysema in the right lung had greatly diminished.

Over the ensuing weeks there was a progressive infiltration into the right lung with hilar gland enlargement. Bronchoscopy was carried out six weeks after admission. No foreign body was seen. A considerable amount of thick, sticky secretion was present in the right main bronchus and the mucosa was swollen, but no blockage could be detected. The left bronchus appeared normal. Two days after bronchoscopy a tension pneumothorax developed on the right side of the chest. This was relieved by removing 200 ml. of air which was under considerable pressure. A week later he again developed a tension pneumothorax which, on this occasion, was accompanied by gross surgical emphysema extending from the neck to the lower limbs, and he died a few days later. The intradermal tuberculin test had been negative up to 1/100 on two occasions a month apart.

At post-mortem examination there was mucopurulent secretion in the right lower lobe bronchus. A cavity was present at the right hilum but it was impossible to tell whether this was a liquefied lymph gland or a cavity in lung tissue. There was a septic bronchopneumonia with multiple abscess formation in the right lower lobe. There was also a cavity in the dorsal segment of the right lower lobe. The right lower lobe was covered with a fibrinopurulent layer and the remainder of the lung was adherent to the chest wall. Histological examination revealed a widespread tuberculous infection of the right lung and infection was also demonstrated in the left lung.

The mechanism producing the tension emphysema in this case appears likely to have been a combination of extrabronchial compression by tuberculous glands and intrabronchial obstruction by mucopurulent secretions. The latter appears to be the factor which precipitated the emphysema and which accounted for its sudden onset and disappearance.

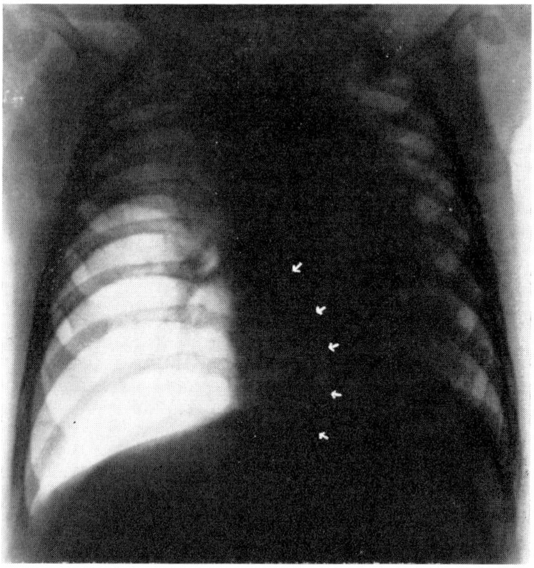

FIG. 8.—Case 5: Obstructive emphysema of the right lower lobe.

Lobar Obstructive Emphysema : Bronchial Obstruction by Mucopus

Case 6. This boy was born at home, birth weight 6 lb. 12 oz. (3,062 g.). He made satisfactory progress for the first four weeks. Five days before admission to hospital he developed an upper respiratory tract infection. Just before admission respiratory symptoms became much more marked with cough, cyanosis and increasing dyspnoea.

On admission on February 13, 1957, his temperature was 101° F. and his respiration rate 60 per minute. There was indrawing of the intercostal spaces and costal margin recession. The left side of the chest was fuller than the right. Coarse crepitations were audible over both lungs, especially the right. Cyanosis was evident and responded to oxygen. The white cell count was 14,000 per c.mm.

Radiological examination showed obstructive emphysema involving the left lung with some displacement of the mediastinum to the right and slight mediastinal pleural herniation, increased aeration of the left lung with widening of the intercostal spaces and depression of the diaphragm (Fig. 9). The right lung showed secondary collapse with patchy consolidation.

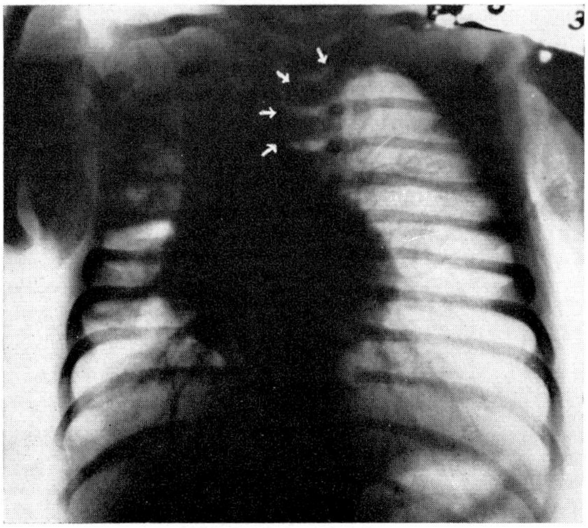

FIG. 9.—Case 6: Obstructive emphysema of the left lung, mediastinal displacement, partial collapse and consolidation of the right lung.

After 48 hours' treatment with penicillin and streptomycin most of his symptoms had disappeared, his temperature had become normal and radiographs of the chest showed that obstructive emphysema was no longer present, the lungs showing only minor inflammatory change.

He made an uninterrupted recovery. It appears likely that the obstructive emphysema of the left lung resulted from obstruction of the left main bronchus with mucopus in an infant suffering from pneumonia.

LOBULAR OBSTRUCTIVE EMPHYSEMA

Lobular Obstructive Emphysema : Aspiration of Mucus and Spontaneous Pneumothorax

Case 7. This boy was born at term on October 14 1956. He was very 'mucousy' at birth and was asphyxiated. He was given intragastric oxygen. He remained cyanosed and respiratory movement was accentuated. Crepitations were audible over both lungs. Radiological examination just after birth showed patchy atelectasis throughout both lungs with an area of obstructive emphysema at the left lung base (Fig. 10). Respiratory embarrassment continued and a second radiograph seven hours after the first showed a pneumothorax on the left side. Paracentesis of the left pleural cavity produced a few millilitres of air with some diminution of respiratory distress. On the following day marked respiratory embarrassment recurred and was relieved by aspirating the pleural cavity, when 20 ml. of air under considerably increased pressure were removed. Again there was marked clinical improvement. A few hours later the chest had again to be tapped. Over the next 24 hours his respiratory difficulty progressively diminished and the crepitations which had persisted from birth gradually disappeared. He made a satisfactory recovery and two days after birth there was no longer radiological evidence of pneumothorax.

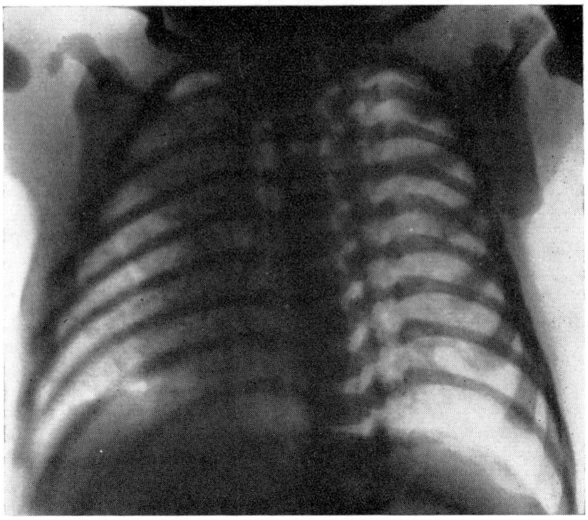

FIG. 10.—Case 7: Lobular obstructive emphysema of the left lower lobe.

Aspiration of mucus into the lungs in this case appeared to have produced obstructive emphysema involving particularly the lower lobe of the left lung. Air had ruptured into the pleural cavity from the over-distended left lung causing a pneumothorax.

Lobular Obstructive Emphysema : Aspiration of Mucus

Case 8. This boy was born at term on April 14, 1956, by spontaneous vertex delivery, the birth weight being 6 lb. 3 oz. (2,806 g.). He was very 'mucousy' at birth. Twelve hours after birth moderate respiratory difficulty was still present, the costal margin receding on inspiration and the anterior chest wall bulging forward. Radiological examination showed hyperaeration of the lungs, particularly on the left side with splaying and horizontal positioning of the ribs, depression of the diaphragm and some mediastinal displacement to the right (Fig. 11).

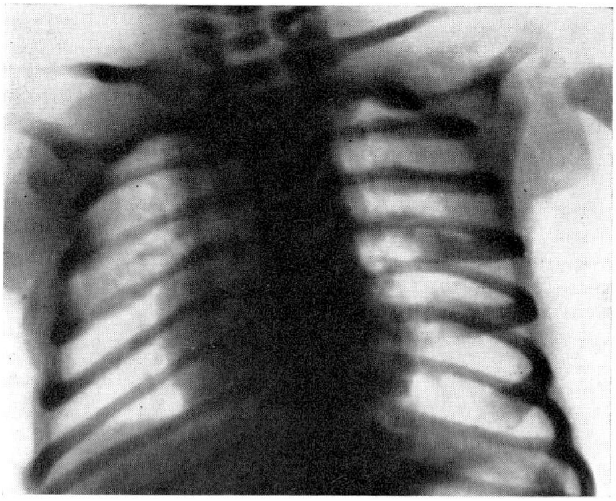

FIG. 11.—Case 8: Obstructive emphysema, especially of the left lung, widening of the rib spaces and slight mediastinal displacement.

A few days later all abnormal physical and radiological signs in the chest had disappeared.

In this case, consequent on aspiration of mucus, there appeared to be widespread tension emphysema with the left lung more affected than the right.

Lobular Obstructive Emphysema : Aspiration of Vomitus

Case 9. This boy was born at term, the birth weight being 7 lb. 4 oz. (3,289 g.). At the age of 11 weeks he developed an acute episode of vomiting. A few hours after the onset of this he was found in his cot collapsed and in obvious respiratory distress. He was admitted to hospital on May 9, 1956, exhibiting marked broncho-spasm and with the chest fully inflated. He died shortly after admission.

Post-mortem examination (Dr. K. Rhaney) showed aspirated vomit throughout most of the bronchial tree, even to the smallest respiratory passages. Most of the lung tissue was acutely over-distended with air and the lungs did not collapse on opening the chest. Histological examination confirmed the emphysema of the lungs and showed no evidence of acute inflammation.

No doubt in this case the vomitus blocked the bronchi in such a way as to obstruct outflow of air but allowed some entry of air on inspiration.

CYSTIC OBSTRUCTIVE EMPHYSEMA

Cystic Obstructive Emphysema : Congenital or Acquired Cyst

Case 10. This boy was born six weeks prematurely on March 4, 1955, the birth weight being 3 lb. 12 oz. (1,701 g.). He fed poorly from birth but apart from that remained reasonably well for two weeks when he developed gastro-enteritis. This illness was complicated by pneumonia. Two weeks later he suffered a second attack of pneumonia from which he again made a satisfactory recovery.

At the age of 3½ months he had a third attack of pneumonia accompanied by a febrile convulsion, and was admitted to hospital. Radiological examination showed an air-containing cyst in the left lung in the posterior basal segment of the lower lobe (Fig. 12).

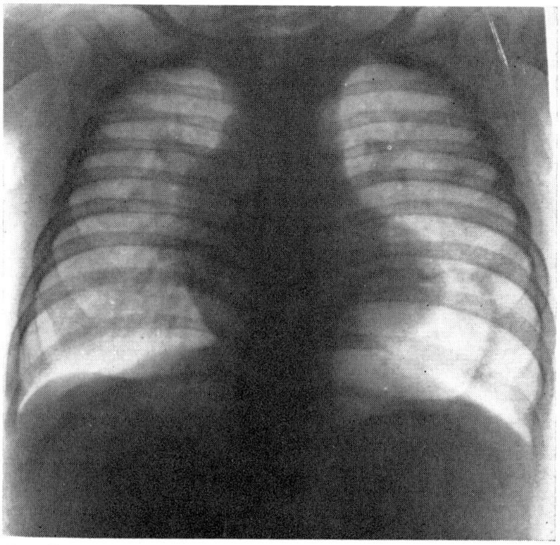

FIG. 12.—Case 10: Congenital or acquired cyst of the left lower lobe.

Clinically he was noted to be intermittently dyspnoeic, particularly on sitting up. The intercostal spaces were markedly indrawn and the costal margin receded on respiration. He had a persistent cough.

Intermittent respiratory embarrassment and indrawing of the chest persisted for four months. The cyst remained unaltered and it was decided to remove it. At operation on November 16, the lower lobe was found to be adherent to the paravertebral gutter and the diaphragm. The lung was freed and the lower lobe was found to contain a large cyst with collapse of surrounding lung tissue. The cyst was removed by resection (Mr. M. Fallon).

On recovery the remainder of the left lung expanded fully, and over a period of a fortnight all abnormal signs disappeared from the chest, except some costal indrawing.

On pathological examination (Dr. K. Rhaney) the cyst was found to be surrounded by lung tissue. A bronchus entered the cyst from the supero-medial aspect, running obliquely through the wall and entering the cavity under a crescentic valve-like fold in the external lining. Macroscopically there was no evidence of pneumonia. Histologically the cyst was found to be of bronchial origin, lined by pseudo-stratified ciliated columnar epithelium.

Deep to the epithelium were bundles of smooth muscle fibres forming a complete layer round the cyst. A bar of cartilage was present in the cyst wall, the surrounding lung was collapsed, and in the hilar region there was some chronic inflammatory change.

It would be difficult to say whether this cyst was congenital and predisposed to recurrent pneumonia or whether it was the result of the attacks of pneumonia. The mechanism whereby it persisted seems clear, however, namely the valvular entry of the bronchus into its wall.

Cystic Obstructive Emphysema : Post-pneumonic Pneumatocoeles

Case 11. This girl was the third child of healthy parents. She was born at full term on May 7, 1953, her birth weight being 7 lb. 13 oz. (3,544 g.). On the second day she began to vomit and on the fourth day the vomitus was slightly bloodstained. An oesophageal hiatus hernia was suspected and on the sixth day a 'lipiodol' swallow was given. This showed that an oesophageal hiatus hernia was present, but during the examination some 'lipiodol' was aspirated into the lungs with the result that inadvertently bronchography was carried out. This showed a normal bronchial tree and the lung fields were clear.

She was nursed in the upright position and the vomiting lessened. She was discharged home on the 23rd day gaining weight satisfactorily. Eight days later she was readmitted to hospital. For the previous few days the vomiting had increased, she had become fevered and her respirations had become grunting and rapid. Physical examination showed a marked impairment of the percussion note over the upper half of the left lung, coarse crepitations over the posterior aspect of the left lung and some mediastinal displacement to the right. The white cell count was 27,000/c.mm. Radiological examination of the chest showed consolidation of the left upper lobe with early formation of multiple bullae. She was given penicillin intramuscularly, 100,000 units four-hourly, and streptomycin, 0·25 g. six-hourly. After two days her condition remained unchanged and on this account she was given oxytetracycline, 50 mg. six-hourly by mouth, in place of the other antibiotics. From sputum obtained by a cough swab coagulase-positive staphylococci were cultured. The diagnosis made was that of staphylococcal pneumonia involving predominantly the upper lobe of the left lung.

Clinically she responded satisfactorily to oxytetracycline therapy but serial radiological examination showed the development of large emphysematous bullae within the substance of the left upper lobe. Over a period of several weeks these progressively increased in size showing evidence of positive pressure (Fig. 13). She developed an obvious asymmetry of the chest with ballooning of the upper part of the left thorax anteriorly, diminished respiratory movement on that side and costal margin recession. On percussion the area of deep cardiac dullness was absent. There was diminished air entry over the left lung.

This infant continued to be nursed in the upright position and despite the large bullae made very satisfactory progress with a normal weight gain and no cough. Her respiration rate varied between 30 and 70 per minute. The bullae persisted unchanged for a period of nine months. At the end of that time they began to diminish in size and disappeared entirely over a period of two months. She has remained well since, over a period of two years, and has had no further respiratory symptoms. The chest radiograph remains quite clear.

Combined Cystic Obstructive Emphysema and Lobar Obstructive Emphysema

Case 12. A boy, the third child of healthy parents, weighed 6 lb. 1 oz. (2,750 g.) at birth. The birth had been normal at full term and there had been no post-natal asphyxia or respiratory difficulties.

When 7 weeks old he suffered from bronchitis and a week later was admitted to an infectious diseases hospital with gastro-enteritis. He was in hospital for three and a half weeks due to slow recovery and poor weight gain. During his stay in hospital his respiration rate rose suddenly one day to 80 per minute, remained at 50 to 80 per minute for two days and then returned to normal. This incident was accompanied by marked tachycardia.

On June 24, 1949, at the age of 6 months, he was admitted to hospital, having been vomiting for three days. He was noted to be only 50% of the expected weight but no respiratory signs were evident. During the first week his respiration rate was occasionally a little rapid. On the tenth day, following a feed, he developed marked tachypnoea accompanied by respiratory distress. At the same time there was an obvious fullness of the right side of the chest compared with the left; there was a hyperresonant percussion note over the right chest anteriorly and there was marked lower intercostal and costal margin recession, the thoracic cage staying fixed in the position of full inspiration. The breath sounds were diminished over the right lung and the apex beat was

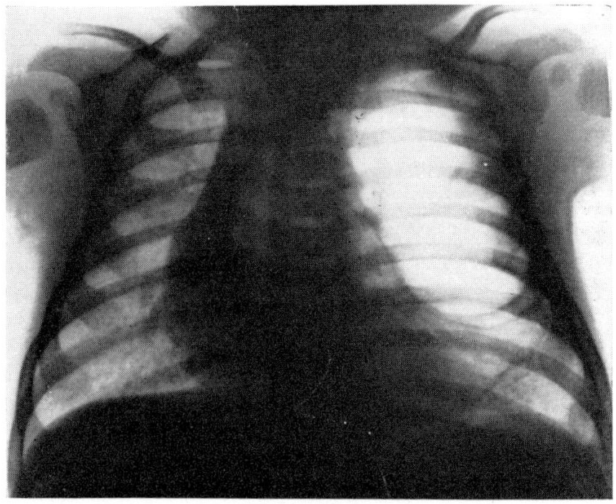

FIG. 13.—Case 11: Fully developed post-pneumonic (staphylococcal) pneumatocoele.

displaced to the left half an inch outside the mid-clavicular line. There was no cough or asthmatoid wheeze. The intradermal tuberculin test was negative up to a strength of 1/1,000. Radiological examination confirmed the presence of obstructive emphysema of the right lung with abnormal radiotranslucency, herniation of the mediastinal pleura into the left hemithorax, cardiac displacement to the left, paradoxical movement of the mediastinum and diminished movement of the right diaphragm (Fig. 14). There appeared to be two air-containing cysts at the region of the right hilum. Thereafter tachypnoea (50 to 100 per minute) and respiratory embarrassment remained constant.

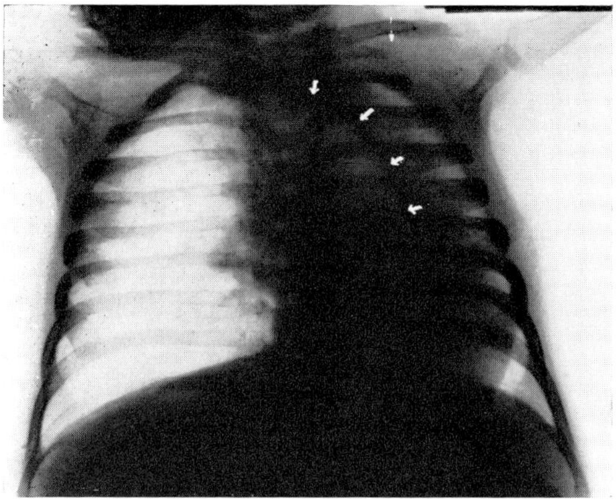

FIG. 14.—Case 12: Obstructive emphysema of the right lung with mediastinal pleural herniation.

A few days later bronchoscopy was carried out (Mr. M. J. Gibson). The lumen of the right main bronchus was seen to be moon-shaped, apparently as a result of external pressure. Thereafter dyspnoea became progressively worse, the child's condition deteriorated and he died three weeks after admission to hospital.

At post-mortem examination (Dr. A. B. Goodall) the right lung was voluminous and occupied the whole of the right half of the thoracic cavity and part of the left half, its left anterior border being 2 cm. to the left of the midline. The heart was displaced to the left, the right border of the heart being to the left of the midline. The left lung appeared small and compressed towards the posterior chest wall. The heart was normal and the ductus arteriosus closed. The innominate artery was very short and the right common carotid and subclavian arteries sprang almost directly from the aorta. The bronchial and intercostal arteries appeared to originate normally. A multilocular mucous cyst was present in the superior mediastinum on the left side behind the oesophagus and the trachea, the largest loculus of this cyst being about half an inch in diameter. On section the gross emphysema of the right lung was confirmed. There was no differentiation of the lung into lobes. At the hilar region within the lung substance there was a cyst ½ in. in diameter and immediately above it a smaller cyst about half this size. These cysts were in close relationship to the right main bronchus, the bronchus passing across the posterior wall of the main cyst in its upper aspect. The cysts contained air. Inflation of the right main bronchus caused air bubbles to appear at a slit-like opening in the antero-lateral wall of the larger cyst. This opening was covered by a flap and the obliquity of the track into the cyst was such that the flap acted as a valve preventing egress of air from the cyst. The left lung was not normally lobulated and there was only a rudimentary interlobar fissure. Lymph nodes were not enlarged.

The spleen weighed 4 g. and the liver 170 g. The left kidney weighed 23 g. and there was a normal left ureter. The right kidney and right ureter were absent. The right renal artery was also absent and there was no right ureteric orifice in the bladder. The pancreas appeared normal.

In this case there appeared to be a double valvular mechanism: an air-containing tension cyst at the hilum exerting pressure on the right main bronchus in such a way that valvular emphysema of the lung resulted.

Discussion

These cases are fairly gross examples of regional obstructive emphysema in infancy and illustrate a variety of pathological conditions in which this disorder may occur.

The classification suggested might be represented schematically in the following way:

REGIONAL OBSTRUCTIVE EMPHYSEMA

Lobar		Lobular	Cystic
Congenital lobar emphysema		Liquor amnii Mucus Mucosal swelling Vomitus } producing bronchiolar obstruction in a regional distribution	Congenital tension cysts Acquired (post-pneumonic) cysts
Foreign body Mucus or mucopus Mucosal swelling Granulation tissue	Intra-bronchial		
Enlarged hilar glands Enlarged heart Extra-bronchial cysts Aberrant blood vessels including ductus arteriosus	Extra bronchial		
Mixed Forms			

It is not suggested that every cause of regional obstructive emphysema is mentioned in the above classification but this classification could probably include within it all forms of regional obstructive emphysema whatever the cause.

Diagnosis

Clinically marked obstructive emphysema is likely to be associated with a bulging or 'blown' chest wall, with a resonant or hyper-resonant percussion note and with diminished air entry over the affected region. There may also be signs of mediastinal displacement and loss of cardiac dullness.

Radiologically obstructive emphysema is most likely to be confused with collapse associated with compensatory emphysema. In obstructive emphysema there is essentially evidence of positive pressure over-inflation of the affected part of the lung so that in grosser degrees there may be downward depression of the diaphragm, splaying of the ribs, anterior bowing of the sternum, mediastinal shift, mediastinal pleural herniation and paradoxical movement of the mediastinum on breathing. In Cases 2, 3 and 5 obstructive emphysema of one lobe was associated with secondary pressure collapse of the adjacent lobe. It is important that such a secondary collapse due to external pressure should be differentiated from primary collapse due to bronchial obstruction and accompanied possibly by some compensatory emphysema. As Robertson and James (1951) have pointed out, primary collapse, in contradistinction to secondary pressure collapse, is associated with elevation rather than depression of the diaphragm, and with a greater degree of radio-opacity than a lobe subject to compression by an adjacent emphysematous lobe. The degree of emphysema in compensatory emphysema is at most only slight. Nor is compensatory emphysema ever associated with the ballooning and mediastinal herniation of obstructive emphysema. It seems to us that the radiological diagnosis of compensatory emphysema is made too often in infancy and childhood on the analogy of adult experience and without sufficient regard to the likelihood of obstructive emphysema at this age and to the factors which indicate its presence.

In its lesser degrees, obstructive emphysema may be difficult to demonstrate radiologically. The contrast between normal and emphysematous lung in regional obstructive emphysema does, however, make recognition easier then in generalized emphysema.

As obstructive emphysema is a functional condition dependent on active respiration, lungs affected by it may return to normal size after respiration ceases, and if the degree of over-inflation has been insufficient to exceed the elastic limit of the lung no abnormality may be revealed at necropsy (Carter, 1940).

General Role of Obstructive Emphysema in Producing Respiratory Symptoms in Infancy

Obstructive emphysema may be a much commoner factor in the genesis of respiratory embarrassment in infancy than is generally realized. Because of the difficulty of recognizing it in its minor degrees and at post-mortem examination, the significant role which it may play in respiratory disease in infancy may have been underestimated.

The extent of respiratory distress is no doubt proportional to the volume of lung affected by the emphysematous process and to the severity of the air tension within the lung. It may be, too, that abnormal pressure changes in the lung disturb the neurological control of respiration by virtue of stimuli transmitted via the vagus nerve in the manner of the Hering-Brauer reflex.

Particularly is obstructive emphysema likely to be of importance in the newborn infant and in the infant with respiratory infection. In the newborn, inhalation of mucus and liquor is so common that it would be surprising if widespread lobular obstructive emphysema did not frequently occur. It appears likely that spontaneous pneumothorax in the newborn infant, as seen in Case 6, results from such a mechanism (Silver, 1939). Davis and Stevens (1930) have demonstrated the presence of pneumothorax radiologically in almost 1% of 702 consecutive newborn babies and Solis-Cohen and Bruck (1934) in approximately 2% of 500 neonates. A much higher proportion must surely develop obstructive emphysema without going on to pneumothorax. Where spontaneous pneumothorax develops there are two possible routes by which the air can reach the pleural cavity from the pulmonary alveoli. It may rupture directly through the visceral pleura of the lung, or it may travel indirectly, rupturing first into the interstitial tissue (Howie and Weed, 1957), tracking thence to the root of the lung (Macklin, 1939) and rupturing through the mediastinal pleura which yields more easily than does the visceral pleura (Hamman, 1939). The latter appears to be the common route. In infection, too, conditions predisposing to obstructive emphysema are likely to be present. Inflammatory swelling and secretions are likely to block the interalveolar pores and the smaller bronchi and bronchioles are likely to be partially obstructed by swelling of their lining mucosa and by inflammatory exudate. From the clinical point of view the over-inflation and bulging of the thoracic cage and the hyper-resonant percussion note seen frequently in respiratory infection in infants are in keeping with the view that in such cases obstructive emphysema is a common and significant cause of disordered respiratory function.

Acute bronchiolitis, in particular, creates conditions favourable for the occurrence of generalized obstructive emphysema (Nelson and Smith, 1945).

In the adult, in contradistinction, obstructive emphysema appears to be an uncommon occurrence, although it has been reported to have resulted from mucous plugs and from carcinoma obstructing the main bronchi (Maxwell, 1940). The infant seems to be much more prone to it and the narrow lumen of the bronchi and greater elasticity of the bronchial walls may be relevant factors. During the period of infancy, too, congenital anomalies of the bronchi are likely to reveal themselves. The possibility of their occurrence should be borne in mind in any infant who exhibits episodic tachypnoea, intercostal indrawing or respiratory embarrassment.

Lobar Obstructive Emphysema

Although in some cases of lobar emphysema, as for example with a foreign body, the check-valve mechanism described by Jackson is clearly evident this is not always so.

In congenital lobar emphysema no obvious valvular mechanism may be evident (White-Jones and Temple, 1954; Holzell, Bennett and Vaughan, 1956). In other cases deficiency of the cartilaginous rings of the bronchial wall similar to that seen in Case 1 has been described (Overstreet, 1939; Fischer, Tropea and Bailey, 1943; Shaw, 1952) and it is postulated that in these undue flaccidity of the bronchial wall allows it to collapse or become distorted during expiration in such a way as to cause obstruction to the egress of air. An association between mucous membrane folds and deficient bronchial cartilage has been reported (Fischer *et al.*, 1952) and mucosal folds alone have been held responsible for obstructive emphysema (Robertson and James, 1951). External pressure on a bronchus by an aberrant artery and by a patent ductus arteriosus has been reported (Robertson and James, 1951; Fischer *et al.*, 1952). Clark, Nairn and Gowar (1956) have brought forward evidence that congenital bronchostenosis may occur and act as a check valve. The bronchial obstruction which in Case 11 resulted from external pressure by a congenital cyst which was itself subject to obstructive emphysema appears to be a unique mechanism.

In congenital lobar emphysema symptoms of dyspnoea, tachypnoea and cyanosis may be present from birth. Frequently they develop or recur within a few days or weeks of birth. Distress may be acute and early recognition may be life saving.

Barsby (1941) reported three cases of obstructive emphysema resulting from pressure by tuberculous hilar glands, and at that time could find only 16 other reports of this condition in the literature. The majority of cases occurred during the first year of life.

Whether or not operative treatment is employed in lobar obstructive emphysema must depend on the cause and nature of the valvular mechanism and the severity of the emphysema. In Case 1, not operated on, congenital lobar emphysema proved rapidly fatal. In Case 2 operative treatment was successful. In Case 3 spontaneous recovery seems likely. Several reports on the value of resection of affected lobes in congenital lobar emphysema have appeared (Leahy and Butsch, 1949; Robertson and James, 1951; Williams, 1952; Fischer *et al.*, 1952; Holzel *et al.*, 1956). Sloan (1953), however, reported four patients who had residual symptoms after lobectomy. Two of these showed radiological evidence of the further development of emphysema in other parts of the lung following operation. Cases of congenital lobar emphysema can recover spontaneously (Caffey, 1953; Holzel *et al.*, 1956). Holzel *et al.* have described a child with congenital lobar emphysema showing symptoms from birth and not operated on who gradually improved as he grew older. At 5 years of age he was in good health and radiologically there was minimal evidence of emphysema. Thus, although resection of the affected lobe in congenital lobar emphysema may be a life-saving measure and is probably indicated in severe cases, it does not follow that operation should be invariably undertaken. The extent and frequency of respiratory embarrassment will probably be the determining factors. Deflation of the lung can be carried out as an immediately pre-operative measure by the introduction of a needle through the chest wall, and in acute respiratory embarrassment this may be a necessary emergency procedure. Although we used this procedure successfully in Case 2 it has not always been found to be of benefit.

In the acquired forms of lobar obstructive emphysema except for that produced by foreign bodies there is probably less scope for operative treatment. A foreign body in a bronchus which cannot be dislodged by coughing or posturing is a clear indication for bronchoscopic removal. Tuberculous granulation tissue which can be clearly visualized on bronchoscopy and which is causing respiratory distress in virtue of obstructive emphysema should probably be removed (Graham and Hutchison, 1947). Thoracotomy for the removal of tuberculous hilar glands exerting pressure on bronchi and causing severe obstructive emphysema may be an operative emergency (Macpherson, 1957). Where, as in Case 6, mucopus and swelling of the mucous membrane are responsible for obstruction, appropriate antibiotic therapy will be the most important factor in treatment.

Lobular Obstructive Emphysema

Considering the various types of emphysema quantitatively, lobular emphysema is almost certainly the most commonly occurring for the reason that aspiration into the lungs in the newborn and infection and bronchospasm in infancy are so common. When severe and massive the clinical features of pulmonary over-inflation resulting from lobular emphysema may be obvious enough. In its lesser forms, however, lobular obstructive emphysema may be less evident clinically. Yet arguing by analogy from the severe generalized lobular obstructive emphysema seen in acute bronchiolitis of infancy and from the severe regional lobular obstructive emphysema present in cases such as 7 and 9 reported here, it is likely that any obstruction of smaller bronchi or bronchioles in infancy by aspirated fluid, secretions, or swelling of the lining mucosa may result in lobular emphysema of varying degree. The development of obstructive emphysema in any lobule is likely to interfere to a greater or lesser extent with its functional capacity.

Cystic Obstructive Emphysema

Conway (1951) has described varieties of lung cyst and discussed the aetiology in the light of the cases which he reported and the literature on the subject. He accepts that congenital cysts can undoubtedly occur but concludes that the majority of lung cysts seen after the first few days of life are acquired. Clark *et al.* (1956) have recently described the successful removal of a lung containing multiple congenital cysts. Successful removal of congenital lung cysts has also been described by Fischer *et al.* and by Conway. There appears little doubt that the congenital cysts in Case 12 were primarily responsible for the fatal lobar emphysema from which the patient suffered, and an attempt at operative removal should have been made.

Post-pneumonic pneumatocoeles, which constitute the main differential diagnosis from congenital cysts usually have a good prognosis and tend to disappear spontaneously. Where, as is so frequently the case, congenital cysts or acquired post-pneumonic cysts are subject to tension emphysema the valvular mechanism seems usually to be that which occurred in Case 10. The tangential opening of the supplying bronchus into the cyst results in a slit-like or flap-like mouth which acts as a valve and whose valvular nature tends to be preserved by the pressure in the cyst (Fig. 1). There is thus a vicious cycle of events maintaining the obstructive emphysema within the cyst. Some factor suddenly breaking this cycle may be responsible for the sudden disappearance of, for example, a post-pneumonic pneumatocoele. Clark *et al.* (1956) have suggested that multiple congenital cysts of the lung can result from the presence of both bronchiolectasis and a check-valve obstruction of the bronchus. In the presence of the increased tension within the lung resulting from the check valve the bronchiolectatic areas distal to the valve expand to form cysts.

Mixed Forms of Regional Obstructive Emphysema

Although it is convenient and possibly useful to classify obstructive emphysema into three main types these may not occur in a 'pure' form. Case 12 illustrates a 'mixed' form in which cystic and lobar emphysema were combined. The assertion of Clark *et al.* (1956) that areas of congenital bronchiolectasis may become cystic in the presence of a check-valve obstruction of a main bronchus causing lobar emphysema suggests another mixed form.

Summary

It is suggested that regional obstructive emphysema can be classified as lobar, lobular or cystic with subsidiary groupings dependent on pathogenesis.

A series of cases in infants is reported illustrating varieties of regional obstructive emphysema. These are classified according to the scheme outlined above.

Diagnosis is discussed and the important role of obstructive emphysema in the production of respiratory symptoms in infancy is emphasized.

The mechanism of production of the various forms of regional obstructive emphysema and their treatment is considered.

REFERENCES

Barsby, B. (1941). *Lancet*, **1**, 627.
Caffey, J. (1953). *Pediatrics*, **11**, 48.
Carter, R. A. (1940). *Radiology*, **35**, 391
Clark, N. S., Nairn, R. C. and Gowar, F. J. S. (1956). *Arch Dis. Childh.*, **31**, 358.
Conway, D. J. (1951). *Ibid.*, **26**, 504.
Davis, C. H. and Stevens, G. W. (1930). *Amer. J. Obstet. Gynec.*, **20**, 73.
Fischer, C. C., Tropea, F. and Bailey, C. P. (1943). *J. Pediat.*, **23**, 219.
Graham, S. G. and Hutchison, J. H. (1947). *Arch. Dis. Childh.*, **22**, 162.
Hamman, L. (1939). *Ann. intern. Med.*, **13**, 923.
Heinbecker, P. (1927). *J. clin. Invest.*, **4**, 459.
Holzel, A., Bennett, E. and Vaughan, B. F. (1956). *Arch. Dis. Childh.* **31**, 216.
Howie, V. M. and Weed, A. S. (1957). *J. Pediat.*, **50**, 6.
Jackson, C. (1930). *J. Amer. med. Ass.*, **95**, 639.
Leahy, L. J. and Butsch, W. L. (1949). *Arch. Surg. (Chicago)*, **59**, 466.
Macklin, C. C. (1939). *Arch. intern. Med.*, **64**, 913.
Macpherson, A. M. C. (1957). In *Symposium of Tuberculosis*, ed. F. R. G. Heaf. London.
Maxwell, J. (1940). *Brit. med. J.*, **1**, 520.
Nelson, W. E. and Smith, L. W. (1945). *J. Pediat.*, **26**, 36.
Overstreet, R. M. (1939). *Amer. J. Dis. Child.*, **57**, 861.
Reinberg, S. A. (1925). *Brit. J. Radiol.*, (B.I.R. Sect.). **30**. 451.
Robertson, R. and James, E. S. (1951). *Pediatrics*, **8**, 795.
Shaw, R. R. (1952). *Ibid.*, **9**, 220.
Silver, H. B. (1939). *Amer. J. Dis. Child.*, **57**, 907.
Sloan, H. (1953). *J. thorac. Surg.*, **26**, 1.
Solis-Cohen, L. and Bruck, S. (1934). *Radiology*, **23**, 173.
Van Allen, C. M. and Soo, Y. C. (1933). *J. clin. Invest.*, **12**, 171.
White-Jones, R. H. and Temple, L. J. (1954). *Arch. Dis. Childh.*, **29**, 248.
Williams, M. H. (1952). *J. thorac. Surg.*, **24**, 522.

AN INBORN ERROR OF METABOLISM WITH THE URINARY EXCRETION OF α-HYDROXY-BUTYRIC ACID AND PHENYLPYRUVIC ACID

BY

ALAN J. SMITH and LEONARD B. STRANG

From the Departments of Chemical Pathology and Child Health, King's College, University of Durham

(RECEIVED FOR PUBLICATION OCTOBER 3, 1957)

We have recently seen a baby girl with gross mental deficiency who had repeated attacks of generalized oedema. She also had an extremely unpleasant, pungent smell due to the presence in her urine of a substance derived from α-hydroxy-butyric acid. So far as we know, this acid has not previously been detected in human urine. The urine also contained phenylpyruvic acid and phenylacetic acid as well as an excess of certain amino-acids.

We believe that the infant had a double metabolic abnormality. One was the familiar defect of phenylketonuria in which a block in the conversion of phenylalanine to tyrosine leads to the accumulation of phenylalanine in the body and to the excretion in the urine of phenylpyruvic acid, phenylacetic acid and other derivatives of phenylalanine (Jervis, 1954). The urinary excretion of α-hydroxy-butyric acid cannot be related to the metabolism of phenylalanine and indicates the presence of another metabolic defect.

Clinical History

Mary D. was the first baby of healthy, unrelated parents, and was born normally in a maternity hospital. She breathed and cried at birth but from the beginning she refused the breast. From the first day of life she had an unusual and unpleasant smell. On the fourth day she developed occasional extensor spasms and was extremely pale, listless and unresponsive to stimuli. She was at that time thought to have a severe cerebral abnormality.

On the ninth day of life she first came under our observation. She was quite flaccid and unresponsive to stimuli. The fontanelle tension was increased and the head circumference was 14 inches. She lay motionless and required tube feeding. The curious smell which had been noticed on the first day of life was still present. It hung about her room and clung to her clothes and the clothes of those who nursed her. It was described by different observers as smelling 'like an oast house', 'like burnt sugar' and 'like dried celery'. The source of the smell was her urine.

Further investigations at this time gave the following results:

Lumbar Puncture. Normal pressure, clear fluid, no cells and protein 120 mg./100 ml.

Subdural Puncture. There was no evidence of subdural collections.

Serum. The urea level was 41 mg./100 ml., potassium 3·1 mEq./l, calcium 5·1 mEq./l and total protein 7·8 g./100 ml.

During the first six weeks of life she improved sufficiently to feed from a bottle and was able to go home. She remained hypotonic and completely unresponsive to stimuli, never taking notice of anything or attempting to raise her head. She had long spells of loud, monotonous crying little affected by sedation.

Between the ages of 5 and 10 months she had frequent episodes of fever, rapid breathing and generalized pitting oedema. There was no evidence of congestive heart failure. The first attack was regarded as due to infection and treated with chemotherapy. Subsequently, however, she often recovered within a matter of 12 to 24 hours from attacks for which no chemotherapy was given.

At 9 months she had grown a small amount of completely white hair. She had also increased in size (weight 20 lb. and head circumference 17 inches) but remained mentally defective and responsive only to painful stimuli. The characteristic smell persisted in the urine throughout life. At 10 months she died at home.

Necropsy Report

Dr. J. Hart-Mercer reported as follows:

The body weighed 7·75 kg. (within normal limits). It was 'well nourished', *i.e.*, the subcutaneous fat was abundant, measuring up to 1·5 cm. on the anterior abdominal wall. The head circumference was 42 cm. (a little small for the age). The scalp hair was very blonde and fine.

The internal appearance showed evidence of terminal inhalation of bilious vomit into the bronchi.

The thymus (12 g.) showed some degree of accidental involution.

There were a few fibrous pleural adhesions in the left interlobar fissure, and marginal emphysema and moderate emphysema bilaterally. Foci of broncho-pneumonia were found in both lungs, particularly in the lower lobes, associated microscopically with pneumococci.

All the chambers of the heart were slightly dilated.

The liver was slightly enlarged (to 284 g.) and microscopically merely showed venous congestion with centrilobular degenerative and atrophic changes in the liver cells.

The spleen weighed 17 g. and was a little smaller than normal. It showed *fleckmilz*, *i.e.*, multiple small foci of recent and developing necrosis affecting irregular areas of pulp and lymphoid tissue. Resembling early infarcts, they were not apparently associated with gross arterial change but recent thrombi were encountered in occasional arterioles.

The kidneys weighed together 133 g., about twice the normal combined weight. The enlargement was bilateral and diffuse, the subcapsular surfaces smooth, the cortices pale. Microscopy showed hypertrophic-looking proximal convoluted tubules lined by unusually tall epithelium. In many of these cells there was hyaline droplet degeneration.

The glomeruli were largely unaltered, but here and there thrombus or thrombus-like eosinophilic material occluded one or more capillary loops.

The cells of the lower nephrons frequently showed lipid droplets in their cytoplasm and occasionally their lumen was distended with hyaline cast material.

The brain weighed 700 g., a little small for the age. Neither externally nor on section was there evidence of gross maldevelopment. Indeed the appearances were almost normal. The width of the white matter in the cerebral hemispheres may have been slightly reduced but the only convincing change was the unduly soft consistency of all parts of the brain.

Microscopic examination showed widespread changes in cerebrum, brain-stem and cord suggesting a nutritional encephalomyelopathy with widespread defect of myelinization.

Examination of Urine

The urine during life was a clear, amber-coloured liquid with the characteristic penetrating smell already described and which did not diminish during storage at 4° C. The reaction was acid to litmus, no albumin was present and no formed elements were found on repeated microscopy.

The first specimen gave a slight reduction with Benedict's qualitative reagent on one occasion which was shown to be due to glucuronic acid.

Phenylketonuria. The addition of a few drops of ferric chloride to the urine gave a fairly persistent emerald green colour which was consistent with the presence of phenylpyruvic acid. The colour was more intense if the urine was acidified, extracted with ether and a drop of ferric chloride added to the extract. The characteristic smell was found to be extracted at the same time; since this did not happen when alkaline urine was similarly extracted it could be concluded that the pungent-smelling substance was acid in nature. The phenylpyruvic acid was quantitatively estimated by a slight modification of the method of Berry and Woolf (1952). A freshly synthesized and purified sample of phenylpyruvic acid (Herbst and Shemin, 1939) was used for the calibration curve. The concentration was found to be 8·96 mg./20 ml. urine or 134·4 mg./24 hours.

Phenylpyruvic acid is an oxo-acid and as further confirmation of its presence it was decided to make 2·4 dinitrophenylhydrazine derivatives of all the oxo-acids in the urine by the method of Cavallini, Frontali and Toschi (1949). The extract of the derivatives from the urine was compared chromatographically with derivatives prepared from a series of oxo-acids. The 2·4 dinitrophenylhydrazine derivative of phenylpyruvic acid was prepared from the freshly synthesized acid by the method of Smith and Jones (1948). The solvent phase of tert-amyl alcohol, 50 parts; ethyl alcohol, 10 parts; water, 40 parts, was used as the developing solvent (Altmann, Crook and Datta, 1951) on Whatman No. 3 paper buffered to *p*H 6·0 or *p*H 7·0. An additional reason for examining these oxo-acid derivatives was the fact that the acids in dilute solution in water have smells somewhat similar to that of the urine.

The keto-acids chosen were α-oxo-butyric, oxo-glutonic, pyruvic, α-oxo-glutaric, acetoacetic, p-hydroxy-phenylpyruvic, oxo-malonic and laevulinic. The spots needed no development since the derivatives were yellow. The phenylpyruvic acid derivatives had an R_F of 0·66 on paper buffered to *p*H 6·0 and 0·60 on paper buffered to *p*H 7·0.

The urine showed only one derivative which had the same R_F as the phenylpyruvic acid on paper at both *p*H 6·0 and *p*H 7·0. This was a useful confirmatory test for phenylpyruvic acid. Nearer the solvent there was a discrete unstained area of the paper which contained a substance with the characteristic smell of the patient's urine. The smell was therefore not due to an oxo-acid. It was easy to demarcate the area by smell and so assign an R_F value of about 0·8 to the unknown colourless substance.

The Identification of the Unknown Substance. In order to identify this strongly smelling non-ketonic, ether-soluble substance, a 25 ml. sample of urine was acidified to *p*H 1·0 with concentrated HCl and extracted three times with 25 ml. ether. The combined extracts were evaporated by a stream of nitrogen and the residue dissolved in a small volume of ether. This extract was compared against a series of aliphatic and phenyl-substituted aliphatic acids by paper chromatography. The developing solvent used was propanol, 60 parts; ammonia, 30 parts and water, 10 parts (Buffs, Peters and Wakelin, 1951). Whatman No. 3 paper was used unbuffered and found to give more discrete spots than the thinner papers. The acids used for comparison were phenylpyruvic acid (freshly prepared), phenylacetic acid, β-hydroxy-butyric acid and α-hydroxy-butyric acid. These derivatives of butyric acid were used because their smell in dilute aqueous solution was very similar to that of the urine. The chromatogram was run overnight (about 12 hours) dried in air and the spots developed by spraying the chromatogram with 'universal indicator' (B.D.H. Ltd.) adjusted to a purple colour with sodium hydroxide (Long, Quayle and Stedman, 1951). A more even spray was obtained when alcoholic potassium hydroxide was used to adjust the colour. The ammonium salts of the acids showed up as red spots on an originally purple background which quickly faded. The urine extract was found to give three acid spots of R_F values 0·56, 0·62 and 0·76. The slowest running spot was equivalent to that of phenylpyruvic acid and the others were equivalent to α-hydroxy-butyric acid which itself gave rise to two spots. The fastest moving spots of both the urine and the pure α-hydroxy-butyric acid (R_F 0·76) possessed the characteristic smell originally noticed in the urine. Pure phenylacetic acid had an R_F of 0·75 and hence was not separable from the α-hydroxy-butyric acid.

As a confirmation of the identity of the smell with α-hydroxy-butyric acid, a sample of the urine extract was allowed to stand at room temperature for a few days during which time the phenylpyruvic acid decomposed. This could be shown by a negative ferric chloride test and chromatographically, but the smell remained just as persistent. This old extract was also run in a different solvent system of butanol, 95 parts; formic acid, 5 parts; saturated with water (Lugg and Overell, 1948). The completed chromatogram was sprayed with 'universal indicator' but dried in air for a longer period than previously. Both the urine and the α-hydroxy-butyric acid gave two spots each of R_F 0·77 and 0·85 but now in each case the smell was associated with the slower moving component.

The method of formation of the smell was investigated by producing further chromatograms of α-hydroxy-butyric acid in propanol ammonia in an atmosphere of cyanide (by placing in aqueous solution of potassium cyanide in a tank) to inhibit oxidation. The area of the fastest moving spot was relatively much smaller than previously. This suggested that the smell was due to an oxidation product of α-hydroxy-butyric acid which had previously been increased in amount during chromatography.

Phenylacetic Acid. In the previous chromatograms one of the spots of α-hydroxy-butyric acid had a very similar R_F value to phenylacetic acid. Although we suspected the presence of the latter substance, proof had not been obtained. This was done by using a different solvent. This solvent was benzene, 40 parts; formic acid, 40 parts; and water, 20 parts (Bray, Thorpe and White, 1950). With it the old urine extract gave spots of R_F 0·23, 0·55, 0·77 and 0·88. The three slower moving spots were the same as those given by α-hydroxy-butyric acid and the fastest moving one was the same as that given by phenylacetic acid. The characteristic smell of the urine was associated with the spots with R_F values of 0·55 and 0·77 and the different smell of phenylacetic acid was associated with the spot of R_F 0·88.

Amino-acids. Routine two-dimensional ascending paper chromatography in phenol-water-ammonia and collidine-lutidine-water (Dent, 1948) was performed on the urine. This showed an excess of phenylalanine, methionine and tyrosine. A further modification consisted of evaporating the urine to dryness under reduced pressure and extracting the amino-acids with acetone. The acetone extract was compared with the other amino-acids by one-dimensional descending paper chromatography with the solvent propanol, 60 parts; ammonia, 30 parts; water, 10 parts. On dipping the dried chromatogram in 0·1% ninhydrin in acetone and drying for five minutes at 100° C., large amounts of phenylalanine, methionine and tyrosine were demonstrated. There was, however, no evidence of α-amino-butyric acid which had been suspected as the source of the α-hydroxy-butyric acid.

All these results were confirmed in post-mortem urine.

Discussion

The child presented a clinical picture similar in some respects to that of phenylpyruvic oligophrenia. Unusual features were marked unresponsiveness to stimuli, muscular flaccidity, recurrent episodes of pyrexia with generalized oedema and a penetrating smell in freshly passed urine. This smell bore no resemblance to that of phenylacetic acid which is commonly associated with phenylketonuria. It effectively masked the smell of that substance which was also in the urine.

The urinary findings established that the baby had a metabolic defect producing phenylketonuria together with another abnormality leading to the excretion of α-hydroxy-butyric acid in the urine. The odour was so characteristic that it should be easy to recognize any further examples of this condition. The smell was probably due to an oxidation or polymerization product of α-hydroxy-butyric acid, since it was reduced in amount on paper chromatography in an atmosphere of cyanide. It was associated with a single spot except in chromatography performed in benzene, 40 parts; formic acid, 40 parts; water, 20 parts, in which two spots with the characteristic smell were found. The α-hydroxy acids tend to polymerize together and to form lactones as shown in Fig. 1 for α-hydroxy-

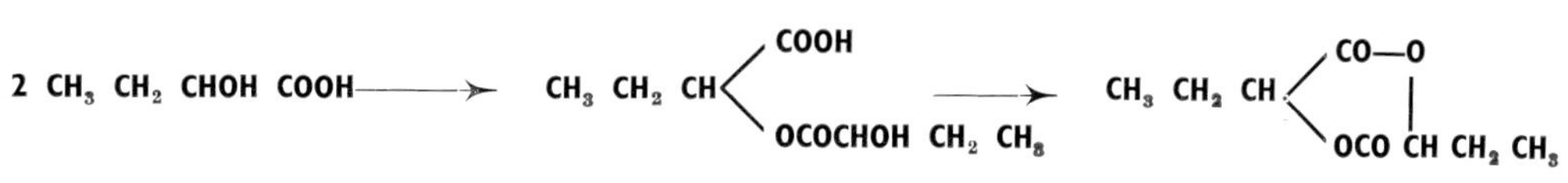

FIG. 1.

butyric acid. This should account for the multiple spots in chromatograms of this substance.

Abnormal excretion products other than phenylpyruvic acid have been detected in the urine of patients with phenylketonuria and are listed by Jervis (1954). These are phenyllactic, p-hydroxy-phenyllactic, phenylacetic, p-hydroxy-phenylacetic and o-hydroxy-phenylacetic acids. The chemical relationships between those substances are shown in Fig. 2 and it is probable that all can be derived from phenylalanine. Of these only phenylacctic acid was detected in the urine of the patient we are discussing. Normally the acids with a hydroxylated benzene ring are derived from tyrosine, but in phenylketonuria it is possible they are derived from hydroxylation of the derivatives of phenylalanine.

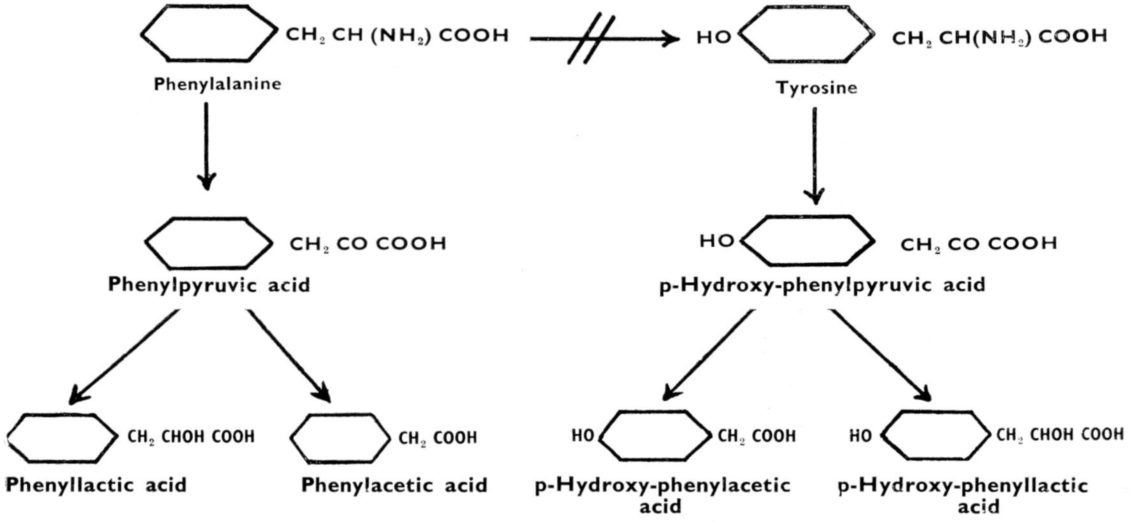

FIG. 2.

The presence of α-hydroxy-butyric acid cannot be explained from this system and its origin in intermediary metabolism must at present remain uncertain. It is unlikely to be formed in the oxidation of fat since this leads to the formation of oxo- and hydroxy derivatives in the β position. A possible source is from α-amino-butyric acid and thence by reduction perhaps by bacteria to the α-hydroxy compound as shown in Fig. 3. This type of hydrolytic deamination is known to take place in bacteria (Baldwin, 1947) and it is possible that bacteria in the renal tract were responsible for it in our patient. No urinary infection, however, was detected and the smell was present in freshly passed specimens, and within a few hours of birth. The amino-acid analogue of α-hydroxy-butyric acid, α-amino-butyric acid, has been shown in human urine (Dent, 1947) but it was not detectable in our patient.

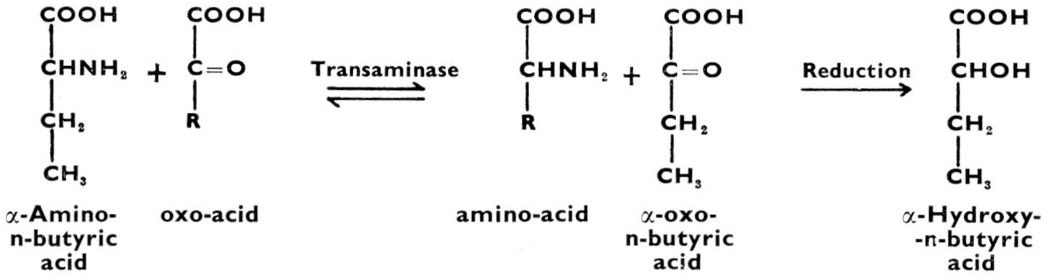

FIG. 3.

α-Oxo-butyric acid may be linked to the metabolism of many other amino-acids as shown by experimentation in mutated bacteria. Carroll, Stacey and du Vigneaud (1949) have shown that α-oxo-butyric acid occurs in the catabolism of homoserine and Lien and Greenberg (1953) have shown that the same compound occurs in the metabolism of threonine. It has also been shown by Umbarger and Adelberg (1951) that α-oxo-butyric acid can be used in the synthesis of isoleucine and valine from simpler substances. So far there has been no evidence of similar mechanisms in humans.

The absence of any signs during life or at necropsy of renal infection and the fact that the distinctive smell was present in fresh specimens of urine incline us against the view that the α-hydroxy-butyric acid was produced wholly or in part by bacterial action. We regard it as more probable that its presence was due to a defect in intermediary metabolism and that this was a major factor in causing the child's illness.

Summary

A child is described in whom a syndrome of mental deficiency and recurrent episodes of oedema were associated with the urinary excretion of α-hydroxy-butyric acid and phenylpyruvic acid.

The presence of α-hydroxy-butyric acid gave rise to an unusual smell.

Phenylacetic acid, phenylalanine, tyrosine and methionine were also present in excess in the urine.

Some possible modes of formation of the α-hydroxy-butyric acid are discussed.

We wish to thank Dr. A. L. Latner for his advice and criticism throughout the course of the investigation, and also Prof. S. D. M. Court and Dr. F. J. W. Miller for help in the preparation of this paper. We are grateful to Dr. J. Hart-Mercer for the necropsy report.

References

Altmann, S. M., Crook, E. M. and Datta, S. P. (1951). *Biochem. J.*, **49**, lxiii.
Baldwin, E. (1947). *Dynamic Aspects of Biochemistry*, p. 213. Cambridge.
Berry, J. P. and Woolf, L. I. (1952). *Nature (Lond.)*, **169**, 202.
Bray, H. G., Thorpe, W. V. and White, K. (1950). *Biochem. J.*, **46**, 271.
Buffa, P., Peters, R. A. and Wakelin, R. W. (1951). *Ibid.*, **48**, 467.
Carroll, W. R., Stacy, G. W. and Vigneaud V. du (1949). *J. biol. Chem.*, **180**, 375.
Cavallini, D., Frontali, N. and Toschi, G. (1949). *Nature (Lond.)*, **164**, 792.
Dent, C. E. (1947). *Biochem. J.*, **41**, 240.
—— (1948). *Ibid.*, **43**, 169.
Herbst, R. M. and Shemin, D. (1939). *Organic Syntheses*, **19**, 1 and 77. New York and London.
Jervis, G. A. (1954). In *Genetics and the Inheritance of Integrated Neurological and Psychiatric Patterns, Res. Publ. Ass. nerv. ment. Dis.*, **33**, 259.
Lien, O. G. and Greenberg, D. M. (1953). *J. biol. Chem.*, **200**, 367.
Long, A. G., Quayle, J. R. and Stedman, R. J. (1951). *J. chem. Soc.*, p. 2197.
Lugg, J. W. H. and Overell, B. T. (1948). *Aust. J. sci. Res.*, Ser. A, **1**, 98.
Smith, F. J. and Jones, E. (1948). *A Scheme of Qualitative Organic Analysis*, p. 37. London.
Umbarger, H. E. and Adelberg, E. A. (1951). *J. biol. Chem.*, **192**, 883.

A CASE OF HARTNUP DISEASE

BY

WALTER HENDERSON

From the County Hospital, York

(RECEIVED FOR PUBLICATION AUGUST 13, 1957)

This new disease was first described last year by Dr. Hart and Professor Dent and their colleagues (Baron, Dent, Harris, Hart and Jepson, 1956) under the title 'Hereditary pellagra-like skin rash with temporary cerebellar ataxia, constant amino-aciduria, and other bizarre biochemical features'.

The name 'Hartnup disease'—after the family then described—was later used in a reference to the syndrome by Harris (1957) and is that at present preferred by the original authors. No further accounts of cases have yet been published in this country and it seemed, therefore, that the following case was worthy of record. A brief reference to two further cases in Holland has been made by Jonxis (1957).

Angela P. was born on July 1, 1947, the second child of healthy, unrelated parents. Her infancy and early childhood were uneventful; she had most of the childhood infectious fevers but otherwise was well and grew normally. In March of 1952 she developed diarrhoea which was treated with a sulphonamide but did not clear up for nearly three weeks.

She was first seen in consultation on May 13, 1952, at the age of 4 years 10 months, on account of recurring attacks of unsteadiness, in some of which she fell and hurt herself. These episodes started shortly after the diarrhoea had cleared up. At about the same time she began to develop a rash on the face and lower parts of the arms. This rash was always made worse by exposure to the sun; it had been diagnosed as sensitivity to sunlight and was being treated with only partial success by protective creams. Her appetite was poor and she was rather temperamental. Apart from a mild ataxia there was little to be found abnormal in the nervous system.

When seen again six weeks later it was clear that there had been some deterioration: she was now unsteady at all times when on her feet, sometimes she felt giddy when walking about and would then sit down if possible; at other times she fell—rather more often to the left than to the right. The rash was as bad as ever and caused her a good deal of inconvenience. These troubles were making her more temperamental and difficult at home. She was admitted to hospital for five days on July 2 1952.

The clinical examination showed a girl of average physique, definitely ataxic whenever she walked. When walking about the ward she would sometimes appear to feel giddy or unsteady and would quickly sit down, but it was clear that she was constantly ataxic. The legs showed no wasting and the tendon reflexes were all slightly exaggerated. The plantar reflexes were flexor. The arms showed definite but mild intention tremor with increased tendon reflexes, but she could feed herself, play with toys and fasten buttons. No sensory disturbance could be made out. There was no papilloedema and no affection of any of the cranial nerves. A radiograph of the skull was normal. The urine showed no abnormalities.

The rash was quite striking, being only on the exposed areas of the body, and was very marked on the back of the neck, most of the face, the backs of the hands and outer surfaces of the arms—strictly to the sleeve level—and the dorsal surface of the feet where exposed through the straps of the sandals, the calves and knees to the lower limit of the dress. The skin in the affected areas was reddened, rough and dry; in a few areas it was thickened. Round the mouth and external nares there was hardening and cracking at the muco-cutaneous junctions.

The child was fretful during her stay, unhappy and anxious to get home. She did not vomit, her appetite was indifferent and she had no headache. No definite diagnosis was reached and she was allowed home.

When she was followed up six weeks later in the middle of August, it was reported that her unsteadiness was much more marked; she could only walk for a few yards and now moved about very little, being especially diffident about going up or downstairs.

Examination showed a more marked ataxia with very unsteady gait; she walked with a rather wide base and could only manage a few steps without support. The deep reflexes were still exaggerated. The arm and hand movements were jerky, there was intention tremor and she could feed herself only with considerable difficulty. The ocular fundi were normal. There was mild nystagmus, not very well sustained, detectable in both lateral directions. Her speech was rather slow and at times she tended to split up words. The rash was slightly more marked. She also had an angular stomatitis, a very slight atrophic glossitis, and a mild vulvitis. The hair was soft and loose, coming out readily when brushed and combed.

In view of the increasing severity of her symptoms she was transferred to The Hospital for Sick Children, Great

Ormond Street, on August 27, 1952, under the care of Dr. P. R. Evans.

Investigation there confirmed the above findings, and the photographs (Fig. 1) show clearly the distribution of the rash. The cerebrospinal fluid was clear and contained no cells; protein was 30 mg. per 100 ml.; sugar, 91 mg./100 ml.; chlorides, 700 mg./100 ml.; and W.R. negative. The urine showed no porphyrins, but there was an increase in the amino-acid content.

Dr. Evans noted that the dermatitis in its appearance and distribution closely resembled that seen in pellagra and suggested that the other symptoms might also be due to vitamin B deficiency.

Treatment was therefore started on September 2 with riboflavin, 3 mg. t.d.s., and nicotinamide, 10 mg. four times daily, by mouth. She was given a high-protein diet, with added brewers' yeast. The skin was treated with cremor calamine.

Within a week of starting specific treatment it could be seen that the ataxia was less marked and the skin lesion definitely improving. After two weeks, improvement had reached the stage where she could walk without support. The deep reflexes were still brisk. She could now feed herself much more readily. After four weeks, a test dose of ultra-violet light still showed some skin sensitivity.

After eight weeks' treatment she had gained 4 lb. in weight. She had apparently quite recovered and was allowed home on October 25, 1952, with instructions to take riboflavine and nicotinamide for a further three months.

A few months later she was reported to be perfectly well, attending school regularly and showing no behaviour difficulties.

Further retrospective enquiry into possible causes of the 'pellagra' syndrome suggested that her diet might have been partly to blame, as she had, for some months before her symptoms developed, lived largely on cornflakes and milk. There seemed to have been an association in time between the attack of diarrhoea and the first appearance of rash and ataxia, and it was felt that this illness and its treatment with sulphonamide over a period of two to three weeks might have interfered with the absorption of vitamins.

The publication by Baron, Dent, Harris, Hart and Jepson (1956) of details of the Hartnup family, and their consideration of two other children described in the British literature as having 'pellagra' seemed to provide an answer to this unresolved diagnostic puzzle. Angela was seen again and a specimen of urine was analysed by Professor C. E. Dent who reported that 'the chromatogram shows a gross disorder of amino-acid excretion, identical with that of our other cases of Hartnup disease'

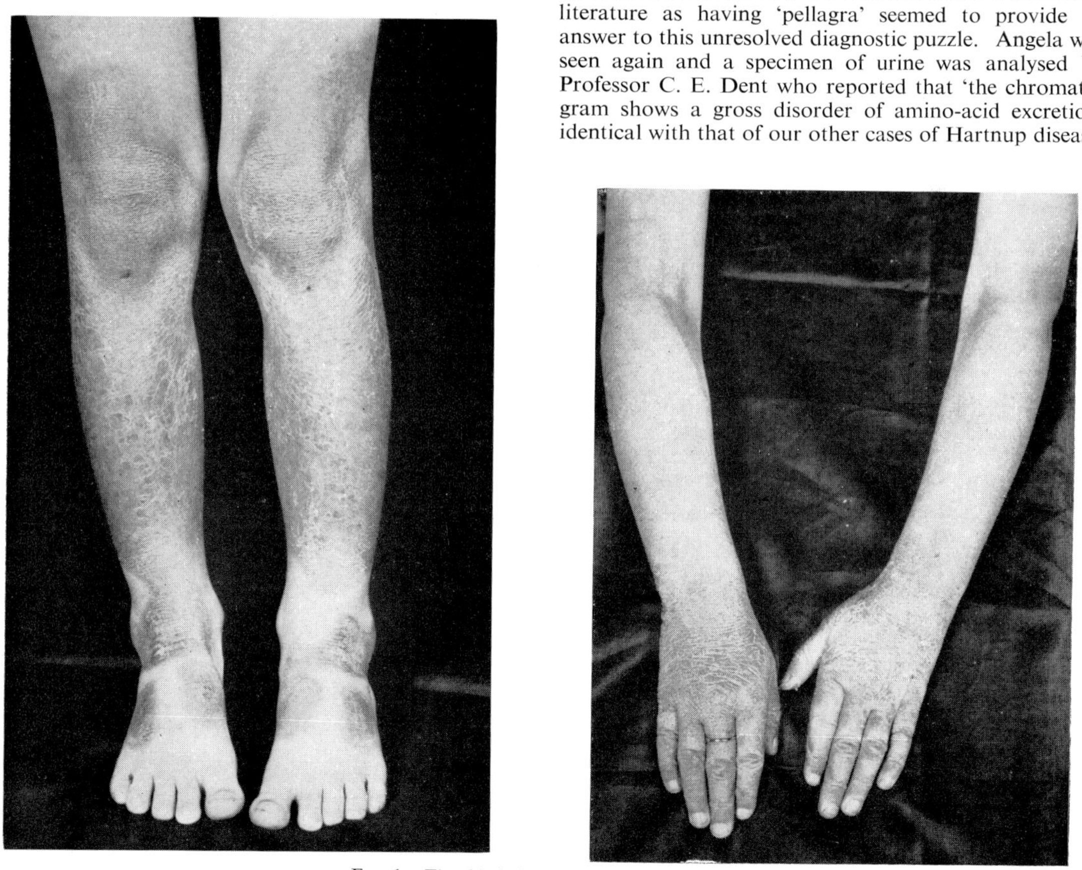

FIG. 1.—The skin lesions (September 1, 1952).

(Fig. 2). 'Indole chromatograms were also carried out (by Dr. Jepson) and showed the usual gross excretion of tryptophan, indican, indolylacetic acid and indolylacetylglutamine in the pattern characteristic of the disease.'

A detailed investigation of the genetic background in this case has been undertaken and a family tree constructed (Fig. 3).

Angela's father died suddenly in 1955 at the age of 44 from a coronary thrombosis. The paternal grandfather died at about 70, and the paternal grandmother at 78. The cause of death is not recorded in either case. The maternal grandfather died at 74 of a coronary thrombosis, and the maternal grandmother at 63 of asthma and bronchitis. One of Mrs. P.'s sisters died at the age of 4 years, and a niece died at the age of 9 months, but in neither case is the cause of death recorded.

The urines of 26 of the 31 living relatives (including aunts and uncles and their offspring) have been tested by Dr. H. Harris for amino-acids but none shows the characteristic chromatogram of Hartnup disease.

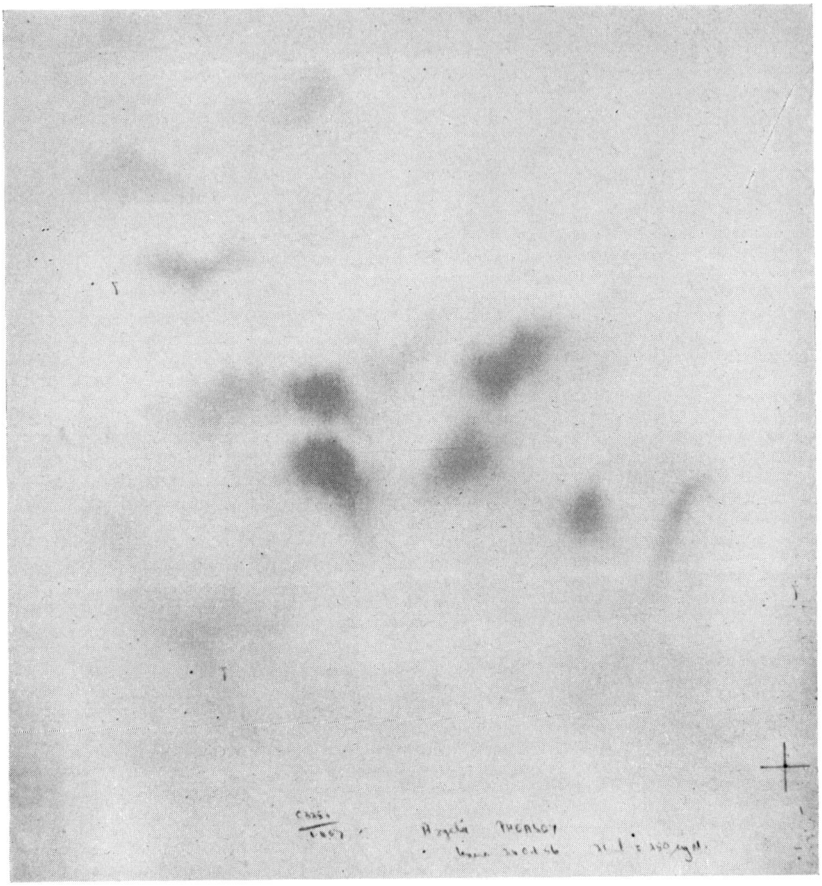

FIG. 2.—Urinary amino-acid chromatogram showing the typical pattern of amino-acid excretion.

At this time, it was noted that she was fit and well, and normally grown for her age. Her I.Q. has not been tested but she shows no evidence of slow mental development. In the intervening three years she had shown no further ataxia and clinical examination of the central nervous system showed no abnormal signs. Her skin, however, continued to show mild sensitivity to sunlight: the backs of the neck and hands readily became reddened and thereafter soon became sore if not treated with calamine lotion. In summer she has to be careful not to expose herself too much in the sun. She has been given no more nicotinamide.

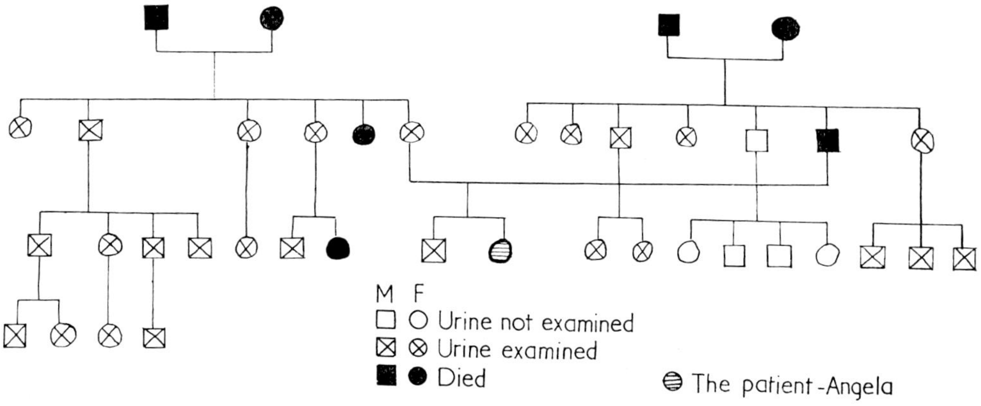

FIG. 3.—The family tree.

Summary

A case of 'pellagra' in an English child of 4½ years is described. There was a very satisfactory clinical response to large oral doses of riboflavine and nicotinamide and recovery appeared to be almost complete.

Subsequent investigation at the age of 9½ years has shown the cause to be the characteristic renal amino-aciduria and other biochemical disturbances associated with Hartnup disease.

I am very grateful to Dr. P. R. Evans for his help in the early stages of this case and to the Department of Medical Illustration, The Hospital for Sick Children, Great Ormond Street, for the clinical photographs; to Professor Dent for his help and encouragement and for permission to reproduce the chromatogram; and to Dr. H. Harris for the family tree.

REFERENCES

Baron D. N., Dent, C. E., Harris, H., Hart, E. W. and Jepson, J. B. (1956). *Lancet*, **2**, 421.
Harris, H. (1957). *Brit. med. Bull.*, **13**, No. 1, p. 26.
Jonxis, J. H. P. (1957). *Ned. T. Geneesk.*, **101**, 569.

DISSOCIATION AS A GUIDE TO DEVELOPMENTAL ASSESSMENT

BY

R. S. ILLINGWORTH

From the Children's Hospital, Sheffield, and the Department of Child Health, the University of Sheffield

(RECEIVED FOR PUBLICATION SEPTEMBER 18, 1957)

In the assessment of an infant's development, in the light of the mother's developmental history and of one's own developmental examination, one considers not only how far one's findings tally with the mother's history, but the relationship of one field of development to another. For instance, if a child's speech development is quite out of step with his motor development, an attempt to determine the reason for it and its significance must be made. Such a departure from the usual relationship of one field of development to another may be termed 'dissociation'. It is a common and important finding which has received little or no attention in the literature. For convenience I shall consider it in different fields of development.

Delayed Motor Development Without Retardation in Other Fields

The commonest cause of delayed motor development in an infant is mental deficiency; but in mental deficiency there will also be retardation in other fields of development such as social behaviour, interest in surroundings, and speech, for no child with isolated delay in motor development can be mentally defective.

Obvious causes of isolated motor retardation are hypotonia and hypertonia. Rare causes include infantile myopathies, diastematomyelia and other purely mechanical defects.

Hypotonia. The causes of hypotonia have been reviewed by Walton (1956, 1957) and need not be recapitulated here. They include amyotonia congenita and allied conditions. Hypotonia sufficient to cause significant motor retardation could hardly be missed. In the developmental history and examination there is a striking dissociation between the grossly retarded motor development and the normal social behaviour. For instance, the child has begun to smile at the usual age (4 to 6 weeks), to vocalize his pleasure two or three weeks later, to take a normal interest in his surroundings, to follow his mother's movements with his eyes (at 2 or 3 months of age), and to turn his head to sound at about 3 months. Later on he has shown excitement at feed times, and has imitated his parents in sounds and simple movements (6 to 9 months). His vocalizations have followed the usual pattern and his speech has developed at the usual time, so that he says three or four words with meaning by 12 months, and has joined two or three words together by 21 to 24 months. On the other hand, he is grossly retarded in head control, and subsequently in sitting, creeping and walking. An illustrative case history is as follows:

When this girl was seen at 13 months her head control was that of a 10-weeks-old baby. The manipulative development was average. She was saying single words with meaning. There was generalized hypotonia, and as the knee jerks were present the diagnosis of congenital hypotonia was made. Subsequently she put words together at 27 months and walked without help at 5 years.

This child has a mild congenital hypotonia with an average intelligence. The normal social and subsequently normal speech behaviour would preclude the suspicion of mental deficiency.

Less easy to assess is the combination of mental deficiency with hypotonia. This is not a particularly common combination, but the complication of hypotonia might well lead to too gloomy a prognosis for intellectual development because of the severe motor retardation. One should look for a glimmer of hope in the relationship of the motor defect to other fields of development. In uncomplicated mental deficiency there tends to be relatively less retardation in motor development than in social behaviour and speech. When there is an additional mechanical difficulty, such as cerebral palsy, that position is reversed. One might find, therefore, that there is very severe motor retardation with only moderate retardation in speech. This would indicate a motor defect with an only moderately low intelligence quotient (I.Q.). The case of cerebral palsy described below is an example.

Acrodynia (pink disease) may present a confusing picture, in that the mother's history indicates that early development was normal, and that deterioration in motor development then ensued.

An 8-month-old child was referred for confirmation of the diagnosis of mental defectiveness. The mother was not able to give a reliable developmental history. The child's head control (when placed in the prone and when pulled to the sitting position) was that of a 4-month-old baby, but he was interested in test objects. His manipulative development was not less than that of an average 8-month-old baby. His grasp of a 1-in. cube was a mature one, with a rapid transfer to the other hand. He was seen to chew. He was markedly hypotonic and other signs of acrodynia were found. He made an uninterrupted recovery and became a normal child.

The dissociation between the delayed motor and normal manipulative and social behaviour showed immediately that this boy could not be mentally defective, but that there should be a mechanical difficulty affecting his gross motor development.

Rickets, which is now hardly ever seen in this country, would give a similar developmental picture, because of the hypotonia with which it is associated.

Severe illness may cause delay in motor development because of the poor muscle tone which it induces while development in other fields is likely to be normal.

Hypertonia. Cerebral palsy presents considerable developmental problems because it is seen in several different forms; there are all degrees of severity, and it is so frequently associated with a low level of intelligence which itself greatly affects the child's development.

The diagnosis of spastic paraplegia can often be made in the older infant on the history alone, provided that the intelligence is average. There is a story of normal social development (smiling by the age of 6 weeks, and so on), with normal manipulative development (voluntary grasping by 5 months), normal speech, but grossly delayed walking. The age of sitting may or may not be normal. The mother may have noticed stiffness of the lower limbs. The diagnosis is confirmed by the physical examination. The following history is an example:

A girl grasped objects voluntarily at 5 months, sat unsupported at 8 months, was helping her mother to dress her at 13 months (by holding her arm out for clothes and the foot out for a shoe) and spoke in sentences at 23 months. She was not able to walk at 5 years. She had a paraplegia with a normal I.Q. (The school medical officer assessed her on the Terman-Merrill scale as 'average' at 5 years without giving a figure.)

A mild degree of paraplegia can easily be missed in the early months.

I observed a child from 10 months of age on account of defective head control. There was no retardation in other fields. I suspected paraplegia, but subsequently decided that the knee jerks were within normal limits. There was no adductor spasm on abducting the hips. I saw the boy repeatedly, and eventually when he was 4 years old found undoubted evidence of mild disease of the pyramidal tracts involving the lower limbs. There was no deformity. He had learned to sit without support at 14 months, to feed himself with a cup at 18 months, and to join words together at 23 months. He was not able to walk at 4 years. At that time his developmental age in fields other than walking was 40 months.

Unfortunately, an average level of intelligence is unusual in cerebral palsy, so that one has the confusing picture of two factors combining to affect and retard development. Here the phenomenon of dissociation is of real value in developmental prognosis. It is particularly important to assess the child's interest in surroundings, his powers of concentration and speech. Whereas a mentally defective spastic child will make little effort to grasp an object, a spastic child of the same age and degree of spasticity but with a good level of intelligence will make determined efforts to grasp. Hence one notes the dissociation between the physical disability and the powers of concentration. If retardation in speech is only slight, severe mental deficiency is impossible: hence it is a most important indication to look for in assessing a child with cerebral palsy. Naturally speech is often retarded by other factors, such as deafness, in the presence of a good level of intelligence, so that no absolute reliance can be placed on the absence of speech as an indication of low intelligence.

A 24-month-old child was referred with a diagnosis of mental deficiency. He began to grasp objects voluntarily at 10 months, but was not able to sit. He began to say words with meaning at 18 months and to join words together at 30 months.

This gross motor delay with only a moderate delay in speech would suggest a severe mechanical disability with only a moderately low I.Q. He had a spastic quadriplegia, and his I.Q. at 5 years was 71.

A possibility to consider on finding isolated motor retardation is the subsequent development of athetoid movements, indicating that the child is in fact suffering from athetosis. It is by no means always the case, however, that motor retardation is found in early infancy in children who will subsequently be shown to be athetoids, for, provided that the I.Q. is average, the motor development in some of these children is normal. One would certainly bear the possibility in mind if there were a history of severe perinatal anoxia, of improperly treated haemolytic disease of the newborn or hyperbilirubinaemia with prematurity.

Other Causes. There remain some cases of isolated motor retardation in which even prolonged observation fails to reveal any sign of organic disease.

A baby, aged 7 months, was referred by a paediatrician because of defective head control. He had been examined with regard to suitability for adoption. On examination his head control (when prone and when pulled to the sitting position) was that of a 3-month-old baby, but his manipulative development was that of a 7-8 month baby. His interest in surroundings and his alertness seemed average. He was able to chew. There were no signs of cerebral palsy. I expressed the opinion that this was merely isolated motor retardation. His subsequent history showed that he spoke single words and sat without support at 1 year, put words together at 18 months and walked without help at 23 months. Subsequent examination showed that he was normal in all respects, with an I.Q. of just over 100.

In view of his prospective adoption, the responsibility of making a correct diagnosis was a big one.

Normal Motor Development with Retardation in Other Fields

One occasionally sees a child in whom motor development is within 'normal' limits but in whom defective social and speech development leads to a diagnosis of mental deficiency. It is not rare to see relatively advanced motor development in mongols in early infancy—a fact noted by Gesell.

I observed a mongol who began to smile at 4 months, to grasp objects voluntarily at 6 months, and to sit unsupported at 7½ months. At this time his interest in his surroundings was very defective. Development then slowed down, and he only began to walk without help at 34 months and to put words together at 69 months. At this age his I.Q. was 28. I saw another mongol who at 8 months was sitting securely without support, quite as well as an average baby; but his interest and concentration were notably defective, and he showed hand regard—normally lost by 16 weeks. His I.Q. subsequently was 30.

A girl sat without support at 7½ months, and walked without help at 21 months. Concentration was poor. She was only able to say six words at 39 months. At five years her I.Q. was 50. Another girl sat without support at 8 months, and walked without help at 17 months, but there was no speech and concentration was poor. There was full sphincter control by 24 months. She began to say single words at 3 years and to put words together at 5. At ten years her I.Q. was 20. Another girl sat without support at 6 months, and walked without help at 18 months, but I was impressed by the aimless hyperkinesis, defective concentration, and delayed speech development. Her I.Q. at 56 months was 52. In none of these cases was there any degenerative disease of the nervous system or deterioration in performance.

Other Variations in Motor Development

One sometimes sees the picture of a 'slow-starter' —a child who is seriously retarded in motor development in the first few weeks and then catches up.

A child with a birth weight of 5,000 g. and a normal perinatal history had a complete head lag at 13 weeks like that of a newborn baby and did not follow with the eyes till 17 weeks or smile till 18 weeks. From that time she made rapid strides in development, and at 25 weeks her head control was that of a 16-week-old baby. She sat without support at 7½ months, and walked without support at 1 year. She was able to say ten words with meaning at that age. Her I.Q. at 5 years was 122.

Some children develop normally for the first few weeks and then develop thyroid deficiency, encephalitis, or signs of a degenerative disease of the nervous system. When these develop suddenly, as in the development of akinetic seizures with hypsarrhythmia (Illingworth, 1955), one sees, shortly after the change has occurred, the unusual picture of normal motor development with grossly defective concentration and interest in surroundings, indicating severe mental deficiency.

Within the field of motor development itself there are occasionally certain unusual variations. Normally a child learns to sit before he creeps. I have seen the reverse happen in a child who had been brought up in an institution, and who presumably had never been given any chance to sit. One commonly sees dissociation between the sitting and standing development: for instance, an 8-month-old child is seen to sit securely, like an average child of the same age, and yet to bear as little weight on the legs as a 2- or 3-month-old child. This is simply due to the mother not allowing him to bear weight on the legs in the erroneous belief that it will weaken or otherwise harm them.

Sometimes the age of sitting unsupported is quite average, while the child is unusually late in walking without help. In all other fields the child develops normally. For instance, a child sits unsupported at 7 months, but cannot walk without help till 18 months or later. As has already been stated, one sees this in cases of paraplegia. In most children, however, there is no organic disease. One factor may be lack of confidence or fear of falls. When a child refuses to walk without help for a long period (for four or five months, for example), simple observation will show that his walking is maturing, and that as soon as he decides to walk alone he is walking well, like a child who has achieved the skill several weeks earlier.

Unusual but isolated advancement in motor development certainly does not indicate a high level of intelligence.

I saw a child sit without support at 4 months, creep (not crawl) at 4½ months, and pull himself to the standing position at 6 months. I expressed the opinion at that time that this was merely an isolated advancement, and that his I.Q. would not prove to be above the average. This was because he was in no way above the average in other fields of development. Although he subsequently walked without help at 8 months, his I.Q. at 5 years was 88. I saw another boy who walked unaided at 8 months, but was not advanced in other fields. His I.Q. at 6 years was 103.

Sphincter Control. Sphincter control is an unimportant field of development from the point of view of assessing a child's intelligence. It is delayed by a variety of organic and semi-organic conditions, and in particular by over-enthusiastic toilet training. In addition, there are very strong familial factors, unrelated to intelligence. When a child with average development in other fields is very late in acquiring control of the bladder, there is nearly always a family history of the same complaint. In mentally defective children one occasionally finds that sphincter control has been acquired at the usual time.

I would pay little attention to a history of unusually early acquisition of control, unless I were really satisfied that the control is truly voluntary, in that the child definitely asks for the chamber when he wants to void. It is easy to confuse the early 'conditioning', which is quite involuntary, with voluntary control.

Eyes, Ears, Manipulation. Unusual retardation in the use of the eyes, ears and hands, in the absence of retardation in other fields, is very rare. It may occur in the presence of obvious physical defects—visual or auditory in the case of the special senses, or of myotonia or other mechanical disability in the case of the hands. Unusual advancement in these fields is of no prognostic importance, though special manipulative aptitude can sometimes be detected in the early months.

Chewing. I find that the age of beginning to chew (average 6 months) is a useful milestone of development, with little variation in children of average development, and invariable retardation in mental deficiency.

I know of only one variation from the average in children of normal development in other fields, and that is related to mismanagement, in the form of failure to give the baby solid foods at an age when he should be given them. When they are introduced some months later (at the peak of the period of negativism), refusal to chew may occur.

Social Behaviour. Isolated lateness in social responsiveness, such as smiling and taking notice, is extremely rare in early infancy. It could be due to a visual defect.

In older infants and young children it is not so rare. I saw a child who was suspected of mental deficiency, because of a complete failure to smile or show facial responsiveness, but found that she was an example of congenital facial diplegia (Möbius syndrome). A child first seen by me at the age of 4 years, and in whom the diagnosis was infantile autism, was said by his mother never to have shown any social responsiveness at all. Development in all other respects had been normal. His I.Q. was average. One sees children with relatively 'normal' development, but with defective concentration and interest (see above). This nearly always signifies mental deficiency.

Unusually advanced social development is a good sign of superior intelligence. It is possible that early smiling might be in part related to a child's pleasant personality, but there is no evidence to that effect. I have seen two children smiling in response to social overture in the first week, and vocalizing in the third week: they had I.Q.'s subsequently in the region of 140.

In later months, unusually good concentration, alertness, determination and interest in surroundings is an important sign of superior intelligence and much more important than advanced motor development. It is unfortunate that it is so difficult to assess it and convert the assessment into figures.

Speech Development. Delayed speech development in the absence of retardation in other fields is never due to mental deficiency. It may occur in children with average or superior intelligence. In the majority of such cases there is either a family history of similar lateness, or there is no discoverable cause. Einstein gave his parents grounds for concern because of his defective speech at the age of 4 years. He was still speaking indistinctly at the age of nine. Other causes of lateness in speech without retardation in other fields include deafness, high-frequency or otherwise. It is never due to 'laziness', and serious harm is done by advising parents to do nothing for such a child unless he speaks properly. He does not speak because he cannot, not because he is too lazy to speak. I firmly believe that the statement repeated from textbook to textbook that delay in speech is due to parents and siblings doing things for a child before he asks for them is a myth. I very much doubt the truth of another oft-repeated statement, that lateness in speech is due to jealousy. All children are jealous, and as lateness in speech is common, it is indeed difficult to prove that lateness in speech is due to jealousy and not to something else. I would only go so far as to say that inability to speak may perhaps be a very rare result of jealousy, but that it cannot be proved. Lateness in speech is never due to 'tongue tie' or to cleft palate, though cleft palate may be associated with a low I.Q. and so with lateness in speech. In this case there would be retardation in other fields too.

Unusual advancement in speech is a reliable sign of superior intelligence. I have never seen it in a child of average intelligence.

The importance of relating the level of speech development to that of development in other fields has already been noted.

Summary and Conclusions

In assessing the development of an infant or young child one should always note the relationship of one milestone of development to another, in order to assess the rate of development, and the relationship of milestones in one field of development to those in another. Not infrequently development in one field is out of step with that in another. This might be termed dissociation. The reasons for this imbalance are discussed.

Isolated delay in motor development may occur without apparent reason, so that the child grows up to be perfectly normal. More often it results from a physical disability, in particular hypotonia or hypertonia. It never signifies mental deficiency.

Relative advancement in motor development in relation to other fields occasionally occurs in mentally defective children. Unusual and isolated advancement in motor development does not mean superior intelligence.

Retardation in social behaviour is of considerable prognostic significance, implying a poor prognosis for intelligence. The degree of retardation in a child with retardation in other fields is of great importance: only slight social retardation with severe motor retardation may occur in the presence of a severe mechanical disability, such as cerebral palsy, with an only slightly lowered intelligence. Advanced social development is a good index of superior intelligence, except that it is difficult to assess in figures.

Isolated delay in speech frequently occurs in children of normal or superior intelligence, and never means mental deficiency. Only moderate retardation in speech in the presence of severe retardation in other fields (as in cerebral palsy) excludes severe mental deficiency. Isolated advancement in speech is a good sign of superior intelligence.

Isolated delay in sphincter control is commonly associated with mismanagement or with familial factors, and is of no importance in developmental assessment. Advancement, relative or absolute, is of little value because of the difficulty in assessing its significance (i.e. whether the control is really voluntary and not mere conditioning).

Delay in chewing may result from mismanagement, and otherwise does not occur alone.

I wish to thank Arnold Gesell, who gave me the opportunity to learn about normal development in his Department.

References

Illingworth, R. S. (1955). *Arch. Dis. Childh.*, **30**, 529.
Walton, J. N. (1956). *Lancet*, **1**, 1023.
—— (1957). *Proc. roy. Soc. Med.*, **50**, 301.

DYSMATURITY

BY

S. SJÖSTEDT, G. ENGLESON and G. ROOTH

From the Departments of Obstetrics and Gynaecology, of Paediatrics and of Internal Medicine, University Hospital, Lund, Sweden

(RECEIVED FOR PUBLICATION AUGUST 23, 1957)

History

The Scottish obstetrician Ballantyne (1902) seems to have been the first to call attention to dysmaturity. He described the dry, parched skin, the long nails, the paucity of the amniotic fluid, the presence of meconium in amniotic fluid, and the advanced ossification in the skull. He found the weight and length of these children to be nearly always above average.

Bossi (1907) gave a description of dysmature infants which in the main agrees with Ballantyne's, but he maintained that they have a reduced amount of subcutaneous fat and that therefore their weight is lower than might be expected.

Bäcker (1915) described dysmaturity and emphasized that dysmature infants are subnormal as far as fat and weight are concerned.

Then, for some time, no attention seems to have been paid to dysmaturity, until Runge (1939, 1942, 1948) gave a detailed description of the dysmature child. He also indicated a method of recognizing the condition in some cases even before delivery. He called attention to the fact that in some women who eventually are delivered of dysmature children the amount of amniotic fluid and concomitantly the circumference of the abdomen decreases successively before delivery. Runge considers dysmaturity to be a sign of placental insufficiency as regards the transport of oxygen as well as other substances. He made no chemical analyses and his conclusion was probably based on the presence of meconium in the amniotic fluid and the loss of weight of the child.

Although no further major studies have been published, it is obvious that German obstetricians have realized the difference between prolonged gestation and dysmaturity, as is evident from Martius' textbook on obstetrics published in 1943.

In other countries, dysmaturity does not seem to have been recognized until Clifford, in 1945, reported 46 cases; he has more recently (1951, 1953, 1954, 1957) described the syndrome and its clinical importance in detail. Like Runge, Clifford considers dysmaturity to be caused by a placental insufficiency and introduces the term 'placental dysfunction syndrome'. However, he has no further proof that a placental insufficiency is the cause of dysmaturity, but seems to base his conclusions on the same clinical grounds as Runge and finds support in Walker's work (1954) on prolonged gestation. Clifford's papers are of considerable importance because he classified dysmaturity in different stages and because he has made the dysmaturity syndrome known to pediatricians. Consequently, the condition has since been the subject of reports from several countries (Taylor *et al.*, 1952; Selander, 1954; Ravera and Bottinelli, 1955; Kunstadter and Schnitz, 1956; and others).

Present Investigation

Definitions. In this investigation, the duration of pregnancy is given in weeks calculated from the first day of the last menstrual period. Thus, for example, if a child is born in the 40th week, this implies that the pregnancy has lasted between 274 and 280 days. If the gestation time exceeded 294 days, we have called this prolonged gestation or prolonged pregnancy.

If the child showed the clinical syndrome which Clifford (1954) designates as the 'placental dysfunction' syndrome, known in German as 'überreif', we use the expression 'dysmaturity' without regard to the duration of pregnancy.

The term 'postmaturity', which is often seen in the literature, is avoided because some authors use it to denote prolonged pregnancy, others to denote dysmaturity, others again to denote both prolonged pregnancy and dysmaturity.

Material. An investigation has been made of 1,171 newborn infants, all delivered at the Department of Obstetrics, University Hospital, Lund, between January 1, 1956, and March 31, 1957.

Only during the later part of the investigation were all children born classified according to dysmaturity. The material was selected, in so far as mostly children with prolonged gestation were included. The selection in these cases was always made before the children were born.

The infants were classified, largely according to Clifford's classification, the day after delivery. This was done by only one of us, who at that time had no information concerning the mother, the duration of pregnancy, the delivery, the amniotic fluid or the placenta. Thus the classification was made only on the basis of inspection and observation of the naked infant.

Normal and premature infants without signs of dysmaturity have been grouped in Stage 0.

Stage 1 corresponds to Stage 1 of Clifford. The skin is cracked, parchment-like and peeling and the arms and legs are thin. The infants are more awake and alert than usual but they may have respiratory distress and a tendency to vomit. The bones of the skull are harder than is ordinarily found.

If the clinical picture just described was less pronounced and there was doubt whether to classify the infants as normal or dysmature, they were placed in Stage 0-1.

Infants who exhibited the signs attributed to Stage 1 in a very marked degree, have been grouped in Stage 2. In addition, the trunk was thin in these cases. In Stage 2, Clifford includes meconium staining of the amniotic fluid, but as the examining doctor did not have any knowledge of the amniotic fluid, this sign was not taken into account in grouping the infants. However, they all had greenish skin, umbilicus or nails. The amount of meconium needed in the amniotic fluid to stain the infants is very small, as shown by Desmond *et al.* (1956). This can also be deduced from the fact that in only half of our Stage 2 cases was meconium staining of the amniotic fluid noted at the time of delivery. Some of the infants also produced meconium stained vomit.

Stage 3 corresponds precisely to that of Clifford. In these infants the trunk and extremities are strikingly thin, moreover they have a rather pronounced dystrophic appearance. The skin peels off in large flakes. The nails and the skin are yellowish in colour.

Great care was taken in order to obtain as reliable information as possible about the time of gestation. Most of the mothers were under observation by the staff during pregnancy and, after labour, their menstrual history was examined in detail by us. Only cases with a regular menstrual cycle have been included and any case in which the duration of pregnancy was at all doubtful has been rejected in the calculation of the gestation time.

Blood samples from the newborn infants were taken from the umbilical cord, which was clamped in two places immediately after delivery. Blood was drawn from either the vein or the arteries and mixed with heparin or sodium oxalate. If not indicated otherwise in the tables, the blood was always drawn from the vein.

The investigation was in two parts, the first covering the period from January 1 to October 31, 1956, and the second from November, 1956, to March 31, 1957. During the first part, 581 infants were investigated in the manner outlined above. However, the series was considered too small and therefore another 590 infants were studied. As both parts of the investigation have given the same results, no detailed statistical analysis of the two series is necessary.

Frequency. Only a few reports on the frequency of dysmaturity are available. Selander (1954) gives a figure of 12·0% from a study of 1,330 infants. If the infants were born more than four days after the calculated date, 20·3% displayed the syndrome. Taylor *et al.* (1952) stated that the incidence of yellow vernix not associated with haemolytic disease —that is, dysmaturity Stage 3, was 1·2%. Ravera and Bottinelli (1955) report that 2·25% of their infants were born more than 14 days after term and often had symptoms of dysmaturity (in 38 out of 42 cases). Kunstadter and Schnitz (1956) investigated 247 infants with a gestational age of 294 days or more and among these found 11 infants showing clinical symptoms consistent with dysmaturity; this gives a figure of 0·4% for infants delivered liveborn. Hinselmann (1957) in 5,258 deliveries had 600 infants with a gestation time of more than 294 days and among these were 42 infants with all or nearly all the signs of dysmaturity—that is, 7·0% of those with prolonged gestation and 0·8% of all the deliveries.

The frequency of dysmaturity in our material is shown in Table 1. The calculation of the frequency has been made only for the period when all of the infants delivered were classified.

TABLE 1

STAGE AND PERCENTAGE DISTRIBUTION OF DYSMATURITY IN 444 NEWBORN INFANTS

Stage of Dysmaturity					
0	0–1	1	2	3	1–3
58·6%	24·8%	14·9%	1·6%	0·2%	16·7%

Thus, the frequency of dysmaturity in our material is 16·7%. The advanced Stages 2 and 3 were only seen in 1·8% of the newborn infants.

Gestation Time. Runge, and later Clifford, pointed out that dysmaturity is usually associated with prolonged pregnancy, but that it may be present even in infants born before term. Selander (1954) gives a dysmaturity frequency of 2·4% for infants born two to three weeks before term and a frequency of 1·1% for infants born more than three weeks before term.

Our material consists of 968 cases (Table 2).

TABLE 2
DISTRIBUTION ACCORDING TO GESTATION TIME (968 CASES)

Stage of Dysmaturity	Duration of Pregnancy in Weeks								
	36	37	38	39	40	41	42	43	≥44
0	3	9	21	103	141	149	42	14	11
0–1		1	5	25	57	77	41	9	8
1	1		2	13	47	61	50	26	12
2				1	2	8	13	6	10
Total	4	10	28	142	247	295	146	55	41

Two hundred and three cases have been excluded because, as already mentioned, the gestation time was uncertain. It should be noted that the frequency displayed in Table 2 does not give a true picture of the dysmaturity distribution as sometimes only infants of mothers with a gestation time of 41 weeks or more were investigated. Thus, the frequency distribution has been somewhat shifted towards the right—that is, towards prolonged gestation. However, the table clearly shows the increased frequency of dysmaturity with increasing gestation time, but it also shows that most of the infants with Stage 2 dysmaturity are born within 294 days.

Parity of Mother and Sex of Infant. Several investigators have shown (Rütte, 1949; Hosemann, 1948; Clifford, 1954; Lindell, 1956; Strand, 1956) that the increase in infant mortality observed in prolonged pregnancy only refers to primiparae. It is, therefore, of interest to study whether dysmature infants are mostly born to primiparae or not. This information is presented in Table 3 together with the sex distribution of the infants.

If Stage 0-1 is included in the dysmaturity group, this syndrome is more frequent among primiparae than among multiparae. A statistical analysis shows that this difference is significant ($0{\cdot}01>p>0{\cdot}001$). With advancing stage of dysmaturity the frequency of boys dominates over that of girls. If again Stage 0-1 is included, this difference is statistically almost significant ($0{\cdot}02>p>0{\cdot}01$).

TABLE 3
SEX DISTRIBUTION AND DYSMATURITY AMONG PRIMIPARAE AND MULTIPARAE (1,171 CASES)

Stage of Dysmaturity	Primiparae		Multiparae	
	Boys	Girls	Boys	Girls
0	100	107	201	196
0–1	61	41	86	80
1	69	55	75	55
2	12	6	15	8
3			4	
Total	242	209	381	339

Age of Mother. Clifford stresses that dysmature infants born of elderly primigravidae must be watched with great care, since experience has shown that foetal morbidity and mortality are high in these cases. It is therefore of interest to study whether the frequency of dysmaturity also increases with the age of the mother. As seen from Table 4 in our material there is no increasing frequency of dysmaturity with advancing age of the mother.

TABLE 4
PERCENTAGE DISTRIBUTION OF MATERNAL AGE

Maternal Age	Stage of Dysmaturity			
	0	0–1	1	2+3
	%	%	%	%
<20	7·0	6·2	7·5	8·9
20–24	22·8	22·4	27·5	17·8
25–29	32·9	35·0	31·0	29·0
30–34	23·5	22·0	19·3	22·2
35–39	10·8	12·3	13·0	15·6
≥40	2·8	1·9	1·6	6·7

Weight of Infant. The growth of the foetus has been the subject of much speculation, particularly in the case of prolonged gestation. Solth (1947), Calkins (1948), McKiddie (1949), Hosemann (1952) and Lindell (1956) state that growth slows down towards the end of pregnancy and then become almost stationary or at least increases very little as gestation proceeds. Some authors (Rathburn, 1943; Freudenberg, 1950) even state that in prolonged gestation the foetus will lose weight. Table 5 gives the weight of the infants for the 921 cases in which the gestation time was between 39 and 44 weeks.

TABLE 5
MEAN WEIGHT IN G. AT TERM AND IN PROLONGED PREGNANCY (921 CASES)

Duration of Pregnancy in Weeks	Stage of Dysmaturity			
	0	0–1	1	2+3
	g.	g.	g.	g.
39	3,320	3,425	3,118	2,600
40	3,440	3,363	3,332	3,140
41	3,675	3,597	3,423	3,230
42	3,708	3,677	3,649	3,233
43+44	3,819	3,761	3,561	3,603

Two curves are given in Fig. 1, one corresponding to Stages 0 and 0-1 considered together, the other to Stages 1, 2 and 3, also considered together. Fig. 1 shows that the mean weight of the normal infants increased continuously from the 39th to the 43rd and 44th week and that this increase was of the same magnitude each week. The mean weight of the dysmature infants was at 39 weeks already some 200 g. less than the mean weight of the normal infants but showed a similar weekly increase from the 39th to the 44th week.

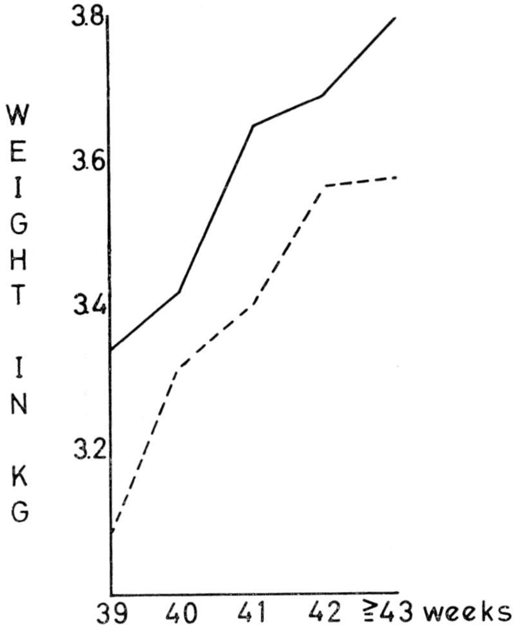

FIG. 1.—Weight curves of normal and dysmature infants.
———— Normal infants, Stages 0 and 0·1
— — — — Dysmature infants, Stages 1, 2 and 3

From a consideration of the gestation times in Table 2 and the weight curves in Fig. 1 two important conclusions can be drawn:

1. Although the frequency of dysmaturity is increased in prolonged gestation, it is not caused by prolonged gestation since evidence of dysmaturity is already manifest before term.

2. Although both normal and dysmature infants increase in weight with increasing gestation time, the difference in the weight curves can explain the apparent decrease in weight in prolonged pregnancy observed by other authors. Because of a steadily increasing proportion of dysmature infants in prolonged pregnancy, the percentage of the normal infants with high weight is gradually reduced, whereas the percentage of the dysmature infants with small weight gradually increases. This causes a flattening of a growth curve which includes all the infants. With great foresight this explanation was hypothetically proposed by Clifford (1957).

The reduced weight which the dysmature infants show as compared with the normal ones indicates insufficient nutrition during a relatively extended period of time, as would be expected in the case of placental insufficiency.

Length of Infant. Most of the above-mentioned authors who have studied the weight of the newborn infant have also studied the length and found that it increases up to and including the 43rd week.

This is confirmed in Table 6 which shows that, according to our data, the infant's length increases irrespectively of dysmaturity until and including the 43rd week. Thus, dysmature infants are of normal length but reduced weight. However, it should be remembered that it is difficult to measure the length of the newborn infant with a satisfactory exactness. The reduction in length which is suggested in the 44th week may not be real because the material is small and only includes 40 infants, and furthermore, in spite of our precautions, the true gestation time may, in some cases, be only 40 weeks instead of 44.

TABLE 6

INFLUENCE OF GESTATION TIME AND DYSMATURITY ON MEAN LENGTH OF INFANT

Gestation Time in Weeks	Stage of Dysmaturity			
	0	0–1	1	2+3
	cm.	cm.	cm.	cm.
37	46·6	47·5	—	—
38	48·8	47·9	50·5	—
39	49·5	49·5	49·0	48·0
40	49·7	49·6	49·6	50·0
41	50·8	50·5	50·3	50·1
42	50·6	50·9	51·1	49·7
43	51·7	51·4	51·0	52·0
≥44	50·2	50·6	51·0	51·1

Oxygen Saturation in Cord Blood. The oxygen saturation in the cord blood during prolonged gestation has been the subject of much discussion. Walker and Turnbull (1953) claimed that the oxygen saturation in the cord blood decreases with advancing gestation time in prolonged pregnancy. However, the number of infants studied was small. Minkowski *et al.* (1953) support Walker's thesis although they find exceptions. MacKay (1957) in a recent study, like Walker's, also from Scotland, of 240 infants, reaches the same conclusion as Walker and Turnbull (1953). But MacKinney *et al.* (1955) studying cord blood oxygen saturation in 594 infants did not find significant differences between mature infants and infants with prolonged gestation. Rooth and Sjöstedt (1957b), investigating 363 infants, found no changes in the oxygen saturation from the 39th week to the 43rd week.

As far as we know, the oxygen saturation in cord blood has not been studied before in relation to dysmaturity, although Runge and most subsequent authors on dysmaturity have considered dysmature infants to be hypoxic.

The oxygen saturation, measured with a Brinkman haemoreflector in the manner already described by Rooth and Sjöstedt (1955) has been measured in the umbilical vein in 210 infants and in the arteries in 165 infants in our series (Table 7).

TABLE 7

MEAN OXYGEN SATURATION IN PER CENT IN UMBILICAL CORD BLOOD

		Totals	Stage of Dysmaturity 0	0-1	1	2
Vein	Number	210	104	35	59	12
	HbO_2		63·7%	58·6%	56·9%	51·1%
Artery	Number	165	79	29	47	10
	HbO_2		38·7%	34·7%	34·6%	24·3%

The oxygen saturation decreases both in the umbilical vein and in the arteries with advancing stages of dysmaturity. Thus, according to our results, in prolonged pregnancy the cord blood oxygen saturation is decreased only if the infant also is dysmature. An infant with no signs of dysmaturity will retain its oxygenation in spite of a prolongation of pregnancy beyond term.

These observations could explain the differing results obtained by the various authors studying the oxygen saturation in the cord blood of infants in prolonged gestation. If the number of infants studied is small, as in Walker's report, the percentage of dysmature children may be much higher than if a sufficiently large number of cases had been studied. Furthermore, there may be a notable difference in the frequency of dysmaturity in different countries.

Haemoglobin in Cord Blood. Walker and Turnbull (1953) found that from the 40th to the 43rd week the amount of haemoglobin in cord blood increased considerably and interpret this as a compensation for the decreasing oxygen saturation. Marks *et al.* (1955) and Rooth and Sjöstedt (1957a) could not confirm these results, both groups finding no increase in the haemoglobin in cord blood during prolonged gestation. MacKay found a slight rise with increasing maturity but the results tended to agree with the results of Marks *et al.*

No studies are available regarding the influence of dysmaturity on the cord blood haemoglobin. We have measured this in 885 infants (Table 8). The technique has been described earlier by Rooth and Sjöstedt (1957a).

The haemoglobin values rise with advancing signs of dysmaturity and this rise is already evident in the intermediate group, Stage 0-1. This increase of haemoglobin in dysmature infants suggests that, *in utero*, they were hypoxic, but it may be only a sign of haemoconcentration.

TABLE 8

MEAN HAEMOGLOBIN IN G. PER 100 ML. UMBILICAL CORD BLOOD (885 CASES)

	Stage of Dysmaturity 0	0–1	1	2
Number	450	205	194	36
Haemoglobin ..	16·1	16·7	16·9	17·0

Plasma Pentoses. The concentration of pentoses in plasma has been studied by Green and his collaborators, among others. Green *et al.* (1949) noted a significant rise in the plasma pentose fractions in battle casualties and believed this to be the result of ischaemia in the injured tissues. In the pregnant woman an increase in the plasma pentose fractions has occasionally been noted. Green *et al.* (1951) consider this to be due to a relative uteroplacental ischaemia.

Using the method of Mejbaum (1939) as modified by Green *et al.* (1951), we have measured the plasma pentoses in the cord blood of 198 infants (Table 9).

The plasma pentoses increase with advancing signs of dysmaturity. This probably indicates a progressive ischaemia and therefore supports our results on the analyses of the oxygen saturation and the haemoglobin in the cord blood.

TABLE 9

MEAN PLASMA PENTOSES IN MG. PER 100 ML. UMBILICAL CORD BLOOD (198 CASES)

	Stage of Dysmaturity 0	0–1	1	2
Number	92	35	58	13
Pentoses	4·6	5·0	5·6	6·5

Protein-bound Hexoses. For more than 50 years the protein-bound polysaccharides in serum have been studied mainly in connexion with diabetes mellitus. Abnormally high values have been found in a number of different pathological conditions. However, no final explanation for this abnormality has been found (Keiding, 1957). The most commonly accepted explanation (Greenspan *et al.*, 1951) is that the protein-bound hexoses indicate tissue destruction. We have measured the protein-bound hexoses in the cord blood of 246 infants and our results are given in Table 10.

The protein-bound hexoses increase with advancing signs of dysmaturity. Even if no definite explanation for this can be given, it points to an increasing pathological process in the infant or in the placenta.

TABLE 10

MEAN PROTEIN-BOUND HEXOSES IN MG. PER 100 ML. UMBILICAL CORD BLOOD (246 CASES)

	Stage of Dysmaturity			
	0	0–1	1	2
Number	48	105	74	19
Hexoses	127·1	127·0	148·5	152·3

Bilirubin. Icterus neonatorum has been the subject of extensive investigations. Most of these studies have been devoted to the serum of the infant's blood after birth; however, others have been concerned with the cord blood as well. Davidson *et al.* (1941) report a mean value of 1·69 mg. per 100 ml. in 94 cases with a range of 0·42 to 3·9. As others before them they found that the higher the cord bilirubin the more intense became the icterus of the infant and the longer it lasted. Schick *et al.* (1942) compared the cord blood bilirubin in prematures, normal infants and overmatures (weight more than 3,800 g., length more than 52 cm.). With increasing maturity the bilirubin was reduced but the differences were so small that no conclusions could be drawn. We have analysed the bilirubin in the cord blood of 446 infants with Jendrassik's method (Table 11).

TABLE 11

MEAN BILIRUBIN IN MG. PER 100 ML. UMBILICAL CORD BLOOD (446 CASES)

	0	0–1	1	2
Number	218	115	103	10
Bilirubin	1·52	1·58	1·86	2·82

Although the differences are not large, there is a gradual increase in the bilirubin values in the cord blood with advancing signs of dysmaturity.

Non-protein Nitrogen. Reports on the NPN in cord blood have been published by Hellmuth (1924), Naeslund (1931), Slemons (1919), Pommerenke (1936) and Lichtenstein (1931). Their values vary between 25 and 40 mg. per 100 ml. of cord blood, and in the umbilical vein the values are slightly higher than in the arteries. Lichtenstein has correlated the NPN with the birth weight of the infant and shown that starting at a weight of 1,500 g., the NPN remains at the same level or 33 mg. per 100 ml. of cord blood.

McCance and Widdowson (1954) studied ten full term or post-mature infants all delivered by forceps. They analysed the urea and found a mean value of 39·9 mg. per 100 ml. of cord blood in six dysmature infants as compared with 30·9 in four normal infants. They took this as an indication that the urea concentration in cord blood is higher among dysmature infants and recommended further investigations.

We have analysed the cord blood of 804 infants for NPN (Table 12).

TABLE 12

MEAN NON-PROTEIN NITROGEN IN MG. PER 100 ML. UMBILICAL CORD BLOOD (804 CASES)

	Stage of Dysmaturity				
	0	0–1	1	2	3
Number	398	209	170	23	4
Non-protein nitrogen	28·8	29·4	29·7	34·7	37·0

The non-protein nitrogen in the cord blood also increases with increasing signs of dysmaturity. This is caused either by a placental insufficiency which prevents the foetus from excreting its NPN through the placenta or by an increase in tissue (notably placental tissue) destruction and subsequent increased production of NPN. Probably both of these mechanisms are of importance at the same time.

Albumin in Urine. Tests for proteinuria have been so consistently positive, especially during the second to fifth day after birth, that albumin in the urine is to be considered a more or less physiological constituent of the newborn infant's urine (Heller, 1913; Franz and Reuss, 1914; Ewald, 1916; Pfaundler, 1924). Ewald found that 75% of the urine samples taken from infants with birth weights below 3·5 kg. reacted positively to the albumin test; furthermore, 69% of the tests on larger infants were positive.

We have tested the urine for albumin using Heller's test on specimens from 577 newborn infants (Table 13). These specimens were taken as early as

TABLE 13

FREQUENCY IN PER CENT OF ALBUMIN IN URINE (577 CASES)

	Stage of Dysmaturity			
	0	0–1	1	2+3
Number	114	208	217	38
Albumin	18%	29%	30%	63%

possible, always within the first three days of life. The urine of all infants with positive albumin tests showed a negative reaction within one week after birth.

The frequency of albumin in the urine of the newborn infant increases with the degree of dysmaturity, showing that these infants are also suffering from an impairment of the renal function.

Glycosuria. Hoeniger (1911) reports the frequent occurrence of reducing substances in infants after complicated deliveries. Lindig (1922) found this in only three cases out of 24 delivered by forceps.

We have, using the glucose oxidase reaction, tested the urine of 577 newborn infants shortly after birth (never later than the third day). (Table 14.)

TABLE 14

FREQUENCY IN PER CENT OF REDUCING SUBSTANCES IN URINE (577 CASES)

	Stage of Dysmaturity			
	0	0–1	1	2+3
Number	114	208	217	38
Reducing substances	0·9%	1·9%	5·1%	10·5%

The frequency of glycosuria also increases with the degree of dysmaturity. In the normal infant glycosuria is rare, but is present in about 10% of the dysmature infants in Stages 2 and 3. Sometimes these infants may even show a clinical picture which resembles diabetes, a case report of which has been presented by Engleson and Zetterqvist (1957).

Discussion

The present study shows the importance of distinguishing between, on the one hand, the gestation time of the infant—that is, whether it is prolonged or not, and, on the other, the state of the infant—that is, whether the infant is normal or dysmature.

We find no untoward effects on the infants due to the prolongation of pregnancy *per se*, but we do find considerable changes in dysmature infants. Unfortunately, this important fact does not yet solve the clinical controversy as to whether labour should be induced or not in a woman who carries her child beyond term. The answer is, of course, that labour should be induced if the infant is dysmature, but this cannot as a rule be verified until after the child is born. If the Ballantyne-Runge sign is present—that is, if the circumference of the abdomen is rapidly reduced late in pregnancy, the child is likely to be dysmature. Foetal electrocardiogram studies (Southern, 1957) also indicate a possible method of diagnosing dysmaturity before birth.

The clinical picture of the dysmature infant is distinct and can be recognized with a little training. It would be advantageous to register all the newborn infants according to dysmaturity. Thus, mortality and morbidity statistics on the neonatal period in different hospitals and countries would be more easily comparable.

Interpretation of Results

The reduced weight, the hypoxia, the increased haemoglobin, and possibly also the increased NPN, indicate a reduction in the diffusion capacity of the placenta. This reduction is probably caused by an ischaemia or destruction of placental tissue, as indicated by the increase in pentoses and protein-bound hexoses, and possibly also by the increased NPN. The increase in bilirubin may be a sign of the increased blood formation and a concomitant increased turnover of the haemoglobin pigments. It may also be due to hypoxic disturbances in the liver function, as the increased frequency of albumin in the urine might be a sign of hypoxic kidney function.

Summary

In order to prevent confusion between the terms 'prolonged pregnancy' and 'postmaturity' the term 'dysmaturity' is introduced to denote the placental insufficiency syndrome.

One thousand, one hundred and seventy-one newborn infants have been classified according to dysmaturity and studied from various aspects.

The frequency of dysmaturity in our series is 16·7% and increases with advancing gestation time; it is also higher for primiparae and male infants. Both normal and dysmature infants increase in weight during gestation, but from the 39th week onwards until delivery the dysmature infants have a mean birth weight 200 g. below that of normal infants. As dysmaturity becomes increasingly severe the oxygen saturation in the cord blood decreases, whereas there is an increase in the haemoglobin, in the plasma pentoses, in the protein-bound hexoses, in the bilirubin and in the non-protein nitrogen.

The more pronounced signs of dysmaturity are also allied to an increased frequency of albumin and glucose in the urine of the newborn infants.

This study was supported by grants from the Swedish Medical Research Council, Stiftelsen Synsvaga Barn and the Association for the Aid of Crippled Children.

REFERENCES

Ballantyne, J. W. J. (1902). *J. Obstet. Gynaec. Brit. Emp.*, **2**, 521.
Bossi, L. M. (1907). *Gynäk. Rundschau*, **1**, 30.
Bäcker, J. (1915). *Ibid.*, **9**, 29.
Calkins, L. A. (1948). *Amer. J. Obstet Gynec.*, **56**, 167.
Clifford, S. H. (1945). *Amer. J. Dis. Child.*, **69**, 327.
—— (1953). *A.M.A. Amer. J. Dis. Child.*, **86**, 319.
—— (1954). *J. Pediat.*, **44**, 1.
—— (1957). *Advanc. Pediat.*, **9**, 13.
——, Reid, D. E. and Worcester, J. (1951). *A.M.A. Amer. J. Dis. Child.*, **82**, 232.
Davidson, L. T., Merritt, K. K. and Weech, A. A. (1941). *Amer. J. Dis. Child.*, **61**, 958.
Desmond, M. M., Lindley, J. E., Moore, J. and Brown, C. A. (1956). *J. Pediat.*, **49**, 540.
Engleson, G. and Zetterqvist, P. (1957). *Arch. Dis. Childh.*, **32**, 193.
Ewald, L. (1916). *Mschr. Geburtsh. Gynäk.*, **43**, 347.
Franz, T. and Reuss, A. von (1914). *Z. Kinderheilk.*, **11**, 193.
Freudenberg, K. (1950). *Arch. Gynäk.*, **177**, 736.
Green, H. N., Hopewell, J. D. and Threlfall, C. J. (1951). *Brit. med. J.*, **2**, 571.
——, Stoner, H. B., Whiteley, H. J. and Eglin, D. (1949). *Clin. Sci.*, **8**, 65.
Greenspan, E. M., Tepper, B., Terry, L. L. and Schoenbach, E. B. (1952). *J. Lab. clin. Med.*, **39**, 44.
Heller, F. (1913). *Z. Kinderheilk.*, **7**, 303.
Hellmuth, K. (1924). *Arch. Gynäk.*, **123**, 57.
Hinselmann. (1957). *Zbl. Gynäk.*, **79**, 597.
Hoeniger, E. (1911). *Dtsch. med. Wschr.*, **37**, 500.
Hosemann, H. (1948). *Klin. Wschr.*, **26**, 118.
—— (1952). In *Biologie und Pathologie des Weibes*, 2nd ed., ed. L. Seitz and A. I. Amreich, Vol. 7, p. 828. Berlin.
Keiding, N. R. (1957). *Protein-bound Carbohydrates and Proteins of Serum from Diabetic Patients*. Copenhagen.
Kunstadter, R. H. and Schnitz, S. E. (1956). *J. Amer. med. Ass.*, **161**, 1551.
Lichtenstein, A. (1931). *Z. Kinderheilk.*, **51**, 748.
Lindell, A. (1956). *Acta obstet. gynec. scand.*, **35**, 136.
Lindig, P. (1922). *Klin. Wschr.*, **1**, 995.
McCance, R. A. and Widdowson, E. M. (1954). *Arch. Dis. Childh.*, **29**, 495.
MacKay, R. B. (1957). *J. Obstet. Gynaec. Brit. Emp.*, **64**, 185.
McKiddie, J. M. (1949). *Ibid.*, **56**, 386.
MacKinney, L. G., Ehrlich, F., Goldberg, I. D. and Cantwell, K. T. (1955). *A.M.A. Amer. J. Dis. Child.*, **90**, 520.
Marks, J., Gairdner, D. and Roscoe, J. D. (1955). *Arch. Dis. Childh.*, **30**, 117.
Martius, H. (1943). *Lehrbuch der Obstetrik und Gynäkologie*. Stuttgart.
Mejbaum, W. (1939). *Hoppe-Seyl. Z. physiol. Chem.*, **258**, 117.
Minkowski, A., Caillebotte, M., Saint Anne-Dargassies, S., Larroche, J. C., Barab, R. and Maille, G. (1953). *Ét. néo-nat.*, **2**, 197.
Naeslund, J. (1931). *Acta obstet. gynec. scand.*, **11**, 293.
Pfaundler, M. von (1924). In *Handbuch der Geburtshilfe*, ed. A. Döderlein, 2nd ed. Vol. 1. Berghmann, Munich.
Pommerenke, W. T. (1936). *J. clin. Invest.*, **15**, 485.
Rathbun, L. S. (1943). *Amer. J. Obst. Gynec.*, **46**, 278.
Ravera, G P. and Bottinelli, I. (1955). *Minerva pediat.* (*Torino*), **7**, 486.
Rooth, G. and Sjöstedt, S. (1955). *Acta obstet. gynec. scand.*, **34**, 442.
——, —— (1957a). *Arch. Dis. Childh.*, **32**, 91.
——, —— (1957b). *Acta obstet. gynec. scand.*,
Runge, H. (1939). *Dtsch. med. Wschr.*, **65**, 541.
—— (1942). *Zbl. Gynäk.*, **66**, 1202.
—— (1948). *Geburtsh. u. Frauenheilk.*, **8**, 401.
Rütte, U. von (1949). *Schweiz. med. Wschr.*, **79**, 1123.
Schick, B., Weiner, S. B. and Reiner M. (1942). *Amer. J. Dis. Child.*, **64**, 655.
Selander, P. (1954). *Acta paediat.* (*Uppsala*), **43**, 587.
Slemons, J. M. (1919). *Amer. J. Obstet. Dis. Wom.*, **80**, 194.
Solth, K. (1947). *Geburts. u. Frauenheilk.*, **7**, 134.
Southern, E. M. (1957). *Amer. J. Obstet. Gynec.*, **73**, 233.
Strand, A. (1956). *Acta obstet. gynec. scand.*, **35**, 76.
Taylor, W. C., James, J. A. and Henderson, J. L. (1952). *Arch. Dis Childh.*, **29**, 442.
Walker, J. (1954). *J. Obstet. Gynaec. Brit. Emp.*, **61**, 162.
—— and Turnbull, E. P. N. (1953). *Lancet*, **2**, 312.

CONGENITAL INTERRUPTION OF THE AORTIC ARCH

BY

BRIDGET V. FOLEY

From the Central Laboratory, Belfast

(RECEIVED FOR PUBLICATION AUGUST 25, 1957)

Complete interruption of the aortic arch is rare, and so far only seven cases appear to have been recorded (Maud Abbott, five cases, 1927; Evans, one case, 1933; Sewart, one case, 1948).

Apart from the rarity of this condition, the present case is recorded because it emphasizes that the clinical recognition of the condition may be complicated where there is persistent patency of the ductus arteriosus, and when an interventricular shunt allows better oxygenated blood to reach the lower part of the body. The case also illustrates, by the coincidence of abnormalities representing disturbances at the same period of development and by the occurrence of a maternal illness at, or about, the same time, the theory that many congenital abnormalities are the result of arrests of development at critical periods of embryonic development.

In infantile coarctation the aorta narrows proximal to the entrance of the ductus arteriosus, and here the diameter of the vessel is less, and usually much less, than that of the subclavian artery. In consequence, the lower part of the body is almost entirely supplied during foetal life by blood from the right ventricle which reaches it *via* the ductus arteriosus. There is no stimulus to develop anastomoses between branches from the aorta above and those below the narrowing. After birth and with the closure of the ductus, the circulation in the lower half of the body is dependent on the flow through the coarctated part of the arch and becomes insufficient. In complete interruption of the aortic arch the lower part of the body is at all times completely isolated from the left ventricle and is supplied by blood from the right ventricle through the patent ductus arteriosus. After birth this is venous blood and even that is only available for the short period that the ductus remains patent.

Clinical History

The mother was 24 years old and her blood group was Rh positive. After a 39-week pregnancy, a baby boy was delivered normally, on December 9, 1956, weighing 2,700 g. He was the second child, the elder, being premature, weighed 1,050 g. at birth, but is at present alive and well.

On the fourth day the infant fed poorly from the breast and supplementary feeding was started. He was then slightly jaundiced. On the sixth day complete artificial feeding was necessary and the baby was tube fed. Later on the same day he appeared ill, was pale and shocked and had a slightly jaundiced appearance. There was no pyrexia or cyanosis. The respirations were grunting and laboured with marked abdominal breathing. The liver and spleen were both palpable. The umbilicus was healing satisfactorily and the fontanelle was not depressed. The heart sounds were normal and no murmurs were heard. There were widespread crepitations over the right lung. The haemoglobin was 80% (Sahli). A radiograph showed a large heart with a shadow on its right border. It was considered that there was some central consolidation of the lung and probably an aspiration pneumonia. Oxygen, 'alevaire' and 'crystamycin' (0·5 ml. twice daily) were administered. In spite of the fact that the infant had never fed satisfactorily the birth weight had not decreased and he now weighed 2,800 g. At 9.30 p.m. on the same day the infant's condition suddenly deteriorated and he died in a few minutes.

Necropsy

The body was that of a well-developed male infant. The skin and conjunctivae had an icteric tinge. There was no pitting oedema. On opening the chest a large heart, with a big right ventricle, occupied the major part of the front of the chest, compressing the left lung posteriorly. The venous drainage was normal. The right auricle was not dilated and opened by a normal tricuspid valve into the right ventricle. This valve showed several cherry red, pin-head-sized cysts on its auricular aspect, the so-called 'congenital cysts'. The right ventricle was large with well-developed muscular walls. There was a patent interventricular septal defect high up in the membraneous portion, measuring 3 mm. by 4 mm. The pulmonary outflow tract was prominent and a large pulmonary artery, normal in position and direction, proceeded from it, giving off a branch to each lung and then, without change in its diameter, continued through the widely dilated patent ductus, to become the descending aorta. This gave origin to the usual thoracic and abdominal branches and divided into the common iliac arteries. The left auricle was not dilated.

There was a defective interauricular septum due to an inadequate and fenestrated septum secundum. The persistently patent slit-like opening measured 9 mm. by 2 mm. The left auricle opened through a normal mitral valve into the left ventricle which was smaller than the right. The aorta originated from the left ventricle. It was a smaller vessel than the pulmonary artery and was guarded by three semilunar cusps normally placed. The coronary vessels arose normally. A normal innominate and left carotid vessel were present and the aorta terminated as the left subclavian artery. There was no communication or strand of fibrous tissue between it and the distal aorta (Figs. 1-2).

The left lung was compressed by the enlarged heart, but the right lung filled the pleural cavity well. The other organs were congested, but were not otherwise abnormal.

Histology

The left lung showed extensive areas of primary non-aeration with some vernix 'squames' and mononuclear cells with foamy cytoplasm. A similar reaction was present in the right lung and the changes in both were consistent with the clinical diagnosis of an 'aspiration pneumonia'. The liver showed focal areas of necrosis with some prominence of myeloid haemopoiesis in relation to the portal tracts. The adrenal had a nest of primitive neuroblasts which measured 1·6 mm. by 0·8 mm. Sections of spleen, thymus, pancreas, kidney and brain showed the changes of acute congestion.

Discussion

To understand the pathology of this condition the embryology should be considered. During the course of development six pairs of aortic arches develop but not all are present at any one time. The period of development of the aortic arches extends throughout the fourth week of intra-uterine life and their transformation mainly occupies the fifth to the seventh week. The first arch appears at the beginning of the fourth week. Second, third, fourth, fifth and sixth arches appear in rapid succession but by the sixth week, when the sixth arch has appeared, the first and second arches are beginning to atrophy. Only towards the end of the fifth week are all the arches open and even the first is atrophic when the sixth is developing. Normally the first, second and fifth arches disappear entirely. The common carotid vessels are formed from the third arches. The fourth left arch forms that part of the arch of the aorta between the origin of the left common carotid artery and the aortic end of the ductus. This is the site of the defect in the present

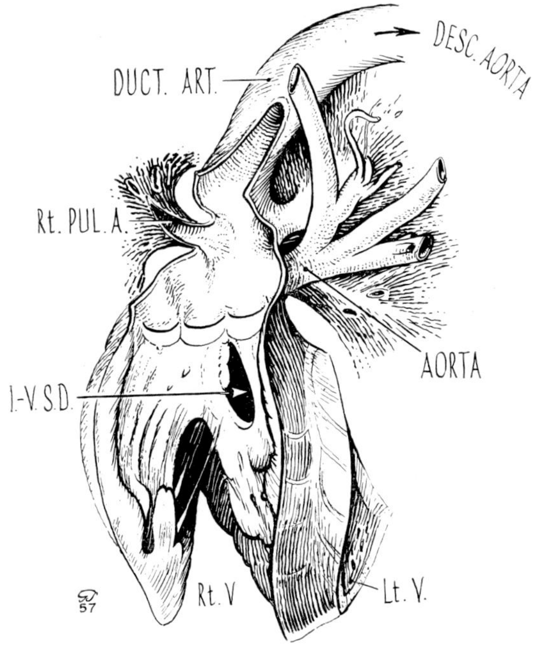

FIG. 1.—The heart showing the continuity of the descending aorta with the pulmonary artery and the interventricular septal defect. DUCT. ART., ductus arteriosus; DESC. AORTA, descending aorta; Rt PUL. A., right pulmonary artery; I-V.S.D., interventricular septal defect; Rt V., right ventricle; Lt V., left ventricle.

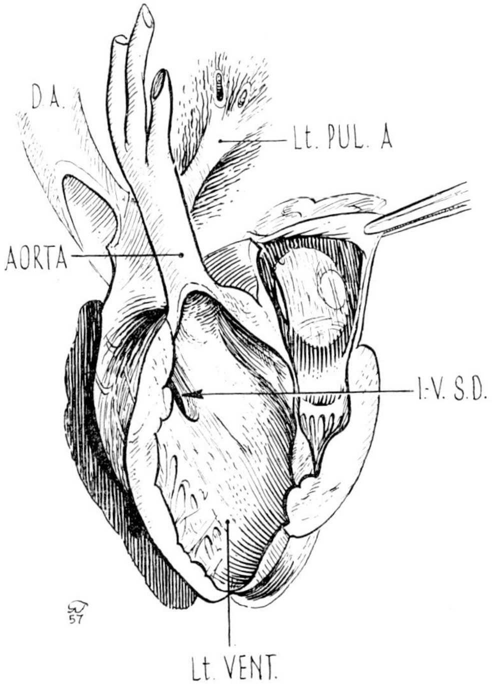

FIG. 2.—The left ventricle showing the aorta giving rise to the vessel of the head and upper extremities.
D.A., ductus arteriosus; Lt PUL. A., left pulmonary artery I-V.S.D., interventricular septal defect; Lt VENT., left ventricle

case, which essentially represents an involution of this portion of the fourth arch similar to the process normally affecting the first, second and fifth arches. Normally the portion of the same left arch distal to the origin of the subclavian artery joins the sixth arch to form the descending part of the arch of the aorta. The sixth arch forms both the pulmonary arteries and the ductus arteriosus, the latter closing in the neonatal period and its remains being identified as a fibrous band.

The interauricular septal formation begins in the fourth or fifth week of intra-uterine life and this is complete, apart from the post-natal closure of the foramen ovale, by the eighth week. In the first two weeks of neonatal life the foramen ovale closes in approximately 80% of infants. The interventricular septal formation begins in the fifth week of gestation and is completed by the eighth week.

In interruption of the aortic arch there is a complete disappearance of a portion of the fourth arch as well as the normal involution of the first, second and fifth arches. In infantile coarctation there is a failure of the structures derived from the arch in the region proximal to the ductus arteriosus to grow or to develop at the same rate as the rest of the vascular system at some period in foetal life.

The cause of any congenital defect is usually unknown, but at the present time environmental influences resulting from maternal illness or metabolic upsets during the first three months of pregnancy must receive most careful consideration. The period from the fourth to the eighth week is most critical with regard to heart development. Many of the known virus infections and obscure febrile illnesses have been implicated from time to time.

In the present case the defects would suggest some upset during the fifth to the sixth week of prenatal life. Careful investigation of the mother's health in the early months of her pregnancy was significant. Conception date could be more or less restricted to March 28, 1956. On April 28 and 29 the patient was ill with headache, vomiting, general malaise and slight pyrexia. The diagnosis of 'sinusitis' was made and only sedatives and analgesics were prescribed. The age of the foetus at this time was four and a half weeks. After a rapid recovery the mother's health was good until May 25, 1956, when she was confined to bed for a few days with a typical influenzal syndrome of headache, prostration, generalized muscle pain and vomiting. The foetal age at this time was eight weeks.

During the fourth-fifth week of prenatal life at a critical stage in the development of the aortic arches and the interauricular septum and just before the formation of the interventricular septum this foetus could feasibly have been subjected to some upset secondary to the maternal illness which resulted in the defects already described. The illness at the eighth week is probably of secondary importance as the cardiac structures are more or less established at this date.

Summary

A case is described of complete interruption of the arch of the aorta in a male infant dying aged 6 days. A patent interauricular and interventricular septum resulted in the absence of clinical cyanosis. The mother had a febrile illness at a critical period in the development of the aortic arch and cardiac septa in the foetus.

I wish to thank Mr. W. R. Sloan, consultant obstetrician, Lagan Valley Hospital, for permission to report this case; Dr. J. A. H. McClelland, the family doctor, for assisting with the ante-natal history; Dr. J. Edgar Morison for his help and advice; and Mr. G. A. Smith who made the illustrations.

REFERENCES

Abbott, M. D. (1927). In Osler, W. and McCrae, T., *Modern Medicine*, 3rd ed., vol. **4**, pp. 772. London.
Evans, W. (1933). *Quart. J. Med.*, n.s. **2**, 16.
Sewart, M. (1948). *Arch. Dis. Child.*, **23**, 63.

NORMAL DIAMETER OF THE HEART IN RADIOGRAPHS OF PRE-SCHOOL CHILDREN

BY

DAVID HEWITT

From the Department of Social Medicine, Oxford University

(RECEIVED FOR PUBLICATION SEPTEMBER 20, 1957)

Over a period of several years children in the Oxford Child Health Survey had a chest radiograph taken at six-monthly intervals. As part of a genetic study measurements of the breadth of the heart shadow have been made on all those children who had brothers or sisters in the Survey. The chest radiograph was dropped from the routine examination some years before the end of the Survey but sufficient measurements have been taken to provide reasonable estimates of the average heart diameter of healthy children up to the age of 5 years. A summary of these measurements is presented here in the hope that it may provide a useful standard of comparison for children in whom enlargement of the heart is suspected.

Possibly the most usual radiographic criterion of normal heart size is the cardiothoracic index (total transverse heart diameter divided by internal diameter of the thorax), a value in excess of 0·50 being taken as *prima facie* evidence of enlargement.

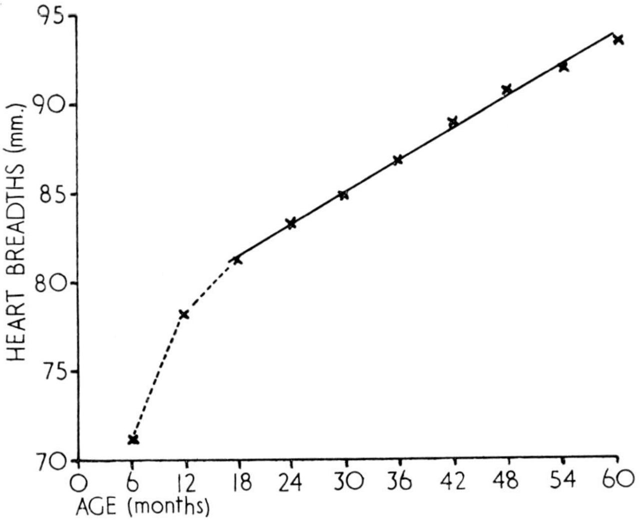

FIG. 1.—Mean radiographic heart diameter of Oxford children aged 6 months to 5 years: mixed series of boys and girls.

However, this ratio has certain disadvantages in early childhood when it is difficult to control the phase of respiration during exposure. In young children also the long axis of the heart is inclined at a much more shallow angle to the transverse axis of the thorax than in later life, so that healthy infants may exhibit a cardiothoracic index well in excess of 0·50. Bakwin and Bakwin (1935) concluded that age-standards for total transverse diameter provide as good a guide to normal heart size as the cardiothoracic index. This index has therefore not been calculated for the Oxford children and the present report is concerned only with absolute measurements.

All films were taken in the anterior posterior direction using a focal-film distance of 4½ feet (1·37 metres). The child was posed sitting in an erect position and an attempt was made to take the picture at full inspiration, although this was not always possible, especially with the younger children. Following Caffey (1945) heart diameter was taken as, 'the sum of the greatest perpendicular distance from the midline of the thorax to the right cardiac margin and the greatest distance from the midline to the left cardiac border'. Measurements were read directly from the film with a transparent rule marked in half-centimetre units.

The apparent diameter on any individual film will, of course, depend to a considerable extent on the phase of the heart-beat at the moment of exposure. In view of the number of children measured at each age this source of variation has probably had a negligible effect on the averages, but, together with other errors, will certainly have inflated the estimated standard deviations and thus broadened the range of 'normal' diameter. This point is discussed below in connexion with Fig. 2.

Mean heart diameters at ten ages are shown in Fig. 1 for all children measured, without distinction of sex. It will be seen that the increase in heart diameter between the ages of 6 and 12 months is about 7 mm. and in the following six months about 3 mm. Thereafter the mean diameter increases very regularly at a rate of between 3 and 4 mm. per year. The linear correlation coefficient between age and mean heart diameter over the range 18 months to 5 years is +0·9986, a degree of correlation which justifies the use of a fitted regression line for estimating normal diameters in this age range. Such a line is also shown in Fig. 1.

The means and standard deviations at each age for boys and girls separately are shown in Table 1. Throughout the first five years of life the mean breadth is greater for boys than for girls by an amount which ranges from $2\frac{1}{2}$ to $4\frac{1}{2}$ mm. but which may reasonably be regarded, after allowance for sampling fluctuations, as a fairly constant $3\frac{1}{2}$ mm. The standard deviation also tends to be greater for boys than for girls by an amount which, on average, is slightly more than proportional to the difference in means. However, for practical purposes, the coefficient of variation

$$\left(\frac{\text{standard deviation}}{\text{mean}} \times 100\right)$$

may be regarded as the same for each sex and, over the ranges 18 months to 5 years it may also be regarded as constant from age to age at about 6·2%.

These regularities in the data make it possible to draw a simple channel for the normal heart diameter of healthy young children, and this has been done in Fig. 2. The boundaries of this channel have been drawn at distances of two standard deviations above and below the mean, that is, they should include rather more than 95% of measurements based on individual films of healthy children. In particular, rather less than 1 in 40 radiographs of

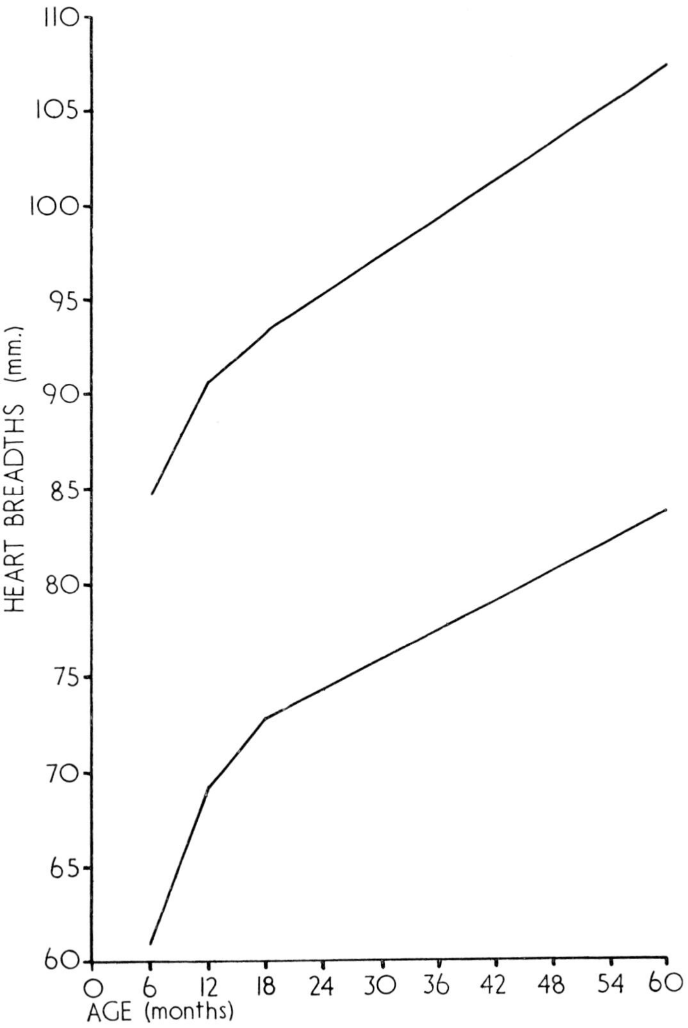

FIG. 2.—Normal channel of heart growth in young children. Approximately 95% of films of boys taken under the stated conditions should yield measurements between these limits. To compare a girl's heart diameter with these standards first add $3\frac{1}{2}$ mm.

TABLE 1

MEAN AND STANDARD DEVIATION OF RADIOGRAPHIC HEART DIAMETER OF OXFORD BOYS AND GIRLS AGED 6 MONTHS TO 5 YEARS

		Age in Months									
		6	12	18	24	30	36	42	48	54	60
Boys	No. measured	98	106	101	94	74	73	69	67	56	47
	Mean (mm.)	73·2	79·8	82·7	84·8	86·9	87·9	91·2	92·2	93·8	96·1
	Standard deviation	6·2	5·2	5·2	5·1	4·8	6·1	5·5	5·8	6·4	6·1
Girls	No. measured	104	113	102	97	85	83	74	67	60	60
	Mean	69·4	76·7	79·7	81·6	83·2	85·4	86·8	88·8	90·3	91·4
	Standard deviation	5·4	5·2	5·1	4·9	5·1	5·7	5·4	5·4	5·0	5·3

healthy children taken under the stated conditions should show a heart diameter greater than that indicated by the upper line. The figure has been drawn for use as a standard for boys, but it may also be used to assess girls' measurements if these are first increased by 3½ mm. The channel is strikingly wide: a heart diameter of 84 mm. could be regarded as just within normal limits both at 6 months and at 5 years. However, as stated above, the true range of variability will have been somewhat exaggerated as a result of certain errors inherent in the measurements. From calculations based on successive measurements of the same children it can be inferred that the channel might have been narrower by about one-fifth if the measurements from which it is derived has been free from error. If several films of the same child exhibit heart diameters outside the limits of Fig. 2, or with an average outside them, there is, of course, a much stronger presumption of abnormality than when an isolated film falls outside these 95% limits.

No attempt has been made here to incorporate an allowance for general body size, but it must be borne in mind that children who are markedly large or small for their age must be expected to have rather larger or smaller hearts. In the present study it has been found (on the basis of assessments combining successive measurements of the same children) that heart diameter at a given age is correlated with body weight to the extent of +0·437. There is also a normal tendency for large or small hearts to run in a family, the sib-sib correlation of heart diameter in the Oxford data (again based on a combination of successive measurements) being +0·367.

Bakwin and Bakwin (1935) have published radiographic measurements of the heart diameters of a group of New York children taken at monthly intervals during the first year of life. Their figures emphasize the relatively rapid growth of the heart during the earliest months of life: the average gain in the first six months was 19 mm. (from 49 to 68 mm.) compared with only 7 mm. (from 68 to 75 mm.) in the remainder of the first year. Thus, the gain between the ages of 6 months and 1 year was the same as found in the present study, although the New York children (who were described as coming from 'very poor homes') had slightly narrower hearts on average than post-war Oxford children of corresponding age. (After allowing for a slight difference in magnification the margin is about 2 mm.) The heart measurements of Denver children given by Maresh (1948) for children from the age of 4 years onwards are based on posterior anterior exposures and therefore cannot easily be compared with the present series. However, they agree with the Oxford measurements in showing a greater average heart diameter for boys than girls at the ages of 4 and 5 years, and also a similar degree of correlation with height and with weight.

Summary

Measurements of chest films taken in the course of the Oxford Child Health Survey have been used to set up approximate standards of normal heart diameter for children aged 6 months to 5 years.

All the films used in this study were taken by Miss Eleanor Roberts and Miss Margaret Barnes. I am indebted to Dr. W. Pennybacker for advice on the measuring technique. The Oxford Child Health Survey is supported by a grant from the Medical Research Council.

REFERENCES

Bakwin, H. and Bakwin, R. M. (1935). *Amer. J. Dis. Child.*, **49**, 861.
Caffey, J. (1945). *Pediatric X-Ray Diagnosis*. Chicago.
Maresh, M. M. (1948). *Pediatrics*, **2**, 382.

THE CHANGING AETIOLOGY OF ERYTHEMA NODOSUM IN CHILDREN*

BY

JOHN LORBER
From the Children's Hospital, Sheffield

(RECEIVED FOR PUBLICATION SEPTEMBER 9, 1957)

In his Bradshaw Lecture for 1944, Professor Bruce Perry (Perry, 1944) reviewed the historical aspects of the aetiology of erythema nodosum and later Doxiadis gave a more detailed account in his monograph on the subject (Doxiadis, 1951). It has been shown that erythema nodosum is a hypersensitivity reaction and the main triggers which elicit this reaction are certain bacterial and fungal infections. The relative importance of the various aetiological agents is influenced by geographical and racial factors as well as by the age of the patient. Their importance may also vary from time to time. Erythema nodosum was often in the past thought to be a manifestation of rheumatic fever, but this theory has long been disproved. In this country, tuberculosis and beta-haemolytic streptococcal infections are the only known important factors in children.

In recent years, only two large series of cases have been published in Great Britain and both of these emphasized the overwhelming importance of recent tuberculous infection. Perry found that of 67 children with erythema nodosum seen in the Bristol region 50 (75%) were tuberculin positive and 29 (43%) showed evidence of active primary tuberculosis. Only 11 children had a clear-cut history of pharyngitis; nine of these were tuberculin negative and skin tests showed that four were sensitive to streptococcal mucoproteins. The incidence of tuberculous infection was even higher in Doxiadis' (1949) 100 children who were seen in Newcastle-upon-Tyne and in Sheffield between 1947 and 1949. All his patients were tuberculin tested and 88% were positive, and 59 (67%) showed evidence of active tuberculous infection. Tuberculous complications developed within three months after the appearance of the erythema nodosum in eight children. A possible streptococcal aetiology has not been excluded for Doxiadis' patients, as tests for evidence of recent streptococcal infection were not performed. It must be remembered, however, that in those days it was much easier to demonstrate tuberculous infection than streptococcal infection by laboratory means.

Present Investigation

Material. In view of the recent considerable decline in the incidence of childhood tuberculosis in our community (Lorber, 1953) it seemed of interest to review the cases of erythema nodosum in children seen in Sheffield in more recent years. For this purpose, the records of all the 89 children under 15 years of age who were found to have erythema nodosum and who attended the Children's Hospital, Sheffield, during a period of six years from January 1, 1951, to December 31, 1956, were used. Of these, 40 were under the care of Dr. T. Colver. In addition I obtained permission to include cases seen by Dr. R. R. Gordon of the City General Hospital, Sheffield, and by Dr. H. R. Vickers and Dr. I. B. Sneddon of the Department of Dermatology, the Royal Infirmary, Sheffield. These sources added a further 16 cases for study making a total of 105. No further cases have been found after searching the records of the various Sheffield Hospitals and of the Chest Clinic.

Age and Sex Incidence. Erythema nodosum was seen in four children under 2 years of age. There were three peak years with 12 cases at 2 years, 17 cases at 9 years and 11 cases at 10 years. Otherwise, the frequency of the condition was very similar at each year of life, with an average of six cases (Fig. 1). Twenty-seven (26%) children were under 5 years of age, 42 (40%) were between 5 and 10 years of age and 36 (34%) were 10 to 15 years of age (Table 1).

There were 48 boys (46%) and 57 girls (54%). There was an interesting and progressive gradient

* Based on a paper delivered to the Paediatric Section of the Royal Society of Medicine on April 26, 1957.

in sex incidence in different age groups (Table 1). Under 5 years of age there were more boys than girls

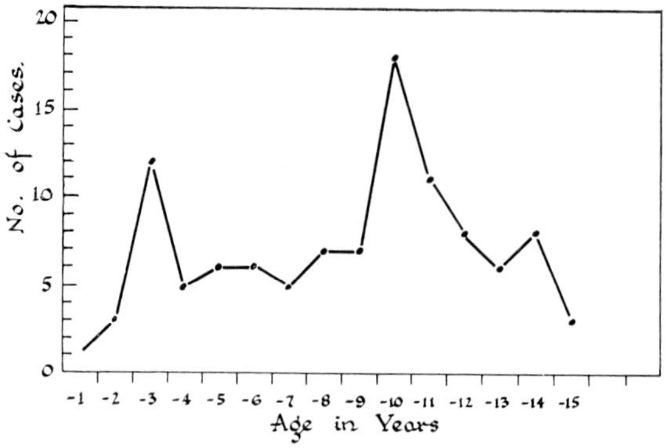

FIG. 1.—Age distribution of erythema nodosum.

TABLE 1

AGE AND SEX INCIDENCE
ERYTHEMA NODOSUM IN SHEFFIELD INVESTIGATION, 1951-56

Age in Years	Total	Females Number	%	Males Number	%
– 5	27	10	37	17	63
–10	42	23	55	19	45
–15	36	24	67	12	33
Adults	55	52	94	3	6
All ages	160	109	68	51	32

(17 boys to 10 girls), between 5 and 10 years of age boys were a little less often affected (19 boys to 23 girls) and between 10 and 15 years there were twice as many girls as boys (12 boys to 24 girls).

In 55 adult patients seen by Dr. Vickers and Dr. Sneddon during the same period 52 (94%) were women.

Aetiology

Tuberculosis. All children were tuberculin tested and a radiograph of the chest was obtained. The tuberculin tests used were the jelly test (without flour paper) and the Mantoux test in varying strengths from 1 to 100 T.U. old tuberculin (1/10,000-1/100).

A positive skin test was found in 65 children (62%) as a result of natural infection. Five other children were also tuberculin positive but these had recently been vaccinated with B.C.G. and form another group. Thirty-five children (33%) were tuberculin negative (Table 2).

TABLE 2

TUBERCULIN TEST REACTIONS IN CHILDREN WITH ERYTHEMA NODOSUM

Tuberculin Test Reaction	Number	%
Positive	65	62
Positive (B.C.G. vaccinated) . .	5	5
Negative	35	33
All cases	105	100

There was a decreasing incidence of tuberculous infection during the six years of this study. Whereas in 1951 to 1953, 73% of 49 children were tuberculin positive as a result of natural infection, in 1954 to 1956 this proportion fell to 51% of 56 cases. There was also a fall in the absolute number of tuberculin positive cases from 36 in 1951 to 1953 to 29 in 1954 to 1956 (Table 3).

TABLE 3

INCIDENCE OF TUBERCULOUS INFECTION IN CHILDREN WITH ERYTHEMA NODOSUM

Year	Number of Cases	Tuberculin Positive Number	%	Active Tuberculosis Number	%
1947-49*	100	88	88	59	59
1951-53	49	36	73	27	55
1954-56	57	29	51	19	34

* Doxiadis, 1949.

The incidence of tuberculous infection was practically the same in boys and girls (62%). Tuberculosis, however, was much commoner in younger than in older children. Of 29 children aged 2 to 5 years, 25 (86%) were tuberculin positive; of 52 under 9 years of age 37 (71%) and of 53 of 9 years or more only 28 (53%) were tuberculin positive (Table 4).

TABLE 4

INCIDENCE OF TUBERCULOSIS IN CHILDREN WITH ERYTHEMA NODOSUM ACCORDING TO AGE AND SEX

	0–8 Years					9–14 Years				
	All Cases	Tuberculin Positive		Active Tuberculosis		All Cases	Tuberculin Positive		Active Tuberculosis	
		Number	%	Number	%		Number	%	Number	%
Boys	30	21	70	17	57	18	9	50	8	44
Girls	22	16	73	13	60	35	19	54	8	23
Total	52	37	71	30	58	53	28	53	16	30

Children with Active Primary Tuberculosis. A positive tuberculin reaction does not necessarily indicate that the erythema nodosum was due to the tuberculous infection, unless tuberculin conversion coincided in time with the eruption and other possible causes were excluded. Unfortunately, in most cases there was no record of the tuberculin status before the skin eruption. It was possible, however, to divide the 65 tuberculin positive children into two groups: in 46 (43%) there was clinical and radiological evidence of a recent and active tuberculous process, and in the remaining 19 the only evidence of the tuberculous infection was the positive skin test.

The proportion of children with active primary tuberculosis was 55% in 1951 to 1953 (27 of 49) and only 34% (19 of 56) in 1954 to 1956 (Table 3). As might be expected, younger children with a positive skin test more often had an active tuberculous lesion. In children under 9 years of age 58% had active lesions as compared with 30% of all children aged 9 years or more. Among 35 girls aged 9 years or more only eight or 23% had an active tuberculous infection (Table 4). In this group there was a big difference between the incidence of active tuberculosis in the two sexes.

All the 46 children (25 boys and 21 girls) with definite active primary tuberculosis had non-calcified primary complexes or enlargement of the hilar lymph nodes in radiographs of the chest. In no case was the hilar enlargement bilateral. In 18 of those who had been followed up for a sufficient period calcifications were subsequently demonstrated. Significant contact with an active case of tuberculosis was either already known or was found to have occurred immediately prior to the onset of the erythema nodosum in 22 cases. In five cases, tubercle bacilli were cultured from gastric washings. This is a minimal figure, as children were often not admitted to hospital and gastric washings were not a routine procedure. Ten of the 46 are known to have developed important tuberculous complications within nine months of the eruption. These were tuberculous meningitis in three, bronchopneumonia in one, arthritis of the hip in one, pleural effusion in three and phlyctenular conjunctivitis in two (Table 5).

Children with Inactive Tuberculosis. It is not possible to calculate precisely the expected incidence of positive tuberculin reactors in this group of 105 children based on the incidence in the general child population, as the information is not sufficient and the numbers are relatively small. It is likely, however, that the incidence of 18% who showed a positive tuberculin reaction as the only evidence of infection corresponds fairly well to that in the general child population. Seven of 52 (13%) were under 9 years of age, and 12 of 53 (23%) were over 9 years of age. There was only one child in this group who had definite enlargement of the hilar lymph nodes but he was known to be tuberculin positive 18 months earlier. None of these 19 children are known to have developed tuberculous illness of any type during the period of observation.

B.C.G. Vaccinated Children. Five children who gave a positive tuberculin reaction had been vaccinated with B.C.G. before the onset of the erythema nodosum. One of these, a boy of 14, was vaccinated nine months earlier at school and he converted two months later. His illness followed a sore throat and although his throat swab was negative when he was first seen, the antistreptolysin-O titre was 600 units. A radiograph of the chest was normal. The B.C.G. vaccination was clearly not responsible for his eruption, which was probably due to streptococcal infection.

In the other four vaccinated children the eruption occurred at about the time of tuberculin conversion, but an additional factor was present in three of these, so that the B.C.G. vaccination was not necessarily responsible for the attack. The father of one had active pulmonary tuberculosis and this 18-month-old child was not segregated from him during the period of vaccination. The child developed erythema nodosum only two weeks after vaccination. He then had a normal radiograph of the chest, but two years later a further radiograph showed a shadow consistent with a primary tuberculous complex. This child may well have had a recent virulent tuberculous infection which led to his erythema nodosum.

Table 5

TUBERCULOUS COMPLICATIONS IN 46 CHILDREN WITH ACTIVE PRIMARY TUBERCULOSIS

Meningitis	3
Bronchopneumonia	1
Hip disease	1
Pleural effusion	3
Phlyctenular conjunctivitis	2
Total	10 (22%)

Two 13-year-old girls had been vaccinated at school. One had already had an attack of erythema nodosum four years earlier and the fresh attack was preceded by a severe sore throat. When first seen her throat swab was negative, but an A.S.O. titre was not performed. She had a typical fresh B.C.G. lesion, and a radiograph of the chest was normal. The other girl was vaccinated only three weeks before the erythema nodosum, but she already had a good B.C.G. lesion and gave a positive reaction to 10 units of O.T. A radiograph of the chest was negative. She did have a sore throat a week before the onset of the erythema nodosum, but her throat swab when first seen was negative. The A.S.O. titre was 200 units. The eruption cleared completely, but two weeks later a fresh extensive eruption developed without a preceding sore throat. This time beta-haemolytic streptococci were present in her throat swab. In these two girls either the B.C.G. vaccination or a streptococcal infection or both might well have been responsible for the eruption.

Finally, an infant aged 10 months had a mild eruption of erythema nodosum six weeks after vaccination without any other additional feature. This is the only child in whom B.C.G. was the only known predisposing factor, but streptococcal infection was not excluded by laboratory evidence.

Streptococcal Infection. Of the 35 patients whose tuberculin tests and radiographs were negative at the time of their erythema nodosum, 17 had a sore throat within two weeks before the eruption. Throat swabs were taken at the time of the child's first visit in 15 children, including 11 with preceding sore throats, and beta-haemolytic streptococci were grown in four. In addition, an elevation of the A.S.O. titre was found in six children whose throat swabs were negative or in whom swabs were not taken (titres of 200, 450, 600, 800, 900 and 2,000 units). A recent beta-haemolytic streptococcal infection was therefore demonstrated in ten of these 35 (Table 6). In 19 children in this group no investigations were undertaken to detect such infections. Among 11 children from whom were obtained both throat swabs for culture and blood for A.S.O. titre, there were only two who gave a negative reaction to both tests.

Unfortunately, in most of the tuberculous cases no further investigations were carried out after a positive tuberculin test and other evidence of active tuberculosis was found. Nevertheless, among the 65 tuberculin positive children the eruption was preceded by a severe sore throat in 15, and Lancefield group A beta-haemolytic streptococci were cultured from throat swabs in four of these. Another child had an A.S.O. titre of 500 units. As no throat swab was taken from 45 children and the anti-streptolysin-O titre was only estimated in one, the five proven cases of concurrent streptococcal infections represent a minimal figure. Four of the five had an active tuberculous lesion.

Among the 105 children there were, therefore, 35 (33%) who complained of a preceding sore throat; beta-haemolytic streptococci were found in their throat swabs in nine and a significant elevation of their A.S.O. titre was also found in nine patients. The total with proven streptococcal infection was 17 (16%) (Table 6).

TABLE 6

INCIDENCE OF STREPTOCOCCAL INFECTION IN CHILDREN WITH ERYTHEMA NODOSUM

Type of Case	Total	Pharyngitis	Positive Throat Swab or Elevated A.S.O. Titre*
Tuberculous ..	65	15	5
B.C.G.	5	3	2
Non-tuberculous	35	17	10
Total ..	105	35	17

* 200 units or more.

Rheumatic Fever. Only one child had coexistent rheumatic fever. This boy of 12 developed erythema nodosum and rheumatic fever with carditis following a streptococcal tonsillitis.

Other Diseases. In no child were other associated diseases detected, e.g., sarcoid or meningococcaemia.

Drugs. None of the children received sulphathiazole and no clear evidence is available that drugs played a part in provoking the eruption in any case.

Familial Factors. More than one case of erythema nodosum occurred in three families. In one, a girl of 11 years and a boy of 8 years had erythema nodosum at about the same time following sore throats. Both of these were known to have been tuberculin positive 18 months earlier. In the second the mother developed erythema nodosum before her 2-year-old boy. The boy had an active tuberculous infection which was probably contracted from a tuberculous neighbour.

More interesting is the history of the third family in which three children were affected in the course of six years. This is the only true example of familial susceptibility to erythema nodosum in this series.

The three children, twin brothers and a cousin, lived in the same house. All three were persistently tuberculin negative. One twin developed erythema nodosum at the age of 6, in 1950. The next episode occurred in January, 1953, when the second twin had erythema nodosum following a sore throat. He had beta-haemolytic streptococci in his throat. The first twin then had a second attack in December, 1954, without any apparent predisposing cause. Finally, their first cousin, a girl of 9 years, had erythema nodosum a further 15 months later. She, too, had a proven beta-haemolytic streptococcal throat infection.

Relapses. Six children (5%) had a second attack after the eruption of the first attack had completely faded. Two children had their first attack before 1951 and four during the six years of this study. In three, the second attack occurred between three and five years after the first one. In the three others this happened within four weeks of the first crop. In only one child was active tuberculosis detected at the time of the first attack, but even she had a preceding sore throat. In none of the other cases did tuberculosis play a part, except that two had been vaccinated with B.C.G. not long before their second attack. It is of interest, however, that the twins quoted above, one of whom had two attacks, were subsequently vaccinated with B.C.G. without subsequent erythema nodosum.

Discussion

It is legitimate to conclude from these findings that although tuberculosis is still a very important aetiological factor in erythema nodosum in children, its importance is steadily decreasing. In the last three years little more than half the children had a positive tuberculin reaction and only one-third had active tuberculosis.

Tuberculosis was a far more important aetiological factor in young children among whom 71% had a positive skin test and most of these had active primary tuberculosis. These figures are in contrast with children over 9 years of whom only 30% had active primary tuberculosis.

As B.C.G. vaccinations are increasing in number, we shall have to think of it among the possible causes when confronted with a case of erythema nodosum.

We shall not know the true incidence of streptococcal aetiology until all cases are investigated routinely by throat swabs and the estimation of A.S.O. titres. When we do this we shall probably find many cases of erythema nodosum in which multiple factors operate. This was shown to some extent by the figures which have been presented. The concept of mixed infection or complex aetiology has previously been elaborated by Westergren (1945).

Holmdahl (1950) found in a series of 657 cases that the prognosis of primary tuberculosis was much worse in children with than in those without erythema nodosum. Our smaller series fully confirms his findings. It appears reasonable, therefore, to prescribe a course of treatment with isoniazid plus streptomycin or P.A.S. for children who show evidence of an active primary tuberculosis associated with erythema nodosum.

Summary

In a consecutive series of 105 children with erythema nodosum seen in Sheffield between January 1951 and December 1956, 65 (62%) were tuberculin positive as a result of tuberculous infection, five cases followed B.C.G. vaccination, and 35 (33%) were tuberculin negative.

There was a progressively falling proportion of children with a positive tuberculin reaction. Out of 49 children seen in 1951 to 1953, 73%, and out of 56 seen in 1954 to 1956 only 51% were tuberculin positive. An active primary tuberculous lesion was seen in 46 children (43%) in the whole series. The proportion was 55% in children seen during 1951 to 1953 and 34% in 1954 to 1956. Ten of the 46 children developed various forms of tuberculous diseases (apart from the erythema nodosum and the primary complex) during observation. In 19 children (18%) the only evidence of tuberculosis was a positive skin test.

Five children developed erythema nodosum after B.C.G. vaccination, and in four this occurred at the time of tuberculin conversion. Nevertheless, additional tuberculous or streptococcal infections were present in three of them.

Among 35 tuberculin negative children, 17 complained of a preceding pharyngitis and in ten laboratory evidence of a beta-haemolytic streptococcal infection was obtained; in 19 children no investigations were performed to prove a possible streptococcal aetiology. Such investigations were even less commonly performed in the 65 tuberculin positive children. Nevertheless the eruption was preceded by a sore throat in 15 and streptococcal infection was demonstrated in five. Among the 105 cases there were altogether 17 with a proven streptococcal infection.

Relapse of the erythema nodosum occurred in six cases and multiple cases occurred in three families.

I wish to thank Professor R. S. Illingworth for his criticism; Dr. T. Colver, Dr. R. R. Gordon, Dr. I. B. Sneddon and Dr. H. R. Vickers for permission to study their cases and the many family physicians who referred their patients to us.

References

Doxiadis, S. A. (1949). *Brit. med. J.*, **2**, 844.
—— (1951). *Medicine (Baltimore)*, **30**, 283.
Holmdahl, K. (1950). *Acta tuberc. scand.*, Suppl. 22.
Lorber, J. (1953). *Brit. med. J.*, **2**, 1122.
Perry, C. B. (1944). *Ibid.*, **2**, 843.
Westergren, A. (1945). *Nord. Med.*, **25**, 312

CLINICAL AND BIOCHEMICAL CHANGES DURING EXCHANGE TRANSFUSION

BY

JAMES W. FARQUHAR and HYLTON SMITH

From the Department of Child Life and Health, University of Edinburgh, and the Edinburgh Central Hospital Group Biochemical Laboratory

(RECEIVED FOR PUBLICATION AUGUST 26, 1957)

The development of exchange transfusion has greatly altered the prognosis of haemolytic disease of the newborn and the procedure is now accepted as being essential in cases of any severity. It is carried out wherever the criteria for operation are fulfilled and by operators of varying skill and experience. The difficulties associated with blood transfusion have received increasing attention in recent years, and its employment is beset with problems not only of cytology and serology but of microbiology, biochemistry, allergy, dynamics, religion and race. Some of these are greatly increased by the volume of blood used in exchange transfusion. Considering that the infant may be perfused with stored blood of altered chemistry in quantities of up to three times his own blood volume, it is surprising perhaps that it can be done at all. Hazards such as sepsis, air embolism, portal-vein thrombosis and perforation of the umbilical vein have been described, but are fortunately uncommon. Circulatory overloading is an ever-present danger in the profoundly anaemic infant, and it may be precipitated by conducting the exchange transfusion too rapidly. Deterioration and even death, however, may occur in infants whose pre-operative condition gave rise to no concern. Such clinical deterioration was observed in 40% of the cases transfused by Walker and Neligan (1955), and it did not appear to be related in any simple way to the baby's initial condition, to birth weight, to the technical difficulties encountered or to the rate of exchange. Moreover, Walker (1955) was led to believe, from inquiries received by him, that unexpected death was commoner over the United Kingdom than he had previously thought. Signs of clinical disturbance which had been observed by one of us (J. W. F.) during exchange transfusions at the Simpson Memorial Maternity Pavilion, Edinburgh, between 1948 and 1953, prompted us to undertake a joint study of a series of infants during operation.

Plan of Investigation

In the belief that analysis of serum taken during exchange transfusion would reflect the ability of the newborn infant suffering from erythroblastosis foetalis to maintain a normal serum electrolyte picture, electrolyte balance with reference to calcium and potassium ions has been evaluated.

Methods

Clinical. The technique of exchange transfusion was essentially that described by Farquhar and Lewis (1949). A careful clinical record was kept during the transfusion. This included recording the volume of blood exchanged, heart rate, and the occurrence of clinical incident. The exchange was carried out slowly, and if the patient was not tolerating the procedure the apparatus was flushed with saline and the infant rested for 5–15 minutes. As many as three or four rest periods were necessary for readjustment in some of the more seriously disturbed babies.

Specimens of blood were collected at regular intervals during transfusion. In the first series of cases studied blood was collected at intervals immediately before the administration of calcium gluconate. In the second series blood was collected at intervals immediately before and after the administration of calcium gluconate. In the event of any abnormal incident occurring during transfusion, specimens of blood were collected immediately. During specimen collection, contamination of blood samples with the contents of the polythene catheter was avoided by the following procedure. A few millilitres of the infant's blood was sucked into the syringe and rejected into the waste bucket. By this means any residual donor blood was removed from the polythene catheter. The actual blood specimen was then withdrawn and placed in a centrifuge tube. Specimens were centrifuged soon after clot retraction, and the sera were stored in the refrigerator until analysis.

Analytical. Sodium and potassium were determined by means of the flame photometer; protein by the micro-Kjeldahl procedure (King, 1951); total calcium by the method of Sobel and Sobel (1939), with the modification that the serum was ashed prior to oxalate precipitation in order to eliminate citrate; citric acid by a method devised by one of us (H. S.), the principle depending on the oxidation of citrate to acetone with vanadate, and the subsequent distillation of the liberated acetone into an alkaline solution of salicylaldehyde, forming a coloured complex which was measured colorimetrically.

Simultaneous electrocardiography would have been of much value, but unfortunately no suitable machine was available.

Patterns of Clinical Disturbance Observed

A quite unexpected near-fatality observed during exchange transfusion in 1953 finally provoked these observations.

A mature female infant of 8 lb. 6 oz. birth weight, second of a family, had a cord haemoglobin of 17·4 g. per 100 ml., a cord serum bilirubin of 3 mg. per 100 ml., and a strongly positive Coombs test. There was no splenomegaly and the liver was judged to be normal. Influenced only by the bilirubin level, it was decided to carry out an exchange transfusion. No trouble was anticipated. Aliquots of 10 ml. of blood were exchanged at an average time interval of one minute. Calcium gluconate 0·1 g. was injected at intervals of 100 ml. The operation proceeded smoothly until 430 ml. had been exchanged, when the infant suddenly collapsed and became pale and unresponsive. The heart rate increased from 132 to 152 beats per minute. Calcium was given without effect. Glucose 20% solution was given intravenously quite empirically in a dosage of 6 ml. The baby appeared to improve, but on resumption of the exchange she collapsed again. Glucose was given once more with less convincing effect. The transfusion was then continued much more cautiously and in negative balance to a total of 740 ml.

Of the 19 infants studied, one died during transfusion. Six others showed some clinically recognizable disturbance at some stage of the procedure. The remaining 12 infants were normal throughout. Different patterns of clinical disturbance were observed, and a description of these is essential to the further understanding of the investigation.

Distal Cyanosis. Two babies produced an alarming clinical picture which, probably as a result of modification in technique, was not observed in subsequent transfusions. In both cases (F and R) difficulty was experienced in withdrawing blood during the first 100 ml. of blood exchanged. Persistent efforts were made to overcome this by partial withdrawal and reintroduction of the catheter. In both cases the catheter tip was advanced along the umbilical vein for about 11 cm. and repeatedly encountered some resistance, which was thought at the time to be within the portal circulation. Both babies developed a deep cyanosis of the lower half of the body, and this contrasted dramatically with the pallor of the upper half. Increased venous filling became apparent over the trunk and the veins were noted to drain superiorly. No pitting oedema of the legs was noted. The symptoms disappeared spontaneously in about half an hour. This phenomenon has been designated 'distal cyanosis'.

Retching. Three infants (B, H and J) suffered from repeated retching of mucus. This is a common observation during exchange transfusion, and because of this milder degrees have not been recorded.

Shock. Three infants (B, F and M) presented a clinical picture to which the term 'shock' has been loosely applied. These infants showed some or all of the following features in varying degree. After crying lustily initially on restraint, they became unduly quiet and pale during operation. At least one infant was so pale that the possibility of internal bleeding was considered. The babies were cool and their abdomens became distended. The latter was not due to liver enlargement. They became 'hypotonic' and unresponsive. Little change in heart rate was observed and there was no increase in venous pressure. Case B showed this clinical picture within the first 100 ml. of blood exchanged, but survived an exchange of 600 ml.

Cardiac Failure. Signs of congestive heart failure appeared in one case only (J). This baby suffered from repeated retching during the exchange of the first 200 ml. of blood. He remained irritable, and after an exchange of 700 ml. he was beginning to show evidence of deterioration. Respiration became a little distressed and dyspnoea was obvious after 800 ml. of blood. At this stage the heart rate had increased from a resting rate of 138 to one of 164 per minute. The venous pressure in the portal circulation rose from a resting level of 7·5 cm. to 30 cm. The baby was a little cyanosed, the superficial veins became more obvious and the liver enlarged. Unfortunately the blood specimen taken at this point was lost, but the values found in the preceding one were coexistent with the signs of early cardiac failure.

Acute Non-fatal Collapse. One infant (R) collapsed suddenly and unexpectedly, but he fortunately recovered. He had been well until 470 ml. of blood had been exchanged. He then retched and became apnoeic and deeply cyanosed. The heart sounds were faint and the rhythm was irregular, but his condition gradually improved over a ten-minute period. This has been broadly termed 'acute non-fatal collapse'. Samples of this infant's blood were being taken only at intervals of 200 ml., and the nearest specimen to the incident was taken after 400 ml. of blood had been exchanged.

Death. One infant (I) died during operation. This infant was born with assistance by the breech, was limp at birth and was covered with yellow vernix. The cord haemoglobin was 9·8 g. per 100 ml. and the serum bilirubin 3·5 mg. per 100 ml; there were very many nucleated red cells in a peripheral blood smear and the Coombs test was strongly positive. Both liver and spleen were palpably enlarged. Apart from pallor no abnormality was noted until the infant collapsed and died at 500 ml. Necropsy revealed considerable bilateral tearing of the tentorium cerebelli, and a subtentorial subdural haematoma of such size that the medulla oblongata was flattened antero-posteriorly. Considerable intraperitoneal haemorrhage was also noted. No source of bleeding was found to explain this other than some haemorrhage around the umbilical vein in the region of the anterior abdominal wall. Although no perforation was found, this seemed to be the likely source of intraperitoneal blood loss. The pathological opinion was that the subdural bleeding alone, or with the intraperitoneal haemorrhage, provided adequate reason for the baby's death.

Relationship of Behaviour to Severity of Disease, Birth Weight, Volume and Speed of Exchange

The severity of the haemolytic disease process was classified arbitrarily into three grades: mild (+), moderate (++) and severe (+++) (Tables 1 and 2). In all cases a Coombs test was positive. The mild cases had a cord haemoglobin value greater than 14 g. per 100 ml. and a serum bilirubin of 3 mg. per 100 ml. or less. Neither liver nor spleen was enlarged. The moderately severe cases had a cord haemoglobin value greater than 11·2 g. but less than 14 g. per 100 ml. and the serum bilirubin was 3 mg. per 100 ml. or less. Some enlargement of liver and/or spleen was noted. The severe cases had a cord haemoglobin value of less than 11·2 g. and a serum bilirubin of more than 3 mg. per 100 ml., enlargement of liver and spleen, possibly bruising or oedema, and in one case a birth weight of less than $5\frac{1}{2}$ lb.

The aim of the operation was to employ 80-120 ml. of donor blood per lb. body weight, to use the umbilical route wherever possible and to effect the exchange fairly slowly.

There were cases where only a small volume was exchanged—for example, Case P. This infant was treated in another hospital. Attempts to employ the umbilical vein were unsuccessful and the registrar catheterized the long saphenous vein in the groin. Even here withdrawal was exceedingly difficult, and because the infant was only mildly affected the procedure was abandoned. In all cases the speed of exchange was fairly leisurely by intention, but in some it was prolonged by the technical difficulties encountered. The numbers are, of course, very small, but there is a reasonable distribution of severity. Five cases were mild, seven moderate and seven severe. If those cases which pursued a normal course are considered, four were mildly affected, three were of moderate severity and as many as five severe. Of the clinically abnormal cases, one was mildly affected, four were of moderate severity and only two severe. Of those showing the 'shock' picture, none had severe haemolytic disease. The only death occurred in the severely affected group. Only one other of this group (total seven cases) showed any abnormality, and this was limited to retching.

Regarding the speed of exchange, a total of 6·36 litres of blood was exchanged in the normal group in 1,386 minutes (excluding Cases K and P). The average rate of exchange was 4·6 ml. per minute, In the abnormal group a total of 4·12 litres of blood was exchanged in 968 minutes, so that the average speed of exchange was 4·3 ml. per minute. In the cases showing no clinical disturbance, therefore, the exchange was effected a shade more quickly on the average, but the fact that in the abnormal group intentional delays followed the occurrence of incidents, and so increased the duration of operation a little, must be kept in mind.

Pattern of Serum Electrolytes

Introductory Remarks. Analytical data referring to the cases investigated are charted in Figs. 1 and 2. Fig. 1 shows the individual results obtained from six normal transfusions, while Fig. 2 shows the individual results from seven transfusions at which clinical abnormalities were observed. From reference to the appropriate figures it will be apparent that they depict only the general trend of serum electrolytes during transfusion. It will be appreciated that, since specimens were collected at intervals during transfusion, it is only at these points that electrolytes could be assessed. Fluctuation must have occurred in the periods between collection of specimens, this fluctuation being influenced by movement of electrolytes in and out of the plasma compartment and, of course, by metabolic factors. Nevertheless, if this point be borne in mind in the evaluation of the results, it is believed that the general pattern which emerges from this investigation adequately portrays the effect of infusion of citrated blood upon serum electrolytes.

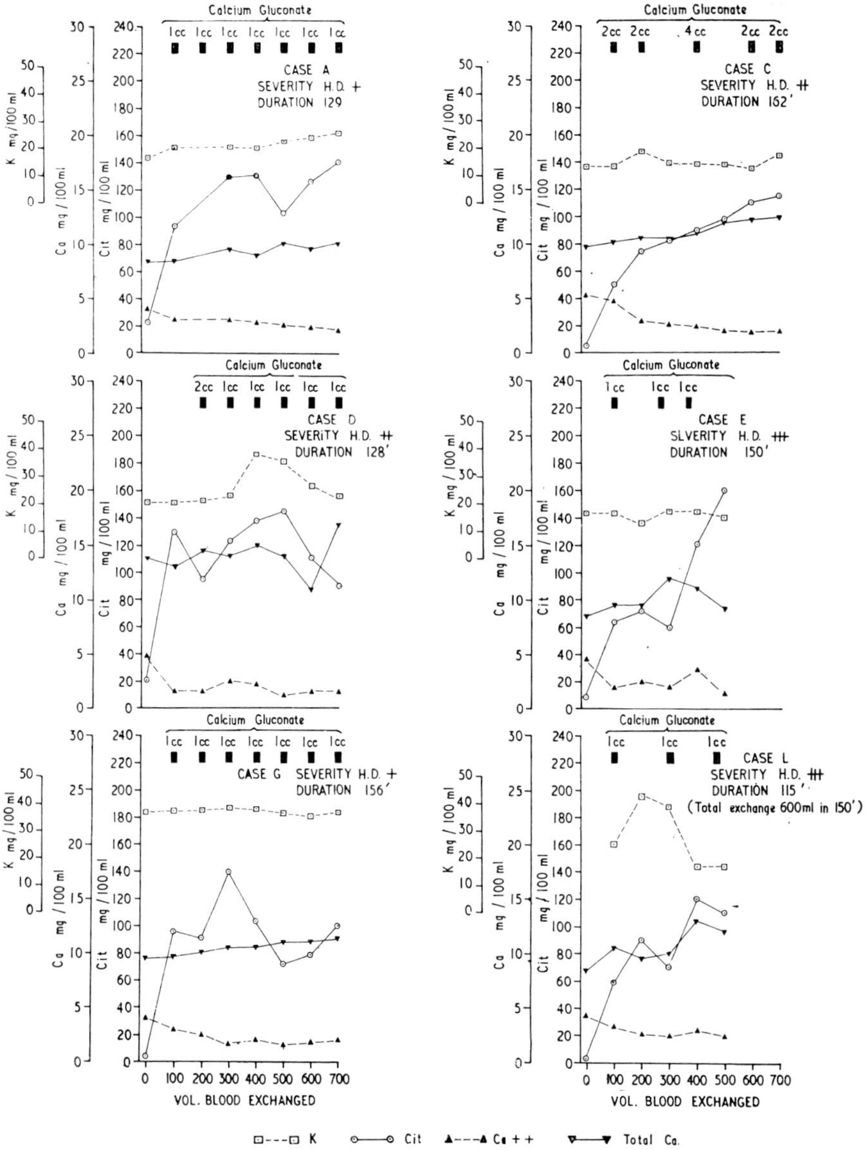

FIG. 1.—Serial serum electrolyte levels during six normal exchange transfusions.

The Group as a Whole. From the outset of the investigation attention was focused on the relationship of four biochemical situations to the clinical behaviour of the baby. These were: the influence of high citrate levels, of calcium-ion depression by citrate, of high serum potassium levels and the mutually reinforcing influences of a high potassium and a low calcium ion upon the heart. These are depicted in Figs. 3 and 4. In each graph every relevant analytical result in the series is included and marked by a symbol which denotes the clinical state of the patient at the time when the sample was taken. In Fig. 3 the coexisting citrate and calcium-ion levels are entered against each other. If high citrate levels *per se* were responsible for clinical abnormality, then the symbols denoting abnormal behaviour should be across the top of the graph. If clinical abnormality were the result of high citrate levels depressing calcium ion, however, then the abnormal cases should be at the top of the graph and towards the left. The upper part of the graph does not in fact contain the abnormal cases, nor do they lie predominantly to the left of the picture. The one death does lie in the top left-hand corner, but otherwise there is reasonable dispersal of the abnormal symbols among those which imply normal behaviour when the specimen was taken. In Fig. 4 the serum potassium levels were plotted against the coexisting levels of calcium ion. If hyperpotassaemia were responsible, then the abnormal cases should lie across the top of the picture, whereas if depression of calcium ion were responsible, then they should lie to the left of the picture. If the offending biochemical upset were coexisting hyperpotassaemia and calcium-ion depression, then the abnormal cases should lie in the top left-hand quadrant. Apart from the important exception that the only death did in fact represent the highest serum potassium level at the lowest calcium-ion level, the other abnormal symbols are scattered across the

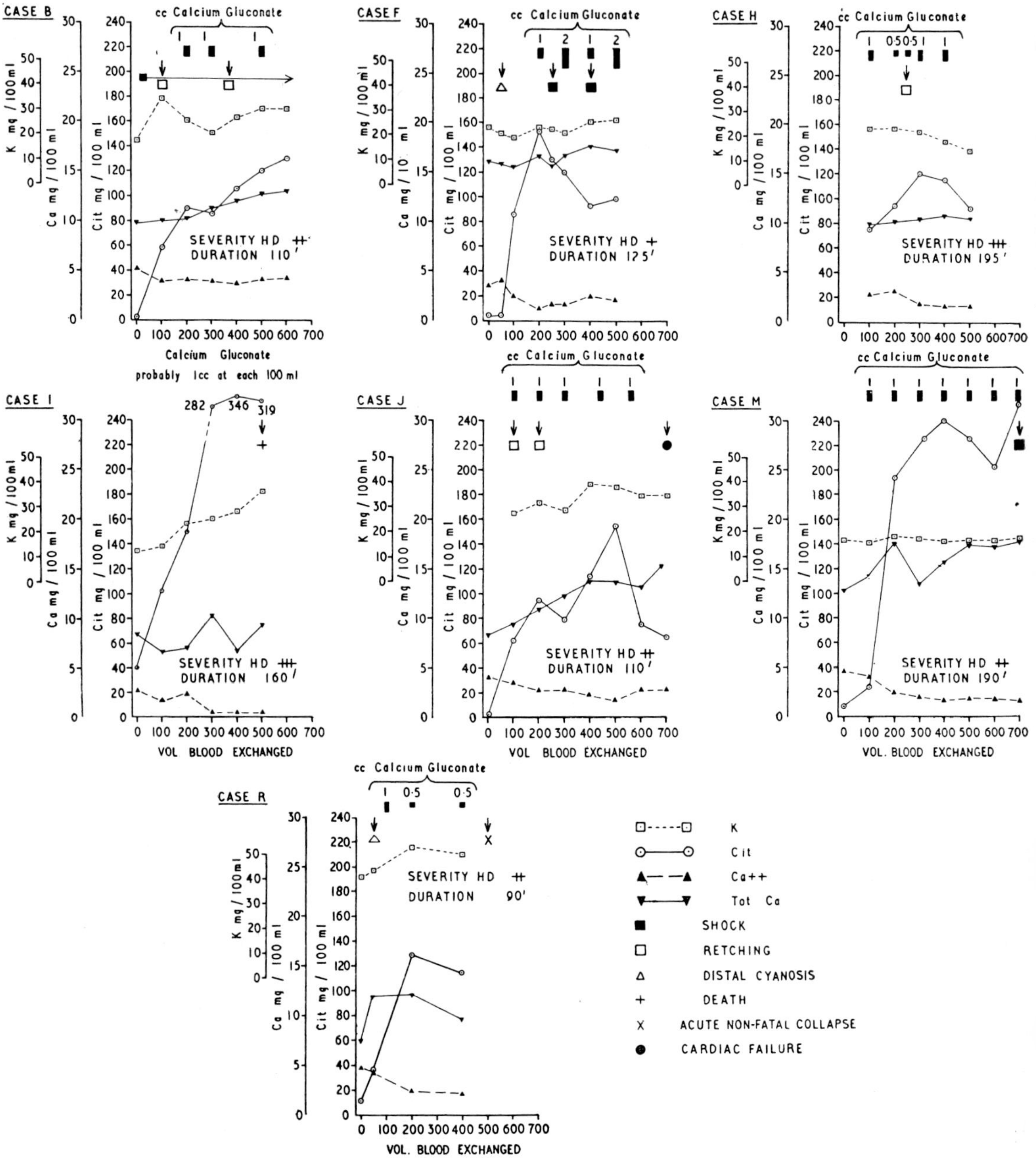

FIG. 2.—Serial serum electrolyte levels during seven abnormal exchange transfusions.

picture and fairly evenly disposed among the normal cases. From these two pictures it is possible to state that, with the exception of the fatal case, there was no relationship in this series of cases between the coexisting biochemical values and the clinical behaviour at the moment of taking the specimen.

It was apparent that a pattern of serum electrolytes during transfusion emerged from this investigation, this pattern being common to all infants whether or not clinical incident was observed. In summary, there appeared to be an increase in total calcium and citrate, a decrease in active calcium ion, and either no change or an increase in serum potassium. Several conclusions have been drawn from these results.

Citrate and Calcium. Great excess of citrate was found in the serum during exchange transfusion, and if, in fact, the formation of calcium citrate *in vivo* were dependent only upon chemical kinetic factors, then all available calcium ion in the plasma of these infants, except for the small amount liberated in the primary dissociation, should have been combined as calcium citrate. That this situation did not exist was apparent from the clinical state of the infants. The physiological environment, then, must be more complex than experiments *in vitro* would suggest, although all the calcium supplied in the form of calcium gluconate appeared to be inactivated immediately after injection (Fig. 5), if it can be presumed that calcium gluconate is completely ionized. The results are illustrated in Fig. 5. The absence of the classical manifestations of hypocalcaemia during transfusion even though subsequent analysis of serum showed a profound depression of calcium-ion concentration, is difficult

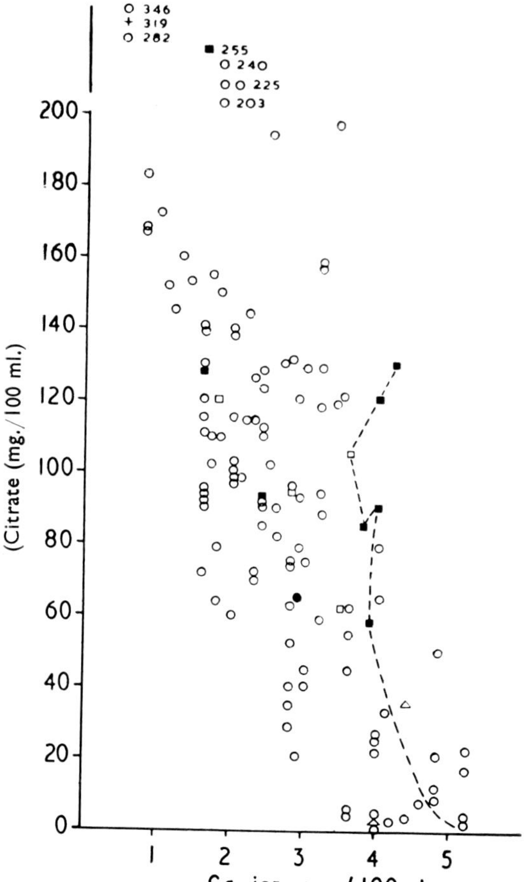

ꟻIG. 3.—Clinical behaviour during exchange transfusion related to plasma values of citrate and calcium ion.

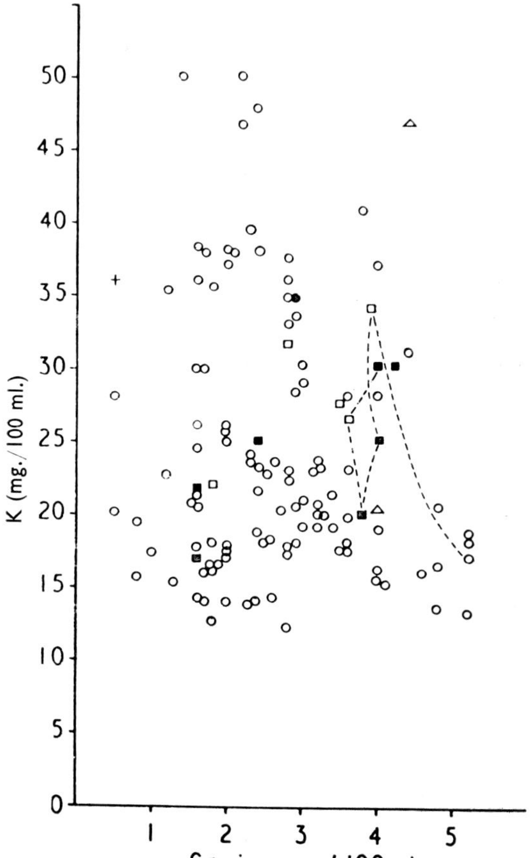

FIG. 4.—Clinical behaviour during exchange transfusion related to plasma values of potassium and calcium ion.

to explain. Since the formation of calcium citrate is known to be a slow reaction, it is suggested that

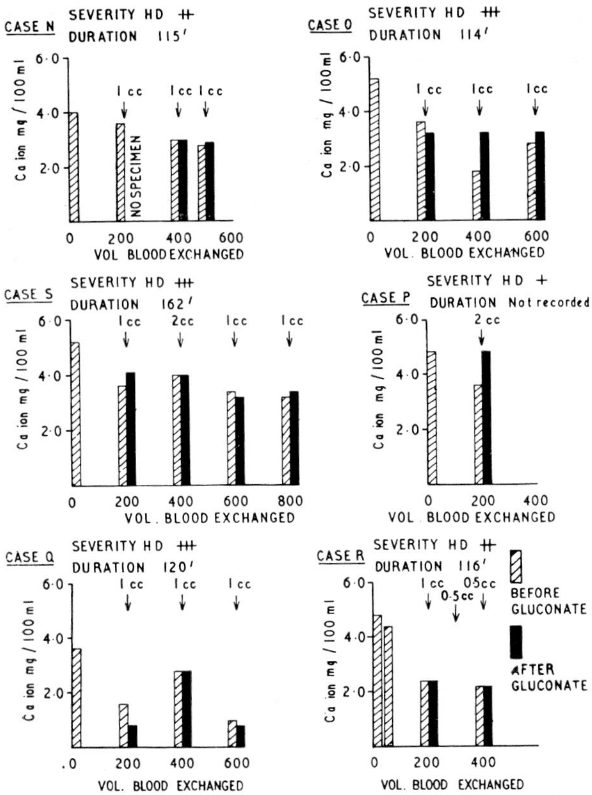

FIG. 5.—Effect of calcium gluconate on serum calcium-ion concentration.

complex formation may have been incomplete during transfusion, but on storage of the serum in the absence of active metabolic factors the reaction between citrate and calcium ions was able to reach completion.

It is claimed that during exchange transfusion the rate of transfusion is the most important factor in the development of hypercitraemia. Table I shows the infusion rate of citrate in this series, and it is apparent that the safety rate recommended by Mollison (1951) was commonly exceeded. There did not appear to be any correlation between the hypercitraemia and the citrate infusion rate, and it is considered significant that hypercitraemia of equal severity developed in both the clinically normal and abnormal groups. All infants showed considerable ability to 'metabolize' infused citrate, even in the presence of alleged hepatocellular immaturity.

It has been postulated that a high serum citrate level in the resting state is indicative of hepatocellular dysfunction. Hypercitraemia was commonly observed in the pre-transfusion state in this investigation. Natelson *et al.*, (1948) quoted the normal range of serum citrate as 1·5 to 6·0 mg. per 100 ml., with a mean value of 3·8 mg. per 100 ml., and in this series the range was 1·4 to 40·0 mg. per 100 ml., with a mean value of 12·6 mg. per 100 ml. The fatal case had a resting serum citrate level of 40·0 mg. per 100 ml., yet post-mortem examination revealed no gross hepatocellular damage. Furthermore, liver enlargement was not a common feature in any of the other cases, but this does not exclude the possibility of a 'metabolic' immaturity existing. Confirmatory evidence of high resting citrate values has been provided by the low level of resting serum calcium ion observed in this series.

TABLE 1

TABLE RELATING RATE OF TRANSFUSION, RATE OF CITRATE INFUSION AND INCIDENCE OF CLINICAL ABNORMALITY

Case	Severity of Haemolytic Disease	Birth Weight (kg.)	Volume of Blood Exchanged (ml.)	Time taken for Exchange (minutes)	Citrate Infused (mg./kg./hr.)	Incident
A	+	3·2	700	129	286	—
B	++	2·9	600	107	397	Shock, retching
C	++	3·3	700	162	202	—
D	++	3·2	700	128	400	—
E	+++	2·5	500	150	356	—
F	+	2·6	500	125	—	Distal cyanosis
G	+	3·5	700	156	293	—
H	+++	2·3	500	195	242	Retching
I	+++	2·7	500	160	218	Death
J	++	3·3	850	110	542	Retching, heart failure
K	+	3·2	300	240	80	—
L	+++	3·0	600	150	385	—
M	++	2·7	700	190	240	Shock
N	++	2·6	500	115	404	—
O	+++	3·8	600	114	302	—
P	+	—	200	Not recorded	—	—
Q	+++	3·2	560	120	303	—
R	++	3·6	470	81	298	Distal cyanosis, acute collapse
S	+++	3·8	800	162	334	—

Potassium. Variations in serum potassium during exchange transfusion were unpredictable. Hill (1954) quoted the normal range of serum potassium in the newborn infant as 17·5 to 21·1 mg. per 100 ml. In this series the normal pre-transfusion range was 13·3 to 40·0 mg. per 100 ml. Table 3 shows that five infants (F, G, K, N, R) had pre-transfusion serum potassium levels above normal, and in these instances either no change or a rise accompanied the transfusion. Of those infants who had a normal pre-transfusion serum potassium level, five (B, D, I, J, L) developed a hyperpotassaemia during transfusion. All these infants were transfused with donor blood with a plasma potassium content of over 30·0 mg. per 100 ml. Except in the fatal case, however, the hyperpotassaemia was not relatable to any particular clinical abnormality, since the phenomenon was observed in both clinically normal and abnormal infants. Furthermore, two infants classified as clinically abnormal (H, M) had a normal serum potassium level throughout transfusion. One point is worthy of note: the plasma potassium level of the donor blood used in the fatal case was 110 mg. per 100 ml., and at death coexisting high potassium and low calcium-ion concentrations were recorded. Whether the high potassium level influenced the onset of cardiac failure could not be ascertained, since electrolyte imbalance was not considered to be the cause of death.

TABLE 2

ANALYSIS OF CASES ACCORDING TO SEVERITY OF HAEMOLYTIC DISEASE

	+	++	+++
Total number of cases	5	7	7
Clinically normal	4	3	5
Clinically abnormal	1	4	2
(*a*) Shocked	1	2	—
(*b*) Retching	—	2	1
(*c*) In cardiac failure ..	—	1	—
(*d*) Acutely collapsed ..	—	1	—
(*e*) Dead	—	—	1

Summary of Biochemical Changes in Abnormal Cases

Fig. 2 illustrates serum electrolyte changes during exchange transfusion in the abnormal cases.

Distal Cyanosis. This was not associated with any particular electrolyte pattern. Symptoms appeared early in the exchange, and at a time when serum citrate was beginning to rise and serum-calcium ion to fall. Both infants had a pre-transfusion hyperpotassaemia, which persisted throughout transfusion.

Retching (Cases B, H, J). This was associated with a hyperpotassaemia, a rising serum citrate level, and a serum calcium ion which was by no means unduly low when compared with other apparently normal transfusions.

Shock (Cases B, F, M). In Case B, shock appeared before any marked change in either serum citrate or calcium ion, but hyperpotassaemia was present after only 100 ml. of blood had been exchanged, and therefore coexisted with the appearance of clinical signs of shock. Case F presented

TABLE 3

CHANGES IN SERUM POTASSIUM DURING EXCHANGE TRANSFUSION

Case	Volume of Blood Exchanged (ml.)							
	0	100	200	300	400	500	600	700
	Serum Potassium (mg. per 100 ml.)							
A	16·2	20·5	—	20·8	20·4	22·7	24·0	25·7
B	17·0	34·0	25·0	20·0	26·5	30·0	30·0	—
C	13·3	13·6	19·0	14·3	14·0	14·0	12·7	17·7
D	20·5	20·5	21·4	23·2	38·0	35·4	26·0	24·4
E	16·1	16·1	13·8	17·4	17·5	15·4	—	—
F	23·1	18·8	22·7	20·6	25·1	26·0	—	—
G	37·0	37·5	38·0	38·4	38·2	36·2	35·7	37·0
H	—	23·0	23·1	22·0	17·8	14·4	—	—
I	12·4	14·0	18·0	20·0	28·0	36·0	—	—
J	—	27·7	31·6	28·3	39·5	38·0	34·8	34·8
K	31·0	36·0	30·0	50·0	—	—	—	—
L	—	20·0	24·5	23·5	18·0	18·0	—	—
M	16·5	15·7	18·2	17·0	16·0	16·5	16·5	17·1
N	28·0	—	28·0	—	29·0	—	33·0	—
O	18·7	—	18·1	—	21·7	—	22·4	—
P	17·7	—	24·3	—	—	—	—	—
Q	19·9	—	21·8	—	17·8	—	17·3	—
R	40·8	—	53·2	—	50·1	—	—	—
S	18·0	—	17·6	—	24·8	—	21·4	19·0
Mean value	21·6	22·9	24·9	24·3	26·0	25·2	26·7	25·0

only a mild hyperpotassaemia. Signs of shock appeared towards the end of the transfusion in Case M. At this time the serum citrate level had suddenly increased to 250 mg. per 100 ml., but serum potassium was within the normal range. Serum calcium-ion level was apparently uninfluenced by the sudden change in citrate, remaining, as it had done throughout the transfusion, at about 2 mg. per 100 ml.

Cardiac Failure (Case J). Heart failure appeared at a point in the transfusion when the serum electrolytes were beginning to return towards normal. The citrate level had fallen substantially, total calcium had reached a peak of 15 mg. per 100 ml., calcium ion had risen by 1·0 mg. per 100 ml., and serum potassium had fallen by 5 mg. per 100 ml. to a level of 30 mg. per 100 ml.

Acute Non-fatal Collapse (Case R). The infant collapsed after 500 ml. of blood had been exchanged, and the nearest sample of blood to this incident, taken at 400 ml., indicated a profound hyperpotassaemia although the serum citrate level was falling and the serum calcium ion was relatively stable at 2 mg. per 100 ml. It is significant that the bottle of donor blood had been changed after 400 ml. had been transfused, and the plasma potassium concentrations in the two bottles were 85·4 mg. and 52·8 mg. per 100 ml. respectively. The plasma potassium value after the exchange of 400 ml. of blood, although high, was actually a little lower than it had been earlier, and a further reduction might have been expected by the time of the clinical incident, in view of the lower plasma potassium content of the second bottle.

Death (Case I). In the fatal case, serum citrate had reached by far the highest level in the series, yet death took place when the citrate level was beginning to decrease. Serum calcium-ion concentration was not measurable, nor had it been for some time before death. At the time of death serum potassium had reached a peak value of 36 mg. per 100 ml. Thus there existed a profound hypocalcaemia and hyperpotassaemia.

Hyperpotassaemia. This was the only constant feature of the abnormal cases, and it was severe in the cases of cardiac failure, acute non-fatal collapse and death. Three apparently normal infants (D, G, L), however, exhibited hyperpotassaemia of similar magnitude.

Conclusion. It is believed that none of the clinical incidents was due entirely to electrolytic imbalance, since similar biochemical changes were common to all the infants of the series. Serum electrolytes reflect the total electrolyte pattern to some degree, but clinical abnormality need not necessarily be the result of a sudden change in plasma electrolytes. Rather it may be due to prolonged exposure of the intracellular environment to a gradually changing extracellular environment. Considered from this point of view, a study of serum electrolytes throughout a transfusion is more important than the assessment of electrolytes at any particular instant in a transfusion. Critical evaluation of the results of this investigation has failed to show a correlation between electrolytic imbalance and clinical abnormality during transfusion, but there is no doubt that all infants undergoing exchange transfusion are exposed to an abnormal biochemical state over a prolonged period.

GENERAL DISCUSSION

Citrate

Hypercitraemia. The possible importance of rising levels of plasma citrate in the production of symptoms during infusion of citrated blood was emphasized by Wexler *et al.* (1949) and Ames *et al.* (1950). The level of citrate was found to rise to a figure 10 to 30 times greater than the pre-transfusion value. This was accompanied by a decrease in plasma calcium-ion concentration. Prolongation of the Q-T interval on ECG tracings was recorded by Ames *et al.* (1950). Although the latter could be attributed to the depression of calcium-ion concentration by citrate, no constant relationship existed between the plasma citrate concentration and the ECG change. Furthermore, the Q-T interval could return to normal in the presence of continued high levels of citrate. These studies were made on convalescent infants. Plasma citrate, total calcium and total protein were determined, and plasma calcium-ion concentration was assessed indirectly by employing the normogram of McLean and Hastings (1935). Several of the babies became irritable during the infusion; their skins were pale and mottled, and a normal skin temperature was not restored by the use of blankets alone. One infant collapsed suddenly and responded only to prolonged resuscitative measures. Another was found dead during transfusion. The authors considered that these acute disturbances were almost certainly the result of acute lowering of plasma calcium-ion level. Critical study of the case records, however, shows no convincing evidence for such a belief and reveals the presence of other factors predisposing to complication. They believed that the absence of reactions in the majority of cases might be explained on the basis of the existence of forces capable of counteracting the calcium-ion-lowering effect of citrate. However, they provide no explanation of why these two less fortunate individuals should have been deficient in this homoeostatic mechanism. More recently Bunker *et al.* (1955) have shown, in a series of 130 adults who received moderate to large volumes of citrated blood, that many patients developed hypercitraemia, and theoretically calcium-ion concentration in the plasma ought to have been seriously depressed. More marked elevation of plasma citrate occurred when transfusion was extremely rapid, prolonged or repeated. Higher levels also occurred where the liver was damaged, and this may be important in the newborn infant with or without haemolytic disease.

The present investigation has demonstrated conclusively that a great increase in serum citrate occurs during the infusion of citrated blood, and it is important to consider the facts which influence this phenomenon. The acid-citrate-dextrose mixture used as an anticoagulant in this country has been criticized and praised for many years. When it was first instituted the dangers of citrate were emphasized, but until the technique of replacement transfusion and massive blood transfusion became common, little attention was focused upon the possibility of citrate intoxication in medical practice. In the infants in this series, amounts of citrate ranging from 738 to 3,413 mg. were infused into a plasma compartment of less than 200 ml. average volume, so that accumulation of citrate under these circumstances could be dangerous. It is believed that citrate in stored donor blood is confined essentially to the plasma. Thus, if the recommended ratio of volume of anticoagulant to blood is strictly adhered to, then the plasma citrate content of the donor blood should be about 600 mg. per 100 ml. It will be appreciated that any marked deviation from the standard technique may result in significant changes in the plasma citrate. Ames particularly emphasized this point when describing an alleged case of citrate intoxication following the infusion of plasma containing 1,536 mg. of citrate per 100 ml. With this in mind Walker and Neligan (1955) recommend the use of packed cells in exchange transfusion.

Speed of Citrate Infusion. Although the plasma citrate level in the donor blood is the first consideration, the rate at which it is infused is obviously important. It is desirable that the rate of transfusion be adjusted so that the homoeostatic mechanisms controlling citrate are able to deal with the citrate as fast as it is being infused. Mollison (1956) stipulates a maximum rate of 260 mg. of citrate per kg. of body weight per hour, but Wexler *et al.* (1949) and Walker *et al.* (1955) freely admit to exceeding this rate without clinical incident. In the present series similar conditions prevailed. Nakasone *et al.* (1954) performed an interesting experiment in which citrate solutions of varying strengths were infused into dogs and the response of cardiac muscle was measured by ECG tracings. They suggested that it was not the actual level of citrate in the perfusate which was the factor precipitating cardiac changes, but rather the cumulative dose of citrate in the animal's body. In other words, hypocalcaemia was induced after the infusion of a critical amount of citrate, whether this was attained over a short period by the infusion of a solution containing a high concentration of citrate or after a longer period with a solution containing less citrate. For this reason the slower the rate of transfusion the less severe the hypercitraemia which will develop. It is suggested that the clinical incidents in this series were not related to the infusion rate of citrate. Reference to Table 1 will show that the safety rate was often exceeded in cases which appeared normal throughout transfusion, yet in other abnormal cases the infusion rate was below the recommended safety rate.

Metabolism of Citrate. It should be borne in mind that reports describing rapid metabolic breakdown of citrate during the infusion of citrated blood are based on observations of plasma citrate concentration during a period when rapid diffusion out of the plasma compartment is occurring. Transfer of citrate to other compartments of body water would account, at least in part, for the disappearance of exogenous citrate out of the plasma water. The average amount of citrate contained in 100 ml. of citrated donor blood is 370 mg. Assuming that no transfer occurred out of the plasma compartment into interstitial water, then the amount of this citrate which would be retained after the exchange of 100 ml. of blood by the technique employed in this investigation would be about 320 mg. In practice, however, a proportion of this would be transferred to interstitial water, and, assuming even distribution throughout the extracellular water, about a seven-fold reduction in the theoretical maximum plasma concentration could be expected. The actual level in the plasma would depend on the degree of transfer of the citrate at the time of collection of the specimen, but it should be within the range of 46-320 mg. per 100 ml. Thus the levels recorded in this series indicate that a considerable portion of infused citrate migrated out of the plasma compartment after each 100 ml. of blood exchanged. Increased intracellular metabolism of citrate was likely to occur under the stimulus of the infusion of citrate. The exact rate of oxidation of citrate in the human being is unknown, but toxic effects appear to depend on dosage and rate of administration. Most tissues contain a specified citric-acid dehydrogenase, the liver and renal parenchyma being the most active sites of metabolism (Thunberg, 1953; Mårtensson, 1940). Wexler observed delayed removal of citrate from plasma in one fatal case which showed gross liver damage at necropsy, and from this evidence he postulated that delayed citrate metabolism might result from impaired liver function. In the fatal case of the present series a similar delayed removal of citrate was observed, yet post-mortem examination revealed no severe liver damage. It is quite possible that a mild degree of metabolic immaturity exists in newborn infants, especially those suffering from erythroblastosis foetalis. This would explain the resting hypercitraemia observed in some cases in this series. It can only be concluded, however, that all infants appeared to have efficient homoeostatic mechanisms for removing infused citrate from plasma.

It is suggested as a hypothesis that all the factors discussed must operate during the infusion of citrated blood. Initially the prevention of severe hypercitraemia by careful adjustment of the donor plasma citrate level and the rate of transfusion can be controlled by the operator. Presumably any infused citrate enters the plasma, and from there it is transferred to interstitial water and finally to the intracellular water, where it is metabolized. Reference to Figs. 1 and 2 will indicate the general pattern of serum citrate during transfusion. The initial dramatic rise to a level between 100 and 160 mg. per 100 ml. may represent a phase in which citrate is essentially confined to the plasma. Once mechanisms controlling transfer out of the plasma compartment become operative it is reasonable to expect a fall in the plasma citrate if the rate of transfer exceeds the rate of citrate infusion in the plasma. This has been confirmed in the present investigation. Fluctuations observed at later stages in the transfusion may reflect the efficiency of intracellular metabolic pathways. Thus a rising citrate in the presence of a constant rate of citrate infusion suggests some impairment of function (Cases I, M). Conversely, a falling serum citrate level suggests efficient metabolism, while a fluctuating citrate level may be indicative of sudden changes in the citrate intake with which the intracellular metabolic processes are unable to cope. All except two infants (I, M) were able to metabolize infused citrate very efficiently. If citrate intoxication were the causative factor in some or all of the clinical incidents in this series, then it is difficult to explain the fact that serum citrate levels of a similar magnitude did not precipitate incidents in the normal infants.

Citrate-induced Hypocalcaemia. The high serum citrate recorded in this investigation should have induced severe hypocalcaemia. The theoretical implications are that all available calcium ions in the plasma of infants undergoing transfusion should be inactivated, but the results indicate that, although significantly reduced, this reduction was not complete except in the fatal case. Two explanations are proposed. First, citrate was present in the plasma in high concentration, but there was no evidence to show whether the whole or part of it was present in an active ionic form. In fact an inactive molecule, possibly bound to protein, may have existed. Such complexes are known to exist in the case of protein and glucose and the lipoproteins. Under such circumstances only ionized citrate would be available for reaction with calcium and other cations. Secondly, the formation of calcium citrate is not an instantaneous reaction, and this might explain the apparent discrepancy between the absence of clinical manifestations of tetany, even though subsequent analysis of serum showed a profound depression of calcium ion. During transfusion calcium citrate formation may have been incomplete, whereas on storage of the serum in the absence of enzyme action, reaction was allowed to reach completion in the presence of excess of citrate ion. Whatever the explanation, analysis revealed that complete inactivation of calcium ion in serum did not occur. There was no evidence to confirm the finding of others (Lansing and Scott, 1942) that significant mobilization of calcium ion occurred from intracellular sources, nor did it appear that the injection of calcium gluconate was effective in elevating calcium ion in serum. On clinical grounds, Walker and Neligan (1955) abandoned the use of gluconate, and they did not observe tetany in a series of 272 transfusions.

Herlitz (1942) observed active tetany in infants whose plasma calcium-ion level had fallen below 3·5 mg. per 100 ml., yet even with serum calcium-ion levels below 2·0 mg. per 100 ml., classical tetany was not seen during this investigation. The absence of clinical abnormality is not inconsistent with a reduction in calcium ion, as the factors governing neuromuscular irritability are complex, and the maintenance of a normal state of irritability may have been due to compensatory mechanisms. The exact means by which tetany is brought about has not yet been elucidated, but the original work of Ringer and Loeb (discussed in any standard textbook of physiology) might elucidate the problem. They postulated a delicate equilibrium between the cations of the serum, and any disturbance of this equilibrium, such as a decrease in calcium, magnesium or hydrogen ions or an increase in sodium, potassium or hydroxyl ions, causes hyperirritability of the tissues. It has been shown in this series that an increase in potassium and a decrease in calcium ion occurred in serum, thus favouring the development of neuromuscular hyperirritability.

It has been demonstrated that citrated blood is weakly acid in reaction, and the infusion of such a medium would favour the production of a metabolic acidosis. This problem is at present under investigation by Walker (personal communication, 1956), but no results have been reported to date. Increase in hydrogen-ion concentration would tend to compensate for the coexisting hypocalcaemia and hyperpotassaemia in terms of neuromuscular irritability. For example, Mudge and Vislocky (1949) observed that the acidosis of chronic renal disease was not specifically related to a change in acid-base equilibrium, but was associated with a decrease in intracellular potassium and a rise in intracellular sodium. In this investigation perfusion of donor blood did not significantly alter the infants' sodium level in the face of a virtual replacement of their blood and a donor plasma concentration around 400 mg. per 100 ml. Since renal excretion of sodium must have been negligible during transfusion, diffusion or transfer of excess sodium out of the plasma compartment must have occurred. Is it reasonable to postulate that at least some of this sodium entered the intracellular water, possibly reflecting that some movement of potassium into the extracellular water had occurred?

Potassium

The leakage of potassium from red blood cells during storage is a well-known phenomenon (De Gowin *et al.*, 1940), and the significance of this was emphasized by Mollison (1951). Toxic levels of potassium in blood plasma are associated with cardiac arrest, and in fact the injection of potassium citrate solution into the coronary circulation has been used experimentally to produce elective temporary cardiac arrest (Melrose *et al.*, 1955). In the adult the transfusion of one or two pints of blood does not greatly affect the recipient's plasma potassium concentration, but the situation is different during exchange transfusion in a newborn infant, where one pint of blood is equivalent to about twice the infant's blood volume. The influence of transfusion upon serum potassium concentration in eight infants was studied by Miller *et al.* (1954). Hyperpotassaemia was present, particularly when the donor blood had been stored for a week or longer. No convincing proof was offered that the high potassium levels were harmful to these infants. Sudden unexplained death in two infants also prompted the investigation carried out by Campbell (1955). Hyperpotassaemia was present in three of four deaths in the series, but comparably high figures were recorded in infants who had shown no abnormality. Although the levels were potentially lethal, Campbell was unable to ascribe the deaths with certainty to hyperpotassaemia. Some success was obtained with insulin in maintaining more normal potassium levels, and the author's experience of comparative morbidity and mortality in comparable control and test groups is awaited with interest.

Serum potassium levels recorded in the present investigation indicated that 60% of infants developed a hyperpotassaemia either before or during transfusion, but these changes were common, even in the asymptomatic infants. Rise in plasma potassium level during exchange transfusion is influenced by the intake of potassium in the donor plasma, the ability of the renal mechanism to excrete excess potassium and the efficiency of intracellular 'metabolic' sites in removing potassium from the plasma. It was apparent in this investigation that the development of hyperpotassaemia was closely related to the infusion of donor blood. The incidence of hyperpotassaemia was high when the donor plasma potassium level exceeded 30·0 mg. per 100 ml. As in the case of citrate, however, the high serum potassium levels were not relatable, surprisingly, to the rate of transfusion. Thus the development of hyperpotassaemia may be due to accumulation of potassium rather than to the potassium concentration of the perfusate. In the adult renal excretion of potassium is a most important homoeostatic mechanism preventing potassium intoxication, but, since renal immaturity is an accepted phenomenon in the newborn, their ability to excrete excess potassium is doubtful. In fact the mean normal urine output in the first 24 hours is about 20 ml., so that the maintenance of a normal serum level during transfusion must depend upon mechanisms other than renal. One of these must be the transfer of potassium from the plasma to other compartments of the body water. Simple distribution within the extracellular water will result in a seven-fold decrease in the concentration of any exogenous potassium which is confined initially to the plasma. The serum potassium concentration *per se* does not necessarily reflect the state of cellular potassium, and it is not justifiable automatically to associate a high serum potassium level with a toxic accumulation of potassium in body water. In fact Tarail and Elkinton (1949) have shown that a cellular deficiency of potassium may exist in the presence of a high serum potassium level. Although this would explain the absence of potassium intoxication in the cases in this investigation with a high serum potassium level, it is difficult to imagine in infants suffering from erythroblastosis foetalis. These infants are exposed to a severe haemolytic process which starts *in utero*, and it is possible that in the absence of a renal homoeostatic mechanism these infants are in a state of positive potassium balance. This fact tends to be confirmed by the high incidence of resting hyperpotassaemia.

Experiments (Joseph *et al.*, 1939; Fenn, 1939; Houssay *et al.*, 1936; Eichelberger, 1941) have shown that the intravenous injection of soluble potassium salts results in the accumulation of potassium within the liver cells, and this process is enhanced by the simultaneous infusion of glucose solution. Presumably potassium enters the intracellular space of the hepatic cells during hepatic glycogenesis. This is suggested as a working hypothesis in the present investigation. The liver is only a temporary site, but it serves as a means of preventing potassium intoxication in the absence of renal regulating mechanisms. The liberation of potassium during glycogenolysis inevitably occurs, but at a rate which allows adequate renal excretion of potassium by the maturing renal tissue.

Coexistent Hypocalcaemia and Hyperpotassaemia

The biochemical abnormality observed in this investigation was the coexisting hyperpotassaemia and hypocalcaemia. The danger of simultaneously rising potassium and falling calcium-ion levels in the blood was described by Guest (1952). Protection of dogs against normally lethal concentrations of potassium may be provided by the intravenous injection of calcium (Winkler *et al.*, 1939). Modification of the effects of potassium intoxication in children by the administration of calcium salts was claimed by Govan and Weiseth (1946). Latent tetany in a group of adults with coexisting hypopotassaemia and hypocalcaemia was rendered manifest by the slow intravenous infusion of potassium salts even though the final plasma potassium level did not exceed the usual normal range (Engel *et al.*, 1949). More recently Levine *et al.* (1952) have claimed that hypocalcaemia may actually potentiate the electrocardiographic signs of hyperpotassaemia. None of these facts was confirmed in this investigation. There is some suggestion that the hyperpotassaemia may have precipitated heart signs in the cases of acute non-fatal collapse, cardiac failure and death, but completely asymptomatic infants presented a hyperpotassaemia of similar magnitude. The evidence is strong in favour of profound electrolytic imbalance in the fatal case, although the actual cause of death was found to be haemorrhage. It appears that there is no association between the clinical disturbance observed during exchange transfusion and the changes which undoubtedly occur in plasma electrolytes.

Other Possible Explanations of the Clinical Disturbances

Circulatory Stress

Interference with Postnatal Readjustment of Circulation. The picture of differential cyanosis of the distal half of the body is most alarming. Only two such cases have been seen by J. W. F. and both occurred in this series. In each great difficulty had been met in withdrawing blood and much time had been spent manipulating the catheter. On the first occasion the development of some venacaval obstruction was considered, and the spontaneous resolution of the disturbance was witnessed with relief. The production of a temporary veno-arterial shunt through a patent ductus arteriosus must be considered. Increasing experimental evidence is becoming available that the ductus arteriosus does not close within a few minutes after birth. The careful studies of lambs by Dawes *et al.* (1954) and Born *et al.* (1956) at Oxford have shown that in that animal the closure takes place over hours, and is dependent on changes in oxygen tension and the release of sympathetic amines.

The occasional observation of cyanosis of the lower part of the body of newly born babies stimulated Eldridge *et al.* (1954) to carry out oxygen saturation studies upon arterialized capillary blood from the right hand and foot of healthy newborn human infants; 14 studies were made on 12 subjects. Of the 14 studies, eight showed significantly lower values in the foot than in the hand. In all five studied from one to three hours after delivery the oxygen saturation of blood from the foot was significantly lower than in the hand, indicating the presence of a veno-arterial shunt to the lower part of the body. Three of the five infants studied from three hours to three days after birth showed lower blood oxygen-saturation values in the foot than in the hand. None of the four infants who were older than three days showed significant oxygen-saturation differences. One baby who had a significant difference at two hours which persisted at two days showed no difference between hand and foot values by the fifth day. Should these studies be confirmed, then exchange transfusion is being carried out at a time when the ductus may be open functionally and when it may be the site of a veno-arterial shunt.

From this it is but a step to the fact that the increase in pressure in the right side of the heart which may occur during exchange transfusion may increase the right-to-left shunt through the ductus and give rise to visible cyanosis in the distal half of the body. The increased pressure might be the result of a weakened myocardium going into failure, of excessively rapid transfusion or of partial spasm of the great abdominal veins which would act normally as a blood reservoir. Such an explanation is not entirely satisfactory, however. If the cyanosis were the result of a veno-arterial shunt through the ductus, it is surprising that it appeared in the very early stages of operation, that it did not become progressively more noticeable and that it resolved although operation was continued. Perhaps the withdrawal of the catheter for a few centimetres was responsible, as the blood flow which had been directed through the ductus venosus to the vena cava close to the heart would then be subjected to the cushioning effect of the portal circulation. Even if this were so, a major difficulty still remains. There was no doubt that the superficial veins over the front of the abdomen became much more obvious and that they drained upward over the chest. They did not constitute convincing evidence of occlusion of the inferior vena cava, but they suggested it. Catheterization of the umbilical vein takes the catheter tip to the inferior vena cava at 12-14 cm. from the abdominal wall (van Loghem *et al.*, 1949). When obstruction is encountered at 10-11 cm., the catheter may have turned into the portal circulation and the withdrawal of blood may be very difficult or even impossible. Catheterization of the ductus venosus is not easy, but from a knowledge of the length of polythene tube introduced into these two infants the catheter tips must have lain in the ductus venosus or in the portal circulation. 'The fact that veins are capable of constriction may be observed by anyone who attempts to insert a cannula into one without due care' (McDowall, 1938). The ductus venosus is a foetal vessel which is in process of establishing or maintaining functional closure at the time when an exchange transfusion is being carried out. Irritation by a catheter could be expected to intensify the muscular constriction. The vessel is relatively short and it enters the inferior vena cava.

As a possible explanation for a very curious phenomenon it is suggested that spasm spreading to the greater vessel and producing partial occlusion merits consideration. Resolution of the physical signs might then follow partial withdrawal of the catheter and relaxation of the vena cava. Sphincter mechanisms exist on the great veins of some mammals. The dog has one on the hepatic vein, and the common seal has one on the posterior inferior vena cava (Harrison and Tomlinson, 1956). No reference can be found to the existence of any such structure in the human embryo at any point in development. Spasm of the inferior vena cava of animals may occur, however, as a reflex phenomenon in the absence of any recognizable sphincter. The fact that the vena cava of the horse could be made to constrict by stimulating the abdominal sympathetic was recorded by Valentin (1839). Splanchnic stimulation can cause constriction of the inferior vena cava (McDowall, 1938), and the portal vein can be made to constrict similarly (Burton-Opitz, 1913). Furthermore, Neil (quoted by McDowall, 1956) has obtained records of post-ganglionic sympathetic activity in fibres supplying the superior and inferior venae cavae. Such impulse discharge is markedly increased reflexly by such a remote procedure as the perfusion of the carotid-body areas with blood of low oxygen saturation. With spasm of the vena cava in mind, radiological studies employing a contrast medium were planned for such further cases as might be encountered, but none has occurred.

Even if both these explanations should be incorrect, the phenomenon, of which there may be milder unobserved degrees, reminds the paediatrician that he is producing acute dynamic changes in a circulatory system which is undergoing simultaneous adaptation to extra-uterine life. Following the occurrence of the second case the catheter tip has never been inserted for more than 7-8 cm. from the abdominal wall. The employment of less rigid catheter material may have some advantage (Tizard, 1957).

Speed of Exchange. The development of signs of cardiac failure during exchange transfusion is not uncommon, but, apart from the unknown importance of the coexisting hyperpotassaemia and reduced calcium ion in Case I, the other biochemical findings in the series were unassociated with cardiac failure. The mechanical stress of exchange transfusion must be considerable. When a 7 lb. baby receives an 80 ml. per lb. body weight exchange he is subjected to a constant withdrawal and replacement of from 3% to 7% of his blood volume every two to three minutes for $1\frac{1}{2}$ to 2 hours. This takes place in a subject whose myocardium may be unhealthy before operation is begun and who may have other weak points in the circulatory system. The spleen, for example, may rupture either spontaneously or during exchange transfusion. In 1949 an exchange transfusion by the umbilical route was carried out by one of us (J. W. F.) on a severely affected baby of 5 lb. weight. Twenty-ml. aliquots of blood were used and all seemed well until 380 ml. had been exchanged. The infant then collapsed suddenly and died in a few moments. The catheter was clamped *in situ*, and at necropsy its tip was found in the inferior vena cava near the right atrium. The right side of the heart was extremely dilated. No other abnormality was found and the death may be attributed to the author's inexperience.

The deterioration observed so commonly by Walker and Neligan (1955) was thought to be unrelated to the initial condition of the infants, the birth weight, technical difficulties encountered or the rate of exchange. Yet at least one of their subjects was so delicately balanced that the injection of only 10 ml. at one point in an exchange transfusion dramatically converted an apparently well baby into a dead one. The effect of the too-rapid transfusion of anaemic patients was described by Starling (1918) as being like an overloaded heart-lung preparation. Venous pressure rises and cardiac output falls. Referring to what Wiener (1943) has described as 'speed shock', the *British Medical Journal* (1955) points out that the circulatory collapse is related, not to the properties of the stored blood, but to the total volume given and the speed of administration. The ability of children to tolerate relatively faster transfusion than adults was mentioned by Andrews and Coleman (1957), but their subjects were aged 4 years or more.

The need for care and experience in carrying out exchange transfusion has been stressed by Philipsborn *et al.* (1956). They found from the literature that most exchange transfusions were carried out in from one to two hours, and decided to investigate the effect of rapid exchange transfusion in pups. The operation was carried out on healthy mongrel pups through the femoral artery and employing their own heparinized blood. They discovered that much larger aliquots of blood could be used with safety than had been anticipated, and that the vascular trees of puppies could be expanded or contracted by as much as 25% without significantly altering the venous or arterial pressures or provoking changes in the ECG.

Circulatory equilibrium could be maintained under challenges far exceeding those which ordinarily occur during exchange transfusion. When two of the puppies were subjected to additional stress (barbiturate overdosage in one and exsanguination shock in another), however, they were less able to face the challenge of rapid exchange transfusion. There are obvious differences between the animal experiment and the human operation. The experiment employed healthy puppies receiving their own warm heparinized blood by the femoral artery, whereas the operation is carried out on human infants who have been the victims of a pathological process for some weeks and possibly involving the circulatory system, and who receive cool or cold stored citrated blood by the portal circulation.

Whatever the part played by excessive speed in the production of symptoms during exchange transfusion, the surgical principle of gentleness in operating is likely to be less upsetting to an infant than haste and undue manipulation. Where signs of distress appear they frequently subside if the baby is left undisturbed for five or ten minutes, and if cardiac failure is definitely present a small venesection may be carried out with advantage. Clinical deterioration may take place, however, in the absence of the classical signs of cardiac failure. The descriptive term 'shock' has been applied here to those infants who become cold, pale and limp, who develop varying degrees of abdominal distension and whose breathing may be accompanied in expiration by a faintly audible, murmuring whine. The pallor may be so striking that intraperitoneal haemorrhage is suspected. The condition was recognized by Walker and Neligan (1955), who also described it as shock and who recommended the giving of more blood as treatment. In the present investigation the clinical disturbance was unaccompanied by a single biochemical pattern.

Increasing Blood Viscosity. Variation in the viscosity of the blood influences the load carried by the heart (Whitby and Britton, 1953). Any increase in blood viscosity is naturally harmful when it increases the work thrown on a heart with reserves of strength seriously diminished by disease (*Lancet*, 1942). The immediate cause of death from haemolytic disease within 12 to 24 hours of birth is cardiac failure, for which the best immediate treatment is venesection and oxygen administration (Mollison, 1956). The viscosity of blood increases with increase in the haematocrit. For these reasons the wisdom of using packed or sedimented red cells for exchange transfusions may be doubted where the infant's original haematocrit is low and the haematocrit of the donor blood is appreciably higher. The transfusion of anaemic patients was found by Evans (1942) not to increase whole-blood viscosity, but he transfused with whole blood and the procedure was not comparable in volume or speed with exchange transfusion. No observations on changes in blood viscosity during exchange transfusions with whole blood and with sedimented cells have been found. If the viscosity does in fact rise with a rising haematocrit, then this would provide an objection to the routine exchange of the profoundly anaemic patient's blood with aliquots of sedimented cells. It is acknowledged, however, that if high-output cardiac failure is to be avoided in such infants the haemoglobin value may need to be raised to some extent. This may be done without employing sedimented cells for the whole operation, and it should be done slowly. Any residual anaemia may be corrected later by scalp-vein transfusion when the patient's immediate survival has been assured. At the Simpson Memorial Maternity Pavilion emphasis has always been placed upon leisurely exchange with whole blood and upon the judicious maintenance of a negative balance between withdrawal and replacement in severely affected babies. Rising blood viscosity would be unlikely to bear any relationship to the clinical disturbance of mildly affected infants during exchange transfusion. The blood viscosity of such cases may in fact fall during operation.

In practice, however, there is probably less difference than might be thought between the blood from which the supernatant plasma has been decanted and whole blood which is allowed to stand undisturbed throughout the operation. Recent observations on blood containers in Edinburgh (Cumming, 1957) have shown how very difficult it is to maintain anything like an even suspension of cells in the standard glass transfusion bottles even when these are intermittently inverted.

Cooling

Chilling of the baby during exchange transfusion has been thought to be responsible for some of the abnormalities observed. The rectal temperatures of infants receiving blood at 70°-80° F. have been shown to fall from 97°-99° to 94°-96° in 21 cases studied by Marting *et al.* (1955). Cooling of this degree might occur in newborn infants exposed on a table for two hours unless careful precautions such as those described by Corey *et al.* (1955) are taken to avoid it. Four of the 21 infants, however, showed signs of shock after about 250 ml. had been exchanged. Their blood was noted to be poorly oxygenated, and this was attributed to hypothermia. Two of the four babies died. As a result of their investigation Marting *et al.* produced a glass helix which was immersed in a thermostatically controlled water-bath and through which the donor blood was heated briefly on its way to the baby. The blood reached the infant at a temperature of 96°-100° F. Following this innovation the rectal temperatures of further infants studied were maintained, and their condition was claimed to be better than that of the infants who had received cool blood.

A dramatic description of cardiac arrest during exchange transfusion was given by Pew (1955). An infant with moderately severe haemolytic disease received an umbilical exchange transfusion with very fresh citrated blood. Shortly after 350 ml. had been exchanged the heart stopped suddenly. The infant's chest was opened and the heart massaged. Normal cardiac rhythm was restored after about two minutes. The exchange transfusion was continued and the exposed heart kept under observation. As blood was injected the heart was noted to slow and to be 'definitely cool'; indeed the bradycardia became so profound that further cardiac massage and the intracardiac injection of adrenaline were required. Normal rhythm was again restored; the exchange transfusion was carefully completed and the chest repaired. The total serum calcium concentration shortly after cardiac arrest was only 5·7 mg. per 100 ml. The baby showed some twitching when convalescent. The calcium was not recorded, but the sign disappeared when calcium gluconate was given. No information was provided about the speed of operation or where the tip of the catheter lay. Cooling was considered to be the possible precipitating factor. The first bottle of blood had been adequately warmed, and the crisis developed soon after the second, unwarmed, bottle had been brought into use.

The local application of cold to the front of the chest produces a slow heart rate, diminished systolic output and increased blood pressure (McDowall, 1956). Extracorporeal cooling of dogs down to temperatures of 26° C. will not precipitate cardiac arrest, but the injection of very cold blood close to the heart can provoke auricular fibrillation (Delorme 1957). This would be particularly dangerous if it occurred in an infant with a devitalized myocardium and whose heart was receiving rapidly recurring influxes of 10-20 ml. of blood under pressure.

Autonomic Stress

The catheterization of the umbilical vein and the shunting to and fro of blood in the portal circulation may be more disturbing than has been thought previously. Walker and Neligan (1955) gained the impression that excessive traction on the umbilical cord during manipulation of the catheter produced vomiting. There is no doubt that the prodding of obstructions within the portal circulation makes the baby retch and he commonly regurgitates. Distension of the portal circulation by rapid transfusion may also precipitate this trouble. Such reflex stimulation was undoubtedly the cause of retching in this small series. Operations in the upper abdomen in relation to diaphragm and peritoneum may provoke hiccup, vomiting and shock. Exchange transfusion evokes dynamic changes in a region richly supplied with both afferent and efferent autonomic nerves and may be expected to give rise to some disturbance.

Inexperience

The experience of those conducting exchange transfusions varies widely. There is more to the procedure than exchanging 10 ml. aliquots of blood. In a surgical team it is unlikely that an operation carrying a comparable mortality would always be left to the house-surgeon or an inexperienced registrar. Yet junior staff may be left unsupervised to carry out an exchange transfusion in the belief sometimes held by senior staff inexperienced in this procedure that normal skill and common sense are all that is required. The apprenticeship to be served by the would-be operator of exchange transfusion is neither short nor easy, and even after many successes the experienced may be humbled by failure. It is interesting to note that Walker and Neligan (1955) had a low mortality, and yet Walker (1955) in a personal communication stated that, taking the country as a whole, the problem of unexpected death was more common than he had previously thought. This suggests that where both skill and experience were available the mortality was lower than in other areas where experience was less. Precisely this view has been expressed by Walker and Mollison (1957). They have shown from national figures that an appreciable number of infants dying of haemolytic disease had received exchange transfusions which were inadequate in volume, and that the actual number of deaths from haemolytic disease in England and Wales was in excess of the estimated annual mortality. Walker and Mollison (1957) calculated that some hospitals might be conducting an exchange transfusion as infrequently as once in four or five months. In such circumstances experience and team-work are hard to obtain. As many as 150 more affected infants might be saved annually if they were to receive exchange transfusion from experienced operators. We also believe that both the morbidity and mortality associated with exchange transfusion may be reduced by experience, and that the latter can be achieved best by centralizing treatment. Smaller obstetric or paediatric units might therefore have to sacrifice their occasional opportunities of carrying out the procedure, but many would be prepared to do so for the sake of the child. In the towns around Edinburgh a number of hospitals make a practice of sending the affected mother to the Simpson Memorial Maternity Pavilion for delivery, and for treatment of the child should that be necessary. By doing so they assure the infants of very early treatment by a team which possesses reasonable experience.

Conclusions

Various clinical disturbances may be observed during exchange transfusion in the infant suffering from haemolytic disease. Exchange transfusion produces considerable change in the patients' plasma electrolytes. The citrate level increases, potassium frequently increases and the calcium-ion level falls irrespective of the total serum calcium. The changes in serum electrolytes were shared by infants who were disturbed and by those who showed no abnormality. The depression of calcium ion can be neither prevented nor corrected by injecting calcium gluconate in the dose employed in this study. Other possible causes of clinical disturbance have been suggested. Evidence for them has not been sought in this study. They include such factors as interference with the circulation during the period of post-natal readjustment, excessive speed of exchange, changing blood viscosity, manipulation of the catheter within the abdomen, the injection of cool blood and, above all, inexperience on the part of the operator.

We wish to express our thanks to Professor R. W. B. Ellis and Dr. C. P. Stewart for their encouragement during this work, and to the former for his constructive criticism of the paper. We are grateful also to those registrars who took samples of blood and kept careful clinical records during some of the exchange transfusions.

The biochemical data included in this paper formed part of the Ph.D. thesis submitted successfully by H. S. to the University of Edinburgh.

References

Ames, R., Syllm, I. and Rapoport, S. (1950). *Pediatrics*, **6**, 361.
Andrews, L. G. and Coleman, D. J. (1957). *Brit. med. J.*, **1**, 19.
Born, G. V. R., Dawes, G. S., Mott, J. C. and Rennick, B. R. (1956). *J. Physiol. (Lond.)*, **132**, 304.
British Medical Journal (1955), **2**, 1493.
Bunker, J. P., Stetson, J. B., Coe, R. C., Grillo, H. C. and Murphy, A. J. J. (1955). *J Amer. med. Ass.*, **157**, 1361.
Burton-Opitz, R. (1913). *Quart. J. exp. Physiol.*, **7**, 57.
Campbell, W. A. B. (1955). *Arch. Dis. Childh.*, **30**, 513.
Corey, E. L., Wood, J. B., Donegan, C. C. and Birdsong, M. (1955). *J. Pediat.*, **47**, 216.
Cumming, R. A. (1957). Personal communication.
Dawes, G. S., Mott, J. C. and Widdicombe, J. G. (1954). *J. Physiol. (Lond.)*, **126**, 563.
De Gowin, E. L., Harris, J. E. and Plass, E. D. (1940). *J. Amer. med. Ass.*, **114**, 850, 855.
Delorme, E. J. (1957). Personal communication.
Eichelberger, L. (1941). *J. biol. Chem.*, **138**, 583.
Eldridge, F. L., Hultgren, H. N. and Wigmore, M. E. (1954). *Science*, **119**, 731.

Engel, F. L., Martin, S. P. and Taylor, H. (1949). *Bull. Johns Hopk. Hosp.*, **84**, 285.
Evans, P. (1942). *Lancet*, **1**, 162.
Farquhar, J. W. and Lewis, I. C. (1949). *Ibid.*, **1**, 953.
Fenn, W. O. (1939). *J. biol. Chem.*, **128**, 297.
Govan, C. D. and Weiseth, W. M. (1946). *J. Pediat.*, **28**, 550.
Guest, G. M. (1952). *Amer. J. Dis. Child.*, **84**, 638.
Harrison, R. J. and Tomlinson, J. D. W. (1956). *Proc. zool. Soc. Lond.*, **126**, 205.
Herlitz, G. (1942). *Acta paediat. (Uppsala)*, **30**, 153.
Hill, F. S. (1954). *Practical Fluid Therapy in Pediatrics.* Philadelphia.
Houssay, B. A., Marenzi, A. D. and Gerschman, R. (1936). *Rev. Soc. argent. Biol.*, **12**, 434 ; ref. quoted by Fenn : Houssay, B. A. and Marenzi, A. D., *Rev. Soc. argent. Biol.*, **13**, 139 (1937).
Joseph, M., Cohn, W. E. and Greenberg. D. M. (1939). *J. biol. Chem.*, **128**, 673.
King, E. J. (1951). *Micro-analysis in Medical Biochemistry*, 2nd ed., p. 45. London.
Lancet (1942), **1**, 176.
Lansing, A. I. and Scott, G. H. (1942). *Anat. Rec.*, **84**, 91.
Levine, H. D., Vazifdar, J. P., Lown, B. and Merrill, J. P. (1952). *Amer. Heart J.*, **43**, 437.
Loghem, J. J. van, Bolhuis, J. H. van, Soeters, J. M. and Veeneklaas, G. M. H. (1949). *Brit. med. J.*, **2**, 49.
Mårtensson, J. (1940). *Acta physiol. scand.*, **1**, Suppl. 2, p. 59.
Marting, F. L., Wagoner, S. C. and Wilson, V. C. (1955). *Amer. J. Dis. Child.*, **89**, 289
McDowall, R. J. S. (1938). *The Control of the Circulation of the Blood.* London.
—— (1956). *Ibid.* Supplemental Volume.
McLean, F. C. and Hastings, A. B. (1935). *J. Biol. Chem.*, **108**, 285.
Melrose, D. G., Dreyer, B., Bentall, H. H. and Baker, J. B. E. (1955). *Lancet*, **2**, 21.
Miller, G., McCoord, A. B., Joos, H. A. and Clausen, S. W. (1954). *Pediatrics*, **13**, 412.
Mollison, P. L. (1951). *Blood Transfusion in Clinical Medicine.* Oxford.
—— (1956). *Ibid.*, 2nd ed. Oxford.
—— (1957). Annual Meeting British Paediatric Association (to be published).
Mudge, G. H. and Vislocky, K. (1949). *J. clin. Invest.*, **28**, 482.
Nakasone, N., Watkins, E., Janeway, C. A. and Gross, R. E. (1954). *J. Lab. clin. Med.*, **43**, 184.
Natelson, S., Pincus, J. B. and Lugovoy, J. K. (1948). *J. clin. Invest.*, **27**, 446.
Pew, W. L. (1955). *J. Pediat.*, **47**, 645.
Philipsborn, H. F., Miller, R. A. and Traisman, H. S. (1956). *Ibid.*, **49**, 67.
Sobel, A. E. and Sobel, B. A. (1939). *J. biol. Chem.*, **129**, 721.
Starling, E. H. (1918). *The Linacre Lecture on the Law of the Heart.* London.
Tarail, R. and Elkinton, J. R. (1949). *J. clin. Invest.*, **28**, 99.
Thunberg, T. (1953). *Physiol. Rev.*, **33**, 1.
Tizard, J. P. M. (1957). Personal communication.
Valentin, G. (1839). *De functionibus nervorum cerebralium et nervi sympathici.* Huber, Berne.
Walker, W. (1955). Personal communication.
—— (1956). Personal communication
—— and Mollison, P. L. (1957). *Lancet*, **1**, 1309.
—— and Neligan, G. A. (1955). *Brit. med. J.*, **1**, 681.
Wexler, I. B., Pincus, J. B., Natelson, S. and Lugovoy, J. K. (1949). *J. clin. Invest.*, **28**, 474.
Whitby, L. E. H. and Britton, C. J. C. (1953). *Disorders of the Blood.* 7th ed. London.
Wiener, A. S. (1943). *Blood Groups and Transfusion.* 3rd. ed. Springfield (Illinois).
Winkler, A. W., Hoff, H. E. and Smith, P. K. (1939). *Amer. J. Physiol.*, **127**, 430.

TREATMENT OF PERSISTENT ENURESIS WITH THE ELECTRIC BUZZER

BY

IAN G. WICKES

From the North Middlesex Hospital and South-East Essex Group

(RECEIVED FOR PUBLICATION SEPTEMBER 17, 1957)

The treatment of enuresis has largely defeated physicians in the past. Some have readily acknowledged this and have pinned their faith on the child growing out of it. Others have used numerous drugs with varying success; since there is a tendency towards spontaneous improvement, and since inert pills are partly effective by suggestion, it has been difficult to assess what specific effect, if any, a particular drug possesses. Psychiatrists have tended to attribute the disorder to infantile regression and have sought, by child guidance techniques, to readjust the child's interpersonal relationships; they have turned a blind eye to the symptom itself, a wise move since it so seldom disappears with such therapy. Nevertheless there is a widespread belief that enuresis is purely psychogenic, a belief which is illustrated by a common mis-spelling 'eneuresis'—as if the condition were a neurosis. Undoubtedly nervous factors influence enuresis (as with epilepsy and asthma) but it is equally true that the cure of bedwetting will often greatly improve the child's emotional state, indicating that the anxiety is secondary, in part at least.

The treatment of enuresis was revolutionized when it was discovered by chance that an apparatus for signalling to the parents that their child had a wet bed and needed changing also had the property of training the child to become dry. Pfaundler (1904) used a quilted pad for the purpose, Mowrer (1938) improved the apparatus by including a relay, and Seiger (1946) first described a metal and rubber pad that could be dried. Subsequently Davidson and Douglass (1950) reported 20 cases in deprived children with 15 cures; Seiger (1952) reported a series of 106 cases, 94 becoming dry for two months or longer, in the majority of cases after less than one month's treatment. Geppert (1953) reported a series of 42 cases with 38 successes using a similar method. Crosby (1950) used the conditioning method but instead of a bell or buzzer he used electrodes attached to the genitalia and loin so that at the start of micturition 'a stimulus, capable of variation to any devised intensity, is applied to the patient'. His results were successful in 52 out of 58 cases.

In view of the intractable nature of enuresis the above results seem almost too good to be true. It is certainly surprising that the medical profession has not adopted the method to any extent in Great Britain, but commercial firms have exploited the treatment on a large scale offering it direct to the public without the supervision of a physician. Only one small series (in deprived children) has been reported and occasional letters (Gillison, 1956) have appeared in the medical press supporting the method. In some quarters there is considerable resistance to it as evidenced by the reply in the *British Medical Journal* (1957) in which the writer, after describing many largely ineffective and blunderbuss remedies, goes on to refer to the conditioning method as 'rather a crude type of therapy'! Since ignorance and prejudice envelop the subject it seemed desirable to collect a series of persistent intractable enuretics to observe how they responded to this form of treatment.

The Apparatus and its Use

One of the reasons why this treatment has not been popular amongst doctors is because of the lack of availability of sets. For some years one firm has been hiring sets for a sum which far exceeds that which the average hospital patient can afford. Recently another manufacturer has begun to produce one which sells at less than half that sum. I have been fortunate in that the father of a former patient has been producing efficient sets which have been sold at less than one-fifth the cost of hiring. Furthermore, through the generosity of the Chamberlain Foundation, I have been able to lend a similar set free of charge to those parents who were unable to buy one.

The apparatus consists of an alarm unit containing a buzzer, light, relay and 6-volt battery together with two flexible leads that can be clipped on to two fine metallic rectangular gauze mats about 16 × 20 in. The mats are best secured on the bed by slipping each into a pocket obtained by sewing a pillowcase to a drawsheet along its three closed sides to make a double open-ended pocket. The child, preferably devoid of pyjama trousers, lies above the linen sandwich containing the mats. The alarm unit stands on a table or chair close to the bed and is switched on at bed time. The alarm is actuated when the circuit is completed by urine that has soaked through the layers to reach the lower of the two mats. Occasionally a 'dry ring' is obtained if the mats inadvertently touch (frayed ends of wire may traverse the intervening material) or if the patient sweats profusely. Conversely, the alarm may fail to sound if a clip becomes dislodged by a restless sleeper. Normally, however, a teaspoonful of urine will suffice to start the buzzer and this, by awakening the child, will bring an end to micturition and will eventually, in favourable cases, prevent the act starting at all. The size of the wet patch indicates how quickly the child has awakened. In a typical response the size of the patches diminishes as the training takes effect but sometimes the child is such a heavy sleeper that all the patches remain large because he is not awakened by the buzzer (another member of the family may have to switch it off). In such cases a louder bell can be plugged into the set or dexamphetamine can be prescribed as well but these additional measures are seldom required. When the alarm sounds and the child awakens he is instructed to switch it off, get up and finish passing urine. In very bad cases it is desirable to re-set the apparatus using a dry drawsheet ensemble but in the majority one alarm per night is sufficient.

The Series

In the past five years over 500 enuretic children have been referred to my out-patient clinics. Many of them have responded to simple forms of therapy and many others have recovered spontaneously but gradually a hard core of resistant cases accumulated. They were treated with the electric buzzer, the only criteria for selection being that they were old enough, sufficiently severe, and resistant to other forms of therapy. There were only nine omissions from a consecutive series of 109 cases selected for treatment and provided with an apparatus: in four the parents refused to report progress, in two the children (aged 10 and 12) refused to use the apparatus, in two the parents were too stupid to be able to work it and in one the boy stopped wetting before the set was put into use.

The series therefore consists of 100 persistently enuretic children consecutively supplied and treated with a conditioning apparatus. It is important to emphasize that inclusion was by enrolment rather than by completion of treatment. Since the successes are usually rapid, a better rate of cure could have been obtained by discarding those in whom the treatment is incomplete.

Age. There has been a tendency to provide older children with this treatment partly because they have usually resisted many others and partly because they are more likely to cooperate. A few young ones have been included, usually because they had inherited a set after an older sibling had completed treatment. In general, however, the use of an apparatus under the age of 7 has not been recommended and it will be seen from Table 1 that 74 fall within the 7-13 bracket, 14 being younger and 12 older than this group.

Sex. There is general agreement that males predominate in any series of enuretic children and this has been the case here. Only 19% were girls.

TABLE 1

AGE AT START OF TREATMENT AND SEX

Age in Years	Total	5–7	–9	–11	–13	–15	–17	17+
Male ..	81	12	18	19	22	7	2	1
Female ..	19	2	4	8	3	2	—	—
Total ..	100	14	22	27	25	9	2	1

Onset. In the vast majority enuresis had been present since birth and the longest dry spells (if any) before treatment had seldom exceeded one week. In five cases enuresis had begun, after a long period of dryness, at the age of 4 years or older; in two others it had been very infrequent until the age of 5. Four mothers stated that there had been a dry spell at least six months long between the ages of 1 and 3 years—a difficult fact to explain. Two boys had been dry for four and five months respectively after treatment with a conditioning apparatus obtained elsewhere; they were therefore relapses but entered this series as new cases because their parents could not afford to hire a second apparatus.

Family History. For the purpose of this enquiry, enuresis was regarded as having been present if bedwetting had occurred above the age of 5 years. A positive history in a close relative (parent or sibling) was obtained in 47 cases (one or both parents in 30, one or more siblings in 17, parent and sibling in ten). The history relating to enuresis in the patients' parents was not complete in 18 cases but in six a more distant blood relative had been affected. A negative history in near relatives was obtained in 35 cases with complete records but in 22 of these it was positive in more distant relatives (aunts, uncles and first cousins). These findings indicate that about 50% of cases have a positive family history and a further 30% have blood relatives affected by the disorder.

Intelligence. In this series the great majority were of average intelligence. Eight were above, nine were below and one was educationally subnormal.

Nervous State. Parents were asked if the child had any other nervous troubles. In 30 they were absent and in 70 they were present, being very severe in five. (In an unselected series of children starting school 50% were stated to be nervous, but this is a younger age group.)

Investigations. All the children were medically examined and their urine tested. Twenty-eight of the first 50 cases in the series and 17 of the second 50 had been fully investigated by means of micturating cysto-urethrograms, cysto-urethroscopy, pyelography, etc. This falling off in zeal for investigation was due to a change of policy whereby latterly only failures were investigated. In two cases this was refused.

Previous Treatment. Almost every patient had failed to respond to weeks or months of drug therapy which had extended for over one year in 29 and was continuous for five years in one. Three were referred from child guidance clinics and one other had failed to respond to that kind of treatment. One successful case had previously attended a faith healer for many months. As already stated, two had relapsed following this form of therapy.

Results

It soon became apparent that successful cases usually responded rapidly. This led us to use the total number of wet nights during the third month as a criterion of early response which subsequently proved to be a reliable index of the final outcome.

TABLE 2

EARLY RESPONSE CORRELATED WITH SEVERITY OF ENURESIS

Total No. Wet Nights During 3rd Month	Total	Severity of Enuresis Before Treatment (Approximate Proportion of Wet Nights)			Group	
		<50%	50%–75%	75%–100%	Charity	Private
Nil ..	44	5	15	24	25	19
1–3 ..	10	2	1	7	6	4
4–6 ..	14	2	3	9	10	4
7+ ..	17	1	3	13	12	5
Abandoned	7	1	3	3	5	2
Not known	8	2	2	4	4	4
Total ..	100	13	27	60	62	38

In Table 2 the early response is correlated with the frequency of wetting when treatment was first started. Infrequent wetting means that the training effect is seldom applied. Hence children who were wet appreciably less than 50% were not treated in this way and those in this group did rather less well than the average. In the worst group the results are also suboptimal because concealed within it were several children who were wet more than once each night and hence had further to go to become dry. The best results were therefore obtained in the group with 50 to 75% wet nights at the outset, for 59% had fewer than four wet nights in the third month compared with 54% and 50% in the other two groups.

Also in Table 2 a distinction is made between those who bought an apparatus and those who borrowed one free of charge. The latter group included many with very low social standards which perhaps explains why they achieved less good results. Taking all the cases which were wet fewer than four times during the third month, there were 23 out of 38 (60%) who bought their own sets compared with 31 out of 62 (50%) who borrowed one.

TABLE 3

LATE RESULTS CORRELATED WITH EARLY RESPONSE

Total No. Wet Nights During 3rd Month After Starting Treatment	Total	Final Assessment (4 mth.–2 yr.)			
		Dry	Occasionally Wet	Improved	Failed
Nil	44	38	5	—	1
1–3	10	7	3	—	—
4–6	14	3	5	4	2
7+	17	1	1	3	12
Abandoned	7	—	—	—	7
Not known	8	1	1	2	4
Total	100	50	15	9	26

In Table 3 the late results are correlated with early response. The successful 65 cases have been followed up for a period ranging from four months to well over one year; it exceeded six months in 43 cases of which 15 were followed up for more than one year.

Of the 50 cases finally classified as 'dry', 38 became completely dry before the third month of treatment began, whereas only one was ultimately cured when the number of wet nights in the third month exceeded seven.

In addition to the 50 dry cases, 15 children have been classed as 'occasionally wet'. They had on an average one or two wet nights per month after treatment was completed. As might be expected, the early response tended to be less rapid in this group.

The nine classified as 'improved' each showed a marked reduction in the amount of wetting but at the final assessment there was still appreciable wetting. Thus one child was wet 19 times during the first week of treatment but steadily improved so that in the 32nd week he was only wet twice.

Eighteen of the failures failed to respond appreciably. One responded at first but then relapsed and continued to wet frequently; he lived in a very poor home and had no bed of his own. To these failures must be added seven in whom the treatment was abandoned before the end of the third month, making a total of 26 failures.

Younger children did slightly better than older ones, the average age of the successful cases being 9 years compared with 11 years for the 26 failures.

There were too few children of below average intelligence from whom to draw definite conclusions but the impression has been gained that those with lower intelligence respond less rapidly.

Relapses. There were nine cases in which relapses requiring a refresher course occurred and eight responded rapidly and completely. One had been completely dry for nine months before relapsing. No doubt as further time passes other relapses will require treatment. In most cases the relapse was clearly related to an infection, fatigue or anxiety over examinations at school. Even some of the children classified as 'dry' experienced an isolated wet night in such circumstances but they were very rare.

Pattern of Response

The mechanism of the treatment is clearly one of training; in a favourable case the number of wet nights steadily diminishes and at the same time the size of the wet patch gets smaller indicating that the child is waking up more quickly. This is well illustrated by the following typical case history:

L.C., a boy aged 11 years, had never had a dry night all his life. He was of average intelligence, not nervous, a restless sleeper; his maternal grandmother, mother and brother had all been bedwetters. Drug therapy had not helped him. His response was as follows:

Weeks	Wet Nights	Size of Patch
1st	7 (twice one night)	3 large
2nd	4	All small
3rd	2	Both small
4th	1	Small

The set was then removed from his bed and he has been followed up for eight months but has never since been wet. Occasionally he has to get up in the night to pass urine.

Some children find that they have to get up at night in order to keep dry but as their confidence increases the necessity diminishes. If, however, they are ill or tired they may fail to do so and wet the bed. Forty-one successful cases replied to a questionnaire which revealed that 27 never got up in the night, eight occasionally did and six usually or always did. Some parents who were enuretic in childhood still had to get up to micturate each night indicating that nocturnal frequency persisted.

Failures

It would be tedious to give details of all the failures. Probably lack of cooperation is the commonest cause; thus of the eight in whom no detailed reports for the first three months were available, four were failures. Parents were usually to blame and in a few cases treatment was started in hospital in an effort to avoid this. In one case treatment had to be abandoned because the county M.O.H. forbade us to treat him in the residential home where he lived because a psychiatrist advised against this form of therapy and recommended an alarm clock instead! One juvenile delinquent was responding well in hospital but absconded before treatment was completed because he learned that he was wanted by the police. Two mothers were definitely psychotic. Very heavy sleepers were not awakened but this was sometimes overcome by administering dexamphetamine for a time as well. In one case this failed and so did vibrators attached to his forehead; perhaps an electric shock would have roused him but it was not considered justifiable. Some were awakened but failed to be trained so that the number of wet nights did not diminish though the bed was less soaking. In three cases an initial response was followed by a return to the original frequency suggesting an active resistance to the treatment, probably emotionally determined. We aimed at keeping the child on the set until four consecutive dry weeks had been achieved but one educationally subnormal girl aged 13 refused to use it for more than one week and a boy complained that the neighbours heard the buzzer and he resented the publicity that this entailed.

Conclusion

The fact that a favourable response was rapidly obtained in 65 out of 100 severe enuretics speaks for itself. The marked improvement in the mental outlook of these cases was most gratifying. Several parents reported that their children were happier and more confident now that their enuresis had been eliminated. It is clear that a great deal of the associated anxiety was secondary to the enuresis and disappeared with it. There can be no doubt that psychological aetiological factors have been greatly exaggerated in this disorder, though they certainly play a part in aggravating it. Probably they are of the same degree of importance in enuresis as in asthma, migraine and epilepsy, disorders, incidentally, with which it is frequently associated. In my opinion it is fully justifiable and very rewarding to tackle the symptom directly by the conditioning method, a triumph for therapeutic behaviourism.

Summary

One hundred intractable severe persistent enuretics have been treated by the conditioning method.

There were 81 boys and 19 girls aged 5-17 years.

Fifty responded rapidly and completely, 15 dried up almost completely, nine improved markedly but slowly and 26 were failures.

The pattern of response and the reasons for failure are described.

A positive family history was obtained in 47 and more distant relatives were enuretic in a further 28 cases but the records were not all complete.

Successful cases frequently showed definite improvement emotionally. The importance of psychological factors in causing enuresis of this type has been greatly exaggerated.

Relapses were mainly provoked by infections, sometimes by fatigue and anxiety.

I am most grateful to the Chamberlain Foundation for so generously providing me with sets to lend to patients unable to afford to buy one. The Foundation distributed them through the International Office Service, Ltd., 30 City Road, London, E.C.1.

I am also indebted to Mr. M. P. Curwen, statistician, St. Bartholomew's Hospital, for his help with the presentation of the results.

REFERENCES

British Medical Journal (1957). **1**, 1017.
Crosby, N. D. (1950). *Med. J. Aust.*, **2**, 533.
Davidson, J. R. and Douglass, E. (1950). *Brit. med. J.*, **1**, 1345.
Geppert, T. V. (1953). *J. Amer. med. Ass.*, **152**, 381.
Gillison, T. H. (1956). *Brit. med. J.*, **1**, 1174.
Mowrer, O. H. (1938). *Amer. J. Psychol.*, **51**, 163.
Pfaundler, M. (1904). *Verh. Ges. Kinderheilk.*, **21**, 219.
Seiger, H. W. (1946). *J. Pediat.*, **28**, 733.
—— (1952). *Ibid.*, **40**, 738.

RECURRENT ABDOMINAL PAINS: A FIELD SURVEY OF 1,000 SCHOOL CHILDREN

BY

JOHN APLEY and NORA NAISH

From the United Bristol Hospitals

(RECEIVED FOR PUBLICATION AUGUST 16, 1957)

What sort of children are they who complain of recurrent abdominal pains, and how do they compare with children who do not suffer from such pains? Because patients referred to hospital are inevitably pre-selected, we have tried to answer these questions by a survey of 1,000 unselected children at primary and secondary modern schools.

One of us throughout the survey, and sometimes both, attended routine school medical examinations at Bristol from January, 1955, to June, 1956. A few children not accompanied by a parent were excluded; the remainder were asked if they suffered from bouts of abdominal pain.

Nature of Investigation

Children with Pains. In our series we included every child who had had at least three bouts of pain, severe enough to affect his activities, over a period of not less than three months, with attacks continuing in the year preceding the examination. In taking the history, which was obtained from the mother as well as the child, we went into considerable detail regarding home life and the family as well as the child's personal history. The school headmasters and headmistresses helped greatly by providing reports on behaviour, intelligence and attainments.

Children with pains were examined clinically, but ancillary investigations were not undertaken (it is intended to publish separately a complementary investigation of hospital cases). The single exception was electro-encephalography (E.E.G.), for which facilities were made available at a convenient centre.

Control Series. Detailed information on the same lines, *i.e.*, personal and family history, as well as clinical examination and E.E.G., was obtained from a proportion of the children living in the same districts and attending the same school medical examinations, but not found to be complaining of abdominal pains. As a rule the child who happened to be next on the list after one with pains was chosen for the control series. The numbers were, however, considerably increased by adding further children as often as time permitted, and by including a small number of those below school age who by chance had come with their mothers.

Incidence

When 1,000 children with their mothers had been questioned the investigation was stopped. The numbers obtained are summarized in Table 1.

TABLE 1

CASE MATERIAL

	Total	Boys	Girls
Preliminary Questioning	1,000	528	472
Detailed Questioning and Examination:			
Recurrent abdominal pains*	108	50	58
Controls	312	155	157

* Thirteen children whose pains had ceased more than a year previously have been excluded here and from the calculations of incidence.

Of the total, 10·8% had recurrent abdominal pains fulfilling our criteria. Girls were affected more often than boys (12·3% to 9·5%).

Age Distribution. There was considerable variation in the incidence of pains at different ages (Fig. 1). There were no complaints of pains in the small number of children below 5 years of age. In boys from 5 to 10 years of age there was a steady incidence of between 10% and 12%, followed after a fall by a late peak at 14 years. In girls the incidence was similar up to the age of 8 years. This was, however, followed by a marked rise, with more than a quarter of all girls of 9 years affected, and subsequently a steady decrease.

Age of Onset. The age of onset of the pains in 118 children is illustrated in Fig. 2. (The total of

118 is made up of 108 children with continuing pains and 13 in whom pains had ceased more than a year previously, less three in whom the age of onset was not known.)

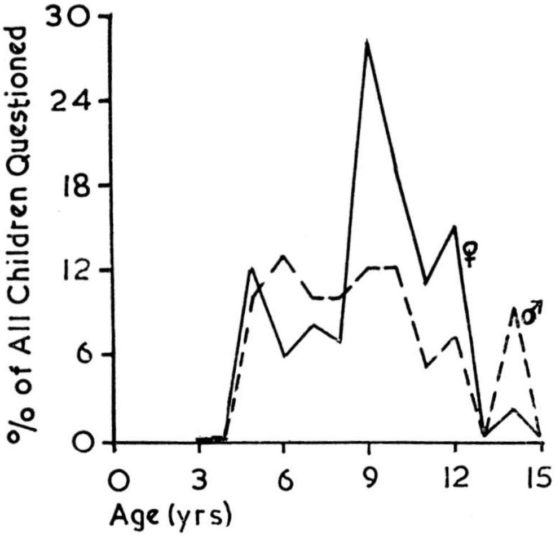

FIG. 1.—Proportion of children affected at each year of age.

In both boys and girls there was a steady rise up to the age of 5 years. In the boys the numbers then fell; but in the girls there was a further striking rise, with pains commencing in a large proportion between 8 and 10 years of age, and none subsequently.

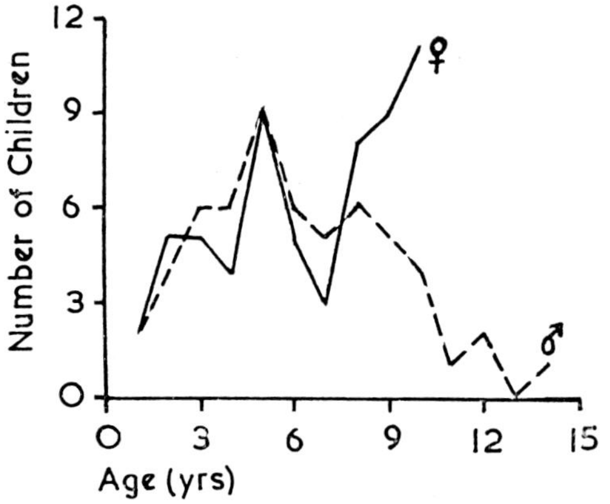

FIG. 2.—Age of onset of pains. (118 children: 57 boys, 61 girls.)

The Pains

A full description of variations in the characteristics of the pains will not be given here. We have found elsewhere (unpublished hospital data) that an accurate description of pain in children is more likely to be obtained during attacks than in the intervals.

In brief, it seemed that in some two-thirds of the children the pain was felt at or round the umbilicus. With only a few exceptions, it occurred in the mid-epigastrium among the remainder. In about a quarter it was severe. The time of occurrence varied greatly. The duration of the pain showed great variability from case to case, and from one bout to another in most children. The frequency of occurrence also varied considerably, from those with a rare (often severe) episode to those who said they nearly always had some (usually mild) pain. About one-fifth showed a tendency to periodicity.

The pains were attributed to many factors. The most common were excitement, worry or 'being worked up', feelings often associated with schooling. One girl had a severe attack on the day after she lost a pound note which a neighbour gave her to buy cigarettes. As 'cures', soda-water, defaecation and the doctor's medicine came low in the list. Rest was often thought helpful, but in most cases the pains just got better.

Table 2 summarizes the disturbances associated with attacks of pain.

TABLE 2

DISTURBANCES ASSOCIATED WITH ATTACKS OF PAIN

	%
Pallor	38
Vomiting	22
Fever	11
Headache	23
Subsequent sleepiness or lethargy	26

The association was scored only if it occurred commonly or invariably. Several might occur together, and in a fifth of the cases (often those with severer pains) the combination of abdominal pain, vomiting and headache, and sometimes fever, was recorded. There were in addition 13 children who had bouts of headache and vomiting without abdominal pains.

As between the isolated abdominal pain and the combination of many disturbances, there seemed to be a gradation from case to case, which made any clear-cut grouping unprofitable. In any individual child the pattern tended, however, to be more or less constant, though with occasional variations in severity.

Family History

The child is an inseparable part of his family, and we were particularly interested in comparing the families of children with pains against those without pains. Table 3 summarizes some relevant data from the family histories.

TABLE 3
DATA FROM FAMILY HISTORIES

Complaints of other Members of Family	Percentage in Children With Pains	Without Pains
Recurrent abdominal pains	46	8
Peptic ulcer	10	3
Appendicectomy	8	3
Migraine	14	3
Nervous breakdown	10	2
Fits	6	3

We have included only the immediate family, *i.e.*, parents and siblings, though the data of more distant relations showed similar trends. In the diagnoses listed we have not attempted to be precise, since the sources of our information were non-medical. Thus, under 'peptic ulcer' we included only those in whom there was said to have been a haematemesis or operation, or radiographic confirmation; under 'migraine' we included all severe headaches; and under 'nervous breakdown' disorders severe enough to have caused a serious disruption of normal life. Mothers accounted for two-fifths of those members of the family affected by recurrent abdominal pains, fathers a slightly smaller proportion, and brothers and sisters the remainder.

A marked preponderance of the disorders listed was found in the families of children with abdominal pains, though the figures for 'fits' are too small to be statistically significant. It is clear that the families of these children have an enhanced tendency to abdominal and 'nervous' disorders. In other respects, including psychosis and serious behaviour disorders, the numbers were very small and we found no obvious differences from the controls.

An additional item was the proportion of 'broken homes', *i.e.*, where one or other parent was dead, or had left home, or there had been a divorce or legal separation. We recorded a 'broken home' in 4% of the children with pains, as, rather unexpectedly, against 7% of the controls.

Child's History

Some noteworthy differences also emerged when we compared the histories of children with and without abdominal pains (Table 4).

TABLE 4
DATA FROM PERSONAL HISTORIES

	Percentage in Children With Pains	Without Pains
Appendicectomy	5	0·3
Tonsillectomy	24	26
Frequent headaches	14	5
Bilious attacks	12	5
Habitual constipation	5	3
Fits	2	6
Asthma	6	2

Appendicectomy in the control series was rare (1 in 312). The histories of five children with recurrent abdominal pains in whom appendicectomy was performed were obtained and are summarized herewith.

Case 1. Colicky pains for nine months. 'Normal looking appendix' removed. Pains recurred.

Case 2. Pains for several months. Operation because of tenderness in R. iliac fossa. Normal appendix removed. Pains recurred.

Case 3. Pains for several years. 'Mildly infected appendix' removed. No further pains when seen two years later.

Case 4. No previous pains. Operation at 2 years of age. Acutely inflamed appendix (and pelvic abscess) removed. Recurrent abdominal pains during the ensuing seven years.

Case 5. Four attacks of abdominal pain in two years. In the fifth attack pain became localized for the first time to the R. iliac fossa, with overlying rigidity. Acutely inflamed retro-caecal appendix removed. No further information available.

Tonsillectomy was the only other operation done with any frequency; the incidence was almost identical in the two groups.

The children with abdominal pains suffered more than the controls from headaches and from so-called bilious attacks. The comparative figures for constipation, fits, asthma and allergic conditions in general were too small to warrant conclusions. The history of other physical disorders showed no significant differences between the two groups.

Physical Assessment

We assessed the children of both groups by recording items like physique, posture, height, weight, colouring, palpable lymph nodes, condition of the teeth and tongue, and all abnormalities found on routine clinical examination. The average weights of the younger children with pains were less by 1 to 2 lb. than those of the controls; the numbers of older children were too small for definite conclusions. In other respects, including height, there were no apparent differences.

Intelligence

For the assessment of intelligence we relied on school reports, based on the child's ability, progress and attainments. On this basis children are allocated to one of the school educational 'streams'. We have presumed that errors inherent in such a method are equally applicable to both groups of children and do not affect the validity of a comparison between them. Table 5 shows that the two groups are almost identical.

TABLE 5
INTELLIGENCE ASSESSMENT

Educational Stream	Percentage in Children With Pains (No: 120)	Without Pains (No: 221)
A	20·8	21·2
B	28·3	28·0
C	32·5	32·1
D	16·6	16·3
E	1·6	2·2

Emotional Disturbances

From information given by the parent, schoolmaster and child, we compared the frequency with which some common complaints which might reasonably be attributed to emotional disturbances occurred in the two groups of children. Table 6 shows those groups in which there was a significant difference.

TABLE 6
SOME EXPRESSIONS OF EMOTIONAL DISTURBANCE

Disturbance	Percentage in Children With Pains	Without Pains
Undue fears	27	10
Nocturnal enuresis	20	8
Sleep disorders (including nightmares)	39	18
Appetite difficulties	37	21

Among appetite disorders we inquired particularly about milk-drinking habits, because of the suggestion that excessive milk drinking may be associated with abdominal pains. We found that children with pains tended to drink not more, but rather less than the controls. In other respects, like nail-biting and tics, there were no apparent differences.

Personality

From the information available we tried to group the children with or without pains according to their personality traits. The findings are summarized in Table 7.

TABLE 7
PERSONALITY TRAITS

Trait	Percentage in Children With Pains	Without Pains
Normal, average, good ..	51	80
Hostile, anti-social, unreliable	5	5
Aggressive, quarrelsome, jealous	6	2
Passive, negative	4	5
Highly-strung, fussy, excitable	21	4
Anxious, timid, apprehensive	13	4

As compared with the controls, many more of the children with pains tended to be highly-strung, fussy, excitable, anxious, timid and apprehensive. We formed an impression of over-conscientiousness in many children with pains, and also in their parents. More of these children, too, were said to be 'bad mixers' (23% as compared with 15% of the controls).

Electro-Encephalography

With the cooperation of the parents we took this opportunity of obtaining E.E.G.s from many children without pains and comparing the findings with those of children in the same range of ages but with recurrent abdominal pains. E.E.G.s were obtained from 202 school children without pains and 97 with pains (Table 8). The reports, both on children with abdominal pains and on the controls, were made by Dr. E. C. Turton without knowing into which group they fell.

TABLE 8
REPORTS ON ELECTRO-ENCEPHALOGRAMS

E.E.G. Record	Percentage in Children With Pains (No: 97)	Without Pains (No: 202)
Normal	74	74
Normal but immature for age	12	9
Organic abnormality	0	0·5
Localized slow activity ..	0	0·5
Focal spikes	4	1·5
Epileptiform	10	14·5

In the epileptiform group were included all definite and borderline cases, whether in resting or evoked (photic stimulation and hyperpnoea) records. The classification of normal records was based on accepted descriptions for children (*e.g.*, Henry, 1944). Children with a history of fits were included: there were two with abdominal pains (neither had had fits for several years) and 12 without pains (including three continuing under treatment for fits).

Discussion

Incidence. The high incidence of recurrent abdominal pains in our unselected school population confirms the impression that this is one of the commonest of childhood complaints. Our material was drawn from working and lower middle class families, in a thriving town with a population approaching half a million and negligible unemployment. We have no means of comparing the incidence with that in either agricultural communities or in the higher social and financial scales.

Naturally, the incidence must vary according to the criteria used in the selection of cases. Ours were chosen with the object of ruling out trivial and transient disturbances, on the one hand, and, on the other, serious organic disorders which would be expected to have become manifest in the time limit we set. The series of children with pains proved similar to another series of children referred to hospital with the same complaint (unpublished data). The significant differences found were that in children attending hospital because of abdominal pains the proportion with severe pains is slightly higher, there are more 'only children', and there are proportionately fewer girls in the pre-pubertal age-group.

On these grounds we consider that our conclusions are, in the main, applicable to the vast numbers of children with this common complaint.

Age Incidence. The age incidence and the age of onset of pains in our series set some interesting problems which remain to be solved. In the early years the curves for both sexes are similar, suggesting that the underlying factors are the same for both. It is of interest that the peak occurs at the age when schooling commences. From the age of 8 years the pattern diverges markedly in the two sexes, and the onset of puberty in girls might be postulated as an additional factor. From our data we cannot confirm or refute this possibility. As between girls with or without pains, there was no disparity in the time of development of secondary sex characters; and the number in whom the menarche had occurred was so small as to be non-contributory.

Organic Disorders. It is obviously important to determine or eliminate organic disease as a cause, though in many large published series the proportion of children with a demonstrative causative organic disorder has been shown to be small. In the present study, on clinical examination we found no appreciable physical differences between children with or without pains, other than a slight disparity in average weight. Even this may reasonably be related to the appetite disturbances which are commoner in children with abdominal pains.

The figures for epileptiform abnormalities in the E.E.G.s of our two groups lend no support to the notion that the recurrent abdominal pains which are so common in childhood are an expression of epilepsy without fits.

Emotional Disorders. Under this heading fall the significant differences between our groups of children with or without pains. Children with certain types of personality seemed commonly affected. They were timid, nervous, anxious or over-conscientious—just the types of children in whom emotional disturbances would be expected to develop. In children with an underlying predisposition school or other difficulties often seemed to have a 'trigger effect' in evoking pains.

Family History. High though they are, our figures for the incidence of abdominal pains in the families are almost certainly an underestimate. We have found elsewhere that the proportion of positive replies increases if the number of interviews is increased and the parents are given better opportunities to remember. But even as they stand the figures illustrate the continuing thread of disorder in successive generations. Our data contribute nothing to the fascinating problem of why perhaps only one among several children, with a common family background, should develop abdominal pains.

The relatively high incidence not only of functional but also of organic abdominal disorders in the families of children with pains is of great interest. Is it that these 'abdominally minded' families are more thoroughly investigated? Have these families a predisposition to abdominal disorders of different sorts? Does functional disorder develop into organic disease? In this connexion we mention two parents who, like their children who were in our series, had complained of abdominal pains in childhood, and who now suffer from peptic ulcer in adult life. Similar examples will probably occur to most doctors, but they must be considered and weighed against the high frequency both of abdominal pains in childhood and of peptic ulcers in adult life.

Conclusions

We set out to compare children complaining of recurrent abdominal pains against children without them, in a large, unselected group of school children. In our survey three subsidiary points were established: *First*, the high incidence of recurrent abdominal pains, especially at certain ages and particularly in girls. *Second*, the high incidence of abdominal and certain other complaints in the families of affected children. *Third*, the negative evidence of any physical association with the pains, and the positive evidence of frequent emotional disturbances.

Children with abdominal pains tend to fall into certain categories as regards personality and emotional patterns, so much so that often one can forecast which children are likely to develop the symptoms. Often when difficult situations are imminent, as at the beginning of school terms or examinations, the occurrence of pains can be correctly predicted. As compared with other children, those with pains tend to be anxious, timid, fussy and over-conscientious, taking the ordinary difficulties of life (especially of school life) too much to heart.

We gratefully acknowledge our indebtedness to Dr. A. L. Smallwood, Senior School Medical Officer, and other School Medical Officers in the Bristol area, and to the Chief Education Officer and his staff, including the headmasters and headmistresses who cooperated so generously and made our survey possible, and to Dr. E. C. Turton for the E.E.G. reports.

REFERENCES

Henry, C E. (1944). *Monogr. Soc. Res. Child. Dev.*, **9**, No. 3 (Serial No. 39).

SALMONELLA MENINGITIS

BY

KENNETH C. WATSON

From the Department of Pathology, University of Natal, and King Edward VIII Hospital, Durban, South Africa

(RECEIVED FOR PUBLICATION AUGUST 19, 1957)

Meningitis due to organisms of the salmonella group is a relatively uncommon condition but is of importance because of the very high mortality rate which has been recorded. The first case of meningitis due to this cause was reported by Ghon (1908) and was due to *Salmonella paratyphi B*. The literature since that time has been reviewed by several authors including Bahrenburg and Ecker (1937) who reported 34 cases, Ramón Guerra, Peluffo, Laguarda and Aleppo (1939), Henderson (1948) and Beene, Hansen and Fulton (1951). Henderson (1948) has produced the most comprehensive review of the subject and quotes 144 cases, including three of his own, due to *S. panama*, *S. newport*, and *S. typhi-murium* respectively. The report by Beene *et al.* (1951) includes a further 87 cases not referred to by Henderson. These include 17 cases due to *S. typhi* which Henderson specifically excluded from his review. These authors also include a case of their own due to *S. montevideo*, the first recorded case due to this organism.

Three epidemic outbreaks in newborn infants have been reported. Guthrie and Montgomery (1939) discuss 12 cases due to *S. enteritidis*. In each one there was diarrhoea with vomiting, convulsions, coma, and a fatal termination. Post-mortem examination showed a purulent meningitis associated with catarrhal enteritis. Curbelo and Martinez Cruz (1941) reported 21 cases in newborn infants in an explosive-type outbreak in Cuba. Here the causative organism was *S. havana* and again there was a fatal outcome in each patient. High and Spaulding (1946) recorded a further outbreak involving ten infants, due to *S. panama*, again with a 100% fatality rate.

During the past 18 months four cases of salmonella meningitis have been encountered in this hospital. Two of these have been due to species of salmonella not previously reported as having been found in the cerebrospinal fluid, namely, *S. johannesburg* and *S. heidelberg*.

Reports of Cases

Case 1. M.P., a female Bantu infant aged 11 months, was admitted to hospital with a history of loss of appetite and general malaise. The child had recently had an attack of whooping cough complicated by bronchopneumonia and had apparently not fully recovered. No further details were obtainable from the relatives.

On examination, the child appeared listless and apathetic. The temperature was 103·0° F. and the pulse rate 130 per minute. The skin showed some signs of dehydration but the anterior fontanelle was tense and bulging. There was marked neck stiffness and Kernig's sign was positive. The deep reflexes were equal and brisk. The ocular fundi appeared normal. Examination of other systems was essentially negative. Shortly after admission the child had a number of generalized convulsions.

Lumbar puncture showed a turbid fluid under greatly increased pressure. Queckenstedt's test gave a normal response. The fluid had the following composition: protein, 200 mg. %; sugar, 10 mg. %; globulin (Pandy's test), greatly increased; chlorides, 670 mg. %; lymphocytes, 120 per c.mm.; polymorphonuclear leucocytes, 620 per c.mm. A Gram stained film of the fluid showed the presence of many Gram negative bacilli. Culture of the fluid resulted in the isolation of an organism of the salmonella group. Further examination of it showed its antigenic structure to be IV, V, XII : r—1, 2, 3, which is that of *S. heidelberg*. Sensitivity testing *in vitro* by the dried disc method showed the organism to be sensitive to chloramphenicol, streptomycin and the tetracycline group of antibiotics.

Treatment was begun on the day of admission with 0·25 g. of streptomycin intramuscularly followed by 0·25 g. twice daily. Chloramphenicol, 125 mg., was also given intramuscularly followed by 125 mg. every six hours. During the subsequent ten days there was little change in the clinical state. The cerebrospinal fluid four days after admission was sterile. In view of the poor response, chloramphenicol was discontinued after ten days and tetracycline, 125 mg. intramuscularly every six hours, was given instead. Again there was no improvement under this regime and culture of the cerebrospinal fluid in the third week of illness gave rise to a heavy growth of *S. heidelberg*. There was a gradual deterioration in the infant's condition and death took place one month after admission. Permission for necropsy was refused.

Case 2. M.D., a male Bantu infant aged 5 months, was admitted with a history of diarrhoea of one month's duration. No further clinical history was obtained. The child was in a state of coma with a temperature of 102·6° F. and a pulse rate of 126 per minute. There was a pronounced squint and marked neck stiffness with a positive Kernig's sign. Examination of the lungs showed signs suggestive of bronchopneumonia. Examination of other systems was negative.

Lumbar puncture on admission showed a turbid fluid under increased pressure. The fluid had the following composition: protein, 500 mg. %; chlorides, 670 mg. %; sugar, 47 mg. %; globulin, marked excess; polymorphonuclear leucocytes, 800 per c.mm. and lymphocytes, 120 per c.mm. Gram stained films showed large numbers of Gram negative bacilli. Culture of the fluid resulted in the isolation of an organism of the salmonella group. Subsequent antigenic analysis showed its structure to be as follows: I, IX, XII : g, p-, which is that of *S. dublin*.

The child died some 20 minutes after admission. Necropsy examination showed an extensive purulent meningitis. There was a moderate degree of fatty change in the liver and areas of bronchopneumonic consolidation were present in both lungs.

Case 3. S.J., a 4-month-old female Bantu infant, was admitted to hospital with a two weeks' history of diarrhoea accompanied by vomiting. No further details were available from the relatives apart from the fact that she had been in hospital one month previously with a similar complaint.

The child was in a moribund state. The temperature was 103·2° F. and pulse rate 126 per minute. The respirations were rapid and coarse crepitations were present in the right mid-zone. The anterior fontanelle was tense and bulging. The eyes were deviated to the right side and there was a marked degree of neck retraction and some degree of opisthotonos. Kernig's sign was positive. Both upper and lower limbs were very rigid. The deep reflexes were brisk. The pupils were equal, central and reacted to light. The spleen was palpable one finger breadth below the costal margin. Examination of other systems was negative.

Lumbar puncture was performed but only a small quantity of fluid was obtained by aspiration. Queckenstedt's test indicated the presence of a block. Examination of the fluid revealed a large number of polymorphonuclear leucocytes and numerous Gram negative bacilli. There was a marked excess of globulin but insufficient fluid was available for further biochemical investigation. Culture of the fluid resulted in the growth of an organism which on further investigation was found to be a salmonella with the following antigenic structure : I, XL : b—e, n, x. This is the antigenic formula of *S. johannesburg*. The organism was sensitive *in vitro* to chloramphenicol, streptomycin and the tetracycline group of antibiotics.

On admission the child was given 500,000 units of penicillin intramuscularly. Following the report of a probable salmonella infection chloramphenicol therapy was begun the next day with 250 mg. intramuscularly and then 250 mg. every six hours. Streptomycin, 0·5 g., was also given intramuscularly. The child's condition was critical, however, and death occurred the following day. Permission for necropsy was refused.

Case 4. T.X., a 3-year-old female Bantu child, was admitted to hospital with a history of having had a convulsion during sleep a few hours earlier. The convulsion had involved all limbs equally and since then the child had been in a state of coma. Before the onset of the convulsion the child had apparently been quite well. No previous history of convulsions was admitted and the past medical history was negative.

The child was in coma with a temperature of 105·0° F. and pulse rate of 118 per minute. She was having almost continuous convulsive movements involving all four limbs but especially marked on the left side. The head was rotated to the left. The pupils were dilated and did not react to light. There was no evidence of neck retraction and Kernig's sign was negative. The deep reflexes on both sides were brisk and the plantar responses were flexor in type. There was bilateral purulent conjunctivitis. Examination of other systems was negative.

Lumbar puncture revealed a purulent fluid under increased pressure containing: protein, 500 mg. %; chloride, 700 mg. %; sugar, 70 mg. %; globulin, marked excess; polymorphonuclear leucocytes, large numbers. Gram stained films showed many Gram negative bacilli. Culture of the fluid resulted in the isolation of an organism giving the biochemical reactions of a salmonella. This organism, however, was in a rough phase and all attempts to obtain the smooth state were unsuccessful. Consequently the antigenic formula is in doubt. The organism was sensitive *in vitro* to chloramphenicol, streptomycin, and the tetracycline group of antibiotics.

Chloramphenicol, 250 mg., was given intramuscularly followed by a similar dose every six hours. During the following few days the child developed marked signs of meningeal irritation with neck retraction and a positive Kernig's sign. There was little improvement in the clinical state for a period of some three weeks during which time she remained pyrexial. The causative organism was still present in the cerebrospinal fluid one week after admission but the fluid became sterile on the tenth day. After three weeks there was a gradual slow recovery complicated at one stage by the development of measles. The child was discharged three months after admission apparently cured.

Discussion

Salmonella organisms infecting the leptomeninges give rise to an acute purulent meningitis. In infants the clinical course of illness is often rapid and is more often associated with diarrhoea and lesions in the gastro-intestinal tract than is the case with older children and adults. However, just as in other forms of meningitis, the classical signs of meningeal irritation may be lacking in the infant and thus render the diagnosis more difficult. This was the case in our fourth patient where on admission there was nothing to indicate the presence of acute meningitis.

Age Incidence of Salmonella Meningitis. The age incidence of salmonella meningitis shows that there is a striking tendency for the very young to be affected. Table 1 shows the age distribution in 138 patients. This includes some of the patients reported by Henderson (1948) together with subsequent reports where the age group was available and including the four cases reported here.

TABLE 1

AGE INCIDENCE OF 138 CASES OF SALMONELLA MENINGITIS

Number of Cases	Age Groups				
	New-born	Less than 3 Months	3/12–1 Year	1–15 Years	15+ Years
138	55	31	26	14	12

The above figures show that 112 of the 138 cases (81%) occurred in infants under the age of 1 year and all but 12 occurred in children under the age of 15. The reason for this age distribution is not clearly apparent since the pathogenesis of salmonella meningitis is incompletely understood, but it is largely in keeping with certain other forms of meningitis such as the tuberculous and influenzal varieties. However, infection by salmonella organisms, where the clinical manifestations are confined to the gastro-intestinal tract, does not appear to be more common in children than in adults. It seems probable that the organism is carried to the meninges via the blood stream and it has been suggested that the high rate in infants is due to the preceding birth trauma rendering the tissues more susceptible to infection. This may be a factor in certain cases such as that reported by Neter (1944) where meningitis developed in a child aged three years who had had hydrocephalus since birth. Such a theory, however, does not explain the occurrence of outbreaks amongst newborn infants. In these it may be that certain inherent characteristics of the organisms themselves may be concerned in the localization in the meninges. It has also been suggested that salmonella infections of the meninges may follow other types of infection of the central nervous system due to a lowering of the local tissue resistance. In the 144 cases reviewed by Henderson (1948) five followed an attack of meningococcal meningitis and two others occurred during the course of treatment of syphilitic infections of the central nervous system. This hypothesis of decreased tissue resistance is one that is extremely difficult to prove or disprove. It is one which has been supported by Zinsser, Enders and Fothergill (1939) but it has lost much of its popularity in recent years. Neter (1944) has suggested that salmonella bacteraemia and meningitis may follow other types of infection such as otitis media, pyelitis and malaria. In our Case 1 the onset was preceded by an attack of whooping cough. It has also been suggested that the gastro-intestinal tract of the infant is more permeable to bacteria than that of the adult but again no satisfactory support for this hypothesis is available. One important factor is probably the well-known inability of the infant to produce a satisfactory antibody. Consequently, organisms gaining access to the blood stream are presumably in a more favourable position to reach the meninges and cause infection than in the adult where antibody formation is better.

Incidence of Various Salmonella Species. Table 2 shows the distribution of 151 salmonella species isolated from the cerebrospinal fluid and includes the four cases reported here in addition to those discussed by Henderson (1948). In addition to those shown in Table 2 the following species have been reported in isolated examples in the literature: *S. bovis-morbificans*, *S. bredeney*, *S. manhattan*, *S. paratyphi C*, *S. blegdam*, *S. montevideo* and *S. dublin*.

TABLE 2

SALMONELLA SPECIES IN 151 CASES OF SALMONELLA MENINGITIS

Salmonella Species	Number of Cases
S. paratyphi B	22
S. paratyphi A	7
S. enteritidis	45
S. cholerae-suis	8
S. typhi-murium	13
S. panama	17
S. havana	21
S. london	1
S. eastbourne	1
S. oranienburg	1
S. newport	2
S. anatum	1
S. derby	1
S. bareilly	1
S. loma-linda	1
S. new-brunswick	1
S. johannesburg	1
S. heidelberg	1
S. dublin	1
Undetermined	5

We have not included cases of meningitis due to *S. typhi* in this discussion. Although typhoid fever is extremely common in this part of the world, where we have had experience of some 400 cases in the past few years, we have not yet seen a case of true typhoid meningitis. Many patients with typhoid fever present with signs of meningeal irritation but the cerebrospinal fluid is usually normal or shows only a very slight increase in the number of cells.

The distribution of salmonella types in Table 2 is probably not altogether accurate in certain respects. Up to 1935 only four salmonella species had been reported from the cerebrospinal fluid, namely, *S. paratyphi B*, *S. enteritidis*, *S. paratyphi A* and *S. cholerae-suis*. Lack of knowledge concerning the antigenic structure of the salmonella group would explain this failure to recognize other types. The increasing number of reports of salmonella species in the cerebrospinal fluid not previously identified makes it probable that any salmonella species, including many which are primarily pathogenic to animals, may localize in the meninges and cause meningitis.

Prognosis in Salmonella Meningitis. The death rate from this condition is high and particularly so in infants as compared with older children and adults. The introduction of broad spectrum antibiotics may materially alter the death rate in the future but so far experience with this form of treatment has been restricted by the small number of cases available. The incidence of sequelae is uncertain but is probably the same as that found in other forms of acute purulent meningitis. Table 3 below shows the number of deaths in relation to age group in a series of 143 cases where the age was known.

TABLE 3

NO. OF DEATHS RELATED TO AGE IN 143 CASES OF SALMONELLA MENINGITIS

Age	Number of Cases	Number of Deaths	Percentage Died
Newborn–30 days ..	67	63	94·0
30–90 days	20	17	85·0
90 days–1 year	26	23	88·4
1–15 years	18	12	66·6
15+years	12	9	75·0

The figures in certain of the age groups are too small to be significant statistically but if we consider the number of deaths in children over and under one year it will be seen that there were 21 deaths in 30 cases (70%) in the former group and 103 deaths in 113 cases (91%) in the latter age group. If we subject these results to analysis by the χ^2 test the probability (P) value for χ^2 is greater than 3·84 which indicates a significance difference between the death rates at the 5% level.

In addition to the association of deaths with age groups, the number of deaths in relation to the type of salmonella involved is of interest. Table 4 shows the number of deaths in 133 cases due to seven different salmonella species.

TABLE 4

NO. OF DEATHS RELATED TO SALMONELLA SPECIES IN 133 CASES OF SALMONELLA MENINGITIS

Salmonella Species	Number of Cases	Number of Deaths	Percentage Died
S. paratyphi B ..	22	13	59·0
S. paratyphi A ..	7	5	71·4
S. enteritidis ..	45	45	100·0
S. cholerae-suis ..	8	6	75·0
S. typhi-murium ..	13	13	100·0
S. panama	17	14	82·3
S. havana	21	21	100·0

All the cases of *S. enteritidis*, *S. typhi-murium* and *S. havana* infection proved fatal whereas as high a recovery rate as 41% is recorded in the 22 cases of *S. paratyphi B* infection. This finding does not seem to be related to age distribution since the number of cases in children under one year, due to *S. enteritidis*, is not statistically greater than those due to *S. paratyphi B*. Table 5 shows the relative age distribution of these two types of infection. It would appear that not all salmonella species have the same effect on the host though what factors may be responsible for the greater pathogenicity of some types as compared with others are at present unknown.

TABLE 5

DISTRIBUTION OF *S. PARATYPHI B* AND *S. ENTERITIDIS* WITH RESPECT TO AGE

Organism	Age Groups					Total
	Newborn–30 Days	30–90 Days	90 Days –1 Year	1–15 Years	15+ Years	
S. paratyphi B	6	6	3	3	3	21
S. enteritidis ..	13	8	14	7	2	44

Treatment of salmonella meningitis is at present unsatisfactory. Following the introduction of sulphonamides a number of cures were reported and recovery has also been attributed to the effect of streptomycin (Pearlman and Gordon, 1949). Padnos and Goldin (1951) also reported recovery in a case due to *S. bareilly* which was treated with intravenous aureomycin. Most salmonella strains are sensitive *in vitro* to the tetracycline drugs and they reach the cerebrospinal fluid in adequate amounts. It remains to be seen, however, whether they will effect a reduction in the mortality rate from this disease.

Summary

Four cases of meningitis due to salmonella infections are reported. Two of these were due to salmonella strains not previously isolated from the cerebrospinal fluid, namely *S. johannesburg* and *S. heidelberg*.

Salmonella infections of the meninges occur most commonly in infants in whom there is a higher death rate than in adults or older children. Prognosis may depend on the type of salmonella responsible for the infection as well as the age group.

I wish to thank Dr. P. Klenerman, Paediatrician to King Edward VIII Hospital, for permission to quote from the case notes of the patients in her charge.

REFERENCES

Bahrenburg, J. H. and Ecker, E. E. (1937). *J. infect. Dis.*, **60**, 81.
Beene, M. L., Hansen, A. E. and Fulton, M. (1951). *Amer. J. Dis. Child.*, **82** 567.
Curbelo, A. and Martinez Cruz, J. A. (1941). *Arch. Méd. Inf.*, **10**, 170.
Ghon. (1908). Bericht über den XIV Internationalen Kongress für Hygiene und Demographie. Berlin, 1907, Vol. 4, p. 21.
Guthrie, K. J. and Montgomery, G. L. (1939). *J. Path. Bact.*, **49**, 393.
Henderson, L. L. (1948). *Amer. J. Dis. Child.*, **75**, 351.
High, R. H. and Spaulding, E. H. (1946). *Amer. J. Dis. Child.*, **72**, 181.
Neter, E. R. (1944). *Arch. intern. Med.*, **73**, 425.
Padnos, E. and Goldin, M. (1951). *J. Pediat.*, **38**, 85.
Pearlman, L. N. and Gordon, A. S. P. (1949). *Canad. med. Ass. J.*, **60**, 483.
Ramón Guerra, A., Peluffo, E., Laguarda, M. and Aleppo, P. L. (1939). *Arch. Pediat. Urug.*, **10**, 669.
Zinsser, H., Enders, J. F. and Fothergill, L. D. (1939). *Immunity: Principles and Application in Medicine and Public Health*. New York.

CALCIFIED MESENTERIC LYMPHANGIOMA

BY

R. L. BISHTON, C. P. SAMES and HUGH R. E. WALLIS
From The Royal United Hospital and St. Martin's Hospital, Bath

(RECEIVED FOR PUBLICATION SEPTEMBER 2, 1957)

Levene, Walker and White (1956) reported two cases of mesenteric lymphangioma which presented as acute abdominal emergencies. They reviewed the published work, and showed that this is a rare condition. The following case is reported as an interesting complication of this disease.

Case Report

Paul R., aged 12, had from the age of 5 years recurrent attacks of central abdominal pain. These were accompanied by feelings of nausea and fullness in the epigastrium. The pain was colicky in nature, associated with constipation and relieved to some extent by the passage of flatus. At first the attacks occurred at intervals of five or six weeks, and they lasted for 24 hours. By the time he was 12 they had become less frequent but more severe, and vomiting occurred.

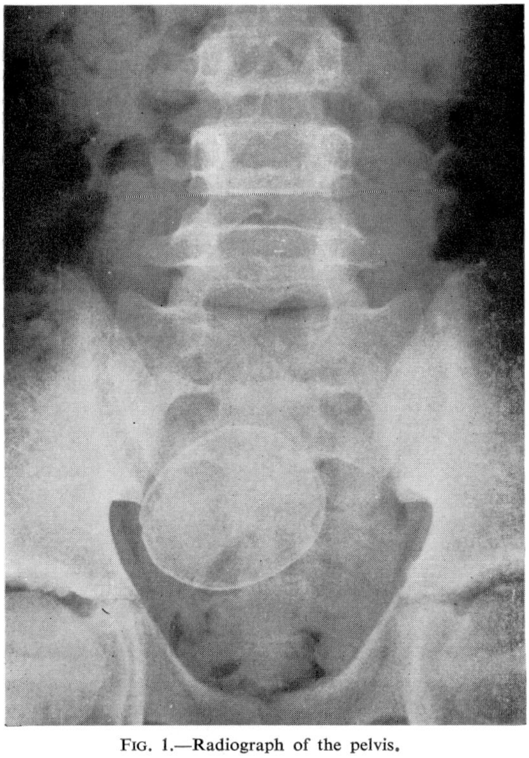

FIG. 1.—Radiograph of the pelvis.

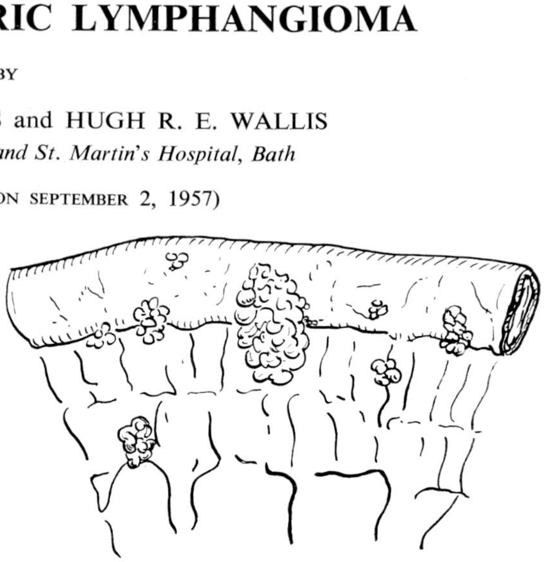

FIG. 2.—A portion of the jejunum seen at operation (about hal actual size).

On examination of the abdomen there was no physical abnormality, but rectal examination revealed a large, mobile, spherical mass which could be balloted in the abdomen. The blood picture and urine were normal. A tuberculin test was negative. A radiograph showed a calcified mass in the pelvis (Fig. 1). A barium enema revealed no communication with the large bowel.

Laparotomy was undertaken (C.P.S.), and there was found to be a little cloudy fluid in the peritoneal cavity. The surface of the jejunum and most of the ileum showed extensive engorgement of the lymphatics, which in many places had formed collections of lymphatic cysts (Fig. 2). At the distal end of the ileum there was a large, round, hard mass lying in the mesentery, but attached to the bowel wall (Fig. 3). The tumour was excised together with 4 cm. of the ileum, and an end-to-end anastomosis was performed. In addition, a small nodule was taken from the mesentery for the purpose of histology. The patient made a good recovery. Three months later he was very well and had no abdominal pain or nausea.

Pathology Report (R.L.B.)

The mesenteric nodule was a fatty nodule 0·5 cm. in diameter and consisted of fibro-fatty tissue in which were many dilated lymphatic spaces. No other lesion was seen

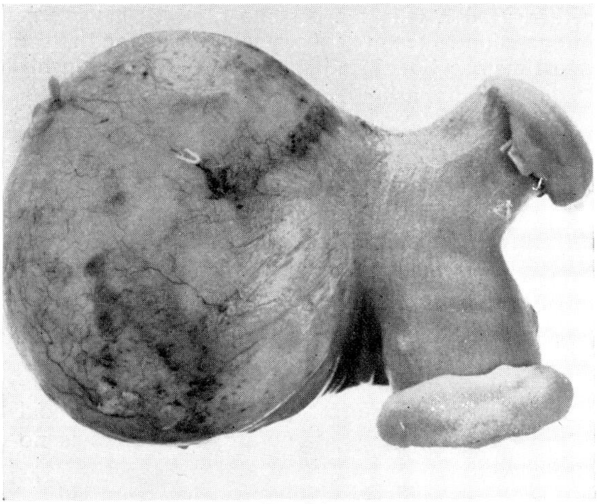

FIG. 3A.

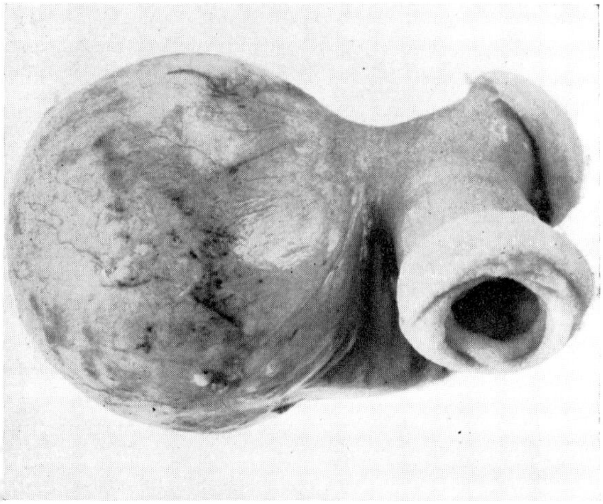

FIG. 3B.

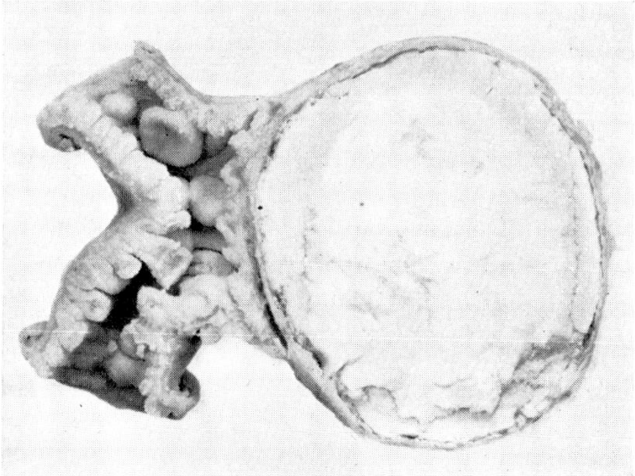

FIG. 3C.

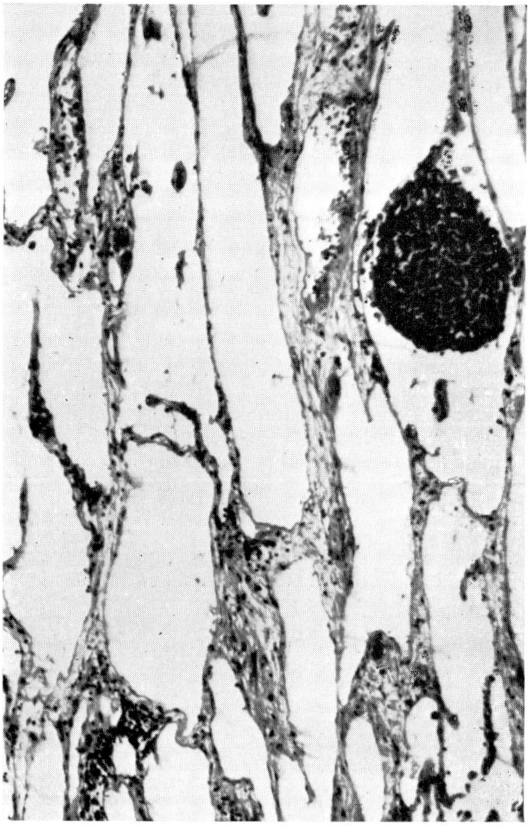

FIG. 4.—Section of mesentery showing lymphangiectasis with some lymphoid aggregates (×120).

FIG. 3.—A and B: Cyst and attached bowel. C: Cut surface of specimen showing polypoidal mucosa of small bowel (actual size).

and the diagnosis was considered to be lymphangiectasis of the mesentery.

The main specimen was a segment of small intestine 4 cm. long with a spherical hard mass 4·5 cm. diameter attached just to one side of the mesenteric border. On bisection with the aid of a saw, the mass consisted of uniform cream necrotic material (resembling caseation) with a thin peripheral calcified shell. On the external surface of the tumour there were a few tiny transparent cysts containing clear fluid and measuring 1 mm. in diameter. The attached bowel showed two small polypoid lesions of the mucosa, but there was no ulceration. No lymph nodes were found in the mesentery.

The contents of the 'cyst' were necrotic and consisted of droplets of sudanophilic fat, much of it being birefringent. There was no iron pigmentation such as would be expected from old haemorrhage. The wall of the cyst consisted of dense fibrous tissue with some calcification; it had no connexion with the muscle of the bowel. In the mesentery there was a lymphangiectasis accompanied by a few small lymphoid aggregates (Fig. 4). The intestinal polypi showed a lymphangiectatic condition in the submucosa.

The final diagnosis was of mesenteric cyst with lymphangiectasis of the mesentery and small intestine.

Family History

No similar condition has been observed in any of the patient's relatives. About a year later his younger brother, aged 7, fell on a bar and ruptured his spleen. An operation to remove it became necessary and at the same time the bowel and mesentery were thoroughly examined. No signs of lymphangiectasis were seen.

Discussion

The nature of the attacks, the feeling of fullness and the relief from passing flatus, suggest that there was an element of subacute obstruction. Since the cyst has been removed there has been much improvement, and there are no symptoms referable to the condition. As a matter of interest a fat balance was carried out after the operation. This gave a normal result, with 91·5% absorption. The blood cholesterol level was 150 mm. %, and the total fatty acid 194 mg. %. It seems, therefore, that there is no interference with fat absorption.

This appears to be the first case recorded of calcification in a lymphangiectatic cyst.

We wish to thank Dr. K. Reeves, who referred the case, Mr. T. Schofield, F.R.C.S., for information about the patient's brother, Mr. N. Swain for the print of the radiograph and Mr. G. W. Griffin, F.I.M.L.T., for the photomicrograph.

REFERENCE

Levene, M., Walker, P. A. and White, T. A. (1956). *Arch. Dis. Child.*, 31, 502.

SWEAT TEST FOR THE DIAGNOSIS OF FIBROCYSTIC DISEASE OF THE PANCREAS

REPORT OF A FATALITY

BY

K. A. MISCH and H. M. HOLDEN

From the Department of Pathology, Lister Hospital, Hitchin, and the Children's Annexe of the Luton and Dunstable Hospital, Luton

(RECEIVED FOR PUBLICATION SEPTEMBER 8, 1957)

The recognition of the electrolyte disturbance in the sweat of patients with fibrocystic disease by Darling, diSant' Agnese, Perera and Andersen (1953) led Shwachman, Leubner and Catzel (1955) to devise a simplified method of obtaining sweat for biochemical assay.

In this method the patient is placed in a plastic bag up to the neck and covered with a blanket, the sweat being collected in a weighed square of gauze which is covered with a piece of impermeable sheeting and strapped to the back. The recommended time is 30-90 min., depending on the rate of sweating.

The test is now widely used. In spite of the theoretical risks no serious ill effects from it have been reported. We have had the unfortunate experience of a death following its use, which we record as a reminder of its potential danger.

Case Report

A boy, aged 13 months, was admitted to hospital on account of failure to thrive, backwardness and diarrhoea with bulky and offensive stools, for an unknown period. Delivery and the neonatal period had been normal but he sat up late, and was unable to get into a sitting position at the time of admission. He appeared in a neglected condition and the home conditions were bad. Apart from his low weight, flabby musculature and slight ichthyosis of the skin, physical examination revealed no abnormality.

The Wassermann reaction, chest radiograph and Mantoux test were negative, and the blood count was normal. The stools were pale, bulky, greasy and offensive; no pathogens were isolated. The duodenal fluid was slightly alkaline and showed tryptic activity to a titre of 1 : 32 (gelatin film method of Harrison, 1947). As this suggested pancreatic impairment, pancreatin granules were given with each meal. There was a rapid general improvement with increase in weight (5 lb. (2·25 g.) in four weeks) and he started to walk.

Although the child was now well, because of the apparent pancreatic impairment a Shwachman test was performed (after sedation with 1 ml. of paraldehyde) by the method described above but using hot water bottles to promote sweating. The test lasted two hours. The result, an increase in the weight of the gauze by 0·2 g., with complete absence of chloride and sodium, was equivocal, and it was decided to repeat the test a week later. The patient was sedated with chloral hydrate gr. 3 (0·05 g.) and, as this had no effect, paraldehyde 0·75 ml. As little sweat had been obtained in the previous test, the period of collection was extended to three hours under the same conditions as before. Throughout the patient's general condition appeared satisfactory, though on removal from the bag he appeared anxious and restless. This was attributed to the discomforts of the test. Half an hour later he vomited copiously. On examination then he was unconscious and pale with a hot, moist skin, and a temperature of 104° F. (40·3° C.) in the axilla. Respirations were irregular; pupils equal and reacting to light; deep reflexes normal. Under treatment with tepid sponging, subcutaneous and intravenous fluids and a mega unit of penicillin the temperature fell to 100° F. (37·6° C.) but the general condition deteriorated; the pupils became temporarily unequal and deep reflexes were absent. The pulse rate rose to 160-200 per minute. Death occurred in coma 14 hours after conclusion of the test.

Necropsy

This was performed five and a half hours after death and showed a well-developed boy with a somewhat rough skin, but without external abnormalities. Throughout the body there were scattered small and some larger flame-shaped haemorrhages mainly involving skeletal muscle and internal organs, especially marked on the pericardial and left septal surfaces of the heart, the omentum and the kidneys, and there were patches of haemorrhage in the well-pigmented adrenals. The lungs were uniformly and extremely congested, firm, and deep red. The gastro-intestinal tract, liver, bile passages, pancreas and ducts were macroscopically normal. The spleen was slightly enlarged (45 g.), firm, and of a deep red with sharply demarcated large Malpighian corpuscles. Generalized mild but not abnormal lymphoid tissue hyperplasia was noted with enlarged tonsils and adenoids and a generalized mild lymphadenopathy. The thymus was normal (24 g.).

Examination of the skull showed the meninges tense but not congested, the brain bulging with flattened convolutions and a pressure cone of the cerebellum. A small grey nodule, 3-4 mm. in diameter, was noted projecting from the tuber cinereum close to the infundibulum to the left of the midline.

Sectioning of the brain (1,200 g.) showed dry, pale, bulging surfaces suggesting interstitial oedema. A small petechial haemorrhage was seen in the floor of the fourth ventricle. No further nodules were found.

Histology

Sections of the pancreas revealed no evidence of fibrocystic disease, and serial blocks of the terminal centimetre of the main duct showed no obstruction. The acinar cells were filled with secreting granules. The lungs showed extreme congestion only, with no abnormality of structure. The liver was normal apart from very scant round-cell infiltration of the portal tracts. Tonsils, cervical and abdominal lymph nodes, spleen and intestine confirmed slight generalized non-specific hyperplasia of the lymphoid tissue. No sign of an inflammatory reaction was seen in brain and meninges. Sections of cerebral cortex, corpus striatum and hypothalamus confirmed the oedema and showed a few small scattered capillary haemorrhages. The nodule on the tuber cinereum was a small lipoma of the pia mater. The abdominal skin showed hyperkeratosis, deficiency of the stratum granulosum and normal but inactive sweat glands (lumina closed).

Bacteriology

Films and cultures of the cerebrospinal fluid and spleen revealed no micro-organisms.

Pathological Summary

Heat stroke. Mild ichthyosis. Incidental finding: lipoma of meninges.

Comment

The necropsy findings, cerebral oedema and scattered body haemorrhages, taken in conjunction with the sequence of events, bears out the diagnosis of heat stroke, although the highest body temperature recorded, the first to be taken, and when the collapse had already occurred, was only 104° F. (40·3° C.) in the groin.

The method of obtaining sweat as devised by Shwachman is a simple and most useful diagnostic procedure but the potential danger of interference with the normal heat regulation of the body ought to be clearly recognized. At an external temperature of over 90° F. (32·2° C.) evaporation of sweat is almost the sole means of maintaining the normal body temperature (Best and Taylor, 1955). In the original experiments by Darling *et al.* (1953) a room heated to 90° F. was used to promote sweating, but in the Shwachman test the enclosure of the body by a plastic bag prevents any evaporation and permits a dangerous hyperpyrexia to occur. Patients with fibrocystic disease are known to sweat excessively and the danger of heat exhaustion due to excessive loss of electrolytes has been recorded by Kessler and Andersen (1951). This, however, need not be considered here as it bears no relation to hyperthermia. It is of interest though that the only fatality in their series occurred in an infant which was brought to the hospital during a heat wave wrapped up in a thick woollen blanket, thus preventing heat loss, and having a temperature of 106° F. (41° C.).

The simple screening test of Shwachman and Gahn (1956) which merely requires the placing of a hand on an agar plate incorporating silver chloride and an indicator, might be used more widely to demonstrate the increase of chloride in sweat of patients with fibrocystic disease. In its interpretation the possibility of a doubtful result ought to be borne in mind. We have found one false negative in a severely ill child in which fibrocystic disease of the pancreas was confirmed at necropsy. The polythene bag test should be limited to doubtful cases and when performed due regard must be given to the possibility of hyperthermia, and frequent recordings must be made of the body temperature. The duration of the test should be limited to the time specified by Shwachman and additional heat by hot water bottles or electric blankets should be avoided.

Summary

A fatality due to heat stroke following Shwachman's test involving the collection of sweat for the diagnosis of fibrocystic disease is reported. The potential danger of the test is emphasized.

We wish to thank Dr. C. G. Fagg at whose suggestion this case is being reported, Dr. H. Haber for his advice on the skin sections, and H.M. Coroner, Mr. J. H. Hoare, for permission to publish.

REFERENCES

Best, C. H. and Taylor, N. B. (1955). *The Physiological Basis of Medical Practice*, 6th ed., p. 734. London.
Darling, R. C., diSant' Agnese, P. A., Perera, G. A. and Andersen, D. H. (1953). *Amer. J. Med. Sci.*, **225**, 67.
Harrison, G. A. (1947). *Chemical Methods in Clinical Medicine*, 3rd ed., p. 506. London.
Kessler, W. R. and Andersen, D. H. (1951). *Pediatrics*, **8**, 648.
Shwachman, H., Leubner, H. and Catzel, P. (1955). *Advances in Pediatrics*, Vol. 7, p. 249. Chicago.
Shwachman, H. and Gahn, N., (1956). *New Eng. J.Med.*, **255**, 999.

PAEDIATRIC PATHOLOGY CLUB

Proceedings of the Third Annual Meeting

The third meeting of the Paediatric Pathology Club took place at the Children's Hospital, Sheffield, on November 8 and 9, 1957. Sixty members and guests attended.

Dinner was taken at the George Hotel, Hathersage, on the evening of Friday, November 8. There followed a discussion on pyelonephritis at which the principal speakers were W. W. Payne (London), R. C. B. Pugh (London), R. B. Zachary (Sheffield), A. M. MacDonald (Glasgow), B. I. Ivemark (Stockholm), K. B. Rogers (Birmingham), and A. G. Marshall (Wolverhampton).

The afternoon of Saturday, November 9, was taken up with a discussion of the National Perinatal Mortality Survey and a report by Dr. N. Brown on the pilot survey at Bristol.

Summaries of Original Papers

P. S. MacFarlane (Glasgow). 'Haemolytic Anaemia associated with Acute Renal Damage in Infancy.' Eight cases, in which a severe haemolytic anaemia was associated with renal damage, were described. The recent frequent association of what are rare diseases in infancy, may be of significance and the possibility that this is a new syndrome must be kept in mind.

The striking red cell morphology with frequent 'burr' cells was demonstrated.

Seven cases progressed to fatal uraemia in spite of adequate treatment of the haemolysis. At necropsy one case showed confluent cortical necrosis, five cases acute necrotizing glomerulitis and one case a severe tubular lesion with less severe glomerular damage. One case recovered.

This series suggests that the haemolytic anaemia does not cause the renal damage or *vice versa*, but rather that the two are concomitants and that a common ætiology is to be sought. The 'burr' cell phenomenon was present in two cases before a significant rise in blood urea had taken place.

There is no convincing evidence of an antigen-antibody reaction and the fundamental aetiology remains obscure.

R. C. B. Pugh (London). 'Pyelonephritis.' The term 'pyelitis' is probably unjustified as in nearly every case of so-called pyelitis there is also involvement of the renal parenchyma.

In a series of 150 necropsies in children, pyelonephritis was found in ten cases. Of these, six children had an underlying deformity of the urinary tract and in two cases pyelonephritis complicated tuberculosis.

An analysis of eight fatal cases of posterior urethral valves showed that in all there was pyelonephritis, which led to the development of renal rickets in two cases and to hypertension in the four older children.

When considering the morbid anatomical changes in pyelonephritis, the description of Weiss and Parker cannot be bettered, although a distinction should be made between the disease in neonates and in slightly older children, in whom the changes are very similar to those seen in adults.

The appearance of vascular lesions in pyelonephritis is also important especially as they resemble intrinsically those seen in hypertension. However, their distribution is different as they are confined to the scarred areas in pyelonephritis but occur in both the scarred and non-scarred areas in pyelonephritis complicated by hypertension.

The cases of glomerulonephritis, nephritis, pyelonephritis and nephrosis that occur in the neonatal period are a complex and as yet incompletely understood group.

N. O. Ericsson and B. I. Ivemark (Karolinska Institutet, Stockholm). 'Renal Dysplasia and Pyelonephritis in Infants and Children.' Clinical, radiological and pathological examinations were performed on 34 children, 30 of whom showed infections of the urinary tract. Eight were under 1 year of age, and 26 of them from 1 to 11 years. Malformations of the urinary tract predominated, 16 patients having ureterocele and nine ectopic ureters, an inevitable composition of paediatric material, as cases with no such malformations rarely undergo operation. Thirty-one females, and three males were encountered, a sex distribution due to the female predominance in pyelonephritis and ureteric malformations rather than in renal dysplasia. No preponderance of left-sided abnormalities was found.

The specimens were grouped in three categories. (1) *Dysplastic* (15 specimens) malformed kidneys with numerous primitive ducts resembling the mesonephric duct. Thirteen showed pyelonephritis. (2) *Presumably dysplastic* (16 specimens) mostly hydronephrotic kidneys with few medullary ducts ('medullary dysplasia') and primitive cortical 'ductules', resembling mesonephric ductules. All specimens displayed severe pyelonephritis. (3) *No obvious renal dysplasia* (three specimens). Ductules: no medullary dysplasia. Striking inflammatory changes.

The microscopic findings suggest abnormal budding of the ureter to be the underlying cause of the dysplasia. The cortical ductules described may be evidence of renal dysplasia—possibly residual mesonephric tubules or abnormal proliferation of ureteric buds. Concomitant inflammation in all patients surviving more than seven days is an indication that renal dysplasia is an important predisposing element in the pyelonephritis of infancy and childhood.

C. G. PAINE (Sheffield). 'Changes in the Placenta with Particular Reference to Essential Hypertension and Pre-eclamptic Toxaemia.' A description of the normal ageing changes in placental tissue was given. This related to the villous stroma which was converted from primitive mesodermal tissue to adult fibrous tissue, the arterioles of the villous stalks which changed from primitive blood spaces to relatively thick, muscular walled tubes to deal with the increasing volume of foetal blood, the villous blood vessels with special reference to subtrophoblastic sinusoid formation in the late weeks of pregnancy, and the syncitiotrophoblast which started as a thick plastic multinuclear structure, and finished as a thin membrane capable of rapid metabolite exchange at full term. A description was given of the distribution of lipoid with normal syncitium.

The normal changes were compared with those seen in essential hypertension affecting pregnancy, and in pre-eclamptic toxaemia. In the former condition, thromboses and fibrin deposition in the overlying decidua were associated with local intervillous fibrin deposition and infarct formation, and with premature ageing of the villous blood vessels and stroma, such that subtrophoblast sinusoid formation was limited. In pre-eclamptic toxaemia, syncitial atrophy was accompanied by a diminution in lipoid. It was considered that this was related to the diminution in pregnandiol excretion which occurs in pre-eclamptic toxaemia.

J. BEVERLEY (Sheffield). 'Stress and Pathogenicity of Toxoplasma.' Evidence was produced that most toxoplasma infection in animals and humans remains subclinical. Instances from the literature of clinical grade infections in various species were cited to illustrate that such factors as cold, concomitant infections, captivity, infancy, pregnancy, injury and endocrine imbalances may have contributed to the severity.

A strain of toxoplasma, isolated from a rabbit, was found to be only feebly pathogenetic for non-pregnant mice, causing them to lose weight from the ninth to the 15th days after inoculation, but they completely recovered. When the same strain, in the same doses, was injected into other mice so that the peak of the illness occurred at different stages of pregnancy it was found that injection 11 to three days before pregnancy caused abortion with 17% of mothers dying; injection during the first 12 days of pregnancy caused abortion or full term still-births, or live births which soon died, and the maternal mortality was 55%; injection between the 13th and 16th day resulted in live litters which were not reared and no maternal mortality; and inoculation between the second and 12th day of lactation rarely caused neglect of the litters but a 92% maternal mortality around the time of weaning.

J. H. ALLAN (Sheffield). 'The Mineralization of Enamel in Developing Teeth.' Ground sections of human deciduous teeth, ranging in development from 26 weeks *in utero* to 18 months after birth, were examined in plane polarized light, and the following pattern of mineral accretion deduced.

1. Following the commencement of enamel organic matrix formation, a primary, fairly diffuse deposition of mineral matter occurs along a narrow zone at the incisal amelo-dentinal junction. From this latter area, the amount of mineral matter falls in a regular manner towards the periphery of the enamel.

2. In the peripheral enamel a secondary deposit then occurs, producing slightly better mineralized zones in the cervical region and just deep to the enamel surface. This secondary deposit results in an area of slightly lower mineral content being present in the centre of both labial and lingual enamel.

3. A final deposition then starts on the lingual side of the incisal amelo-dentinal junction and expands cervically and peripherally, gradually obliterating the primary and secondary deposition patterns. This final deposition, which initially advances parallel to the organic matrix incremental lines, gradually alters its direction until it is almost parallel to the enamel surface.

These results support the view that all the main phases of enamel mineralization proceed peripherally from the amelo-dentinal junction, not cervically from the incisal surface.

J. L. EMERY, G. H. JOWETT and MORAG S. MACDONALD (Sheffield). 'Post Natal Changes in the Glomeruli of the Kidney.' Kidneys from 235 children aged 26 weeks *in utero* to 13½ years were described.

The glomeruli were classified according to six stages of maturity. The percentages of these six stages were related to age.

A reproducibility survey showed that there had been a subconscious change in standards of classification during the period of the survey, but the following conclusions appear valid.

1. Primitive forms may persist until 4 to 6 months of age, but some of these may be abnormal.

2. The majority of glomeruli are of mature type from 6 years onwards, but it is not until after 12 years of age that all are of adult form.

3. A very wide individual variation in the rate of glomerular maturation was found.

In addition, various case reports were given.

BOOK REVIEWS

A Primer of Paediatrics. By ELCHON HINDEN; Foreword by K. H. Tallerman. (Pp. xv+356. 25s.) London: Macdonald. 1957.

This new book is designed for the senior student and family doctor and it is intended as an introduction to paediatrics.

There are three sections—from conception to 4 weeks of age, from 4 weeks to 2 years and from 2 years to puberty—and in each section both normal child care and children's diseases are considered. The subdivision into age groups thus clearly segregates neonatal paediatrics from, for example, the school health service, or prematurity from tuberculosis. The different subjects are discussed in a down-to-earth manner and the writing is in the first person; this, combined with the fact that there are no references to distract the attention, gives a comfortingly familiar style to the prose.

This book truly is an introduction to paediatrics and above all to paediatrics for the family doctor. It makes no excursions into controversy, it seeks no great scientific heights, nor is any subject dealt with very exhaustively. These are not the avowed purposes of the book, which is to act as a first presentation of paediatrics and in this object it can fairly be said to be successful. Throughout the text there is an abundance of sound commonsense views, sometimes expressed didactically, sometimes a little tenuous. The lack of an index will detract from its usefulness as a book to be consulted. For anyone about to start a study of paediatrics it can be wholeheartedly recommended as an introduction to what paediatrics is about. It is not a long book and every medical student starting his paediatric clerkship would benefit enormously if he were sent away for two or three days to read 'A Primer of Paediatrics' as though it were a novel. The text, which reads very easily, would make this a pleasure as well as instructive and would give a conception of paediatrics which no other book at present available is capable of doing.

Diabetes Mellitus: With Emphasis on Children and Young Adults. By T. S. DANOWSKI. (Pp. xxiv+510; illustrated. 108s.) London: Baillière, Tindall and Cox. 1957.

This book, according to the author, was originally intended to deal with diabetes in children, but it has been enlarged to embrace a presentation of the fundamental alterations in metabolism which occur in diabetes mellitus.

The first part is entitled 'Biochemical and Hormonal Aspects', and in the six chapters devoted to this section an attempt has been made to make a comprehensive survey of the main knowledge on carbohydrate metabolism and of the factors which affect it—hormonal, dietetic and experimental. The task the author has set himself is a very ambitious one and to condense all the relevant information into six chapters has necessitated a degree of condensing which makes it very hard reading. He includes, however, a considerable amount of literature for those who wish to go further into the matter.

The next part deals with 'Manifestations, Diagnosis and Therapy' and here the author varies between recounting the experiences gained from his own clinic and that culled from the enormous literature already existing on diabetes. The first chapters of this, on incidence, type of onset, heredity, the methods to be adopted in making the diagnosis, etc., are excellent. The following chapters, however, to some extent go over the same ground as has already been covered in Part 1 and he again discusses the question of how insulin acts, what happens when glucose is given, the effects of glucagon, epinephrine, etc., and one feels that these chapters could have been very much shortened with considerable advantage. When dealing with the actual therapy, the author attempts to adopt a mid-way position between the ultra-strict school of treatment and those who allegedly adopt a 'laissez faire' method of treatment. The reviewer found it rather difficult to appreciate exactly where the author stood in this matter. However, it is quite obvious that it is impossible to write a description of a therapy which has to vary with each patient, and it is probable that many apparent differences between different methods of treatment are largely non-existent in actual fact. He finishes this section with a chapter on the regulation of hydrogen ion concentration of body fluids, which seems quite out of place.

Part 3, entitled 'Developmental Aspects and Complications', merely continues the story of the treatment of diabetes. The first chapter deals with such matters as diabetic acidosis and coma and the various factors that cause them, the symptomatology and a theoretical discussion of the methods of treatment. The next chapter once again discusses the various factors, such as the metabolism of sugar which may lead to ketosis, and for a third time discusses the adrenocortical system, electrolytes, *p*H, etc. It is only in the following chapter that the actual treatment is dealt with. Again in these three chapters, there is considerable repetition of previous work and in the reviewer's opinion, they could well be condensed into one chapter.

The next two chapters deal with somatic growth and development of the juvenile diabetic—personality, emotions and scholastic performance, etc. These are unfortunately relatively short chapters and the reviewer would have liked to have had a rather fuller account of the author's own experiences in his clinic as well as the well-documented summaries that he gives of the literature. The next chapter deals with the vascular, ocular and renal changes and only 13 pages are devoted to this in a book which contains nearly 500 pages. As this particular problem is the one which looms most menacingly over the adolescent diabetic, it is disappointing that a much fuller treatment of this subject is not given.

The final chapters deal with the gastro-intestinal tract and liver, fertility and pregnancy, and a final short one on neuropathy, insulinogenic lipodystrophy and necrobiosis lipoidica in diabetics.

In the reviewer's opinion, the very praiseworthy attempt of the author to combine the physiological, experimental and clinical approaches to diabetes into one book has been only a partial success. It has made the book rather difficult to read, and for those who are rather more interested in the clinical aspects of diabetes in children, much of the book is unrewarding. The clinical sections of the book are somewhat uneven, but on the whole are good, and one of the best aspects of this book is the excellent bibliographies which are given at the end of each chapter. The book is well presented and there are only a few typographical errors. There is an excellent table of contents and a good index.

The Diagnosis and Treatment of Endocrine Disorders in Childhood and Adolescence, 2nd ed. By LAWSON WILKINS. (Pp. xxvi+526; illustrated. £6 12s. 6d.) Oxford: Blackwell Scientific Publications; Springfield, Illinois: Charles C. Thomas. 1957.

This book, first published in 1950, was quickly and universally recognized as a classic text. Endocrine disorders, apart from cretinism and diabetes, are rare in childhood and only a specialist working in a great city with the resources of a famous general hospital around him could have studied adequately the natural history of endocrine disease in childhood. When Lawson Wilkins started his endocrine clinic at the Harriet Lane Home nearly 20 years ago endocrinology was practically limited to observational records, and, as chemistry, physics and biology made their astonishing contributions, Wilkins was ready to apply these new methods to endocrine disease in childhood. In this second edition of his fine textbook he generously acknowledges the work of the 17 associates who have worked with him from 1938 until today. To read this list of distinguished names is to recognize how much fundamental work in endocrinology he has inspired and sponsored. Not included in the list of associates are Money and the two Hampsons, who at his instance, have made important psycho-sexual studies which are fully described in the new edition. Their fundamental conclusion is that the sex rearing (up to 2 years), and not gonadal, hormonal or chromosomal sex, determines the psycho-sexual orientation and that to change the sex of rearing is an invitation to disaster. In those fields in which the author is most interested this edition is not only up to the minute, but a little in advance of Greenwich mean time. It includes, for example, important discussions of the mental prognosis in hypothyroidism (Smith, D. W., Blizzard, R. M. and Wilkins, L., *Pediatrics*, 1957, **19**, 1011) and the sex chromatin pattern in testicular disorders (Grumbach, M. D., Blanc, W. A. and Engle, E. T., *J. clin. Endocrinol. Metab.*, 1957, **17**, 703) which have just reached the library tables in this country.

This edition is larger by 140 pages than the first edition, but it retains the same splendid factual and pictorial quality. The chapter on diagnostic methods has been rewritten and is now a comprehensive summary of the available techniques, though English readers will regret that there is no mention of Norymberski's 17-ketogenic assay which is still giving good service in laboratories here. Methods of investigation of thyroid function are excluded from this chapter and it might save space in future editions if the whole of this chapter were broken up and redistributed. There is some repetition of information; for example, the effect of A.C.T.H. on the output of steroids in adreno-cortical hyperplasia is given three times on pages 69, 305 and 333. With the multiplication of new methods there will be an opportunity in the next edition for a division of available diagnostic techniques into categories—essential, useful and research. There is no discussion as to whether I^{131} should be used in young children, a matter which has occupied British workers (*Arch. Dis. Childh.*, 1956, **32**, 166). The 80 pages devoted to the thyroid is the best account of thyroid disease in children in any textbook. The author gives good evidence for his belief that the mental and neurological deviations in cretinism are the direct result of thyroxine deficiency and not due to an associated congenital defect. In the treatment of thyrotoxicosis in childhood, preference is given to the use of anti-thyroid drugs rather than to surgery. Generous reference is made to papers by British authors (both in this section and throughout the book), but there is no mention of the observation of P. R. Evans (*Pediatrics*, 1952, **41**, 706) on the vertebral changes in hypothyroidism. Paediatricians will turn eagerly to the account of adrenocortical hyperplasia, for most of the dramatic advances in this field have been the work of the author and his associates. In the maintenance treatment of congenital virilism he recommends 25-75 mg. of intramuscular cortisone every third day and two to five DCA pellets of 125 mg. each by implant in the salt-losing type with the addition of 2 to 3 g. of sodium chloride daily. The need to watch height increments in these children as well as 17-ketosteroid output is emphasized.

Dwarfism and the problems of disturbed growth are still in the observational stage, and they will remain static subjects until growth-hormone assays are possible in man, so there is little that is new to be related here. The author has retained the same height standards as in the first edition which, adapted from Engelbach's tables of 25 years ago, are now 1 to 3 in. below the 50 percentiles in children over the age of 5 years in the most recent and reliable surveys. The chapters on calcium and phosphorus metabolism and on carbohydrate metabolism have been largely rewritten and are now worthy of the rest of the work. All readers will be grateful for two lucid chapters on deficiencies and deviations of sexual development—a subject made more confusing by the method of chromosomal sexing devised by Barr. The genetic explanations of these disorders are not yet complete, but the author produces a series of satisfactory hypotheses which are consistent with the known facts.

This book is essential reading for paediatricians, for there is much information here collected which cannot easily be discovered elsewhere. Lawson Wilkins' work has added lustre to the great traditions of the Johns Hopkins Hospital.

ABO INCOMPATIBILITY AND HAEMOLYTIC DISEASE OF THE NEWBORN

BY

G. H. VALENTINE

From the St. Thomas Elgin General Hospital, St. Thomas, Ontario, Canada

(RECEIVED FOR PUBLICATION NOVEMBER 5, 1957)

Since the work of Boorman, Dodd and Trinick (1949), incompatibility in the ABO system has been recognized with increasing frequency as a cause of haemolytic disease. Robinson, Phillips and Prystowsky (1951), Shumway, Miller and Young (1955), Davidsohn (1956) and others have written on this condition. And yet haemolytic disease due to ABO incompatibility is much less widely known than that due to Rhesus incompatibility. The failure widely to recognize ABO disease may be due to several reasons. Chiefly it is due to the fact that it is usually not a serious condition. In its severe degree it is uncommon. In its common form it is so slight as scarcely to be recognized. So the disease is held to be rare. Belief that a disease is rare leads to a lessened vigilance in its detection, and it is remarkable how once a disease is found to be not uncommon how quickly it becomes commonplace. Then again, that elegant test, the direct antiglobulin test of Coombs, which so readily detects haemolytic disease in blood group incompatibilities other than ABO, is usually negative by the more usual techniques. By the special technique of Rosenfield (1955), however, it may be shown to be positive. With heterospecific pregnancies with A or B incompatibility, antibodies are by definition present in the blood of the mother, although where disease is present they are believed to be of a different nature from the 'natural' antibody. In Rhesus disease the presence of antibody with Rhesus incompatibility indicates disease. It is not necessarily so in ABO disease. Moreover, no immune antibody may be detectable ante-natally in ABO disease, although it may appear after delivery. Unlike Rhesus disease, ABO disease cannot be anticipated by ante-natal testing with any certainty. Finally, it may be that the term 'physiological jaundice' makes for a too easy road to diagnostic apathy, and one that is trod too often.

It is stated by Davidsohn (1956) that ABO haemolytic disease appears in 1 in 3,000 random pregnancies and by Gunson (1956) that it accounts for 15% of all cases of haemolytic disease of the newborn. Certainly it is generally believed to be less common than disease due to Rhesus incompatibility. However, Rosenfield (1955) found laboratory evidence of abnormality attributable to ABO incompatibility in 38 cord blood specimens of 1,480 random samples.

The present small survey purports to show that clinically recognizable ABO haemolytic disease is a common condition and that it may quite often need close watching and active treatment.

Survey and Findings

This survey, conducted in a hospital which serves a population of about 60,000 of mixed European descent, deals with the period August 1, 1956, to July 19, 1957. During this time there were 1,000 live births. It is the universal practice in this locality for deliveries to be in hospital. The survey therefore covers 1,000 random live births.

During the period under review all babies judged to show the slightest jaundice within the first 24 hours after birth were reported. It was found that minimal jaundice was difficult to detect in artificial light, and it is more than likely that some escaped investigation if they became jaundiced but slightly at night toward the end of the 24-hour limit set by the terms of the survey. Nevertheless, in 1,000 live births, 21 babies were found to be recognizably jaundiced within 24 hours. Six were found to have haemolytic disease due to antibody anti-D and one to be due to anti-E, and these are excluded from the series. Fourteen babies with jaundice believed not due to Rhesus disease were investigated. It should be emphasized that no baby who became jaundiced within 24 hours is excluded from the investigation apart from the seven in whom D or E incompatibility was found. Nothing was known about the blood groups of mother or baby until early jaundice had prompted investigation.

Table 1 relates to the parity of the mother, the birth weight in pounds and ounces and the time of onset of the jaundice in hours after birth. It will be noted that in three instances first babies were involved and that one came within the World Health Organization definition of prematurity. Cases 2 and 3 were dizygotic twins of the same blood group, A. There was no difference in sex incidence. The time of onset of the jaundice varied between four and 23 hours with a mean of 14 hours. The smaller babies did not become jaundiced earlier than those of larger size.

Table 2 refers to the initial bilirubin estimation and to the maximal bilirubin estimation. Bilirubin estimations were not done at night if the jaundice did not seem to be deepening rapidly, nor were they repeated if the initial level was low and the baby not becoming more icteric.

It will be seen that we were able just to detect jaundice at a level of 4 mg. % but it was our experience that it did not become easily visible until a level of about 6 mg. % was reached. In three cases the maximal bilirubin reached the figure of 20 mg. % or over, and in these babies exchange transfusions were done. In one case, Case 6, three exchanges were required to keep the bilirubin at a safe level. The average time for the onset of jaundice in these three cases was 14 hours, which does not differ from the series as a whole.

Table 3 shows the first haemoglobin level determined after the jaundice was first reported. In no case was the haemoglobin below 15 g. %, and in the majority it was considerably higher. The most severely jaundiced did not have lower haemoglobin levels than the remainder. In twelve instances it is recorded that splenic enlargement was specifically sought. In two only was it found.

Table 4 shows the presence or absence of spherocytes in a stained smear and the osmotic fragility of the red cells in venous blood expressed as the percentage concentration of sodium chloride in which haemolysis is first apparent.

In eight instances spherocytosis is recorded as being present. It is remembered that it was also present in two further cases, Cases 2 and 3, but there is no written record of this. All cases showing spherocytosis showed haemolysis in concentration of 0·60% saline, or greater, but those showing the most obvious spherocytosis were not those with the greatest fragility. Reticulocyte counts were done in only nine of the 14 babies. In only three was the count above the normal of 4·35% (Washburn, 1941) for this age group.

Table 5 shows the reaction on a slide of the whole blood of the baby when mixed with complement inactivated normal AB serum compared with the same serum with the addition of bovine albumin (Witebsky, 1954). Thirteen of the 14 babies had blood which agglutinated with normal AB serum within 90 seconds. One baby showed no reaction where reaction might have been expected. In five there was agglutination also in the AB serum with bovine albumin.

Experience with this test has shown that it is most difficult to interpret with confidence. The agglutination may be very fine and scarcely visible. It is easily confused with rouleaux formation. The time limit of 90 seconds must be strictly enforced or false positive results will be found. Incorrect readings in our hands have been too frequent to make the test really valuable.

The direct antiglobulin test of Coombs was performed in the 14 babies in the series. In only one, Case 4, was macroscopic agglutination seen with a test carried out as described by Zuelzer and Cohen (1957).

Table 6 shows the blood groups of the babies compared with those of their mothers. It will be seen that in every one of the 14 cases of babies becoming jaundiced within the first 24 hours an incompatibility, O-A or O-B, was found. In 12 A was the incompatible, in two it was B. No attempt at subgrouping into A_1 or A_2 was made.

Table 7 shows the ABO phenotype distribution in 50 mother-child pairs randomly selected in our area. For clarity, those where incompatibility of A or B exists are marked with an asterisk. It is seen that such incompatibility was present in 10 births out of 50. If this finding is compared with Table 6 a marked and highly significant difference is obvious. That every mother in the series was group O and every baby either group A or B can scarcely be due to chance.

It might be argued that 50 random mother-child combinations is too small a number to rule out a peculiar bias in blood group distribution, but the percentage of compatible and incompatible pairs in that small number is almost identical with the number which would be expected on the basis of the ABO gene frequencies. This calculation was made and resulted in the expectation of 81% compatible mother-child pairs, assuming that mating is random and unrelated to blood groups.

Table 8 shows the maximal bilirubin level in relation to the D factor of Rhesus of the babies and their mothers. It is seen that of 14 babies jaundiced in the first 24 hours no less than seven were d/d: in common parlance, they were Rhesus negative. Using tables (Mainland, 1948) giving the confidence limit for small samples, it can be shown that this

TABLE 1

MATERNAL PARITY, BIRTH WEIGHT AND TIME OF ONSET OF JAUNDICE

Case No.	1	2	3	4	5	6	7	8	9	10	11	12	13	14
Parity of mother ..	1	2	2	1	2	2	3	3	1	2	2	4	9	2
Birth weight (lb. oz.)..	7·2	6·8	4·15	8·10	6·6	6·10	8·5	6·14	6·4	6·5	8·9	8·14	6·13	6·4
Onset of jaundice (hr. P.N.) ..	4	18	22	6	20	23	7	11	12	8	18	10	9	20

TABLE 2

INITIAL AND MAXIMAL BILIRUBIN ESTIMATIONS

Case No.	1	2	3	4	5	6	7	8	9	10	11	12	13	14
Initial bilirubin (mg.%)	6·5	8·0	5·0	8·6	11·9	13	7·0	7·5	9·2	7·0	11·3	6·4	4·0	8·6
Maximal bilirubin (mg. %)	6·5	9·0	5·0	8·6	14·6	25·0*	7·0	22·0*	10·3	20·0*	14·0	6·4	16·2	8·6

* Exchange transfusion.

TABLE 3

INITIAL HAEMOGLOBIN LEVELS

Case No.	1	2	3	4	5	6	7	8	9	10	11	12	13	14
Haemoglobin (g. %) ..	19·5	18·0	18·5	20·0	17·0	20·0*	18·5	17·0*	16·0	16·5*	16·5	19·5	15·0	19·0

* Exchange transfusion.

TABLE 4

SPHEROCYTOSIS AND OSMOTIC FRAGILITY IN BABIES

Case No.	1	2	3	4	5	6*	7	8*	9	10*	11	12	13	14
Spherocytosis ..	—	?	?	++	+	+	+	—	+	—	—	+++	+	+
Osmotic fragility (% sodium chloride)	0·64	0·64	0·60	0·60	0·80	—	0·80	0·52	0·84	0·56	0·56	0·60	0·60	—

* Exchange transfusion.

TABLE 5

WITEBSKY TEST REACTIONS

Case No.	1	2	3	4	5	6*	7	8*	9	10*	11	12	13	14
Reaction in AB serum	+	+++	+	+	+++	+	+	+	0	+++	+	+	+++	+
Reaction in AB serum + albumin ..	0	+	0	+	0	+	+	0	0	0	+	0	0	0

* Exchange transfusion.

TABLE 6

BLOOD GROUPS OF MOTHERS AND BABIES

Case No.	1	2	3	4	5	6*	7	8*	9	10*	11	12	13	14
ABO:														
Baby	A	A	A	A	B	A	A	B	A	A	A	A	A	A
Mother	O	O	O	O	O	O	O	O	O	O	O	O	O	O
Rhesus:														
Baby	D	D	D	D	d/d	d/d	d/d	d/d	d/d	d/d	D	d/d	D	D
Mother	d/d	D	D	D	D	d/d	D	d/d	D	D	D	d/d	D	D

* Exchange transfusions.

TABLE 7

ABO PHENOTYPE DISTRIBUTION IN 50 RANDOM MOTHER-CHILD PAIRS

ABO phenotype	O-O	O-A	O-B	A-O	A-A	B-O	B-A	B-B	AB-O	AB-B	AB-AB
No. of pairs	11	6*	2*	6	18	1	2*	1	1	1	1

* Incompatibility of A or B.

TABLE 8

RHESUS D FACTOR IN MOTHER AND BABIES AND MAXIMAL BILIRUBIN LEVEL

Case No.	1	2	3	4	5	6*	7	8*	9	10*	11	12	13	14
Rhesus:														
Baby	D	D	D	D	d/d	d/d	d/d	d/d	d/d	d/d	D	d/d	D	D
Mother	d/d	D	D	D	D	d/d	D	d/d	D	D	D	d/d	D	D
Bilirubin, maximal ..	6·5	9	5	8·6	14·6	25	7	22	10·3	20	14	6·4	16·2	8·6

* Exchange transfusion.

TABLE 9

BLOOD GROUP OF BABY AND ANTIBODY LEVEL IN MATERNAL BLOOD

Case No.	Baby ABO	Mother Anti-A	Mother Anti-B	Nature of Antibody
1	A	—	—	—
2	A	320	40	Both resistant to neutralization. Anti-A eluted from baby's cells.
3	A	320	40	Both resistant to neutralization. Anti-A eluted from baby's cells.
4	A	40	20	Both weakly immune. Findings not too conclusive.
5	B	40	320	Anti-B is strongly immune. Anti-A weakly so.
6	A	—	—	—
7	A	640	80	Only anti-A is of immune variety.
8	B	640	80	Both antibodies strongly immune.
9	A	640	80	Both antibodies strongly immune.
10	A	640	160	Both antibodies of immune variety.
11	A	—	—	—
12	A	1,000	320	Both of immune variety. Blood taken 6 weeks after delivery.
13	A	160	40	Both antibodies of immune variety.
14	A	320	20	Anti-A is strongly immune. Blood taken 6 weeks after delivery.

observed distribution of Rhesus negative babies with jaundice and AB incompatibility is a departure from the expected in a population such as ours at a low level of significance (significant at 5% level, but scarcely so at 1% level). It will also be noted that the three babies requiring transfusion were Rhesus negative (d/d), and that the average maximal bilirubin value in this series was higher for the Rhesus negative (d/d) babies than for the D positive infants. The mean difference was 5·3 mg. %, the standard error of difference 3·20. In this small series the difference between the maximal bilirubin levels of the D positives and the Rhesus negatives (d/d) was not significant.

Table 9 illustrates the level of antibodies found in the blood of the mother. Except where indicated in the table blood samples were taken two to four days after delivery. The antibody titrations were most kindly carried out at the Ortho Research Foundation, Raritan, New Jersey, under the direction of Dr. Phillip Levine, whose comments are given in brief.

Antibody studies were carried out on the blood of the mothers of 11 of the 14 babies in the survey. It will be seen that a high titre of immune antibody is present against the factor carried by the baby with a frequency which seems far too high for it to be the result of mere chance or of immunization unrelated to the pregnancy. However, in Case 4 the antibody levels were not very convincing, while in Case 8, where the baby was group B, immune anti-A was present in a titre of 1:640 and immune anti-B in a titre of 1:80 only.

Discussion

Investigations on the cases presented here are in some instances incomplete, but the following facts clearly emerge. The slightly lower birth weights of those requiring treatment was not a significant difference. There was no difference in the average time of onset of the jaundice in those in whom the jaundice later became severe. Late onset did not mean mild disorder. The Coombs test was positive in one baby, but this was one with a low level of bilirubin throughout. The initial haemoglobin level was no lower in those threatened with kernikterus than in the others, nor was splenic enlargement a feature of severe disease. Spherocytosis was present or absent in mild and in severe cases alike, as was an increased osmotic fragility of the red cells. Agglutination of the baby's cells in AB serum was found in the three severely affected babies, but it was also found in most of the others, including that with the lowest bilirubin. A reticulocyte count of 11% was found in one of those with marked icterus, but a similar count was found also in one of the mildest of the series. Immune anti-A was found in a titre of 1:640 in one of the babies with severe jaundice, but it was present in the same titre in a baby whose bilirubin never rose above 7 mg. %. Incompatibility of group B was present in a severe case, but was present also in a case of only moderate severity.

There was thus, in this series, no difference between the cases with severe jaundice and those with mild jaundice apart from the degree of jaundice itself.

The 14 cases where ABO incompatibility existed appeared to represent a uniform picture of the same disease manifesting itself in greater or less severity. There was no way of forecasting which would become an anxiety and which would cause no alarm. All need close watching.

The true incidence of ABO disorder is difficult to determine. Rosenfield (1955) found laboratory evidence in 38 specimens of 1,480 cord blood samples collected at random. It appeared that the disorder was present in the babies of 11% of mothers who lacked A or B when this was possessed by the foetus. The high degree of significance in the present small series for the frequency of incompatibility compared with that expected suggests that these cases, selected purely because they were clinically jaundiced, were indeed examples of ABO haemolytic disease. If this be accepted, we found ABO haemolytic disease to be clinically recognizable in one in every 71 births and likely to be present in 7% of mother-child pairs where A or B incompatibility exists.

An arbitrary limit of 24 hours was set for the onset of jaundice coming within this review. When one sees that of the 14 cases believed to have ABO haemolytic disease, four first showed jaundice at 20 hours or over, one immediately suspects that many cases of jaundice with onset after 24 hours may in fact be examples of haemolytic disease. This we have found to be so. It is clear, however, that the disorder does not always appear, in form detectable by known methods, every time that incompatibility exists. Why this curious selection occurs is at present unknown. It is likely that a combination of circumstances must exist before the disorder is manifest. It appears (Zuelzer and Cohen, 1957) that babies of subgroup A_2 escape altogether and that full maturity of the antigenic potential of A_1 is not developed in the newborn. It may be that in some babies the immune antibody does not cross the placental barrier or is neutralized in so doing by the A or B substances in the placental tissue. It may be that there is an antigenic fraction associated with, but not identical with the A and B antigens, which is present in some but not in others. Unger and Wiener (1954) have demonstrated a factor C in the ABO system, and to this factor they attribute ABO haemolytic disease. If the group O mother of a baby of group A had, herself, a mother who was of group A and a secretor one could see that she, while herself a foetus, could develop tolerance to the A antigen from being subjected to A in intra-uterine life. Were this to happen one could imagine that such a mother would not herself have a baby with ABO haemolytic disease for, to her, the A factor would no longer be antigenic. Probably there is no single explanation of why the disorder does not always appear when conditions seem to be fulfilled for its appearance.

In this survey a discrepancy at a low level of significance is noted between the incidence of Rhesus negativity in mother-child incompatible babies affected with ABO haemolytic disease and what would be expected from the random distribution. If this difference be real it is difficult to explain. Until a larger series proves or disproves the significance of this observation it would be idle to speculate further.

Some would discount the levels of antibody titrations presented in Table 9, saying rightly that many normal people who have never received inoculation with human blood or tissue products may have a high level of immune anti-A or anti-B. Nevertheless, taken in conjunction with other evidence, it does not seem that the titres found here can really be disregarded.

It is a matter for regret that we did not use the test for free homologous antibody using adult cells of the same group as the baby. At the time this survey started the value of this test (Zuelzer and Cohen, 1956) was not realized. We are now employing this test using the A or B cells of the baby's father for, if his baby is affected, he will himself possess cells upon which free antibody in the baby's serum will react; that reaction being detected by the indirect Coombs test.

Summary

From 1,000 unselected live births all babies showing jaundice in the first 24 hours were investigated. Twenty-one such babies were found. Seven were diagnosed as being examples of Rhesus haemolytic disease and these are excluded from this series. Fourteen were considered to have ABO haemolytic disease, and for this evidence is presented.

ABO haemolytic disease can occur in clinically recognizable degree as often as once in every 71 births and may arise in 7% of AB incompatible mother-child pairs. It is thus about three times more common than haemolytic disease due to Rhesus incompatibility.

There is always a reason for jaundice within 24 hours of birth. The diagnosis of 'physiological jaundice' should not be invoked to explain such a happening.

My thanks are profoundly due to many: to the nursery nurses for their unfailing enthusiasm and vigilance, to the doctors who permitted me to see their patients, to the laboratory technicians for their most painstaking work at all hours and to the staff of the medical records department. I am also most grateful to the Ortho Research Foundation and to Dr. Phillip Levine for the reports on the antibody titrations and to Dr. Carol Buck of the University of Western Ontario for the statistical examinations.

REFERENCES

Boorman, K. E., Dodd, B. E. and Trinick, R. H. (1949). *Lancet*, **1**, 1088.
Davidsohn, I. (1956). *Obstet. Gynec.*, **8**, 318.
Gunson, H. H. and Goodfellow, Alice M. (1956). *Mod. Med. Can.*, **11**, 1.
Mainland, D. (1948). *Canad. J. Res. (E)*, **26**, 1.
Robinson, G. C., Phillips, R. M. and Prystowsky, M. (1951). *Pediatrics*, **7**, 164.
Rosenfield, R. E. (1955). *Blood*, **10**, 17.
Shumway, Clare N., Miller, G. and Young, L. E. (1955). *Pediatrics*, **15**, 54.
Unger, L. J. and Wiener, A. S. (1954). *J. Lab. clin. Med.*, **44**, 387.
Washburn, A. H. (1941). *Amer. J. Dis. Child.*, **62**, 530.
Witebsky, E. (1954). Proceedings of the Fourth International Congress of the International Society of Hematology. New York.
Zuelzer, W. W. and Cohen, Flossie. Sixth International Congress of the Society of Hematology. Boston, 1956.
——, —— (1957). *Pediat. Clin. N. Amer.*, May, p. 405.

THE DISAPPEARANCE OF FOETAL HAEMOGLOBIN IN CONGENITAL CYANOTIC HEART DISEASE

BY

M. K. COGHLAN and M. C. JOSEPH

From the Department of Child Health and the Interdepartmental Laboratory, Guy's Hospital, London

(RECEIVED FOR PUBLICATION NOVEMBER 5, 1957)

Children with congenital cyanotic heart disease become adapted to some extent to anoxaemia. A well-recognized response is an increase of haemoglobin concentration; this increase might also be accompanied by a change in the type of haemoglobin formed. Foetal haemoglobin is more favourable than adult haemoglobin for oxygen uptake, and postnatal anoxaemia might promote the production of foetal haemoglobin in significant amounts. The observations reported here were made to test this hypothesis.

Adams (1952) found that in a group of 19 infants and children with congenital cyanotic heart disease foetal haemoglobin did not persist in greater amounts than in a group of normal children and adults. The range of age of the cyanosed group was wide and included infants, children, adolescents and an adult aged 30 years, but their control group did not include any infants, the youngest patient being 4 years old, and the oldest 70 years. Their mean values in the cyanosed and control groups (6% and 3%) exceeded the accepted upper limits of 1% to 2% in normal children and adults (Singer, Chernoff and Singer, 1951; Zannos, 1953; Huisman, Jonxis and Dozy, 1955; Jonxis and Visser, 1956).

We used the optical method of Brinkman and Jonxis (1935), with modifications (White, 1956), to estimate the proportion of foetal haemoglobin from 24 full term normal infants. We found this to be a mean value of 72% with a range of 59% to 88%; this closely agrees with figures given by Schulman, Smith and Stern (1954) and Walker and Turnbull (1955). No foetal haemoglobin was demonstrated in the blood of four normal adults.

The same method was then used to determine the proportion of foetal haemoglobin present in 25 infants and children aged from 6 weeks to 8 years with Fallot's tetralogy; the cyanosis in most of these patients was severe. During the same period 22 infants and children formed a control group.

Method

Heparinized venous blood (2·5 to 5 ml.) was collected and the cells were washed twice with 0·85% sodium chloride and then once with 1·2% sodium chloride. The cells were then mixed with distilled water, frozen overnight and subsequently allowed to thaw at room temperature. After the addition of shredded asbestos, the stroma was removed by spinning for one hour at 3,000 r.p.m.; 0·2 ml. of the supernatant fluid was then added to 4·6 ml. of ammonium hydroxide in a cuvette and, using a Gallenkamp photometer with an Ilford 608 (red) filter, an initial reading D_0 was taken. Then 0·2 ml. of normal sodium hydroxide was added with rapid stirring and readings were taken over the next 10 minutes at 10-second intervals, the time interval being gradually lengthened to one minute. If foetal haemoglobin was present, readings were continued for up to three hours, the final reading being $D\alpha$ The amount of haemoglobin remaining undenatured at time (t) was calculated from the formula:

$$\text{Amount of foetal haemoglobin present} = \frac{D_t - D\alpha}{D\alpha - D_0}$$

These figures were then plotted on semi-logarithmic paper using time as the abscissa and the curve obtained was extrapolated backward to cut the ordinate at a figure representing the amount of foetal haemoglobin originally present in the sample.

Results

Foetal haemoglobin was not found in any infant or child over 7½ months old in the cyanotic or in the control groups. Variable amounts of foetal haemoglobin were found in infants under 7½ months. During this period 21 estimations were made in five cyanosed and in three control infants (Table 1).

The degree of cyanosis in the five infants was severe. All were full term infants except J.H. whose birth weight was 3 lb. 1 oz. and gestation period 34 weeks. Foetal haemoglobin was not found in two infants (M.W. and P.C.) at 22 weeks, and in a further four infants (M.S., S.H., A.M. and R.S.) at 26 weeks; at this time only J.H. had foetal haemoglobin present (9%) and this was not detectable at 30 weeks.

TABLE 1

PERCENTAGE OF FOETAL HAEMOGLOBIN IN CYANOSED AND CONTROL INFANTS

		Age in Weeks						
		6	10	14	18	22	26	30
		%	%	%	%	%	%	%
Cyanotic Group	J.H.	61	40	24	22	21	9	0
	M.S.	—	—	—	10	—	0	—
	M.W.	44	—	—	—	0	—	—
	S.H.	—	18·5	—	—	—	0	—
	D.B.	—	—	—	7·8	—	—	—
Control Group	P.C.	64	—	—	—	0	—	—
	A.M.	54	—	—	23	—	0	—
	R.S.	—	32	—	—	—	0	—

Discussion

The oxygen curve of foetal haemoglobin lies to the left of that of adult haemoglobin, provided that the pigment is in the corpuscles (Leibson, Likhnitzky and Sax, 1936; McCarthy, 1943). This increased affinity of foetal haemoglobin for oxygen is most marked at the higher oxygen tensions. Thus, the presence of a high proportion of foetal haemoglobin is favourable for oxygen intake. Walker and Turnbull (1953, 1955) have stated that the rise in total haemoglobin which they have observed in the anoxic foetus at term was mainly due to an increased production of foetal haemoglobin. As term approached they found a rise in total haemoglobin which was proportional to a fall in oxygen saturation of the blood in the umbilical vein. Recently Rooth and Sjöstedt (1957) were unable to confirm this correlation.

Persistent postnatal anoxia usually causes a rise in total haemoglobin, thereby increasing the amount of oxygen available to the tissues; an increase in the proportion of foetal haemoglobin would augment this by further increasing the oxygen uptake in the lungs. Furthermore, at birth the mechanism for the formation of foetal haemoglobin is still active (Schulman *et al.*, 1954) and under the stimulus of persistent anoxia, foetal haemoglobin would be readily formed.

The figures for J.H. (Table 1) show that, from 14 to 27 weeks, the percentage of foetal haemoglobin remained the same while during the same period the total haemoglobin rose from 9·2 g. % to 17·5 g. %. This suggests that during this time the production of foetal haemoglobin was at least maintained.

It should be pointed out that although the method used had the disadvantage of being relatively inaccurate for amounts of foetal haemoglobin below 10% it was especially suitable for accurate measurement of larger amounts. However, foetal haemoglobin did not persist in significant amounts beyond 30 weeks in the children and infants whom we studied and the foetal pigment disappeared at about the same rate in both the cyanotic and control groups.

Summary

Blood from 25 infants and children with cyanotic congenital heart disease was tested quantitatively for foetal haemoglobin. Twenty-two normal infants and children of similar age were studied over the same period. Foetal haemoglobin was not found in any child over the age of 7½ months in either group.

We thank Dr. P. R. Evans and Dr. R. C. Mac Keith for their helpful criticisms. Some of the patients studied were under the care of Sir Russell Brock to whom we are grateful. We acknowledge with thanks advice given by Dr. J. C. White, Hammersmith Postgraduate School of Medicine, on the technique of estimation.

REFERENCES

Adams, F. H. (1952). *J. Pediat.*, **40**, 42.
Brinkman, R. and Jonxis, J. H. P. (1935). *J. Physiol. (Lond.)*, **85**, 117.
Huisman, T. H. J., Jonxis, J. H. P. and Dozy, A. (1955). *Biochem. Biophys. Acta.*, **18**, 576.
Jonxis, J. H. P. and Visser, H. K. (1956). *A.M.A. J. Dis. Child.*, **92**, 588.
Leibson, R. G., Likhnitzky, I. I. and Sax, M. G. (1936). *J. Physiol. (Lond.)*, **87**, 97.
McCarthy, E. F. (1943). *Ibid.*, **102**, 55.
Rooth, C. and Sjöstedt, S. (1957). *Arch. Dis. Childh.*, **32**, 91.
Schulman, I., Smith, C. H. and Stern, G. S. (1954). *A.M.A. J. Dis. Child.*, **88**, 567.
Singer, K., Chernoff, A. and Singer, L. (1951). *Blood*, **6**, 413.
Walker, T. and Turnbull, E. P. N. (1953). *Lancet*, **2**, 312.
——, —— (1955). *Arch. Dis. Childh.*, **30**, 111.
White, D. D. (1956). Personal Communication.
Zannos, L. (1953). *Acta paediat. (Uppsala)*, **42**, 305.

BASOPHILIC LEUCOCYTES IN CHILDREN IN HEALTH AND DISEASE

BY

ROSS G. MITCHELL

From the Department of Child Health, University of St. Andrews, Dundee

(RECEIVED FOR PUBLICATION NOVEMBER 5, 1957)

The presence of basophilic leucocytes (basophils)* in human blood was first established by Ehrlich (1891). These cells differ from other polymorphs by their slightly smaller size, by the metachromatic staining reaction of their granules, and by their slower rate of motility (Sabin, 1923). Probably less is known about the basophils than about any of the other formed elements in the blood, mainly because they are very scanty in the peripheral blood and because until 1953 there was no satisfactory method of counting them accurately. Counts based on examination of blood smears are unreliable unless very large numbers of cells are counted and consequently in most studies of the variations of leucocytes in disease the basophils have been ignored or dismissed in a few words as of no significance. In his monograph on mast cells, Michels (1938) gathered most of the information about basophils available at that time and the inaccuracy and contradictions of many of the earlier papers are readily apparent on reading this review, in which the author stigmatized much of the previous literature as 'worthless'. The few standard paediatric textbooks which do more than mention the existence of basophils merely remark on the lack of information available. For example, Nelson's *Textbook of Pediatrics* (Nelson, 1954) states that 'basophils occur in small numbers in the blood of children. Their function is unknown and they appear to have clinical significance only in that they are consistently elevated in chronic myelogenous leukemia in children'.

Recent evidence that basophils contain heparin (Behrens and Taubert, 1952; Martin and Roka, 1953) and histamine (Graham, Lowry, Wheelwright, Lenz and Parish, 1955; Code and Mitchell, 1957) throws fresh light on the function of these cells, while the introduction of a chamber-counting method by Moore and James (1953) has made it possible to measure even small changes in the numbers of circulating basophils with considerable accuracy. It therefore seemed worth while to undertake a study of these cells in the blood of children in order to determine more accurately the changes which occur in response to disease. The three diseases chosen for study were lobar pneumonia, acute rheumatism, and anaphylactoid purpura (Schönlein-Henoch syndrome), as examples of common acute diseases of varied aetiology in children.

The basophils were also counted in the blood of 67 healthy children, in order to obtain some indication of the normal variations.

* 'Basophil' should correctly be spelled 'basiphil' since it is derived from the Greek word βάσις (basis) but the spelling 'basophil' has become established in the literature.

Methods and Procedure

The method used was essentially that described by Moore and James (1953), except that 0·075% toluidine blue (B.D.H.) was used instead of 0·05% as recommended. The stain was adjusted to *p*H 7·75 with sodium hydroxide and filtered before the addition of saponin, which was made up as a 30% solution in 50% ethyl alcohol. Basophils, eosinophils and total leucocytes were counted simultaneously in the same counting chambers, all the counts being made by the author.

Free-flowing capillary blood obtained by finger-prick was used and all counts were made between 12 noon and 2 p.m., in nearly every case just before a meal. The only exception to this was that the initial counts in acutely ill children were made as soon as possible after admission to hospital, regardless of the time of day. Counts were made daily for the first five days after admission, at one week, and thereafter twice weekly.

The erythrocyte sedimentation rate (E.S.R.) was determined by a modification of Cutler's micro-method, except where otherwise indicated.

Healthy Children. The healthy children had been admitted to hospital for the treatment of some minor anatomical abnormality, in the great majority of cases an inguinal hernia, and a smaller group who were admitted to a short-stay children's home for social reasons, usually because the mother was in hospital. There were also a few enuretic children in whom full investigation had revealed no physical cause of the symptom. None of the children had a history of allergic diseases.

Lobar Pneumonia. Cases of pneumonia had to satisfy the following criteria: (*a*) onset of symptoms within the previous four days; (*b*) leucocytosis of over 12,000 per c.mm.; (*c*) pyrexia of at least 100° F.; (*d*) radiological evidence of pulmonary consolidation.

Eleven cases of pneumonia were studied, and all were treated with penicillin injected intramuscularly; two children (Cases 4 and 5) had a sulphonamide drug in addition. Ten of the children made a rapid and uninterrupted recovery while one seriously ill child (Case 8) did not respond to penicillin but rapidly recovered when treatment was changed to oral tetracycline on the fifth day.

Acute Rheumatism. To be included, cases of acute rheumatism had to satisfy the following criteria, which also fulfil the requirements for the diagnosis of rheumatic fever laid down by Jones (1944): (*a*) duration of symptoms for one week or less; (*b*) leucocytosis; (*c*) pyrexia; (*d*) migrating polyarthritis; (*e*) presence of a significant cardiac murmur; (*f*) E.S.R. above 50 mm. in the first hour. Nine children with acute rheumatism were studied; they were treated with salicylates in a dose of approximately 1 gr. per lb. per day, and an initial course of penicillin by intramuscular injection lasting one week.

Anaphylactoid Purpura. Children with anaphylactoid purpura were included in the study if they showed the specific exanthem (Gairdner, 1948), purpura of the characteristic distribution, and one or more swollen, painful joints. No child who had had a previous attack was included. Six children satisfied the criteria (Cases 22 to 27); except where indicated the only treatment given was a course of intramuscular penicillin lasting one week. Because of the interval which usually elapsed before the child was sent into hospital it was not always possible to make the first basophil count at the beginning of the disease, but it was made within a week of onset in five children and within two weeks in the sixth (Case 27). When the first count was made, however, all the children had fresh purpura and acute joint manifestations or acute abdominal pain with tenderness and muscle guarding.

Results

Healthy Children. Counts of basophils, eosinophils and total leucocytes were made on a single occasion in each of 67 healthy children. There were 46 boys and 21 girls, their ages ranging from 6 months to 12 years. The mean basophil count for the whole group was $45\cdot0\pm2\cdot5$ per c.mm., with a standard deviation of $\pm20\cdot1$ and a range from 13 to 94 per c.mm. The mean count for the boys was $45\cdot6\pm3\cdot1$ (S.D. $\pm21\cdot3$) and for the girls $43\cdot6\pm3\cdot5$ (S.D. $\pm17\cdot5$). When the children were grouped according to age, the mean counts were as follows:

Age (years)	No.	Basophils per c.mm.
-1	7	44·0
1-2	9	45·3
2-3	10	44·7
3-5	13	46·7
5-8	14	44·4
8-12	14	44·5

The basophil count thus does not alter significantly throughout childhood.

The mean eosinophil count for the whole group was $245\cdot8\pm22\cdot7$ per c.mm., with a standard deviation of $\pm185\cdot5$, and the mean total leucocyte count was 8,390 per c.mm.

In general the eosinophil count tended to be low when the basophil count was low and high when it was high, but there were many exceptions and the numerical relationship between the two types of cell was not a close one.

Lobar Pneumonia. The results of serial basophil counts in the 11 children with lobar pneumonia are shown in Fig. 1 and Table 1. In all cases the basophil count was low on the first day, none being over 20 per c.mm. Clinical recovery was associated with a rapid rise in the basophil count to reach a maximum during the second week, when no count of less than 50 per c.mm. was recorded. Thereafter the numbers of basophils began to fall; the counts were not continued after the third week because the patients were then discharged. As can be seen from Fig. 1, the curve of the mean eosinophil counts was similar to that of the mean basophil counts, and as would be expected the total leucocyte count rapidly fell to normal. In the severely ill boy (Case 8) whose illness did not respond to penicillin, the number of basophils remained low for the first four days but increased rapidly when tetracycline was given, reaching 135 per c.mm. on the 17th day.

Acute Rheumatism. Of the nine children who fulfilled the diagnostic criteria, eight (Cases 12 to 19) pursued an uncomplicated course to recovery and

TABLE 1

SERIAL BASOPHIL COUNTS IN 11 CASES OF LOBAR PNEUMONIA

Case No.	Age (years)	Days 1	2	3	4	5	7	10	14	17	21	24
		(Basophils per c.mm.)										
1	7	16	25	37	34	38	41	66	104	78		
2	3¼	13	34	38	42	44	46	78	70			
3	6¼	20	28	31	31	43	75	100	63	63		
4	7	19	31	25	25	29	38	55	58	53		
5	2¼	6	13	25	47	45	72	63	61	64		
6	3	19	31	37	38	46	56	74	56			
7	2½	19	25	45	41	46	72	53	56			
8	8¼	0	0	6	13	22	47	66	110	135	103	55
9	2¾	12	19	31	45	42	49	91	116	52		
10	5	12	16	31	53	52	87	91	69	66		
11	9	17	25	29	30	44	40	63	79	70		
Mean		14	22	30	36	41	57	73	77	73		

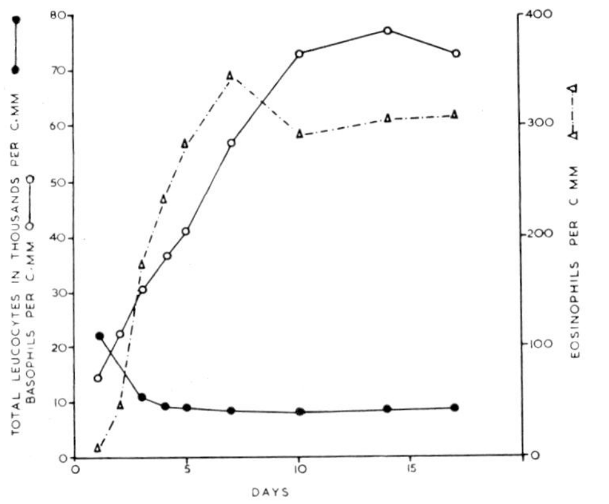

FIG. 1.—Mean basophil, eosinophil and total leucocyte counts in 11 cases of lobar pneumonia.

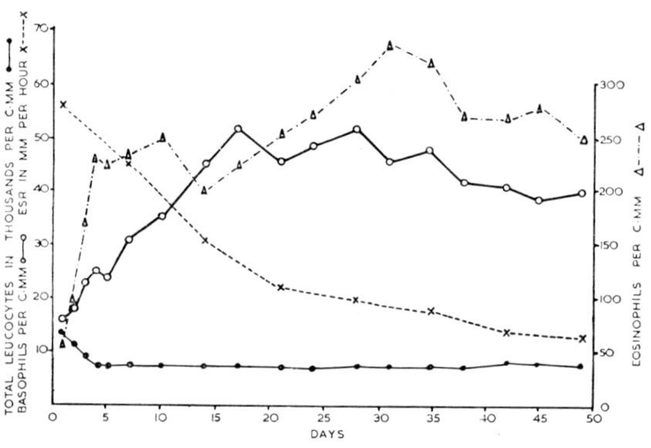

FIG. 2.—Mean basophil, eosinophil and total leucocyte counts and mean erythrocyte sedimentation rates in eight cases of acute rheumatism.

TABLE 2

SERIAL BASOPHIL COUNTS IN EIGHT CASES OF ACUTE RHEUMATISM

Case No.	Age (years)	Days 1	2	3	4	5	7	10	14	17	21	24	28	31	35	38	42	45	49
		(Basophils per c.mm.)																	
12	12	1	9	9	19	25	31	38	42	47	32	30	35	25	28	29	30	—	28
13	10	6	13	16	17	13	13	19	27	29	22	31	34	30	22	20	19	21	19
14	7½	30	22	27	28	38	37	28	28	42	49	—	59	—	63	52	48	50	56
15	11½	29	25	31	34	25	29	28	47	55	48	56	60	41	50	38	34	42	37
16	10	3	6	9	13	19	25	28	36	38	31	28	35	39	44	44	41	29	31
17	7	20	17	13	18	13	20	48	63	50	39	39	45	37	42	31	29	25	33
18	11	16	22	44	44	41	45	36	59	70	63	71	61	64	53	42	42	39	41
19	10	19	27	31	25	19	44	54	55	81	87	86	90	83	85	82	87	69	73
Mean		16	18	23	25	24	31	35	45	52	46	49	52	46	48	42	41	39	40

the changes in numbers of basophils are recorded in Fig. 2 and Table 2. As in the cases with pneumonia, the initial count in every case was low, none being above 30 per c.mm. In most cases the count remained low during the first week, rose gradually to reach a maximum in the third, fourth or fifth week, and thereafter fell slightly to a more or less stationary level. Counts were not continued beyond the seventh week of the illness as the children were usually sent home or transferred to a convalescent home on recovery.

The E.S.R. in all cases diminished steadily as recovery proceeded, being below 15 mm. per hour in six of the eight cases by the seventh week, and reaching this level soon afterwards in the other two. During the initial period of recovery (Figs 2 and 3), when the basophil count was rising to a maximum level, there was an inverse relationship between the

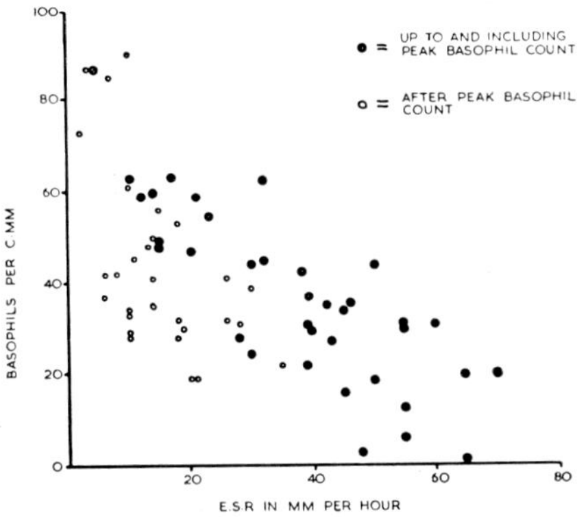

FIG. 3.—The relationship between the basophil count and the erythrocyte sedimentation rate in eight cases of acute rheumatism.

basophil count and the E.S.R. but this relationship ceased as the basophil count began to fall.

The ninth child with acute rheumatism was a boy of 9 years old who had a relapse during his illness and is therefore considered separately (Fig. 4, Case 20).

The basophil count was 25 per c.mm. on admission six days after the onset of symptoms. The pyrexia, leucocytosis and joint pains quickly subsided and after a few days the basophil count began to rise steadily, reaching 81 per c.mm. on the 17th day. During the same period the E.S.R. was gradually falling. At the end of the fourth week in hospital, however, there was a sudden recurrence of joint pains and pyrexia; the basophil count fell to 16 per c.mm. and the E.S.R. increased again. Salicylate dosage was increased, and the symptoms disappeared; the basophil count again began to rise, reaching 63 per c.mm. before levelling off at 50 per c.mm. Concurrently the E.S.R. fell to normal and the child thereafter made an uninterrupted recovery.

One further child with acute rheumatism who had no polyarthritis, and therefore did not fulfil the criteria, was nevertheless included in the study because she had severe carditis, subcutaneous nodules and a previous history of rheumatism so that the diagnosis could not be in doubt.

She was a girl of 11 years (Fig. 4, Case 21) who had had an acute attack of rheumatism two years previously from which she had made a good recovery. Five days before the first basophil count, she vomited and complained of abdominal pain. Pyrexia developed and on admission she was seriously ill with slight cyanosis, tachycardia, leucocytosis of 19,000 per c.mm., and an E.S.R. of 145 mm. in the first hour (Westergren). Subcutaneous nodules were palpable over the occipital region. Systolic and diastolic murmurs were audible at the heart apex and a radiograph of the chest showed considerable cardiac enlargement. The basophil count was 19 per c.mm. Treatment with salicylates and antibiotics resulted in some improvement; the E.S.R. after 10 days had fallen to 100 mm. per hour and the basophil count had risen to 55 per c.mm. During the next 14 days, however, the child's condition deteriorated, the apex beat moved out into the axilla, the E.S.R. rose again to 121 mm. per hour and the basophil count fell to 28 per c.mm. In view of this deterioration, treatment with cortisone was started; this resulted in disappearance of basophils from the peripheral blood and a fall in the E.S.R. to 10 mm. per hour, and coincided with clinical improvement. Two weeks after starting cortisone, however, she developed acute pharyngitis; the basophil count rose to 48 per c.mm. and the E.S.R. to 25 mm. per hour. With recovery, the basophil count again fell to a very low level, and the E.S.R. returned to normal. The dose of cortisone was gradually reduced, and when it was only 50 mg. per day, the basophil count began to rise, and the curve thereafter showed the gradual rise and fall with levelling off between 30 and 40 cells per c.mm., which has been demonstrated in recovery

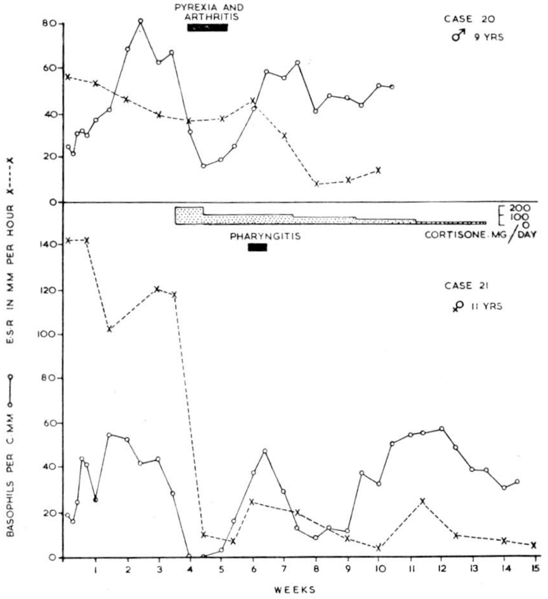

FIG. 4.—Serial basophil counts and erythrocyte sedimentation rates in two cases of acute rheumatism with complications.

from uncomplicated acute rheumatism. On reducing the dose of cortisone the E.S.R. showed a slight rise but quickly fell again to normal, and the child made a steady and uneventful recovery.

This case therefore illustrates a reversal of the usual inverse relationship between the basophil count and the E.S.R. as a result of the action of cortisone in reducing the E.S.R. and lowering the basophil count.

Anaphylactoid Purpura. Because of the variable course of the disease, the six children with anaphy-

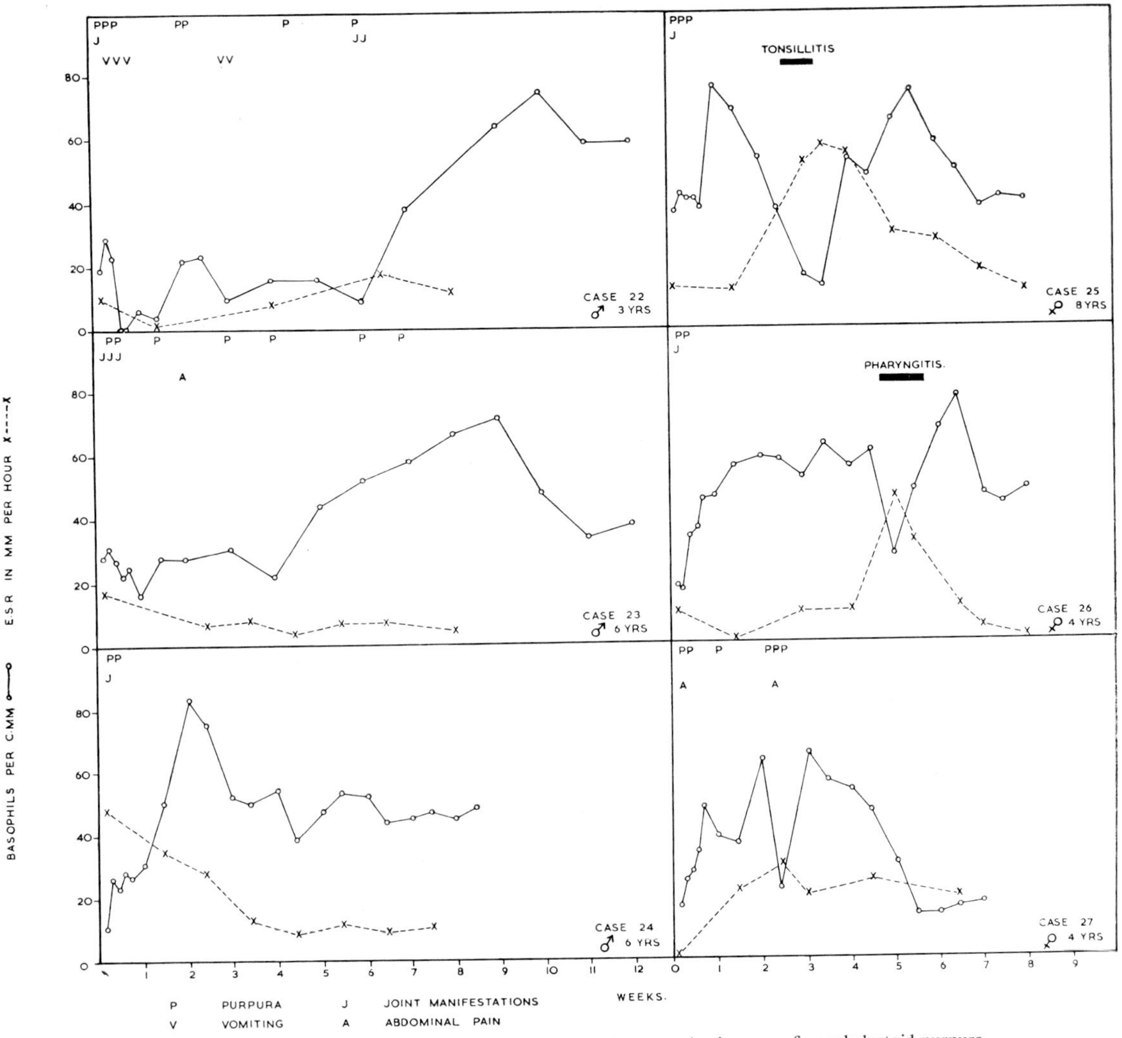

FIG. 5.—Serial basophil counts and erythrocyte sedimentation rates in six cases of anaphylactoid purpura.

lactoid purpura could not be treated as a single group for analysis of the results and the data for each child are therefore presented separately (Fig. 5).

In Case 22, the child was severely ill with vomiting and haematemesis, and fresh purpura continued to appear during the first six weeks. The basophil count remained low during this period, falling even lower during episodes of acute vomiting, and during a recrudescence of joint symptoms in the sixth week. With recovery the number of basophils increased steadily to a maximum count of 75 per c.mm. and then decreased a little and remained fairly stationary. Case 23 showed a similar series of events although the child was not so ill and recovery began about the fifth week. In spite of an uninterrupted clinical recovery this boy continued to have occasional slight purpura without any effect on the basophil count, which rose steadily to a maximum of 72 per c.mm. and then levelled off. In both Cases 22 and 23 the E.S.R. was low throughout the illness.

In Case 24 recovery was rapid and uninterrupted, with no further purpura or arthritis after the first few days. The basophil count rose rapidly from 11 per c.mm. on the day of admission to 83 per c.mm. at the end of two weeks and thereafter fell to about 45 per c.mm. The E.S.R. was high initially, possibly indicating a mild respiratory infection, and fell steadily as recovery progressed. Cases 25, 26 and 27 were each characterized by initial recovery, followed by a relapse or complication, succeeded again by recovery. In case 25 there were no further manifestations of the disease after the first few days and the basophil count rose quickly to 76 per c.mm. During the third week it fell rather rapidly and acute tonsillitis developed with pyrexia and an elevated E.S.R. Treatment with penicillin resulted in subsidence of the fever and inflammation, followed by a fall in the E.S.R. and a rise in the basophil count to reach 75 per c.mm. once again. Thereafter the count fell gradually to level off at about 40 per c.mm. Case 26 showed a similar course of events with an initial rise of the basophil count to a level of about 60 per c.mm., and a rapid drop to 28 per c.mm. in the fifth week, coincident with an acute attack of pharyngitis associated with an elevated E.S.R. With recovery from the acute infection, the E.S.R. fell and the basophil count rose to a maximum of 78 per c.mm. before levelling off between 45 and 50 per c.mm.

In Case 27 there was abdominal pain with fresh purpura on admission, when the basophil count was found to be 17 per c.mm. After two days the symptoms subsided and the basophil count rose to 63 per c.mm. at the end of the second week. During the third week there was a fresh outbreak of purpura with further abdominal pain, and the basophil count fell sharply to 22 per c.mm. Thereafter recovery was uninterrupted, the basophil count rose again to 65 per c.mm. and then fell gradually to a level of about 15 per c.mm.

In spite of the variable course pursued in this disease, therefore, there is a pattern in the basophil response. The count is low in the acute stage, and rises during recovery. A relapse or an intercurrent infection is usually associated with an abrupt fall in the numbers of circulating basophils, which may be the first indication of such a setback.

In anaphylactoid purpura, the occurrence of purpura cannot always be correlated with the clinical condition, and fresh crops of purpura may appear from time to time long after apparent recovery. Similarly the basophil count could not be related to the occurrence of purpura, but reflected rather the general clinical state. It was particularly noticeable that an acute episode of haematemesis with shock could result in the immediate disappearance of circulating basophils, as in Case 22; whereas the number of basophils might steadily increase in spite of recurring purpura, as in Case 23. Only in Case 27 did the recurrence of purpura appear to be associated with an abrupt fall in the basophil count, but there was abdominal pain as well, indicating a more severe disturbance than purpura alone.

In general the eosinophil counts followed the trend of the basophil counts, in so far as the numbers of eosinophils diminished during episodes of acute illness and tended to increase in the recovery phase. The counts were, however, much more variable and sudden and unaccountable fluctuations often took place without coincident changes in the basophil count or the clinical state.

Discussion

Basophil Counts in Healthy Children. The difficulty of selecting normal children for leucocyte counts has been pointed out by Sturgis and Bethell (1943). Relatively mild infections, such as are common among apparently healthy school children, may cause fluctuations in the leucocyte count, while increased eosinophil and basophil counts have been reported in chronic tonsillar enlargement and chronic sinusitis respectively (Bunting, 1914; Rud, 1947). It was therefore decided to study healthy children in hospital rather than in the schools or at home, because a thorough clinical examination could be made which would ensure the absence of minor infections. For this reason the number of healthy children is small but may nevertheless present a more accurate standard of health than a cross-section of the school population. The preponderance of boys is due to the greater frequency of inguinal hernia in boys than in girls.

The numbers of basophils in the peripheral blood of these healthy children are similar to those found in the blood of adults by the method of Moore and James (1953). Thus the mean count of $45 \cdot 0 \pm 2 \cdot 5$ per c.mm. does not differ significantly from the mean counts of 46·7 per c.mm. found in 36 men by Moore and James, 41·0 per c.mm. in 30 men and women by Angeli, Tedeschi and Cavazzuti (1954), and $44 \cdot 8 \pm 2 \cdot 4$ per c.mm. in 96 men and women by Rorsman (1957a), while the range from 13 to 94 per c.mm. is similar to the ranges of 11 to 107 recorded by Moore and James and of 9·3 to 112·5 recorded by Angeli and his colleagues. After the characteristic rise and fall in the basophil count in the immediate newborn period (Mitchell, 1955) the count remains at the same level throughout childhood, an observation which confirms the work of Kato (1935). Neither Angeli and his colleagues nor Rorsman found significant sex differences in their series of basophil counts and similarly in the present study no difference between the counts in boys and girls was found. Although the number of children is too small to fix the extreme limits of normal, basophil counts below 10 per c.mm. or above 110 per c.mm. should be regarded as probably abnormal, although for any one individual the limits of normal may be very much narrower. It is apparent that the criteria suggested by Alder (1923), namely, that an increase or decrease of more than 15 cells from a mean value of 35 cells per c.mm. should be regarded as pathological, are far too limited.

Basophil Counts in Disease. The ill children to be studied were carefully selected in order to exclude those who were only mildly ill or in whom the diagnosis was in doubt. Thus all the children included were moderately to severely ill and presented a 'textbook picture' of the disease concerned. This was considered to be important in determining the characteristic changes in the basophil count for each disease.

The results indicate that in the three acute diseases studied, the circulating basophils are scanty or absent during the acute phase, increase in number during recovery and are plentiful during the immediate convalescent phase of the illness. Similar changes occur in the numbers of eosinophils, a pattern of response to acute infection which is well established (Wolman, 1951; Weiner and Morkovin, 1952). With full clinical recovery the numbers of basophils return to normal levels; counts have not been continued long enough to determine whether further changes occur during the later stages of convalescence.

Basopenia. The finding of low basophil counts in the acute stages of disease is in accord with some of the earlier reports based on counts of basophils made from blood smears. Thus Arneth (1920) stated that basophils disappeared almost completely from the peripheral blood in influenza and Benjamin and Ward (1932) reported that, although individual counts were inaccurate by their method, there was generally a fall in the number of basophils during the febrile phase of measles, with a rise during convalescence amounting to basophilia during the second week. Whitby and Britton (1953) state that basophils may disappear altogether in acute infections. On the other hand Dible's textbook of pathology (1950) states that 'the proportion and number of basophil leucocytes in the blood are practically never affected by disease, if we except myeloid leukaemia and a slight increase in polycythaemia vera'.

There have been few reports based on accurate counting methods. Mallek (1955) and Labendzinski (1956) found low counts in some acute infectious diseases such as typhoid fever and bacillary dysentery, with a rise during recovery. Their technique involved the haemolysis of red cells and staining of basophils in a thick drop of blood, and was therefore an improvement on the older methods, but still lacked the precision of a counting chamber method. Rorsman (1957a), using a modification of the method of Moore and James (1953), found a mean basophil count of only $8 \cdot 1 \pm 2 \cdot 7$ per c.mm. in 22 cases of urticaria; no such basopenia was found in cases of asthma (Rorsman, 1957b).

Low basophil counts in the present series were generally accompanied by eosinopenia, a characteristic phenomenon of stress. It seems reasonable therefore to attribute the diminution in the number of basophils to the stress of the acute disease, since it is an apparently non-specific reaction common to several diseases of varying aetiology. On this view, it might be expected that other forms of stress would also cause basopenia. Camerada and Leo (1955) have shown experimentally that thyroxin causes a decrease in the numbers of basophils as well as of eosinophils, although it must be said that these authors attributed the effect to a specific action of thyroxin. Fig. 6 shows the results of serial basophil counts on a boy of 10 years with hyperthyroidism and a girl of 20 months with hypothyroidism. The basophil count was low in the acutely thyrotoxic state and rose to normal levels on treatment with thiouracil, whereas the basophil count was abnormally high in the cretin, and fell to normal levels after treatment with thyroid was started, with the usual delay of 10 days or so in the response to this hormone. These illustrative cases lend support to the view that the low basophil counts observed in acute disease are the result of non-specific stress. If such is the case cortisone should cause a disappearance of the basophils from the circulating blood stream, as it does with eosinophils, and this effect has in fact been demonstrated (Code, Mitchell and Kennedy, 1954). It might be argued that the very low basophil counts found in urticaria by Rorsman (1957a) were due to stress, but here the situation is rather different because urticaria is common to a heterogeneous collection of conditions in many of which there is evidence of disordered histamine metabolism (Rose, 1941; Adam, Hunter and Kinnear, 1950). Rorsman's patients had no general systemic disturbance so that the very low counts observed are more likely to have been peculiar to urticaria and not the result of a non-specific stimulus.

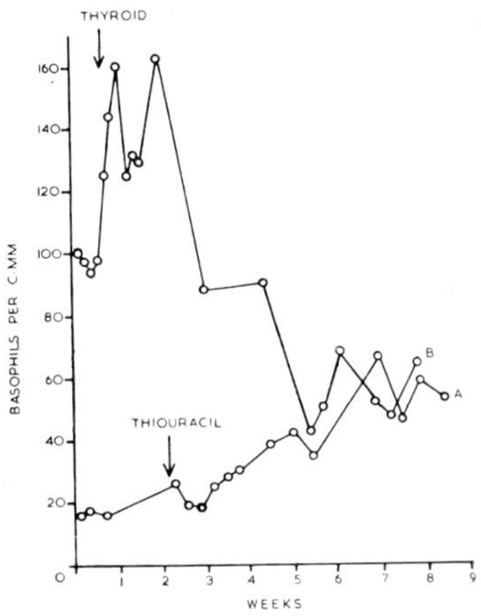

FIG. 6.—Serial basophil counts in (A) a boy with hyperthyroidism treated with thiouracil and (B) a girl with hypothyroidism treated with thyroid extract.

Basophilia. The present work indicates that there

are increased numbers of circulating basophils during the phase of recovery from an acute disease. Increases in the numbers of basophils are more readily observed by differential counts from blood smears than decreases, and therefore although earlier reports on the incidence of low basophil counts were often uncertain and conflicting, there is a larger and to some extent more reliable collection of evidence that the basophil count may be increased in certain diseases. Thus it is established that there may be very considerable numbers of circulating basophils in leukaemia and in polycythaemia (Ehrlich, 1891; Alder, 1923; Doan and Reinhart, 1941). Although extremely high counts have been recorded in leukaemia, even as high as 163,000 basophils per c.mm. (Joachim, 1906), the highest count so far recorded by the present writer was 237 basophils per c.mm. in a boy of 3 years with acute leukaemia, who had 400,000 leucocytes and 419 eosinophils per c.mm. When the total leucocyte count fell to 30,400 per c.mm. one week after starting treatment with mercaptopurine, the basophils fell to 17 per c.mm. and the eosinophils to 25 per c.mm., while at two weeks the leucocyte count was 4,800 per c.mm. the basophils were 9 per c.mm. and the eosinophils had disappeared completely. This suggests that mercaptopurine may have a greater effect than irradiation on the basophils in leukaemia, since there is evidence that these cells are resistant to radioactive agents (Doan and Reinhart, 1941; Johansen, 1955), with the possible exception of radioactive phosphorus (Turchini and Kein, 1955).

Apart from these diseases of the blood-forming organs, an increase in the number of circulating basophils has been reported in other blood diseases, such as chronic haemolytic anaemia and chlorosis (Alder, 1923), and in diseases of the skin (Canon, 1892; Klausner and Kreibich, 1913). Bunting (1914) reported that the basophils are increased in early Hodgkin's disease, but thought that this might be due to chronic sinusitis, which according to this author is constantly associated with an increased number of basophils. Graham (1920) reported increased numbers of basophils in a patient infected with hookworms. Nevertheless, as recently as 1951, Muir's *Textbook of Pathology* observed that 'there is no condition known which regularly calls forth a basophil leucocytosis'.

Bigart (1902) and Rubinato (1907) reported that in cirrhosis of the liver there were greatly increased numbers of circulating basophils, amounting to as much as 20·6% of the total leucocyte count in one case, an observation of some interest since high levels of blood histamine have recently been recorded in this disease (Mitchell, Butt and Code, 1954).

As with the initial basopenia, the basophilia during recovery from acute disease cannot at present be related to any function of the basophils, but is probably a non-specific response to the earlier stress.

Clinical Value of Basophil Counts. The eosinophil count is of some use as a guide to progress in an acute infection (Hain, 1951; Whitby and Britton, 1953), and the greater consistency of the basophil count suggests that it might be of even greater value. Moreover, the demonstrated relationship between the basophil count and the E.S.R. indicates a possible use for the basophil count in the prognosis of acute rheumatism, since a steady increase in the number of circulating basophils has the same significance as a steadily falling E.S.R. Unfortunately the limiting factor is the wide range of normal values, compared with the small range of normal for the E.S.R. The basophil count is remarkably constant in the healthy individual but the normal level is not usually known when a patient is seen in the acutely ill stage. Occasionally the basophil count performed daily has proved of value, when a sudden fall in the number of basophils has been the first indication of a relapse, preceding clinical manifestations by a day or more. Nevertheless increasing experience of basophil counts in a variety of clinical conditions indicates that not enough is known about the factors which may influence the count to permit its use as a reliable clinical test at present.

Functions of the Basophil. In the early years of this century there was much discussion on the relationship of the basophils (mast cells of the blood) to the mast cells of the tissues, but by the late thirties enough information had accumulated to enable Michels (1938) to state that 'in mammals the two types have nothing in common save the basophilic metachromatic staining granules'. This statement must be modified today, since the tissue mast cells, like the basophils, contain both heparin and histamine (Jorpes, 1946; Riley and West, 1953). Nevertheless, the balance of evidence still favours the view that the two types of cell are distinct.

At various times the basophils have been regarded as degenerating lymphocytes, as unripe eosinophils, and even as 'a vestigial remain analogous with the appendix' (Phillips, 1953), but they are now generally accepted as mature granulocytes fully equivalent to the eosinophils and neutrophils (Michels, 1938). There may, however, be a functional relationship between basophils and eosinophils, since they have certain properties in common such as their response to stress or to cortisone (Code *et al.*, 1954; Hamerston, Elveback, Halberg and Gully, 1956). Moreover, there is evidence that while basophils are the main reservoir of histamine in the blood, the eosinophils also sometimes carry histamine, providing additional histamine-carrying capacity which is readily available when the occasion arises (Code and Mitchell, 1957).

It seems reasonable to assume that the content of such potent substances as heparin and histamine bears some relationship to the function of the basophil, although there may be other, possibly more fundamental, activities. Tötterman (1948) searched for evidence of an increased tendency to haemorrhage when increased numbers of basophils were present in the peripheral blood, but was unable to demonstrate that such basophilia predisposed to bleeding. This is perhaps not surprising, since Angeli and his colleagues (1955) showed experimentally that the intravenous injection of heparin caused an increase in the number of circulating basophils, and that the period of maximum augmentation of the basophil count coincided with the most rapid diminution in anti-coagulant activity of the injected heparin, an effect which they attributed to a specific regulatory action of the basophils. Wintrobe (1951) considered that basophils might function in inflammation by delivering anticoagulants to facilitate absorption or to prevent clotting of blood and lymph in the obstructed tissue. The chemical studies of Turchini and Kien (1955) led them to believe that in the presence of disease the synthesis of heparin in the basophils is disturbed so that precursor substances are liberated which are necessary for the elimination of toxic products.

As far as histamine is concerned, Graham and her colleagues (1955) suggested that the basophils may be a source of a limited amount of the amine which is immediately available wherever needed to tide over the period before the arrival of more adequate supplies from the tissue mast cells. It is possible, on the other hand, that the basophils are simply a safe means of transporting a potentially toxic substance pending its destruction or excretion.

It is apparent that in spite of recent progress we are still a long way from answering what Riley (1954) has called the 'riddle of the mast cells', and the answer is unlikely to be found until the larger problems of the physiological significance of heparin and histamine in the body have been solved.

Summary

The circulating basophils have been counted in 67 healthy children and in 27 acutely ill children throughout the course of their illness.

The counts in healthy children were not significantly different from those found in adults by other authors, and the mean count did not vary significantly throughout childhood.

In the three acute diseases studied, lobar pneumonia, acute rheumatism, and anaphylactoid purpura, the number of circulating basophils was always low in the acute stage and high during the stage of recovery. These are regarded as non-specific changes in response to the stress of the acute disease.

Serial basophil counts give some indication of the progress of the disease but are not sufficiently reliable to be of practical clinical use at present.

Possible functions of the basophils are discussed.

I am grateful to Professor J. L. Henderson for his encouragement and criticism.

References

Adam, H. M., Hunter, R. B. and Kinnear, T. W. G. (1950). *Quart. J. exp. Physiol.*, **36**, 49.
Alder, A. (1923). *Folia haemat. teil I. Arch. (Lpz.)*, **28**, 249.
Angeli, G., Tedeschi, G. and Cavazzuti, F. (1954). *Prog. med. (Napoli)*, **10**, 742.
——, ——, —— (1955). *Minerva med. (Torino)*, **46** (**2**), 752.
Arneth, F. (1920). *Berl. klin. Wschr.*, **57**, 109.
Behrens, M. and Taubert, M. (1952). *Klin. Wschr.*, **30**, 76.
Benjamin, B. and Ward, S. M. (1932). *Amer. J. Dis. Child.*, **44**, 921.
Bigart, M. (1902). *C.R. Soc. Biol. (Paris)*, **54**, 1529.
Bunting, C. H. (1914). *Johns Hopk. Hosp. Bull.*, **25**, 173.
Camerada, P. and Leo, P. (1955). *Rass. med. Sarda*, n.s. **6**, 163.
Canon, P. (1892). *Dtsch. med. Wschr.*, **18**, 206.
Code, C. F. and Mitchell, R. G. (1957). *J. Physiol. (Lond.)*, **136**, 449.
——, —— and Kennedy, J. C. (1954). *Proc. Mayo Clin.*, **29**, 200.
Dible, J. H. (1950). Dible and Davie's *Pathology*, 3rd ed. London.
Doan, C. A. and Reinhart, H. L. (1941). *Amer. J. clin. Path.*, **11**, 1.
Ehrlich, P. (1891). *Farbenanalytische Untersuchungen zur Histologie und Klinik des Blutes.* Berlin.
Gairdner, D. (1948). *Quart. J. Med.*, n.s. **17**, 95.
Graham, G. S. (1920). *J. exp. Med.*, **31**, 209.
Graham, H. T., Lowry, O. H., Wheelwright, F., Lenz, M. A. and Parish, H. H. Jr. (1955). *Blood*, **10**, 467.
Hain, K. (1951) *Pediatrics*, **7**, 408.
Hamerston, O., Elveback, L., Halberg, F. and Gully, R. J. (1956). *J. appl. Physiol.*, **9**, 205.
Joachim, G. (1906). *Dtsch. Arch. klin. Med.*, **87**, 437.
Johansen, C. (1955). *Nord. Med.*, **53**, 212.
Jones, T. D. (1944). *J. Amer. med. Ass.*, **126**, 481.
Jorpes, J. E. (1946). *Heparin in the Treatment of Thrombosis*, 2nd ed. London.
Kato, K. (1935). *J. Pediat.*, **7**, 7.
Klausner, E. and Kreibich, C. (1913). *Folia haemat. teil I. Arch. (Lpz.)*, **15**, 347.
Labendzinski, F. (1956). *Sang*, **27**, 432.
Mallek, D. (1955). *Pol. Tyg. lek.*, **10**, 1400.
Martin, H. and Roka, L. (1953). *Acta haemat. (Basel)*, **10**, 26.
Michels, N. A. (1938). In *Handbook of Hematology*, ed. H. Downey, London.
Mitchell, R. G. (1955). *Arch. Dis. Childh.*, **30**, 130.
——, Butt, H. R. and Code, C. F. (1954). *J. clin. Invest.*, **33**, 1199.
Moore, J. E. III and James, G. W. III (1953). *Proc. Soc. exp. Biol. (N.Y.)*, **82**, 601.
Muir, R. (1951). Muir's *Textbook of Pathology*. Revised by D. F. Cappell, 6th ed. London.
Nelson, W. E. (1954). *Textbook of Pediatrics*, 6th ed. Philadelphia.
Phillips, W. (1953). In *Medicine*, ed. H. G. Garland and W. Phillips, London.
Riley, J. F. (1954). *Lancet*, **1**, 841.
—— and West, G. B. (1953). *J. Physiol. (Lond.)*, **120**, 528.
Rorsman, H. (1957a). *Acta derm.-venereol. (Stockh.)*, **37**, 121.
—— (1957b). Personal communication.
Rose, B. (1941). *J. Allergy*, **12**, 327.
Rubinato, J. (1907). *Folia. haemat. (Lpz.)*, 4, Suppl. p. 198.
Rud, F. (1947). *Acta psychiat. (Kbh.)*, Suppl. 40.
Sabin, F. R. (1923). *Johns Hopk. Hosp. Bull.*, **34**, 277.
Sturgis, C. C and Bethell, F. H. (1943). *Physiol. Rev.*, **23**, 279.
Tötterman, G. (1948). *Acta med. scand.*, **130**, 176.
Turchini, J. and Kien, L. K. van. (1955). *Rev. belge. Path.*, **24**, 520.
Weiner, H. A. and Morkovin, D. (1952). *Amer. J. Med.*, **13**, 58.
Whitby, L. E. H. and Britton, C. J. C. (1953). *Disorders of the Blood*, 7th ed. London.
Wintrobe, M. M. (1951). *Clinical Hematology*, 3rd ed. London.
Wolman, I. J. (1951). *Quart. Rev. Pediat.*, **6**, 287.

INTRAPERITONEAL BLOOD TRANSFUSION IN CHILDREN IN ACCRA WITH SPECIAL REFERENCE TO THE TREATMENT OF KWASHIORKOR

BY

SUSAN B. G. OFORI ATTA

From the Princess Marie Louise Hospital, Accra, Ghana

(RECEIVED FOR PUBLICATION NOVEMBER 11, 1957)

The giving of blood to small children presents particular difficulties to medical practitioners in West Africa. Equipment is often inadequate and the time required to ensure the success of the transfusion can often be ill-spared from numerous other hospital and out-patient duties. In addition, the children are usually ill-nourished and dehydrated and intravenous therapy is a major undertaking to those unpractised in paediatric techniques. Waite, Colucci and Glaser (1956) recorded the successful transfusion of blood by the intraperitoneal route in young children and this appears to be a simple and rapid procedure which, if successful, would be of the greatest benefit to practitioners and their young patients in West Africa. This method has been used in Accra and, to date, 43 intraperitoneal blood transfusions have been given to 36 children with clinically satisfactory results. In this paper the methods utilized are outlined and the results briefly discussed. Details of 15 transfusions which have been given to 11 malnourished babies are given.

Methods

The majority of the children were suffering from marasmus, marasmic kwashiorkor or kwashiorkor. Intercurrent infection and multiple infestations were common. The patients with florid signs of kwashiorkor with oedema were treated with skimmed milk alone or skimmed milk with soya bean flour and/or fish until the oedema disappeared (the child then looking the picture of marasmic kwashiorkor) before transfusion was given.

The usual routine in saline and albumin grouping and compatibility tests was followed and the results confirmed by an indirect Coombs test. All the children were rhesus positive (anti-D). In Accra the incidence of the sickle-cell and haemoglobin C traits is in the region of 19% and 10% respectively and the blood with these traits is normally stored and utilized by the transfusion service (Edington, 1956). It was not, however, employed for intraperitoneal transfusions excluding one instance in which S trait blood was given intraperitoneally to one sickling negative baby and the subsequent appearance of the sickling positive cells in the peripheral circulation was studied.

The patients were prepared as for paracentesis abdominis. (In Ghana special care has to be taken in the examination of the liver, spleen and bladder.) The patient was propped up and the abdominal wall and peritoneum 2 inches below and lateral to the umbilicus was anaesthetized with 1% novocaine. The usual routine giving set with a 20-gauge needle was employed and the blood allowed to drip through the set before the needle was inserted into the peritoneal cavity. The amount usually given was 20 ml. per lb. body weight and the rate of flow was regulated to 30 drops per minute. A cover of penicillin was given during the transfusion and sedation when required. Following transfusion a course of antimalarial therapy was prescribed to obviate the possibility of transmitting malaria.

Results

Three of the 39 children transfused died. The minimum period between transfusion and death was two days and the maximum 20 weeks. In no instance was the transfusion thought to be implicated in the cause of death. Necropsies were performed on all three children. A child suffering from severe marasmus died two days after transfusion. Necropsy revealed the cause of death to be marasmus and bronchopneumonia. The free blood in the peritoneal cavity was fluid and uninfected and no adhesions were noted. Haemolysis had not occurred. A second child, an orphan, aged 4 months and weighing only 4 lb. 10 oz., had been fed entirely on maize gruel from the age of 2 days. Death occurred 12 weeks after the transfusion and a necropsy established that the cause was hydronephrosis, pyelonephritis, interstitial pneumonitis and malnutrition. The peritoneal cavity contained a few black specks in the paracolic gutter but was otherwise normal. A third child died 20 weeks after transfusion. The peritoneal cavity was free from infection and adhesions.

From the results of these necropsies it would appear that the introduction of compatible blood into the peritoneal cavity is unlikely to lead to complications in later life.

The infants in general withstood the procedure well: only one severe reaction occurred and that was in the sickling negative infant who received sickling positive blood. The complications observed after transfusion were abdominal distension in 27 cases (this was usually mild, gave no cause for anxiety and cleared up within 48 hours), mild pyrexia in 26 cases, and one abdominal haematoma which resolved spontaneously. There were no cases with melaena, bowel symptoms or jaundice.

The sickle-cell negative patient who received compatible sickling positive blood (20 ml. per lb. body weight) showed the most severe reaction—the temperature rose to 102·8° F. and vomiting, restlessness and abdominal distension occurred. These symptoms regressed spontaneously at the end of four days. The eventual response to transfusion in this patient was considered, however, to be eminently satisfactory. The rate of appearance of the sickling positive cells in the peripheral blood of the patient was studied and the results are shown in Table 1.

TABLE 1

PERCENTAGE OF SICKLING POSITIVE CELLS (S) APPEARING IN PERIPHERAL BLOOD OF NON-SICKLING INFANT

Day*	S Cells	Day*	S Cells	Day*	S Cells
	%		%		%
1	Scanty	49	9	70	0·2
2	Scanty	53	8	71	0·1
4	1	56	8	73	0·5
9	4	58	7	73	Scanty
21	15	60	5	74	Nil
28	12	69	1	75	Nil

* Day following transfusion.

From Table 1 it appears that, following intraperitoneal blood transfusion, the transfused cells reach their greatest concentration in the peripheral blood two to four weeks after transfusion. No sickling positive cells were detected in the peripheral blood at the end of 74 days. No explanation can be given for this. The recipient did not appear to be suffering from a haemolytic anaemia and, as the average life of the erythrocyte is 120 days and as sickle-cell trait cells are known to survive normally, it was expected that the sickled cells would be detected for a longer period.

The clinical response of the patients to blood

TABLE 2

CLINICAL DETAILS OF 11 BABIES SUFFERING FROM SEVERE MALNUTRITION TREATED BY INTRAPERITONEAL BLOOD TRANSFUSIONS

Case No.	Age (months)	Weight on day of Transfusion (lb.)	(oz.)	Condition	Hb. before Transfusion (%)	Hb. after Transfusion (%)	Result	Remarks
1	8	9	4	(Failure to thrive) Marasmus	60	85	Discharged	
2	4½	5	4	Marasmus	57	70	Died after 12 weeks	
3	14	11	3	Marasmic kwashiorkor	40* 65	60 78	Discharged	Slow progress
4	12	11	0	Marasmic kwashiorkor	55	83	Discharged	
5	5	7	2	(Failure to thrive) Marasmus	45 60	67 90	Discharged	Attack of malaria before 2nd transfusion
6	9	8	1	Marasmus	53	75	Discharged	
7	44½	22	11	Marasmic kwashiorkor	55	79	Discharged	
8	12	10	2½	Kwashiorkor	44	67	Discharged	
9	30 T	11	1	Kwashiorkor	55	71	Discharged	
10	18	13	0	Marasmic kwashiorkor	50 63	70 81	Died 20 weeks after transfusion	Two attacks of malaria before 2nd transfusion
11	about 10	9	1	Kwashiorkor	45 69	68 80	Discharged	Slow progress

* Where two figures appear under haemoglobin before and after transfusion, the top figure refers to the first transfusion and the lower figure to the second transfusion.

transfusion was good. Brief details of 11 severely malnourished patients who had received 15 transfusions are given in Table 2.

It is difficult to assess the results of treatment in kwashiorkor, and controlled studies were not possible. Clinically, however, the babies appeared to benefit immensely from the transfusion (Figs. 1 and 2) and, perhaps most important, the nursing staff were most enthusiastic about it as a method of treatment. Not only did the transfusion increase the haemoglobin level of the blood but it appeared to increase the child's resistance to intercurrent infection, the incidence of which, especially of staphylococcal infection, was lower in these children. The rate of recovery was also usually greatly accelerated. Four patients, however, showed a comparatively slow response and in these cases transfusion was repeated in six weeks when a rapid recovery ensued.

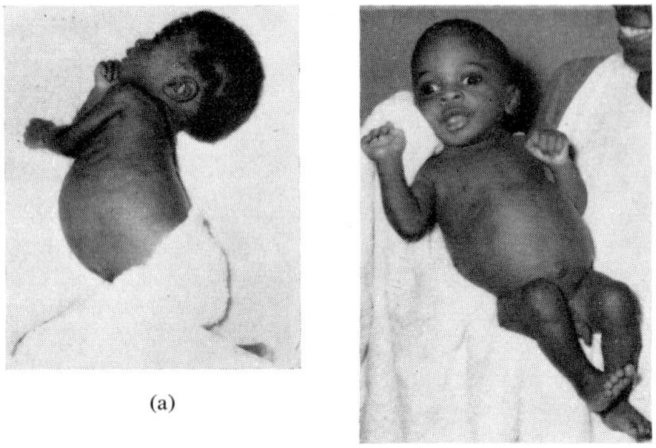

(a) (b)

FIG. 1.—Case 5. Boy aged 5 months, (*a*) before treatment: marasmus; weight 7 lb. 2 oz. and (*b*) after treatment.

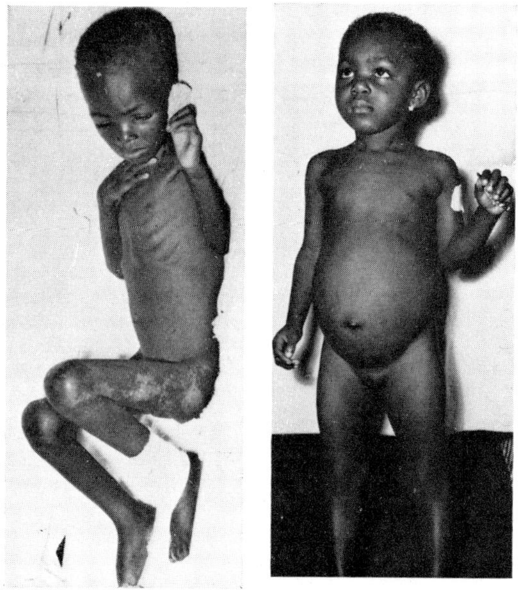

(a) (b)

FIG. 2.—Case 7. Girl aged 44½ months, (*a*) before treatment: marasmic kwashiorkor; weight 22 lb. 11 oz. and (*b*) after treatment.

Comment

In the malnutritional syndromes seen in Accra the most important single factor lacking in the diet is protein and it would appear that the giving of blood is a simple and rapid method of remedying this deficiency. Hitherto blood has not been used in the treatment of marasmus and kwashiorkor in Accra in view of the technical difficulties involved, and also because it is only recently that blood has become readily available for transfusion. The intraperitoneal transfusion provides a simple and safe method of giving blood to these patients. Clinically the infants have responded well to this form of therapy. It is regrettable that full biochemical investigations could not be undertaken in each case but time and staff were lacking and it is hoped that in the future a more intensive investigation can be done. Meanwhile, however, it has been shown that intraperitoneal blood transfusion is a useful and simple therapeutic measure in West Africa.

Summary

Intraperitoneal blood transfusion has been found to be a safe and simple method of treatment. Erythrocytes are absorbed from the peritoneal cavity into the peripheral circulation. Abdominal complications are unlikely to occur in later life.

My thanks are due to the Chief Medical Officer, Ghana, for permission to publish, to Dr. G. M. Edington for advice and details of the necropsies, to the nursing staff of the Princess Marie Louise Hospital and to the staff of the Medical Research Institute, particularly Mr. Sackey.

REFERENCES

Edington, G. M. (1956). *W. Afr. med. J.*, n.s. **5**, 71.

Waite, M. E., Colucci, D. D. and Glaser, J. (1956). *Amer. J. Dis. Child.*, **91**, 561.

TRAUMATIC SUBPERIOSTEAL HAEMATOMA OF THE FEMUR IN THE NEWBORN

BY

ROSS G. MITCHELL and K. RHANEY

From the Department of Child Health, University of St. Andrews

(RECEIVED FOR PUBLICATION DECEMBER 2, 1957)

Subperiosteal haemorrhage usually accompanies fracture of a long bone at birth. The occurrence at birth of a subperiosteal haematoma without fracture was not widely recognized until attention was drawn to the condition by Snedecor, Knapp and Wilson (1935), who called it 'traumatic ossifying periostitis'. A few other reports of this type of birth injury were subsequently published under such titles as periosteal stripping (Burman and Langsam, 1939), neonatal contusion (Caffey, 1945) and ossifying haematoma (Brailsford, 1948), and the subject was later reviewed by Snedecor and Wilson (1949). The number of reported cases is still small, and no pathological studies have yet been published; we therefore present two cases, one of which was examined at necropsy.

Case Reports

Case 1 (M.H. 52/343). A first-born female child was born at term, her weight being 7 lb. 10 oz. (3·5 Kg.). She presented as a frank breech in the left sacro-anterior position. To effect delivery the left leg was brought down with some difficulty, the right following more easily. The baby appeared normal at birth but on the third day it was noted that she was not moving the left leg as freely as the right and that there was slight pitting oedema of the left foot. On the following day the distal end of the left femoral shaft was tender and felt thicker than normal. The infant's general condition was good and radiographic examination of the affected femur revealed no abnormality. (Fig. 1). At one week the thickening of the femur was more pronounced and there was radiological evidence of subperiosteal 'ossification' around the shaft which gradually increased (Figs. 2 to 5). The infant's general progress was quite satisfactory and she was discharged from hospital on the thirteenth day. At the age of 16 months radiological examination of the femur showed no abnormality (Fig. 6).

Case 2 (D.R.I. 54/274). A female infant weighing 8 lb. (3·6 Kg.) was born at term, the pregnancy being the mother's eighth. The mother was admitted in labour, with the infant presenting as a transverse lie, the arm having prolapsed into the vagina. Internal version was carried out with some difficulty and was followed by breech extraction. Following delivery the infant's condition was poor and she was kept in oxygen for 24 hours. During the first few days she was lethargic and fed slowly. It was noted that she was not moving her legs, and examination indicated that there had been severe injury to the spinal cord: there was slight costal indrawing, a patulous anus through which meconium constantly dribbled, and flaccid paralysis of both legs, though strong stimulation resulted in a withdrawal reflex. Radiological examination of the legs on the fourth day showed no evidence of injury to the bones (Fig. 7).

Towards the end of the first week pitting oedema of both legs developed and on the eighth day she was admitted to a paediatric ward in Dundee Royal Infirmary where the clinical findings were confirmed. By the end of the second week the oedema had diminished and there was now slight thickening of the distal end of the right femoral shaft. Radiological examination showed an opacity round the cortex of the femur, and this subsequently increased in size and density (Figs. 8 to 10). The oedema of the legs had completely disappeared when the infant was 3 weeks old although there was no appreciable diminution of the paralysis. Despite the severity of the birth injuries the infant fed well and seemed contented. An unexplained pyrexia developed at the age of 3 weeks. It was not associated with a leucocytosis and the blood was sterile on culture; radiological examination showed a small patch of atelectasis at the apex of the right lung. Intermittent pyrexia up to 105° F. continued for five weeks despite treatment with streptomycin and chlortetracycline, but the infant gained weight steadily, began to take notice and made slight spontaneous movements of the legs. The intermittent pyrexia subsided at the age of 8 weeks, but in the meantime costal indrawing had increased, and 10 days later the infant suddenly died from respiratory failure.

SUMMARY OF NECROPSY. The spinal cord showed gross destruction from approximately C 7 to T 3. The damaged segments were shrunken and stained with altered blood pigment. The lungs showed hypostatic congestion and oedema; the major intra-pulmonary bronchi contained mucopus and much of the right lung was collapsed. The other organs showed no abnormality

Figures 1 to 6. Serial radiographs of the left knee in Case 1.

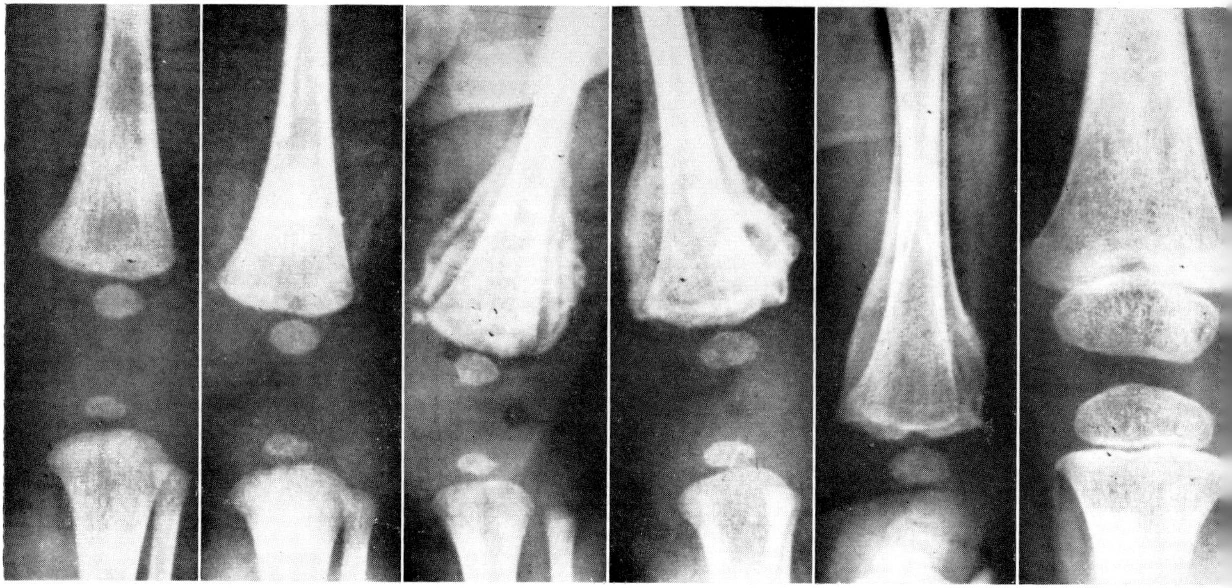

FIG. 1.—4 days. FIG. 2.—7 days. FIG. 3.—14 days. FIG. 4.—21 days. FIG. 5.—35 days. FIG. 6.—16 months.

FIG. 1.—No abnormality visible on fourth day after birth.

FIGS. 2-5.—Appearance and subsequent increase of subperiosteal ossification round lower end of femur.

FIG. 6.—At 16 months the ossified haematoma has disappeared completely and femur appears normal.

on macroscopic and histological examination. The right femur which showed no gross abnormality was removed and examined histologically.

HISTOLOGY OF RIGHT FEMUR. Transverse sections of the distal part of the shaft (Figs. 11 and 12) showed that part of the surface was covered by a layer of new subperiosteal bone which was less sclerotic than the original cortex. The new bone enclosed a relatively large space, surrounded by scar tissue and filled with degenerated blood and fibrin and fragments of dead bone but these had not excited any osteoclastic activity. The scar tissue contained many histiocytes laden with haemosiderin but showed no evidence of pyogenic inflammation. The cortex of the original shaft appeared to be thinner beneath the new layer than it was elsewhere but showed no other abnormality.

Discussion

Clinical Features. Subperiosteal haematoma of a long bone in a newborn infant is almost invariably the result of trauma during birth. It should be suspected when there is a history of difficult delivery, particularly if internal version has been performed, and there is limitation of movement of a limb, possibly pain on passive movement, and swelling of soft tissue. Careful palpation will usually reveal tender thickening around the affected bone. At this stage, radiological examination may show the soft tissue swelling but will probably reveal no bony abnormality. However, the diagnosis will be confirmed by the radiological changes which appear after the first week (Figs. 1-10). In the absence of clinical signs of injury, minor degrees of subperiosteal haemorrhage may easily be overlooked; thus, Snedecor and Wilson (1949) found evidence of the condition in no less than three of 50 consecutive breech deliveries when routine radiographs of the limbs were taken on the 7th day of life. In their experience the distal end of the femur is most commonly involved although the proximal end and the tibia may be affected. Involvement of the humerus has also been reported, usually when delivery has been by the vertex (Scaglietti, 1938).

Injury to the epiphysis is quite commonly associated with subperiosteal haematoma but was not present in either of our cases. Both lesions occurred together in two of the 11 cases of injury to the long bones at birth reported by Snedecor and Wilson (1949) while four had epiphyseal damage alone.

Pathogenesis. Subperiosteal haemorrhage is probably produced by manual traction on a limb combined with torsion (Snedecor *et al.*, 1935) and hence

Figures 7 to 10.—Serial radiographs of the right femur in Case 2.

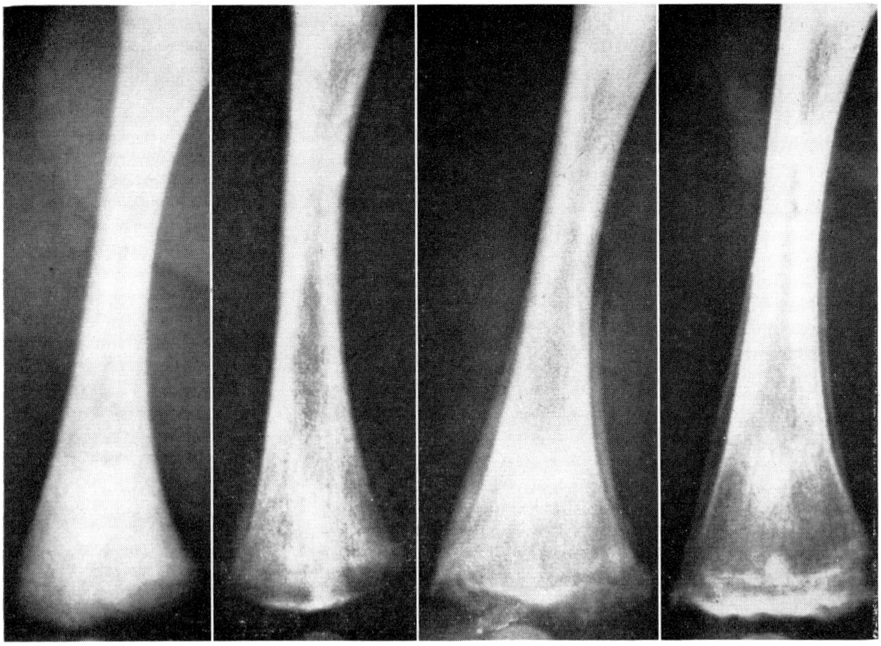

FIG. 7.—4 days. FIG. 8.—17 days. FIG. 9.—22 days. FIG. 10.—32 days.

FIG. 7.—No abnormality visible on fourth day after birth.

FIGS. 8-10.—Appearance and subsequent increase of ossification in subperiosteal haematoma.

(The opacity immediately above the epiphyseal centre in Fig. 9 is an artefact.)

is most likely to occur in a difficult internal version and in an assisted breech delivery.

Stripping of the periosteum from the shaft of a long bone is believed to occur much more easily in the foetus and newborn than in the adult (Macewen, 1912; Caffey, 1945). This impression appears to have been confirmed by investigation at necropsy (Barmeyer, Alderson and Cox, 1951) and it is therefore reasonable to assume that forcible periosteal stripping during delivery injures or tears the numerous blood vessels that are known to enter the bony cortex from the periosteal layer (Ham, 1953) giving rise to a subperiosteal haematoma which is presumably followed by the formation of callus and new subperiosteal bone. This belief is supported by the histological findings in Case 2, particularly by the evidence that bleeding had occurred at the site of the new subperiosteal bone. However, the presence of fragments of dead bone within this new subperiosteal layer indicates that bone injury, albeit of minor degree, has accompanied periosteal stripping and various possible explanations for this have obviously to be considered. A gross fracture of the shaft can reasonably be excluded, and we believe that direct manual compression during obstetrical manipulation is unlikely to cause necrosis of the dense cortical bone of the femoral shaft in a mature infant, though it might crush the more delicate trabeculae, many of them radially arranged (Ham, 1953), of immature cortical bone. The most probable explanation is that periosteal stripping was accompanied by avulsion of fragments of cortical bone as well as by subperiosteal haemorrhage, for our investigations at necropsy in the newborn have shown that the periosteum of the femur, though easily stripped from most of the shaft, is more firmly attached to the metaphysis and is inseparable from the bone and its muscle attachments along the linea aspera. It is also possible, of course, that devitalization of cortical bone follows injury to its blood supply from the periosteum (Ham, 1953). Avulsion of bone appears to have been regarded by Caffey (1956) as the explanation of 'chip fractures' accompanying new subperiosteal bone formation in relation to the tibia of an infant aged 3 weeks.

Differential Diagnosis. A presumptive diagnosis of subperiosteal haematoma may reasonably be made when clinical evidence of injury to a long bone is found after a difficult delivery, and is followed by the appearance and subsequent regression of the characteristic radiological changes. When these changes are slight, they may be confused with the double contour of the long bones that is sometimes seen in normal infants; the latter, however, is seldom visible during the first month of life and occurs

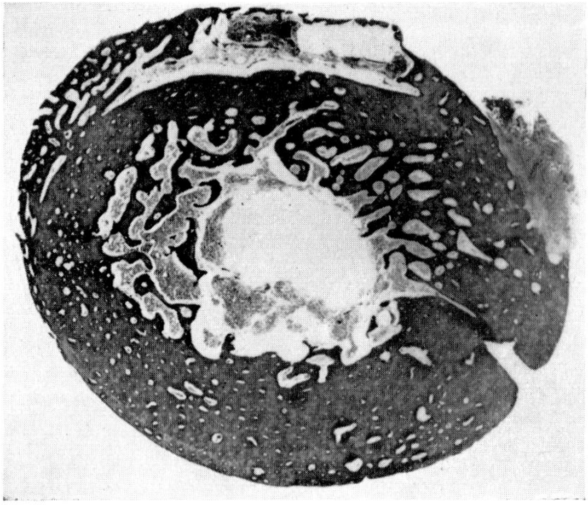

FIG. 11.—Case 2: Histology of femur. Transverse section of shaft showing layer of new subperiosteal bone on part of surface. A space within the new bone is filled with bone debris and altered blood. (Some of this debris has fallen out of the section during preparation.) H. and E. × 11.

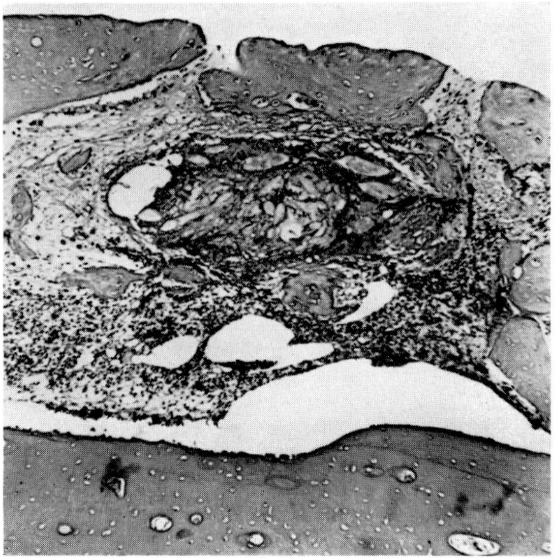

FIG. 12.—Case 2: Histology of femur. New subperiosteal bone under higher magnification showing mixture of necrotic bone and blood enclosed by new trabeculae. H. and E. × 70.

most frequently in small premature infants, usually after a normal birth (Glaser, 1949; Hancox, Hay, Holden, Moss and Whitehead, 1951). Infantile cortical hyperostosis also gives a somewhat similar radiological picture and at one time Smyth, Potter and Silverman (1946) even doubted the existence of ossifying subperiosteal haematoma as a separate entity, believing that the cases so diagnosed were really examples of infantile cortical hyperostosis. In the latter condition, however, there is considerable systemic disturbance with pronounced irritability, loss of weight and fever, several of the long bones are usually involved throughout their entire length, and, characteristically, the mandible and clavicles are affected (Fairbank, 1952). Furthermore, infantile cortical hyperostosis rarely occurs during the first 2 weeks of life although Kitchin (1951) has reported one rather atypical case in a newborn infant, and the condition has been diagnosed radiologically *in utero* (Barba and Freriks, 1953; Bennett and Nelson, 1953). In the second of our two cases of subperiosteal haematoma, prolonged fever suggested yet another possibility, namely, osteomyelitis, but this diagnosis was rejected because ossification preceded the onset of fever, and study of the femur at necropsy showed no evidence of pyogenic inflammation.

When an ossifying subperiosteal haematoma is discovered some weeks or even months after birth, it may be mistaken for a sarcoma or for a manifestation of scurvy (Brailsford, 1948, 1953). Although scurvy may produce an indistinguishable radiological picture, it is usually accompanied by other signs of vitamin C deficiency, and in the absence of these a history of a difficult breech delivery will suggest a presumptive diagnosis of traumatic subperiosteal haemorrhage. It is theoretically possible, of course, that vitamin C deficiency might be a contributory factor in the pathogenesis of subperiosteal haemorrhage following birth trauma, but the mere fact that the haematoma undergoes 'complete resolution' when vitamin C is administered is not proof, as Brailsford (1953) avers, that scurvy has been partly responsible. Neither of the infants we have described showed any sign of vitamin C deficiency and, in the absence of corroborative evidence, it seems unnecessary to invoke scurvy as an additional aetiological factor in the neonatal period. Neither hypervitaminosis A nor syphilis is likely to be confused with subperiosteal haematoma, and both should readily be differentiated by the history and by full clinical investigation. Finally, subperiosteal haematomata may follow comparatively minor injuries in postnatal life and again this is presumably because the periosteum is more loosely attached to the bones than it is in adult life (Barmeyer, Alderson and Cox, 1951; Silverman, 1953; Bakwin, 1956).

Treatment. Subperiosteal haematoma of the newborn requires no treatment. As the bone increases in diameter the subperiosteal layer becomes incorporated in the shaft and the bone eventually assumes its normal contour, though residual thickening may be visible radiologically for many months (Caffey, 1945). However, when there is an associated injury of the epiphysis, orthopaedic treatment may be necessary to prevent permanent disability.

Summary

The clinical and radiological features of traumatic subperiosteal haematoma of the femur in two newborn infants have been described.

In both cases there was a history of difficult breech delivery, with strong manual traction on one of the legs.

Necropsy was performed on one of the infants and examination of the femur showed a layer of new subperiosteal bone enclosing fragments of dead bone and some altered blood.

It is suggested that the subperiosteal haemorrhage was produced by a combination of manual traction and torsion of the limb and that cortical bone was probably avulsed as the periosteum was stripped off the femoral shaft.

The differential diagnosis and treatment have been discussed.

We wish to express our thanks to Professor J. L. Henderson and Professor A. C. Lendrum for their helpful criticism, to Dr. H. G. Morgan who performed the necropsy in Case 2, and to Mr. R. Fawkes for the histological preparations and photomicrographs.

References

Bakwin, H. (1956). *J. Pediat.*, **49**, 7.
Barba, W. P. and Freriks, D. J. (1953). *Ibid.*, **42**, 141.
Barmeyer, G. H., Alderson, L. R. and Cox, W. B. (1951). *Ibid.*, **38**, 184.
Bennett, H. S. and Nelson, T. R. (1953). *Brit. J. Radiol.*, **26**, 47.
Brailsford, J. F. (1948). *Ibid.*, **21**, 157.
—— (1953). *Arch. Dis. Childh.*, **28**, 81.
Burman, M. S. and Langsam, M. J. (1939). *Arch. Surg. (Chicago)*. **38**, 250.
Caffey, J. (1945). *Pediatric X-ray Diagnosis.* Chicago.
—— (1956). *Ibid.*, 3rd ed. Chicago.
Fairbank, T. (1952). *Gt Ormond Str. J.*, 83.
Glaser, K. (1949). *Amer. J. Roentgenol.*, **61**, 482.
Ham, A. W. (1953). *Histology*, 2nd ed. London.
Hancox, N. M., Hay, J. D., Holden, W. S., Moss, P. D. and Whitehead, A. S. (1951). *Arch. Dis. Childh.*, **26**, 543.
Kitchin, I. D. (1951). *J. Bone Jt Surg.*, **33-B**, 248.
Macewen, W. (1912). *The Growth of Bone.* Glasgow.
Scaglietti, O. (1938). *Surg. Gynec. Obstet.*, **66**, 868.
Silverman, F. N. (1953). *Amer. J. Roentgenol.*, **69**, 413.
Smyth, F. S., Potter, A. and Silverman, W. (1946). *Amer. J. Dis. Child.*, **71**, 333.
Snedecor, S. T. and Wilson, H. B. (1949). *J. Bone Jt Surg.*, **31-A**, 378.
——, Knapp, R. E. and Wilson, H. B. (1935). *Surg. Gynec. Obstet.*, **61**, 385.

SUBGLOTTIC HAEMANGIOMA: TWO INFANTS WITH LARYNGEAL STRIDOR

BY

C. A. HOLBOROW

From The Hospital for Sick Children, Great Ormond Street, London

(RECEIVED FOR PUBLICATION SEPTEMBER 24, 1957)

The literature contains records of 18 infants with stridor due to haemangiomata in or just below the larynx. Two of these were reported by Mr. James Crooks in this Journal (Crooks, 1954). Since then he has had three further cases at The Hospital for Sick Children, Great Ormond Street, and I am indebted to him for permission to publish details of two of them, bringing the total number of cases recorded up to 21.

Case Histories

Case 1. (Fig. 1). C.E. was a girl born on January 6, 1956. Laryngeal stridor developed after an attack of acute bronchitis at 6 weeks of age. The stridor continued with intermittent pyrexia, and a laryngoscopy was performed at another hospital when she was 3 months old. The larynx was found to be very red; no web or tumour was seen. The stridor continued despite antibiotics and a month later she was transferred to The Hospital for Sick Children. On examination there was biphasic stridor with rib and suprasternal recession. The child had a good colour and was not distressed. The only other abnormality was a haemangioma of the lower lip. A laryngoscopy was performed under a general anaesthetic. The larynx was red and some subglottic swelling was seen which was thought might be due to infective oedema. Following this examination the stridor was very marked but was relieved by nursing in an atmosphere saturated with water vapour. A respiratory infection delayed further investigation for two months when a further laryngoscopy showed a symmetrical subglottic swelling which appeared to be either inflammatory oedema or a haemangioma. The stridor and respiratory obstruction which followed this examination necessitated a tracheostomy.

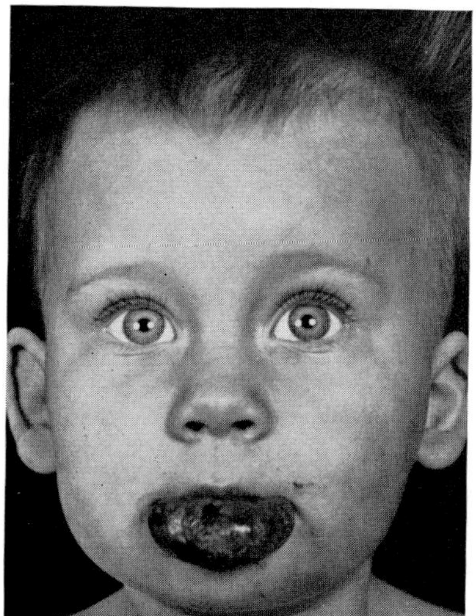

FIG. 1.—Case 1. Child after removal of tracheostomy tube.

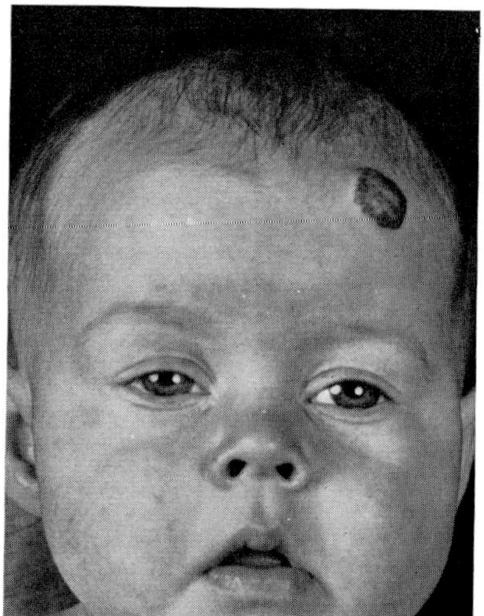

FIG. 2.—Case 2.

Because of the haemangioma on the lip it was assumed that the swelling seen was haemangiomatous and the subglottic region was irradiated by means of deep x-ray (250 R.). The treatment was followed by considerable tracheal obstruction and respiratory distress. A month later laryngoscopy showed that the subglottic swelling was larger, and a biopsy confirmed the diagnosis of haemangioma. A second course of irradiation (200 R.) caused no reaction and one month later an attempt was made to remove the tracheostomy tube under sedation. The child tolerated laryngeal respiration for two days until increasing dyspnoea and stridor compelled the replacement of the tube. Bronchospasm and respiratory infection followed and congestive cardiac failure developed. This was controlled with digoxin and antibiotics and a third course of deep x-ray was then given. The treatment provoked no reaction but the tube was left in place because of a pyrexia due to teething and it was finally removed under sedation seven months after admission. Progress was satisfactory and a later laryngoscopy showed a good airway with only some residual swelling in the subglottic region. The child was discharged home eight months after admission. She has attended for treatment to her lip but has had no more stridor.

Case 2. (Fig. 2.) J.G., also a girl and a second child, was born on February 5, 1957. A laryngeal stridor was first noticed at 6 weeks of age and gradually became worse finally becoming very marked with a cold. There was some feeding difficulty. When seen at another hospital a lateral radiograph of the soft tissues of the neck showed a rounded swelling partly blocking the trachea below the cords. She was transferred to The Hospital for Sick Children and was found to have a biphasic stridor with rib recession. There was, in addition, a small haemangioma of the forehead which, the mother said, had gradually enlarged since birth. Laryngoscopy revealed a rounded swelling arising from the posterior wall of the subglottic region. A biopsy taken from this swelling showed that it was a partly canalized haemangioma. Considerable stridor followed this operation but a tracheostomy was avoided by nursing in a humid atmosphere for 24 hours. The subglottic region was irradiated twice with an interval of two weeks by means of deep x-ray (250 R. and 200 R.). No reactions followed and two days after the second treatment the stridor ceased. A month after admission she was discharged home and has had no subsequent trouble.

Comment

Haemangiomata are malformations rather than neoplasms and canalization accounts for their seeming growth (Willis, 1948). This gradual enlargement was observed in the first case recorded here. The condition is probably not as rare as the few records suggest and reports of a number of cases have appeared recently (Baker and Pennington, 1956). The records are all very similar. Though it has been suggested that this condition occurs more often in males there is no difference in the incidence between the sexes in the small number recorded. Stridor usually becomes apparent during the first three months of life as canalization occurs. It is the presenting symptom. The site of the haemangioma is usually the subglottic region or the upper trachea, though the supraglottic region has been affected and in one case (Baker and Pennington, 1956) the mediastinum and bronchi were involved. In over half the number there were other haemangiomata, usually on the head and neck. The mortality is considerable and nine of the 21 cases have died of respiratory obstruction.

The most satisfactory treatment has, in all cases, proved to be radiotherapy (Suehs and Herbut, 1940; Ferguson, 1944; Kasabach and Donlan, 1945; Crooks, 1954) and though there is some theoretical danger to the developing larynx there are no reports of such damage. The second case described here is the only one recorded where a proven haemangioma has been successfully treated without tracheostomy. The two case histories are an interesting comparison in this respect as the first shows that the hazards of a tracheostomy and the difficulty in removing the tube markedly increase the risk to the child and the time spent in hospital. In many cases, of course, tracheostomy must be performed on admission and an increase in the size of the haemangioma following irradiation may lead to sudden respiratory obstruction. However, provided that everything is in readiness for an emergency operation, the risk of irradiation without an elective tracheostomy appears to be justified.

References

Baker, D. C. and Pennington, C. L. (1956). *Laryngoscope (St. Louis)*, **66**, 696.
Crooks, J. (1954). *Arch. Dis. Childh.*, **29**, 12.
Ferguson, G. B. (1944). *Arch. Otolaryng. (Chicago)*, **40**, 189.
Kasabach, H. H. and Donlan, C. P. (1945). *J. Pediat.*, **26**, 374.
Suehs, O. W. and Herbut, P. A. (1940). *Arch. Otolaryng. (Chicago)*, **32**, 783.
Willis, R. A. (1948). *The Pathology of Tumours.* London.

INTRASPINAL NEUROBLASTOMA IN A NEWBORN BABY

BY

E. ELEFANT, V. VOJTA and V. BENEŠ

From the Third Paediatric Clinic, the Children's Department of the Neurological Clinic of Charles' University and the Neurosurgical Department of the Střešovice Hospital, Prague

(RECEIVED FOR PUBLICATION NOVEMBER 4, 1957)

Intraspinal and spinal cord tumours are quite rare in childhood. Most authors reporting cases of tumours found within the spinal canal use the term 'spinal cord tumour' in a broad sense without regard to whether they are spinal cord tumours proper or of extradural origin. In this paper we refer to an 'intraspinal' neuroblastoma in a newborn infant, and wish to emphasize that though it is intraspinal, yet it is not a tumour of the spinal cord proper, but is situated extradurally.

Anderson (1953) described 21 cases, of which the youngest was 5 months old. Dandy (1925) reported on such tumours in 36 patients of whom five were under 15 years of age. Ford (1944), amongst 70,000 neurological cases in children, found only three spinal cord tumours, the youngest child with this type of tumour being 9 years old. Stookey (1928) analysed 160 cases of spinal cord tumour of which only eight were under 12 years of age. In Elsberg's series (Elsberg, 1925) the youngest patient was 3 years old and Buchanan's youngest patient was aged 3 months (Buchanan, 1950). In the entire world literature, according to Mosberg (1951) and Elefant, Jeklerová and Lesný (1955), altogether 25 cases diagnosed during the first year of life have so far been described. Mosberg's studies have also shown that 75% of all spinal tumours diagnosed during the first year of life consist of lipomas, dermoids, teratoids or teratomas.

Ingraham and Matson (1954) divide intraspinal tumours in children into three groups: (1) congenital tumours, ranging from simple dermoid cysts to highly variable tridermal teratomasi; (2) intramedullary gliomas, including astrocytomas, ependymomas, medulloblastomas and multiform glioblastomas ; (3) extradural extension of paraspinal lesions, including neuroblastoma, reticulum cell sarcoma and lymphosarcoma.

Omitting cases of teratoma, dermoid and tumours associated with developmental anomalies such as spina bifida, meningocoele or sinus pilonides, the present authors were unable to find in accessible literature more than two cases of pure spinal cord tumour diagnosed in the newborn (Katcher, 1952; Parkinson, Medovy and Mitchell, 1954). They therefore consider it appropriate to record the following case.

Case Report

M.L. is the second son of a mother who during the second month of her pregnancy suffered from renal colic and from the eighth month with sciatica-like pains. Normal delivery took place at a maternity hospital on June 23, 1955, of a lively baby weighing 3·580 Kg. and measuring 52 cm. in length. On the 5th day the hospital paediatrician (Dr. R. Nosková) discovered considerable flabbiness of the lower limbs, especially the left, and laxity of the joints. On the following day the condition was worse: the legs were cool, the tonus was lowered, more so on the left side where no reflexes could be elicited. The baby was transferred on the same day to the Third Paediatric Clinic for investigation.

On admission the lower limbs were cool and the soles of the feet cyanotic; Moro's reflex showed no brisk response in the lower limbs. Spontaneous movement of the right leg was weak, and dorsiflexion of the left foot absent; the calf muscles were hypotonic on both sides, more so on the left, and possibly even hypotrophic. The anus was gaping and the perineum around it formed a pouch-like bulge, thought to be due to paresis of the pelvic floor muscles, which when compressed produced a stream of urine. A barium enema and cystoradiography revealed no abnormality. Lumbar puncture on the 15th day produced only a small amount of xanthochromic cerebrospinal fluid with a light admixture of blood. Plain radiographs of the spine showed sinistroscoliosis with maximal curving of the upper lumbar portion. At this level there was also a suspected dilatation of the spinal canal which was particularly apparent in a lateral view. The arches of the 1st and 2nd lumbar vetrebrae were conspicuously thin, and formed an angular kyphosis (Figs. 1 and 2). On the basis of these findings an expansive process within the upper lumbar portion of the spinal canal was suspected (neuroradiologist, J. Jirout).

On July 13, when the infant was 3 weeks old, pneumoperimyelography was carried out (Figs. 3 and 4). Following insufflation of 20 ml. of air by the lumbar route in a

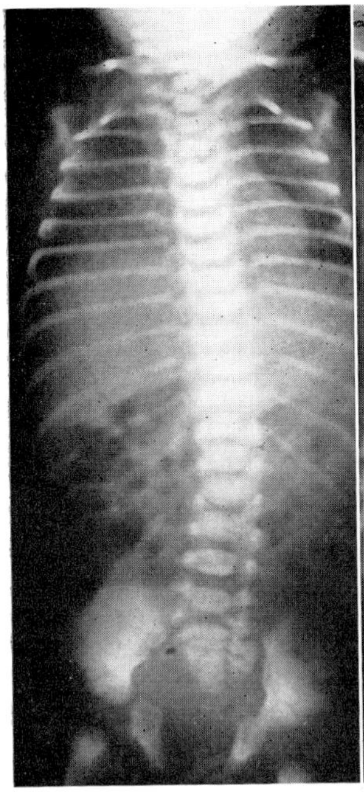

FIG. 1.

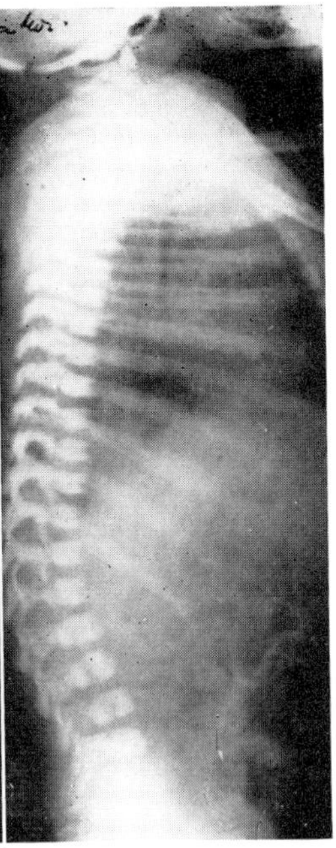

FIG. 2.

FIG. 1.—Plain radiograph of spine (anteroposterior).

FIG. 2.—Plain radiograph of spine (lateral).

FIG. 3.—Pneumoperimyelogram. The air filling extends up to arch of L1 (marked by arrow).

FIG. 4.—Pneumoperimyelogram. On slightly raising pelvis the air filling reaches upper border of arch of L1 (marked by arrow).

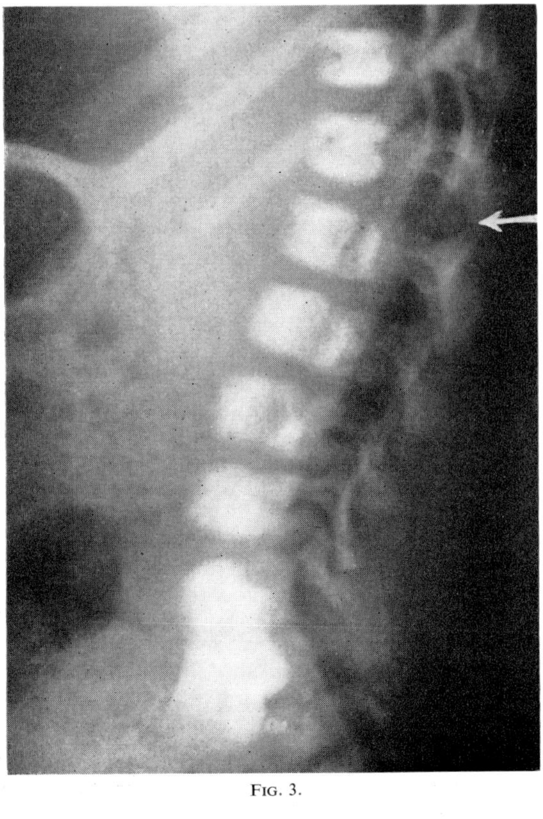

FIG. 3.

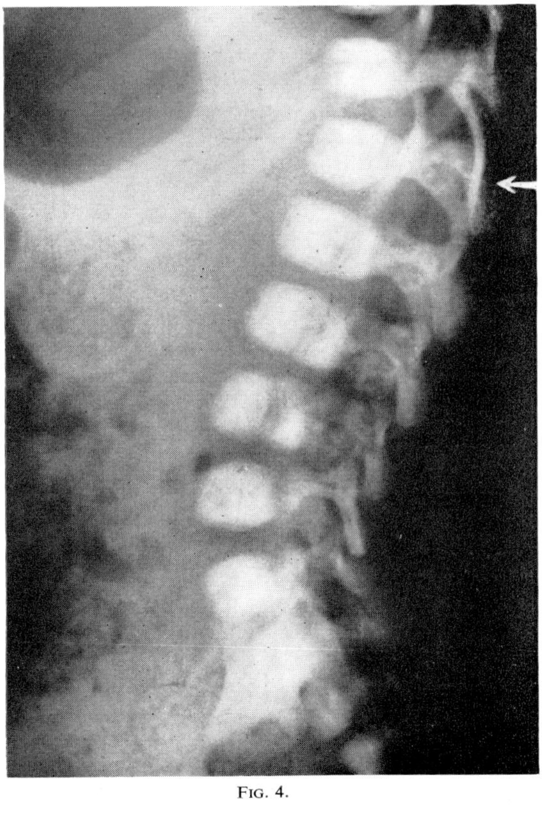

FIG. 4.

lying-down position, the lateral view radiographs revealed an air filling in the sacral and lumbar portions extending cranially up to L2. This is in keeping with pressure changes above L1 (J. Jirout).

At the same time a sample of cerebrospinal fluid was withdrawn and examined: the fluid was blood-stained and, after centrifuging, mildly xanthochromic, with 103 lymphocytes and numerous erythrocytes. Pandy's reaction was ++++, Ross Jones +++, Nonne Appelt +++, and the protein 0·86 g. per 100 ml. A radiograph of the lungs showed a light shadow over the right cardiophrenic angle. The baby was afebrile throughout.

At a neurological examination on July 15 it was found that since the previous examination the movement of the left leg as well as the tone of the calf muscles of both sides had improved. Spontaneous mobility of both lower limbs was symmetrical, though in suspension the right lower limb was more feeble. The reflexes of L5-S2 were absent on both sides. The perineal bulging continued on both sides while the anus was somewhat more gaping than a week earlier. It was decided that the findings were consistent with compression of the cauda.

Improvement in the mobility of the lower limbs was observed after the first lumbar puncture. Since, during a second lumbar puncture, a quantity of dark blood had escaped, a haemangioma was believed to be present, which diminished in size after puncture and so exerted less pressure on the cauda equina. Laminectomy of L1-L2 was recommended.

The baby was operated on at the age of 28 days on July 22, 1955, at the neurosurgical department of the Střešovice Hospital in Prague, and laminectomy of L1-L2 was performed under local anaesthesia. Beneath the arches a bluish violet tissue with a delicate capsule was found, which at first gave the impression that a haematoma beneath the dura mater was present. On closer examination, however, it was found to be neoplastic tissue which it was possible to remove gradually with comparatively little haemorrhage. It had grown practically across the entire antero-posterior dimension of the spinal canal. Not until the greater part of the tumour had been removed could it be established that the pouch of the dura mater was pressed forward and to the left, whereas the remainder of the canal was filled by a tumour which extended even under the arch of T12. The latter arch was also removed but the tumour reached even higher. In the lower part of the tumour there was a cyst the size of a pea filled with a greyish yellow caseous substance. The upper part of the tumour was penetrated through and through by one of the nerve roots, as was confirmed by the response to traction. In view of the extent of the laminectomy and the fact that the baby began to breathe more quickly and the pulse rate to rise, it was decided to discontinue the operation even though the entire tumour had not been removed.

Histological examination of the excised mass was carried out by M. Vorreith who found portions of strongly haemorrhagic tumorous tissue and nerve ganglion. The tumour cells were comparatively small, mostly rounded in shape with a dark nucleus and a well-defined basophilic cytoplasm. In some parts between the islets of cells there was a fibrillary structure, pointing to the neurogenic nature of the tumour. In numerous places the tumour cells constituted rosette-shaped formations. In the portions broken up by haemorrhagic areas there were occasional leucocytic infiltrations and foci of siderophages. Mitoses were not found. He concluded that the findings were consistent with neuroblastoma.

Following the operation the baby was in good condition, drank well and gained in weight. From early in July to early August, 1955, the baby was given radiotherapy: 100R were administered in each of 26 sittings by V. Stašek. During this treatment only once was there a change in the blood count, the erythrocytes falling to 3,760,000, the haemoglobin decreasing to 60% and immature white cells making their appearance.

Before discharge the baby was re-examined neurologically. Signs of affection of the cauda were still present, more so on the left side, but compared with the findings before operation there was pronounced improvement on both sides, especially at the right. Before discharge the baby was thriving satisfactorily and at the age of 3½ months weighed 5·31 Kg.

Of the laboratory and other investigations we record the following results: the blood group was A rh; the W.R. negative; an electrocardiogram revealed tachycardia, but was otherwise normal; a radiograph of the lungs on August 5, 1955, showed elevation of the right diaphragm.

The baby was readmitted for six days on January 22, 1956. The ocular fundi were normal. The blood picture showed 4,490,000 erythrocytes, 74% haemoglobin, 8,300 leucocytes; polymorphs with rod-shaped nuclei 4%, with segmented nuclei 36%; lymphocytes 59%; and monocytes 1%.

At 7 months of age the flaccid peripheral paresis of the lower limbs was still present but the sphincter signs were much improved. As against the earlier picture it was now the right lower limb that was the more affected of the two. A radiograph of the skeleton showed no destructive changes, nor evidence of metastases, and there was no scoliosis; only at the sites of the laminectomy the vertebral bodies were more translucent. At home exercises were being carried out with the baby according to instruction.

The third stay in hospital at the age of 11 months took place between May 25 and June 16, 1956. The baby weighed 10·3 Kg. and measured 76 cm. The circumference of the head was 47 cm., and of the chest 49 cm. The baby had sat up without support from the age of 10 months, was standing and could already walk holding on to the cot. Dentition began at 8 months, speech at 10 months. By this time the anterior fontanelle was closed, the occiput firm, and the operation scar in the thoracolumbar region of the back well healed. The blood picture continued to be normal. A radiographic examination of the chest showed elevation of the central portion of the right diaphragm, while one of the skeleton showed no metastases, and normal ossification of the long bones. The ocular fundi were normal.

At the age of 12 months a further neurological examination showed peripheral hypotonia of the left lower limb. There was a slight pes valgus on the left. When the left lower limbs was moved spontaneously extension of the foot was carried out incoordinately by means of the extensor muscles of the toes; tibialis anterior responded well to stimulation and showed normal tonus. Patellar reflexes were increased on both sides. The plantar reflexes were of the extensor type. The reflexes of L5-S2 were bilaterally decreased. There was a physiological lumbar lordosis. With support the baby stood comparatively firmly, the centre of gravity being transmitted to the right leg. Micturition was streamlike, the flow of urine was promptly halted and did not dribble. away. The anal sphincter was well-contoured though slightly enfeebled; the anal reflex could not be elicited. As far as sensation was concerned, there was a loss of pain sensibility on the right side distally from L4, on the left from L5.

Since the abnormal neurological findings were receding, no further radiotherapy was recommended for the time being. The myelogram showed no tumour cells and the marrow was normal.

The baby began walking without support at 18 months. It was last examined at the age of 20 months, when it weighed 12·75 Kg. It had one regular daily stool and micturition was normal. Its mental development was in keeping with its age. The sensory disturbance in the region of S2-S3 persisted as well as mild hypotonia of the right S1-S2 segments but otherwise the neurological findings had almost returned to normal.

Discussion

It is not intended to deal here with the clinical entity of spinal cord compression as such, which in childhood presents numerous features in common with compression in the adult. It should, however, be recalled that, just as in intracranial tumours, intraspinal expansive processes have their syndrome of hypertension. Apart from changes in the composition of the cerebrospinal fluid (increased protein, xanthochromia), changes in its pressure and disorders in its circulation may help in diagnosis. They are an equally valuable diagnostic help in children even though in the younger ones their evaluation is more difficult because of lack of co-operation. In the younger subjects sensory and root manifestations have a greatly restricted value in determining the levels of localization since here it is a matter of estimating the approximate level of disordered sensation on the basis of the child's general reaction, elicited as painful stimuli passing from a zone of diminished or absent sensitivity, hypoaesthetic or anaesthetic, to a normal or hyperaesthetic one.

On careful examination of plain radiographs of the spine in cases of cord compression, dilatation of the spinal canal, occurring especially in children and confined to a few segments, cannot be missed. Note is taken of the interpedicular distance, flattening of the inner surfaces of the pedicles or their possible disappearance. The changes are greatest at the level of the tumour, below which they decline in magnitude. Another important feature is the change in the normal shape of the spine. At the site of the expansive process the spine is altered in shape over a small area, being straightened as if it were stiff, or there may be a scoliosis confined to a brief segment of the spine (Jirout, 1956). Impressions of the posterior wall of the vertebral body and dilatation of the intervertebral foramina are diagnostically as valuable in childhood as they are in adults. An accurate spatial picture of the boundaries of the expansive process may be obtained with the aid of pneumoperimyelography, which is kinder to the patient than iodine perimyelography.

The authors' own experience as well as that recorded in the literature (Ingraham and Matson, 1954) shows that the most frequent erroneous diagnoses in cases of spinal cord compression are poliomyelitis or amyotonia congenita.

The symptomatology of our present case included a feature which we have not so far come across either in our experience or in the literature. This was paresis of the pelvic floor manifesting itself by a pouch-like bulge, in the differential diagnosis of which a cystic formation within the pelvis had to be excluded.

In view of the clinical signs of compression of the cauda equina and the corresponding changes in the radiographs of the spine, together with the results of pneumoperimyelography, the upper boundaries of the compression were not searched for. Prompt improvement of mobility following operation, even though the entire tumour had not been removed, justifies the belief that it did not extend higher than one segment above that reached at operation. There is reason to believe that early operative intervention on the 28th day of life—the patient being perhaps the youngest ever subjected to such an operation—was responsible for the remarkable disappearance of the clinical signs and the fact that the child is now free from gross motor disability.

The effect of the radiotherapy cannot be unequivocally evaluated in the light of the latest findings on the spontaneous remissions of the malignity in neuroblastoma (Cushing and Wohlbach, 1927; Lehmann, 1932; Farber, 1940). Gross (1953) as well as other workers have found that neuroblastoma treated before the age of 2 years has a more favourable prognosis than those diagnosed later.

Neuroblastoma, one of the most frequent malignant tumours in childhood, originates primarily in paraganglionic areas but often penetrates into the spinal canal via the intervertebral foramina. It is a highly vascular, fairly soft, cellular tumour; it never, however, penetrates the dura mater or nerve sheaths. Its aetiology and pathogenesis are not clearly understood. If signs of rapid progression of the cord compression are present it would be wrong to await the effect of irradiation or other conservative treatment. In such cases laminectomy with complete excision of the intraspinal tumour is called for as soon as possible. Such treatment with subsequent radiotherapy leads to functional restoration. Extensive laminectomies in small children may lead to spinal deformities (lordosis, kyphoscoliosis). By combining surgical measures with radiotherapy, Wittenborg (1950) found that 30% of patients with neuroblastoma survived over three years. In general, however, and with rare exceptions—a survival of 15 years (Lehman, 1932) and one of 17 years (Oberkircher, 1953)—the disease ends fatally within one year. It is noteworthy that Lehman's case was not treated radiologically at all.

Summary

The literature is surveyed on spinal cord compression in children in general and in infants and the newborn in particular.

A case of intraspinal neuroblastoma is described, which was diagnosed in a newborn baby on the eighth day after birth, and treated on the 28th day by laminectomy with partial extirpation of the tumour and post-operative radiotherapy.

A follow-up at the age of 20 months showed very good results from the surgical treatment and possibly also from the post-operative radiotherapy. The child walked safely without support and there were no signs of incontinence or metastases.

The baby was re-examined at the age of 34 months and its neurological condition was found to be unchanged.

To our knowledge it is the third case of pure intraspinal tumour in the newborn recorded in world literature.

References

Anderson, F. M. and Carson, M. J. (1953). *J. Pediat.*, **43**, 190.
Buchanan, D. (1950). *Arch. Neurol. Psychiat. (Chicago)*, **63**, 835.
Cushing, H. and Wolbach, S. B. (1927). *Amer. J. Path.*, **3**, 203.
Dandy, W. E. (1925). *Ann. Surg.*, **81**, 223.
Elefant, E., Jeklerová, J. and Lesný, I. (1955). *Ann. paediat. (Basel)*, **184**, 253.
Elsberg, C. A. (1925), *Tumors of the Spinal Cord and the Symptoms of Irritation and Compression of the Spinal Cord and Nerve Roots. Pathology, Symptomatology, Diagnosis and Treatment.* New York.
Farber, S. (1940). *Amer. J. Dis. Child.*, **60**, 749.
Ford, F. R. (1944). *Diseases of the Nervous System in Infancy, Childhood and Adolescence*, 2nd ed. Springfield, Illinois.
Gross, R. E. (1953). *The Surgery of Infancy and Childhood*, pp. 606-625, 762-769. Philadelphia.
Ingraham, F. D. (1938). *Amer. J. Surg.*, **39**, 342.
—— and Matson, D. D. (1954). *Neurosurgery of Infancy and Childhood.* Springfield, Illinois.
Jirout, J. (1956). *Speciální neuroradiologie*, Státní zdrav. nakladatelství. Praha.
Katcher, A. L. (1952). *J. Pediat.*, **40**, 785.
Koop, C. E., Kiesewetter, W. B. and Horn, R. C. (1955). *Pediatrics*, 16, 652.
Lehman, E. P. (1932). *Ann. Surg.*, **95**, 473.
Mosberg, W. H. (1951). *J. Neurosurg.*, **8**, 220.
Oberkircher, O. J., Staubitz, W. J. and Parmenter, F. J. (1953). *J. Pediat.*, **43**, 177.
Parkinson, D., Medovy, H. and Mitchell, J. R. (1954). *J. Neurosurg.*, **11**, 629.
Schwartz, H. G. (1952). *Ann. Surg.*, **136**, 183.
Stookey, B. (1928). *Amer. J. Dis. Child.*, **36**, 1184.
Wittenborg, M. H. (1950). *Radiology*, **54**, 679.

SOME UNUSUAL FINDINGS IN A FAMILY WITH FRIEDREICH'S ATAXIA

BY

PETER E. SYLVESTER

From the Royal Liverpool Children's Hospital and The Fountain Hospital, London

(RECEIVED FOR PUBLICATION NOVEMBER 11, 1957)

Introduction

Friedreich's ataxia, a hereditary disorder of the nervous system, is characterized by the onset of ataxia of gait, weakness and clumsiness of the limbs, and dysarthria of speech in young patients of either sex. Loss of tendon reflexes, usually combined with extensor plantar responses and impairment of vibration and joint sense, is often found. Nystagmus is common. Complications include mental symptoms, kyphoscoliosis, pes cavus and claw hand. Cardiac complications often terminate the disease. These findings are associated with progressive degeneration of the spinocerebellar and cortico-spinal tracts, the posterior column and Clarke's column.

A family, in which a father and six of his children are believed to suffer from Friedreich's ataxia, is reported because of several unusual features. Notably, optic atrophy and nerve deafness are the most consistent findings, and upper and lower motor neurone disturbances appear more conspicuous than those of the spino-cerebellar system. The rate of progress of the disease varied considerably: one child died within two and a half months of the onset of symptoms, whilst others with muscle wasting appeared to remit during the period of observation.

Before the diagnosis was finally established in the members of this family many conditions were considered. These included tuberculous meningitis, Arnold-Chiari malformation, posterior fossa lesion, spinal tumour, progressive muscular atrophy, peripheral neuritis due to avitaminosis, diphtheria, lead poisoning, toxic myelitis, and syphilis of the nervous system and meninges.

Family History

The medical history of the family preceded the period of observation, 1955-1956, by at least 16 years. The family consisted of the parents and nine children, four of whom died, three of these had nervous symptoms and signs. Both parents were Gentiles and were unrelated. The mother, 45 years, was quite well with no muscular weakness or ataxia. She had a long standing internal strabismus of the left eye but there was neither optic atrophy nor nystagmus. She was not deaf. The father, 44 years, suffered from childhood poliomyelitis which resulted in shortening of one leg. He had severe impairment of hearing, poor vision, bilateral optic atrophy and normal hands. His gait though cumbersome, due to his shortened leg, did not appear ataxic and he walked well unaided. His visual and auditory symptoms were slowly progressive for a number of years. Enquiry into the family tree revealed no history of disease of the nervous system in other members (Fig. 1).

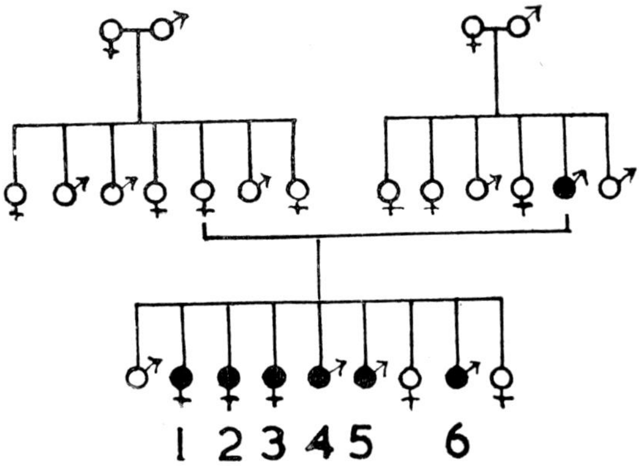

FIG. 1.—The family tree, with case numbers.
● = affected person.

The first child, a boy, not affected with nervous symptoms, was born in 1935 with bilateral talipes. He died of pneumonia at $3\frac{1}{2}$ years. Necropsy revealed a well-nourished child with a large thyroid. Examination of the nervous system was not done.

Three girls and two boys who developed symptoms and signs of nervous disease were born in 1937 (Case 1), 1939 (Case 2), 1942 (Case 3), 1944 (Case 4) and 1946

(Case 5). A daughter, born in 1948, was alive and well, but a son born in 1949 (Case 6) had nervous symptoms and signs. The youngest child, a daughter born in 1951, was unaffected and well.

Three children died (Cases 1, 2 and 5) and necropsies were done on two patients but, unfortunately, war damage destroyed reports and specimens. However, some specimens of Case 1 were obtained from the Pathology Department of Liverpool University and these are available for study. They include cross sections of the mid-brain, pons, medulla, cervical, thoracic and lumbo-sacral cord, and the optic nerve, which have been stained with haematoxylin and eosin, Loyez's and Marchi's methods.

Special investigations were carried out on some of the five patients. The results were as follows: (1) The Wassermann reaction was negative (Cases 2, 3, 4, 5, 6) and in both parents. (2) Toxoplasmosis dye and complement fixation tests (Cases 3, 4, 6) and in the mother were negative. (3) Radiographs of skull and spine (Cases 1, 2, 3, 4, 5) were normal with the exception of Case 3 which showed a slight degree of platybasia. (4) Electrocardiography, normal results (Cases 3, 4, 6). (5) Urinary lead, copper, amino acids and phenylpyruvic acid estimations were within normal limits (Cases 3, 4, 6). (6) Vitamin A absorption was within normal limits (Cases 3, 4, 6). (7) Plasma electrophoresis was normal (Cases 3, 4, 6). (8) Electromyography was normal (Case 6). (9) Muscle biopsy (Case 4) revealed normal muscle. (10) Cerebrospinal fluid appeared normal (Cases 1, 2, 3, 4, 6). If any comment could be made, it was that the sugar content showed a constant tendency towards the low side of normal (between 50 and 60 mg. /100 ml.). (11) The fasting blood pyruvic acid was determined in Cases 3, 4 and 6 after the method of Friedemann and Haugen (1943). The value was within normal limits (0·5 to 1·1 mg./100 ml.) in Cases 3 and 4 but raised (1·7 mg./100 ml.) in Case 6. An hour after a loading dose of glucose the levels remained within normal limits (1·7 to 2·3 mg./100 ml.) in Cases 3 and 4, but in Case 6 a raised value persisted (3·1 mg./100 ml.). The reason for this was not clear.

All the affected children were born normally and were healthy infants. Milestones (holding up the head, sitting, standing and walking) were passed normally. Up to the onset of symptoms all had been healthy with the exception of Case 2, who had a sacrococcygeal pelvic tumour removed surgically at 9 months, and Case 6, who had a congenital strabismus at 3 years which had been satisfactorily corrected by the time symptoms developed. Cases 3, 4 and 6 suffered minor head injuries but these were not severe enough to cause concussion.

Impairment of vision and hearing were the most constant symptoms in children and father; slow to start, they were gradually progressive. There was no history of middle-ear disease. A similar picture was seen in the optic fundi of the father and Cases 2, 3, 4, 5, and 6. The discs, uniformly pale, stood out distinctly from an apparently normal retina. In Case 2 the left disc was involved but in the others both discs were affected. In Case 1 the fundi were thought to be healthy during life but after death demyelination of the optic nerve was found. Fields of vision (Cases 3, 4) showed peripheral constriction with no central scotoma. Light reflexes, where noted, were present (Cases 2, 4, 5, 6). Tests for the auditory nerve (Rinne and Weber) revealed impairment of bone and air conduction. The tympanic membranes appeared healthy. On this evidence it was assumed that deafness was nervous in origin. The degree of deafness varied; it was slight in Cases 1, 2, and 6, moderate in Case 4 and severe in Cases 3 and 5, causing Case 3 to attend a school for the deaf, where her poor visual acuity restricted her ability to learn lip reading. All the patients learnt to speak, if somewhat monotonously and monosyllabically, and were not considered to be grossly dysarthric.

Four children had nystagmus (Cases 1, 2, 4, 5). In Case 1 it occurred in all directions, it was horizontal in Cases 2 and 4, and rotatory in Case 5. The facies were expressionless and on smiling the lips were transverse. Other cranial nerves appeared intact, with no other signs of bulbar involvement.

None of the patients had convulsions or tremors. Mentally, they were dull and were either irritable (Cases 1, 5) or apathetic (Cases 2, 6). Acute fright and attacks of clinging to the mother overcame Case 5 periodically.

To add to the misery of this family, the parents often quarrelled about their responsibility for the children's plight. In particular, the father blamed the mother, because of the 'turn in her eye', which he considered to be the cause of the children's eye trouble, and as a result he often sought the companionship of other women thereby creating a further difficulty.

Other physical findings are listed in Table 1.

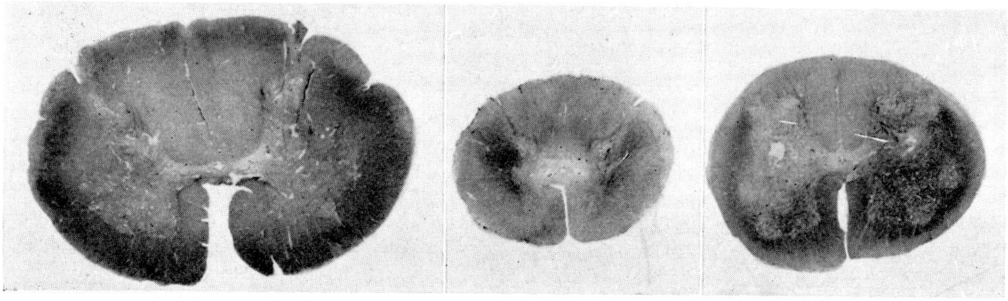

FIG. 2.—Demyelination of posterior columns, dorsal and ventral spino-cerebellar tracts in sections of cord at cervical, thoracic, and sacral levels. Loyez ×5.

TABLE 1

PHYSICAL FINDINGS IN FAMILY WITH FRIEDREICH'S ATAXIA

Case No.	1	2	3	4	5	6
	Female	Female	Female	Male	Male	Male
Age of onset (in years) ..	$2\frac{1}{2}$	$7\frac{3}{4}$	9	9	5 1/6	5 1/6
Symptoms: presenting	Fatigue	Impaired hearing	Impaired hearing	Failing vision	Difficulty in fastening buttons, turning doorknobs	Leaning on things for support
subsidiary	Weakness and leaning on things for support. Rolling of eyes. Unsteadiness of hands when holding objects	Weakness of hands. 'Pins and needles' in hands, feet. Unsteadiness in walking, with stiff legs, high steppage	Unsteady gait. Poor vision. Headaches	Deterioration in hearing	Deafness. Irritability. Muscle weakness. Difficulty in walking: often toppled forward. Failing vision	Difficulty in fastening belt clasp
duration	Died within $2\frac{1}{2}$ mth. from 'demyelinating myelitis'	Died 19 mth. later from 'toxic polyneuritis'	4 yr.	1 yr.	Died $3\frac{1}{2}$ yr. later from pneumonia	8 mth.
Past history	Healthy	Sacrococcygeal tumour removed at 9 mth.	Minor head injury	Minor head injury	Healthy	Minor head injury. Congenital strabismus at 3 yr.
Motor Function: Posture	Dorsal kyphosis	Normal	Lordosis	Scoliosis. Pes cavus	Claw hand	Slumped forward in sitting position
Tone	Poor in arms	Increased in legs	Normal	Normal	Increased in legs	Poor all limbs
Power	Weakness both arms	Weakness of grip	Good	Good	Weakness arms and legs	General weakness
Wasting	None	Marked in small muscles, hands, deltoids	None	Deltoids and spinati, hands	Deltoids with scapular and thenar muscles	Supra and infra-spinati
Fibrillation	Not noted	None	Deltoids	Quadriceps	None	Spinati
Sensory Function: Tactile sensitivity ..	Not tested	Normal	Normal	Normal	Not tested	Not tested
Pain sensitivity	,,	,,	,,	,,	,,	Normal
Joint position	,,	Not tested	,,	,,	,,	,,
Vibration sense ..	,,	Normal	Absent in ankles	Absent in ankles	,,	,,
Reflexes: Plantar	Extensor	Bilateral extensor	Normal	Normal	Left extensor	Normal
Abdominal	Absent	Present	Present	Present	Present	Present
Deep	Not tested	Increased especially in legs with knee clonus	Absent ankle jerks	Diminished	Diminished but increased left leg	Normal
Coordination: Finger to nose test ..	Not tested	Normal	Normal	Intention tremor right hand	Not tested	Normal
Heel to knee	,,	Not tested	,,	Normal	,,	,,
Rombergism	,,	Positive	Positive	Positive	,,	Negative

Histology

Examination of the sections from Case 1 showed that degenerative changes were most marked in the cord (Fig. 2) where symmetrical demyelination involved the tracts of Goll and Burdach, the anterior and posterior spino-cerebellar tracts and the cortico-spinal tracts. Demyelination could be discerned in the area of Monakow and lateral aspect of the restiform body in the medulla, but the pyramids and the medial lemnisci appeared intact. The normal orderly arrangement of the axons was replaced by many irregular distended spaces. Towards the periphery of the involved tracts the contents of many of these spaces stained with osmic acid. Axis cylinders were difficult to define and it was not possible to say whether they were reduced in number. The anterior and posterior nerve roots stained with osmic acid.

The entire grey matter of the cord was congested, there was no oedema or perivascular cuffing. Two haemorrhagic cystic spaces had formed in the postero-lateral regions of the grey matter in the sacral cord. The walls of the vessels in the cord and meninges appeared normal and so did the meninges.

There was widespread damage of nerve cells. Some stained densely, the nucleus being eccentric and the chromatin network lost. Others appeared swollen and contained a feebly stained and eccentric nucleus, the chromatin being either arranged around the periphery of the cell or completely absent. Satellitosis was observed around some of the swollen cells.

Areas showing nerve cell damage included the grey matter of the cord (in one thoracic section they were completely absent), the cuneate nucleus, the Vth nerve nucleus, and the substantia nigra. Both anterior and posterior horns of the cord were affected as well as Clarke's column. Glial cells appeared increased in both grey and white matter.

Concentric demyelination was seen in the optic nerve.

Two sections of the cord and one of the optic nerve were stained by Holzer's method. By this means an increase of glial tissue was demonstrated in the posterior columns, the posterior spino-cerebellar tracts, the anterior horns, Clarke's column and in the optic nerve.

No abnormality could be detected in the vestibular nuclei and the trapezoid bodies. The auditory pathway could not be studied in the limited number of sections available. The superior and medial accessory olivery nuclei, the pontine nuclei, the Xth and XIIth nerve nuclei appeared normal.

Discussion

Diagnosis. Even when it became clear that the disorder was heredo-familial, its nature remained uncertain because the clinical picture varied so much. Bogaert (1948) observes that the more complex a heredo-degenerative disease seems anatomically, the more it appears to merge with other groups. For this reason familial amyotrophic lateral sclerosis was diagnosed in Cases 3, 4, 5 and 6 because signs of upper and lower motor neurone disease were prominent. However, posterior column loss (Cases 3, 4), nystagmus (Cases 4, 5) and intention tremor (Case 5) cast doubt upon this diagnosis.

Greenfield (1954) discusses the association of Charcot-Marie-Tooth and Roussy-Levy syndromes with Friedreich's ataxia because their pathological features are similar in some respects. The points of clinical similarity with these syndromes in the present family are 'main-en-griffe' (Case 5), reduction of the deep reflexes (Cases 3, 4, 5), spinal deformities (Cases 1, 3, 4), remissions (Case 6) and degeneration in dorsal columns, pyramidal and spino-cerebellar tracts and loss of cells in Clarke's column. Points of difference are the presence of nystagmus, intention tremor and absence of characteristic wasting of the peroneal and anterior tibial muscles.

Friedreich's ataxia was considered the most likely diagnosis in the light of all the symptoms and signs of the patients and the histopathology of Case 1.

Optic Atrophy and Nerve Deafness. Optic atrophy is not uncommon in Friedreich's ataxia; Sjögren (1943) found an incidence of 12%. The form varies, as in other hereditary ataxias. A retinal type, in which there is degeneration of the retina and choroid with an increase in pigmentation was described by Franceschetti and Klein (1948), and designated 'tapeto-retinal degeneration'. Neuritis of the optic nerve head and retrobulbar neuritis may also be seen. André-van-Leeuwen (1948) suggested three varieties of this form.

The first shows typical retrobulbar neuritis in which vision is rapidly diminished, sometimes considerably, there is a central scotoma and temporal pallor of the disc. Peripheral fields are usually little affected. Sometimes lesions extend beyond the papillo-macular bundle when there is deficiency in the peripheral fields of vision. The age of onset is 30 to 40 years.

The second shows rapid onset of optic nerve degeneration with considerable loss of vision almost to the point of complete blindness. The disc is pale and there is considerable shrinkage of the visual fields. In less advanced cases central as well as peripheral vision may be lost. This type usually comes on about puberty although it may appear congenitally or in early infancy.

The third shows loss of vision of less sudden onset with peripheral constriction of the visual fields which is seen more typically in the spino-pontocerebellar degenerations. Pallor of the discs may be complete or confined to the temporal halves. Sometimes, a discordance between loss of central and peripheral vision may be noticed. Even when a central scotoma is present it may be uncertain whether it is due to retrobulbar neuritis. At other times the picture is that of a slowly progressing optic atrophy. The age of onset is variable and the course slow. The findings in the present family resembled this third type.

Atrophic changes in the papillo-macular bundle of the optic nerve, chiasma and tracts was described by Bogaert in an 11-year-old child with Leber's disease, who died of cerebral haemorrhage and whose cord showed lesions of similar type to those found in Friedreich's ataxia.

André-van-Leeuwen comments that, exceptionally, optic atrophy may precede other nervous symptoms. Sometimes it appears simultaneously, but mostly it follows other symptoms, often by a number of years.

Nerve deafness is much rarer than optic atrophy and their combination is unusual. Bogaert (1948) describes three brothers who suffered from Friedreich's ataxia, two of whom had central deafness and optic atrophy, in whom he regards inheritance as recessive. Unfortunately, necropsies were not carried out, but, in another type of hereditary ataxia, Nyssen and Bogaert (1934) described lesions in a brother and sister in whom there was demyelination of the optic chiasma and degeneration of the primary and secondary pathways of the cochlear system. Degenerated fibres were traced through the restiform body, cochlear nucleus, superior olivery nucleus, trapezoid body, Monakow's bundle and the medial lemniscus to the corpora quadrigemina and internal geniculate body. The cord was not examined. The limited number of sections in the present family made it impossible to compare accurately the histological findings; there was no degeneration of the trapezoid bodies, the medial lemnisci or superior olivery nuclei, but demyelination was present in Monakow's area and the restiform body. Urich, Norman and Lloyd (1957) in studying the auditory pathway of a 10½-year-old girl, who suffered from Friedreich's ataxia, found widespread loss of cells in the central cochlear nucleus. Deafness was not detected clinically but audiometric studies were not done.

Matthews (1950) reported deaf-mutism in three siblings with symptoms and signs of Friedreich's ataxia. A fourth sibling with similar peripheral signs was not a deaf mute.

Clinical evidence of involvement of the vestibular branch of the VIIIth nerve (loss of caloric reaction) was found by Guillain, Mollaret and Aubrey (1935) in 18 cases of Friedreich's ataxia. They found nerve deafness to be rare. They claim that vestibular investigation in Friedreich's ataxia may have some diagnostic value.

Montandon (1948) discusses the auditory, anatomical and pathological implications in hereditary ataxias, and concludes that most lesions causing deafness commence in the labyrinth and may be so slight as to escape detection unless sought carefully by audiometry. The degenerative process tends to spread centrally and when this occurs central deafness masks labyrinthine deafness.

General Comments. Pathogenesis is discussed in most textbooks of neurology and by Greenfield (1954) and will not be repeated here.

The genetic basis of Friedreich's ataxia is beyond doubt. It may be transmitted by dominant or recessive genes. In the present family it is dominant. Some idea of the frequency with which each type occurs is given by Bell (1948) who analysed the findings in 500 pairs of siblings thought to be recessive in origin and 144 pairs thought to be dominant. From the analysis it was found that the age of onset in both groups was similar and that there was a marked tendency for siblings of one family to present symptoms at the same period of life. This last fact may have practical prognostic implications for unaffected and much older siblings, but in the present family in which there are two young unaffected siblings, conclusions on this point cannot yet be drawn.

Matthews suggested that when deaf mutism occurs it may be due to the chance association of two genes. It seems more likely that all the clinical and pathological findings are due to the same process and are attributable to the same causal factor. Diverse anatomical changes in the nervous system, similar to those found in Friedreich's ataxia, have been caused in animals by vitamin A deficiency (Mellanby, 1934) and it seems reasonable to deduce that one gene acting in some similar manner might be responsible for all findings.

Summary

The clinical findings in a family, consisting of a father and six of his children believed to suffer from Friedreich's ataxia, are presented. An unusual feature is the presence of optic atrophy and nerve deafness.

Histological findings in the cord, medulla and midbrain are described.

My thanks are due to Professor N. B. Capon and Dr. R. W. Brookfield for access to their case records at the Royal Liverpool Children's Hospital, and to Dr. J. S. Elwood who helped me with the histology. My colleagues at the Fountain Hospital were kind enough to offer helpful criticism.

References

André-van-Leeuwen, M. (1948). *Rev. oto-neuro-ophtal.*, **20**, 43.
Bell, J. (1948). *Treasury of Human Inheritance.* Vol. 4. London.
Bogaert, L. van (1948). *Modern Trends in Ophthalmology*, Vol. II, edited by Arnold Sorsby, London.
Franceschetti, A. and Klein, D. (1948). *Rev. oto-neuro-ophtal.*, **20**, 109.
Friedemann, T. E. and Haugen, G. E. (1943). *J. biol. Chem.*, **147**, 415.
Greenfield, J. G. (1954). *The Spino-Cerebellar Degenerations.* Amer. Lect. Ser. No. 244. Oxford.
Guillain, G., Mollaret, P. and Aubrey, M. (1935). *Rev. neurol. (Paris)*, **63**, 36.
Matthews, W. B. (1950). *J. Neurol. Neurosurg. Psychiat.*, **13**, 307.
Mellanby, E. (1934). *Nutrition and Disease.* Edinburgh and London.
Montandon, A. (1948). *Rev. oto-neuro-ophtal.*, **20**, 181.
Nyssen, R. and Bogaert, L. van (1934). *Rev. neurol. (Paris)*, (II), 321.
Sjögren, T. (1943). *Klinische und erbbiologische Untersuchungen über die Heredoataxien.* Copenhagen. Also in *Acta Psychiat. Neurol. (Kbh.)*, Suppl. **27**.
Urich, H., Norman, R. M. and Lloyd, O. C. (1957). *Confin. Neurol. (Basel)*, **17**, 360.

A CASE OF INTRACRANIAL DERMOID CYST ASSOCIATED WITH THE KLIPPEL-FEIL DEFORMITY AND RECURRENT MENINGITIS

BY

A. PETER ROBERTS
From the Children's Hospital, Birmingham

(RECEIVED FOR PUBLICATION OCTOBER 1, 1957)

Intracranial dermoid cysts are rare: of 2,023 verified intracranial tumours recorded by Cushing (1932) there were 15 examples, including epidermoid cysts. In many cases there is an associated congenital dermal sinus. The following is presented as a typical case.

Case Report

D.H. is the second child of healthy parents, the elder child being normal. He was first referred to the Children's Hospital in July, 1954, at the age of 4 weeks because of diarrhoea and vomiting. This was thought to be dietetic in origin, and the only abnormal finding was the presence of the Klippel-Feil deformity, which was confirmed by radiological examination (Fig. 1).

Ten months later he was admitted with acute bronchitis, and examination at that time revealed a small mobile lump in the occipital region. This was considered to be a fibroma.

He then remained well for 15 months until August, 1956, when he was readmitted with a two-day history of refusal to eat, vomiting and drowsiness. He was extremely irritable and crying more than usual, especially if disturbed.

On examination owing to his spinal deformity it was not possible to confirm any neck stiffness. There was no papilloedema.

Lumbar puncture yielded a cloudy fluid containing 3,250 white cells per c.mm., most of which were polymorphonuclear. The protein content was 700 mg. %, the sugar 6 mg. % and the fluid was sterile on culture.

A diagnosis of probable meningococcal meningitis was made: he was treated with penicillin and sulphadimidine and his progress was satisfactory.

Soon after returning home vomiting recurred. He was crying continuously, banging his head and he was noticed to have photophobia. Two weeks later he was readmitted and on this occasion his cerebrospinal fluid contained 1,350 cells per c.mm., of which 75% were polymorphonuclear. The protein content was 60 mg. %, sugar 27 mg. %, and again the culture was sterile. No cause for the relapse of his meningitis was found and he was treated with a course of chloromycetin, and later given a course of tetracycline. Serial lumbar punctures showed a progressive improvement in his cerebrospinal fluid, and coincidently his general condition improved.

Following discharge he remained well for a further seven months, when he was readmitted with a history of vomiting and crying for five days; on examination he had an upper respiratory tract infection, and the cerebrospinal fluid was found to be normal. He was discharged home but within a few days started vomiting. He again had photophobia, his mother thought he had been having

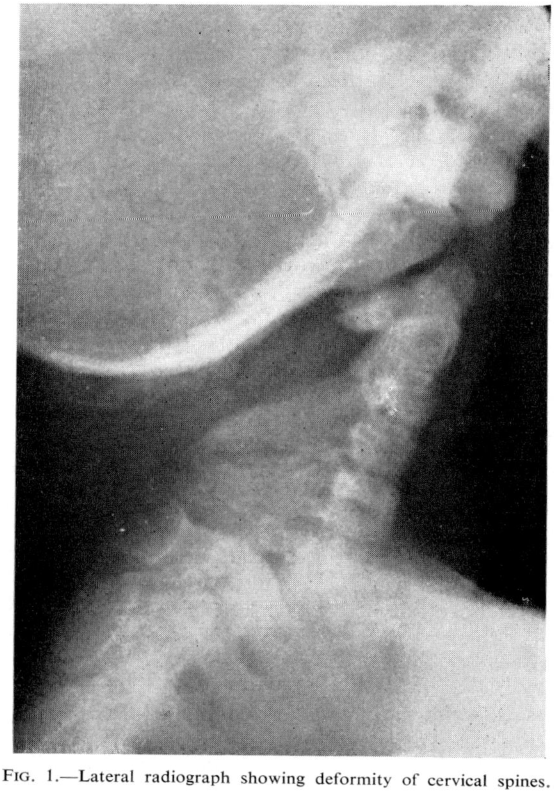

FIG. 1.—Lateral radiograph showing deformity of cervical spines.

headaches, and the history suggested that he probably had a convulsion on the night before his readmission two weeks later. On examination he was found to have gross bilateral papilloedema. There was now a soft circumscribed swelling just below and to the left of the extended occipital protuberance. Examination of the skin overlying the swelling showed a small pore from which hairs protruded.

A plain radiograph of the skull showed a small bony defect in the occipital bone just to the left of the midline (Fig. 2).

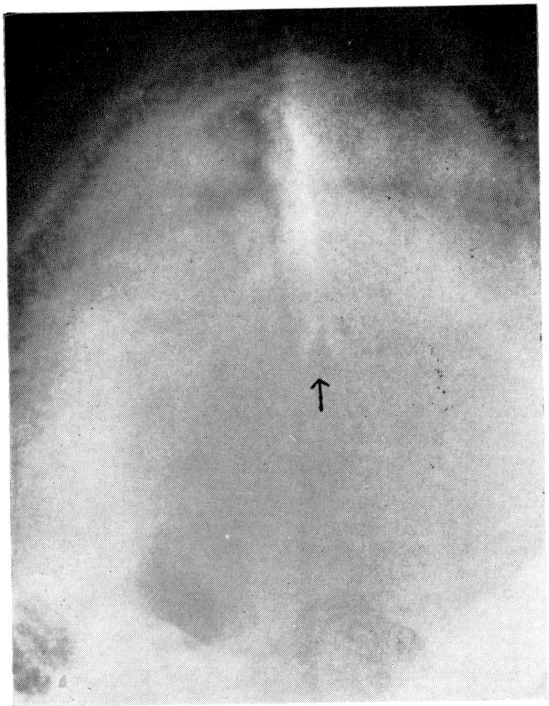

FIG. 2.—Radiograph of skull showing bony defect in occipital bone.

A ventriculogram showed symmetrically dilated but undisplaced lateral ventricles. The third ventricle was dilated and the aqueduct of Sylvius was kinked (Fig. 3). Some air passed through into the fourth ventricle which was not enlarged. The air passed freely down the spine but on returning to the skull most of it accumulated just below the foramen magnum. The findings were considered to be consistent with a mass in the posterior fossa.

The cerebrospinal fluid obtained by ventricular puncture contained 2 cells per c.mm. and less than 10 mg. % of protein.

A pre-operative diagnosis of a dermoid cyst of the scalp associated with a congenital dermal sinus leading to an intracranial dermoid cyst was made, and a craniotomy performed on May 3. The scalp dermoid was excised and a sinus tract was found passing through the occipital bone into the posterior fossa just below the torcular. The dura was found to be very adherent at this point. On opening the posterior fossa a large cystic dermoid was found in the midline. Anteriorly the thin wall of the cyst had become adherent directly to the surrounding brain, and as it was not possible to remove the cyst intact the contents were first aspirated. The cyst was lined with a fairly thick wall of typical glistening desquamated epithelium, and in addition contained a hair. The collapsed cyst was then removed.

The fluid aspirated from the cyst contained numerous pus cells and degenerate Gram positive cocci: it was sterile on culture.

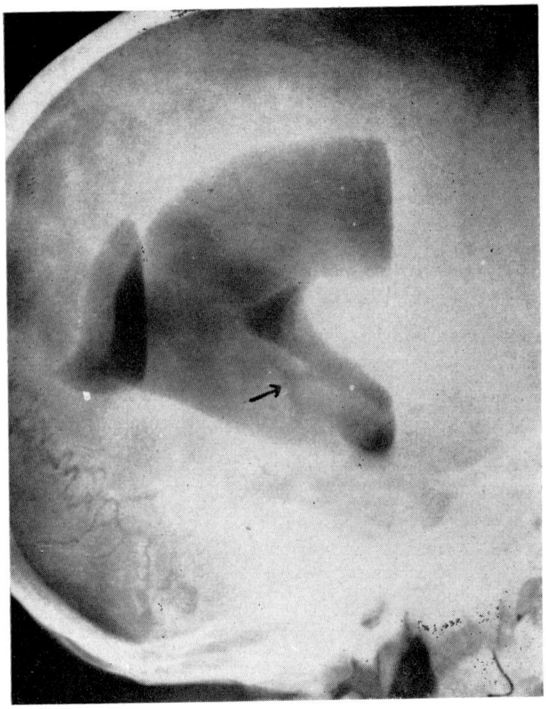

FIG. 3.—Ventriculogram demonstrating kinking of aqueduct of Sylvius by mass in posterior fossa.

Post-operatively he was given a course of tetracyline and his recovery was uneventful.

Pathological Report. The specimen consisted of a stalk of fibrous tissue, 3·75 cm. in length, with a cystic mass at either end. The larger of these cysts was incomplete but appeared to have been approximately 4 cm. in diameter. It had a thin but substantial membranous wall and contained pearly flakes of keratin. A solitary curly hair, 1·4 cm. long, lay within the cyst near its attachment to the cord. The smaller tumour at the other end of the cord was irregular in shape and measured 1·75 cm. in maximum diameter. It had a more fibrous wall, and contained yellowish-brown material and also one or two fine hairs.

A transverse section through the interconnecting cord showed no visible lumen but a firm solid structure of fibrous appearance 2 mm. in diameter.

Histology. The intracranial part of the specimen showed a cavity lined by keratinizing squamous epithelium. A few cerebellar folia attached to it showed patchy degeneration of Purkinje cells but otherwise appeared normal. There was no dural tissue separating the two, but the pia-arachnoid was thickened and infiltrated with lymphocytes and polymorphonuclears (Fig. 4).

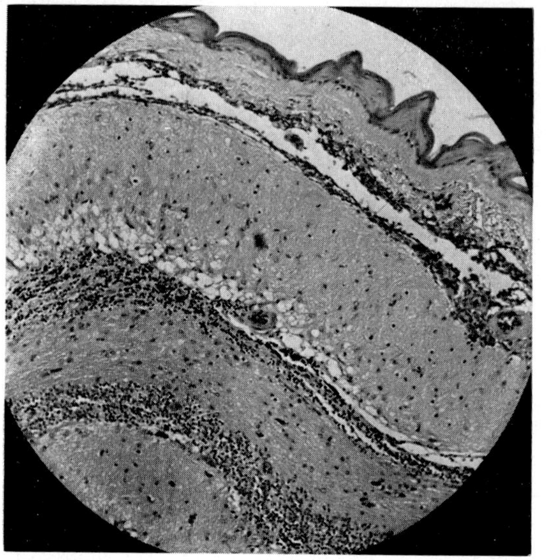

FIG. 4.—Photomicrograph showing intracranial cyst wall and patchy degeneration of adjacent brain tissue. No dural tissue is present. Haematoxylin and eosin × 50.

A section through the stalk showed a solitary remnant of a piece of hair embedded in a core of fibrous tissue (Fig. 5).

The extracranial mass consisted of granulation tissue heavily infiltrated with acute and chronic inflammatory cells. It contained many fragments of hairs with conspicuous foreign-body giant cells, and also some keratinous debris. The diagnosis was of an intracranial dermoid cyst.

Discussion

During recent years there have been several papers reporting cases of congenital dermal sinus but the majority of these have been situated in the spinal axis (Cardell and Laurance, 1951; Perloff, 1954; Haworth and Zachary, 1955; Amador, Hankinson and Bigler, 1955).

Mount (1949) first described two cases of intracranial dermoid cyst associated with congenital dermal sinus. In both cases the cyst was infected forming an intracranial abscess.

Matson and Ingraham (1951) described 10 cases in which there were intracranial complications of congenital dermal sinuses. In nine of their cases the intracranial extension of the sinus was in the posterior fossa, and in the other case there was an infected dermoid cyst in the frontal fossa.

Logue and Till (1952) reviewed the literature and found 25 cases of posterior fossa dermoid cysts to which they added a further seven cases. Of these 32 cases, 22 had no dermal sinus or only an incomplete sinus. Of the remaining 10 cases with a complete sinus there were seven in which the dermoid cyst was intradural and three were extradural.

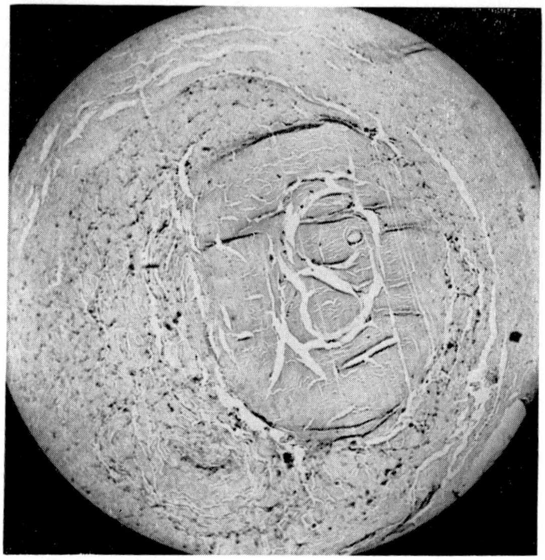

FIG. 5.—Photomicrograph of section through stalk showing a hair embedded in core of fibrous tissue. Haematoxylin and eosin × 42.

More recently, Tytus and Pennybacker (1956) in their paper entitled 'Pearly Tumours in relation to the Central Nervous System' have described a further 43 cases of epidermoid and dermoid tumours. In their series there were eight cases in which the tumour was situated in the midline subtentorially, and of these, three were associated with dermoids of the scalp together with dermal sinuses. One of their patients also had multiple fusion defects of the vertebral column.

The site of the congenital dermal sinus opening is usually marked by a skin dimple, or the sinus may terminate in a cystic swelling in the scalp as in the case presented here. It is situated in the midline, either over the occiput or over the bridge of the nose.

On close inspection hairs may be seen protruding from the mouth of the sinus.

Intracranial dermoid cysts occur most frequently in the posterior fossa, but may also occur at the base of the brain or within the ventricles.

In a child with a congenital dermal sinus a plain radiograph of the skull will invariably demonstrate a small bony defect.

Histologically the cyst wall is made up of squamous epithelium. The contents may be hair, teeth, bone, sebaceous material, masses of squamous epithelium and cholesterin crystals.

Complications frequently occur and fall into two groups: (1) The dermal sinus forms a natural tract, which allows infection to enter the central nervous system resulting in either an intracranial abscess or meningitis. (2) The intracranial cyst may enlarge and cause direct pressure effects on the brain, or it may cause signs and symptoms of raised intracranial pressure.

With regard to the treatment Matson and Ingraham (1951) state 'The treatment of choice is surgical excision of the entire dermal sinus tract from the skin surface to its deepest projection, including all cystic expansions, before infection has occurred or at least at a time when no infection is present'.

In the case presented here there was also the Klippel-Feil deformity. This is known to be associated with other congenital abnormalities of the central nervous system, among which Illingworth (1956) has mentioned 'cholesteatoma' of the cerebellum. This tumour is now considered to be epidermoid in origin.

Summary

A case of recurrent meningitis due to an infected intracranial dermoid cyst is reported. The condition was associated with a congenital dermal sinus and the Klippel-Feil syndrome.

In any obscure case, and particularly any recurrent case of meningitis, it is recommended that a careful search should be made for any evidence of a congenital dermal sinus.

I wish to thank Dr. C. G. Parsons for permission to publish this case, and Mr. E. Turner for details of the operation and for his helpful advice. I should also like to thank Dr. K. B. Rogers for the bacteriological investigations, Dr. R. Astley for the radiographic findings, Dr. A. H. Cameron for the histological reports, Mr. J. G. Williamson for the photographs and Mr. D. R. Paton (Royal Hospital, Wolverhampton) for the photomicrographs.

REFERENCES

Amador, L. V., Hankinson, J. and Bigler, J. A. (1955). *J. Pediat.*, **47**, 300.
Cardell, B. S. and Laurance, B. (1951). *Brit. med. J.*, **2**, 1558.
Cushing, H. (1932). *Intracranial Tumours.* Springfield, Illinois.
Haworth, J. C. and Zachary, R. B. (1955). *Lancet*, **2**, 10.
Illingworth, R. S. (1956). *Arch. Dis. Childh.*, **31**, 8.
Logue, V. and Till, K. (1952). *J. Neurol. Neurosurg. Psychiat.*, **15**, 1.
Matson, D. D. and Ingraham, F. D. (1951). *Pediatrics*, **8**, 463.
Mount, L. A. (1949). *J. Amer. med. Ass.*, **139**, 1263.
Perloff, M. M. (1954). *J. Pediat.*, **44**, 73.
Tytus, J. S. and Pennybacker, J. (1956). *J. Neurol. Neurosurg. Psychiat.*, **19**, 241.

SIRENOMELIA: SYMPUS DIPUS ("MERMAID")

BY

HUGH JOLLY and EDITH M. LAMONT

From the South Devon and East Cornwall Hospital, Plymouth

(RECEIVED FOR PUBLICATION NOVEMBER 5, 1957)

Hendry and Kohler (1956) have recently reviewed the condition of sirenomelia, and in view of its rarity it was thought that a further case record would be of value.

Case Record

The mother, a primigravida of 18 years, had a normal pregnancy, she was rhesus negative, and had no antibodies. The infant was delivered as an extended breech on July 6, 1957, four weeks before term, and weighed 3 lb. 14 oz. (1·76 Kg.). Grunting respirations occurred as soon as the child was delivered and these continued for several minutes, while the heart continued to beat for one hour. Immediately after delivery the child cried and the toes were seen to move.

External Examination. At necropsy a well-preserved sirenomelus of uncertain sex, 17½ inches long, was seen (Fig. 1). The upper limbs appeared flattened antero-posteriorly, and the wrist, metacarpo-phalangeal and interphalangeal joints were readily hyperextended. The pelvic girdle was about two-thirds the expected diameter. A small, shallow dimple was present over the top of the coccyx, and another dimple, immediately below it, represented an imperforate anus. External genitalia were not present, nor was there any urethral orifice. The lower limbs were fused in their whole length and were rotated so that the patellae were on the lateral aspect of the leg. Movement at the knee was possible in a forward direction only. The fused feet were inverted, with the soles anterior, the heels posterior, and the great toes lateral. Eight toes were present, but the smallest was in the midline, on the posterior aspect, and was not visible from the front.

The pinnae were misshapen and placed a little lower than normal. They did not contain cartilage.

Internal Examination. The head and neck were normal. In the thorax, a tracheo-oesophageal fistula was present half-way between the larynx and the bifurcation of the trachea. The upper end of the oesophagus ended blindly, and was wider and thicker than the lower part which emerged from the anterior aspect of the trachea and continued normally. The trachea was normal except for the small aperture leading into the oesophagus. The lungs were poorly expanded. The inter-lobar fissures were normal except for the right transverse which was represented by a fibrous band. The thorax was otherwise normal.

In the abdomen, the spleen, pancreas, liver and biliary passages were normal; the only abnormal part of the alimentary canal was the sigmoid colon, which ended blindly in a bulbous swelling lying in the left iliac fossa.

The adrenal glands were large, occupying an area equal

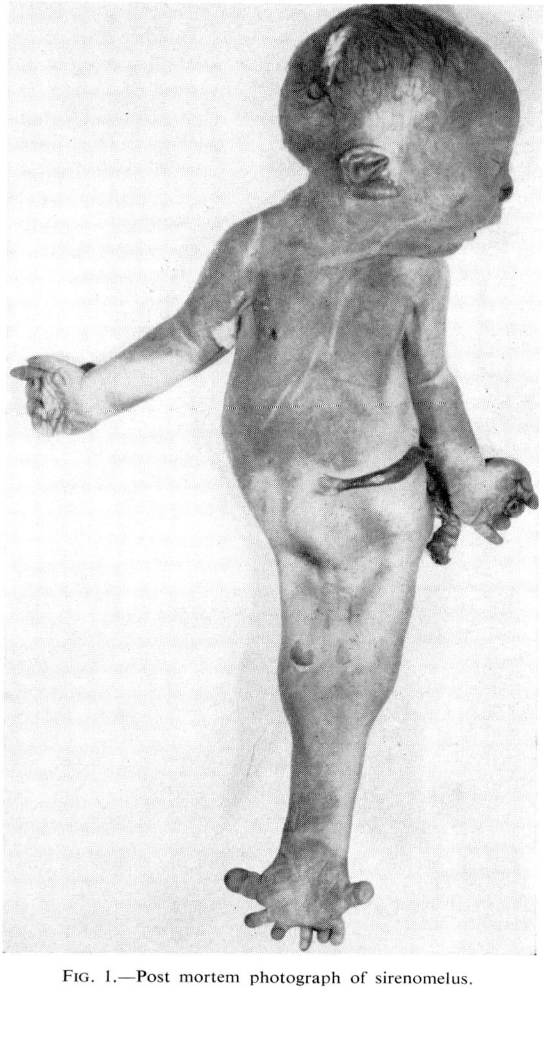

FIG. 1.—Post mortem photograph of sirenomelus.

to that normally occupied by the kidneys. A spherical body, 4 mm. in diameter, situated immediately inferior to the left adrenal gland, was shown histologically to be a rudimentary kidney. No ureters were present but a tubular structure was present on each side below the level of the kidney, attached to a gonad and ending blindly in the skin of the inguinal region (Fig. 2). Histological

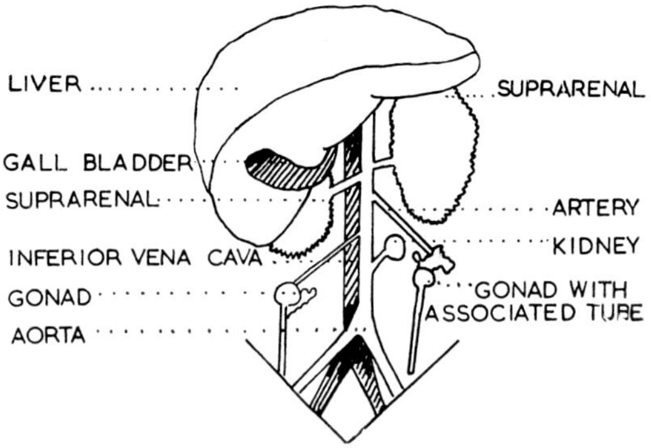

FIG. 2.—Diagram of posterior abdominal viscera.

examination of the gonads showed embryonic seminiferous tubules in the form of solid rods some of which showed early lumen formation, corresponding to the fifth month of development, while cell nuclei examined from several sites showed a female chromatin pattern.

No other pelvic organs were present. The great vessels in the trunk appeared normal, but there was only one artery in the umbilical cord.

MUSCULATURE OF PELVIS AND LOWER LIMBS (Fig. 3). The only internal pelvic muscles present were iliacus and psoas on either side. An unidentified muscle ran between the two greater trochanters. Muscle fibres, arising from both surfaces of the transverse processes of the lower three segments of the sacrum, fused just inferior to the tip of the coccyx, to form a median muscle, whose tendon was inserted into the morphological lateral condyle of the right tibia. The hamstrings were absent. The quadriceps attachments were normal except for an extra branch of the patellar tendon on the left, which ran infero-medially, to be inserted into the tarsus. The deeper fibres of vastus lateralis formed a cruciate arrangement posterior to the knee-joint, and a few of these fibres formed a slender median muscle, whose tendon was attached to the tarsus. The anterior tibial group of muscles (on the posterior aspect of the lower limb) was abnormal and no muscles arose from the anterior aspect of the lower legs. An interosseus muscle arising from the central fibula ran laterally to each tibia.

Radiographic Examination (Fig. 4). The head, neck and upper limbs were normal. There were seven cervical vertebrae, 13 thoracic vertebrae and paired ribs, and six lumbar vertebrae, five sacral segments directed more posteriorly than usual, and a coccyx. In the pelvis, a median bony ridge represented the fusion of the right and left conjoined rami of the ischium and pubis, thus causing the acetabula to face postero-laterally. In the conjoined lower limbs, two separate femora and two tibiae were present, while a median bone, equal in width to the tibiae, lay posterior to them and was thought to represent a fusion of the fibulae. Three centres of ossification were seen in the tarsus, and eight toes were present.

Discussion

In sirenomelia, the developmental abnormality in the lower limbs appears to be a failure of the medial rotation which normally takes place in foetal life. Consequently the anterior aspect of the limb is directed laterally and the fibulae come to lie medial and posterior to the tibiae. This medial position of the fibulae is a characteristic finding in the condition and in our case there is only a single median bone which from its width and muscle attachments is thought to represent a fusion of the fibulae. The failure of rotation causes the soles of the feet to be directed anteriorly and the great toes to be on the lateral aspect of the feet, and results in the peculiar fish tail shape of the fused feet. There is similar failure of rotation of the thighs so that the greater trochanters are directed posteriorly.

Malformations of the urinary tract are usual in

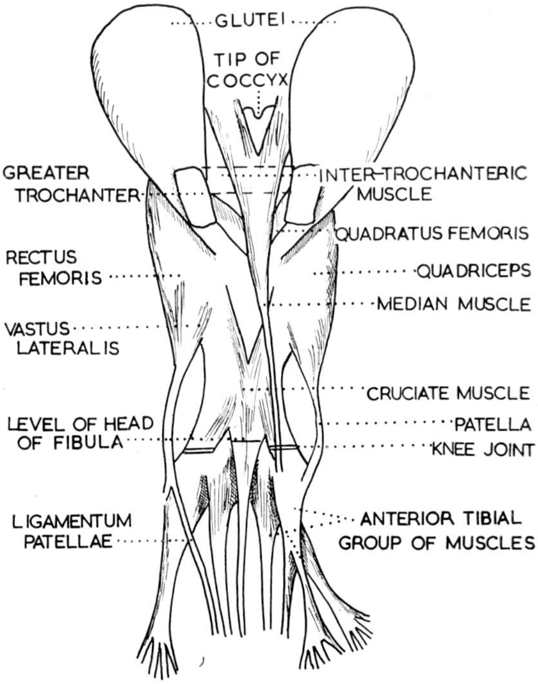

FIG. 3.—Diagram of musculature of pelvis and lower limbs.

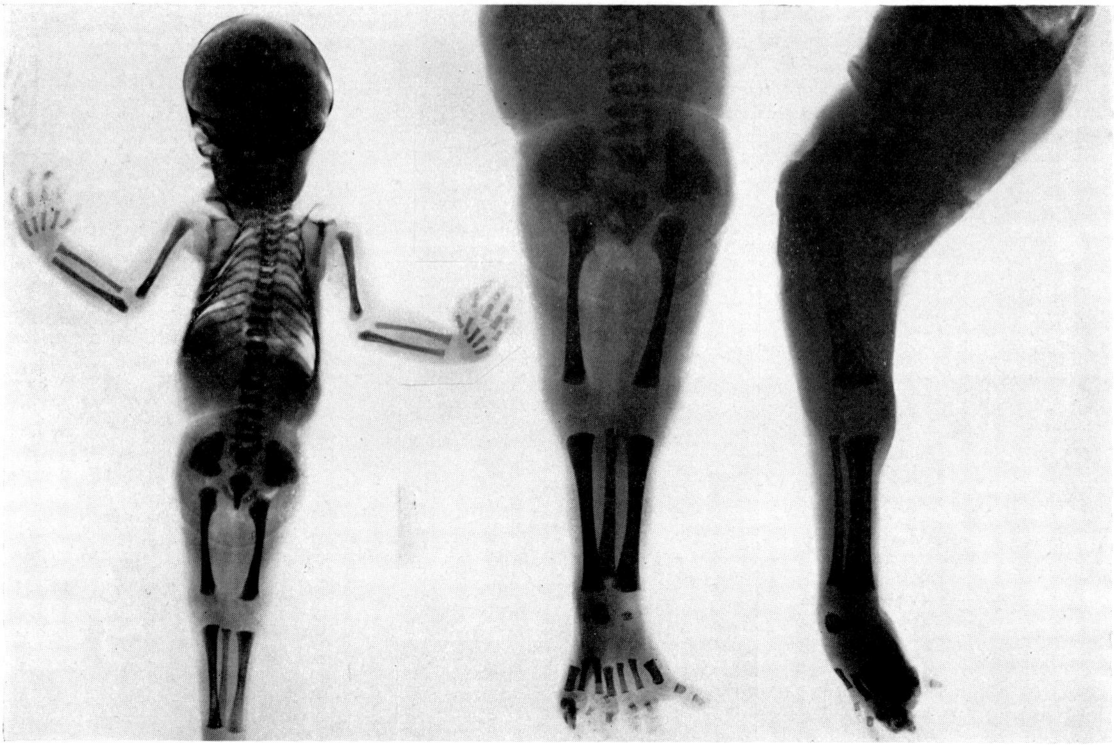

FIG. 4.—Anterior and lateral radiographs of skeleton. The extra vertebrae, the median pelvic bone, the posterior tilt of the sacrum, the posterior fused fibulae, and the fused feet are well shown.

this condition and in this case the only existing part of the urinary system was a single rudimentary left kidney.

Contrary to popular mythical beliefs, the majority of infants with sirenomelia have male gonads as in this case. The nuclear chromatin pattern is less specific to the condition so that little can be deduced from the fact that the pattern was female.

In this case, as in others, only one artery was present in the umbilical cord, while an added feature was the presence of a tracheo-oesophageal fistula.

Summary

A further case of sirenomelia is recorded in view of recent interest in the subject.

We are indebted to Dr. M. R. Thomas for assistance with the necropsy. We are also grateful to Detective Constable R. V. Dallen for the photograph and to Chief Constable J. F. Skittery for providing this facility.

Reference

Hendry, D. W. and Kohler, H. G. (1956). *J. Obstet. Gynaec. Brit. Emp.*, **63**, 865.

GARGOYLISM: CLINICAL, RADIOLOGICAL AND HAEMATOLOGICAL FEATURES IN TWO SIBLINGS

BY

S. B. GRIFFITHS and M. FINDLAY

From the Department of Pathology, University of Natal, and King Edward VIII Hospital, Durban

(RECEIVED FOR PUBLICATION NOVEMBER 5, 1957)

Gargoylism is a rare disease. The complete form of this condition is easily recognized, but incomplete cases occur, and some of these are confused with the Morquio-Brailsford type of chondro-osteo-dystrophy. Most of the recorded cases have been in infants and children, and the early manifestations of this disease are well described by Caffey (1952). Fairbank (1951) states that, as a rule, gradual deterioration takes place and that the child dies before growth is complete. The expectation of life is much greater in incomplete varieties. Lindsay (1950) emphasizes the frequency with which the cardiovascular system is involved. The average age of gargoyle patients dying of cardiac failure is approximately 11 years, with a range of from 1 to 29 years. Cardiac hypertrophy is a striking feature, and there are pronounced lesions in the valves and the coronary arteries. He states that extra-cardiac factors probably contribute to cardiac embarrassment. The most important of these are thoracic deformity and chronic interstitial pneumonitis; the latter appears to be secondary to chronic nasopharyngeal inflammation. Extensive reviews of the clinical and radiological features of this condition are available. It is therefore unnecessary to repeat them.

The two cases to be reported seem to be the first described in non-whites in South Africa. The only cases previously reported from South Africa by McDonald and Opie (1951) and Jackson (1951) have been in individuals of European extraction. Townsend-Coles (1955) has noted three cases in children of the Northern Sudan.

Case Reports

Case 1. An Indian male, known as 'Tweedledum', was first admitted to King Edward VIII Hospital on August 30, 1954, at the age of 11 years. He was of stunted growth, height 3 ft. 8 in. (Figs. 1 and 2). He was deaf and dumb, but of a happy disposition. He had a large dolichocephalic type of head on a very short neck. The facies were heavy, with a depressed bridge to the nose. His respiration was snorting, with open mouth, and he had a profuse nasal discharge. The tongue constantly protruded: the tricuspid teeth were irregular and not in a straight row. The abdomen was protuberant, with everted umbilicus. Hirsutes was evident. There was gross hepatomegaly, but no splenomegaly. He could not extend the elbows freely, and could not raise the arms straight above the head. Flexion of all joints was full. The hands were claw-like. There was no obvious spinal deformity. Reflexes were all present, and motor power was good. There was no clouding of the cornea. The fundi were normal. There was no cardiomegaly; the pulse was 80 and regular. The heart sounds were closed.

LABORATORY EXAMINATIONS. The cerebrospinal fluid was normal. The serum cholesterol was 173 mg. %. The serum calcium was 11·1 mg. %. The serum alkaline phosphatase was 19 K.A. units. Kolmer complement fixation tests on blood and cerebrospinal fluid were negative. The haematological features will be discussed separately.

Case 2. An Indian male, known as 'Tweedledee', was aged 10 years at the time of admission with his brother and was slightly taller. He had an identical configuration, and exhibited very similar features. Hirsutes was marked (Figs. 1 and 2). He was mentally alert, showing an eager interest in his surroundings and was always the instigator in the two's activities. He exhibited night blindness. He was not completely deaf, and was able to speak, though not very distinctly. There was no clouding of the cornea and the fundi were normal. He had signs of upper respiratory catarrh. There was no cardiomegaly.

Laboratory findings were very similar to those of his brother and were non-contributory.

Radiological Features

These were almost identical in the two siblings. The radiographs illustrated are those of Case 1.

Skull. This showed some degree of hydrocephalus, with a dolichocephalic configuration. The pituitary fossa

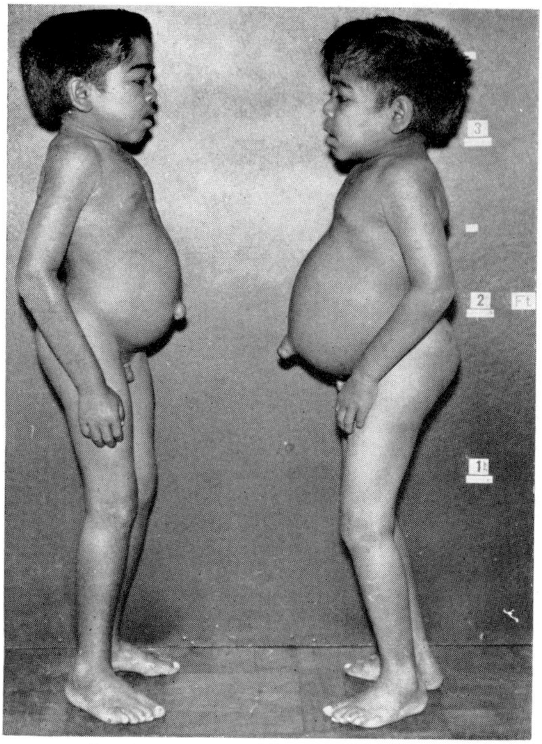

FIG. 1.—The brothers, aged 10 and 11 years.

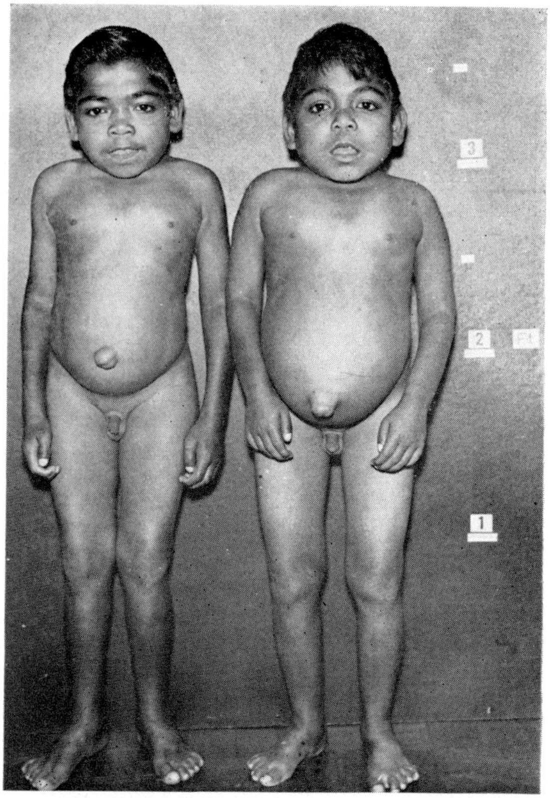

FIG. 2.—The brothers, at the same age as in Fig. 1.

was not obviously enlarged, but the posterior clinoid processes were long (Fig. 3). There was some bulging of the temporal regions. The mandibles appeared slightly enlarged.

Spine. Some of the dorso-lumbar vertebrae were biconvex, and a few vertebrae showed very slight beaking at the lower anterior angles. There was no abnormal kyphosis, and no hypoplasia of the vertebral bodies.

The ribs appeared thicker than normal. The glenoid fossae were shallow.

Upper Limbs. The long bones appeared somewhat tubular, the diaphyses being about the same width as the metaphyses. There was bowing of the radii, and the distal ends of the metaphyses of the radii and ulnae sloped towards each other. Ossification of the wrist bones and carpal bones was delayed. The metacarpals and phalanges were tubular, with a thin cortex, and there was slight pointing of the proximal ends of the metacarpals. The terminal interphalangeal joints of both hands were flexed (Fig. 4).

Lower Limbs. The capital femoral epiphyses were flattened, and there was a coxa valga deformity. The acetabula did not appear shallow. The cortex of the

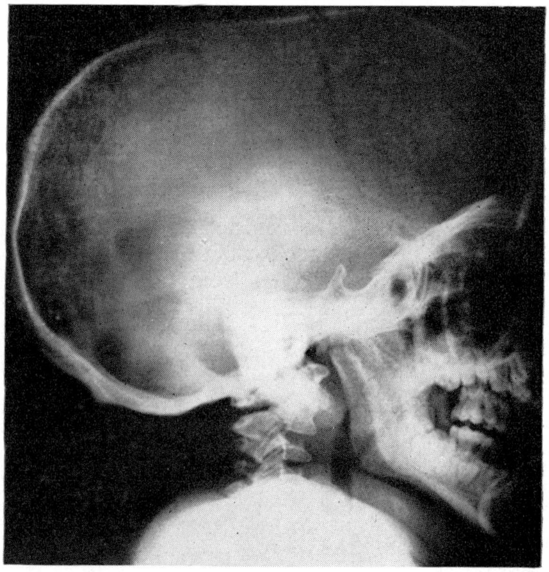

FIG. 3.—Dolichocephalic skull, with elongated posterior, clinoid processes.

lower ends of the femora was thinned and the bones had a shape similar to that seen in Gaucher's disease. The feet showed slight changes similar to those of the hands.

Heart and Lungs. There was some increase of the pulmonary vascular shadows, and prominence of the pulmonic arc. There was no enlargement of the heart at the first examination (Fig. 5). On re-examination approximately two years later cardiomegaly was demonstrated, with marked increase in the prominence of the pulmonic arc, suggesting cor pulmonale (Figs. 5 and 6).

Although the clinical features of these cases are well developed and diagnostic, the radiological features are relatively slight. Retardation of growth is not marked. The upper limbs are not shortened, and the degree of deformity of the shafts of the long bones is not striking. The vertebral changes are very much less obvious than in many reported cases. All the findings, however, are in conformity with the changes described in gargoylism.

FIG. 4.—Showing the flexed terminal interphalangeal joints, the tubular shape of the phalanges and metacarpals, the pointed bases of the metacarpals, the abnormal slope of the distal metaphyses of radii and ulnae and bowing of radii.

FIG. 5.—No cardiomegaly; slight increase of the pulmonary vascular shadows and slight prominence of pulmonic arc.

FIG. 6.—Cardiomegaly with marked increase in prominence of pulmonic arc.

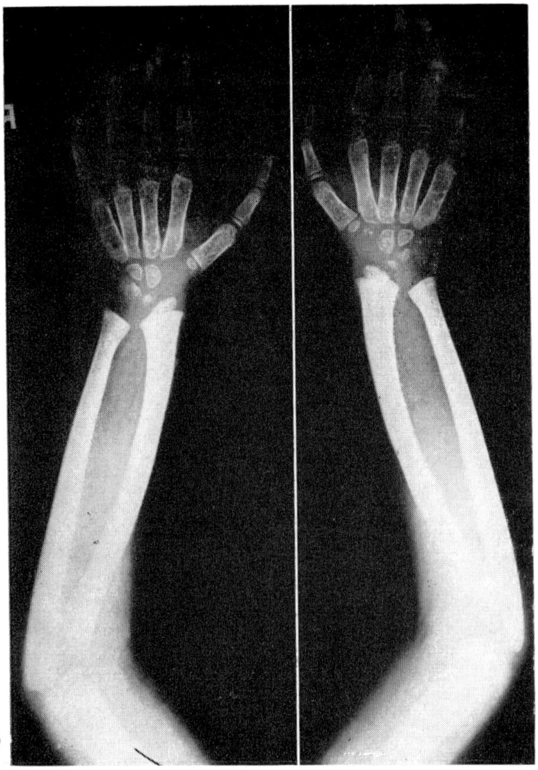

FIG. 4.

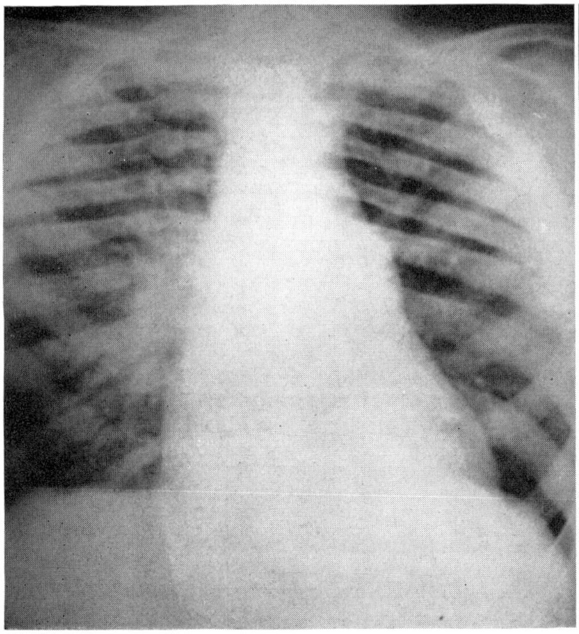

FIG. 5.

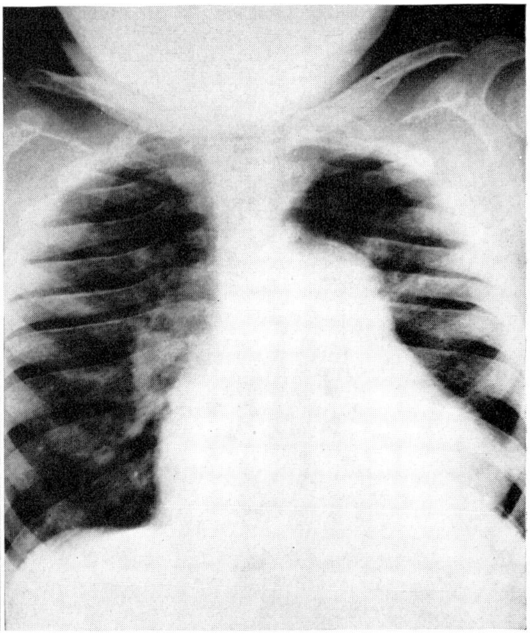

FIG. 6.

Haematological Findings

The peripheral bloods of the two cases were virtually normal. Alder's (1939) anomaly, which consists of a purple staining granulation of the cytoplasm of the polymorphonuclears, lymphocytes and monocytes, was searched for but was not found. This, however, is not surprising as, in spite of some reports, only a moderate number of cases of gargoylism show any abnormality of the white cells of the circulation (McKusick, 1956; Reilly and Lindsay, 1948).

Sternal punctures were performed on both patients. Great difficulty was experienced in piercing the extremely tough skin over the sternum, but good samples of marrow were obtained. The marrow particles were of normal cellularity and leucopoiesis and erythropoiesis were normal. Again Alder's anomaly was not observed, in spite of a prolonged search. The most striking feature of the films, which were stained by the May-Grunwald Giemsa technique, was the presence of numerous large cells distended with many very dark purple-staining masses of varying size. These granules, the largest of which were 1-2μ in diameter, almost completely obscured the outline of the cells, and partially obscured the nuclei. Similar masses of granular material were also found lying free, presumably originating from cells ruptured in smearing. The cells containing these granules were considered to be histiocytes and are shown in Fig. 7.

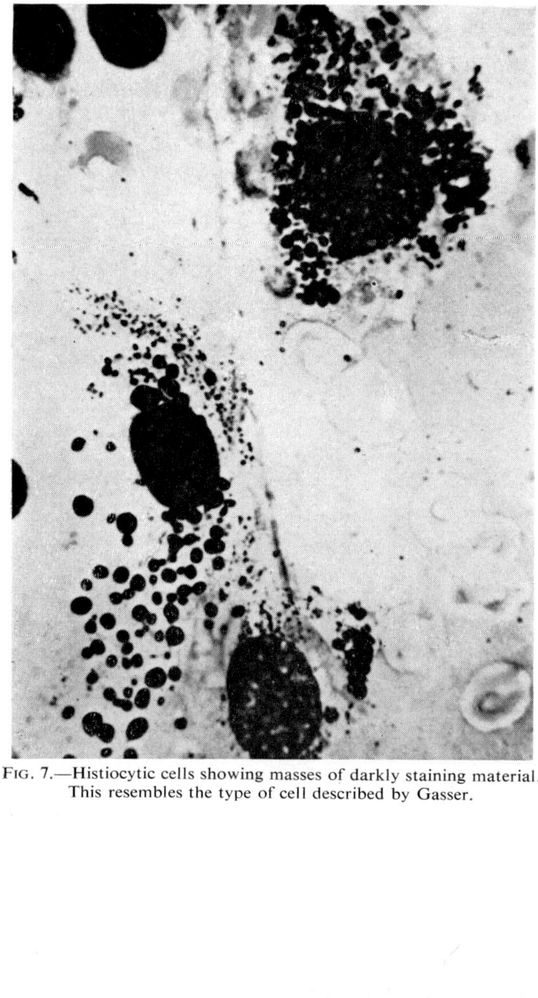

FIG. 7.—Histiocytic cells showing masses of darkly staining material. This resembles the type of cell described by Gasser.

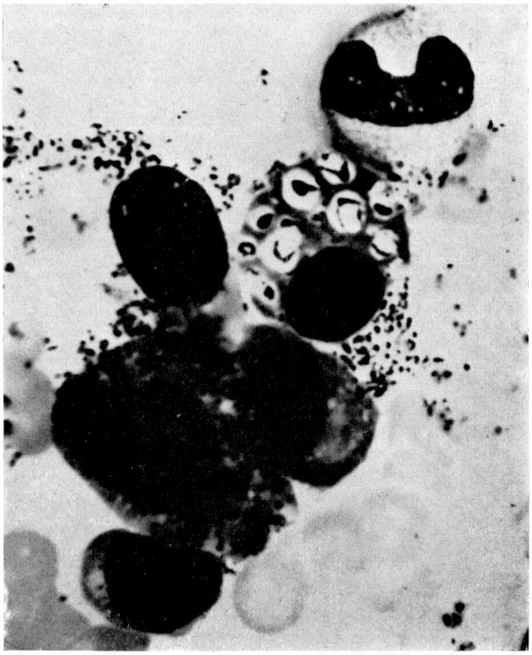

FIG. 8.—Ring-like bodies in clear vacuoles found in cytoplasm of plasma cells.

They were found in the marrow of both patients and are considered to be identical with those described in a case of gargoylism by Gasser (1950).

In addition to this abnormality, further extraordinary inclusions were observed. They were dark purple-staining ring-shaped bodies approximately 1μ in diameter with clear centres, which were found in vacuoles in the cytoplasm of cells, believed to be plasma cells. They are shown in a microphotograph (Fig. 8).

We were unable to trace reports of similar findings in the literature, and we consider them to be quite distinct from the inclusion bodies described previously as occurring in gargoylism.

These cells were present in the marrows of both cases. In September, 1956, the bloods of these cases were re-examined by Dr. J. Duncan-Taylor who found the same phenomena in the bone marrow. Attempts to stain the granules and the ring-like bodies using Nile-blue sulphate and the periodic acid-Schiff method on formol vapour fixed material were unsuccessful. At no time was the material allowed to come in contact with alcohol or xylol and the preparations were examined under water.

Progress

The brothers were under observation for two and a half years, and had been in and out of hospital many times. 'Tweedledum', the elder, had three attacks of bronchopneumonia in 18 months, and developed chronic heart failure. He became dyspnoeic at rest. There was slight ankle oedema. The liver was enlarged to the umbilicus, and there was some enlargement of the spleen. The blood pressure was 120/90 mm. Hg. An electrocardiogram showed right ventricular strain and hypertrophy. The heart became enlarged, with the apex beat in the fifth interspace between the nipple line and the anterior axillary line. There was a blowing systolic murmur at the apex, conducted to the axilla. The pulmonary second sound was accentuated with a soft systolic murmur. He died in March, 1957, from acute cardiac failure. Permission for necropsy could not be obtained.

'Tweedledee', the younger, was always admitted to hospital with his brother because they were inseparable, He has had one attack of bronchopneumonia in the last 18 months. He is not in congestive cardiac failure, and has not developed cardiomegaly. He has dyspnoea on slight exertion. Hepatomegaly is fairly marked, but there is no sign of splenomegaly.

The mother of the children has recently been interviewed, but she was a bad witness, and little information could be obtained as to the earlier history of the siblings. She had two normal children, one about 19 years and the other 9 years old.

Aetiology and Pathogenesis

The aetiology and pathogenesis of this comparatively rare disease is a matter of controversy. The term lipochondrostrophy suggested by Washington (1937) indicated the current view that the disease was a disorder of lipid metabolism associated with skeletal deformities. In a recent review by Creveld (1953) it is still classified amongst the lipoidoses, although current work suggests that the abnormal substance present in the tissues is not a lipoid. The disease was considered to be a lipoid storage disease by Ellis, Sheldon and Capon (1936) and by Henderson (1940).

The essential lesion of the disease is the accumulation, in various parts of the body, of cells containing an abnormal substance, and the bizarre clinical features of the disease can be attributed to the resulting disturbance of structure and function of the affected tissue. The chemical composition of this stored material has been the subject of several recent papers but its nature is still undecided. One of the difficulties is that only a small number of cases have had biopsies or autopsies performed, and no investigator has had material from more than three or four cases to examine. It is possible that the condition is a syndrome which may be caused by the accumulation of more than one substance, thus accounting for the varying results reported. This would also account for the variation in the clinical features of some reported series; and there is increasing recognition of 'incomplete' forms, some of which can only be differentiated with difficulty from similar conditions such as Morquio-Brailsford disease (Kammerer, Mathis and Wackenheim, 1955).

The injection of macromolecular substances of varying chemical nature into experimental animals can produce extensive anatomical changes (Hueper, 1942) but so far the syndrome of gargoylism has not been produced.

Lindsay, Reilly, Gotham and Skahen (1948) thought that the stored material in gargoylism was a glycogen-protein complex. Brante (1952), in a study based on three cases in which he isolated a lipid and a non-lipid fraction, thought the disease was mucopolysaccharidosis. Uzman (1955) reported the isolation of a polysaccharide and a glycolipid fraction. He considered the disease was not caused by the accumulation of these substances, but as a result of a defect in the synthesis of polysaccharide which is known to be intimately concerned with the synthesis of collagen.

Even if it is accepted that the symptomatology of the disease is due to a metabolic defect, there is also evidence that hereditary factors are important in its development. The usual influences which increase the incidence of foetal abnormalities have not been shown to operate in this disease. Maternal age, trauma, disease or state of parity are unimportant. An endocrine factor functioning either directly or as a potentiating influence has been suggested by some (Kammerer *et al.*, 1955), but there is little to substantiate this. Most authors agree that there is a high incidence of families with more than one affected child. Lindsay *et al.* (1948) cite the family described by Böcker (1943) in which there was an affected child in each of four generations who were direct descendants of one unaffected woman. There was also one girl showing signs of Morquio disease in the third generation. Halperin and Curtis (1942) considered that the occurrence of affected individuals could be explained by its being determined by a single autosomal gene. Jervis (1950) in whose series 26 of the 85 families studied had two or more affected members, considered that the numbers were consistent with the condition being due to a single recessive gene. This would only hold if there was a high incidence of cousin marriages. In 11 of 103 families the parents were cousins. A sex linked form has been described (Millman and Whittick, 1952) and single members of binovular twin pairs have been affected, while the other twin has been unaffected. (Lindsay *et al.*, 1948). There is thus strong evidence for gargoylism being a hereditary defect, and McKusick (1956) goes as far as to say that there are at least two genotypes of this disease which can be distinguished clinically.

The two cases described show a remarkable similarity to each other, but whilst the clinical picture closely resembles the classical descriptions of the disease, the radiological features are less marked than might be expected. The blood findings, too, are unusual, and have not hitherto been described. This again emphasizes the probability that different types of the disease exist. Possibly there are different underlying mechanisms which can produce closely similar syndromes.

Summary

Gargoylism in two brothers is described. They appear to be the first cases of this condition recognized in individuals of Indian extraction. The clinical, radiological and unusual haematological findings are described and discussed. Granular inclusions in the bone marrow histiocytes were present, and hitherto undescribed ring-shaped inclusions were present in the plasma cells of the bone marrow.

We wish to thank Dr. S. Disler, Superintendent of King Edward VIII Hospital, for permission to publish these cases, Dr. Rossiter, under whose care they were admitted, and Mr. C. R. Stuart, of the Department of Pathology, University of Natal, for the photographs.

References

Alder, A. (1939). *Dtsch. Arch. klin. Med.*, **183**, 372.
Böcker, E. (1943). (Cited by Lindsay *et. al.*) *Z. Kinderheilk.*, **63**, 688.
Brante, G. (1952). *Scand. J. clin. Lab. Invest.*, **4**, 43.
Caffey, J. (1952). *Amer. J. Roentgenol.*, **67**, 715.
Creveld, S. van (1953). *Advances Pediat.*, **6**, 223.
Ellis, R. W. B., Sheldon, W. and Capon, N. B. (1936). *Quart. J. Med.*, n.s. **5**, 119.
Fairbank, H. A. T. (1951). *An Atlas of General Affections of the Skeleton.* Edinburgh.
Gasser, C. In discussion of paper by Alder, A. (1950). *Schweiz. med. Wschr.*, **80**, 1097.
Halperin, S. L. and Curtis, G. M. (1942). *Amer. J. ment. Defic.*, **46**, 298.
Henderson, J. L. (1940). *Arch. Dis. Childh.*, **15**, 201.
Hueper, W. C. (1942). *Arch. Path. (Chicago)*, **33**, 267.
Jackson, W. P. U. (1951). *Arch. Dis. Childh.*, **26**, 549.
Jervis, G. A. (1950). *Arch. Neurol. Psychiat. (Chicago)*, **63**, 681.
Kammerer, T., Mathis, M. and Wackenheim, A. (1955). *Presse méd.*, **63**, 1386.
Lindsay, S. (1950). *Brit. Heart J.*, **12**, 17.
——, Reilly, W. A., Gotham, T. J. and Skahen, R. (1948). *Amer. J. Dis. Child.*, **76**, 239.
McDonald, R. and Opie, W. H. (1951). *S. Afr. med. J.*, **25**, 725.
McKusick, V. A. (1956). *J. chron. Dis.*, **3**, 360.
Millman, G. and Whittick, J. W. (1952). *J. Neurol. Neurosurg. Psychiat.*, **15**, 253.
Reilly, W. A. and Lindsay, S. (1948). *Amer. J. Dis. Child.*, **75**, 595.
Townsend-Coles, W. F. (1955). *Arch. Pediat.*, **72**, 283.
Uzman, L. L. (1955). *A.M.A. Arch. Path.*, **60**, 308.
Washington, J. A. (1937). In Brennemann's *Practice of Pediatrics*, Vol. IV. Hagerstown, Maryland.

HYDRANENCEPHALY (HYDRENCEPHALY)

BY

L. CROME and PETER E. SYLVESTER

From the Neuropathology Department, The Fountain Hospital, Tooting, London

(RECEIVED FOR PUBLICATION SEPTEMBER 30, 1957)

The terms 'anencéphalie hydrocephalique' and 'hydroanencéphalie' were first used by Cruveilhier (1829, 1862), although the condition appears to have been described even earlier by Breschet (Breschet, 1823, quoted by Kobelt, 1938). The designation was later abbreviated to 'hydranencephalie' ('Hydranenkephalie' in its original German spelling) by Kluge (1902) and Spielmeyer (1905). The subject has been reviewed by Lange-Cosack (1944) and, more recently, by Moser (1952), who collected 32 recorded cases. Many authors still refrain, however, from using the term, presenting similar cases as 'hydrocephalus', 'ox-bladder brain', 'Rindenblasen-porencephalie', 'hydro-microcephaly', 'porencephaly', 'schizencephaly', and so on. Some of the current textbooks do not even mention 'hydranencephaly', while, on the other hand, new cases are being reported (Watson, 1944; Hamby, Krauss and Beswick, 1950; Najman, 1953; Thelander, Shaw and Piel, 1953; Olive and Du Shane, 1953; Hallervorden and Meyer, 1956).

In this condition the cerebral hemispheres are replaced by thin-walled sacs containing cerebrospinal fluid. Its extreme form is incompatible with prolonged survival, and most of the reported cases have been either stillborn or children dying in early infancy. One of the two cases presented by Lange-Cosack, living to 1 year, was allegedly the oldest on record.

While few of these young infants are likely to come under the care of mental deficiency authorities, some, with 'partial hydranencephaly', if such a term be permitted, may live longer and be seen more frequently with low-grade mental defect. We feel justified, therefore, in reporting the following case of hydranencephaly which occurred in a consecutive series of 300 autopsies performed chiefly on low-grade mentally defective children at the Fountain Hospital. If not extreme, the condition may be difficult or impossible to differentiate from related encephalopathies, particularly from hydrocephalus, and this is illustrated by a brief presentation of two further cases, showing some features of hydranencephaly.

Case 1. The patient, the first-born child of healthy parents aged 25 and 24 with no family history of mental or neurological illness, was delivered normally after a pregnancy lasting eight months. He weighed 2·8 kg. at birth and was apparently normal. He developed a cold on the third day and it was noticed then that he never slept more than a few hours at a time.

Constant screaming and the fact that the patient 'took no notice' by the time he was 3 months old caused the parents to seek advice. His head circumference was then 33 cm. with the fontanelle slightly bulging even when not crying. The muscle tone in the limbs, but not in the neck and back, seemed good. The eyes tended to deviate downwards and to the right and the pupils reacted sluggishly to light. Fundal examination, difficult in the circumstances, revealed scattered discrete pigmentation. The left disc was pale and there was a large pale patch near the right disc. He failed to pass any of the usual milestones of development—sitting, crawling, standing, talking or gaining sphincter control. The head gradually increased, never exceeding, however, the limits of normal —42 cm. at 2 years.

Home care became increasingly difficult and he was admitted to the Fountain Hospital at 2 years 9 months, when he was assessed as an idiot with a mental age of 1 month. He weighed 11·4 kg. and lay supine and helpless in his cot. The anterior fontanelle was patent but the skull was normal in shape and size. He could move his limbs and often bit his hands till they bled. Muscle tone was increased in the legs; the knee and ankle jerks were present and both plantar responses were extensor. The abdominal reflexes were absent. He was apparently blind and had marked nystagmus. Both pupils were semi-dilated and reacted sluggishly to light. Ophthalmoscopy confirmed the previous findings of retinal scarring with multifocal pigmentation. His hearing was doubtful. Cardiovascular, respiratory, alimentary and genito-urinary systems were normal.

Routine laboratory investigations such as the W.R., Mantoux and toxoplasmin skin tests were negative. (No other serological tests for toxoplasmosis were done.) Radiological examination at 3 years 9 months showed osteoporosis of the sella turcica and non-united cranial sutures. Later he was found to have a congenital dislocation of the left hip.

During his 18 months' stay in hospital he had several episodes of respiratory infection, vomiting and diarrhoea, and developed measles. He also suffered from petit mal attacks which gave way later to major fits, mostly diurnal, occurring two to four times a month for the last ten months of his life. He made no mental or physical improvement and died of bronchopneumonia at 4½ years.

Pathological Findings

Necropsy. The subject was an extremely dehydrated and emaciated boy weighing 8·9 kg., with regular features and a profuse growth of fine hair over the face and trunk. The head measured 50·5 cm. in circumference. A naevus was present on the left calf, but there were no other external deformities. The trachea and bronchi contained thick secretion and the lungs showed hypostatic congestion, and focal consolidation with 'geographical' surface markings. A few petechiae were present on the pleural surface. All other organs, excepting the brain and eyes, appeared normal.

Microscopical examination of the lungs revealed a combination of lobular collapse with partial infective atelectasis, and inhalation pneumonia. Some alveoli adjoining the areas of collapse were filled with amorphous debris, others contained phagocytic cells of varying size. These had small, darkly-staining nuclei and irregularly outlined, sometimes enormously distended, vacuolated and reticulated cytoplasm. Plasma-cell infiltration was present round the margins of some of the areas of collapse and inhalation pneumonia.

Central Nervous System

The cerebral hemispheres were incised on opening the skull and it was therefore impossible to ascertain whether any of the considerable amount of fluid was subdural. The brain (Fig. 1), emptied of cerebrospinal fluid, weighed 210 g. The left cerebral hemisphere (13·5 × 9 × 5·2 cm.) was represented over the greater part by a paper-thin, transparent sac, marked on its surface by attenuated blood-vessels. Only the posterior and basal portions of the occipital and temporal lobes were more solid, measuring up to 0·4 cm. in thickness. The right hemisphere was better preserved. Its medial surface was also paper-thin, but the rest averaged 0·8 cm. in thickness. While the thinnest parts of the hemispheres were smooth, more solid areas presented a characteristic microgyric pattern, varying from flat 'morocco-leather' to coarser 'cobble-stone' markings. Where it could be measured, the ratio of grey to white matter was about 2 to 1. The internal surface of the hemispheres was smooth and glistening, showing, however, many irregularly distributed nodular elevations of up to 0·2 cm. in diameter. The distended ventricles communicated by a circular central opening (Fig. 2), 4·3 cm. in diameter, the anterior margin of which was formed by the thin fornices. The corpus callosum could not be identified. The basal ganglia were recognizable, the caudate nucleus

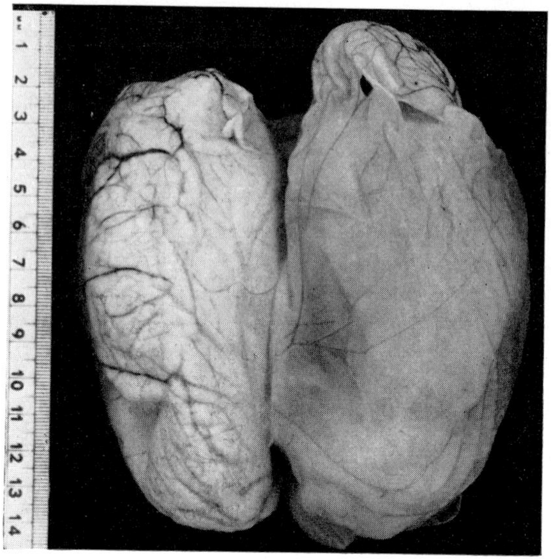

FIG. 1.—Case 1: dorsal view of brain with attenuated vessels on the surface of a dilated and diaphanous left ventricle which has been distended with a balloon.

being relatively large. A thin, elongated connexus thalamicus was stretched across the greatly dilated third ventricle.

The cerebellum, flattened from above downwards, was

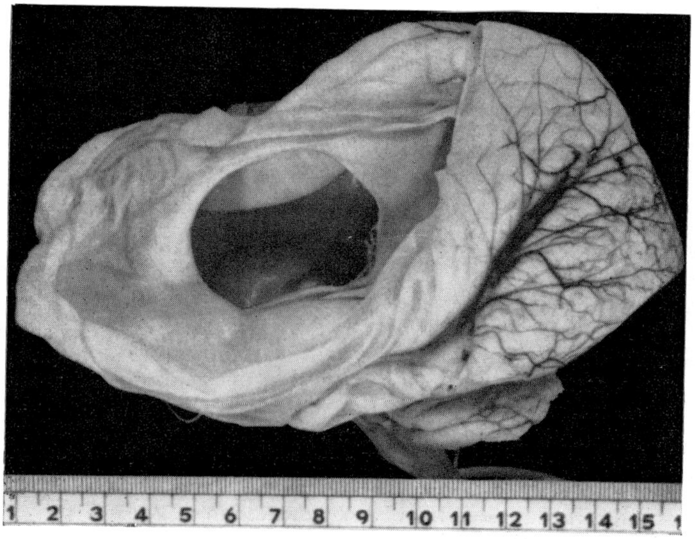

FIG. 2.—Case 1: a large foramen of Monro and dilated lateral ventricles revealed through an incision in the left cerebral cortex.

small, weighing with the brain-stem 42·0 g. The pattern of the arbor vitae was blurred and many folia were narrow. In the brain-stem, the aqueduct of Sylvius was minute and the pyramids absent. The blood-vessels, cranial nerves (with the exception of the optic nerves) and the spinal cord appeared to be normal.

The Eyes. The eyes (Fig. 3), equal in size, measured 2·2 cm. in diameter. Both showed pronounced, cupped macular scarring with pigmentation in and around the scars. Each of the macular scars was larger than the disc, showing 'grease-spot' translucency when held to the light. Scattered pigmentation and smaller scars were also present elsewhere, being more marked in the temporal halves of the globes. The cornea, anterior chambers, irides, ciliary bodies and sclerae seemed normal. The optic nerves were small.

Microscopy

After prolonged fixation in formalin, representative blocks of the cerebral hemispheres, basal ganglia, brain-stem, cerebellum and spinal cord were embedded in celloidin and in paraffin. Sections were stained by the usual neurological and general histological methods. Frozen material was also used as required.

The meninges were essentially normal. Arteries were thin-walled in the subarachnoid space over the hydranencephalic areas, and slightly thickened over the more solid parts of the brain. The external part of the cortical molecular layer was densely gliosed and showed capillary proliferation in some of the better preserved parts (Fig. 4), the glial cells and fibres tending towards parallel orientation to the surface. In places, the glial tissue projected ridgewise into the subarachnoid space.

The cytoarchitectonic structure of thicker portions of the cortex may be summarized as follows. It was most normal in the hippocampus where the molecular and pyramidal-cell layers, the alveus and fascia dentata were clearly identifiable. The arrangement elsewhere was greatly disturbed, bearing no relation to normal lamination. Some areas showed

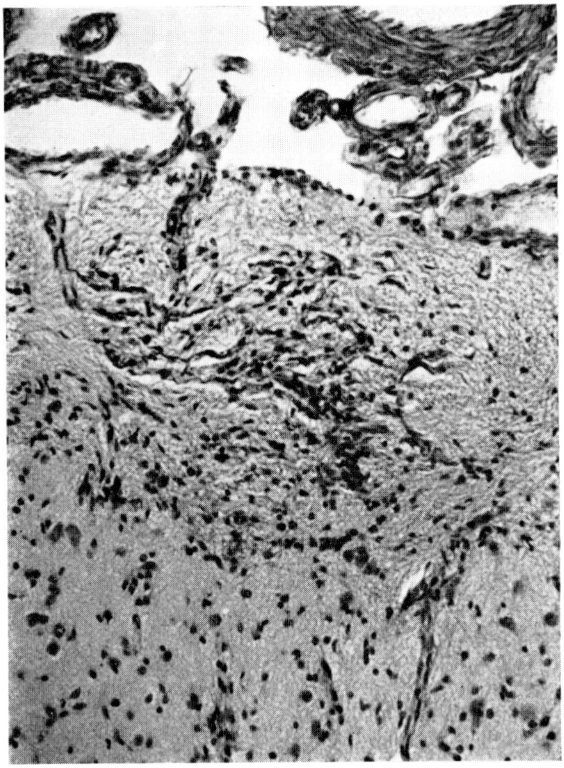

FIG. 4.—Case 1: the external molecular layer of the cortex with glial fibres arranged parallel to the surface. Haematoxylin and eosin × 200.

FIG. 5.—Case 1: cortical microgyria. Haematoxylin and eosin × 30.

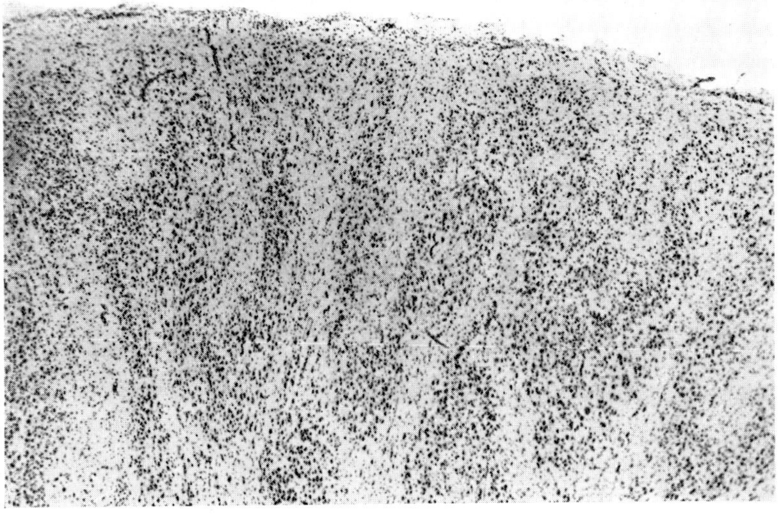

FIG. 3.—Case 1: macular scarring and scattered pigmentation × 3.

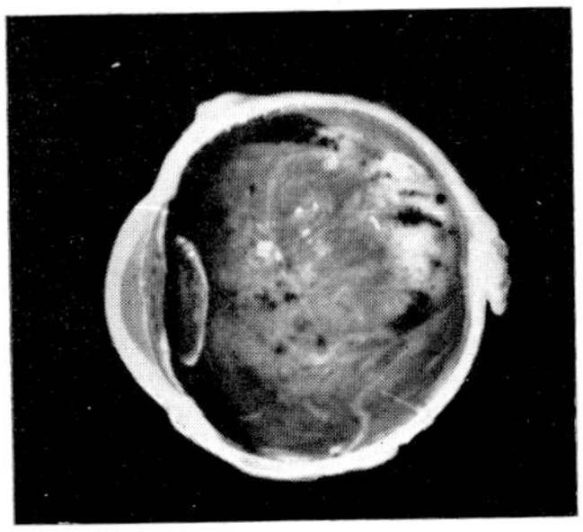

true microgyria (Fig. 5), the superficial garlanded neuronal layer being separated from the deeper grey matter by a sparsely cellular layer. The pattern elsewhere was greatly irregular, defying identification and concise description. Nerve cells varied from area to area: some, in the garlanded superficial microgyric layer were medium-sized pyramids, others were small pyramidal or pleomorphic. Nissl substance stained poorly or not at all. Small delicate bundles of myelinated nerve fibres projected from the main mass of the white matter into the central areas of the microgyric convolutions where these were identifiable. Many irregularly orientated ectopic nerve cells were present in the white matter, forming in its deeper portions small clusters or larger islets, and, particularly near the ventricles, a continuous layer (Fig. 6). These heterotopic

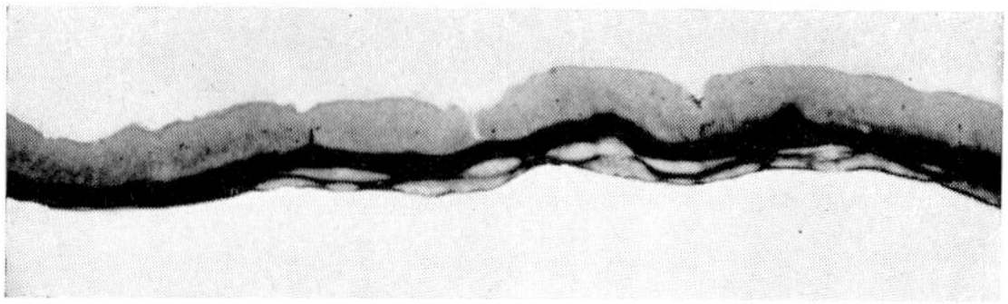

FIG. 6.—Case 1: ectopic grey matter. Heidenhain × 5.

formations of grey matter accounted for the nodular naked-eye appearance of the internal surface of the cerebral hemispheres. Here many of the heterotopic nerve cells showed shrinkage with pyknosis of nuclei and accentuation of dentritic staining. The white matter contained also, near or at the ventricles, many islets and layers of glial cells interspersed densely with particles of calcium (Fig. 7). The latter were mainly extracellular, varying greatly in size. The smallest were dustlike, about 1μ in size, while the largest measured up to 20 to 30μ.

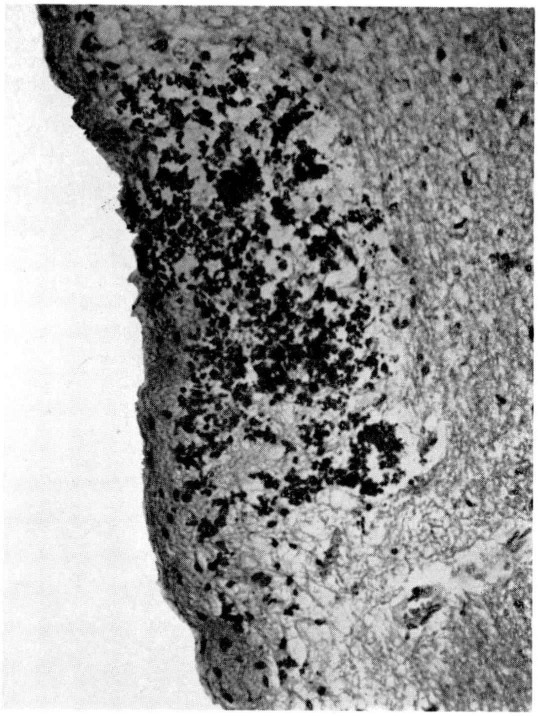

FIG. 7.—Case 1: periventricular calcification. Haematoxylin and eosin × 200.

Most of the ventricular lining, entirely devoid of ependyma, was formed by 12 to 15 rows of glial cells and fibres. In appropriately stained sections this layer showed fibrous gliosis, which was also severe throughout the white matter, particularly in and around the calcified foci, and, as mentioned already, in the sub-pial cortical layer.

The only neutral fat seen was in a few compound granular corpuscles situated in the perivascular spaces, and in some endothelial capillary cells.

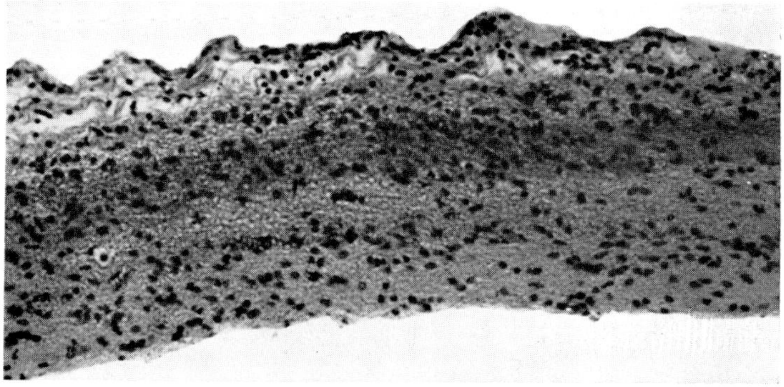

FIG. 8.—Case 1: the cortical membrane composed of partially fused meninges with gliosed cortex. Neurones and ependyma are absent. Haematoxylin and eosin × 200.

The membrane (Fig. 8) enclosing most of the left and a large part of the right hemispheres was formed by partially fused soft meninges externally and a thin uniform layer of glial tissue internally. No stratification of this glial layer could be discerned in thin sections but a certain pattern was visible in appropriately stained thicker sections of celloidin-embedded material. Here the most superficial layer contained few cells and this was followed by a more cellular glial zone, containing also occasional larger degenerate-looking nerve cells and a few compound granular corpuscles. Scanty fragmented and ballooned myelin fibres coursed tangentially in the subjoining layer, which was succeeded internally by irregularly arranged glial cells and fibres. The internal surface was straight and even, showing in a few places foci of linear condensation of four to 10 glial cells.

The basal ganglia were compressed against the base of the skull and the upper part of the striate bodies displaced laterally, presenting, however, little histological abnormality. Normal ependyma lined the entire ventricular system below a point corresponding to the middle of the thalamus. A few ependymal granulations were present. The internal and external capsules were thin on the right side and barely visible on the left. Their myelin stained, however, better than the white matter of the cerebral hemispheres.

Almost the entire cerebellum was microgyric (Fig. 9).

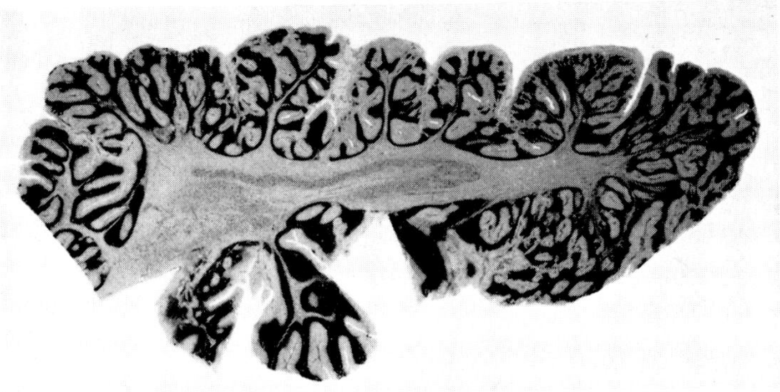

FIG. 9.—Case 1: cerebellar microgyria. Heidenhain × 3½.

Straight or slightly curved tapering streaks of granular and Purkinje cells budded and branched near the surface from stouter and more normally formed folia. Owing to tangential cutting, layers of Purkinje cells were often multiple. The white matter of the cerebellum showed diffuse fibrous gliosis, particularly heavy close to the fourth ventricle, but the dentate and roof nuclei seemed well preserved.

The cerebral peduncles, cortico-pontine fibres and medullary pyramids were rudimentary. The nuclear formations of the brain-stem seemed well developed. A diffuse, fine fibrous gliosis was present throughout the brain-stem, which was most marked around the ventricular and external surfaces. The aqueduct was elongated antero-posteriorly and split into an anterior smaller and posterior larger channel by a bridge of glial tissue in its narrowest portion. Here the widest diameter measured 0·27 mm. and the channel was surrounded by a dense ring of fibrous glia. The constricted portion of the aqueduct widened rapidly with the approach to the considerably dilated fourth ventricle.

The spinal cord showed also diffuse fibrous gliosis, the grey matter being particularly affected. The lateral columns were narrow but showed no discrete areas of demyelination.

Eyes. The retinae and choroid showed widespread focal atrophy varying in extent and severity. Areas of extreme degeneration (Fig. 10) were represented merely by a loose meshwork of fibres containing a few glial cells, with, perhaps, some granules of pigment in the choroid. Moderate degeneration was more extensive, and some normal structural components were usually recognizable in these areas. The retina here was reduced in width, ganglion cells scarce and one or both the nuclear layers depleted of cells. The degree of pigmentation varied greatly, but there was no direct relation between atrophy and pigmentation, some of the most severely degenerated areas showing little or no pigment. The pigment, where present, was mostly extracellular being situated mainly in the external retinal and internal choroid layers, often filling completely elongated spaces. Smaller collections of pigment could also be seen occasionally in the more internal retinal layers. No inflammatory reaction or organisms were present in any of the numerous sections examined.

The neural funiculi of the optic nerves were narrow, and the pial septa thickened.

FIG. 10.—Case 1: retinal atrophy and pigmentation. Haematoxylin and eosin × 200.

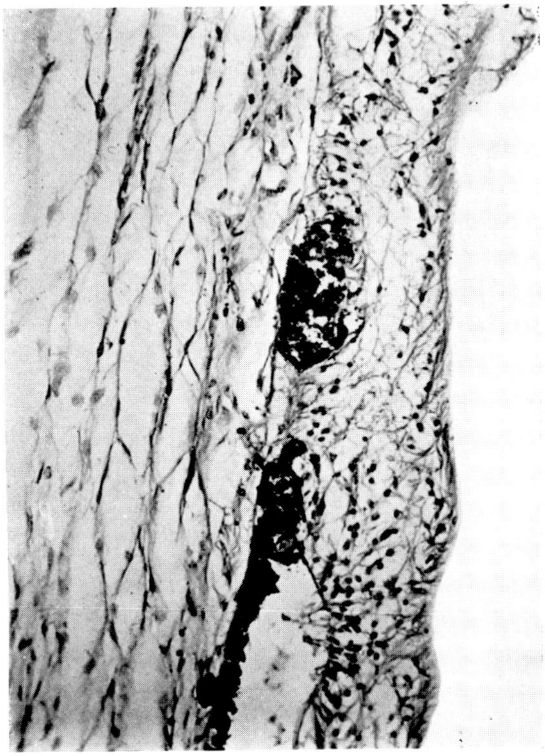

Discussion

Morphology. The size of the hydranencephalic cerebral hemispheres has been inconstant in recorded cases. Some, particularly of older patients, have been large, others normal or frankly micrencephalic. The cardinal feature is absence of all or the greater part of solid cerebral tissue. Where any remains, it is usually found in the basal aspects of the occipital and temporal lobes. This was explained by Lange-Cosack by the greater participation of the vertebral, as contrasted with the carotid arteries, in the supply of these areas. The basal ganglia and the rostral parts of the mid-brain are also absent or degenerate in the most severe cases. Formations below this level are usually substantially intact, showing merely agenesis of the long descending tracts. An exception was cystic change in the cerebellum in a case published by Thelander *et al.* (1953).

The meninges, hydranencephalic membrane and remaining brain tissue are often frankly haemorrhagic, reddish or brownish in colour, showing haemosiderin pigment histologically. Proliferation of phagocytic and meningeal cells, and the presence of fibrin, leucocytes and glial cells have also been noted in some cases.

The histological structure of the membrane enclosing the cystic hemispheres is regarded as crucial in differentiating hydranencephaly from hydrocephalus. In hydranencephaly it is formed externally by the arachnoid and pia and internally by a thin layer of glial tissue said to be devoid of nerve cells, axis cylinders or ependymal lining (Lange-Cosack, 1944; Peters, 1951; Moser, 1952), some neural parenchyma being preserved even in extreme instances of hydrocephalus. However, this criterion may not be conclusive. Russell (1949) describes a membrane in hydrocephalus caused by focal herniation of the ventricular wall through one of the deeper cerebral outer sulci with wide separation of the bordering convolutions. This membrane, partly denuded of ependyma, appeared to resemble that in hydranencephaly, although strips of ependymal cells were present in that case.

Some of the earlier workers also found a few degenerated nerve cells in the hydranencephalic membrane (Kluge, 1902; Spielmeyer, 1905; Kobelt, 1938). Moreover, the demonstration of nerve cells and their processes depends partly on the methods employed. While none could be seen in the thin sections of the paraffin-embedded material in our case, other areas embedded in celloidin and cut more thickly showed unequivocal evidence of nerve cells and myelinated nerve fibres. The absence of ependymal lining is likewise regarded as evidence that the membrane is not formed as in hydrocephalus by the peripherally displaced ventricular wall. This, again, may not be unequivocal. The ependymal lining is, as mentioned already, often partially shed in cases of hydrocephalus, and the ventricular wall can be identified in its absence by the characteristically stratified arrangement of glial cells and fibres in such areas. This was clearly present over a large part of the internal surface of the membrane in our case. A condition, similar to human hydranencephaly was, moreover, described in newborn and stillborn calves by Whittem (1957). He found that the membrane in these cases was formed externally by meninges and internally by ependyma, the intervening spaces containing ragged fragments of well-preserved cortical tissue with nerve cells, astrocytes and other elements. It seems, therefore, that although remnants of neural parenchyma are always scarce, they may not be entirely absent in the hydranencephalic membrane. This would depend, presumably, on the degree and duration of the condition.

The fluid in the hydranencephalic hemispheres is usually clear cerebrospinal fluid. It may, however, be turbid or blood-stained, especially in early cases and after ventricular or spinal puncture.

Stenosis around the foramina of Monro was present in one of Lange-Cosack's cases, and atresia of the Sylvian aqueduct in a case described by Watson. In another instance (Hurowitz, 1936), whose classification is uncertain (*vide infra*), there was no communication between the cerebral cysts and the anterior part of the aqueduct, which was split into many narrow channels. Many of the recorded cases have not been fully examined but some block in the cerebrospinal fluid pathway, functional or anatomical, is frequent; thus Beswick (1948) and Hamby and his colleagues (1950) failed to recover in the cerebrospinal fluid obtained by lumbar puncture dye injected earlier into cerebral ventricles in most cases where this procedure was tried. Aqueductal stenosis was present in our case, the lumen being approximately a quarter of the narrowest width of the normal (0·1 cm.) reported by Sutton (1950), but it is uncertain whether this was the sole cause of the accumulation of the fluid above it.

As expected from the relatively long survival, our case showed more preservation of cerebral tissue especially on the right side, than in other recorded instances. It presented, in addition, microgyria, periventricular calcification and chorioretinopathy with pigmentation, the aetiological significance of which will be discussed below. Similar retinal changes were present in two of the hitherto reported cases (Hamby *et al.*, 1950; Beswick, 1948). 'Microgyria' was mentioned by Kluge in his case, but it is impossible to decide from his description whether this was true microgyria, as in ours.

Aetiology, Pathogenesis and Classification. It seems generally agreed that hydranencephaly results from destruction and resorption of preformed solid cerebral tissue commencing before birth. The possible pathogenetic mechanisms have been fully discussed by Lange-Cosack (1944) and Becker (1949), both favouring ischaemia as the mechanism of the condition and Lange-Cosack suggesting further that this follows compression of the foetal carotid arteries by the umbilical cord or amniotic adhesions. Becker was able to produce comparable unilateral changes in newborn puppies by the injection of a mixture of paraffin and olive oil at a melting point of 40° C. into one of the carotid arteries. The ensuing changes were, successively, necrosis, resorption, and, after nine months to one year, smooth-walled cavitation enclosed by a 'hydranencephalic' membrane. He thought that compression of the carotids might lead first to thrombosis, all intra-arterial traces of which would disappear in time. A case of unilateral cystic degeneration associated with recanalized thrombosis of the middle cerebral artery was reported by Meyer (1949). While this may well be the explanation in some cases, it is difficult to reconcile with the lack of mention of arterial thrombosis in any other of the recorded cases. Moreover, cerebral arteries of hydranencephalic infants observed at craniotomy or by means of angiography by Hamby and by Thelander and their colleagues were patent and, apparently, normal. It is certainly difficult to relate the distribution of the changes in our case to any known arterial pattern.

Congenital syphilis was present in two of the 17 cases reviewed by Lange-Cosack. In an infant aged 20 days presented by Kluge, hydranencephaly was associated with meningo-encephalitis of obscure aetiology. Hallervorden and Meyer noted severe maternal trauma during pregnancy in four of the recorded instances, mentioning focal meningeal inflammatory exudate in their own case. The morphological features of our case, 'hydrocephalus', cerebral calcification and macular scarring with pigmentation, also suggest infection, *i.e.*, toxoplasmosis. Although this could not be confirmed, the diagnosis need not be ruled out by the negative skin test (Sabin and Feldman, 1949) or the absence of identifiable organisms in the no-longer active lesions examined at autopsy. The presence of true microgyria indicates a disturbance occurring before the sixth month of gestation (Crome, 1956).

It seems unlikely that the aetiology and pathogenesis of hydranencephaly are identical in all cases. Thus, very similar changes may set in even post-natally, as in the case described by Kopp (1912) where an entire cerebral hemisphere was converted into a hydranencephalic cyst following severe head injury at the age of 3 years. In a case reported by Globus (1921) as porencephaly, but having certain features of hydranencephaly, there was some histological evidence of inflammation and the author suggested that the condition had been caused by an encephalitis originating in intra-uterine life. It has also been suggested that such changes may result from birth injury (Schwartz, 1927), but this opinion was challenged by later workers on the grounds that the condition is often fully developed in newborn and stillborn infants, and that in some other cases, the patients are, unlike cases of birth injury, relatively symptom-free in the immediate post-natal period.

Typical hydranencephaly can be distinguished from the many variants of cystic encephalopathy, in which cavities are smaller and usually multiple, and from porencephaly in which narrow clefts or funnel-shaped defects traverse all or most of the cortex and white matter. However, there is no unanimity in the use of these terms and less typical forms of hydranencephaly are likely to be classified into one of the above groups.

The relation of hydranencephaly to hydrocephalus presents some difficulty. On account of the frequent evidence of preceding cerebral destruction and resorption, hydranencephaly is regarded as an extensive variant of encephaloclastic porencephaly, quite distinct from hydrocephalus, by most of the recent authors (Lange-Cosack, 1944; Peters, 1951; Moser, 1952). On the other hand, raised intracranial pressure, cranial enlargement, and functional obstruction of the cerebrospinal fluid have been frequently observed in hydranencephaly. These have been interpreted as evidence of hydrocephalus developing secondarily as a complication of hydranencephaly.

The problem depends partly on definition. The term 'internal hydrocephalus' usually refers comprehensively to any excessive accumulation of fluid in the ventricular system. The causes are diverse and include obstruction of the cerebrospinal fluid pathway, oversecretion of fluid or failure of its absorption (Russell, 1949). In other cases hydrocephalus may be a part of a complex of developmental abnormalities. It is likely, for example, that parts of the cerebral vesicles which fail to develop offer less resistance to transient rise in intraventricular pressure than the less abnormal ones, and that localized ventricular dilatation, so frequent in cases of cerebral malformation, may arise in this manner. Ventricles may also dilate passively (hydrocephalus '*ex vacuo*') following atrophy, scarring or resorption of the overlying tissue. If severe and extensive, such destruction may result in hydranencephaly.

Thus, viewed in the light of current definitions, the distinction between hydranencephaly and hydrocephalus would seem to be one of degree, particularly since some of the morphological criteria on which it is largely based have, as stated already, certain limitations.

It may be argued, however, that cases with primary atrophy and destruction of the ventricular wall and periventricular tissue ('encephaloclastic hydrocephalus') should not be included in the general group of hydrocephalus. If so, considerable difficulty will often be encountered in distinguishing between primary and secondary atrophy. The reason for the frequency of raised intra-cranial pressure and of signs associated with it (*vide infra*) in hydranencephaly also remains to be elucidated, although some periventricular and aqueductal stenosis was demonstrated in a few of these cases.

Moreover, some of the less typical variants of hydrocephalus which are common among mental defectives may present certain hydranencephalic features as illustrated by the following two cases.

Case 2. This girl, the younger of two siblings with a family tree free from mental or nervous illness, was born after a normal pregnancy and labour. She failed to develop mentally and was admitted to the Fountain Hospital at 6 months of age. At that time she was characteristically microcephalic with a head circumference of 27 cm. The fontanelles and sutures were closed and the skull showed ridging over the sagittal and lambdoid sutures. The scalp was loose and transversely folded. The only other external abnormalities were two raised vascular naevi, one over the scapula and the other upon the back of the left hand. She had *grand mal* attacks, screamed frequently and failed completely to develop mentally. Routine laboratory tests were negative. During her stay in hospital she had several attacks of respiratory infection, succumbing to one following measles at 16 months.

Necropsy findings, confirmed microscopically, were bronchiolitis, focal collapse and infective atelectasis, and pulmonary oedema.

The brain (Fig. 11), looking like a periwig, was even smaller (116 g. with cerebrospinal fluid) than would be expected from the smallness of the skull (34 cm.) and there was much fluid in the subdural space. The cerebral hemispheres (Fig. 12) above a horizontal plane corresponding approximately to the middle temporal gyri were converted to fluid-filled sacs enclosed by a paper-thin membrane. Conspicuous, somewhat tortuous vessels, coursed over the membrane, the lower half of which was rough on its external surface. The internal lining of the membrane was smooth and glistening. The transition from the upper membranous to the lower solid part of the brain was clear-cut. The latter (Fig. 12) showed microgyria above, and a smooth surface with broad gyri and short, shallow sulci upon its inferior and basal aspects. The anterior commissure was present, the foramina of Monro dilated, the fornices thin and the

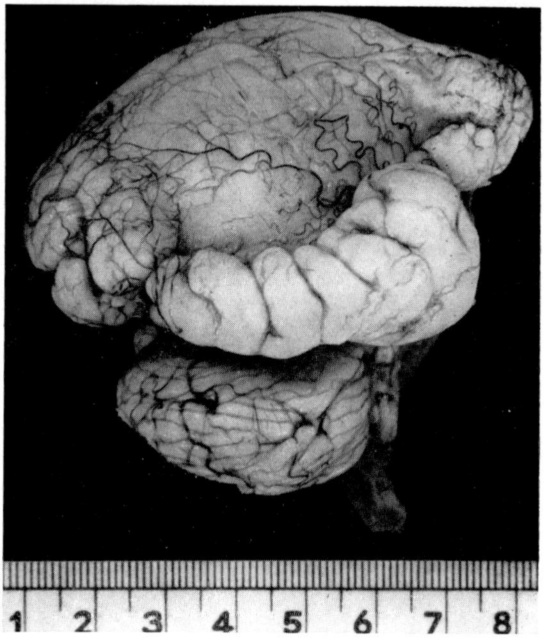

FIG. 11.—Case 2: lateral view of brain with 'periwig' appearance.

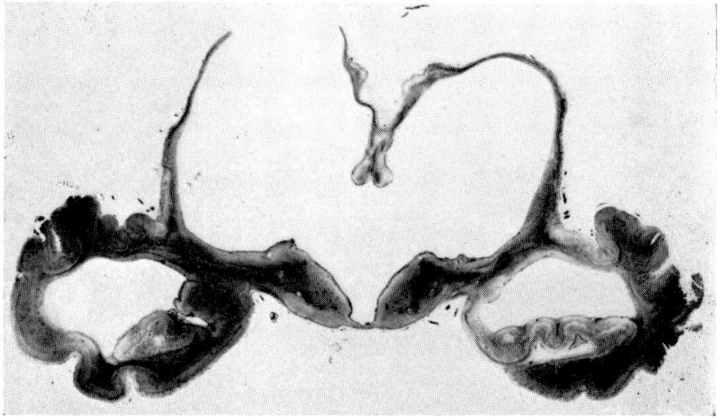

FIG. 12.—Case 2: microgyria and thin cortex in coronal section of entire brain. Heidenhain × 1⅓.

corpus callosum rudimentary. The choroid plexuses in the lateral ventricles were large. The third and fourth ventricles, with the aqueduct, were dilated. The cerebellum, together with the brain-stem, weighed 42 g. The pyramids were absent, and the inferior olives prominent. The optic and oculomotor nerves were thin. Other cranial nerves and basal blood-vessels seemed normal.

The histological appearances were similar to those in Case 1. The thin membrane was formed by soft meninges and a layer of glial tissue mostly devoid of ependyma. The arachnoid was, however, unlike Case 1, irregularly thickened, fibrosed and deficient in places. There was excessive collagenization and proliferation of blood vessels penetrating the glial layer from the meninges. No recognizable nerve cells or myelin fibres were present in the membrane, which showed focally dense fibrous gliosis and many accumulations of glial cells. Considerable neuronal loss and fibrous gliosis were present in the basal ganglia. Some of the cerebellar folia were thin and poorly cellular, but showed no definite microgyria.

COMMENT. While this case presented obvious hydranencephalic features, there were also significant differences. No history of raised intracranial pressure was suggested clinically or by the morphological findings. In particular the intraventricular pathway was patent. The sharp transition from the inferior solid to the membranous upper part of the brain was striking, and the picture as a whole dominated by pronounced micrencephaly. The findings can be best interpreted as hydrocephalus following uneven pallial agenesis, complicated later by meningeal fibrosis and widespread cerebral gliosis. Morphologically, the condition can be best classified as hydrocephalus with severe micrencephaly.

Case 3. This boy, the first child of a 24-year-old healthy unmarried mother, was born at term by Caesarean section performed for an abnormal lie. The birth weight was 4 kg. Normal milestones were not attained. At 4 months, he began to show signs of hydrocephalus, the head circumference being 46 cm. at 6 months. He was admitted to the Fountain Hospital when 16 months old as a hydrocephalic idiot with spastic quadriplegia and bilateral optic atrophy. The head circumference at that time was 58 cm. and this increased by 1·3 cm. during the next five years. Routine laboratory tests were normal. He failed to advance, developing flexor contractures of the limbs, frequent respiratory infections, and eventually dying at 7 years 3 months of bronchopneumonia—confirmed at necropsy.

Translucent meninges covered an abnormally shaped brain (Figs. 13 and 14), weighing 850 g., in which there was great thinning of the cortex in the occipital region (3-4 mm.) and temporal lobes (0·5 mm.). Below the inferior temporal sulci and extending on to the inferior surface of the lobes the gyral pattern was lost, being preserved elsewhere in the brain. The depth of sulci varied from area to area being greatest in the parietal regions, shallow over the thin temporal or occipital cortex. The sulci were wide and deep in the frontal areas. The cerebellum (with brain stem) weighed 126 g., and showed, bilaterally, around the horizontal fissure

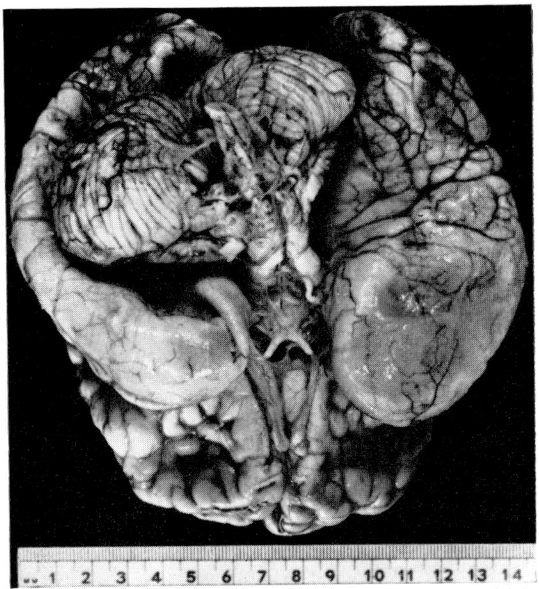

FIG. 13.—Case 3: ventral view of brain with thin temporal lobes.

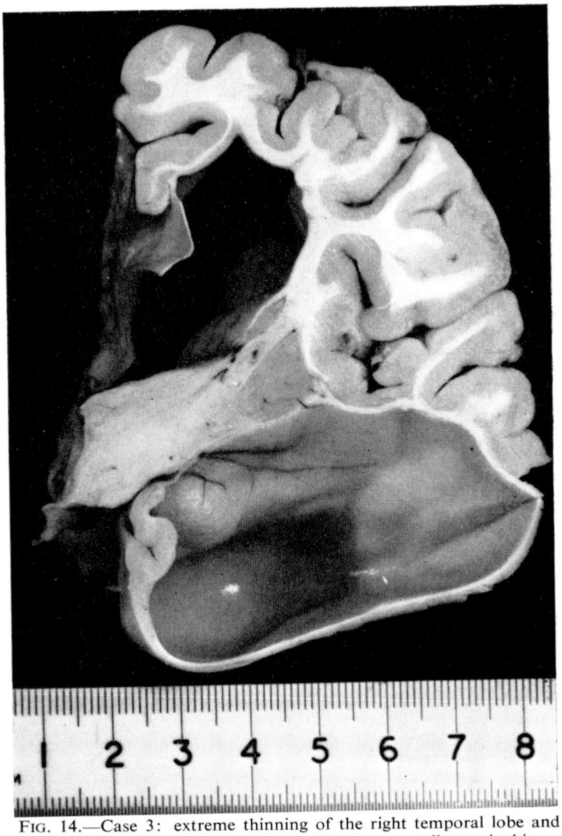

FIG. 14.—Case 3: extreme thinning of the right temporal lobe and dilatation of the lateral ventricle. The corpus callosum is thin.

several atrophic and yellow discoloured folia. The ventricular system, including the aqueduct of Sylvius (Fig. 15) was greatly dilated. The ventricular lining was smooth except in the fourth ventricle where it had an 'ox-tongue' roughness. The entire corpus callosum was thinned. The pyramids were small. Choroid plexuses and blood vessels appeared normal with the exception of those vessels over the thinned temporal lobes, which were reduced in number and calibre. The optic nerves were small and firm but other cranial nerves appeared normal.

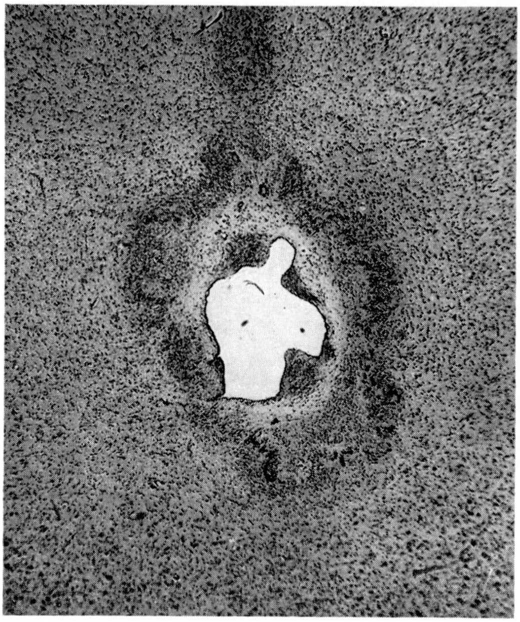

FIG. 15.—Case 3: ependymal granulations and increased gliosis of the aqueduct of Sylvius. Nissl × 25.

Save for lesser stratification of glial cells and the presence of haemosiderin, the membrane (Fig. 16) representing the thinned temporal cortex was similar to the preceding cases. A few degenerated neurones, some of which were calcified, were present in it. In other areas, laminar structure was preserved even in the thinned occipital cortex. Haemosiderin was present in the cerebellum and adjacent meninges, being most marked in the atrophic folia which showed also loss of Purkinje cells and demyelination. Periventricular gliosis was increased throughout, and in the basal ganglia, the aqueduct, and the fourth ventricle, there were many coarse ependymal granulations. The cortico-spinal tracts were small.

COMMENT. Unlike Case 1, the intraventricular pathway in this instance appeared sufficiently patent. Pronounced ependymal granulations suggest past infection, and haemosiderin deposits indicate old haemorrhage. Either or both these factors may have played a significant part in the pathogenesis.

Unlike Cases 1 and 2, there was no evidence of an embryological defect such as microgyria or micrencephaly.

This case is not an uncommon example of communicating hydrocephalus, but the structure of the membrane fulfils the morphological criteria of hydranencephaly (Lange-Cosack).

Despite all the unresolved difficulties, it seems useful to retain a special descriptive term for cases with unequivocal features of hydranencephaly, though this is not, perhaps, the happiest designation. Cruveilhier employed it to describe what he believed to be a combination of anencephaly and hydrocephalus, but this is not really the case. Anencephaly is now known to be a distinct and obvious malformation in which the calvarium is not formed and the brain is represented by a disordered hamartomatous arrangement of vascular and immature neural tissue, often described as 'area cerebrovasculosa'. Although a transitional case showing certain features of both hydranencephaly and anencephaly has been described by Hurowitz, it remains unique and seems different from all other instances of hydranencephaly, in which the skull is complete and the brain is not hamartomatous.

It seems preferable, therefore, to avoid the suggestion of anencephaly in the designation, and 'hydrencephaly' is, perhaps, a better term.

Clinical Features

It appears from a perusal of the literature that a few cases of hydranencephaly show cranial enlargement at or soon after birth, and occasional neonatal

FIG. 16.—Case 3: the thin gliosed membrane of the temporal cortex with normal meninges. Haematoxylin and eosin × 50.

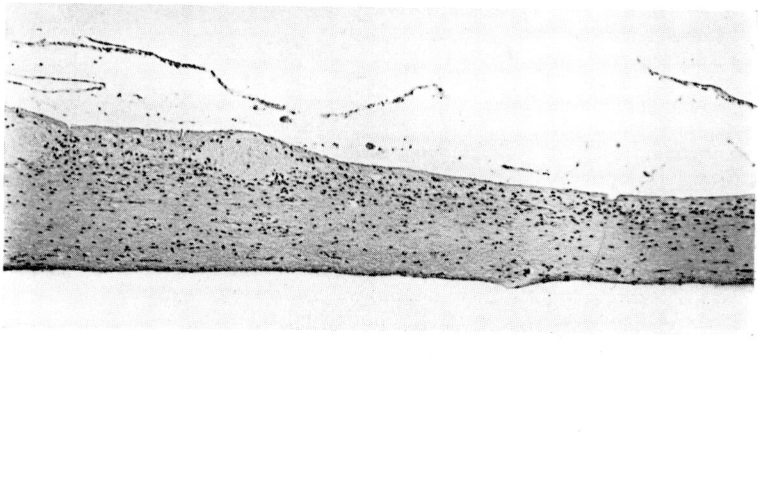

jaundice has also been recorded. Usually, however, the newborn is normal in appearance and behaviour for the first days or weeks. Feeding difficulty, frequent screaming and hypothermia are common later, and these are followed by incoordinate eye movements, strabismus and nystagmus. The optic discs are pale; light reflexes may be present or absent. Movements of limbs are usually present and tendon jerks are brisk. In a few weeks or months the head begins to enlarge, intracranial pressure rises and signs of hyper-irritability develop. A 'cracked-pot' sound is often elicited. The pressure of the cerebrospinal fluid is raised and the fluid often shows excess of protein. Spasticity becomes apparent, and many forms of convulsion and tremor occur. The patients are sometimes anaemic. Failure of mental development is increasingly obvious. Transillumination of the skull is a useful and safe diagnostic procedure (Strasburger, 1910; von Bókay, 1923), a reddish reflection being often seen not only over the skull, but through the retinae and ears. The electroencephalogram may be quite flat and the ventriculographic appearances are diagnostic.

Lange-Cosack distinguished two groups of hydranencephaly. Patients in the first, with the greater loss of cerebral tissue and involvement of subcortical centres, are severely disabled and show disturbance of autonomic regulation. They do not survive beyond the first month. The subcortical centres are not involved in the second group, and patients deteriorate less rapidly. It appears, therefore, that the clinical features may enable severe cases to be diagnosed correctly in life. Nevertheless, it is doubtful whether the clinical features are always sufficiently clear-cut to distinguish less severe hydranencephaly from other forms of hydrocephalus. Hydranencephalic patients living long enough to be classed as mentally defective, as our Case 1, could be expected to present even more frequently with atypical features.

Summary

Hydranencephaly is a congenital condition in which the cerebral hemispheres are replaced by thin sacs containing cerebrospinal fluid. Characteristically, the sac wall consists of pia and arachnoid overlying the glial layer—all that remains of the cerebral cortex and white matter.

Hydranencephaly is a descriptive term not implying, on the evidence available, specific aetiology, pathogenesis or clinical features which would always distinguish it from other severe variants of hydrocephalus or porencephaly. It is unfortunate that, etymologically, the term suggests a combination of hydrocephalus and anencephaly, since it is in fact unrelated to anencephaly, hence 'hydrencephaly' is more appropriate.

These conclusions are reached by a review of the literature and the study of a fairly typical case of hydranencephaly in a $4\frac{1}{2}$-year-old epileptic idiot and of two hydrocephalic cases presenting partial features of hydranencephaly.

Toxoplasmosis was suggested by the findings in the first case but this could not be verified.

We are indebted to our colleagues at the Fountain Hospital for access to their case records and their helpful criticism.

References

Becker, H. (1949). *Dtsch. Z. Nervenheilk.*, **161**, 407, 446.
Beswick, W. F. (1948). *N.Y. St. J. Med.*, **48**, 2364.
Bókay, J. von (1923). *Mschr. Kinderheilk.*, **25**, 43.
Crome, L. (1956). *J. Path. Bact.*, **71**, 335.
Cruveilhier, J. (1829). *Anatomie pathologique du corps humain*, p. 1. Paris.
—— (1862). *Traité d'anatomie pathologique générale*, Vol. 4, p. 75. Paris.
Globus, J. H. (1921). *Arch. Neurol. Psychiat. (Chicago)*, **6**, 652.
Hallervorden, J. and Meyer, J. E. (1956). In *Handbuch der speziellen pathologischen Anatomie und Histologie*, p. 222, edited by O. Lubarsch, F. Henke and R. Rössle, Berlin, Band 13. Teil 4.
Hamby, W. B., Krauss, R. F. and Beswick, W. F. (1950). *Pediatrics*, **6**, 371.
Hurowitz, J. (1936). *Schweiz. Arch. Neurol. Psychiat.*, **38**, 207.
Kluge, H. (1902). *Z. Kinderheilk.*, **23**, 208.
Kobelt, W. (1938). Thesis, Univ. Heidelberg.
Kopp, J. (1912). *Dtsch. Z. Chir.*, **116**, 226.
Lange-Cosack, H. (1944). *Arch. Psychiat. Nervenkr.*, **117**, 595.
Meyer, J. E. (1949). *Z. Kinderheilk.*, **67**, 123.
Moser, E. (1952). *Ann. paediat. (Basel)*, **179**, 193.
Najman, E. (1953). *Ibid.*, **181**, 249.
Olive, J. T. and DuShane, J. W. (1953). *Amer. J. Dis. Child.*, **85**, 43.
Peters, G. (1951). *Spezielle Pathologie der Krankheiten des zentralen und peripheren Nervensystems*, p. 194. Stuttgart.
Russell, D. S (1949). *Observations on the Pathology of Hydrocephalus, Spec. Rep. Ser. med. Res. Coun. (Lond.).* No. 265.
Sabin, A. B. and Feldman, H. A. (1949). *J. Pediat.*, **35**, 296.
Schwartz, P. (1927). *Ergebn. inn. Med. Kinderheilk.*, **31**, 165.
Spielmeyer, W. (1905). *Arch. Psychiat. Nervenkr.*, **39**, 807.
Strasburger (1910). *Dtsch. med. Wschr.*, **36**, 294.
Sutton, D. (1950). *Brit. J. Radiol.*, **23**, 208.
Thelander, H. E., Shaw, E. B. and Piel, J. J. (1953). *J. Pediat.*, **42**, 680.
Watson, E. H. (1944). *Amer. J. Dis. Child.*, **67**, 282.
Whittem, J. H. (1957). *J. Path. Bact.*, **73**, 375.

THE WENCKEBACH PHENOMENON AND AURICULAR-VENTRICULAR DISSOCIATION IN CHILDREN

BY

M. H. SHNIER

From the Department of Paediatrics, Baragwanath Hospital, Johannesburg

(RECEIVED FOR PUBLICATION NOVEMBER 26, 1957)

The Wenckebach type of heart block is characterized by a progressive lengthening of the P-R interval until A.V. conduction fails and a beat is dropped. This form of heart block was first described as a clinical entity by Wenckebach (1899) on the basis of radial arteriograms. Since then, this phenomenon has been seen in a variety of conditions including digitalis poisoning, rheumatic fever, tonsillitis and other febrile conditions, diphtheritic and other forms of myocarditis and myocardial infarction. It is not uncommon in adults but few case descriptions refer to children.

Sprague and White (1927), when describing cases of heart block under the age of 30 years, make brief reference to a group of children showing this phenomenon. They described a transient Wenckebach phenomenon in a girl aged 16 years following tonsillectomy and a post-operative cold and more severe grades of heart block in children suffering from diphtheria and rheumatic fever. Zimdahl (1951) and Kuhn, Donoso and Sapin (1954) each described the cases of two children in whom the Wenckebach phenomenon complicated cardiac catheterization. Langen (1956) reported the phenomenon in two 19-year-old youths in whom no cardiac lesion could be found. Ehrentheil, Alimurung and Massell (1952) on analysis of 107 electrocardiograms showed a relationship between sinus arrhythmia and the Wenckebach phenomenon.

A.V. dissociation exists when the auricles and ventricles beat independently. According to Wood (1946) this condition occurs when in nodal rhythm retrograde conduction is completely blocked while forward conduction remains unimpaired. As the rate of discharge from the sinus node is usually slower than that from the A.V. node, the ventricles beat faster than the auricles. Occasionally, however, the auricular rate may be the faster (Magri, 1953).

As in the Wenckebach phenomenon, rheumatic fever, diphtheria, acute febrile states, myocarditis and myocardial infarction may be associated with A.V. dissociation.

This paper presents the case histories of five children with cardiac arrhythmia. Two of these cases are examples of the Wenckebach phenomenon and three cases are examples of A.V. dissociation.

Case Histories

Case 1. A 4-year-old African child was in good health until five days before admission to hospital when she developed an irritating cough. Soon after this, diarrhoea and vomiting commenced associated with anorexia, fever, vague abdominal pains and headache.

Examination revealed a thin undernourished child. Her temperature was 103° F. The pulse rate varied between 50 and 100 beats a minute and was unaffected by respiration. The volume was poor. The heart was not clinically enlarged and no murmurs were audible. The remainder of the clinical examination was essentially negative and the child was investigated as a case of pyrexia of unknown, possibly influenzal, aetiology.

An electrocardiogram recorded 12 hours after admission (Fig. 1a) shows the Wenckebach phenomenon (the first and last complexes) and 2:1 A-V block. This arrhythmia persisted for 96 hours with periods of 2:1 A-V block (Figs. 1b and 1c) and the classical Wenckebach phenomenon (Fig. 1c and 1d).

LABORATORY INVESTIGATIONS. The haemoglobin was 15·8 g./100 ml. with a leucocyte count of 9·000/c.mm. (60% neutrophil polymorphs, 6% monocytes, 29% lymphocytes, 5% eosinophils). The sedimentation rate was 50 mm. per hour (Westergren). The serum sodium was 135 mEq./l. and the serum potassium was 5·7 mEq./l. No pathological organisms were found in the blood, stools or urine. Agglutination tests for typhoid fever and complement fixation tests for viral diseases were negative.

The fever abated 48 hours after admission but the child remained distressed until the fifth day of illness when she improved dramatically. This improvement coincided with a return to normal cardiac rhythm (Fig. 1e).

This patient was observed for a further two months during which period her electrocardiogram continued to show a normal rhythm (Fig. 1f).

Case 2. An African boy, aged 9 years, had been in good health until four days before admission to hospital.

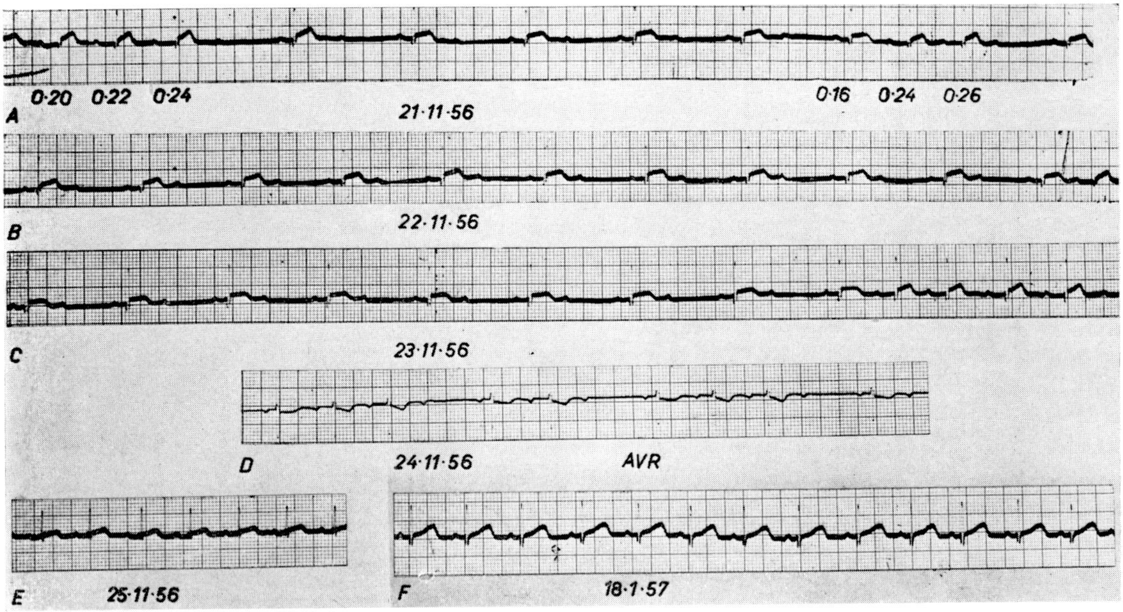

FIG. 1.—Case 1. Pyrexia of unknown, possibly influenzal, origin. Fig. 1a: (standard lead II) classical Wenckebach phenomenon tracing in the first and last three complexes with 2:1 A.V. block which may be considered as extreme form of this phenomenon. Fig. 1b: 24 hours later, a 2:1 A.V. block, which was unaltered the next day (Fig. 1c). Fig. 1d: (lead AVR) a day later, classical Wenckebach phenomenon tracing. Figs. 1e and 1f: normal tracings four days and two months after initial tracing.

He then developed pain in the chest accompanied by a severe cough productive of green mucoid sputum. He had also noticed increasing breathlessness and swelling of the feet.

Examination revealed a dyspnoeic child with dependent oedema to the level of the sacrum. The pulse rate was 120 beats a minute and the volume was full. The blood pressure was 100/75 mm. Hg. The maximum cardiac impulse was located in the 6th intercostal space over the anterior axillary line and suggested left ventricular hypertrophy. A grade III systolic murmur was heard at the mitral area replacing the first heart sound and was conducted into the axilla. The pulmonary second sound was slightly accentuated and clearly split. Crepitations were audible at the bases of both lungs. The liver was palpable 4 fingerbreadths below the costal margin.

LABORATORY INVESTIGATIONS. The haemoglobin was 15·3 g./100 ml. with a leucocyte count of 7,800 per c,mm. (41% neutrophil polymorphs, 4% monocytes, 55% lymphocytes). The E.S.R. was 8 mm. per hour (Westergren), the antistreptolysin titre was 1/200 units and the C reactive protein was ++++. The diagnosis was acute rheumatic carditis with congestive cardiac failure.

During the first 12 hours the child received 1·0 mg. of digoxin orally divided into three doses given 4-hourly. During the next 12 hours he was given three doses of 0·125 mg. and thereafter was maintained on 0·125 mg. twice daily. In addition he was given a low salt diet and received a mercurial diuretic by intramuscular injection on alternate days. On this therapy his pulse rate slowed from 120 to 96 beats a minute. A month later he complained of nausea and vomiting and dropped beats were noticed. Digoxin was discontinued and potassium chloride g. 3 daily was given by mouth. Three days later when cardiac failure was again apparent, digoxin therapy was recommenced without recurrence of the arrhythmia.

Electrocardiographic studies concomitant with the onset of nausea and vomiting (Fig. 2a) showed P-R intervals of 0·28 seconds with occasional dropped beats. The dropped beats occurred at random without lengthening of the preceding P-R intervals. The P-R intervals following a dropped beat were shortened to 0·24 seconds while the electrocardiograms recorded 24 and 72 hours later (Figs. 2b and 2c) showed that the P-R intervals varied in length from 0·28 to 0·32 seconds before a dropped beat occurred.

A return to normal rhythm was recorded four days after the arrhythmia was first noted (Fig. 2d).

Case 3. A 9-year-old African boy had suffered, since the age of 6 years from repeated attacks of pain in the chest, back and feet with periodic swelling around the ankles. His exercise tolerance remained good until four weeks before admission to hospital, when breathlessness occurred on exertion. His symptoms gradually increased until he was immobilized by dyspnoea and a generalized swelling of his whole body.

On examination the child was dyspnoeic with dependent oedema to the level of the sacrum. The jugular veins

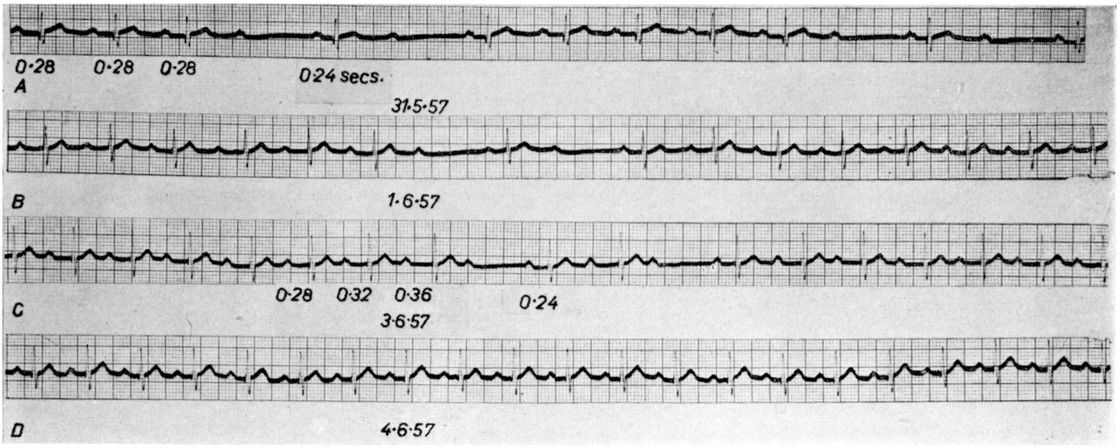

FIG. 2.—Case 2.—Rheumatic carditis on digoxin therapy. All tracings are from standard lead II. Fig. 2a: Mobitz block, constant P-R interval of 0·28 seconds going into a 2:1 A.V. block. P-R intervals following dropped beats are shortened to 0·24 sec. Fig. 2band c: slight variations in P-R interval 0·25-0·32 sec. before dropped beat, i.e. form of varying Wenckebach phenomenon. P-R intervals following dropped beats are shortened to 0·24 sec. Fig. 2d: normal tracing four days after initial tracing.

were engorged to 2 in. above the sternal angle and the liver was enlarged to three fingerbreadths below the costal margin. The maximum cardiac impulse was located in the 6th intercostal space in the anterior axillary line and was characteristic of left ventricular hypertrophy. A grade III systolic murmur, completely replacing the first heart sound was heard at the mitral area and a blowing diastolic murmur radiating from the base of the heart down the left sternal border was also present. The pulmonary second sound was accentuated and split. All the pulses were palpable, regular in rate and collapsing in quality. The left side of the chest was dull to percussion and there was bronchial breathing over the apex of the left lung.

LABORATORY INVESTIGATIONS. The haemoglobin was 11·5 g. per 100 ml. and the E.S.R. was 49 mm. in one hour (Westergren). The C reactive protein was ++++. Urine analysis was negative. A radiological examination of the chest showed cardiac enlargement and consolidation of the whole of the left lung. An electrocardiogram demonstrated bifid P waves of left auricular enlargement. The diagnosis was left lobar pneumonia and congestive cardiac failure with established aortic and mitral incompetence.

He received 0·5 mg. of digoxin orally followed by three 8-hourly doses of 0·25 mg. and a maintenance dose of 0·25 mg. daily. In addition he received 1 ml. of a mercurial diuretic on alternate days. As improvement was slow, the maintenance dose of digoxin was doubled to 0·25 mg. twice daily. Some 28 days later he complained of abdominal pain and vomited. His pulse was found to be irregular and an electrocardiogram (Fig. 3a) revealed a rate of 75 to 100 cycles a minute with well marked sinus arrhythmia. The P waves occurred at regular intervals but bore no relationship to the QRS complexes, showing A-V dissociation.

This dissociation could be temporarily abolished by injecting 0·25 g. of potassium chloride intravenously as is demonstrated in Figs. 3b and 3c which represent the beginning and end of a continuous tracing. A further 0·25 g. of potassium chloride given intravenously produced nodal rhythm (Fig. 3d), which reverted 10 minutes later to A-V dissociation. Fig. 3e taken 18 hours later, and Fig. 3f taken three days later, show a normal tracing with a constant P-R interval of 0·14 seconds.

Case 4. An African child aged 8 years complained of a severe cough, high fever, a stabbing pain in the chest and dyspnoea at rest which commenced 24 hours before admission to hospital.

He was orthopnoeic and the respiratory excursions were obviously limited by pain. The right side of his chest moved poorly on respiration and was dull to percussion. Crepitations, bronchial breathing and diminished air entry were heard over the right base and midzone. The pulse was irregular due to sinus arrhythmia. The heart was not clinically enlarged and a grade II systolic murmur was heard at the mitral area. A diagnosis of right lobar pneumonia was made.

He was treated with 6-hourly intramuscular injections of 500,000 units of penicillin. Two days later the temperature fell to 98° F. and the pulse rate from 120 to 80 beats a minute. Four days after admission the child was still distressed despite the resolution of the infection. An electrocardiogram at this stage shows a ventricular rate of 60 cycles a minute with A-V dissociation (Figs. 4a, 4b and 4c). The P-P and P-R intervals varied in length, the P waves being periodically lost in the QRS complexes. The next day (Fig. 4d) the rate was 54 cycles a minute with sinus arrhythmia present. The A-V dissociation had however disappeared and this return to normal rhythm coincided with a marked clinical improvement.

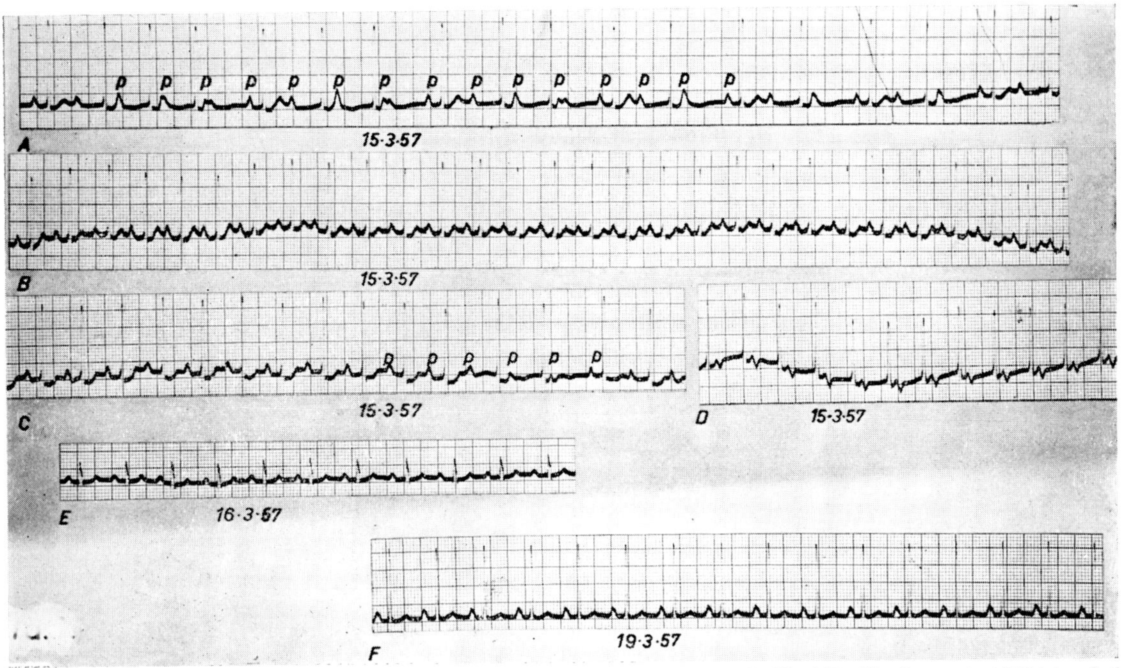

FIG. 3.—Case 3. Rheumatic carditis with left lobar pneumonia. All tracings are from standard lead II. Fig. 3a: constant P-P interval of 0·48 sec. with heart rate of 75 to 100 cycles min. P waves bear no relationship to QRS complexes, showing A.V. dissociation. Fig. 3b and c are beginning and end of continuous tracing during intravenous injection of 0·25 g. of potassium chloride showing tachycardia of 136 cycles/min. with abolition of A.V. dissociation which recurs five min. later (Fig. 3c). Fig. 3d: tracing during intravenous injection of further 0·25 g. of potassium chloride showing that nodal rhythm has replaced A.V. dissociation. Fig. 3e and f: normal tracings 18 hours and two months later.

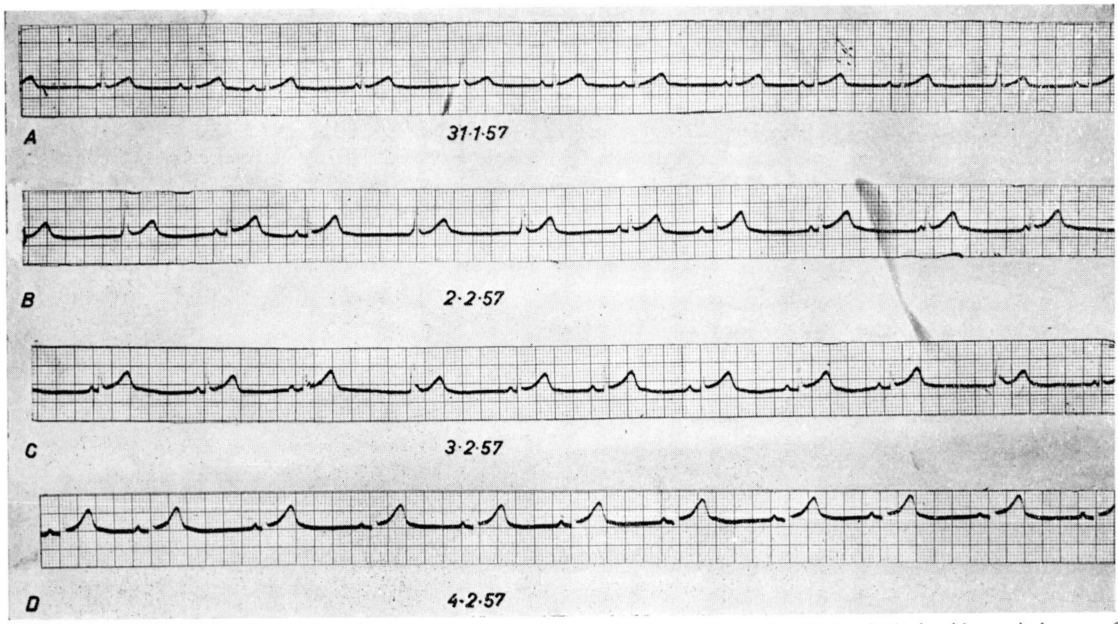

FIG. 4.—Case 4. Lobar pneumonia. All tracings are from standard lead II. Figs. 4a, b and c: sinus arrhythmia with ventricular rate of 60 to 75 cycles/min. P-P intervals vary in length and P waves are periodically lost in QRS complexes. This is tracing of A.V. dissociation. Fig. 4d is tracing taken next day and shows disappearance of A.V. dissociation.

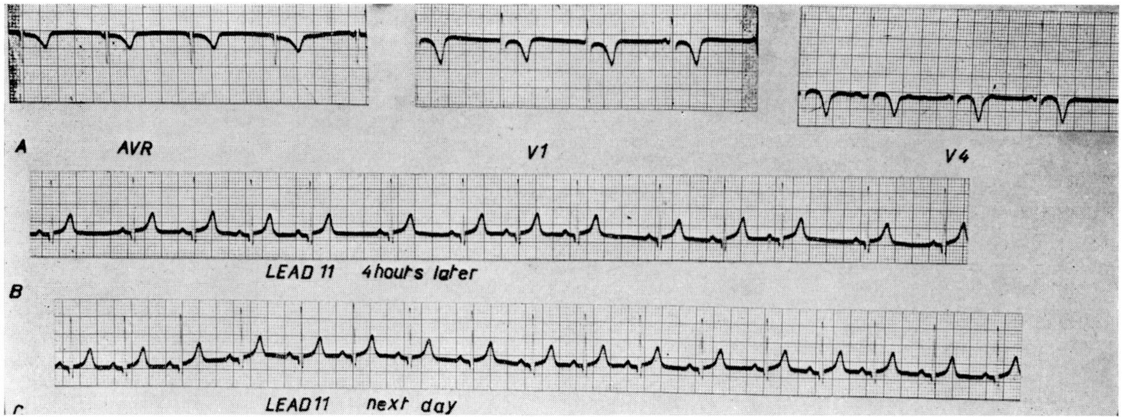

FIG. 5.—Case 5. Belladonna poisoning. Fig. 5a: leads AVR, VI and V4 show A.V. dissociation with P waves moving in and out of QRS complexes. Fig. 5b: standard lead II, taken four hours after preceding tracing and shows A.V. dissociation replaced by sinus arrhythmia. Fig. 5c: standard lead II, normal tracing taken next day.

Case 5. An African staff nurse related the following story about her son aged 8 years.

He had been perfectly well until the night before admission to hospital when he awakened in a state of extreme mental excitement and confusion. His mother found him dashing around his room terrified of the snakes and trains which he claimed were rushing at him. She noticed that he was flushed, his pupils were dilated and his mouth was dry. He had to be strapped down for the night and a doctor called to see him the next day, gave him an intramuscular injection of 'somnifane'. He slept for about three hours and awoke still confused. It was ascertained that he had not had access to drugs but that he might have eaten some berries when playing in the fields.

On examination he was restless, exhibiting quick nervous movements. His skin was hot and flushed, his pupils were widely dilated and reacted to light. His mouth was dry and he was hallucinated. His reflexes were brisk. Clinical examination of the heart revealed no abnormalities and a diagnosis of belladonna poisoning was made.

An electrocardiogram taken because of his irregular pulse is shown in Fig. 5. In the first tracings leads A.V.R., V1 and V4 are shown as they are the only available records. In these leads the P waves can be seen moving in and out of the QRS complexes showing A-V dissociation. A tracing taken four hours later (Fig. 5b) showed well-marked sinus arrhythmia, while the tracing taken on the following day (Fig. 5c) was normal.

Discussion

In childhood arrhythmias occur most commonly with rheumatic heart disease and in patients maintained on high doses of digitalis. In this series arrhythmias were observed in two cases during digitalis therapy given for cardiac failure following rheumatic carditis, in two cases they were associated with acute infections, while the fifth case was associated with belladonna poisoning.

There are very few case reports (Blumgart and Gargill, 1930) of children who showed transitions from A.V. dissociation to sinus arrhythmia. This sequence is shown in Case 5 (Figs. 5a-c), and was associated with belladonna poisoning.

Blumgart and Gargill (1930) demonstrated a distinct relationship between sinus arrhythmia and A-V dissociation. They showed that when the P-P interval lengthens, shortening of the P-R time results. Extreme prolongation of the P-R interval results in a ventricular escape which may manifest itself as A-V dissociation. In this condition the ventricular rate is usually faster than the auricular rate and the P waves fall progressively closer to and are finally lost in the QRS complexes. When the P-R intervals become sufficiently prolonged, a conducted impulse from the auricles may occur, namely, ventricular capture, before A-V dissociation may once again be established.

Many theories have ben advanced to explain these disturbances in cardiac rhythm. Organic interruption of A-V conduction (Mobitz, 1923) has been blamed, as well as exaggerated susceptibility to fatigue of the conducting system (Ehrentheil *et al.*, 1952), and disturbances in conduction just before the A.V. node. Whatever the mechanism, the disturbances in the present series of cases were all of a temporary nature and disappeared when the primary disease was treated.

In the two cases of acute infection and the case of belladonna poisoning which responded to treatment, the heart returned to normal rhythm within one to four days after the primary disease had abated. These children subsequently remained well and active. Where the primary disease caused marked cardiac damage as in the two cases of rheumatic fever, the patients remained ill with a poor exercise tolerance. The prognosis in these cases depended upon the primary disease rather than the changes in cardiac rhythm. It was, however, observed that all five cases remained distressed during the periods of arrhythmia despite improvement of the primary condition. Clinical improvement coincided with the disappearance of the abnormal rhythm. It is therefore felt that the presence of such electrocardiographic abnormalities suggests the need for strict bed rest while dealing with the primary disease.

A lesson learnt from these cases is that any child suffering from an acute infection who does not make a good clinical recovery when the infection has abated, warrants an electrocardiographic study.

An attempt was made in Case 3 to abolish or modify the arrhythmia by the intravenous use of potassium chloride. This case and that of belladonna poisoning were the only two which reverted to normal rhythm within the short space of 18 hours.

Summary

The case histories and electrocardiograms of five children showing disturbances in cardiac rhythm are described. Three children showed A-V dissociation and two demonstrated the Wenckebach phenomenon.

Case descriptions of cardiac arrhythmias in children are rare. Those records appearing in the literature are associated with rheumatic fever, digitalis poisoning and diphtheria.

The prognosis in these cases is related to the primary condition rather than to the electrocardiographic findings.

The suggestion is put forward that cardiac arrhythmias in children should be treated by careful nursing and bed rest.

My thanks are due to Dr. I. Frack, the superintendent of Baragwanath Hospital for permission to publish these case records and to Dr. E. Kahn and Dr. S. Wayburne in whose wards these cases were treated. I am indebted to Dr. L. Schamroth for his valuable help and criticism and to Dr. A. Barnett and Dr. J. Theunissen who helped in the investigations of Cases 2 and 3. I am indebted for the photographs of the electrocardiograms to Mr. Schewitz of the Witwatersrand Medical School.

References

Blumgart, Herman L. and Gargill, Samuel L. (1930). *Amer. Heart J.*, **5**, 437.

Ehrentheil, Otto F., Alimurung, M. M. and Massell, B. F. (1952). *Amer. Heart J.*, **43**, 228.

Kuhn, Leslie A., Donoso, Efraim and Sapin, Samuel O. (1954). *Ibid.*, **48**, 280.

Langen, C. D. de (1956). *Cardiologia (Basel)*, **29**, 77.

Lemann, I. (1953). *Ann. intern. Med.*, **7**, 779.

Magri, G. (1953). *Acta cardiol. (Brux.)*, **8**, 529.

Mobitz, W. (1923). *Dtsch. Arch. klin. Med.*, **141**, 257.

Sprague, Howard B. and White, Paul D. (1927). *Med. Clin. N. Amer.*, **10**, 1235.

Wood, Paul (1956). *Diseases of the Heart and Circulation*, 2nd ed., p. 222. London.

Wenckebach, K. F. (1899). *Zeitschr. f. klin. Med.*, **37**, 475.

——— (1906). *Arch. Anat. Physiol., Lpz.*, **30**, 297.

Zimdahl, W. T. (1951). *Amer. Heart J.*, **41**, 204.

A SALT WASTING SYNDROME IN INFANCY

BY

DONALD B. CHEEK and JOHN W. PERRY
From the Royal Children's Hospital, Melbourne

(RECEIVED FOR PUBLICATION OCTOBER 14, 1957)

A continued loss of sodium and chloride is a well-known phenomenon which occurs during the course of uncontrolled adrenal insufficiency. Such losses are of serious consequence and in children lead to a failure of growth and development, to asthenia and infection. It is well recognized that many of the symptoms of adrenal insufficiency are due to the disturbance in mineral metabolism, and it is not surprising, therefore, that other conditions where excessive amounts of salt are lost from the body occasionally give rise to a picture that resembles, in many respects, adrenal insufficiency. In passing, we can mention fibrocystic disease of the pancreas, hydrocephalus with arachno-ureteric drainage, patients with heart disease who are hypersensitive to mercurial diuretics, cerebral salt wasting, pink disease and salt losing nephritis where there is advanced destruction of the renal parenchyma and tubular resistance to salt-retaining steroids.

This communication considers a case which does not seem to fit into any of the categories in the above list. It is that of an infant, studied over a five-month period, who demonstrated a renal salt wasting condition in the face of otherwise normal kidneys and normal adrenal function and acid-base balance. It will be shown that this salt wasting defect was resistant to desoxycorticosterone acetate and we suggest that the defect may be due to a refractory state on the part of the tubules to endogenous salt-active steroids or mineralo-corticoids.

Methods

Sodium and potassium concentrations for serum, sweat and urine were determined on a direct reading flame photometer (Domingo and Klyne, 1949), or by a direct reading E.E.L. flame photometer. Chloride determinations, serum *p*H, carbon dioxide content, total body water, total body chloride, were all measured by methods set out in a previous communication (Cheek, 1957). To determine total chloride the volume of distribution of bromide was measured and a micro diffusion method was used as described previously (Cheek and West, 1955). Here the diffusion units of Öbrink (1955) were used (obtained from Rudolf Grave Company, Stockholm, Sweden). These units obviate the need for fixative and for subsequent prolonged washings of the units and increase the accuracy of the method. The variation between duplicate determinations of serum bromide was less than 1%. Before the calculation of the extracellular volume index from the bromide space, 10% of the injected bromide was deducted from the total injected, to allow for the entrance of 8% of injected bromide into the red blood cells and for the fact that the volume of distribution of bromide is 1-2% greater than the chloride space. This correction has been applied previously (Cheek, 1954). Recent work indicates that in the rat almost all the intracellular chloride of the body is in red cells; hence it may be that the corrected Cl or Br space in man is a good approximation to true extracellular volume.

Sweat was collected following a pharmacological stimulus similar to a method described (Mauer and West, 1956). Urinary 17-ketosteroid excretion, and corticosteroid excrction were assayed by accepted procedures (Medical Research Council Committee on Clinical Endocrinology, 1951; Reddy, 1954). To assess urea clearance, urine was collected over a 24-hour period according to the technique described by Landis, Elsom, Bott and Shiels (1935).

Case Report

F.C., a male infant, aged 3 months, was the first-born of parents who had been previously in good health. The mother was admitted to the maternity hospital during the last two months of pregnancy because of an excessive gain in weight, hypertension and albuminuria. Labour was induced and the baby was born two weeks prematurely, weighing $5\frac{1}{2}$ lb. Labour was not difficult and delivery was uneventful. The infant was breast fed for two and a half months but failed to gain satisfactorily. A dried milk mixture was tried temporarily but at the age of 3 months he was brought to the Royal Children's Hospital because of poor feeding, unsatisfactory weight gain and cyanotic attacks. The cyanotic attacks had been noticed during the previous month, and were not associated with feeding. They were not accompanied by sweating or change in respiration but did seem to occur on hot summer days. The infant's weight at 1 month of age was 6 lb. 11 oz., at 2 months, 7 lb. 11 oz. and on admission at 3 months, 8 lb. 2 oz.

Course in Hospital. It was found that the infant took his feeds poorly and that he preferred milk to glucose water. During the first three weeks routine investigations were carried out, and the weight of the infant fell progressively. It became clear that the baby did not maintain satisfactory hydration. The haemoglobin was 11 g. per 100 ml. The following investigations revealed no abnormality: subdural taps; lumbar puncture; radiographs of the skull and chest; examination of the urine including microscopic examinations of centrifuged deposits; and a Mantoux test. The blood urea was normal, but once, at a time when the child was poorly hydrated, a level of 67 mg. % was recorded. However, radiographs of the kidneys and intravenous pyelography demonstrated normal findings and a subsequent urea clearance test showed that the infant had normal renal function. Restriction of fluid on more than one occasion produced a urine of 1,020 specific gravity which suggested a satisfactory concentrating ability. A urine chromatogram revealed no abnormal amino acid excretion. No evidence of a congenital heart lesion was found.

On the twenty-second day following admission and at a time when hydration was unsatisfactory, serum electrolyte concentrations were determined (Table 1). Next day the fluid intake was increased by giving 5% glucose solution by gavage, and on the 24th day the infant had a grand mal convulsion and continued to appear dehydrated and cyanosed with sunken eyes and poor skin turgor. The serum sodium and chloride concentrations dropped to low levels (Na 124 mEq/l. and Cl 75 mEq/l.). Intravenous therapy was at once started: a blood transfusion was followed by 400 ml. of isotonic saline and 3 g. of NaCl 24-hourly were added to the feeds. Desoxycorticosterone acetate (DOCA) was given intramuscularly at a dosage of 2 mg. 24-hourly. The response was dramatic, hydration at once improved and body weight increased for the first time. The infant became alert and active and the milk intake rose appreciably.

Two oral glucose tolerance tests showed a flat blood sugar curve but the result of an intravenous test was normal. Radiographs of the adrenal gland showed no calcification and 24-hour urine collections made before steroid therapy contained normal amounts of 17-ketosteroids and corticosteroids. (Adrenal function tests will be discussed presently.) The serum sodium concentration remained near 135 mEq/l. while DOCA and 3 g. of sodium chloride were given 24-hourly (Table 1).

On the 43rd day of study, DOCA was discontinued, but the weight still increased. On the 48th day, salt was stopped and the weight, fluid intake, and serum sodium concentration fell. Dehydration recurred and intravenous saline was again given and 3 g. of salt were again added to the milk. The increase in weight over the next period was not so remarkable. On the 63rd day, DOCA (2 mg.) was recommenced, to see if there would be any increase in the rate of weight gain. There was not, and on the 69th day the steroid was discontinued.

On the 78th day of study, salt was stopped and again the fluid intake, weight and serum sodium concentration fell (130 mEq/l.). Hypotonic dehydration returned. For the next week some special investigations were carried out (see below) and on the 86th day salt was again added to the milk feedings, but in the increased amount of 5 g.

TABLE 1

SERUM ELECTROLYTE CONCENTRATION ACCORDING TO NATURE OF TREATMENT

Day of Study	Na_S (mEq/l)	Cl_S (mEq/l)	K_S (mEq/l)	CO_2 Content	*p*H	Blood Urea (mg. %)	Treatment (per 24 hr.)
22	137	102	5·6			19	Nil
24	124	75	5·0				Increased H_2O intake
30	135	91	5·0			22	NaCl 3 g. DOCA 2 mg.
40	134	102	4·7				NaCl 3 g. DOCA 2 mg.
48	130	105	4·5				Nil
58	136	90	5·9				NaCl 3 g.
72	145	93	6·4				NaCl 3 g.
78	130	97	4·8	24·0	7·36		Nil
87	143	98	5·5	22·4	—		NaCl 5 g.
99	122	96	5·0	19·0	7·40		DOCA 4 mg.
105	138	100	5·5	23·3	7·36	22	NaCl 5 g.
120	142	108	4·2	21·8	—		NaCl 5 g.
127	144	110	5·0	23·0	7·35		NaCl 5 g.
134	150	105	5·1	24·0			Nil

in the 24 hours. Weight increased rapidly by more than 1 lb., hydration was restored and the serum sodium concentration rose to 143 mEq/l. For the next week there was no further increase in weight.

On the 93rd day, salt therapy was replaced by 4 mg. of DOCA 24-hourly. With this treatment weight did not decrease further, but hydration seemed poor as evidenced by the sunken eyes and poor tissue turgor. The infant became lethargic and disinterested in feeding. After six days of steroid therapy his serum sodium concentration had fallen to 122 mEq/l. DOCA was then stopped and replaced by 5 g. of sodium chloride in the milk. Well-being returned and the infant began to thrive again. His serum sodium concentration rose to normal levels.

He was discharged to the Out Patients' Department on the 105th day and examined at weekly intervals. On the 133rd day of study, salt (5 g. 24-hourly) was discontinued but the patient continued to progress satisfactorily (Fig. 1). At 8 months of age he appeared normal but undersized. His weight ($15\frac{3}{4}$ lb.) fell on the third percentile of the weight chart.

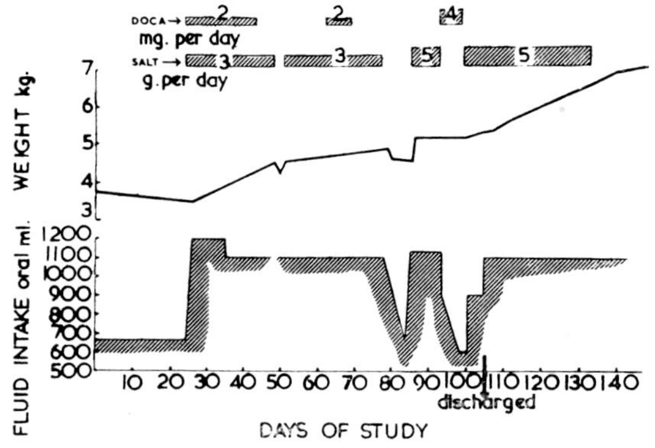

FIG. 1.

Special Investigations. In Table 2 the results of investigation of steroid excretion are recorded. Repeated determination of 17-ketosteroid and 11-oxysteroids in the urine demonstrated normal excretion and the response following 25 mg. of ACTH (gel) per day for a three-day period was also normal. The Thorn eosinophil test was performed and disclosed normal function in so far as the eosinophil level dropped progressively from 150 to 11 cells per c.mm. over a three-hour period. On the previous day, two spot counts had revealed 233 and 166 cells per c.mm. These tests with ACTH were carried out during the 78th to 85th day when no therapy was being given. Also during this period, when the weight had reached a low level, determination of electrolyte intake and urine output was made (81st day). The sodium, chloride, and potassium intake was 13·7, 15·8 and 16·5 milliequivalents per day respectively while the urine output contained 12·3, 15·9 and 8·4 milliequivalents for sodium, chloride and potassium. Hence the intake and urine output for sodium and chloride closely paralleled one another, and if we consider the expected skin losses for these electrolytes (about 2 milliequivalents per day) the data suggest a negative balance for sodium and chloride. However, balance data derived from such a short period cannot be regarded as very significant.

TABLE 2

EXCRETION LEVEL OF URINE STEROIDS ACCORDING TO NATURE OF TREATMENT

Day of Study	Corticosteroids (mg. per 24 hr.)	17-Ketosteroids (mg. per 24 hr.)	Treatment (per 24 hr.)
24	2·9	0·18	Nil
52–57 (4-day collection)	1·2	0·19	NaCl 3 g.
82	0·9	0·17	Nil
83–6 (3-day administration)	—	—	ACTH 25 mg.
86	7·7	0·66	NaCl 5 g.

Data for sweat electrolyte concentrations are set out in Table 3. It can be seen that there was no excessive loss of electrolyte from the skin, in fact, the values for sodium and potassium, when the patient was receiving no treatment, are at the lower limit of normal (Cooke, Pratt and Darrow, 1950). When DOCA and/or salt was given the value for sweat sodium was slightly lower.

TABLE 3

SWEAT ELECTROLYTE CONCENTRATIONS ACCORDING TO NATURE OF TREATMENT

Day of Study	Na (mEq/l.)	K (mEq/l.)	Treatment (per 24-hr.)
36	11·4	20·6	DOCA 2 mg. NaCl 3 g.
51	16·4	18·0	Nil
55	11·1	14·4	NaCl 3 g.

While the serum sodium concentrations fluctuated with the addition to or subtraction of salt from the food (Table 1)—DOCA exhibiting no sodium retaining effect—the data for serum chloride, carbon dioxide content and hydrogen ion concentration suggest that there was no gross departure from a normal state of acid-base balance.

In Table 4 are recorded the urine sodium and potassium concentrations before and after an intravenous injection (2·5 mg.) of water soluble DOCA. It would seem from these investigations that no appreciable sodium retaining effect was exhibited by the steroid.

In Table 5 data for patient F.C.'s total chloride, extracellular volume and total body water at various stages of treatment are presented. By difference we can record the status of intracellular hydration. For comparison with F.C. we have listed the normal range of values for the corresponding weight of a normal infant, and, for contrast, those of an infant with adrenal hyperplasia and insufficiency and dehydration.

TABLE 4

Na/K RATIO IN URINE BEFORE AND AFTER 2·5 MG. DOCA I.V. (93rd DAY)

Flow (ml./30 min.)	Na(mEq/l.)	K(mEq/l.)
4·8	71	26
4·2	80	26
3·3	90	27
→I.V. DOCA 2·5 mg. 4·0	100	27
5·7	104	27

Patient F.C. had a significantly low total body chloride and calculated extracellular volume while on no treatment (48th day), or following six days of DOCA (4 mg. 24-hourly) (98th day). Total body water was not low in the first instance but normal. Since no weight was lost 4 mg. of DOCA were substituted for salt therapy on the 93rd day, it could be assumed that total water was also normal at that juncture. The data suggest that in both of these periods there was an increase in cell hydration. Three weeks after discharge (127th day) data for total chloride and water and extracellular volume were again obtained. The total chloride and extracellular volume were slightly low but within normal limits.

The infant with adrenal hyperplasia and dehydration showed a reduction of total chloride and extracellular volume. The total water was reduced and the calculated index for intracellular volume also appears low.

From these results it seems that the fluid volume changes in patient F.C. resemble those found in simple sodium loss.

Discussion

The investigations of infant F.C. lead us to the tentative conclusion that there can be in infancy a salt wasting syndrome that is not directly related to the adrenal gland or to gross renal disease. We are aware that, in chronic nephritis with destruction of renal nephrons, a renal tubular salt wasting syndrome can arise which is resistant to DOCA, as Thorn, Koepf and Clinton (1944), have clearly demonstrated. However, the routine methods of revealing disease of renal nephrons carried out in the case of patient F.C. supported the belief that renal function was normal and urine chromatography did not indicate a tubular defect in amino acid metabolism. On the other hand, investigation into adrenal function disclosed no abnormality. The serum potassium concentration was never grossly elevated, nor was there an obvious disturbance in acid-base balance. The sweat concentration in patient F.C. was not elevated as it is in Addison's disease (Conn and Louis, 1950). Such findings suggest that patient F.C. was not deficient in endogenous mineralo-corticoid. The urine steroid excretion before and following ACTH showed a normal pattern of response and the Thorn eosinophil test was also normal. At the completion of this study the patient was normal emotionally and mentally and there was no reason to believe that disease of the central nervous system was present.

In a patient with adrenal insufficiency with salt wasting one might expect that the withdrawal of salt and a high dosage of DOCA (4 mg. 24-hourly)

TABLE 5

TOTAL CHLORIDE AND VOLUME MEASUREMENTS IN INFANT F.C. (SALT-WASTER) COMPARED WITH NORMAL VALUES AND WITH THOSE IN INFANT H.O. WITH ADRENAL INSUFFICIENCY

Infant	Weight (Kg.)	*Total Cl (mEq/l.)	E.C.V.† (ml.)	T.B.W.‡ (ml.)	State of Intracellular Hydration	Treatment (per 24 hr.)
F.C. (salt-waster)	4·5	166	1,240	3,000	+	No NaCl for 24 hr.
Normal	4·5	183-203	1,530-1,710	3,081-3,239		
F.C. (salt-waster)	5·2	172	1,420		?+	After 6 days DOCA (4 mg.)
Normal	5·2	205-225	1,720-1,900			
F.C. (salt-waster)	6·35	272	1,970	4,500		NaCl 5 g.
Normal	6·35	271-291	2,300-2,480	4,340-4,561		
H.O. (Adrenal insufficiency; hyperplasia)	5·6	152	1,370	2,720	—	
Normal	5·6	217-237	1,830-2,010	3,822-4,018		

* For infants of 2-9 Kg., Cl_t = 30·7 weight (Kg.) + 55·0 (SD±10 mEq/l.) (Cheek, 1954).
† E.C.V. = Bromide space corrected for intracellular Br (10%). See p. 252.
‡ T.B.W. = Total body water. Normal values and range derived from data of Friis-Hansen (1957).

would lead to uninterrupted progress. One would not expect deterioration and a fall of serum sodium concentration nor would one expect to find, following such high steroid dosage, a reduction of extracellular volume and loss of total body chloride with a probable increase in cell hydration. Yet these are the changes that took place and, furthermore, intravenous administration of water soluble DOCA did not alter the urine sodium/potassium ratio. It seems reasonable to believe that patient F.C. was not sensitive to DOCA at the level of the renal tubules, and that the therapeutic agent that did guarantee well-being was additional sodium chloride. It is probable that the addition of 3 g. of NaCl was not optimal and that 5 g. per day was more beneficial. Progress in weight and serum sodium concentrations support this belief. Jaudon (1946, 1948) described what he believed to be a fractional insufficiency of the salt and water hormone of the adrenal gland in the early period of life. Asthenia, failure to thrive, cyanosis, failure to maintain hydration, were characteristic of his group of infants. But Jaudon also reported low urinary steroid excretion, hypoglycaemia, a dramatic response to DOCA without salt, and acidosis, none of which were observed in patient F.C.

It would seem from our observations that we may be dealing with renal tubules that are refractory for a time to salt-retaining steroids. The diminished extracellular volume in patient F.C. should have initiated an increased production of aldosterone (Bartter, Liddle, Duncan, Barber and Delea, 1956) which in turn should have enhanced renal tubular reabsorption of sodium. It would seem that this was not the case. Yet the low sweat sodium values suggest an adequate endogenous production of salt-retaining steroids. So we arrive at the suspicion that the renal tubules were sensitive neither to endogenous nor exogenous salt-retaining hormone.

The finding of a flat oral glucose tolerance curve on two occasions while the intravenous curve was normal was of interest. In adrenal insufficiency the gastric absorption of glucose is delayed, but this phenomenon is due to coincidental salt depletion and not to lack of cortical hormone (Althausen, Anderson and Stockholm, 1939; Clark and MacKay, 1942).

While we have been unable to find any similar case reports in the literature, Payne (1954) states that he believes a renal tubular salt wasting condition occurs in infancy and that it is resistant to DOCA. He states that such a condition can threaten for a time the life of an infant but after several weeks spontaneous recovery takes place. The condition was thought not to be related to adrenal insufficiency. It is felt that the present paper supports this contention but further patients and scientific data will be necessary for study before one can accept these findings as representative of a new syndrome. Although the routine renal investigations are normal one cannot be positive that parenchymal disease is not present and is yet to become manifest.

Summary

The case is presented of an infant who failed to thrive and to maintain hydration satisfactorily. He was found to have a renal salt wasting defect. Adrenal and kidney function and acid-base balance were found to be normal. Low sweat electrolyte levels were taken as evidence of adequate production of mineralo-corticoid.

This deleterious clinical situation could be reversed by raising the serum concentration to normal with the addition of 5 g. of sodium chloride to the milk intake. When the patient was off salt or on DOCA only, the serum sodium concentration, the extracellular volume and the total chloride fell or were low and the clinical condition deteriorated. DOCA had no effect on the urinary sodium/potassium ratio.

If electrolyte concentration of sweat is a satisfactory index of endogenous mineralo-corticoid production, then this child's salt wasting condition may be related to a transient disturbance in the response of the renal tubules to this hormone.

We are most grateful to Dr. Robert Southby, the Senior Physician responsible for this patient, for allowing us to undertake these investigations, and to Dr. Ian Robinson for much practical help. Urine steroid determinations were undertaken through the assistance of Miss Anne Moore.

References

Althausen, T. L., Anderson, E. M. and Stockholm, M. (1939). *Proc. Soc. Exp. Biol. (N.Y.)*, **40**, 342.
Bartter, F. C., Liddle, G. W., Duncan, L. E., Barber, J. K. and Delea, C. (1956). *J. clin. Invest.*, **35**, 1306.
Cheek, D. B. (1954). *Pediatrics*, **14**, 5.
—— (1957). *Ibid.*, **19**, 68.
—— and West, C. D. (1955). *J. clin. Invest.*, **34**, 1744.
Clark, W. G. and MacKay, E. M. (1942). *Amer. J. Physiol.*, **137**, 104.
Conn, J. W. and Louis, L. H. (1950). *J. clin. Endocr.*, **10**, 12.
Cooke, R. E., Pratt, E. L. and Darrow, D. C. (1950). *Yale J. Biol. Med.*, **22**, 227.
Domingo, W. R. and Klyne, W. (1949). *Biochem. J.*, **45**, 400.
Friis-Hansen, B. (1957). *Acta paediat. (Uppsala)*, **46**, Suppl. 110.
Jaudon, J. C. (1946). *J. Pediat.*, **29**, 696.
—— (1948). *Ibid.*, **32**, 641.
Landis, E. M., Elsom, K. A., Bott, P. A. and Shiels, E. (1935). *J. clin. Invest.*, **14**, 525.
Mauer, A. M. and West, C. D. (1956). *Amer. J. Dis. Child.*, **92**, 160.
Medical Research Council Committee on Clinical Endocrinology .. (1951). *Lancet*, **2**, 585.
Öbrink, K. J. (1955). *Biochem. J.*, **59**, 134.
Payne, W. W. (1954). *Postgrad. med. J.*, **30**, 476.
Reddy, W. J. (1954). *Metabolism*, **3**, 489.
Thorn, G. W., Koepf, G. F. and Clinton, M. (1944). *New Engl. J Med.*, **231**, 76.

ANOREXIA AND SEVERE INANITION ASSOCIATED WITH A TUMOUR INVOLVING THE HYPOTHALAMUS

BY

HELEN KAGAN

Paedriatric Service, Bikur Holim Hospital, Jerusalem, Israel

(RECEIVED FOR PUBLICATION SEPTEMBER 4, 1957)

Anorexia in childhood is a common complaint, resulting as a rule from infectious processes, systemic diseases, metabolic disturbances, or, in healthy children, from quantitative or qualitative over-feeding. There are, however, occasional cases in which none of the above-mentioned factors can be held responsible.

The purpose of this paper is to report the case of an infant suffering from obstinate anorexia since birth, which subsequently proved to be related to a hypothalamic lesion.

Case Report

E.B., a 3-months-old female baby of Turkish-Jewish parentage, was admitted to the Paediatric Service of the Bikur Holim Hospital on November 3, 1955. The parents who were not related were in good health, as was an older sister, aged 2½ years. The baby was delivered at full term after an uneventful pregnancy, weighing 3,200 kg. The baby was breast-fed, the feed being supplemented by a cow's milk formula. From birth onwards it had a very poor appetite; it took both the breast and the bottle most unwillingly and in small amounts, and occasionally vomited. Its weight remained practically stationary. The child behaved normally, smiling and taking some interest in its surroundings.

State on Admission. The infant looked emaciated (weight 3,400 kg.), but it smiled readily and followed light. The head was symmetrical and had a circumference of 37 cm. The anterior fontanelle measured 3 × 2·5 cm. and was somewhat depressed. The visceral organs were without abnormalities, except for a right-sided hernia. The neurological and ocular examinations were negative. Body temperature was normal.

Laboratory Examinations. Analysis of the urine was negative. Results of a blood count were as follows : red blood cells, 4,200,000 (haemoglobin, 10·0 g. per 100 ml.), white blood cells, 8,400 (segmented neutrophils 34%, rod-shaped neutrophils 4%, eosinophils 1%, monocytes 4%, lymphocytes 58%); blood chemistry showed: urea 29 mg. %, sugar 98 mg. %, calcium 9·4 mg. %, NaCl 671 mg. %); total proteins 6·8% (albumin 4·5%, globulin 2·3 %), CO_2 combining power was 52 vol. %; liver function tests were negative. A Mantoux text (1:1,000) was negative. Paper chromatography of the urine showed a normal amino-acid pattern. The stools were of normal colour and consistency; they were negative for parasites and ova. The duodenal juice contained trypsin.

Radiographic examinations of the chest, stomach and duodenum gave negative results.

In view of the child's poor appetite it was fed seven times a day. Yet, throughout its stay in hospital, it fed very poorly and vomited once or twice a day.

There were, however, a few periods lasting from three to seven days during which there was no vomiting. No appreciable weight gain occurred, the child weighing 3,550 kg. on December 12.

Thirty-nine days after the child's admission (December 12), vertical, horizontal and rotating nystagmus were suddenly noted. As far as could be ascertained, no other abnormalities referrable to the central nervous system were present. On December 24, the fontanelle had become tense, bulging and was enlarged to 5·5 × 5 cm. The baby's eyes had by then the typical 'setting sun' appearance. A lumbar puncture yielded a transparent fluid which contained 11 leucocytes per c.mm. and had a pressure of 220 mm. A Pandy's test showed sugar 53 mg. %, NaCl 827 mg. %. A pneumoencephalogram performed on December 28 showed that both lateral ventricles were markedly enlarged. The pressure of the cerebrospinal fluid at that date was 330 mm. and the reaction to Pandy's test was ++. The head circumference had increased to 41 cm. and the fronto-occipital diameter was 17 cm. A diagnosis of a communicating hydrocephalus was made and the child was transferred to the neurosurgical department of the Hebrew University-Hadassah Medical School.

On January 23, 1956, Dr. E. Peiser operated on the baby. After resection of the 5th lumbar vertebral arch, an anastomosis between the subarachnoidal space and the peritoneal cavity was performed with a partial removal of the omentum.

Following the operation the head circumference decreased from 41 cm. to 40 cm., and the bulging fontanelle subsided, but the child's general condition remained poor and it continued stubbornly to refuse food.

On January 31, eight days after the operation, the bulging of the fontanelle reappeared, the head circumference increased to 42 cm., the fontanelle measured 7×7 cm. A lumbar puncture yielded little fluid under low pressure. The child's condition rapidly deteriorated, and she died on February 2.

Necropsy (Professor M. Wolman, Department of Pathology, Hebrew University-Hadassah Medical School). At autopsy, evidence of extreme malnutrition, and signs of the above-described operation were noted. The peritoneal cavity contained 180 ml. of chylous fluid.

BRAIN. Externally, the membranes of the lower part of the brain were markedly thickened and gelatinous. The gelatinous part stretched from the sella turcica to the anterior aspect of the pons and continued down to the spinal cord. The arachnoid of the cisterna magna was most markedly thickened and contained greyish patches 2-4 mm. in diameter, and about 1 mm. in thickness. Coronal sections through the brain showed severe internal hydrocephalus, most marked in the lateral ventricles with thinning of the brain cortex to between 2-8 cm. The third ventricle was found filled with a gelatinous mass adherent on all sides to the walls except for its upper part (Fig. 1). The mass was greyish and homogeneous, was not sharply demarcated from the brain tissue of the hypothalamic regions, and was continuous with the meninges. The tumour occupied the middle portion of the third ventricle and did not invade the posterior part and the pineal recess. The fourth ventricle and the Sylvian aqueduct were not enlarged.

MICROSCOPIC STRUCTURE OF THE TUMOUR (Fig. 2). The microscopic structure of the tumour differed in the various areas. In some places it had a net-like appearance with small compact nuclei, spheroidal or oval, often lobulated or twisted, surrounded by eosinophilic cytoplasm (Fig. 3). Delicate dendritic processes, with little arborization, emerged from the cytoplasm of some of these cells and gave the tissue its reticular appearance. Between these processes capillaries and thin collagen bundles were found. The tissue space between the processes did not stain. In phosphotungstic-acid-haemotoxylin-stained sections most processes stained purple.

In other areas the tumour was much more cellular (Fig. 4). The cells had mostly vesicular, fusiform nuclei with rounded ends. Most of the chromatin was situated at the nuclear membrane. The cytoplasm of these cells was scanty and stained lightly with eosin. From both ends of the cytoplasm emerged long, delicate processes with very little arborization. In some places the tissue appeared loose with few cells and with a polar arrangement of the nuclei which lay parallel to each other. In these areas the amount of blood vessels and collagen was small.

The tumour infiltrated the brain tissue without clear demarcation and in the infiltrated tissue a marked gliotic reaction was present. In the meninges the tumour infiltrated the proliferated connective tissue of the leptomeninges.

The two main types of cells in this tumour could be identified as piloid astrocytes and oligodendrocytes; accordingly the tumour was considered to be a mixed astrocytoma and oligodendroglioma.

Discussion

The presenting sign of the case reported here was an obstinate anorexia with subsequent lack of weight gain which existed from birth until the child's death at the age of almost 6 months. At the age of 4½ months, signs suggestive of a space-occupying intracranial lesion appeared. At autopsy an astrocytoma, presumably originating in the hypothalamus and extending into and blocking the third ventricle, was found. Since during life and at autopsy no other functional or organic abnormalities were detected, a causal relationship between the hypothalamic lesion and the anorexia had to be assumed.

The role of central nervous centres in the pathogenesis of emaciation has been acknowledged for some time. Gull (1874) described a syndrome of extreme inanition due to a morbid mental state which he termed anorexia nervosa and which is to date by some attributed to hypothalamic lesions. On clinical grounds, anorexia nervosa can hardly be differentiated from Simmonds' pituitary cachexia. The latter disease entity which commonly arises from adenohypophyseal failure was later found to occur also in patients with an intact pituitary, but with tumours or inflammatory processes in the region of the third ventricle (Richardson, 1939; Glanzmann and Wegelin, 1942). The claim that the same symptomatology may be produced by disturbances in any part of the functional unit pituitary-hypothalamus (Zondek, 1923) therefore seems perfectly justified. It is substantiated by experimental observations to the effect that both hypophysectomy (Paulesco, 1907; Smith, 1927) and hypothalamic lesions (Bailey and Bremer, 1921) may lead to profound cachexia.

Russell (1951, 1957) described a syndrome presenting in infancy or early childhood with severe emaciation despite an initially normal or even enhanced food intake, and accompanied by locomotor hyperactivity, over-alertness or even euphoria, initial growth acceleration, hypotension and hypoglycaemia. Hypothalamic tumours, almost always astrocytomas, were established as the pathological basis of the morbid phenomena. The emaciation was attributed to an abnormal energy expenditure resulting mainly from hyperactivity and hypermetabolism.

The present case resembles the syndrome described by Russell with regard to age, the presenting clinical manifestation, emaciation, and the source and

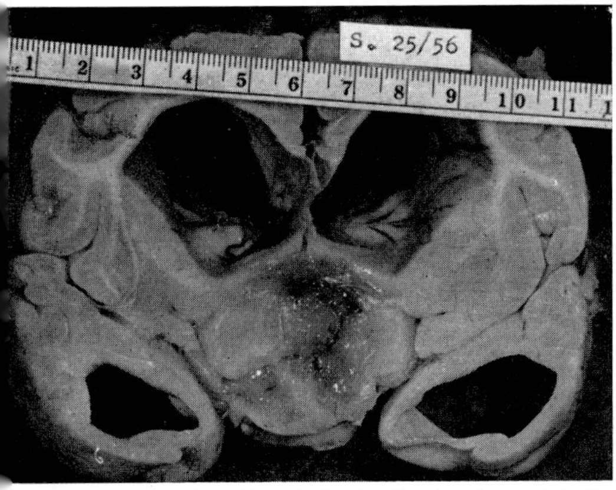

. 1.—Coronal section through brain showing internal hydrocephalus and tumour mass filling dilated third ventricle.

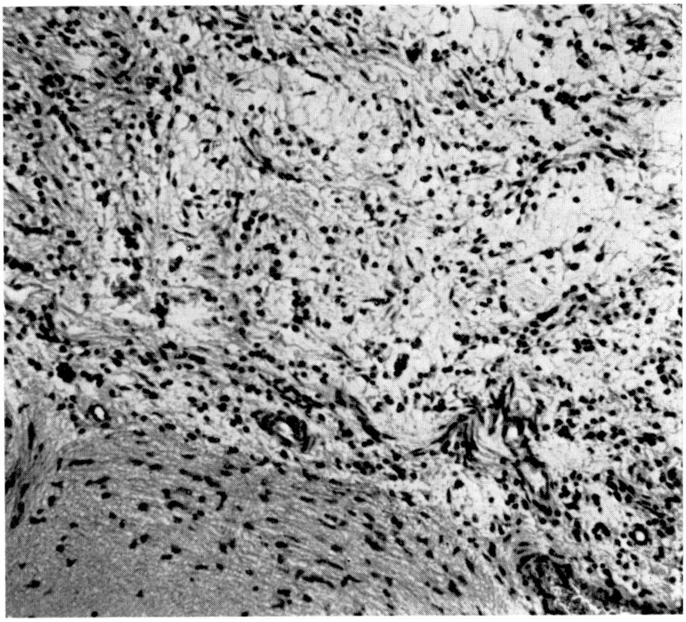

FIG. 3.—Tumour infiltration of meninges, showing net-like appearance of tumour with spongy areas surrounded by more compact bands. At bottom, surface of medulla. H and E. × 140.

. 2.—Tumour structure : fibrillary and bipolar astrocytes lying in bundles with many dilated capillaries. H. and E. × 150.

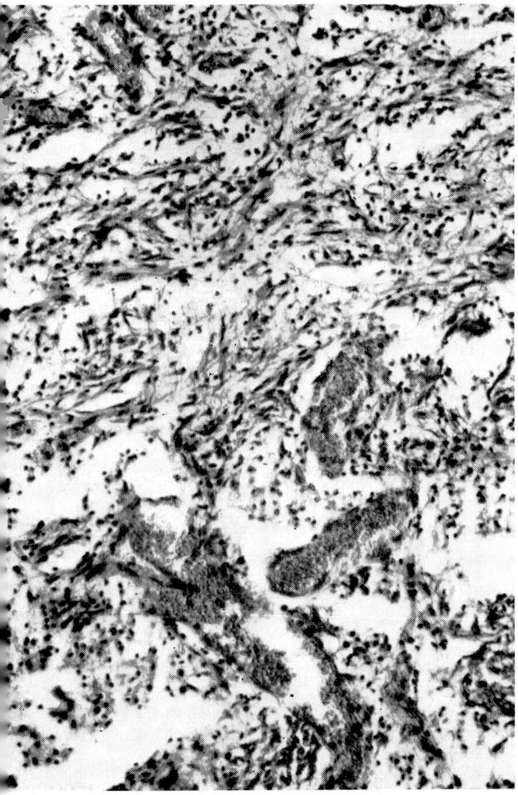

FIG. 4.—A highly cellular area of tumour consisting almost entirely of fibrillary astrocytes.

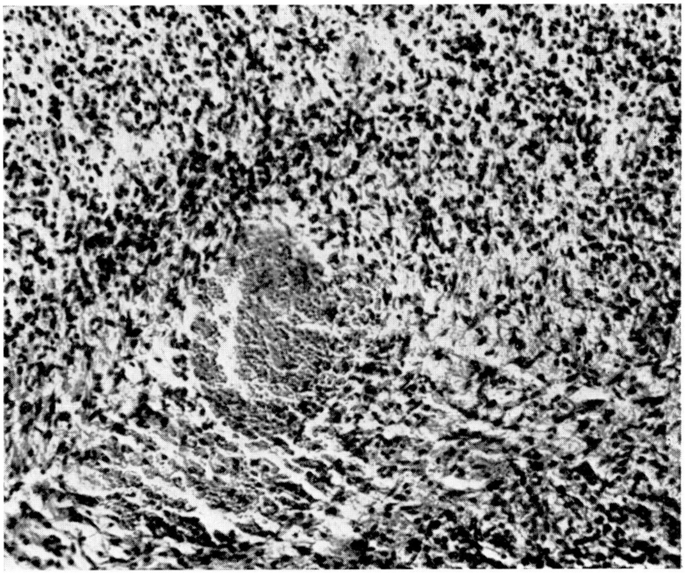

nature of the underlying pathological lesion. However, it differs from Russell's syndrome by the absence of the accompanying clinical criteria of the lesion and the presence of a very marked anorexia which dominated the symptomatology from the very beginning. Consequently it should be regarded as another variety of the multiple hypothalamic syndromes known to exist.

Hypothalamic obesity has been studied, both clinically and experimentally, much more extensively than hypothalamic emaciation. An essential mechanism of both was recently clarified by Brobeck and his group (Brobeck, Tepperman and Long, 1943; Anand and Brobeck, 1951). Electrolytic lesions in the ventromedial nuclei of the hypothalamus produced in rats and cats voracious hunger and subsequent obesity, whilst bilateral lesions in the extreme lateral portions of the lateral hypothalamus inhibited food intake to the point of starvation. It may be assumed that damage to hypothalamic feeding centres may also upset the delicately balanced regulation of food intake in man. Cases are on record in which the appearance of uncontrollable hunger with associated weight gain or of complete anorexia with associated weight loss could be causally related to hypothalamic lesions (Heaney, Eliel, Joel and Stout, 1954; Zondek and Leszynsky, 1956). Heaney's report concerned a child suffering from lymphatic leukaemia who suddenly developed voracious hunger and gained 4 kg. in 20 days. Necropsy revealed a leukaemic infiltrate in the hypothalamus. This case may well be regarded as the counterpart of our present one and both as clinical reflections of Brobeck's animal experiments.

Regardless of these theoretical considerations we may conclude that hypothalamic tumours should be suspected in infants and young childen in whom a thorough clinical investigation fails to account for a failure to gain weight, or for the onset of sudden weight loss, with or without accompanying anorexia. As Russell pointed out, a long time may elapse before the growing tumour produces signs of increased intracranial tension or other neurological signs. In the present case the cerebral nature of the disease process was unfortunately not suspected until the tumour had obstructed the third ventricle.

From a perusal of the literature it appears that this patient is the youngest patient with an astrocytoma on record. The youngest patient recorded in a series studied by Zuelch (1956) was 4 years old when the first symptoms appeared, while Russell's youngest patients were 3 months of age. In the present case complete lack of appetite with resulting failure to gain weight was evident from birth, and it may be concluded that the astrocytoma was of a congenital nature.

Summary

The case is reported of an infant who suffered from birth from severe anorexia with subsequent failure to gain weight. At the age of 4½ months signs referable to an internal hydrocephalus appeared, which were only temporarily relieved by drainage of the subarachnoidal space into the peritoneal cavity. About a month later the child died. Autopsy revealed an astrocytoma originating in the hypothalamus and extending into and finally blocking the third ventricle.

In view of the persistence of anorexia since birth and the absence of any other cause either during life or at autopsy it is postulated that the astrocytoma was congenital in nature.

I wish to thank Professor H. Zondek and Dr. J. Leszynsky for their advice, and Professor M. Wolman for the pathological-anatomical examination.

References

Anand, B. K. and Brobeck, J. R. (1951). *Proc. Soc. exp. Biol. (N.Y.)*, 77, 323.
Bailey, P. and Bremer, F. (1921). *Arch. intern. Med.*, **28**, 773.
Brobeck, J. R., Tepperman, J. and Long, C. N. H. (1943). *Yale J. Biol. Med.*, **15**, 831.
Glanzmann, E. and Wegelin, C. (1942). *Schweiz. med. Wschr.*, **72**, 1401.
Gull, W. (1874). *Trans. clin. Soc. Lond.*, 7, 22.
Heaney, R. P., Eliel, L. P., Joel, W. and Stout, H. (1954). *J. clin. Endocr.*, **14**, 829.
Paulesco, N. C. (1907). *J. Physiol. Path. gén.*, **9**, 441.
Richardson, H. B. (1939). *Arch. intern. Med.*, **63**, 1.
Russell, A. (1951). Proceedings 22nd Meeting British Paediatric Association. *Arch. Dis. Childh.*, **26**, 274.
—— (1957). Extract from *Excerpta med. Sect. VIII Sixth Internat. Congr. neurol.* (Bruss.), 1957.
Smith, P. E. (1927). *J. Amer. med. Ass.*, **88**, 158.
Zondek, H. (1923). *Die Krankheiten der endokrinen Drüsen.* Berlin.
—— and Leszynsky, H. E. (1956). *Brit. med. J.*, **1**, 197.
Zuelch, K. J. (1956). *Die Hirngeschwulste in biol. und morphol. Darstellungen.* Leipzig.

ACUTE SPINAL EPIDURAL ABSCESS: A CASE IN AN INFANT WITH RECOVERY

BY

R. G. RUSHWORTH and P. B. MARTIN
From Guy's-Maudsley Neurosurgical Unit, and the Belgrave Hospital for Children, London

(RECEIVED FOR PUBLICATION OCTOBER 26, 1957)

Acute spinal epidural abscess is a neurosurgical emergency in which early diagnosis and prompt treatment are essential if permanent cord damage is to be avoided. For this reason, this uncommon condition has become well-recognized in recent years, and many full accounts have appeared. However, most of the patients described have been adults, and the following case is reported to illustrate the difficulties of diagnosis in a baby before the appearance of neurological signs.

Case Report

P.S. was born on April 11, 1955, and was three weeks overdue. The birth weight was 8 lb. 8 oz. and the delivery was normal. There was some neonatal skin sepsis, presumably staphylococcal in origin. At the age of 11 weeks he was admitted to the Belgrave Hospital for Children with a pyrexial illness, and a disinclination to move the left arm which was held in Erb's position. No other physical signs were found on admission, and he moved the arm normally after 24 hours. The pyrexia later proved to be due to a staphylococcal pneumonia and empyema, and after a desperate illness he recovered completely.

On July 16, 1956, he was again seen at the Belgrave Hospital, the mother complaining that he had seemed unwell for about two days. He had felt hot, and had screamed whenever he was lifted with her hands beneath his armpits or placed on his back. The feeds had been taken well, there had been no vomiting, and the bowels had been open normally. In February and May, 1956, he had two attacks of fever and irritability each lasting about two days.

On admission the temperature was 100·6° F., pulse 120 and respirations 25 per minute. The child was fretful and did not seem to be in any great pain while lying quietly, but he often screamed when picked up. No localized tenderness was detected to account for this. He was teething and the throat was mildly injected. The cardiovascular and respiratory systems were normal. There was no neck stiffness, and there were no abnormal neurological signs. The spleen was slightly enlarged, but apart from this the abdomen was normal.

Laboratory investigations were carried out: W.B.C. was 7,600/c. mm. (neutrophils 40%), film was normal; E.S.R. was 20 mm. in one hour; a patch test and throat swab were negative; radiographs of the spine, chest, pelvis and abdomen were all normal.

The day after admission his condition was unchanged. The next evening his temperature had risen to 103° F. and the respirations had become more rapid. At 3 a.m. on July 19 he began to twitch and appeared about to convulse, and lumbar puncture was performed that morning. The fluid was clear, but the pressure was not recorded as it fluctuated with the child's crying. The fluid showed: W.B.C. 140/c. mm. (91% polymorphs), R.B.C. 30/c. mm., protein 300 mg. %, sugar 83 mg. %. A blood-culture taken at this time later grew *Staphylococcus aureus*.

It was clear that the child was suffering from an infective process, and despite the absence of focal signs it was considered essential to exclude a cerebral abscess. The child was therefore transferred to the Guy's-Maudsley Neurosurgical Unit. On admission there on July 19 he was irritable and crying, and he looked very ill. The temperature was 102·4° F., pulse 134 and respiratory rate 34 per minute. There were no localizing signs of infection and no abnormal neurological signs. He cried when touched or disturbed, but this was not more noticeable when the back was examined. He resented neck flexion, but there was no neck stiffness, and Kernig's sign was not present.

Ventriculography was performed which excluded a cerebral abscess or other space-occupying lesion. Preliminary lumbar puncture gave clear fluid under a pressure of 30 mm., and specimens of cerebrospinal fluid were taken for examination from the right ventricle and from the cerebral subarachnoid space. The results were: lumbar, protein 350 mg. %, W.B.C. 90/c.mm.; right ventricle, protein 55 mg. %, W.B.C. 5/c.mm. As these figures clearly indicated a cerebrospinal fluid block, cisternal puncture was carried out and 2 ml. of Ethiodan (ethyl-*p*-iodophenylundecoate (B.D.H.)) introduced. This was found to be held up largely at the foramen magnum, but it ran in a thin stream down as far as the seventh cervical vertebra, where the obstruction was complete (Fig. 1). To determine the lower limit of the block, a further 2 ml. of Ethiodan were introduced by lumbar puncture. This ran up as far as the fifth thoracic vertebra, at which level there was complete obstruction

(Fig. 2). The appearances were those of an extradural lesion. During the screening procedure the child lay face downward, and he seemed to find this posture particularly uncomfortable. He cried and struggled to turn over. collection of pus was found. It lay mainly to the left, and had pushed the dura to the right. Further pus was found at T1, which proved to be the upper limit. The laminectomy was continued up to include C7 and C6.

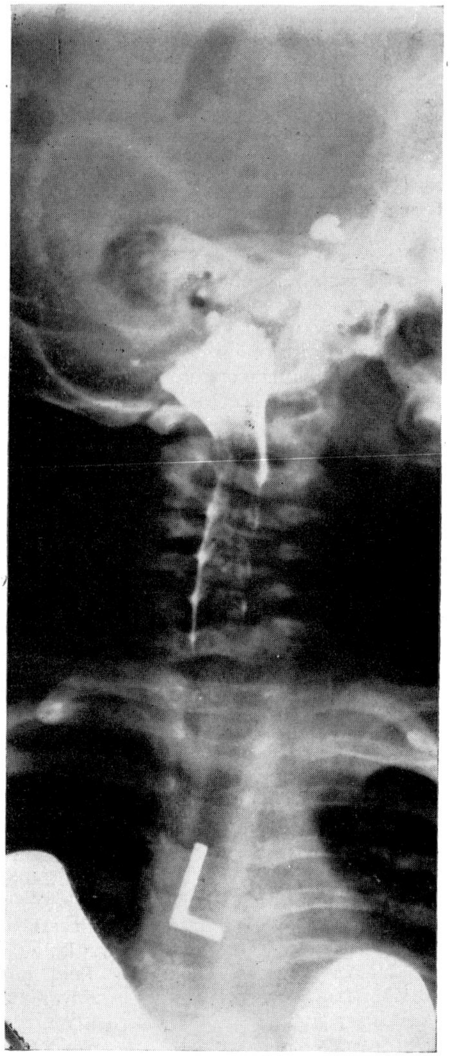

FIG. 1.

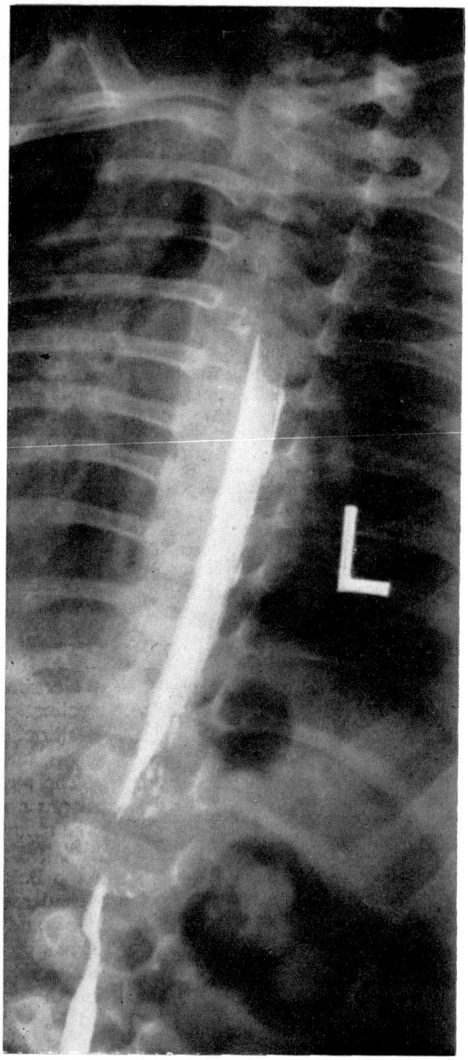

FIG. 2.

Myelographic appearances. In Fig. 1, contrast medium introduced by the cisternal route is seen to be held up for the most part at the foramen magnum, a little running down in a thin stream as far as the seventh cervical vertebra. In Fig. 2, the flow of the lumbar contrast medium is completely blocked at the fifth thoracic vertebra.

A history of repeated staphylococcal infections and the present pyrexial illness suggested epidural abscess as the most likely cause of the block. Laminectomy was therefore performed immediately. The spines and laminae of the third and fourth thoracic vertebrae were removed without any abnormality being encountered, but when the removal was carried up to T2 a large A drainage tube was inserted and the wound closed.

Penicillin and streptomycin had been given before operation, and these antibiotics were continued pending sensitivity tests. The organism was identified as a coagulase-positive staphylococcus which was resistant to penicillin, and this was accordingly changed to terramycin administered systemically, and chloramphenicol instilled locally via the tube.

After some initial anxiety, when the child's temperature rose to 104° F., recovery was rapid and the wound healed perfectly. No neurological signs appeared in the post-operative period, and he began to walk while in hospital. It was thought advisable to continue systemic antibiotic treatment for four weeks, and he was discharged six weeks after the operation. He has remained perfectly well to date (15 months).

Discussion

Infection of the spinal epidural space is always secondary to infection elsewhere in the body, either adjacent or remote. The mode of involvement of the space is obvious enough when the focus is near the involved area, such as an infected rib, but more difficult to understand when spread occurs from some distant site. The metastatic pathway must be either lymphatic or haematogenous, the organism lodging in the epidural tissue and giving rise to an abscess. This child met the staphylococcus very early in life, and it must be presumed that between the repeated episodes it lay dormant somewhere in the body.

Staphylococcus aureus has been the organism responsible for acute spinal epidural abscess in almost all reported cases (Heusner, 1948; Hulme and Dott, 1954). According to Neale (1936) this organism possesses a special affinity for the metastatic invasion of loose fatty areolar tissue of the type which fills the epidural space. The site of the invasion depends upon anatomical considerations. Dandy (1926) pointed out that the spinal epidural space was only present dorsal to the spinal nerve attachments, the dura anteriorly being in contact with the vertebral bodies and their ligaments. In the cervical region the space is only a potential one as far down as the seventh vertebra, but then it begins to deepen and is 0·5-0·75 cm. in depth between the fourth and eighth thoracic vertebrae. It becomes shallow again from the eleventh thoracic to the second lumbar vertebra, and thereafter attains its greatest depth. Consequently an epidural abscess is rarely found above the fourth thoracic vertebra, and is commonest in the lower thoracic and lumbar regions. Dandy considered that local trauma was an important inciting agent in the development of haematogenous infection. An alternative view of the mechanism of invasion of the epidural space was put forward by Browder and Meyers (1937). They considered that haematogenous spread first occurred to a vertebra, the epidural space then being secondarily involved from this focus of infection. No evidence of vertebral involvement was seen in the present case, either in the *x*-rays or at operation, but it could have been so small as to be invisible. Once the abscess is established, the spinal cord is in grave danger. Not only is it subjected to direct compression but the infection may also bring about extensive damage by producing thrombosis of its blood-vessels. In the latter case, the most severe neurological signs may occur very suddenly indeed.

The early symptoms in adults are remarkably uniform. There is a pyrexial illness, localized back pain of the most agonizing intensity, and radicular pain. Familiarity with this picture should make the diagnosis possible before neurological signs appear, but, in a young child with a pyrexial illness and no neurological signs, the condition might well be overlooked if attention is not drawn to the back. Although in this case no local tenderness was found, it was thought in retrospect that significance should be attached to the mother's observations on the type of handling which caused him to scream, and to our own observation of his discomfort when he lay face downwards or was picked up. The features which are of diagnostic importance may then be briefly summarized: (1) A history of infection which may have been weeks or months beforehand. Boharas and Koskoff (1941) found the average interval in 85 cases to be 4·2 weeks, but in one case it was as long as three years. (2) Trauma to the back. (3) An unexplained pyrexial illness. (4) Tenderness of the spine. This may be present on physical examination, or may be suggested by the child's disinclination to lie on its back or face downwards.

If an epidural abscess is suspected, lumbar puncture should be performed with caution, and with frequent removal of the stilette and aspiration as the needle is advanced. Pus in the epidural space may be encountered giving the diagnosis, but if the needle is inadvertently passed through the abscess into the subarachnoid space, then meningitis may result. When the subarachnoid space is tapped, the likely finding is a partial or complete spinal block, with the characteristic manometry and protein elevation. There is a moderate pleocytosis.

There are few reports in the literature of myelography as a diagnostic aid. In adults, although the site of the abscess may be determinable by clinical testing, it seems reasonable to perform this investigation to ascertain its exact level and extent. It should be noted though, that lumbar myelography may prove difficult if a second lumbar puncture has to be done to introduce the contrast medium. The initial diagnostic puncture lowers the pressure of the cerebrospinal fluid, which will already be low if spinal block is present, and when a needle is introduced for the second time an unsatisfactory flow of the fluid is obtained. In these circumstances the contrast medium is very likely to go between the arachnoid and the dura instead of into the subarachnoid space. It was these considerations that underlay the selection of the cisternal route for introduction. Lumbar myelography then proved to be necessary in addition, and was fortunately successful. In the case of P.S., the apparent block was much longer than the extent of the abscess, which may have been due to an associated arachnoiditis.

The treatment is immediate laminectomy and evacuation of the abscess, a small tube drain being inserted to the site before closing. There is no need to leave the wound open. The appropriate antibiotic should be given systemically and locally. The results are excellent if operation is performed before the onset of neurological signs (Heusner, 1948). Operation is urgently required at this stage, for, as has been pointed out, cord damage may come on with great rapidity. If signs of this have already appeared, then permanent paralysis or death is almost certain.

Summary

The case is described of a 15-month-old baby in whom an acute spinal epidural abscess was successfully treated without residual symptoms. The importance of early diagnosis is emphasized, for, if laminectomy and drainage are performed before the onset of neurological signs, complete recovery is to be expected. Once spinal cord damage has taken place, however, then permanent neurological deficit or death is almost certain. The diagnostic difficulties and pathology of the condition are discussed.

We are indebted for permission to report this case to Dr. Mary Wilmers of the Belgrave Hospital, and to Mr. P. H. Schurr, under whose care the child was admitted to the Guy's-Maudsley Neurosurgical Unit. We would like to thank Mr. Murray A. Falconer, Director of the Unit, for his help and advice in the preparation of this paper, and Dr. R. D. Hoare for assistance with the radiological aspects and for permission to reproduce the myelograms.

References

Boharas, S. and Koskoff, Y. D. (1941). *J. Amer. med. Ass.*, **117**, 1085.
Browder, J. and Meyers, E. (1937). *Amer. J. Surg.*, 37, 4.
Dandy, W. E. (1926). *Arch. Surg. (Chicago)*, **13**, 477.
Heusner, A. P. (1948). *New Engl. J. Med.*, **239**, 845.
Hulme, A. and Dott, N. M. (1954). *Brit. med. J.*, **1**, 64.
Neale, A. V. (1936). *Bgham med. Rev.*, **11**, 4.

COW'S MILK ALLERGY IN INFANCY

BY

W. DAVIES

Assistant Paediatrician, East Glamorgan Hospital

(RECEIVED FOR PUBLICATION OCTOBER 7, 1957)

It appears that, in this country, allergy to cow's milk, manifesting itself in infancy, is still regarded as a rarity. Borman (1953) describes milk sensitivity in infancy as a rare condition and the only case report in the available British literature is that of Brodribb (1944). The purpose of this paper is to present the clinical findings in one infant in whom the diagnosis of milk allergy appears to have been proved and to summarize the features described in the literature.

Case Report

C.C.L. (No. 29911), a male first infant, whose father had suffered from seasonal allergic rhinitis for several years, was born on January 6, 1957. He was seen on February 2, 1957. After a normal pregnancy he was delivered at full-term, weighing 8 lb 2 oz., and was entirely breast fed up to five days before admission. During this period he had been contented, was feeding well and had apparently gained weight. At this time, his mother decided to change to artificial feeding because her milk supply was diminishing. A half-cream preparation of dried milk was used. Four days later, he became reluctant to take his feeds, vomited frequently and developed a widespread rash. His mother remarked that he looked ill, seemed apathetic and listless, but cried if disturbed or if attempts were made to feed him. His stools, previously formed, now became loose, frequent (six to eight in the previous 24 hours) and were noticed to contain mucus. He was admitted to hospital.

On admission, he weighed 8 lb. 13 oz., and showed clinical evidence of mild dehydration with slightly inelastic skin and rather sunken eyes. His whole body was covered with a bright red rash, erythematous on the trunk and limbs and urticarial on the face and scalp, with a tendency, in places, to ring formation. His palms and soles were a uniform bright scarlet colour. A soft systolic bruit was audible to the left of the sternum but no other abnormal physical signs were detected. He was afebrile and his heart-rate was 132 per minute. During the examination he passed a watery, green stool containing a good deal of mucus.

He was then offered feeds of half-strength Hartmann's solution which he took eagerly without vomiting. When seen again 16 hours later, the rash had completely disappeared and he appeared more contented and well hydrated. A provisional clinical diagnosis of cow's milk allergy was then made.

The results of laboratory investigations were as follows: stool cultures on three successive days were negative for the enteric, dysentery and type-specific *E coli* groups. No pathogenic organisms grew from blood cultures. There was a faint trace of albumin in the urine, but it was free from deposit and on culture was sterile. A radiograph of the chest was clear. A blood count showed haemoglobin, 76%; red blood cells, 3,900,000 per c.mm.; white blood cells, 15,800 per c.mm.; polymorphs, 38%; eosinophils, 18%; lymphocytes, 41%; and monocytes, 3%. W.R. and Kahn tests on maternal blood were negative.

Stained films prepared from the mucus found in his stools showed large numbers of eosinophil cells. A scratch test using cow's milk produced an immediate urticarial weal, 1·5 cm. in diameter.

After 24 hours on clear fluids, he was offered feeds of expressed breast milk obtained from the breast milk bank at St. David's Hospital, Cardiff. These were taken eagerly without vomiting, his stools became normal and during the first few days he gained 8 oz. in weight, and appeared to be a normal contented infant. On February 13, he was again offered the same preparation of half-cream dried milk and, within a few hours, he became extremely reluctant to take a feed, vomited repeatedly and again passed frequent, loose stools. A faint roseolar rash appeared on his trunk and face and his weight fell to 8 lb. 10 oz. Feeds of half-strength Hartmann's solution were again taken quite eagerly.

On February 17 it was decided to restart feeds of expressed breast milk and again, within a few hours, his symptoms had cleared. His subsequent progress was completely satisfactory and on March 7 he weighed 10 lb. 4 oz. It was then decided to try the effect of feeding him with a soya-bean preparation known as Soyolk, composed of:

		%			%
Fat	..	20	Glucose	..	5·7
Protein	..	41	Ash	..	4·8
Carbohydrate	..	18·59	Fibre	..	2
Moisture	..	7	Calcium	..	0·2
			Phosphate	..	0·71

For a few days, these feeds were taken quite well but he gradually began to lose weight, became irritable, vomited occasionally and passed loose, bulky, and offensive stools. On March 14, expressed breast milk feeds were restarted and his weight began to increase again. On March 31 he weighed 11 lb. 1 oz., on April 24, 12 lb. 4 oz. and on May 19, 13 lb. 5 oz.

On April 2, oral hyposensitization to cow's milk was attempted, starting with one drop daily and doubling the dose each day. On April 9 he was taking 1 dr. daily and, subsequently, the dose was increased by 1 dr. daily. No untoward effects were noted until April 13 when he was taking 5 dr. His stools then became rather loose and the dose was not increased until they were more formed on April 25. No further difficulties were encountered and by May 20 he was taking four-hourly feeds, each of 8 oz. of cow's milk, without any abnormal symptoms or signs (Fig. 1).

He has since progressed quite satisfactorily. On September 6, 1957, he weighed 17 lb., was taking cow's milk, rusks and cereals without difficulty. His stools were well-formed and free of mucus. The cow's milk scratch test now produced an area of erythema slightly less than 1 cm. in diameter.

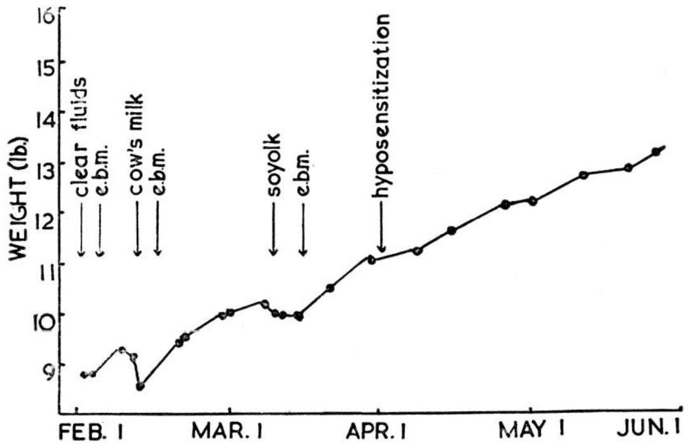

FIG. 1.—Effect of different types of feed on infant C.C.L.'s weight gain.

Discussion

Diagnosis. The findings in the patient described here seem to leave no doubt as to the correct diagnosis. Collins-Williams (1954) states that where a diagnosis of gastro-intestinal allergy is postulated the following criteria must be satisfied:

(1) The history must be compatible with the diagnosis of allergy. (2) A specific allergen must be determined. (3) Symptoms must appear within a reasonable time after ingestion of the allergen. (4) Symptoms must disappear within a reasonable time after exclusion of the food from the diet. (5) Symptoms must return when the food is reintroduced. (6) The food must be one commonly tolerated without difficulty by most people. (7) The diagnosis must be supported by other allergic manifestations to the same allergen, e.g., urticaria. (8) The diagnosis is supported by other known allergies in the same patient. (9) Positive findings in other diagnostic procedures such as blood and gastro-intestinal eosinophilia, positive radiological findings, gastric or sigmoidoscopic examination, effects of drugs and results of skin tests would be of confirmatory value.

Most authorities stress that the diagnosis is essentially a clinical one and that skin tests are unreliable.

Clein (1954) reports that, in a series of 206 patients sensitive to cow's milk, there were two or more allergic persons in the same family in 175 cases and one allergic parent in 168 cases. Kane (1957) describing 102 patients found a family history of allergy in 80%.

Incidence. Figures obtained from the literature seem to vary considerably. Clein (1951) states that one in 15 infants are allergic to cow's milk in some degree. Collins-Williams (1956) in a series of 3,000 patients aged from birth to 15 years seen in private paediatric practice, but excluding all those referred with possible allergic symptoms, found an incidence of 0·3%. He also quotes other observers as giving figures varying from less than 0·1% to 7%.

Pathogenesis. Kane (1957) reports that the intestinal tract of a young infant is more permeable to intact protein than that of older children and adults. Collins-Williams (1955) feels that the milk-sensitive infant falls into one of four categories: he may be sensitized to the factor common to both cow and goat lactalbumin or to the species specific factor of cow lactalbumin alone. With either of these categories there may be sensitization to casein as well. Finally, and much less frequently, he may be sensitized to casein alone. This would explain the well-known observation that some cow's-milk sensitive infants fail to improve on a diet of goat's milk.

Brodribb (1944) felt that the allergen appeared to be either lactalbumin or lactoglobulin. As both occur together in the preparation of dried milk the exact identity seemed to be of little practical importance.

Clein (1954) stressed that the symptoms could be explained on the basis of the usual pathological changes occurring in allergy: oedema of mucous membranes, spasm of smooth muscle and excess mucus secretion.

Tudor (1956) states that unless the child is sensitive to the lactalbumin of cow's milk, goat's milk is not a successful substitute because the casein is identical in cow's milk and goat's milk. It seems, therefore, that any of the proteins occurring in cow's milk may act as the allergen.

Glaser (1956) quotes investigations which seem

to confirm that, while human and cow lactalbumin are completely species specific, this is not so in the case of animals as closely related as the cow and goat. However, lactalbumin is markedly heat labile since there is a decrease in antigenic reactivity even at 60° C., which becomes progressively more marked as the temperature is increased. This would explain why evaporated cow's milk, in which the lactalbumin is practically completely denatured by heat is often as satisfactory as goat's milk in the feeding of milk-sensitive infants. Casein, however, is relatively heat stable, no change being noted in its antigenic activity until the temperature reaches 100° C. The changes then taking place probably explain why superheated cow's milk is occasionally tolerated by cow's milk sensitive infants.

Symptoms. The age of onset of symptoms varies with the time of starting cow's milk feeding but Clein (1954) reported that symptoms appeared in 82% during the first four months and in 89% during the first year of life. The symptoms attributed to milk allergy vary widely and are summarized in Table 1.

Investigations. Laboratory and radiological investigations can only be of confirmatory value in the diagnosis which is essentially a clinical one. Frequently, all such tests are found to be within normal limits.

Treatment. The essential treatment is to remove the offending allergen from the infant's diet and to replace it with a food which provides the necessary basic requirements for adequate growth. Glaser (1956) suggests that in some mild cases boiled or evaporated cow's milk may prove satisfactory; goat's milk is also worthy of trial but, in a high proportion of cases, results are disappointing. He regards human milk as ideal but dismisses it as impracticable because of the difficulty and expense involved in obtaining an adequate supply. The same author has found Nutramigen, a hydrolysed casein preparation, disappointing but agrees that other authorities have had considerable success with it. He also states that it is possible to use a food prepared with strained meat as the protein base.

Various foods prepared from the soya bean have been reported for several years as containing all the

TABLE 1

PERCENTAGE INCIDENCE OF SYMPTOMS ATTRIBUTED IN THE LITERATURE TO COW'S MILK ALLERGY

Symptoms	Kane (1957) (No. 102)	Clein (1951) (No. 140)	Rosenblum and Rosenblum (1952) (No. unknown)	Clein (1954) (No. 206)
	%	%	%	%
Eczema	74			44
Vomiting and diarrhoea	20		15	
Irritability ; colic	37	29	5	31
Asthma	1			7
Recurrent rhinorrhoea	2			13
Vomiting		39	8·3	
Diarrhoea		24	31·6	22
Mucus in stools		6		
Blood in stools		5		
Anorexia		4		3
Diarrhoea and colic			16	
Diarrhoea, vomiting and colic			20	
Pylorospasm				33
Cough, croup, etc.				17
Constipation				4
Urticaria ; angio oedema				1
Apathy, cyanosis, collapse				2
'Very unhappy all the time'				19

Other clinical features which have been attributed to cow's milk sensitivity include haematemesis, coeliac syndrome, ulcerative colitis, regional enteritis, enuresis, convulsions, headache, migraine and behaviour disturbances.

Bigler (1955) stresses that the picture may vary from a very mild upset to a severe illness and that symptoms may last from a few months up to several years. The infant may become desensitized spontaneously as happens in other forms of allergy.

amino-acids necessary for the normal growth and development of the human infant, but recently it has been suggested that they may be slightly deficient in methionine. In our patient, a trial of Soyolk was made but, because of difficulty in feeding and the passage of loose, bulky stools, it was quickly discontinued. Glaser (1956) reports that such symptoms occur frequently for the first few days and suggests that the preparations should be tried at half strength at the beginning. It is possible that persistence with this type of feeding might have led to greater success in our patient.

Oral hyposensitization has frequently been reported as being unsatisfactory, but it was a worthwhile and simple procedure in this case.

Conclusions

Abt (1912) mentioned that some infants have an idiosyncrasy to cow's milk which produces 'toxic symptoms and injuries to the baby'. Since then numerous reports have been published on the subject in foreign literautre but, in this country, the condition is still regarded as a rarity. The patient described here appears to be a fairly obvious example of cow's milk sensitivity; there have been reports of even more acute cases such as infants dying of anaphylactic shock. Although it should be accepted that such acute types are by no means common, a more careful search might well lead to the discovery of the relatively minor forms of the disease. The first essential step in diagnosis is elimination of cow's milk from the diet. This would be simplified considerably if a food similar to Nutramigen were easily available in this country.

Summary

An example of sensitivity to cow's milk in an infant is described and the available literature summarized. In this patient, replacement of the cow's milk by human milk and subsequent oral hyposensitization produced satisfactory results.

I am grateful to Dr. P. T. Bray and Dr. D. A. Williams for their help and advice in the preparation of this paper.

References

Abt, I. A. (1912). *Chicago med. Rec.*, **34**, 115.
Bigler, J. A. (1955). *Pediat. Clin. N. Amer.*, **2**, 503.
Brodribb, H. S. (1944). *Arch. Dis. Childh.*, **19**, 140.
Clein, N. W. (1951). *Ann. Allergy*, **9**, 195.
—— (1954). *Pediat. Clin. N. Amer.*, **1**, 949.
Collins-Williams, C. (1954). *Bull. Hosp. sick Child. Toronto*, **3**, 68.
—— (1955). *Ann. Allergy*, **13**, 415.
—— (1956). *J. Pediat.*, **48**, 39.
Glaser, J. (1956). *Allergy in Childhood.* 1st ed., p. 444. (Amer. Lect. Ser. No. 272). Springfield, Illinois.
Kane, S. (1957). *Amer. Practit.*, **8**, 65.
Norman, A. P. (1953). 'Allergy.' In Moncrieff, A. and Evans, P. (Editors). *Diseases of Children*, Garrod, Batten and Thursfield's 5th ed. Vol. **1**, p. 856. London.
Rosenblum, A. H. and Rosenblum, P. (1952). *Pediatrics*, **9**, 311.
Tudor, R. B. (1956). *J.-Lancet*, **76**, 245.

FRANK BERIBERI IN A 4-MONTH-OLD INFANT

BY

TADEUSZ GIZA and JERZY ARMATA

From the Children's Clinic, formerly in the Jagiellonian University of Cracow

(RECEIVED FOR PUBLICATION NOVEMBER 5, 1957)

Case History

A boy, S.A. 4785/344, aged 4 months, was admitted to the Clinic on February 14, 1957. He was the third child of healthy parents and was born without complications after a normal pregnancy, weighing 4 Kg. The developmental pattern was normal and he never had any illnesses. He was breast-fed till he was 3 months old and he was then given a butter-flour mixture, prepared from overmilled wheat meal. No juices were regularly added, nor any vitamins supplied.

The illness started suddenly with anorexia. The baby was disinclined to feed from the bottle, milk was regurgitated, but not water. He was restless and whining. Constipation, diminished excretion of urine, hoarseness and stiffness of the neck occurred. Two days before admission the child was pale, dyspnoeic, drowsy and had developed diarrhoea.

Upon admission the patient looked acutely and gravely ill. He was cyanosed, there was extreme tachycardia and respirations were 80 to the minute and grunting in character. Nevertheless he was obviously a well-developed and well-nourished child. He weighed 7·1 Kg. and was 67 cm. long. His temperature was normal.

Physical examination revealed rachitic craniotabes, tense and bulging fontanelle, opisthotonos, distension and pulsation of the cervical veins and bilateral loss of the patellar reflexes. There was definite cardiac enlargement in all diameters, with the apical impulse in the left anterior axillary line. Heart sounds were muffled and distant, of poor quality, and the second pulmonic sound was accentuated. A marked gallop rhythm was present. The liver was palpable two fingerbreadths below the right costal border.

Laboratory findings were as follows: Tuberculin skin tests were negative. Wassermann reaction of the blood and cerebrospinal fluid was negative. The erythrocyte sedimentation rate was normal. Examination of the peripheral blood showed haemoglobin 62%, red blood cell count 4·3 million, white blood cell count 10,680, with 35% polymorphonuclears, 3% band forms, 61% lymphocytes and 1% monocytes. The total serum protein was 6·45 g. per 100 ml., albumin 5·41 and globulin 1·04 g. per 100 ml.; serum calcium 9·9 mg. % and phosphate 4·7 mg. %. The cerebrospinal fluid showed a cell count of 4 lymphocytes per c.mm., 20 mg. per 100 ml. total protein and 70 mg. per 100 ml. sugar.

Routine urine analysis was normal. However, testing for phenylpyruvic acid by adding a few drops of 10% ferric chloride solution to the urine acidified with dilute sulphuric acid, produced an intense dark bluish green colour.

A radiograph of the chest showed a generally enlarged cardiac shadow with an enlarged right atrium and with a loss of muscular tone (Fig. 1). The radiographic

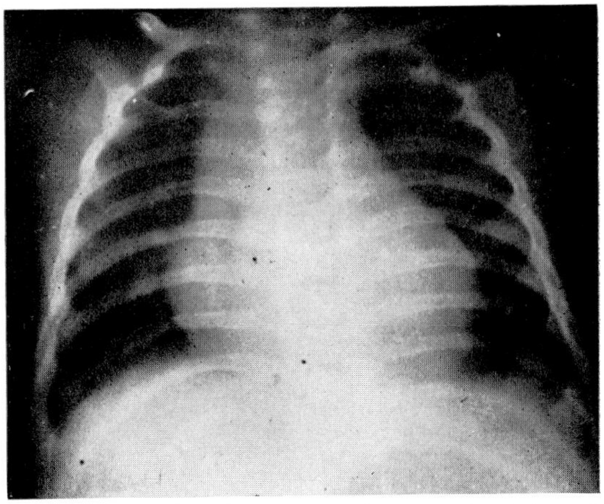

FIG. 1.—Radiograph of chest showing enlarged cardiac shadow with increase of right atrium and loss of muscle tone.

examination of the skull and long bones disclosed evidence typical of rickets.

The electrocardiogram revealed a left ventricular preponderance with shortening of the P-R interval, a prolonged Q-T interval and inversion of T in the praecordial leads (Fig. 2).

As far as the differential diagnosis was concerned, the dominating symptoms were those of acute cardiac insufficiency. Various possible diagnoses were entertained initially. For instance the cardiac type of infantile paralysis the more so as the patellar reflexes were abolished; fibroelastosis; after the onset of neurological signs, rhabdomyoblastosis, which, associated with tuberous sclerosis, gives the so-called Bourneville's disease; and lastly diphtheria, in spite of the lack of any suggestive history or findings.

The definitive recognition came *ex iuvantibus*. A dramatic change in the apparently hopeless condition

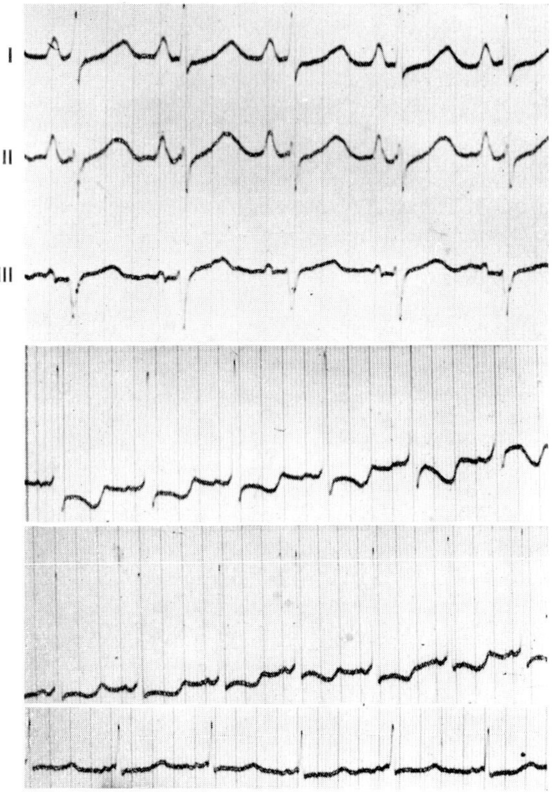

FIG. 2.—Electrocardiogram in case of frank beriberi in infant.

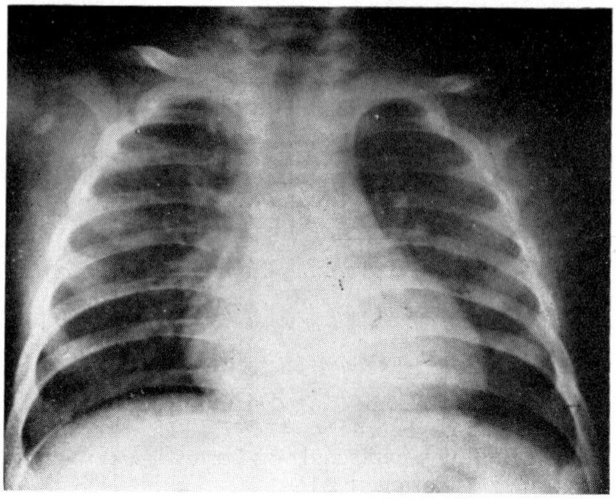

FIG. 3.—Radiograph showing heart within normal limits after two weeks' administration of vitamin B_1.

of the patient following the administration of vitamin B_1 on the third day after admission anticipated the diagnosis.

Forty-eight hours after the intramuscular administration of thiamine, in a dose of 50 mg. daily, the appetite returned rapidly and also the normal skin colouration. The dyspnoea disappeared and respirations dropped to 40 to the minute, the pulse decreased to 120 per minute and there was a progressive decrease in all dimensions of the heart, the sounds of which became louder and clearer. The knee-jerks reappeared on the seventh day. In the second week the heart returned to its normal limits (Fig. 3) and phenylpyruvic acid could no longer be found in the urine. From this time on vitamin B_1 was continued orally. The boy was discharged 23 days after admittance.

Discussion

Special mention should be made of the excretion of phenylpyruvic acid in the urine of this patient. He was a full-term baby and did not receive a high protein diet. His mental development did not seem to be affected, his hair was rather dark, the sclerae white and there was no muscular hypertonicity, tremor or patchy eczema; he excreted a pale urine containing no reducing properties, and there was no dark staining on his diapers; there was no suggestion either from the history, physical examination or from radiographs of the long bones to suggest scurvy. We consider therefore that phenylpyruvic oligophrenia, tyrosyluria of premature infants, alcaptonuria and vitamin C deficiency, all four of them conditions sometimes associated with phenylpyruvic acid in the urine, were excluded.

As we could not relate phenylpyruvic acid excretion to any of these four disorders, we suppose, though possessing no certain proof, that pyruvic acid, present in excess in the tissues during vitamin B_1 deficiency may be conjugated with phenyl radical either in the liver or kidneys and then excreted in the urine. It is well known that phenols are detoxified in the liver by conjugation with sulphuric acid or organic acids. Moreover, Closs and Fölling (1936) have demonstrated the presence of phenylpyruvic acid in the urine of rats suffering from artificially produced hypothiaminosis.

Summary

A 4-month-old infant fed on a butter-flour mixture, prepared from overmilled wheat meal, developed frank beriberi with cardiac enlargement and circulatory failure, a grunting cry and loss of the patellar reflexes. All these symptoms disappeared after giving him large doses of vitamin B_1.

This appears to be the first case of true infantile beriberi reported in Europe.

REFERENCE

Closs, E. and Fölling, A. (1936). *Z. phys. Chem.*, **254**, 258.

WILLIAM HEBERDEN'S CASES OF ANAPHYLACTOID PURPURA

BY

ARTHUR ROOK

From Addenbrooke's Hospital, Cambridge

(RECEIVED FOR PUBLICATION SEPTEMBER 9, 1957)

Of William Heberden (1710-1801) Dr. Wells, in a letter to Lord Kenyon, wrote, 'Dr. Heberden, my Lord, stands in a manner alone in his profession. No other person, I believe, either in this or any other country, has ever exercised the art of medicine with the same dignity or has contributed so much to raise it in the estimation of mankind'. Heberden's modesty, integrity and scholarship earned him the admiration of his contemporaries and the affectionate respect of his biographers. In his writings he recorded accurate observations of disease in a simple lucid style. He contributed many papers to the Philosophical Transactions of the Royal Society and to the Medical Transactions of the College of Physicians. He is now remembered particularly for his descriptions of chicken pox, angina pectoris and the nodes in osteo-arthritis.

His 'Commentaries on the History and Cure of Diseases' was published by his son William Heberden in 1802, the year after his death, first in Latin and later in English. The Commentaries were built up gradually from notes taken from day to day during his active professional life. They were revised each month and expanded or modified until 1782, after which year no significant alteration was made. Chapter 78 of the Commentaries, entitled 'Purpureae Maculae', includes two brief case reports.

> 'A boy, four years old, for several days had swellings rise on his knees, legs, thighs, buttocks, or scrotum. The part affected was not discoloured, and when at rest, was easy, but could not be moved without some degree of pain. Together with these swellings there appeared red spots sometimes round, sometimes angular, a quarter or half an inch broad, which on the second day became purple, and afterwards yellow, just as it happens from a bruise. The child continued perfectly well in all other respects. These swellings ceased to appear in about ten days; but the red spots continued coming out a few days longer.
>
> 'Another boy, five years old, was seized with pains and swellings in various parts, and the penis in particular was so distended, though not discoloured, that he could hardly make water. He had sometimes pains in his belly with vomiting, and at that time some streaks of blood were perceived in his stools, and the urine was tinged with blood. When the pain attacked his leg, he was unable to walk; and presently the skin of his leg was all over full of bloody points. After a truce of three or four days the swellings returned, and the bloody dots, as before. These dots became paler on the second day, and almost vanished on the third. The child struggled with this uncommon disorder for a considerable time, before he was entirely freed from it.
>
> The first of these boys immediately grew better after being gently purged: the other took a decoction of the bark for several days without any manifest good effect.'

These children were certainly suffering from anaphylactoid purpura. Gairdner (1948) gives Willan (1808) the credit for the first description of a patient with this syndrome. Neither Heberden nor Willan differentiated the syndrome from other forms of purpura but Heberden clearly described the association of the skin lesions with gastro-intestinal symptoms, joint pain and haematuria. Although Schönlein (1837) and his pupil Henoch (1874) are rightly commemorated for establishing the syndrome as a distinct entity, Heberden's admirable clinical description does not deserve the neglect which has been its fate.

REFERENCES

Gairdner, D. (1948). *Quart. J. Med.*, **41** (n.s. 17), 95.
Henoch, E. (1874). *Berl. klin. Wschr.*, **11**, 641.
Schönlein, J. L. (1837). *Allgemeine und specielle Pathologie und Therapie*, 3rd ed., Vol. 2, p. 48. Freiburg.
Willan, R. (1808). *Cutaneous Diseases*. London.

BOOK REVIEWS

The Year Book of Pediatrics. Edited by SYDNEY S. GELLIS. (Pp. 469. $7.50.) Year Book Publishers, Chicago. 1957-58.

The Year Book of Pediatrics for 1957-58 is in the tradition and up to the standard of its very competent predecessors. The notice taken of non-American activities has been rising over the years and in the present volume more than one third of the articles abstracted are not American; thus a much broader picture of the year's work in children's medicine is presented. In a mixed bag such as this, providing something for everyone, the quality of the work abstracted will inevitably be variable, yet for anyone wishing to see what has gone on in paediatrics in the past year this book will be more valuable than any other; and if the invited comments by selected experts which follow some of the abstracts are as irritating as ever, they are in the tradition of this Year Book and one must presume that there is a demand for them in some quarters or they would not be there.

Paediatrics. Supplement 1957. Edited by WILFRID GAISFORD and REGINALD LIGHTWOOD. (Pp. v+157; 45 figures. 35s.) London: Butterworth. 1957.

This is the second supplement of Paediatrics for the Practitioner. It contains original contributions by various specialists, on gamma-globulin and immunity, prophylactic immunization, steroid therapy, skin tuberculosis, congenital heart disease, funnel chest, cysts of the neck, the testes and penis, and galactosaemia. In addition there is a further Noter-up or Bringer-up-to-dater which entirely replaces the previous edition.

The volume is as factual and practical as those preceding it and the presentation maintains the high standard set. It makes one miserable to note that the combined price for the set of volumes is now £14 10s. 0d.

Pediatric Profiles. Edited by BORDEN S. VEEDER. (Pp. 267.) St. Louis : C. V. Mosby. 1957.

As the illustrious men of their day die they leave behind them many forms of memorial. Not least of these perhaps is the enduring memory which lingers in the hearts and minds of those who knew them. A later generation may read their writings and they may also be known by one or other alteration they have made to the subject or discipline they adorned. But scientific writing tends not to evoke the personality of the writer, nor does a ward block named after someone conjure up to a younger generation a picture of the man whose memory it honours. In order that succeeding generations should know something not only of the scientific contributions of the great but also something of their personalities the *Journal of Pediatrics* in 1953 started to acquire and publish a series of word pictures of great paediatricians, written by people who had known them intimately. Thirty of these have now been collected in this volume entitled *Pediatric Profiles*, in which worldly achievements are incidental and subordinate to the character and personality of the subject.

The original idea was that only Americans should be included and that they should be not still living, but as the Editorial Board of the *Journal of Pediatrics* progressed, however, they realized that some men who had exerted a national influence on American paediatrics were not in fact Americans, and the scope of the subject matter had to be widened to include some British and Continental paediatricians; we thus find Jacobi, the first President of the American Pediatric Society, next to Sir Thomas Barlow, while Abt is followed by Jundell of Sweden, Still, Poynton, Cooley and Brennemann. What a series of subjects for their authors !

Pediatric Profiles will find a welcome wherever the discipline of paediatrics is followed. To the existing generation, many of whom will remember some of the characters depicted in the book, memories will be re-awakened vividly, while coming generations of paediatricians will find first-hand appraisals of the personalities of men whose work will be bound to influence their daily lives and doings. The book ends with two nostalgic little pieces of what has been called anecdotage, one on paediatrics in Vienna at the turn of the century by Bela Schick and the other by the editor, Veeder, an account of his first National Pediatric Meeting in Washington in 1910.

Orthopedic Surgery in Infancy and Childhood. By Albert Barnett Ferguson, Jr. and five other contributors. (Pp. xii+508; 504 figures. 120s.) London: Baillière, Tindall and Cox; U.S.A.: Williams and Wilkins. 1957.

This book aims to fulfil the need for a comprehensive text-book of the surgery of the locomotor system (excluding fractures) as applied to children.

The authors are to be congratulated on the success of their venture and particularly on their presentation of those aspects of the subject which are controversial. In general their practice is in accord with that of orthopaedic surgeons in this country and such differences as exist are in emphasis rather than of a fundamental nature.

The readers of this journal will find much to interest them in this book which concentrates more on principles of management than on details of surgical treatment. Most of the common orthopaedic conditions are well described and rarities mentioned in sufficient detail to satisfy the needs of those not primarily concerned with this speciality.

Physicians will probably appreciate the concise and clear account of disorders of calcium and phosphorous metabolism contributed by Klein. The section on generalized disorders of the skeleton by Ferguson, although using some terms unfamiliar to British readers is stimulating and pursues an aetiological theme convincingly and with conviction. There is a balanced review of indications for treatment in cerebral palsy and when surgical measures are mentioned emphasis is on the few well-tried and successful procedures such as triple arthrodesis, and even these are discussed in a cautious way. The many operations described which have a theoretical rather than a practical application are rightly left out.

The illustrations are excellent and help both to clarify and amplify the text. The bibliography is well chosen and affords a good introduction to further reading in those subjects which in a book of this nature must be covered briefly. This book should be in the library of every orthopaedic and paediatric hospital and department, but its price, £6, will probably exclude it from the personal collection of many paediatricians and surgeons. This is a pity.

Chirurgie Préventive de la Tuberculose Ostéo-articulaire. By R. Kaufmann. (Pp. 174; 49 figures. Fr. fr. 2,000.) Paris: Doin. 1958.

The author begins 'when this work appears, M. Blondin will have proved before the Academy of Surgery that we know how to cure and above all prevent caries of the vertebrae. Osteolysis which precedes caries is a non-specific reversible state following infection of the adjacent soft parts. Once they have been drained the bone becomes normal'. The primary lesion is lymphatic and the author advises excision of the diseased lymphatic glands and abscess leaving the wound open. Despite endless repetition and the obvious sincerity of the author the reviewer remains unconvinced. It would have been better to include more evidence instead of referring the reader to seven previous publications. Despite these criticisms it is a refreshing book which stimulates thought on a subject which seemed to be cut and dried.

Cryptorchism. By Charles W. Charny and William Wolgin. (Pp. viii+140; 28 figures. 45s.) London: Cassell. 1957.

This book covers the whole field of cryptorchidism except for intentionally making only brief reference to its endocrine aspects.

The various causes of non-descent are considered. The gubernaculum appears to play little or no part. The importance of short testicular blood vessels is stressed. Failure of development of the processus vaginalis and its descent into the scrotum is usually accompanied by descent of the testicle. Excluding gross endocrine disorders there are two main causes of non-descent of the testicle: mechanical difficulties or an inherent incapacity of the testicle to respond to normal gonadotrophic stimuli.

The chapter devoted to pathological findings forms the kernel of the book. These findings have been obtained by testicular biopsies done at operation and to check treatment by operation and by chorionic hormone. The opinion is given that the follow-up of a series of cases is almost valueless without serial biopsies, although, of course, it is realized that seminal analyses afford assessment in cases of bilateral cryptorchidism. It appears that little histological difference exists before the age of 9 or 10 years between the scrotal and non-scrotal testis. The degree of pathological change depends more on the age of the patient than the degree of descent. With the histological material available it was not possible to determine the relative importance of congenital testicular deficiency and the effect of unfavourable environment on the testicle. The histology investigations confirm the previously established findings that in the adult unilateral cryptorchidism allows normal libido, potentia and fertility whilst in bilateral cases it is often only the fertility that is absent.

The second part of the book deals with symptomatology, complications, diagnosis and therapy. The authors' study of the literature and their own experience confirm that many complications are commoner in the undescended testicle than in the normal. Of especial importance are trauma, torsion, associated hernia and malignancy—besides, of course, infertility. It appears that the undescended testicle is about 33 times more liable to become malignant than is the scrotal. It also appears that the intra-abdominal testicle is four times more liable to malignancy than is the inguinal type. The malignancy is usually a seminoma. The point is made that when this occurs in a testicle that has been brought down by orchidopexy, the inguinal lymph nodes should be excised as well as the testicle and its coverings. The authors found very little evidence that psychic disturbances occurred frequently or played an important part.

Possible treatment by gonad-stimulating hormone (chorionic gonadotrophin) followed by androgen is discussed. Great importance is given to the avoidance of overdosage because of the likelihood of harming the other (scrotal) testis. The authors could not be counted as strong supporters of this sort of therapy; they do point out, though, that such treatment differentiates testicles that will and will not descend without operation. The authors attach no value to this therapy as a pre-operative measure to facilitate the operative technique.

They refer briefly to the various techniques of orchidopexy and stress the importance of adequate mobilization of both the testicular vessels and the vas deferens.

Basing their opinion on the histopathology of biopsy specimens which indicates the changes of physiological puberty as beginning at about 9 or 10 years of age, the authors feel that all treatment by hormones or by operation can safely be left until that age. As stated above they accept the use of hormones as a diagnostic and a therapeutic guide but no more. Regarding orchidopexy, in unilateral cases it is felt that the value of this operation is open to question. In these patients fertility is already assured by the other scrotal testis and investigations have shown very poor results of spermatogenesis following orchidopexy. Furthermore, in some cases total atrophy has followed operation. Thus in prepubertal patients orchidopexy is not recommended.

The patient should be watched. Certainly in adults there can be no reason for doing an orchidopexy. In bilateral cases orchidopexy before the age of 10 years is advised as it is the only hope of preventing certain sterility.

If in the repair of a hernia satisfactory orchidopexy is impossible or if the testis is found to be unusually small, then it should be removed provided the other testis is normal.

The results of treatment by gonadotrophins and by operation are reviewed as is the literature. It is pointed out that descent of the testicle into the scrotum is of itself not evidence of successful therapy. It is spermogenesis that is so important to aim for.

The material is well presented. The microphotographs are good and the references and bibliography excellent. These features make for pleasant reading of matters that require to be much more widely known.

The Lower Urinary Tract in Childhood. By S. R. Kjellberg, N. O. Ericsson and Ulf Rudhe. (Pp. ix.+298; 265 figures. 126s.; 18.00$.) Chicago: Year Book Publishers; London: Interscience Publishers. 1958.

This is primarily a radiological monograph and fully upholds the very high standard which we have come to expect from Swedish publications in this field. The illustrations are so numerous and well-reproduced that this volume will undoubtedly become an indispensable work of reference for x-ray departments undertaking urological investigations in children. Good chapters on anatomy and physiology preface the discussion of pathological conditions, but in the latter the text is so sparsely scattered amongst the illustrations that the thread of the argument is sometimes hard to follow. It is interesting to note that, as in other centres where radiography is given precedence over endoscopy, these authors lay great emphasis upon the role of urethral valves as a cause of urinary obstruction and enuresis, while 'bladder neck obstruction' is regarded as rare. The chapter on ectopic ureterocoele is particularly valuable, as might be expected from Dr. Ericsson's previous studies.

Clinical Application of Hormone Assay. By John A. Loraine. (Pp. xii+368; 305 figures. 30s.) Edinburgh and London: E. & S. Livingstone. 1958.

Since the war hormone assays have passed increasingly into the province of the clinician and the clinical research worker; they are no longer confined to the physiologist concerned with pure research, or the pharmacologist attached to a drug house. Clinical problems have brought their own peculiar difficulties to assay work, the chief of which are the minute quantities of the hormones present, as a rule, in biological fluids, and the extreme complexity, i.e., impurity, of the fluid which has to be tested. That these problems have been posed but by no means solved is illustrated by the fact that in five of the nine chapters which deal with bio-assays in this book, the author concludes with the statement that the available techniques are inadequate for routine application in the clinical field and that further work is necessary in methods of extraction of the hormones from blood and urine.

A chapter is devoted to every hormone, except the thyroid, the parathyroid and the gastro-intestinal hormones, and each contains a brief description and evaluation of the possible methods of assay, with a summary of the principal findings in normal and in pathological conditions. The physician who is interested in endocrinology will find the book easy to read and entirely lacking in complicated diagrammatic speculations which often confuse rather than clarify. The specialist will find in it an excellent and critical introduction to work in each field, with frequent suggestions as to what needs to be done.

It is a commonplace that biochemical methods should, if possible, replace biological methods, and this is particularly true in the clinical application of hormone assay. Clearly biological work can hold its own where fundamentally new discoveries are concerned, but the doctor is concerned with an individual patient and the superiority of chemical methods in this report is unquestionable. This is brought out very well by Dr. Loraine in his chapter on the oestrogens. The concepts which emerged from the earlier biological work have not, in the main, been challenged by the subsequent chemical studies, but what the latter have produced are firm figures by which the normal can be distinguished from the abnormal.

Infant Feeding and Feeding Difficulties, 3rd ed. By Philip Evans and Ronald Mac Keith. (Pp. viii+293; 66 figures. 16s.) London: J. & A. Churchill. 1958.

For the third edition of this now well-established handbook on infant feeding Dr. Mac Keith alone is responsible. There is evidence of revision in all parts of it and perhaps most noticeably in the chapters on practical manoeuvres and the physiological aspects of lactation. The section on diets has been extended to include modern work on inborn errors of metabolism.

That a third edition has been called for seven years after the book originally appeared is at once an indication of the advances which have been made in infant feeding in this period and of the popularity of the book.

Les Regimes du Nourrisson Bien portant ou Malade. By P. Delthil. (Pp. 346. Fr. fr. 3,350.) Paris : G. Doin. 1957.

The publishers comment that there are few practical books on infant feeding, that the best of them date from more than 30 years ago and do not represent present ideas and that the comprehensive treatises do not give clear enough guidance. Dr. Delthil's book is 330 pages long, well-printed and clearly set out and may well be a considerable advance on what has been available in French up till now. However, as far as the present ideas on infant feeding in Scandinavia, North America and Great Britain are concerned, it is far from up to date. This might represent a justifiable French decision not to follow fashions popular in other countries but that is not a complete answer. The attitude represented here is not only old-fashioned but is also inefficient, just as ours was 30 years ago. For example, insufficiency of breast milk is said to be revealed by falling-off of the weight curve, pallor and lack of tissue firmness of the child, sometimes by digestive troubles, false diarrhoea or vomiting. Do not French babies announce their hunger by crying? Test weighing is recommended, it being said that in the second month it should be '110 grms to 120 grms' and in the third month '125 grms to 135 grms'. Do not French babies vary widely in their individual needs? The section on breast feeding is too brief and, although it includes a table of amino-acids contained in breast milk, it does not refer to the draught reflex, knowing about which is an 'éclatante' aid in helping mothers to breast feed successfully. There is nothing about the prevention of cracked nipples and, in saying it is sometimes necessary to suspend suckling, no mention is made of the need to express the milk to avoid engorgement when suckling is omitted. A proper knowledge of the physiology and detailed management and difficulties of breast feeding would be a better way of increasing the number of women successfully breast-feeding than the remedy the author recommends, which is, 'Convinced of the striking superiority of breast milk, doctors should proclaim it incessantly and devote themselves to a continued propaganda'. One could make minor criticisms; for example, under renal acidosis, anorexia is mentioned as an important symptom but renal acidosis is not given when the causes of anorexia are discussed.

Dr. Delthil was formerly Chéf de Laboratoire at the Hôpital des Enfants Malades. Whether he is now in practice I do not know. However, there are doctors in Paris who know what immense practical help knowledge of the physiology of lactation and child-centred management, instead of mechanical management of the individual child's feeding, can give. I am inclined to suggest that one of the small English text books on infant feeding adapted by a French paediatrician might be found of greater practical value than this particular work. I am sorry to say this for there is much that is very good and very acceptable in the book but the author seems to me to have missed the chance of including the last 20 years' advances in the practice of successful infant feeding.

Treatment of the Child in Emotional Conflict. By HYMAN S. LIPPMAN. (Pp. x+298. 45s.) London: McGraw Hill. 1956.

Some such book as this should be read by every paediatrician in training. Child guidance is an established adjunct to child health, and the report of the Commission of Child Guidance in this country visualizes considerable extension of this policy. Although the general pattern of all child guidance is similar, the underlying psychiatric and psychological principles in each particular clinic are to a large extent dependent on the training and principles of the consulting psychiatrist in charge. This book is a concise, straightforward exposition of the full Freudian outlook on child guidance. It is written in plain English for the intelligent, but not specially trained, medical personnel, and it is only necessary to become fully acquainted with the precise meaning of such terms as 'ego', 'super-ego', 'id', and a few others, to be clear of the meaning of every page. Since its psychological orientation is totally Freudian, as developed for child guidance by Melanie Klein, Susan Isaacs, Aichorn and others of a rather closely knit group of workers, it will certainly not meet with universal acceptance by paediatricians or child guidance workers in this country. Nevertheless, every page is written with such seriousness and such intensity of understanding and sympathy for the sufferings of the emotionally disturbed child, and so much of it has universal application, that it might well be read with equally responsive understanding by all those engaged in child health work.

The book is divided into seven sections: the first, of four chapters, discusses the general symptoms of emotional complications in childhood and the kind of influences it may exert on mental growth and development. It also takes the reader through the general arrangements and methods of therapy, the working and the staffing, of a particular child guidance clinic in the United States. The following four sections deal successively with four major clinical groupings of emotionally disturbed children, namely, the 'Neurotic Child', the 'Child with Personality Problems', the 'Child who "Acts Out"', and lastly the 'Child with a Tenuous Hold on Life'. Each of these major divisions of from three to six chapters, takes the reader through particular individual types of maladjustment illustrated by brief appropriate extracts from case notes. The last section discusses in general terms the prevention of social and emotional maladjustment and defines some of the wider aims of child guidance.

The author is obviously convinced that with adequate psychotherapy, that is with therapy often lasting over two or three years, but sometimes very much less, children who would otherwise grow up with such maladjustment as to make their adult life burdensome to themselves and others, can eventually be salvaged sufficiently to grow up reasonably well-adjusted human beings. This is a considerable claim, particularly when one reads some of his fearful case notes. But what he does not make quite so clear is how successful a widely distributed network of child guidance clinics will prove to be in dealing with the day-to-day maladjustment of quite a large proportion of the child population. If adult maladjustment has its roots in childhood, which is widely accepted, this latter problem is of vast importance and would be the decisive justification for the large and expensive set up that exists in America and to a lesser extent in this country.

Deafness, Mutism and Mental Deficiency in Children. By LOUIS MINSKI. (Pp. viii+82; 14 figures. 12s. 6d.) London: William Heinemann. 1957.

The main theme of this book is the importance of distinguishing between deafness, mental deficiency and emotional disturbance in children with severe delay in speech development. A brief account is given of two residential units set up by the author to investigate and treat such cases and there are additional sections on deafness in children and psychological testing.

For such a short book there is too much inessential material. For example, almost one-third of the book is devoted to psychological testing, while most of the results of the author's important original work are compressed into some 15 pages. Would not a paper confined to the original work and published in a weekly journal have served the author's purpose better?

It is unfortunate that the earlier Australian figures on the risk of congenital defects following rubella in pregnancy should be quoted, now that prospective investigations have shown them to be fallacious.

These are, nevertheless, minor criticisms and should not be allowed to hinder the promotion of such a worthy cause.

L'Enfant Inadapté. Rôle Médico-social du Médecin. By L. Michaud and D. J. Duché. (Pp. 316. Fr. fr. 3,600.) Paris: G. Doin. 1957.

In this book the possible origins of maladjustment are considered in a most comprehensive manner. The authors' concept of maladjustment differs from ours, for they use it to mean the child who is at a social disadvantage from both physical and mental handicap. The physical causes are dealt with in great detail and hardly a condition has been omitted, but little emphasis is placed on the relative frequency or importance of different diseases, the rare and the commonplace being given equal attention. As to the developmental-psycho-educational aspects these are dealt with in their own particular fashion. There is no 'school' view-point advocated and their eclecticism is all embracing from Melanie Klein to leucotomy. The value of a work of this kind is limited, particularly when our knowledge of where and how things go wrong socially and physically in children's lives is so abundant. As a general review it has a place for those beginning to study children but its unevenness detracts from its otherwise potential value.

Cleft Palate and Speech, 4th ed. By Muriel E. Morley. (Pp. xx+271; 86 figures. £1 7s. 6d.) Edinburgh and London: E. and S. Livingstone. 1958.

That this book has appeared in four editions since it was first published 13 years ago speaks well for its all-round excellence. The title *Cleft Palate and Speech* is a well chosen one because it indicates the theme which runs throughout the book, that treatment must be directed primarily towards achieving the happy result of perfect speech, and that such an object can only be attained by close cooperation between various experts, including surgeon, orthodontist and speech therapist. The book is particularly valuable in this respect and enables each to understand the work of the others, thus coordinating their efforts towards the common goal.

The subject matter is extremely comprehensive and is presented clearly and scientifically. The opening chapters encompass the embryology, anatomy and inheritance of cleft palates. The difficult and controversial subject of the mechanism of palatopharyngeal closure is very reasonably presented, and is followed by the management and surgical treatment. The chapter on the development of surgery will help many readers to orientate themselves in the history of the various procedures and to understand current trends. To most speech therapists who have not been able to watch and study surgical methods themselves this account will be of considerable help. Speech and speech therapy are discussed in the latter half of this book.

There is much that is new in this edition and it is obvious that the author has kept abreast of the surgical development in this field. This book must be essential to all speech therapists and is one which could be read with profit by all concerned with the treatment of cleft palates.

Fluoridation of Public Water Supplies. Report of the Commission of Inquiry, 1957 (appointed by the Governor General of New Zealand). (Pp. 240. 8s.) Wellington: Departmental Fluoridation Committee, Department of Health. 1957.

This report shows clearly that the fluoride content of water in New Zealand should be increased. The amount of dental caries is at present devastating and could be halved. The Commission has found that no harm need be anticipated from this measure. The spectre of chronic fluoride poisoning has been laid with reasonable certainty. Justice has been done to the scientific evidence; moreover, by public hearings it has been seen to be done to the Papatoetoe Anti-fluoridation Society, the New Zealand Organic Compost Society and other representatives of man's right to water, however natural.

While few Cockneys would care to exert their right to imbibe Father Thames in his natural state, this report serves to remind us that the fluoride content of much British water is still inadequate.

PAEDIATRICS IN WESTERN NIGERIA

BY

MALCOLM MACGREGOR

Sometime Lecturer in Paediatrics, University College, Ibadan

(RECEIVED FOR PUBLICATION NOVEMBER 15, 1957)

Introduction

The aim of this article is to present to the reader a broad view of the work of a general hospital in West Africa in its relation to the health of children. Facts and impressions were accumulated by the author during a year's sojourn in Nigeria, too short a time no doubt for a penetrating survey of local problems, but, possessed of the clinical potential of a flourishing and well-esteemed young hospital, long enough for a responsible survey of the main topics confronting workers in Child Health in West Africa. Practice in Africa is bewildering and refreshing to an English doctor, and requires a fresh approach adapted to experiences in new realms of pathology.

Several published descriptions have focused attention on the University College Hospital, Ibadan, during its growth (*vide British Medical Journal*, 1956). Now it is completed and possesses facilities that are unexcelled in tropical Africa. Built beside a teeming Nigerian city, a centre both of commerce and administration, and closely in contact with a university already of considerable renown, the new hospital is exceptionally favoured in its circumstances and associations.

In the waiting period while the new hospital was being built, the medical staff, who were already assembled, were occupied in creating a corporate hospital unit and at the same time in providing the local population of Ibadan with the fuller medical services that such an unexampled mustering of doctors and nurses made possible. These new facilities were grasped with alacrity, and in no sphere more willingly than by parents for their children. It was during this interregnum that the subject matter of this paper was collected. The base hospital was then the Adeoyo Hospital in the middle of the old town, a group of single storied buildings closely encircled by primitive dwelling houses, recently vacated by the Ibadan District Council to furnish the nidus of the University Hospital organization. The little renovation that was possible was done, and soon this primitive and unkempt small hospital became imbued with a mood of energy and promise, so that its achievements far over-reached its material restrictions. The children's ward consisted of a congested room with a balcony, together able to contain some 35 infants and children under 12 years of age. In this ward fulminating gastro-enteritis was treated beside broncho-pneumonia, septic ulcers beside extensive exposed burns, typhoid beside malaria and tuberculosis amidst them all. The frequency of cross infection can only be roughly guessed, but was certainly not very great, as instanced by the fact that diarrhoea seldom developed in hospital even in long-stay patients. Perhaps we owed this to the sunlight and free circulation of air in a ward with constantly open doors and windows. An element of squalor is inseparable from work in these circumstances, but the first affronted reaction to bed linen grey from use and re-use, to the one ward lavatory of hole-in-floor type which served for patients, staff and visitors, to the 'sluice room', a square cell with a tap and a hole in the wall from which the effluent flowed outside in a rather ill-defined way, and to the chicken which continued defiantly to inhabit the out-patient verandah, passed when one realized that these were unalterable but temporary conditions, and that ill results from them were so much less than might be imagined.

Social Aspects. Ibadan is the chief town of the Yoruba tribe by whom Western Nigeria is largely peopled. Easy-going, generous and intelligent, the Yorubas have constructed a community based upon peasant agriculture but centred upon towns. They live in urban concentrations often of considerable size, but for part of the year retire to their farms at a distance to work the land. Consequently there is a fluidity about the population, making census figures for an area inaccurate. Peasant society is largely polygamous and responsibility for wives and children is only partly borne by the husband, with the result that the women make themselves as far as possible economically independent by petty trading, for which they possess enormous aptitude. Market stalls tended by blue-turbanned and vociferous womenfolk are a prime ingredient of Yoruba-land.

In Ibadan there are reputed to dwell some half a million people. It is a sprawling town of mud-built dwellings with corrugated iron roofs intermingled with substantial brick villas and modern emporia. It is fringed by a new growth of fine buildings in a modern tropical idiom, and by reservations of dwelling houses with extensive gardens. Open drains through the town convey sewage and stormwater. Ibadan streets at all times are a press of sound and life, thronged with pedestrians, bicycles and impatiently hooting motor traffic, a witness to the liveliness and vigour of its many-faceted society, which contains Indian, Lebanese and European communities as well as African.

Uncomprehending of the methods and beliefs of practitioners of Western medicine, the common people have, notwithstanding, been quick to recognize its capabilities, particularly since the advent of potent chemotherapeutic drugs. Attempts at rational exposition of the causes of disease and the aims of treatment encounter customs, fears, superstitions and taboos that among the illiterate are a complete bar to understanding. The following account of popular beliefs in Ibadan is based upon a recent article (Omololu, 1956). Diseases, Dr. Omololu says, are always caused by the wrath of spirits, by worms, or by the machination of enemies. Education modifies but does not efface this concept. The conception of micro-organisms causing disease has never been entertained in Yoruba-land. In a polygamous society the ground is fertile for suspicion and culprits are easily found. At a more advanced level, certain poorly-defined notions of pathology are used as comprehensive explanations of a wide range of disorders. A past history of urethral discharge, for example, is regarded as infallible evidence of gonorrhoea and may be held responsible for any urinary, joint or skin symptom. 'Black blood' may be regarded as the cause of an illness whose manifestations range from malaria to vitamin B deficiency and to impotence. A change of blood is indicated and a good doctor knows that injections rather than dietary advice or mixtures can best accomplish the change. It is well-known that injections are the most potent remedies available for almost anything.

Yoruba-land is extremely conscious of its gastro-intestinal tract and in consequence any symptom arising from it is presented forthwith. A patient might fail to mention that he has dyspnoea, but not that he has a coated tongue or that he has vomited. Diarrhoea, dysentery and piles are to the common people synonymous and may be used to denote anything from frequent stools to pruritus ani. One may never take it for granted that the patient has the slightest idea of the meaning of the word he is using; rather it is safer to assume that he is conscious of something amiss in a roughly specified region of the body. A person who complains of constipation for example cannot even be assumed not to have diarrhoea. Intestinal worms are almost omnipresent and the popular mind has conferred upon them an almost unlimited potential for evil. Any digestive upset, increased peristaltic movement, or irritation anywhere in skin or scalp is laid at their door.

The father is dominant in the Yoruba family and his availability and mood are important in deciding whether or not one of his children shall attend hospital. Whether he lives with the mother or not, his consent must be obtained before the child can be brought into hospital. If this is not done the wife by general consent can be divorced with ignominy. Generally speaking, in their devotion to their children, in their courage in breaking with the past, in their efforts to cooperate with doctors, whatever the difficulties, and in their uncomplaining tolerance of discomforts and delays, the young Nigerian mothers deserve measureless praise. For those better-educated girls, increasingly under the influence of English speaking cultures, who have made a monogamous marriage and are yet bonded by birth to a Yoruba manner of life, there is an intolerable conflict at every turn, especially in the raising of their children. A danger is that they will reject their heritage in favour of the meretricious attractions of suburban English culture.

Children are fed almost universally on the breast and lactation is a more abundant and more efficient process than in Britain, rarely attended by complications of engorgement or sore nipples. Manual expression of breast milk occasions no difficulty. At six months or after the output often decreases, and, as it is common to breast feed for one or two years, this is an important influence in retarding growth. Feeding at the breast is entirely on demand and the baby, slung in a girdle on his mother's back, is close enough to be sure that his needs are not overlooked (Fig. 1). Weaning, which occurs late, is likely to be to 'pap' (a paste of maize flour) with occasional meat soup (a dilute vegetable broth, not of much nutritive value, containing dried fish, peppers, palm oil and small quantities of meat). This diet is subsequently varied by the addition of yam and cassava, beans and plantains. Eggs and milk are not in the diet, nor are meat, fish or fresh fruit in any adequate amount. Consequently symptoms of protein deficiency are wide-spread and are aggravated when early withdrawal from the breast is necessary or if illness makes extra demands upon metabolism. Tradition as much as economics is responsible for this ill-balanced diet, and striking benefits are seen if parents can be prevailed upon to give preference to naturally-occurring rich protein foods such as beans, dried fish, ground-nuts and guinea corn, rather than to the time-honoured starchy yams and cassava. The admission of children to hospital has some educative value here and it is hoped that parents will profit from hospital precept and admonishment in the subsequent management of their children (Fig. 2).

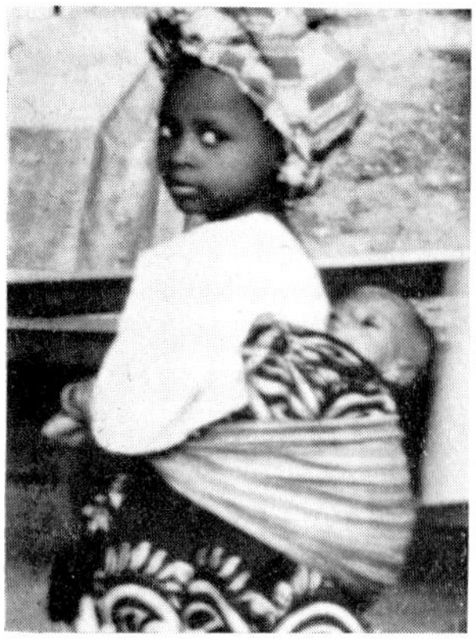

FIG. 1.—Carrying a baby.

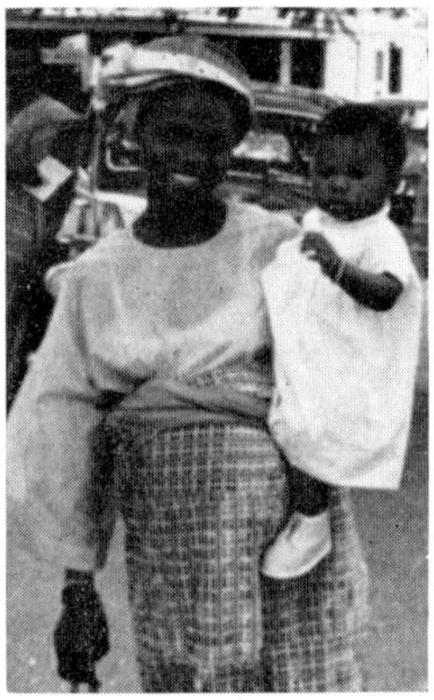

FIG. 2.—Mother and child from infant welfare clinic.

On the whole the Yoruba peasantry is a clean people and standards of personal hygiene are good despite the fact that some methods of child care, such as the early management of the umbilical cord, seriously conflict with European ideas. The babies are mainly overdressed, except for diapers which are non-existent among the uneducated. No attempt is made to inculcate early control of sphincters, which seriously complicates sanitary arrangements for large out-patient clinics. Messes of all sorts are disposed of rapidly by Yoruba women, usually being wiped up by some article of their own clothing; failing that, lifted by hand and thrown to the ground outside.

The educated section of the community is bilingual, English being used for everyday communication. Among the illiterates, the main source of the hospital attenders, an ability to speak English is exceptional. The language problem is further complicated by numerous minority groups from other parts of Nigeria, who dwell in and around Ibadan. Yoruba is a difficult tonal language, requiring a flair to master it; a great part of the hospital work is carried on through interpreters. Although to work through an interpreter is probably less of a constraint in paediatrics, when histories are already at second hand, than in other branches of medicine, the intervention of a third mind is a great hindrance to speed and accuracy. Time-wasting confusion results from a search for detail, with the result that question and answer have to be reduced to rudimentary exchanges, paring away much that is valuable and that might facilitate diagnosis. Interpreters engaged in utilitarian repetitive conversations become desultory and inexact, or at worst provide the answers that they surmise the doctors are expecting. Sympathetic contact with the patients, so vital to indoctrination of novel ideas, is often a struggle to achieve and consultations can too easily become bleak and irritable under the twin pressures of haste and obscurity. Fortunately the strongly developed African sense of humour is often able to bridge the gap and to build an enduring bond of sympathy.

Statistics. The University College Hospital is a very busy one (Figs. 3, 4). If we take the month of August, 1956, at random, approximately 8,000 new out-patients attended the hospital and a quarter of these attended the paediatric department. In all, 23,000 out-patients came to the hospital during the month, and about 300 children attended daily. In the same month, 121 children were admitted to the 36 beds of the children's ward, as against 200 admissions to 131 adult medical and surgical beds in the hospital in the same period. There was therefore a relative preponderance of sick children.

During 1956, 1,881 children were admitted to the children's ward of Adeoyo Hospital. The diagnoses of these children are listed in Table 1, together with some figures concerning mortality. No less than 488 (26%) of these children died. There were approximately 300 more males than females in this series and the male death rate (24% contrasted with 28%) was rather lower than the female. The male preponderance was considerably accentuated in admissions for tetanus, and for diarrhoea at all ages, whereas a significant female preponderance was evident in admissions for protein malnutrition.

When discussing the age distribution of the patients it is important to remember that statements of age by parents are very inaccurate. Dealing as we are with large numbers it is probable that inaccuracies in the one direction are roughly

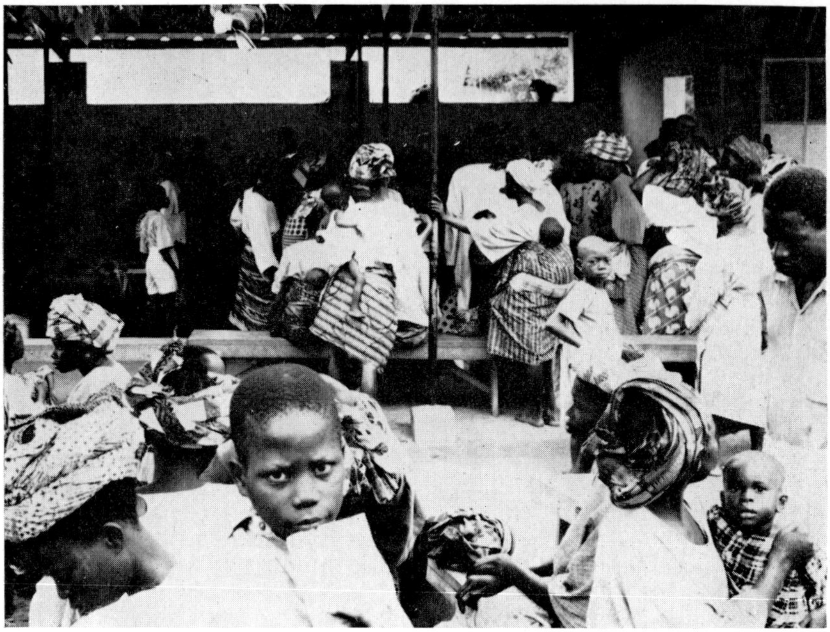

FIG. 3.—Outside the Children's Clinic.

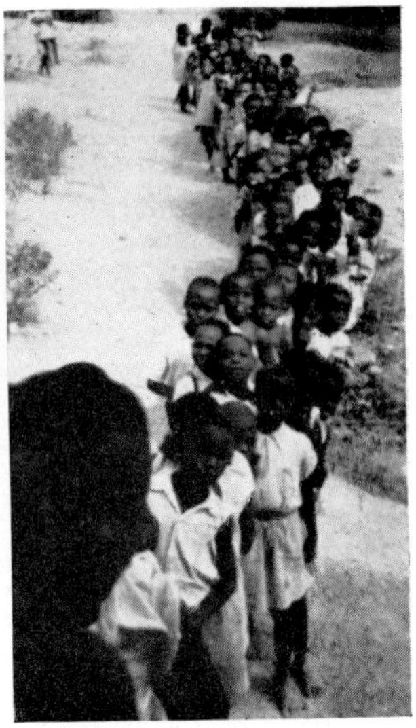

FIG. 4.—Waiting their turn.

balanced by inaccuracies in the other, but the further one gets from birth, the more conjectural are the recorded ages. With this proviso, it appears that one half of the children were under 1 year old, one third between 1 and 3, and one fifth older than this. In this series the death rate according to age

TABLE 1

ADMISSIONS TO CHILDREN'S WARD, ADEOYO HOSPITAL, 1956, ANALYSED ACCORDING TO DIAGNOSIS, AND LISTED IN ORDER OF FREQUENCY

Diagnosis	Total Number	Deaths	Mortality (%)	Sex Ratio M : F
Pneumonia	309	111	36	1·1 to 1
Diarrhoea and vomiting	243	74	30	2·05 to 1
Anaemia	223	29	13	1·3 to 1
Protein malnutrition	157	54	35	0·89 to 1
Tuberculosis	113	33	30	1·3 to 1
Trauma (including burns)	104	7	7	1·3 to 1
Other alimentary disorders	102	12		
Tetanus	95	58	61	2·0 to 1
Other respiratory disease	82	8		
Protozoal and helminth infections	81	14		
Unexplained and unclassified illness	80	46	57	1·2 to 1
Infections of skin, lymph glands, and subcutaneous tissues	78	13		
Other acute specific infections	69	19	28	0·94 to 1
Diseases of nervous system	53	9		
Diseases of genito-urinary system	44	10		
Diseases of bones and joints	38	1		
Purulent meningitis	36	13	36	1·06 to 1
Tumours	31	4		
Other nutritional and deficiency diseases	24	3		
Cardiac and circulatory disease	23	8		
Neonatal diseases	17	7		
Diseases of liver	13	2		
Diseases of eyes	11	2		
Poisoning and idiosyncrasy to drugs	9	3		
Other blood disorders	8	3		
Diseases of endocrine system	2	0		
Total (after correction for multiple diagnoses)	1,881	488	26	1·36 to 1
Total males	1,090	265	24·5	1·17 to 1
Total females	791	223	28·5	

remained constant at 30% up to 6 years, and after that fell steeply. Just over one half of the total deaths occurred in infants (i.e. less than 1 year old).

Selection of Cases for Admission. Children were admitted nearly always for treatment, seldom for investigation only. A strict criterion was that, irrespective of diagnosis, the treatment could not be given as an out-patient. Priority was given to the desperately ill and to acute surgical emergencies. A few children from the surgical waiting list were admitted each week and a few others by the ophthalmic surgeon, gynaecologist and dermatologist from their clinics. The proportion of infants to older children was regulated to some extent by the number of infant cots available. The upper age limit was about 12 years, but was determined also by whether or not the child was too tall to lie comfortably in a small bed. Less direct influences were the willingness or otherwise of parents to accept admission (few in fact refused), and the reputation of the hospital for treatment of particular clinical entities. In general, where it is plain that treatment of a condition is effective, patients will come. The converse is also true. Geographical factors change the emphasis on certain diagnoses; Ibadan has a reputation as a healthy district, and the incidence of many diseases is undoubtedly greater elsewhere in Nigeria. On the other hand, community diseases such as tuberculosis and gastroenteritis may be unduly common in this huge congested township.

Examination of Patients. For the practitioner accustomed to fair-skinned children there is much to learn about the interpretation of physical signs of illness in Africans. Assessment of mucosal colour, jaundice, skin disorders, intelligence and indeed the recognition of an ill child all require experience. At first, judgment of a child's age is often at fault by as much as 3 years. Heights and weights grossly beneath the normal for the chronological age are very common (Fig. 5). Walters (1956) found that children in Ilobi, a village in South West Nigeria, were some 10% shorter in height than English children and that over the first 5 years of life they were about 20% lighter in weight. Racial differences in physique play a part in this, but undoubtedly more important in keeping the children back are undernutrition and ill-health. Children attending out-patients for example might have weights of 15 lb. or even less at the age of 3 or 4.

Many African children, of course, especially those from better homes, are at every age physically comparable with European, and it is perhaps just this spread from super-normality to the most remarkable physical retardation that makes age assessment so difficult. Newly born babies are also small, with birth weights averaging 1 lb. or so below what is customary in England. Their range of skin colour is very great, and includes a shade of yellow-brown difficult to distinguish from a rather deep neonatal jaundice. Certain common symptoms of childhood carry different implications in Nigeria from those they have in Britain. Pallor for example is likely to be due to malaria or to sickle cell anaemia, oedema to protein malnutrition or nephrosis, abdominal pain to dysentery or ascariasis, jaundice in the newborn baby to septicaemia, and in the older child to a crisis of sickle cell disease, while convulsions, one of the commonest reasons for seeking help, are much more ominous than they are here. In the respiratory field alone is the range of diagnoses closely comparable to that in England. An enormous morbidity from whooping cough, bronchopneumonia and tuberculosis is common to the children of both countries.

The death rate in the children's wards is horrifying by European standards and exceeds the total of deaths in all other departments of the hospital.

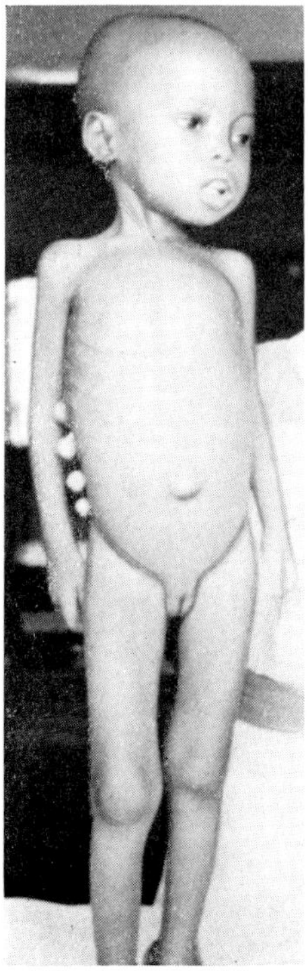

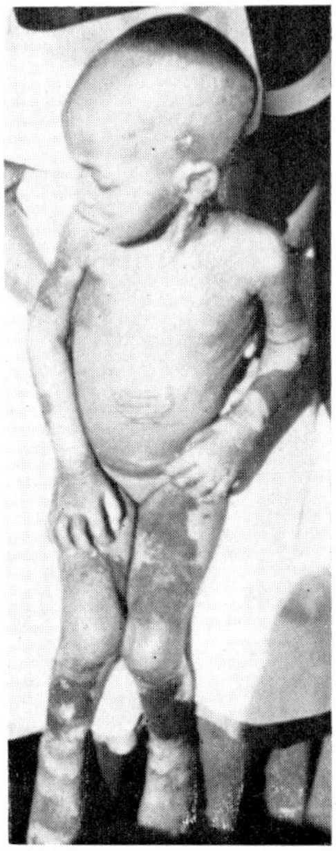

FIG. 6.—Skin changes in protein malnutrition.

FIG. 5.—Five-year-old child.

The greater number of deaths occur within 24 hours of admission, and malnutrition, gastro-enteritis, broncho-pneumonia and tuberculosis account for most of them.

Clinical Discussion

There follows a commentary upon the illnesses that were encountered. They are considered under the headings, and in the sequence, of Table 1.

Pneumonia. This was the commonest reason for admission to hospital and was the greatest single cause of death in the whole series. Two thirds of the cases were in infants, and of the remainder most were in the 1 to 3 year age group. Among the latter, the mortality was even higher than in infants, probably because this is also the age group of protein malnutrition. A bacteriological diagnosis was not often made, but most cases were believed to be broncho-pneumonia of the usual catarrhal origin. Staphylococcal aetiology was inferred on several occasions because of the radiographic appearances. A short fulminating illness, often accompanied by diarrhoea, was the most common mode. Some of the patients in whom the illness ran a more protracted course may have been suffering from whooping cough. The prevalent local method of force-feeding weakly babies by hand certainly accounted for some aspiration pneumonias. Convulsions were always of serious prognosis; they were not obviously due to oxygen lack, and meningeal infection was always excluded. A better clinical response to one antibiotic rather than another was not demonstrated, and the most frequent treatment was with penicillin and streptomycin combined. Two cases were mongols.

Very many cases of pneumonia were treated as out-patients, and because they were less severe the outlook was much more favourable. Those admitted to hospital were either suffering from a virulent infection or were in such a bad condition that they could not stand even a moderate illness.

Diarrhoea and Vomiting. Two thirds of these were infants, and about a quarter of them died. Many were admitted in an extremely dehydrated state. Gastro-enteritis following upon prolonged underfeeding frequently provided us with an emaciated child to whom diarrhoea was the last straw. Nevertheless, one cannot feel content with the results of hospital management of gastro-enteritis. The diarrhoea itself usually ceased fairly quickly with the usually accepted regime of parenteral fluids and chemotherapy. Electrolyte disturbances were corrected, but in many cases the child remained gravely ill and perished on the third or fourth day at a time when hydration was adequate and the known biochemical disturbances had been fully corrected. Much thought was given to the reason for these failures, and vitamin deficiency, hypocalcaemia, adrenal failure and hypoglycaemia were all excluded after experiment. Profound cerebral effects seemed to follow dehydration in many of these babies, who would have convulsions and subsequently remain in a blank immobile state with alteration in muscle tone and a tendency to muscle twitching which was ominous and not properly understood. Lumbar puncture was unrevealing. A number suffered from tetany during the recovery phase, and when tested, the serum calcium was found in such cases to be low. Pathogenic organisms were scarcely ever isolated from the stools, and the bacteriology of infantile gastro-enteritis in Nigeria has not yet been properly classified. As already remarked there was a striking preponderance of males among these patients.

Diarrhoea is probably the commonest symptom with which a young child is brought to hospital. Most out-patients were not very ill, and could be quickly restored by simple treatment, in practice usually a kaolin mixture and an anti-malarial drug. The majority were probably in fact symptomatic diarrhoeas, and not true enteric infections. Others, of course, were suffering from protein malnutrition, and usually revealed themselves as such by their failure to improve and by other signs. True bacillary dysentery was not uncommon in out-patients and responded so well to sulphonamides that such cases seldom got into hospital.

Anaemia. The infants in this group were usually suffering from some respiratory or alimentary illness, and were discovered because of their extreme pallor. Babies with haemoglobin levels of from 10% to 40% were admitted and transfused. They did very well, spending only one night in hospital in most cases, and seldom seemed to require further replenishment. The nature of the anaemia is unsolved. Dr. R. Hendrickse has studied these Ibadan babies with particular attention, and is of the opinion that in most of them the anaemia is due to the effects of malaria. It is doubtful if it is due to haemolysis alone, and there must be an individual idiosyncrasy as these cases were random among infants in the same environment and exposed to the same risk. Their nutritional state seemed irrelevant. The anaemia was usually normochromic, and iron deficiency, although it was not excluded by serum iron levels, is probably not an important contributory agent. Most were less than 6 months old. Dr. Hendrickse found that some of them could be made to reconstitute their own haemoglobin without transfusion, if they were given anti-malarial drugs only. Combination with broncho-pneumonia was common and accounted for some of the deaths. Others died because their anaemia was too profound to be treated in time, and one or two died of the cardio-vascular effects of transfusion.

In older children the aetiology was mixed: iron deficiency, post-infective anaemia, malarial anaemia and no doubt certain cases of sickle cell anaemia, although we have tried to classify these separately. As already mentioned, protein malnutrition does not seem to be a cause of profound anaemia in this population.

No less than 53 cases of sickle cell anaemia were admitted during the year. They were fairly evenly scattered in age throughout childhood. Most of them were admitted in crisis, that is to say with a low haemoglobin, fever and a tinge of jaundice, and with pain or even swelling around the joints. The blood often showed a high leucocytosis with a high nucleated red cell count. The spleen was large and sometimes tender. The swellings around the bones were sometimes inflammatory and this was especially true of the spindle-shaped swellings of the fingers and toes from which pus due to a salmonella organism was sometimes extracted. Jaundice seemingly of an obstructive type occurred in a number of these children, most probably due to a hepatitis. The diagnosis of sickle cell anaemia was confirmed by finding in the laboratory sickling of all red cells within 24 hours, accompanied by a filamentous form of red cell distortion. More accurate diagnosis was obtained by electrophoretic identification of the haemoglobin. There was further support for the diagnosis in the skull contour and in characteristic x-ray alterations in the trabeculation of the bones, although these signs were not invariable. A family history was also helpful. In Western Nigeria the incidence of sickle cell trait is 24%, while sickle cell anaemia occurs in 0·3%. The combination of sickle cell haemoglobin and haemoglobin C occurs in 1%.

We performed Tallquist haemoglobin estimations whenever children seemed unduly pale. Much anaemia of intermediate severity was treated empirically with chloroquine and iron, and a response could be obtained in most cases. In Ilobi, Walters (1956) found haemoglobin averages of 9·2 g.% in the 0 to 1 year age-group, and of 10 to 11 g.% in the 2 to 9 year age-group.

Protein Malnutrition. Although this figured only as the fourth commonest reason for admission, it was in many ways the most important disorder that we were called upon to treat because of its high mortality and its extreme prevalence in less severe forms, and also because it is preventable. The peak period for the disturbance is between 1 and 3 years, and more than half our in-patient examples fell into this age-group. A quarter of them were between 3 and 6, and only 14 were under 1 year old. After 6 years the incidence fell away sharply. The older children showed a slightly higher death rate, and at all ages a preponderance of females was noticed and this was not explained. Protein malnutrition formed a backcloth to all the illness we treated during the year; minor evidence of it was continually noted, and it was not used as a primary diagnosis unless the disease was gross. Even among this group, accompanying diseases figured largely. Pneumonia, tuberculosis, diarrhoea, anaemia and sepsis were the most important of these.

Early manifestations of the disease were oedema of the feet, and lassitude and fretfulness with some diarrhoea. Changes in the pigmentation of the skin came next (Fig. 6), and an extension of oedema. There might be some discolouration of the hair. In bad cases there was gross generalized oedema tending to spare the serous cavities, and a typical mosaic dermatosis on the limbs.

Some other bad cases were miserably emaciated with trophic skin changes but without oedema. In every case there were the characteristic hypoproteinaemia and dietary history as confirmatory points. Persistent watery diarrhoea, common to nearly all cases, aggravated their ill-health. Anaemia, though sometimes gross, did not seem to be a constant symptom, and a haemoglobin level of about 60% was average. These were most unpredictable children to treat, many dying suddenly during the first week in hospital. There would often be no warning of this, and one would be surprised to find that a child who was apparently improving had died during the night. There was a particular tendency to die within the first 48 hours after admission, which seemed greater than could be accounted for by the fact that these children were brought to hospital only when they were in an advanced stage of the disease. Treatment consisted of a graduated introduction of high-protein milk; graduated because too early feeding with concentrated protein exaggerated the diarrhoea and worsened the condition. Nevertheless, we have wondered if the abrupt change from their native high carbohydrate diet to this thin, semi-fluid one played a part in the early death of some of these cases. Education of parents in the best use of available foods was also a vital part of treatment.

Those who did not die improved quite rapidly and had a diuresis at about the end of the first week, and there was subsequent weight gain and restoration of vigour. Many were able to go home at the end of the second week, and were followed up at a Nutrition Clinic. The importance of routine radiographs of the chest in these cases came to be recognized because many of them, even though infected with tuberculosis, failed to give a positive tuberculin reaction in their malnourished, anergic state.

Tuberculosis. Tuberculosis is the commonest reason for admission of patients to the adult medical wards, but only comes fifth in frequency in children. It is, nevertheless, a serious and important disease, as witnessed by the 113 cases who were admitted during 1956. Pulmonary primary infection was, of course, far and away the commonest manifestation, and the brunt of the severe infections fell on young children. There were 17 cases of tuberculous broncho-pneumonia and four cases of miliary tuberculosis among this group. An association with protein malnutrition was common, and the two diseases together are a serious hazard to life. Tuberculous pleural effusion does not seem to be very common, and only two in hospital (and two other out-patients) developed this complication. There were three cases of tuberculous pericarditis with effusion, and one of tuberculous polyserositis. Abdominal tuberculosis, mainly the ascitic form of peritonitis, contributed 10 cases, and one of these showed a pseudo-chylous effusion.

Meningeal tuberculosis seemed to affect a lower age-group than is customary in the United Kingdom. Half of the cases were under 1 year old. Our cases of meningitis did very badly in spite of the use of all forms of chemotherapy, and in many cases cortisone as well.

It is a clinical impression that the glandular element of the primary complex within the chest assumes larger proportions than with English children. Very considerably broadened mediastina were common, but parenchymatous infiltration in the lung was frequently inconspicuous.

Tuberculous superficial lymphadenitis did not account for many admissions, but we noticed a proneness to large axillary tuberculous buboes, apparently not due to a superficial skin focus in the affected limb; in fact many had co-existing disease in the chest. Superficial tuberculosis seems very uncommon, which is the reverse of what one would expect, seeing that so many children have skin sores, and so many adults have open tuberculosis.

In considering tuberculous bone disease one notices at once the remarkable preponderance of Pott's disease of the spine. This accounts for the majority of tuberculous bone lesions at all ages, and begins sometimes in infancy. Spinal caries admitted to hospital had nervous complications as a rule. In such cases, costo-transversectomy with evacuation of paraspinal abscesses was often performed. The prognosis for return of nervous function below the site of disease was quite good in reasonably early cases, though some paraplegia proved irreversible. The policy adopted by Mr. P. Konstam, who was in charge of the surgical management of most of them, consisted in partially immobilizing the spine in a plaster of paris jacket and then treating the child as an ambulant out-patient, unless nervous complications were present. At the same time, of course, the child received chemotherapy. The results of this regime are to be the subject of a report by Mr. Konstam, but it may be said that these simple measures have been rewarded with striking success, and that firm healing with abundant perispinal calcification is achieved in a comparatively short time. Isolated cases of tuberculous hip or knee disease were seen, but were not common.

In a seven-month period, August, 1956 to February, 1957, 253 new children were referred to the weekly tuberculosis clinic. Of these 158 were deemed to have active tuberculosis. A number of other children who were referred to a surgical tuberculosis clinic with glandular or bone lesions, have escaped this inventory. Post-primary lung lesions were present in 11. Phlyctenular conjunctivitis seems to be a common addition to the tuberculous picture, and once established the tendency to reactivation with intercurrent infections persists for a long time. A good deal of corneal damage in children is caused in this way. On the other hand erythema nodosum was seen only twice in the year. Suspicion of a false positive Heaf test was created in five cases, all in very young children in whom after considerable observation no evidence of tuberculosis infection past or present could be found. The Heaf test in each case was positive Grade I. Non-specific tuberculin reactions have been discovered as causing confusion in the Heaf testing of African children, and the subject is discussed by Henshaw (1955).

If disease of the same severity is compared, these Nigerian children with tuberculosis appeared to progress under treatment at least as well as English children. Out-patient chemotherapy was used for all cases of primary tuberculosis with symptoms. Streptomycin was reserved for the more seriously ill, so that P.A.S. and isoniazid were given to the majority. It was gratifying to see the rapid reduction in toxaemia, and the gain in weight. Conditions were such that investigation of contacts could not be carried out.

We carried out a small study of children attending the general out-patients at the Adeoyo Hospital. New cases were Heaf tested on their first attendance and the result read three days later. Results were only obtained on 350 children. The proportion of Heaf positives was as follows:

Age (years)	%
Under 1	4
1–3	14
3–6	23
Over 6	53

These were of course ailing children and a highly selected group, but the sample affords some indication of the level of primary infection in the Ibadan population.

Trauma. Burns and scalds, the most important diagnosis under this heading, made a considerable contribution to the work of the children's ward. The 47 cases in the year were evenly distributed over the ages up to 6 years; there were few after that. Most occurred around the domestic hearth, from clothing catching alight or more often from scalding fluids falling upon the children. A small group was due to a local method of reviving cases of convulsions by hot applications to the feet. Management of burns in the open ward might be expected to lead to serious cross-infection, but in fact this was not so. They were treated by the open exposure method and early skin grafting was carried out where necessary. The incidence of complications was surprisingly low, undoubtedly lower than it would be in an open ward in the United Kingdom. In part this may be due to the rarity of the streptococcus. Blood transfusions were necessary for many of these children, and all of them were nursed under mosquito netting to keep off flies. Four died, a mortality of 8%. Some remained in hospital for relatively long periods of six to eight weeks.

Other Alimentary Disorders. Between 1 and 6 years of age many Ibadan children suffered from cancrum oris. The disease starts as a marginal gingivitis with bleeding gums, after which infection encroaches upon the bony alveolus. A destructive osteomyelitis of the jaw begins and the infection then spreads outwards from this area to contiguous soft tissues, which are eroded. Within a matter of a few weeks there may be a large necrotic area which continues to extend until checked by treatment. The process responds very sensitively to penicillin and extension ceases as soon as this treatment is begun. Nevertheless, a long time is necessary for separation of the dead tissues, which may include a large bony sequestrum, as well as soft tissues sometimes composing the whole thickness of the lip or cheek. Great deformity arises therefore in some children who have been treated for severe cancrum oris, and the plastic repair of this is formidable. Most of the children with cancrum are in a state of reduced nutrition and may be anaemic, but the process itself does not seem to cause much, if any, general illness. In out-patients many children are seen with the premonitory symptoms of cancrum oris, namely bleeding gums, foetor oris and marginal gingivitis, and these symptoms can be brought to an end quickly with a few procaine penicillin injections.

A common surgical condition is intussusception, which in Nigeria mainly affects boys aged from 3 to 10 years. The symptoms are those of subacute intestinal obstruction and it is readily diagnosed and corrected.

Among other conditions that call for comment were five cases of Hirschsprung's disease. This disorder is evidently one that must be taken account of in Nigeria. On the other hand congenital intestinal atresia was only seen twice. Several cases of partial aplasia of the abdominal musculature, without renal abnormality, were seen and may be related in cause to exomphalos, which was observed to be one of the commoner congenital malformations, and to umbilical hernia which is very prevalent indeed. During the year, there was only one case of appendicitis in a child and no case of congenital pyloric stenosis.

Tetanus. Tetanus was the third greatest cause of death in children in this hospital series. In the adult medical wards this disease is the chief cause of death by a considerable margin. Neonatal tetanus comprised two thirds of our total cases. A very large number of infants born in hospital go home within a few hours, and are therefore submitted to the same methods of cord dressing during the early days of life as befalls those born at home. Nevertheless none of our babies with tetanus were born in hospital, and this suggests that liability to this disease depends upon the way in which the cord is severed at birth, and not upon the applications subsequently used. The mortality in newborn babies with tetanus was 77%. Mortality rates are closely related to the day of life on which the first symptoms develop (Fig. 7).

Various regimes of treatment for the newborn were tried through the year, some elaborate, some fairly simple. We still seek a simple routine of universal application which does not require exacting nursing or vigilant medical observation. Most of the deaths occurred after the first few days, the infant entering upon a cold, inanimate, oedematous state with shallow respirations. Another mode of dying occurred during the third week, with a high swinging temperature and finally hyperpyrexia.

Only a quarter of older children with tetanus died, and the risk of death became progressively less with increasing age, up to adolescence. It was often difficult to decide upon the site of entry of the tetanus organism. Chronic otorrhoea was several times suspected to have given access to tetanus.

Active immunization of the population has not been started. Anti-tetanic serum is used routinely in out-patients for wounds and abrasions. We saw a death in a child from anaphylaxis after this.

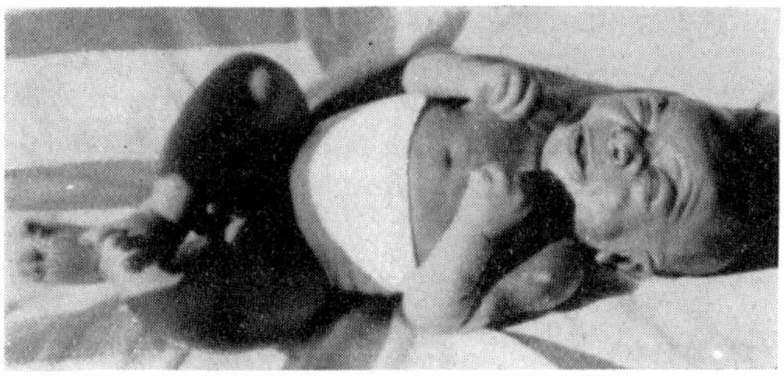

FIG. 7.—Neonatal tetanus.

Other Respiratory Disease. Retropharyngeal abscess was a condition of which we had to be continually mindful; there were seven cases in the year. Another interesting entity was a hyper-acute pharyngitis with a plentiful soft yellow exudate, grave toxaemia and pronounced cervical adenitis with neck swelling. Although these cases (of which we had three, all of whom died) so closely resembled diphtheria, this organism was not isolated from any, nor in fact was any organism incriminated. In one, exudate appeared to involve the larynx and a tracheotomy was performed with temporary relief.

The common cold and upper respiratory disease generally (with the exception of otorrhoea) were not much of a problem. Chronic nasopharyngitis in children, so familiar in England, was practically never seen. Sinusitis was rare. The brunt of the widespread respiratory catarrhs fell upon the bronchi and lungs.

Both acute otitis media and otitis externa are common among Ibadan children of all ages. Recurrent otorrhoea with chronic perforation of the drums is one of the more frequent reasons for attendance. The discharge can be suppressed in most cases by a week of procaine penicillin, to obtain which they come to out-patients. There were many cases also of acute laryngitis, and tracheotomy cases were a commonplace. Chronic respiratory illnesses, whether asthma, bronchiectasis or fibrotic lung were scarce.

Protozoal and Helminth Infections. The incidence of malarial parasitaemia in random samples of the population is fairly accurately known in this area; for example Walters (1956) found in Ilobi the following percentage of malarial parasitaemia:

Age (years)	%
0–1	50
2–4	76
5–9	76

P. falciparum was far the commonest, and a mixture of *P. malariae* and *P. falciparum* next. Occasional *P. ovale* infections were seen. The adult parasite rate was approximately 30%. In Ibadan school children, Garlick (1956) found in the age group 5 to 7 years, 84% parasitaemia (77% *falciparum*, 20% *quartan* and 3% *ovale*; the number of mixed infections was considerable). In out-patient work with children, malaria is very common and heavy parasite densities even in infants were frequently discovered. Infection was quickly overcome with treatment. Patients ill from other causes often also developed malaria and one had to be ready to accept a sudden temperature as an indication for anti-malarial treatment in children in and out of hospital.

Though it is clearly desirable, it was not found possible in 1956 routinely to stain blood films of all children with fever on admission to hospital. It follows therefore that a majority of the cases classed here as malaria were clinical, or presumed, and this presumption was based on a rapid subsidence of symptoms after anti-malarial treatment. A common story was fever and convulsions of sudden onset in a young child, who was semi-comatose and collapsed when admitted. Response to chloroquine was dramatic and consolidated the clinical diagnosis. Although an initial convulsion is common with a malarial infection, true cerebral malaria in a child was not proved to my satisfaction in any case.

Amoebic dysentery was not very common among Ibadan children, but, when present, was usually the cause of severe illness. There were in fact seven deaths in 16 cases. There were only two cases of amoebic hepatitis.

Ascaris infestation is almost universal and seems to cause very few symptoms unless the child is unfortunate enough to become obstructed by a mass of worms in the intestine. This happened twice in this series and both children required laparotomy and worm removal. Whether the abdominal pain that is a common complaint in out-patients is ever related to ascaris infection is debatable. There seems little point in eradicating average worm infestations because of the certainty of return within a short time in this environment. Stool examinations were made on only a few in-patients, and neither there nor in routine reports on out-patients were the ova of hookworm (unlike round and whip-worm) frequently mentioned. This infestation does not appear to be a significant factor in the common anaemias of Ibadan children. Guinea worm is common but there is no effective hospital treatment. For this reason perhaps, fresh cases of guinea worm were not often seen, but late effects, such as abscess formation, sterile cystic collections around the track of the worm, cheloid scarring and sometimes radiographic demonstration of calcified guinea worms were noted many times.

Unexplained and Unclassified Illness. The frequency of obscure and fatal illness is one of the most tantalizing aspects of tropical paediatric practice. Fever with repeated convulsions and ensuing coma was a particularly familiar grouping of fatal symptoms. Such cases, if they did not rapidly respond to anti-malarial drugs, had a bad prognosis. Meningitis was excluded in all of them. In a number necropsies were performed without finding a cause for death. The picture was clinically that of acute encephalitis. More than half these cases died.

Infections of Skin, Lymph Glands and Subcutaneous Tissues. Superficial septic infections were a very important cause of morbidity in children. Of this group of 64 hospital in-patients, one third were newborn infants. In these the complications of umbilical sepsis were the main trouble. It can be truly said that trivial umbilical infections were not often seen, but that dangerous infections were not infrequent. Cellulitis spreading from the navel, and sometimes extending into the pelvic tissues, occurred 11 times and tended to be fatal. *E. coli* was the usual pathogen. Another form of cellulitis that was seen in babies affected the scalp, spreading with alarming rapidity to produce islands of necrosis of the whole thickness of the scalp, leaving large raw areas to be repaired.

At all ages, these children are very subject to multiple subcutaneous abscesses. So-called acute pyomyositis, from which a bacterial causative agent can rarely be recovered, was seen only once; it is a condition mainly confined to young adults. There were two cases of a curious low-grade retro-orbital cellulitis which were not satisfactorily explained or treated. A suppurative lymphadenitis of the iliac glands was a disabling and not unusual condition.

Staphylococcus pyogenes was responsible for the great majority of these septic conditions. Among in-patients it was found in 1956 that 60% of the staphylococci in the Adeoyo Hospital were resistant to penicillin, and among out-patients 35%. About a quarter of in-patients and one seventh of out-patients, moreover, were infected with aureomycin-resistant strains of staphylococcus.

In out-patients, skin sepsis of all kinds accounted for as many attendances as any other condition. Furunculosis about the head and shoulders, to which infants seem especially susceptible, impetigo, pemphigus, cellulitis and abscesses of all kinds were commonplace. Fortunately the *in vivo* response to penicillin seemed better than would be expected from the laboratory figures for drug sensitivity, and most skin sepsis could still be controlled quickly by a daily injection of procaine penicillin for three to four days, supplemented where necessary by incision. Among older children, tropical ulcers around the ankles (Fig. 8), with moist red bases and exuberant edges, were very common, and although no specific organism was isolated, the response to penicillin and eusol dressings was favourable and rapid.

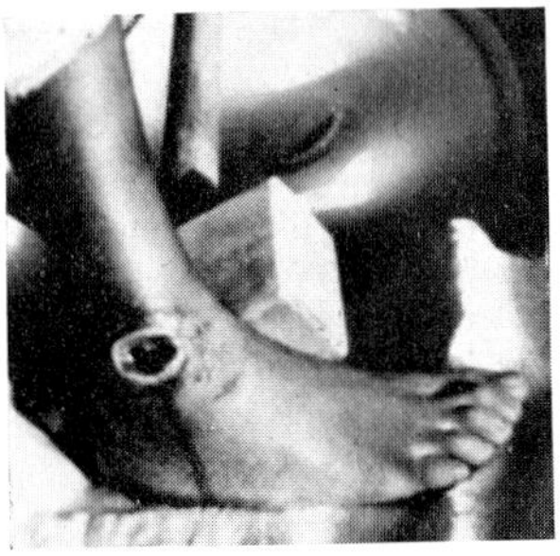

FIG. 8.—Tropical ulceration.

Other Acute Specific Infections. Organisms of the *Salmonella* genus appear to be widespread in the

Ibadan area, and can be recovered from a number of domestic animals and from lizards. We encountered infections at all ages in childhood. Clinical presentations varied from very subacute to the most severe illnesses. There were seven proven cases of infection by *B. typhosus*, and three of these died. *Salmonella* was recovered from certain cases of septicaemia in infancy, at which stage it is one cause of infective jaundice of the newborn.

Possibly the most interesting group were those five cases (all of whom were under 18 months old) who had a salmonella osteitis. Other examples were seen among out-patients. This is a lesion almost confined to young children with sickle cell anaemia. The bones chiefly affected were the small ones of hands and feet; in two the scapula was involved. A feature of this osteitis was its quiet presentation, and the absence of any systemic illness. The disorder appeared to be self-limiting and recovery complete. A typical x-ray picture in which osteolysis predominates can probably be recognized. This association has been reported before in the Belgian Congo, in Jamaica and in the United States, *vide* Golding (1956).

Whooping cough was the only one of the common infectious diseases of English children that proved at all common in Ibadan during 1956. Those admitted nearly all had broncho-pneumonia and ran a long course; they were mainly infants. Several infants severely ill with whooping cough developed an encephalopathy which was usually fatal. Such a child would have convulsions, with steadily diminishing awareness and a progressive rigidity of the limbs. The cerebrospinal fluid was normal. Two points were helpful in out-patient diagnosis of whooping cough. First, a tendency to a more generalized oedema than is usual in English children with a paroxysmal cough. Secondly, a tendency to haemoptysis, presumably due to rupture of pharyngeal veins. This was a common reason for bringing a child to hospital, and was almost diagnostic of whooping cough. Cases of secondary yaws were occasionally seen in out-patients, but positive Wassermann reactions were present in only 0·8% of the age group 5 to 9 years, contrasted with 8% in a group of adult males. No case of clinical syphilis was identified.

Diseases of Nervous System. Bizarre syndromes suggesting acute encephalitis were frequent. One, of sudden onset, occurred in epidemic form (see Wright and Morley, 1958). Children with this syndrome were afebrile, and, though rather somnolent, mentally clear. Wild alternating horizontal movements of the eyes occurred spontaneously, as well as violent agitation of the trunk and limbs on attempting to sit up, or even to raise a leg or arm. There was no disturbance of the C.S.F., and fortunately all the cases recovered in the space of a few days and were left with no immediate sequels.

There were other cases who came in with convulsions and remained unconscious with various pyramidal signs, and in some but not all there was a pleocytosis in the cerebrospinal fluid.

A most interesting group comprised seven children with roughly similar symptoms, in whom there was a sudden onset of hypotonia and weakness of a part of the skeletal musculature. Tendon reflexes were preserved or exaggerated. Flaccidity was so profound that in a bad case the child could not even sit up or hold the head steady. In some there was elevation of cell count or protein level in the cerebrospinal fluid. There were no sensory changes, and these children tended to recover but might relapse. The picture was complicated, however, by the fact that hemiplegia occurred in at least one of them and was permanent, while in others flaccid palsy of one or more limbs persisted. One of these children died of respiratory failure. A number of children were observed who had the permanent residua of illnesses that sounded like encephalitis. Some had convulsions, some mental backwardness, as well as a group with parkinsonism and other basal ganglionic disorders, including oculogyric crises, suggesting a kinship with encephalitis lethargica. The label 'acute poliomyelitis' must be used with caution, but we saw some children who developed flaccid palsies of a number of muscle groups in the limbs during a febrile illness with a mixed pleocytosis in the cerebrospinal fluid, and in some out-patients an isolated flaccid palsy of the limbs of abrupt onset underwent the same sequence of gradual but often incomplete recovery that we are familiar with in poliomyelitis.

It is difficult to say if mental deficiency of primary type is more or less common than in Britain. There are certainly many examples. During the year about 10 mongols were seen. Much mental deficiency is acquired after inflammatory processes in the nervous system, and we diagnosed one defective child on clinical grounds as a case of toxoplasmosis. Two cases of microcephaly were seen. I did not see a cretin during the year. A number of cases of primary cerebral agenesis with palsy were also seen.

Recurrent convulsions in children are not a reason for bringing them to out-patients in Ibadan; in Britain such cases form an important part of clinic work.

Diseases of Genito-Urinary System. Nephrosis is one of the big clinical problems among Ibadan children but it is not encountered much in adults. Such cases present as a Type 2 nephritis, with proteinuria and oedema, without cell deposit in the urine, nor any nitrogen retention. Some of them go on to develop hypertension and azotaemia in a year or more. Some seem to remit quickly and spontaneously, and it was my impression that these remissions were assisted by using penicillin in the first stages. The prognosis for recovery may be better than in British children and several returned as far as can be judged to normal, without residual proteinuria, within a year. A large number continue to run a fluctuating course in out-patients, and their eventual fate remains to be seen. There is nothing in the preceding history of these children that appears to account for the onset of nephrosis. A few start as young as 2 years, but most have been between 3 and 6. Whether the reputed association between quartan malaria and nephritis has any relevance is a matter worth investigating. The infection rate among this group of oedematous children was very low, which contrasts with their susceptibility to pneumococcal infections in Great Britain. Type 1 nephritis, though encountered, was unusual.

Diseases of Bones and Joints. Acute osteomyelitis in young children was very common. A multifocal infection involving simultaneously many bones in several limbs, usually without much systematic upset except some fever, was a frequent and interesting condition. Sometimes there was an associated septic arthritis, or subcutaneous abscesses. The staphylococcus accounted for the majority, but as already mentioned, *Salmonella* was a common pathogen when the child also suffered from sickle cell anaemia. Radiographic changes were early and gross. The mandible was sometimes involved, and the ribs, but predominantly the limb bones. The fairly benign course is reflected in the single death out of 26 cases. Nevertheless, it was often weeks before pus ceased to form at the site of bony swelling, and several patients ran through a wide range of antibiotics before recovery. With the exception of occasional sequestrectomy, surgical measures were seldom necessary; even where sinuses formed, eventual healing occurred. Amyloid disease was not seen in any child during the year.

Acute septic arthritis affected children under 3 years of age. Very often it was an extension of a neighbouring osteomyelitis, but sometimes the joint involvement was primary and the process was then frequently multiple. Surprisingly, intense pain was rarely present and again we were struck by the comparative absence of constitutional illness. These children did well after aspiration of pus from the joints and appropriate chemotherapy; most of them too were infected with the staphylococcus.

Purulent Meningitis. There were 36 cases of acute meningitis and a causative organism was not identified in 15 of them. Preliminary out-patient treatment with penicillin or a sulphonamide may have been sometimes given, but even so the failure rate seems surprisingly high. Of those we did identify, eight were due to *Haemophilus* (seven of these under 1 year old), and another eight to *Pneumococcus* (six of whom were infants). Two infants died of *E. coli* meningitis. In the whole series there was only one meningococcal infection, but possibly this organism was one of those that failed to grow in culture. However, it is well-known that meningococcal meningitis is a scourge in the drier northern parts of Nigeria, and is much less prevalent in the South. With 13 deaths, we cannot be very proud of our results. Many of the cases were advanced when we got them. There was one case of *Ps. pyocyanea* meningitis, and one due to *Haemophilus bronchisepticus*.

Tumours. This group differed little from what might be encountered in a British children's hospital. The strawberry naevus, so common in British babies, was not seen during the year. There were examples of nasopharyngeal lymphosarcoma and bilateral ovarian carcinomata, both of which seem to be of relatively high incidence around Ibadan.

Other Nutritional and Deficiency Diseases. A large number of our patients were chronically underfed. It was only where the resulting emaciation was of such a degree as to require urgent admission to hospital that they appear in this analysis. There were 18 such cases. Very often the mother was herself in poor condition and attempting to feed twins. If she believes that her breast milk is insufficient a very watery maize pap is provided as a supplement, and on this it would be difficult to gain weight. As important as deficiency in food is deficiency of water, and many of these malnourished babies were dehydrated; another reason for their admission. Some marasmic infants, with no other cause than underfeeding, would weigh no more than 7 or 8 lb. at a year old. Vomiting from underfeeding does not seem to happen as in Britain. In fact, vomiting in babies, whether with gastro-enteritis, feeding difficulties or parenteral infections, was strikingly infrequent.

Of the vitamin deficiencies, only two were recognized. These were rickets and riboflavin deficiency. The latter was seen as soreness of the tongue with angular stomatitis. Rickets is not very uncommon in Ibadan children, as Jelliffe (1955) has previously pointed out. Most cases were picked up in infants of about 3 months old. A number of these had been premature, and others shielded from the light as for example by their mothers being in purdah. The main pathogenesis, in fact, was prematurity with overclothing. Some florid examples were seen, but easily corrected with calcium and vitamin D.

Cardiac and Circulatory Disease. No case of acute rheumatism was recognized in 1956. Congenital heart disorders were probably encountered less frequently than in a comparable child population in the United Kingdom. For example, no severely handicapped heart case was seen among the 6,000 hospital births in the year. There were seven cases of what we have termed 'cardiomegaly with heart failure'. Broadly speaking, there are two varieties of this obscure malady, which is common among both children and adults in the locality. The first group consists of rather quiet hearts that are generally enlarged and that present first with congestive failure. There are few or no murmurs and the failure can be compensated after rest in bed and the use of digitalis, but the life of the child is subsequently very precarious and his exercise tolerance severely restricted. Follow-up is not long enough to establish how long these children live after this sequence has taken place. In the other group the hearts are also large, but there is a severe lesion of the mitral valve which is always incompetent and sometimes stenosed. Invariably there are signs of pulmonary hypertension. Some of these too, have been in failure, but others have come to light only when the children were examined for other disorders. That this is an acquired disorder is virtually certain. Nearly all are upwards of 3 years old. There was nothing suggestive of acute rheumatism in these children, who were afebrile, not anaemic, not ill, and younger at onset than is the case with European acute rheumatism. One died in what appeared to be an exacerbation of a chronic cardiopathy, and at necropsy some pericarditis was found, besides endomyocardial fibrosis with thickening and distortion of the mitral valve and the adjacent endocardium. Both the clinical and post-mortem appearances are precisely those of endomyocardial fibrosis as first described by Bedford and Konstam (1946) and in more detail by Williams, Ball and Davies (1954) in East Africa. This is the commonest form of heart disease of young people in tropical Africa. Its aetiology is still quite obscure. Certain other cases of this disorder were seen and followed in out-patients. There is little that one can do to help, though it is of course important to map the natural history of this disease in childhood, but we did get the impression that digitalis was useful for some of the patients who were on the brink of congestive failure.

Neonatal Diseases. Seven infants, all aged less than a week, were admitted with a very deep jaundice and two of these died. The local causes of neonatal jaundice have not been elucidated. Some babies, I think, were merely suffering from physiological jaundice aggravated by an inadequate fluid intake. Others may have been cases of infectious jaundice such as are recorded elsewhere in this analysis. Although we made some attempt to exclude haemolytic disease of the newborn by Coomb's tests and never discovered it, one cannot be sure that there were not examples of this disease among our infants. The very high level of rhesus-positive blood groups among this population makes the chance of rhesus incompatibility between mother and child much lower than in Britain.

Immaturity at birth is a great addition to the many physical dangers attending the growth of an African child. Premature birth is nevertheless a very frequent event in Africa. During the year under review 169 infants (not included in the table of admissions) were reared in a premature nursery attached to the Maternity Department. All of these weighed under 2,000 g. ($4\frac{1}{2}$ lb.) at birth, and comprised about one half of all infants born in hospital in this weight category. (Of the 6,000 annual births in hospital some 850 were under 5 lb. birth weight.) Two thirds of these premature births were twin births (the incidence of twinning is $4 \cdot 2\%$ of all births). It may be said that in the early weeks by using the simplest methods it is possible to obtain in Africa survival rates nearly as gratifying, weight for weight, as in Europe or America. The figures are improved because the gestation period of an African baby of given birth weight has usually been longer than that of the European. Most were spontaneous premature deliveries. There was a lessened risk of death within the first 48 hours of life by comparison with European figures, possibly accounted for by the infrequency of lethal congenital malformation, of haemolytic disease of the newborn, of the alveolar membrane syndrome and of severe chilling after birth. In spite of a congested nursery and a rapid turnover, sepsis occurred in only 14% of babies; it was mainly as in Britain of skin and eyes. In spite of the tropical climate the temperature of small babies tended to fall, and sclerema neonatorum was several times encountered; chilling was a more frequent event than overheating. We are unfortunately almost totally ignorant of the later career of these babies after leaving hospital.

Diseases of Liver. Cirrhosis of the liver, though an important entity in adult practice in Ibadan, was unusual in children, and there are only four examples in the series. If protein malnutrition had this sequel we would be certain to see more cases in older children.

Diseases of Eyes. Corneal ulceration is not a condition that finds its way into hospital very much, which accounts for the fact that we only list four cases here. Corneal ulcers, however, are a big factor in the morbidity of children in this area, and they happen not infrequently during infectious illnesses, especially if the child's nutrition is reduced. It is distressing to see how many children in the streets have corneal nebulae, and of course in the northern provinces of Nigeria trachoma adds to the high incidence of blindness in West African young people. Phlyctenular conjunctivitis may go on to ulceration, and corneal opacities also derive from this. The sequel to corneal ulcer is only too often perforation and shrinkage of the eye and blindness.

Poisoning and Idiosycrasy to Drugs. Very few cases of poisoning came into hospital. Kerosene came first as an agent with three victims, and then accidentally-swallowed caustic alkali. There was another group who were said to be suffering from 'native medicine poisoning'. Undoubtedly a large number of our children, especially those who had had convulsions, smelt strongly of an ammoniacal mixture containing urine, which is used in Ibadan as a medicine. Just how important this is in producing symptoms I am not sure. Some of these children, certainly, remained limp and unconscious and died. Others, however, smelling no less strongly and appearing no less ill, recovered and it is my feeling that the native medicine really plays a rather insignificant role. Further south, nicotine and other alkaloids are employed in native medicines, and potent agents may sometimes be given to children here, but the onus of proof that these neurological symptoms are a result of attempted treatment rather than of the disease itself still rests with the exponents of this idea.

Final Remarks

Certain conditions commonly met with in European practice were encountered too seldom to figure as important. Examples are streptococcal infections and their complications, asthma and kindred psychosomatic disorders, the collagen disorders and some others already referred to. Certain congenital defects were less common than in England, and no case of congenital pyloric stenosis was seen during the year. Nevertheless, the above account demonstrates that we were not confronted in Nigeria with a continuous parade of children suffering from tropical disease in the generally understood sense, nor was the common paediatric currency of England by any means superseded. Though it was true that more than one pathological condition was often present in our young patients it was seldom difficult to disentangle them, or to determine which was dominant in a given clinical situation. In this respect tropical practice among children is less confusing perhaps than among adults, in whom long-standing processes tend to blur the clinical outline of disease.

When the range of normal in all the territories of clinical and laboratory medicine is as yet unmapped and prevailing methods of treatment for many disorders are so discouraging, a great need exists for the collection of data and for clinical research. The teaching of medical students demands an imaginative adaptation of European techniques to fit the widely different local situation. Besides all this, there is the insistent tumultuous pressure of patients, who by their very numbers have power to submerge the medical staff beneath a horizonless sea of routine. Here is opportunity indeed for those with vision and talent, and many will be needed if standards of paediatrics throughout tropical Africa are to be enabled quickly to rise.

References

Bedford, D. E. and Konstam, G. L. S. (1946). *Brit. Heart J.*, **8**, 236.
British Medical Journal (1956). Editorial. *Brit. med. J.*, **1**, 390.
Garlick, J. (1956). Personal communication.
Golding, J. S. R. (1956). *Ann. roy. Coll. Surg. Engl.*, **19**, 296.
Henshaw, J. E. (1955). *West Afr. med. J.*, **4**, 175.
Jelliffe, D. B. (1955). *Infant Nutrition in the Subtropics and Tropics.* W.H.O. Monograph Series, No. 29. Geneva.
Omololu, O. (1956). *J. Univ. Coll. Hosp. (Ibadan)*, No. 2.
Walters, J. H. (1956). Personal communication.
Williams, A. W., Ball, J. D. and Davies, J. N. P. (1954). *Trans. roy. Soc. trop. Med. Hyg.*, **48**, 290.
Wright, J. and Morley, D. C. (1958). *Lancet*, **1**, 871.

PHLYCTENULAR CONJUNCTIVITIS IN AFRICAN CHILDREN

BY

HARRY STEIN and IDA FREIMAN

From the Baragwanath Hospital, Johannesburg

(RECEIVED FOR PUBLICATION DECEMBER 12, 1957)

Phlyctenular conjunctivitis is a focal inflammatory disease of the conjunctiva characterized by a rounded translucent nodule surrounded by a zone of hyperaemia. The nodule may be single or multiple and is situated on the conjunctiva, close to the corneal limbus. Histologically it is an aggregation of large numbers of lymphocytes and occasional polymorphonuclear cells. Secondary infection, photophobia, blepharospasm and lacrimation are features of this condition.

Phlyctenular conjunctivitis is relatively rare among Europeans, but is still common in non-European communities. In 1947 an American Medical Association investigation committee (Barnett, Fields, Milles, Silverstein and Bernstein, 1947) reported that 20% to 50% of children in Alaskan native villages had corneal scars, due to healed phlyctenulosis. Thygeson (1951) noticed a very high incidence of this condition among Apache Indians of Arizona during the years 1934 to 1938 and among the Negro and Puerto Rican children of New York City before World War II.

At Baragwanath Hospital where we deal with an African urban community living under poor hygienic circumstances we see active phlyctenulosis among the children quite commonly. At the Children's Outpatient Department which is attended by children up to 9 years of age, and where the total yearly attendance of new cases is 40,000, 36 active cases of this condition were seen in a 12-month period. We were particularly interested in elucidating the relationship of these cases to tuberculosis which is rife in the community.

The Present Study

This study was done retrospectively and is based on the records of all cases of active phlyctenular conjunctivitis seen at the Children's Outpatient Department in the 12 months from November, 1955, to October, 1956. There were 36 in all.

The age range among our 36 cases was 1 to 9 years, the majority of them being 4 to 8 years old. A slight preponderance of females, 19, to males, 17, was noted, and there appeared to be no month or season in which the cases presented predominantly. The standard of nutrition was average for urban African children in Johannesburg, except for one child who was so malnourished that he was specifically admitted for this.

All of the 36 cases had radiographs of the chest taken. Unfortunately, due to a fear of the excessively strong allergic reactions to tuberculin which have occurred from time to time in this condition, only 17 of the 36 were tested for tuberculin sensitivity, using the tuberculin jelly patch test. Of these 17 cases 15 showed positive reactions, three of which were severe with blistering and tissue necrosis, and two were negative. The radiological survey showed 22 cases with definite evidence of active or healed tuberculosis and of these, five cases had calcified tuberculous lesions (Fig. 1a and b). Fourteen cases had completely normal chest radiographs. One case had associated erythema nodosum and another case had a tuberculide rash.

Discussion

Price (1948) states that the majority of cases of phlyctenular conjunctivitis occur within the first 5 years of life. In Sorsby's (1942) series the age of maximum liability was from 4 to 10 years. Thygeson's cases occurred most commonly between the ages of 8 to 15 years. Our cases occurred predominantly between 4 and 8 years.

Both Sorsby and Thygeson state that the condition is more common in females. In our cases there was only a slight predominance of females over males. Sorsby noted that this condition presented more commonly in Spring; in our cases there appeared to be no seasonal variation.

Malnutrition, focal sepsis, pediculosis and worm infestation have all been incriminated as aetiological agents from time to time. The findings in this series do not support these views. Thygeson states that phlyctenulosis is most frequent in children from the lower economic strata of society whose diet is most likely to be deficient. Our cases all occurred in a predominantly malnourished society, but only one was severely malnourished, the nutrition of the others varying within the average range.

Most writers stress the aetiological importance of tuberculosis, although there is considerable disagreement about the specific phase of tuberculosis with which it is associated.

Sheldon (1955) states that phlyctenular conjunctivitis and erythema nodosum are benign allergic manifestations of primary tubercle occurring at the time of Mantoux conversion and that their presence indicates early tuberculosis. Holt and McIntosh (1940) state that phlyctenular conjunctivitis may occur at the height of the initial tuberculous infection but that it is more common later and shows a tendency to recurrence and chronicity; they also state that it is invariably a manifestation of tuberculosis and is accompanied by a high degree of allergy. Lightwood and Court (1953) claim that, although there is clearly a relationship between tuberculosis and phlyctenular conjunctivitis, the oft-repeated statement that phlyctenulosis is strictly analogous to erythema nodosum is not true and its onset bears no fixed relationship to the emergence of primary tuberculous allergy; they feel that it is best considered as a response to sensitization by several allergens of which in Great Britain tuberculosis is the most important. Ellis (1956) states that as in the case of erythema nodosum, phlyctenular conjunctivitis is regarded as an allergic manifestation for which tuberculous infection elsewhere in the body is responsible in more than 75% of cases. Whilst non-tuberculous cases may occur and while there appears to be some relationship with malnutrition, it should always be assumed that tuberculosis is an aetiological factor until investigation has proved otherwise.

When Fritz and Thygeson (1951) investigated phlyctenular conjunctivitis in Alaskan Indians and Eskimos they found that all cases of active phlyctenulosis had positive tuberculin reactions, while radiographic evidence of active or inactive pulmonary tuberculosis in a comparative study of two Alaskan villages showed a parallel between the prevalence of tuberculosis and phlyctenular conjunctivitis.

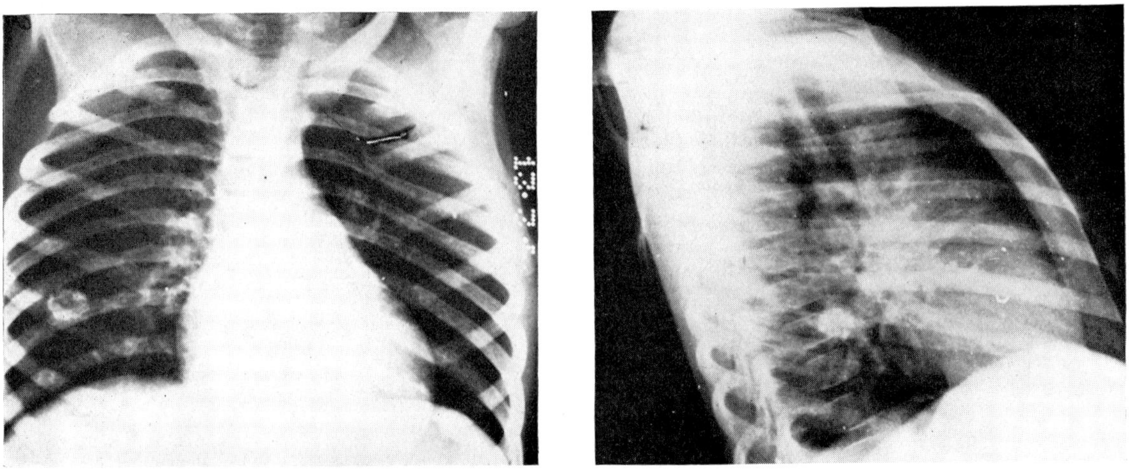

(*a*) *Posterior-anterior view.* (*b*) *Lateral view.*

FIG. 1 (*a*) and (*b*).—Chest radiographs showing calcified primary focus in lungs of patient with phlyctenular conjunctivitis.

Sorsby (1942) writing on phlyctenular conjunctivitis in children and adolescents in England, found that in 592 cases 84·8% were tuberculin positive, as against 15·3% in 900 control cases, and that of 510 cases examined radiologically 72·2% showed evidence of pulmonary tubercle as against 16·1% positive radiographs in 87 controls. The same author investigating the family history of tuberculosis found an incidence of 28·9% in 263 school children with phlyctenular conjunctivitis as opposed to an incidence in the normal school population of 3·7%. The expectation of subsequent overt tuberculosis was statistically higher in the phlyctenular conjunctivitis group.

Damato (1951) reports the cases of 11 children in

Malta who developed phlyctenular conjunctivitis two to six weeks after BCG vaccination and he concludes that this is evidence that phlyctenular conjunctivitis is due to sensitization with tuberculoprotein. He also attributes the lowered general incidence of phlyctenulosis in Malta in recent years to the lowered incidence of tuberculosis brought about by BCG innoculation.

Fritz and Thygeson (1951) consider that phlyctenular conjunctivitis in well-developed tuberculosis may be due either to activation of an already existing focus of tuberculosis which liberates antigenic products into the blood stream or to non-specific vasodilatation caused by secondary bacterial infections of the eye bringing circulating tuberculous antigens to the conjunctivae. They have repeatedly observed the effect of epidemic Koch-Weeks bacillus and pneumococcal conjunctivitis in exciting acute attacks of phlyctenular conjunctivitis in susceptible children.

Our series of cases appears to confirm the view that phlyctenular conjunctivitis is commonly associated with tuberculosis. An interesting finding was that of associated long-standing tuberculous infection as evidenced by calcified lung lesions in five patients. As far as we could determine all the patients were suffering from phlyctenular conjunctivitis for the first time since there was no evidence of old scarring. This suggests that although there is a link between phlyctenular conjunctivitis and tuberculosis, the condition is not necessarily associated with the early hyper-allergic phase of tuberculosis occurring at the time of Mantoux conversion, i.e. approximately six weeks after the initial infection. We feel that this supports the view that phlyctenulosis is not analogous to erythema nodosum and that its appearance bears no fixed relationship to the onset of primary tuberculous allergy.

We wish to thank Dr. E. Kahn (Senior Paediatrician) and Dr. S. Wayburne (Paediatrician) for help in the preparation of this paper, and the Medical Superintendent of Baragwanath Hospital for permission to publish these records. We would also like to thank Dr. M. H. Shnier for the photographs.

REFERENCES

Barnett, H. E., Fields, J., Milles, G., Silverstein, J. and Bernstein, A. (1947). *J. Amer. med. Ass.*, **135**, 500.
Damato, F. J. (1951). *Brit. J. Ophthal.*, **35**, 416.
Ellis, R. W. B. (1956). *Diseases in Infancy and Childhood*, 2nd ed., p. 532. Edinburgh.
Fritz, M. H. and Thygeson, P. (1951). *Publ. Hlth Rep. (Wash.)*, **66**, 934.
Holt, L. E. and McIntosh, R. (1940). *Holt's Diseases of Infancy and Childhood*, 11th ed., p. 333. New York.
Lightwood, R. and Court, D. (1953). In Garrod, Batten and Thursfield's *Diseases of Children*, 5th ed., Vol. 1, p. 804. Edited by A. Moncrieff and P. Evans. London.
Price, D. S. (1948). *Tuberculosis in Childhood*, 2nd ed., p. 186. Bristol.
Sheldon, W. (1955). *Diseases of Infancy and Childhood*, 7th ed., p. 402. London.
Sorsby, A. (1942). *Brit. J. Ophthal.*, **26**, 159.
Thygeson, P. (1951). *Amer. J. Ophthal.* **34**, 1217.

HORMONE EXCRETION IN PRECOCIOUS PUBERTY IN GIRLS

BY

R. D. BULBROOK, F. C. GREENWOOD and A. H. SNAITH

From the Imperial Cancer Research Fund Laboratories, Lincoln's Inn Fields and The Hospital for Sick Children, Great Ormond Street, London

(RECEIVED FOR PUBLICATION JANUARY 29, 1958)

At puberty in girls the sex hormones are secreted in increasing quantities and the clinical signs of puberty follow. In precocious puberty it is generally accepted that the excretion of these hormones will reach adolescent or adult levels but will not be abnormally high as it may be in tumour or hyperplasia of the gonad or the adrenal cortex. Published reports vary depending on the laboratory investigations carried out, and also from case to case (Fischer, 1940; Novak, 1944; Hain, 1947; Seckel, Scott and Benditt, 1949; Lloyd, Lobotsky and Morley, 1950; Lowrey and Brown, 1951; Mossberg, 1951; Paschkis, 1952; Lloyd, 1955). In general, the 17-ketosteroids tend to be a little higher than normal for the chronological age but they rarely reach more than the lower limits of adult levels and may be quite normal. Gonadotrophin determinations are usually positive, but were negative in the cases described by Gross (1940) and by Bronstein, Luhan and Mavrelis (1942). Oestrogen excretion has been measured by biological methods. The results are difficult to evaluate but on the whole oestrogen excretion tends to be low.

The chemical method recently developed by Brown (1955*a*) has made possible the separate estimation of oestrone, oestradiol-17β and oestriol in human urine. This study was therefore undertaken to assess the clinical value of simultaneous estimations of urinary oestrogens, 17-ketosteroids and gonadotrophins in 11 cases of early or precocious puberty. Vaginal smears were also examined. Hormone estimations were carried out on a control series of 15 normal girls in the age range 3 to 10 years.

Methods

Oestrogens. Brown's method (1955*a*) was used to determine the amount of oestrone, oestradiol-17β and oestriol in urine. The accuracy, precision, sensitivity and specificity of this method have been described (Brown, Bulbrook and Greenwood, 1957). The lower limit for the method has been approximated to be 1·0 μg./24 hours for oestrone and oestradiol and 1·5 μg/24 hours for oestriol. Amounts below this have been recorded as zero. It must be emphasized that oestrogen may be present in such urines but in amounts below the calculated limit of sensitivity for the chemical method. For example, in urine from a normal 6-year-old girl the chemical method gave a value for oestrone below the limit of sensitivity and therefore recorded as zero. However, there was good agreement between parallel chemical and biological assays on this urine using the experimental design of Bulbrook, Greenwood and Williams (1957).

Urinary Gonadotrophins. The method of Dekanski (1949) was used to estimate gonadotrophins. The hormone was eluted from kaolin by 20 ml. of N/10 sodium hydroxide in the initial estimations but subsequently elution was carried out at *p*H 11·0 to 11·2 (Loraine and Brown, 1956). The biological test was done on female mice, 21 days old and weighing 10 g. A positive response was an increase in uterine weight of 100% above controls. Three mice were injected at each dose level and doses were adjusted so that a positive response indicated the presence of 5 mouse units or more.

17-ketosteroids. A method similar to that of Holtorff and Koch (1940) was employed to estimate 17-ketosteroids in urine. This method uses aqueous potassium hydroxide and a control reading, and gives higher results than methods using alcoholic potassium hydroxide and the Talbot, Berman and MacLachlan correction (1942).

Vaginal Smears. Vaginal smears were fixed in ether/alcohol and stained with Harris's haematoxylin and Shorr's trichrome stain. They were graded into negative or positive according to the presence of leucocytes and of keratinization of the epithelial cells.

Case Material

Four cases under the age of 3 years are described, none of whom had regular menstrual cycles. A further seven cases, ranging in age from 6 to nearly 11 years, were children who had signs of early puberty but who could not be classified as being definitely outside the normal range for the onset of puberty (Tanner, 1955). Of 39 children attending The Hospital for Sick Children in recent years because of precocious puberty, 29 fell into the latter group. None of the 10 cases in the former group had regular menstrual cycles.

Where possible, urine for oestrogen determination was collected from normal children in the same age groups as the patients described above.

Results

In 15 normal girls in the age range 3 to 10 years no oestrogen was detected in the urine, with one exception, a 7-year-old girl who excreted 2·9 μg./24 hours. In children over the age of 11 years who had breast development and pubic hair, but who had not menstruated, measurable amounts of oestrogen were found (2·9 to 7·1 μg./24 hours).

Oestrogen excretion, 17-ketosteroid excretion, gonadotrophin excretion and the grading of the vaginal smears of the children with early puberty are shown in Table 1.

In contrast to the control group, nine of the cases in this series were excreting amounts of oestrogen above 1·0 μg./24 hours. In seven of the cases, positive vaginal smears were correlated with the finding of oestrogen in the urine, and in three cases negative smears were correlated with the absence of oestrogen. In Case 1 a negative smear was obtained in conjunction with 1·8 μg. of urinary oestriol, while in Case 5 a positive vaginal smear was obtained but no oestrogen was detected in the urine.

Although the number of cases is too small for statistical analysis there appears to be a good association between the vaginal cytology and oestrogen output, although the latter is very low (2·0 to 6·8 μg. total oestrogen/24 hours). Similar results obtained on a large series of women (Young, Bulbrook and Greenwood, 1957) suggest that a very small output of urinary oestrogen, relative to the amounts in menstruating women, cannot be regarded as too low to be of physiological significance.

Case Histories

Case 1. Aged 7 months when first seen, this baby had a blood-stained vaginal discharge at 4 months. This lasted for five days and was followed by episodes three weeks

TABLE 1

OESTROGEN, 17-KETOSTEROID, GONADOTROPHIN EXCRETION AND VAGINAL SMEAR FINDINGS IN GIRLS WITH PRECOCIOUS OR EARLY PUBERTY

Case No.	Age (years)	Oestrone	Oestradiol	Oestriol	Total (μg./24 hr.)	Vaginal Smear	17-ketosteroids (mg./24 hr.)	Gonadotrophins (m.u./24 hr.)
1	7/12	0·0 0·0	0·0 0·0	0·0 1·8	0·0 1·8	Negative Negative	0·7 (0·47±0·16)	Negative Negative
2	1 10/12	0·0 1·3	0·0 0·0	2·2 4·2	2·2 5·5	Positive Positive	2·5 (1·38±0·66)	Negative Negative
3	2	1·8	0·0	3·4	5·2	Positive	1·6	—
4	2 6/12	0·0	0·0	0·0	0·0	Negative	0·9	Negative
5	6	0·0	0·0	0·0	0·0	Positive	2·1 (2·3±0·85)	Negative
6	8 6/12	0·0 1·2	0·0 0·0	0·0 0·0	0·0 1·2	Negative Negative	4·2	Negative
7	10	3·8	0·0	3·0	6·8	Positive	3·7	Positive
8	8	1·9 2·0 1·3	2·1 0·0 0·0	1·7 2·1 4·2	5·7 4·1 5·5	Positive	4·4	Negative Negative Negative
9	10	0·0 1·4 0·0 0·0 0·0	0·0 1·0 0·0 0·0 0·0	0·0 2·2 1·9 2·5 2·1	0·0 4·6 1·9 2·5 2·1	Positive	4·1	Positive 5–20 5–20
10	10		See Fig. 1		11–38	Positive	5·1	Negative 5–20 10–20
11	10 10/12		See Fig. 1		2·6–29	Positive	7·1	10–20

(The figures in brackets give the normal 17-ketosteroid excretion in children of the age groups: 0–1; 1–5; 5–10).

later and again after a further four weeks. Immediately after admission a profuse menstruation lasting eight days began. Development of the breasts and external genitalia beyond the normal was very slight. The nipples were slightly pigmented. There was a single small patch of pigmentation on the abdomen. Subsequently the periods were very irregular with intervals of several weeks or several months; at the present time no loss has been seen for a year. The vaginal smear and a specimen of urine for oestrogen estimation were taken on the second day after the end of the period which occurred in hospital. The vaginal smear was negative and no oestrogen was detected in the urine.

It was not possible to keep the child in hospital but six months later she was re-admitted for 48 hours for urine collection. The vaginal smear was still negative but 1·8 μg. of oestriol were found in the urine. The 17-ketosteroid excretion was at the upper limit of the normal range.

Case 2. This child was admitted to hospital during the first menstrual loss, which persisted for five days, at the age of 1 year and 10 months. On examination, the breasts were moderately developed and a few pubic hairs were present. The height, weight and bone age were advanced by about a year. Subsequent periods occurred after intervals of two, four, and one month, and lasted from one to three days. A second admission was arranged before the next expected period and specimens taken. The vaginal smear was positive and oestrogen was detected in the urine on both occasions. The gonadotrophin estimation was negative.

Case 3. The child was admitted to hospital at the age of 2 years because of vaginal bleeding lasting for one month. The examinations were carried out during the first one or two days following the cessation of the loss. There was no advance in growth, bone age, or breast development, and no pubic hair. It was thought that she was probably not a case of precocious puberty. Examination under anaesthesia revealed no abnormality which could account for the bleeding, however, and the vaginal smear was positive and oestrogen was present in the urine. The 17-ketosteroids were normal. No specimen was obtained for gonadotrophin estimation.

Case 4. This child was admitted to hospital because of congenital dislocation of the hip. At the age of 2½ years she was observed to have pubic hair and minimal breast development. Her growth and bone age was not advanced. The vaginal smear was negative, no oestrogen or gonadotrophin could be detected in the urine. The 17-ketosteroids were normal. This case demonstrates that clinical signs of precocity may be present in the absence of any confirmatory laboratory tests.

Case 5. At the age of 6 years this child had the weight, height and bone age of a child of 8, 10 and 11 years respectively. The breasts were very well-developed. There was no pigmentation of the nipples, no pubic or axillary hair, and the vulva was not developed. On rectal examination, the cervix and uterus were not palpable. There had been no menstrual loss. The vaginal smear was positive in this case although no oestrogen could be detected in the urine.

Case 6. On examination at the age of 8½ years, some breast development had taken place; there was much pubic hair and some axillary hair. No menstruation had occurred. The 17-ketosteroid excretion was just above the upper limit of normal (mean $+2\times$S.D.). Oestrogen was detected in one of two specimens of urine examined.

Case 7. On examination at the age of 10, the height, weight and bone age were in advance of the average by about two years. The breasts were developed and pubic hair was present but menstruation had not occurred. The first period, lasting one day, began five weeks after this examination. Hormone excretion was indicative of puberty; oestrogen and gonadotrophin were present in the urine and the vaginal smears were positive.

Case 8. This child was seen at the age of 8½ years. A few pubic hairs and slight development of the breasts had been noticed for about six months and on one occasion there had been a slight loss of blood for one day. Her height, weight and bone age were all advanced by three or four years. During the next two years she had slight shows of blood, never lasting for more than one day and occurring at intervals of one to three months. Oestrogen was present in three specimens of urine; the vaginal smear was positive and the 17-ketosteroid excretion was just above the normal range for the age. Though gonadotrophin was persistently absent from the urine, it was eventually demonstrated to be present when the patient reached the age of 10 years and regular periods had commenced.

Case 9. When first seen, at the age of 10 years, there had been irregular menstrual loss for a year. The breasts were developed and there was scanty pubic hair. The height was advanced by two years but not the bone age; she was very obese. Weekly specimens of urine were obtained in an attempt to demonstrate cyclical ovarian activity, but the number of specimens available were too few for this. Of five urine specimens, four contained oestrogen. Gonadotrophin was present in the urine.

Case 10. First seen two weeks after the first period, at the age of 10 years; her breasts were developed and pubic hair was present. The height and weight were advanced about four years. Periods have continued at fairly regular monthly intervals. Urine specimens were collected at intervals throughout the cycle and the details of oestrogen excretion are shown in Fig. 1.

Case 11. Breast development was first noticed at the age of 8½ years. Menstruation commenced at 10½ years and continued at regular monthly intervals. When seen at the age of 10 years and 10 months, the height, age, and bone age were those of a girl of 15 years. The cycle of oestrogen excretion is illustrated in Fig. 1.

Certain miscellaneous findings are of interest. In a case of polyostotic fibrous dysplasia, aged 7 years, with early signs of precocious puberty but no menstrual loss, oestriol excretion was 1·6 μg./24 hours; the 17-ketosteroids 1·4 mg., and the gonadotrophins negative. The vaginal smear was negative. In a boy, aged 8, with gynaecomastia of one breast, the oestrogen excretion totalled 4·5 μg./24 hours on one occasion and zero on two others. In one case of idiopathic breast development the vaginal smear was negative, no oestrogen could be detected in the urine, and the 17-ketosteroids were 0·6 mg./24 hours at the age of 15 months; the bone age was advanced six months. Material from a second patient in another hospital was also examined. The vaginal smear was positive; the total oestrogen excretion was 2·7 μg./24 hours, and the 17-ketosteroids were 1·2 mg./24 hours at the age of 3½ years. Gonadotrophin was less than 5 m.u./24 hours. There was apparently no clinical evidence of precocity. Upon enquiry it was learned that breast development regressed after 12 months. The presence of oestrogen in this case suggests that a true precocity was present. In a case of Klinefelter's syndrome in a boy aged 15 with gynaecomastia, gonadotrophin more than 72 m.u. and female genetic sex, the total oestrogens were 4·8 μg./24 hours.

Three normal boys and a girl, in hospital for tonsillectomy, had urines collected on the day of the operation, on the day before and the day following. Although the 17-ketogenetic steroids rose four-fold on the post-operative day, the level of oestrogen excretion was less than 1·0 μg. in all four cases on each of the three days. This result contrasts with similar studies in adult men in whom a rise in oestrogens accompanies the rise of other adrenal steroids following surgical stress.

Discussion

Biological assay results for urinary oestrogen excretion in normal children show considerable variation. For example, Nathanson, Towne and Aub (1941) found levels of up to 5 I.U. of total oestrogen in children of both sexes up to the age of 7 to 8 years, rising to 20 I.U. at the age of 11, and 240 to 382 I.U. in girls between the ages of 13 to 15 years. Dorfman, Greulich and Solomon (1937) found levels of 0 to 25 I.U. in five girls of ages varying from 7 to 12 years, while Pedersen-Bjergaard and Tønnesen (1948) found levels of up to 3 m.u. between the ages of 3 to 12 years. In one of the five cases of precocious puberty described by Hain (1947), the urinary oestrogens were 200 I.U./24 hours, and in the case reported by Gross (1940) they fluctuated between 405 and 12 I.U.; but this is exceptional and in the majority of reported cases oestrogens were absent or less than 10 I.U./24 hours. In his series of nine cases, Novak (1944) reported laboratory results as essentially negative in five; oestrogen levels were 4·4, 4·0,

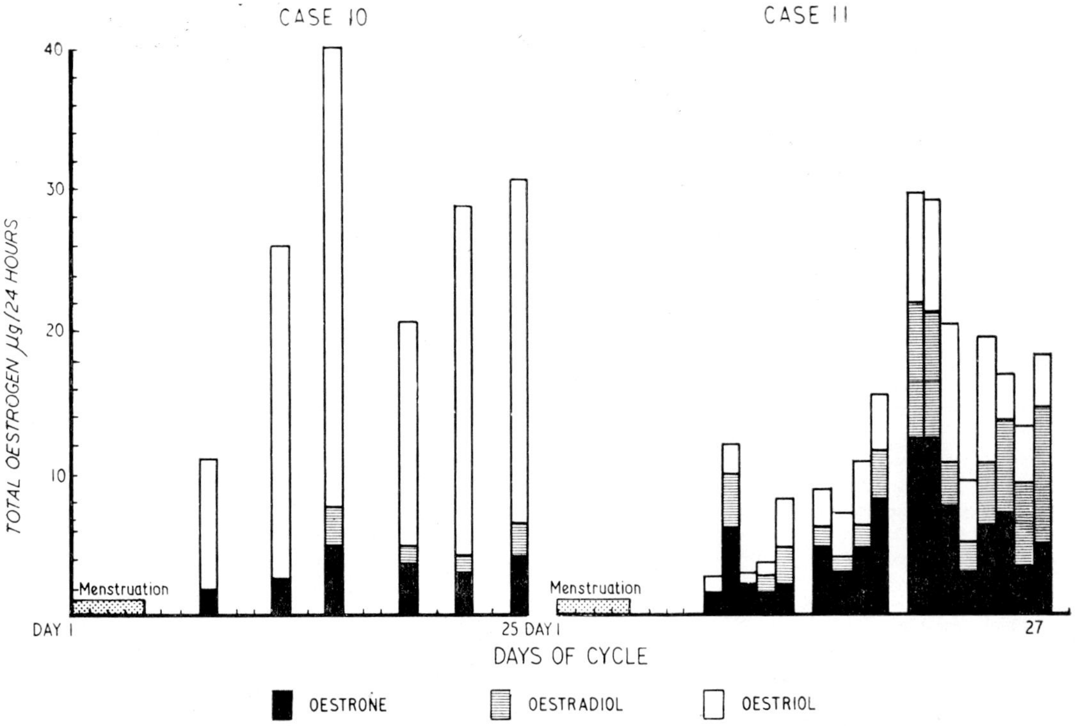

FIG. 1.—Oestrogen excretion during the menstrual cycle. Case 10, aged 10 years; Case 11, aged 10 years 10 months.

and 25·0 I.U. in three, and slightly lower than the normal pubertal level in one.

Although this study is concerned with only a small number of cases of precocious puberty, certain conclusions may be drawn. First, children who have developed certain of the secondary sexual characteristics, advanced growth, breast development and pubic hair, but who have not established regular menstrual cycles, excrete much less oestrogen than adult women (Brown, 1955*b*). It is not known whether the oestrogen excreted by children with precocious puberty is of adrenal and/or ovarian origin. Secondly, oestrogen excretion is nevertheless almost certainly greater in this group than in normal children without any of the signs of approaching puberty. Thirdly, a dramatic rise in oestrogen excretion occurs with the appearance of regular menstrual cycles undoubtedly of ovarian origin. This is illustrated by the two girls, both under 11 years of age, who had regular cycles and who achieved adult levels of excretion. It is probable that there is no essential difference between normal and precocious girls in these respects. It is not possible to say whether an *infant* with regular cycles would show this dramatic rise in excretion since none of the cases described here had the fully developed syndrome. This type of case appears to be uncommon since in Jolly's series of 31 cases only six had had regular cycles before the age of 8 years (Jolly, 1955).

Nathanson *et al.* (1941) reported that about a year and a half before the menarche, oestrogen excretion becomes cyclic in girls, and the intensity of these cycles gradually increases; it is possible that there is a rise and fall in oestrogen and in gonadotrophin excretion in precocious puberty. If this is so, estimations on single 24-hour specimens are necessarily of limited clinical value. Higher values may have existed in our cases and been missed, notably in the three infants who presented with bleeding.

Gonadotrophin was present in the urine of Cases 7, 9, 10 and 11, but absent in Cases 1, 2, 3, 4, 5, 6 and 8. In their extensive study of gonadotrophin excretion by the pre-menarche child, Catchpole and Greulich (1943) estimated the hormone in 24-hour urines every day for at least a month in 16 normal girls. With the approach of the menarche the number of days in which they were able to detect FSH in the urine approximated to 100% while the level of excretion also rose. The results in each case varied with the proximity of the first period. The average time elapsing between the date of the estimations and the date of the menarche in their cases was seven months, while the average percentage of days on which hormones could be detected at a level of 2 m.u. or more was only 43%. In adult women, Levin (1941) found that the daily excretion of gonadotrophin was less than 7·5 m.u. per day during the greater part of the cycle, but peak periods lasting for two days occurred at the mid-cycle when excretion rose to 15 m.u./24 hours in one case and 35 m.u./24 hours in another. It seems probable, therefore, that the absence of gonadotrophin from the urine of some of these cases may be due either to the insensitivity of the test, or to the irregular excretion of the hormone.

Vulval bleeding from local causes may mimic menstrual bleeding if the cause is not obvious on examination. In this event the hormone determinations will be normal but this is insufficient ground for excluding a diagnosis of precocity. If, however, the vaginal smear remains persistently negative, even though further bleeding occurs, it is probable that oestrogen excretion is not raised.

It may be concluded from these results that oestrogen, 17-ketosteroid and gonadotrophin determinations carried out on single 24-hour specimens are not diagnostic of precocious puberty, since completely normal values are not incompatible with the diagnosis. Nevertheless, the results demonstrate quite clearly that oestrogen excretion is usually raised above control levels, associated with a positive vaginal smear. With the present chemical method the error of the determinations at the low oestrogen levels encountered in urine from cases of precocious puberty is very large (Brown, Bulbrook and Greenwood, 1957). It may well be that a more sensitive method which could differentiate with certainty between control levels and the small amounts of oestrogen generally found in precocious puberty might be of diagnostic use. Even with the present method of Brown (1955*a*) the results are useful, especially in conjunction with the 17-ketosteroid values, for, if a gross pathological condition in the gonads or adrenal cortices exists, the figures will probably be high, i.e. well within the adult range (Snaith, 1958). This is unlikely to be the case in precocious puberty, except when the periods are well established and not infrequent.

Summary

Urinary oestrogen, 17-ketosteroid and gonadotrophin determinations have been carried out and vaginal smears examined in 11 girls with precocious or early puberty. While the 17-ketosteroid levels are at the upper range of normal values and the oestrogen levels are above control levels, the results of these estimations are not diagnostic of the condition but are of value in differentiating true precocious puberty from precocity due to pathological conditions involving the gonad or the adrenal, and from non-hormonal vulval bleeding. The results from a control series of 15 normal girls, in the age range 3 to 10 years, are also summarized.

We wish to thank the physicians and surgeons of The Hospital for Sick Children, Great Ormond Street, for permission to study their cases.

References

Bronstein, I. P., Luhan, J. A. and Mavrelis, W. B. (1942). *Amer. J. Dis. Child.*, **64**, 211.
Brown, J. B. (1955*a*). *Biochem. J.*, **60**, 185.
—— (1955*b*). *Lancet*, **1**, 320.
——, Bulbrook, R. D. and Greenwood, F. C. (1957). *J. Endocr.*, **16**, 41.
Bulbrook, R. D., Greenwood, F. C. and Williams, P. C. (1957). *J. Endocr.*, **15**, 206.
Catchpole, H. R. and Greulich, W. W. (1943). *J. clin. Invest.*, **22**, 799.
Dekanski, J. (1949). *Brit. J. exp. Path.*, **30**, 272.
Dorfman, R. I. (1948). In *The Hormones*, Vol. 1, edited by G. Pincus and K. V. Thimann. New York.
——, Greulich, W. W. and Solomon, C. I. (1937). *Endocrinology*, **21**, 741.
Fischer, H. S. (1940). *Amer. J. Obstet. Gynec.*, **39**, 525.
Gross, R. E. (1940). *Amer. J. Dis. Child.*, **59**, 579.
Hain, A. M. (1947). *J. clin. Endocr.*, **7**, 171.
Holtorff, A. F. and Koch, F. C. (1940). *J. biol. Chem.*, **135**, 377.
Jolly, H. (1955). *Sexual Precocity*. Springfield, Illinois.
Levin, L. (1941). *Endocrinology*, **28**, 378.
Lloyd, C. W. (1955). *J. clin. Endocr.*, **15**, 1518.
——, Lobotsky, J. and Morley, M. (1950). *Pediatrics*, **6**, 343.
Loraine, J. A. and Brown, J. B. (1956). *J. clin. Endocr.*, **16**, 1180
Lowrey, G. H. and Brown, T. G. (1951). *J. Pediat.*, **38**, 325.
Mossberg, H. O. (1951). *Acta paediat. (Uppsala)*, **40**, 261.
Nathanson, I. T., Towne, L. E. and Aub, J. C. (1941). *Endocrinology*, **28**, 851.
Novak, E. (1944). *Amer. J. Obstet. Gynec.*, **47**, 20.
Paschkis, K. E. (1952). *Med. Clin. N. Amer.*, **36**, 1711.
Pedersen-Bjergaard, K. and Tønnesen, M. (1948). *Acta endocr. (Kbh.)*, **1**, 38.
Seckel, H. P. G., Scott, W. W. and Benditt, E. P. (1949). *Amer. J. Dis. Child.*, **78**, 484.
Snaith, A. H. (1958). *J. Clin. Endocr.*, **18**, 318.
Talbot, N. B., Berman, R. A. and MacLachlan, E. A. (1942). *J. biol. Chem.*, **143**, 211.
Tanner, J. M. (1955). *Growth at Adolescence*. Oxford.
Young, S., Bulbrook, R. D. and Greenwood, F. C. (1957). *Lancet*, **1**, 350.

URINARY EXCRETION OF 17-KETOSTEROIDS IN CHILDREN

BY

MARGARET PROUT and A. H. SNAITH

From The Hospital for Sick Children, Great Ormond Street, London

(RECEIVED FOR PUBLICATION JANUARY 29, 1958)

Determination of the urinary excretion of 17-ketosteroids (17-oxosteroids) is the most important laboratory test in the investigation of endocrine disorders involving the adrenal cortex and gonads in children. The normal range of excretion varies with the method employed, since non-steroidal pigment may to a greater or lesser degree be measured as 17-ketosteroid. It is important therefore to know the normal range for the method used. This applies particularly to children, in whom excretion rises with age. In this paper normal values for the two most commonly used methods are given as well as figures for the commoner pathological conditions in which 17-ketosteroid excretion is raised. The evaluation of 17-ketosteroid excretion in pathological disorders is discussed.

Methods

Extraction. Twenty-four-hour urines from 73 normal children were extracted as follows. After the volume of the specimen had been measured, 100 ml. were brought to the boil on a hot-plate, and 15·0 ml. of concentrated hydrochloric acid poured down the reflux condenser. Boiling was continued for exactly 10 minutes. The urine was then cooled under the tap and extracted with 2×75 ml. and 1×50 ml. of ether. The ether extract was washed with 2×15 ml. of 10% sodium hydroxide, 1×10 ml. of a saturated solution of sodium hydrosulphite and then with water until the aqueous layer was neutral to litmus. After draining off all the water the ether was dried by adding a little anhydrous sodium sulphate and swirling. The ether was filtered (glass wool) and evaporated on a water bath using an air leak. Extracts were desiccated overnight. Each extract was then dissolved in 2·0 ml. of absolute alcohol and aliquots of 0·20 ml. removed for estimation.

Methods of Estimation. Method 1. Four tubes were set up. The first contained 0·2 ml. of extract, 0·2 ml. of 2·0% m-dinitrobenzene and 0·1 ml. of 5·0 N. aqueous potassium hydroxide; in the second tube 0·2 ml. of absolute alcohol was substituted for m-dinitrobenzene (=control); in the third tube 0·2 ml. of absolute alcohol was substituted for the extract (=reagent blank); in the fourth tube 0·2 ml. of absolute alcohol containing 50 μg. dehydroepiandrosterone was substituted for the extract. The tubes were incubated in a water bath at $25\cdot0\pm0\cdot2$°C. for 60 minutes in the dark and then to each tube was added 10·0 ml. of 70% ethanol. Readings were made in the Spekker (Hilger absorptiometer) using filter 604 and 70% alcohol as blank. Control and reagent blanks were subtracted from the reading. The amount of 17-ketosteroid present in the test was calculated by comparison with the standard reading (fourth tube) and the total for the 24-hour urine derived from this. This method of estimation has been in routine use in this hospital for many years and is similar to that of Holtorff and Koch (1940).

Method 2. In this method of estimation, which employs alcoholic in place of aqueous potassium hydroxide, the correction factor of Talbot, Berman and MacLachlan (1942) recommended by the Medical Research Council (1951) was used. To the first tube was added 0·2 ml. of extract, 0·2 ml. of 2·0% m-dinitrobenzene, and 0·2 ml. of 2·50% potassium hydroxide in absolute alcohol. Appropriate reagent blank and standard tubes were set up. After dilution with 10·0 ml. of absolute alcohol, readings of the test in the Spekker, using the green (604) and violet (601) filters were obtained and after subtraction of the blanks the corrected reading was obtained from the formula of Talbot *et al.* (1942); corrected reading $= \frac{Eg = 0\cdot6\ Ev}{0\cdot72}$

Various methods of correction for non-steroidal pigments were investigated as follows:

Method 3. As in method 2, except that the Hilger Uvispek was substituted for the Spekker, readings being taken at 515 mμ. (in place of the green filter) and 425 mμ. (in place of the violet filter), the above formula being applied.

Method 4. As for method 3, but readings were made at 425 mμ., 515 mμ. and 605 mμ., and the corrected test obtained from the formula of Allen (1950), in which the corrected reading $= E\ 515 - \frac{E\ 605 + E\ 425}{2}$

Method 5. As in method 1 but the Hilger Uvispek was used and the corrected reading obtained as in method 4.

Results

The results for the five methods of estimation are given in Table 1. Only 57 of the 73 urines were estimated by methods 3, 4 and 5. For convenience the means of four age groups with standard deviations are given for methods 1 and 2 in Table 2.

TABLE 1

17-KETOSTEROID EXCRETION IN NORMAL CHILDREN

Age	Method 1	Method 2	Method 3	Method 4	Method 5
weeks					
6	0·67	0·44	0·27	0·14	0·65
,,	0·32	0·23			
months					
3	0·38	0·23			
4	0·51	0·28			
,,	0·36	0·39			
8	0·37	0·10			
,,	0·37	0·21	0·00	·07	0·33
,,	0·37	0·11	0·00	0·9	0·17
years					
2	0·61	0·32	0·16	0·00	0·14
3	1·57	1·50	1·88	2·03	1·66
,,	0·34	0·23	0·02	0·00	0·07
4	2·30	1·70	0·67	0·96	1·00
,,	1·52	0·65	0·42	0·34	0·76
,,	0·75	0·35	0·17	0·06	0·27
,,	1·24	1·03	0·22	0·30	0·75
,,	2·75	1·02	0·20	0·10	0·41
,,	1·50	1·10			
5	1·76	0·77	1·24	0·96	1·40
,,	1·14	0·60	0·18	0·17	0·33
,,	1·63	0·70	0·33	0·00	0·78
,,	0·86	0·30	0·13	0·00	0·29
6	1·78	0·36	0·41	0·15	0·86
,,	2·43	1·73	0·40	0·23	1·64
,,	1·42	0·43			
,,	3·02	1·05			
7	1·10	0·97	0·70	0·48	0·92
,,	3·10	2·70			
8	1·20	0·60	0·21	0·22	0·17
,,	2·60	1·42			
,,	2·70	1·60			
,,	1·40	0·65			
,,	1·55	1·63			
,,	1·60	1·60			
9	2·06	1·50	2·00	1·50	1·00
,,	2·70	1·50	0·66	0·98	1·60
,,	2·78	2·13	1·56	1·41	1·92
,,	4·55	2·05	2·10	1·77	2·99
,,	1·11	0·50			0·16
10	2·60	0·72	1·33	1·50	0·88
,,	2·00	0·87	1·20	1·20	0·54
,,	3·55	2·10	0·60	0·41	2·80
,,	3·00	3·00			
11	3·43	3·28	2·84	2·44	2·94
,,	3·65	2·90	2·82	2·34	3·50
,,	2·60	1·72	0·14	1·05	1·24
,,	3·17	1·38	1·39	1·02	1·11
,,	5·95	4·04	4·22	1·27	3·52
,,	6·70	6·00	3·98	3·85	3·39
,,	4·25	1·95	2·28	2·15	2·30
,,	4·99	3·71	2·54	1·93	3·70
,,	5·40	4·50			
12	2·40	2·70	2·17	2·10	3·40
,,	3·71	5·38	3·21	3·46	3·43
,,	3·46	3·73	1·53	1·77	1·91
,,	9·50	8·10	7·10	6·60	6·20
,,	3·04	2·77	1·46	1·85	3·13
,,	3·48	2·75	2·26	1·70	2·80
13	8·00	5·62	5·11	4·64	4·98
,,		7·00	6·31	5·91	6·71
,,	8·30	7·15	5·50	4·88	6·30
,,	8·50	7·30	3·81	3·56	4·12
14	5·25	5·20	4·45	3·76	4·24
,,	7·11	4·75	4·89	4·40	4·25
,,	5·67	4·12	4·25	4·08	3·90
,,	8·90	8·40	5·72	4·40	7·90
,,	8·50	7·30	5·11	4·24	6·30
,,	5·30	4·50			
15	9·76	8·25	6·78	6·82	7·69
,,	7·08	7·13	6·98	6·46	8·30
,,	6·05		4·26	4·40	3·86
,,	4·34	2·71	3·07	2·77	2·85
,,	8·60	6·70	5·70	5·17	5·70
16	7·31	6·52	6·28	6·08	6·21
,,	5·72	5·30	3·48	3·48	4·31
,,	7·40	6·10	7·30	6·30	7·10

TABLE 2

MEAN EXCRETION OF 17-KETOSTEROIDS IN CHILDREN OF DIFFERENT AGE GROUPS

Age Groups (years)	Method 1 (mg./24 hr.)	Method 2 (mg./24 hr.)
0– 1	0·47± ·16	0·25± ·12
1– 5	1·38± ·66	0·78± ·46
6–10	2·30± ·85	1·38± ·74
11–17	6·03±2·14	4·96±2·06

Discussion

17-ketosteroid Excretion in Normal Children. The urinary excretion of 17-ketosteroids in children has been reported by many authors and results have varied considerably. A comparison of results by various methods has been made by Poli and Fantuzzi (1945). The results quoted for different laboratories by Dorfman (1952), all by the Holtorff and Koch (1940) method, are high compared with the results reported here. The results obtained by method 2 are in closer agreement with results reported by others who have used a similar method. Miller and Mason (1945) found averages of approximately 5·7 mg. in boys and 5·2 mg. in girls for the age group 12-17 years, while Talbot, Butler, Berman, Rodriguez and MacLachlan (1943) found an average excretion of 0·4 mg. at 5 years, and of 1·9 mg. at 10 years. Hain (1947) obtained figures for the 5-10 age group which are somewhat higher, about 3·5 mg. in boys and 2·0 mg. in girls. Bongiovanni (1951) employed aqueous potassium hydroxide, but corrected for the interfering pigments by extracting the developed colour with chloroform, and by this method obtained figures which were comparable with those of Talbot *et al.* (1943).

The three chief causes of variation are probably: (*a*) Differences in the method employed for estimating the 17-ketosteroids after extraction from the urine. (*b*) Differences in the method of extraction. (*c*) Race differences (Barnicot and Wolffson, 1952).

Only the first has been considered here. It is evident from Table 1 that the highest values are obtained by method 1, lower values with method 2, and values which are lower still with methods 5, 3 and 4 in that order. These differences are greater in the lower two age groups, illustrating that what is measured by methods 1 and 2 in these groups is to a greater extent non-steroidal pigment. The much lower results obtained by method 5, compared with method 1, is indicative of the degree to which the results are erroneously high in the latter method. Method 5 is not a valid procedure, however, because when aqueous potassium hydroxide is employed the Zimmerman reaction does not obey Beer's law. Although methods 3 and 4 give lower results than method 2, the latter is a satisfactory routine procedure and superior to method 1. The normal range will vary according to the method of extraction employed, but differences from the results obtained here should not be great provided special purification methods, e.g. Girard's reagent, or chromatography, are not used.

Raised 17-ketosteroid Excretion in Children. The determination of the 17-ketosteroid excretion is of clinical importance in childhood in congenital adrenal hyperplasia, tumours of the adrenal cortex, and precocious puberty. It is not possible to distinguish one condition from the other by the level of excretion. In children of 5 or 6 years with hyperplasia excretion may be as little as 10 mg./24 hours (Table 3, Cases 9 and 12), or approaching 100 mg./24 hours (Table 3, Cases 13 and 32), levels which are more typical, possibly, of adenoma or carcinoma of the adrenal cortex. In all of the cases of adrenal hyperplasia (Table 3), the first 17-ketosteroid determination was abnormally high, i.e. more than the mean $+2\times$standard deviation. In Case 5, the 17-ketosteroids, determined during the first week or two of life at another hospital, were less than 1·0 mg./24 hours and this was passed as normal. It is possible therefore that very low figures may be observed in early infancy and if the diagnosis is thought probable a second specimen should be examined either immediately or in three months' time.

In congenital adrenal hyperplasia the presence of a raised pregnanetriol excretion is diagnostic, but borderline figures may occur here also in the young infant, as in Case 15, in which pregnanetriol excretion was only 0·2 mg./24 hours rising after ACTH to 0·45 mg./24 hours (Case 1, Table 4). (The mean excretion of pregnanetriol in 12 normal children of all ages was 0·04 mg./24 hours with a range of 0-0·18 mg./24 hours.) The raised 17-ketosteroid excretion was therefore of particular significance in this case, especially in view of the fact that the urogenital sinus which was present could possibly have been explained by hormone treatment which the mother had received during the early part of her pregnancy.

It sometimes happens that a child, usually 2 or 3 weeks of age, is admitted to hospital in collapse due to adrenal insufficiency associated with adrenal hyperplasia. Steroid therapy may be commenced immediately and cannot subsequently be withdrawn because of the danger of precipitating a second collapse. Urinary steroid determinations may not, therefore, be carried out, or if they are interpretation may be difficult because of the suppression of the cortex due to the administered hormones. In this event it is important to re-admit the child in order to establish the diagnosis. If suppressive treatment is withdrawn the 17-ketosteroids will be found to rise to a diagnostic level; if suppressive steroids cannot be withdrawn it may be found that the urinary pregnanetriol excretion, though partly suppressed, is still abnormally high. It is important to establish the diagnosis in a case which presents in this way because cases occur in which the plasma electrolytes are

TABLE 3

17-KETOSTEROID EXCRETION IN CONGENITAL ADRENAL HYPERPLASIA, IN BOYS WITH PRECOCIOUS PUBERTY AND IN ADRENOCORTICAL TUMOURS (ESTIMATED BY METHOD 1)

Case	Diagnosis	Sex	Age	17-Ketosteroid Excretion (mg./24 hr.)
			weeks	
1	Adrenal hyperplasia ..	M	2	5·7
2	,, ,, ...	M	4	0·9
3	,, ,, ...	M	9	4·4
4	,, ,, ...	M	10	5·0
			months	
5	,, ,, ...	M	4	7·8
6	,, ,, ...	M	4	2·7
7	,, ,, ...	M	7	8·0
			years	
8	,, ,, ...	M	5	22·7
9	,, ,, ...	M	5	10·3
10	,, ,, ...	M	5	25·3
11	,, ,, ...	M	6	16·9
12	,, ,, ...	M	6	9·1
13	,, ,, ...	M	6½	78·9
14	,, ,, ...	M	9	38·8
			weeks	
15	,, , ...	F	4	2·2
16	,, ,, ...	F	4	3·7
17	,, ,, ...	F	4	7·7
18	,, ,, ...	F	6	3·9
19	,, ,, ...	F	6	7·5
20	,, ,, ...	F	8	5·3
21	,, ,, ...	F	8	4·9
22	,, ,, ...	F	8	2·5
			months	
23	,, ,, ...	F	5	3·9
24	,, ,, ...	F	6	3·8
25	,, ,, ...	F	7	6·4
26	,, ,, ...	F	11	2·8
27	,, ,, ...	F	18	12·6
28	,, ,, ...	F	18	3·1
			years	
29	,, ,, ...	F	2	6·2
30	,, ,, ...	F	4	40·3
31	,, ,, ...	F	5	20·3
32	,, ,, ...	F	8½	29·1
	,, ,, ...	F	10½	129
			months	
33	Precocious puberty ..	M	11	0·3
			years	
34	,, ,, ...	M	3	2·4
35	,, ,, ...	M	4	2·7
36	,, ,, ...	M	10	8·9
37	Adrenocortical adenoma (with virilism)	F	6	3·4—7·5
38	,, ,, ,, ..	F	10	10·0
39	,, ,, ,, ..	F	2	4·1—6·0
40	,, ,, ,, ..	F	5	17·2—20·7
41	Adrenocortical carcinoma (with virilism)	M	2	120 —263
42	Adrenocortical adenoma (with Cushing's syndrome)	M	3	4·2
			months	
43	Bilateral adrenocortical multiple adenomata (with Cushing's syndrome) ..	F	14	3·0

TABLE 4

17-KETOSTEROIDS AND PREGNANETRIOL EXCRETION BEFORE AND AFTER ACTH 10 mg./24 HOURS (CASE 1) AND 40 mg./24 HOURS (CASES 2, 3 AND 4) FOR THREE DAYS

	Case 1	Case 2	Case 3	Case 4
	(*values in mg./24 hr.*)			
17-ketosteroid				
before ACTH ..	2·2	7·3	7·7	30·1
after ACTH ..	3·5	13·8	23·4	39·7
Pregnanetriol				
before ACTH ..	0·2	20·5	14·0	20·0
after ACTH ..	0·4	15·0	37·0	36·8

typical of adrenal insufficiency, though there is no confirmatory evidence of this. In two such cases, both boys, aged 5 and 9 weeks of age, the 17-ketosteroids were raised and subsequently fell. The figures in mg./24 hours were 1·10; 0·85; 0·81; 0·56; and 1·80; 1·13 and 1·00 respectively. It is possible that the 17-ketosteroids were raised as a result of the illness. Such cases might be diagnosed incorrectly as having congenital adrenal hyperplasia. While a provisional diagnosis of hyperplasia can be made on the basis of abnormal plasma electrolyte levels in male infants, and on the presence of a urogenital sinus with or without associated abnormal plasma electrolyte levels in girls, a definitive diagnosis can only be made by the investigation of urinary steroid excretion.

In boys with precocious puberty the 17-ketosteroids may be raised to levels characteristic of the physiological age but are unlikely to exceed 10 mg./24 hours. If 17-ketosteroid excretion is less than 10 mg. a day in a boy, the distinction between the virilizing tumour and precocious puberty must be made on clinical grounds. A raised gonadotrophin excretion would support a diagnosis of precocity, and in adrenocortical tumours the testes are likely to be normal in size for the chronological age. A diagnosis cannot be established on those grounds, however, and special investigations will be required to exclude a tumour.

ACTH tests are of little importance in the diagnosis of congenital adrenal hyperplasia. After administration of ACTH, 20 mg. b.d. for three days, pregnanetriol excretion in a normal child was 0·4 mg./24 hours on the third day. In adrenal hyperplasia pregnanetriol and 17-ketosteroid excretion usually rise after ACTH administration, but this is not invariable (Table 4).

Summary

The excretion of 17-ketosteroids by normal children and by children with congenital adrenal hyperplasia, adrenocortical tumours, and with precocious puberty has been determined. The clinical evaluation of 17-ketosteroid excretion is discussed.

We wish to thank the physicians and surgeons of The Hospital for Sick Children, Great Ormond Street, for permission to study their cases, and the Research Committee for their support.

REFERENCES

Allen, W. M. (1950). *J. clin. Endocr.*, **10**, 71.
Barnicot, M. A. and Wolffson, D. (1952). *Lancet*, **1**, 893.
Bongiovanni, A. M. (1951). *J. Pediat.*, **39**, 606.
Dorfman. R. I. (1952). Ciba Foundation Colloquia on Endocrinology, Vol. 2, p. 160.
Hain, A. M. (1947). *Arch. Dis. Childh.*, **22**, 152.
Holtorff, A. F. and Koch, F. C. (1940). *J. biol. Chem.*, **135**, 377.
Miller, S. and Mason, H. L. (1945). *J. clin. Endocr.*, **5**, 220.
Medical Research Council Committee on Clinical Endocrinology (1951). *Proposed Standard Method of 17-ketosteroid Determination. Lancet*, **2**, 585.
Poli, G. and Fantuzzi, B. (1945). *Minerva pediat.* (*Torino*), **6**, 775
Talbot, N. B., Berman, R. A. and MacLachlan, E. A. (1942). *J. biol. Chem.*, **143**, 211.
——, Butler, A. M., Berman, R. A., Rodriguez, P. M. and MacLachlan, E. A. (1943). *Amer. J. Dis. Child.*, **65**, 364.

THE URINARY EXCRETION OF 17-HYDROXYSTEROIDS IN CHILDREN

BY

R. GARDNER and A. H. SNAITH

From The Hospital for Sick Children, Great Ormond Street, London

(RECEIVED FOR PUBLICATION JANUARY 29, 1958)

The results reported here were obtained as a consequence of routine requests for steroid estimations. Some of the normal figures were obtained privately, but others were obtained from children in hospital, who had no endocrine wasting or similar disorder likely to influence adrenocortical secretion. Most of the requests concerned four types of case: obesity, dwarfism, precocious puberty and adrenal hyperplasia or tumour.

Method

The method of Reddy (1954) was employed. This measures those corticosteroids which have a 17:21-dihydroxy-20-ketone side chain. The two principal glucocorticosteroids which are secreted by the adrenal cortex are hydrocortisone (approximately 85%) and corticosterone (approximately 15%) (Bush, 1953). The principal corticosteroids present in urine are hydrocortisone, cortisone and their metabolites. Both hydrocortisone and cortisone possess the 17:21-dihydroxy-20-ketone side chain, so also do their principal metabolites and therefore these compounds will be measured by the method. Corticosterone lacks the 17-hydroxyl group and it is not measured by this method.

Results

The 17-hydroxysteroids were determined in the 24-hour urines from 94 normal children. The children were divided into two groups, those under 2 years of age, and those over 2. This was done principally because few results were obtained for children at about the age of 2, a most difficult age at which to obtain 24-hour specimens of urine from normal children. The mean excretion of 17-hydroxysteroids in the younger age group was $1 \cdot 2 \pm 1 \cdot 0$ mg./24 hours. In the older group the mean excretion was $3 \cdot 1 \pm 2 \cdot 0$ mg./24 hours (Table 1). The difference between the two groups is highly significant ($P < \cdot 01$). There is no significant difference between the mean figures for excretion for the ages 0-1 year and 1-2 years and the results may be considered as falling into one group. There is probably a rise with age in the older group but the regression is not significant.

Results were obtained from 23 cases of obesity, all of whom were in the older age group. The mean excretion was 3·4 mg./24 hours. In three cases of dwarfism in the younger age group the mean excretion was 0·9 mg./24 hours, and in 15 cases in the older age group it was 2·1 mg./24 hours. In five cases precocious puberty in the earlier age group the mean excretion was 0·7 mg, and in five cases in the older group it was 3·8 mg./24 hours. None of these figures is significantly different from the normal.

TABLE 1

URINARY 17-HYDROXYSTEROID EXCRETION IN NORMAL CHILDREN

Age Last Birthday (years)	Mean 17-hydroxysteroid Excretion (mg./24 hr.)
0– 2	$1 \cdot 2 \pm 1 \cdot 0$
2–17	$3 \cdot 1 \pm 2 \cdot 0$

In the syndrome of congenital adrenal hyperplasia, the excretion of 17-hydroxysteroids is low when determined by paper chromatography (Eberlein and Bongiovanni, 1955). The Reddy method, however, indicates the excretion of normal levels of 17-hydroxysteroids, though in two cases, in brothers, excretion was persistently zero. Furthermore, in three cases to whom ACTH was administered levels rose (Table 2). It must be concluded therefore

TABLE 2

17-HYDROXYSTEROID EXCRETION IN 15 CASES BEFORE AND AFTER ACTH 40 mg./24 HOURS FOR THREE DAYS

Case No.	Diagnosis	Age (years)	17-hydroxysteroids Before ACTH (mg./24 hr.)	17-hydroxysteroids After ACTH (mg./24 hr.)
1	Normal	9	4·3	18·1
2	,, ...	6	8·8	56·5
3	Dwarfism	1	1·3	11·2
4	,, ...	5	0·0	8·2
5	,, ...	6	2·1	17·4
6	,, ...	6	4·8	41·9
7	,, ...	6	1·6	26·8
8	,, ...	8	3·5	26·1
9	,, ...	8	2·9	20·9
10	,, ...	10	4·1	24·2
11	,, ...	11	2·7	31·6
12	,, ...	13½	1·3	9·6
13*	Congenital adrenal hyperplasia	4 *weeks*	2·6	4·7
14	,, ,, ..	2	2·3	9·6
15	,, ,, ..	6½	2·7	12·7

* In Case 13, ACTH 10 mg./24 hours was administered.
The highest figures before and after ACTH are given.

that the compounds measured in this condition are not the same as the compounds excreted by normal subjects.

In six children with dwarfism an ACTH test was carried out. A base line figure was obtained for one or two days prior to the test, and ACTH, 20 mg. b.d. was then administered for three days. Table 2 shows the base line figures and the highest figure obtained after ACTH. Excretion usually declined to the control level on the second day after the last dose of ACTH.

The administration of cortisone will cause a rise in 17-hydroxysteroid excretion. In four adults, 50 mg. of cortisone acetate was administered at 8 a.m. and again at 6 p.m., and the 24-hour urine collection commenced at 8 a.m. on the same day. The excretion of 17-hydroxysteroids by the four individuals was 28·8 mg., 28·2 mg., 26·4 mg. and 24·2 mg. The mean base line figure was 2·4 mg./24 hours.

The 17-hydroxysteroids were determined for the first 19 days after menstruation in a girl aged 11 years. The figures in mg./24 hours were 3·3, 4·3, 14·4, 5·6, 4·3, —, 7·4, 7·7, 7·1, 7·8, —, 7·3, 7·6, 9·5, 9·0, 7·0, 6·0, 7·2, 6·7. It will be observed that, except for the high figure obtained on the third day for which there was no obvious explanation, the level of excretion rises to a peak of 9·5 mg./24 hours, and then declines. This peak of excretion occurred on the day following the peak of oestrogen excretion which was determined concurrently.

In a case of Cushing's syndrome in a boy aged 3½ years, the 17-hydroxysteroids were 3·1 mg./24 hours. In a second case due to bilateral adrenal multiple adenomata, the 17-hydroxysteroids were 9·8 mg./24 hours.

Discussion

The method of Reddy is simpler to perform than the 17-ketogenic method of Norymberski, Stubbs and West (1953). The latter method involves the simultaneous determination of the 17-ketosteroids, but since this result is usually required this is a gain rather than otherwise. In this hospital, however, a method similar to the method of Holtorff and Koch (1940) but different from that employed in the determination of 17-ketogenic steroids has been in use since 1940. An independent method of 17-hydroxysteroid determination was therefore of value. Reddy (1954) gives the normal adult range of 17-hydroxycorticosteroids as 1·1-10·7 mg./24 hours with a mean of 4·7. The smaller excretion in children must be due to size, since blood levels are similar (Ely, Raile, Bray and Kelley, 1954). It is of some importance that the upper limit of normal is lower in children since in Cushing's syndrome the figures may be only moderately raised, or, as in one of the cases referred to here, within the normal range. The difficulties of interpretation of ACTH tests have been discussed by Prunty (1956). Since it is not permissible to experiment with normal children by administering ACTH it is hardly possible to obtain genuine controls, and only two cases to whom ACTH had been given therapeutically were considered to be normal controls (Table 2). The response in Case 2 is striking, and it is of interest that the base line figure here is high. The 17-ketogenic steroids after ACTH in this normal child reached 70 mg./24 hours, a figure which matches the response to ACTH in the cases of Cushing's syndrome due to adrenal hyperplasia described by Prunty.

In the cases of dwarfism (who were given ACTH from the same batch) it is clear that the response is variable, though it is possible that the response varies directly with the base line figures.

The normal excretion of 17-hydroxysteroids in one of the cases of Cushing's syndrome (the 17-ketosteroids were moderately raised) reveals the limitations of laboratory methods in this condition. Since in children tumours of the adrenal cortex and not hyperplasia are usually the cause of the syndrome, it is probably true that laboratory investigations can confirm the clinical diagnosis but cannot exclude it.

The 17-hydroxysteroids may also be of value in the diagnosis of Addison's disease and an ACTH test is of importance here. Otherwise it may be concluded that apart from Cushing's syndrome and Addison's disease, both rare disorders in childhood, the clinical value of 17-hydroxycorticosteroid determinations is limited.

Summary

The urinary excretion of 17-hydroxysteroids by normal children and by children attending hospital for obesity, dwarfism, precocious puberty and adrenal hyperplasia has been determined. The clinical value of this determination is discussed.

We wish to thank the physicians and surgeons of The Hospital for Sick Children, Great Ormond Street, for permission to study their cases, and the Research Committee for their support.

References

Bush, I. E. (1953). *J. Endocr.*, **9**, 95.
Eberlein, W. R. and Bongiovanni, A. M. (1955). *J. clin. Invest.*, **34**, 1337.
Ely, R. S., Raile, R. B., Bray, P. F. and Kelley, V. C. (1954). *Pediatrics*, **13**, 403.
Norymberski, J. K., Stubbs, R. D. and West, H. F. (1953). *Lancet*, **1**, 1276.
Prunty, F. T. G. (1956). *Brit. med. J.*, **2**, 615, 673.
Reddy, W. J. (1954). *Metabolism*, **3**, 489.
Holtorff, A. F. and Koch, F. C. (1940). *J. biol. Chem.*, **135**, 377.

THE PROGNOSIS IN JUVENILE OBESITY

BY

A. G. MULLINS

From St. James's Hospital, Balham, London

(RECEIVED FOR PUBLICATION NOVEMBER 7, 1957)

Juvenile obesity is common. Probably few paediatricians or general practitioners regard it as a serious medical problem. It has not been shown to be associated with high mortality or morbidity rates and, except in the most extreme cases, it is widely regarded as a benign if unsightly condition, usually associated with excessive eating and with tendencies both to improve and to persist. Recently the psychiatric aspects of the condition have aroused interest, and extensive studies have been published (Bruch, 1939, 1940, 1941, 1957; Juel-Nielsen, 1953; Iversen, 1953; Østergaard, 1954).

The exact incidence of juvenile obesity in this country is not known. Johnson, Burke and Mayer (1956) studying a cross-section of elementary and secondary schoolchildren in Boston, found that it occurred in 9% of the boys and in 12·5% of the girls in 6,000 children. It is doubtful whether the incidence is as high in this country. There is evidence that in some parts of the world its incidence is rising. In Germany, Haase and Hosenfeld (1956) found that, whereas its incidence fell enormously during the war, there are now five times as many cases seen in their clinic as in 1939.

A search of the literature failed to reveal any investigation of the ultimate dangers of juvenile obesity.

Obesity in adults is now one of the greatest medical problems in the western world and its dangers have been intensively studied. Obesity is known to shorten the life of animals (McCay, Maynard, Sperling and Osgood, 1941; Hansson, Brännäng and Claesson, 1953; Kennedy, 1951, 1955). For a long time insurance companies have known that among adults accepted for life insurance overweight of all degrees and at all ages is associated with a high mortality and morbidity. The subject has recently been reviewed by Armstrong, Dublin, Wheatley and Marks (1951) and by Marks (1956). Dublin (1953) points out that the relative increase of mortality in the overweight is increasing, since diseases in which mortality is higher in the underweight, chiefly pulmonary tuberculosis and pneumonia, are declining.

Probably the mortality of the obese as a class is even higher than insurance statistics suggest, since the subjects from whom the statistics were obtained were chosen as good insurance risks (Evans, 1952). Sinclair (1954) has said that if you are in middle life or more, your chances of dying early are greater if you are 10 lb. overweight than are your chances of getting carcinoma of the bronchus if you are a heavy smoker. Jolliffe (1953) calculated that if a cure were found for carcinoma, the average life expectancy would be increased by two years, whereas if obesity were cured, it would be increased by four years.

The part played in this state of affairs by persistent juvenile obesity has not been worked out. Few long-term results of treatment in this condition have been published, and authorities differ in their opinions. Gurney (1936) studied 63 fat women and found that eight of them had been obese all their lives and a further four since puberty; thus persistent juvenile and pubertal obesity existed in approximately 19% of his cases. Ellis and Tallerman (1934) state: 'It is well known that the majority of obese children tend to gravitate toward the normal after puberty has been reached.' Le Marquand (1951) found that a large proportion of fat girls traced to adult life either remained fat or became fat again after childbirth. Bornhardt (1936) re-investigated 65 obese children while they were in their teens and found that girls tended to remain obese more frequently than boys. Mossberg (1948) followed up 328 patients who had been admitted to hospital for obesity in childhood and found that the prognosis was worse in girls than in boys. Hering (1938) re-investigated 30 patients, and found that 10 were normal, 10 were 'giants', i.e. both tall and overweight but without giving an impression of obesity, and 10 were still obese. Hässler (1935) obtained similar results. Haase and Hosenfeld (1956) followed up 21 boys and 24 girls who had been treated before the war, and found that in most of them the condition had persisted. Some of them had lost weight at puberty or during the war, but of these, most had again become obese.

Object of Present Work

This investigation was done because, whilst it was observed that obesity is very common among adult hospital medical out-patients and was either directly responsible for their symptoms or exacerbated the diseases for which they attended, the treatment of the condition was only successful in a minority of cases. In view of this it seemed important to study the subject, and to attempt to discover how far obesity in later life is due to persistent juvenile obesity.

Material and Method

The age, sex, height and weight were recorded in 373 patients seen consecutively in the medical out-patient department at St. James' Hospital, Balham, and the results were compared with the standard tables of Kemsley (1952).

One hundred and one patients seen in out-patients who were 20% or more overweight were selected for further study. These are the 'obese' group, and were sub-divided into 'juvenile obese' and 'adult obese' groups according to whether or not they had been known as 'fatty' at school; this was found to be the most practical single criterion.

Fifty patients whose weight was within 20% of normal weight were studied in a similar way. They were chosen primarily for co-operation and intelligence. An attempt to take detailed life and dietary histories from an unselected series of out-patients of normal weight was abandoned and it was decided that, in spite of the differences between the two groups, intelligent and co-operative subjects would provide more valuable information which could later be used for more standardized studies. Thus the two groups can be compared in some respects, but the 'normals' cannot be regarded as 'controls'.

Twenty-one adults who had received medical treatment for obesity during childhood were investigated in the same way, special attention being paid to possible reasons why their obesity had persisted or resolved. This is the 'treated juvenile obese' group.

Seven patients in the 'treated juvenile obese' group and three in the normal group had suffered from juvenile obesity and later become normal. These were classed together as the 'normal juvenile obese' group.

Each patient was asked the history of her weight and its relation to her life-circumstances. An attempt was made to assess her appetite and type of diet and the factors influencing these. Special attention was paid to early and family history, the influence of pregnancy, and to possible medical and psychological factors influencing the condition. In addition, the usual medical history was taken, a full clinical examination was done in every case and any investigations thought necessary were carried out.

An attempt was made to treat all these patients as out-patients. The method of treatment was primarily dietary with the object of accustoming the patients to a bulky low-calorie diet and of re-educating their eating habits rather than of producing rapid and temporary loss of weight. Drugs, chiefly dextroamphetamine sulphate, were used when it did not seem possible to treat the patient by dietary means alone.

Overall Results

Incidence of Overweight. The impression that obesity is common among the patients was confirmed (Fig. 1). Of the 373 medical out-patients 36% of the men and 52% of the women were more than 10% above standard weight. Twenty-six per cent of the men and 44% of the women were

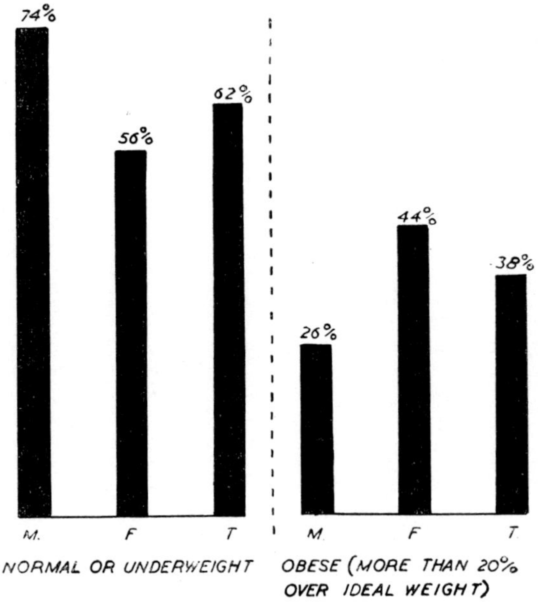

FIG. 1.—Incidence of obesity in 373 medical out-patients. M.=Male; F.=Female; T.=Total.

more than 20% above standard weight, and so were classed as 'obese'. It is interesting to note that a higher percentage of the women (21%) than the men (14%) were also underweight, and that only 26% of the women, compared with 51% of the men were within 10% of standard weight.

Obese Group. Table 1 shows the distribution of age, sex and type of obesity in the 101 obese patients. Of these approximately one third were cases of persistent juvenile obesity and in the remaining two thirds the obesity developed later in life.

TABLE 1

DISTRIBUTION OF 101 OBESE PATIENTS ACCORDING TO AGE, SEX AND TYPE OF OBESITY

Age (years)	Juvenile Obese (32)			Adult Obese (69)			Totals (101)		
	M.	F.	T.	M.	F.	T.	M.	F.	T.
18–19 . .	–	2	2	–	–	–	–	2	2
20–29 . .	–	3	3	3	1	4	3	4	7
30–39 . .	–	2	2	–	6	6	–	8	8
40–49 . .	3	6	9	4	13	17	7	19	26
50–59 . .	–	12	12	9	13	22	9	25	34
60–69 . .	2	2	4	2	11	13	4	13	17
70–79 . .	–	–	–	2	5	7	2	5	7
Total . .	5	27	32	20	49	69	25	76	101

Table 2 and Fig. 2 record the severity of the obesity in the obese group, and show that the condition tended to be more severe in the juvenile obese group than in the adult obese group.

It was not possible to discover the age at onset of the obesity in all the relatives, but the impression gained from those who could remember was that the obese husbands and wives of the obese group tended to become obese after marriage, and that the obese daughters of obese women tended to become obese at the same age as their mothers. There were, however, exceptions to this and one case was seen in which obesity developed rapidly in both mother and son simultaneously.

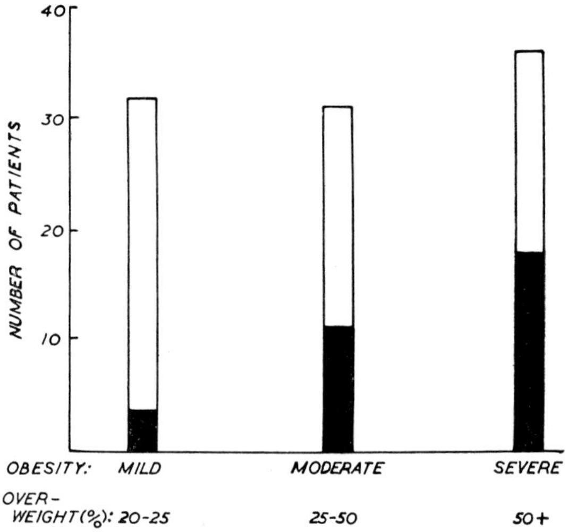

FIG. 2.—Histogram showing proportion of juvenile-type obesity in 101 obese patients. ■ Juvenile obese. □ Adult obese.

TABLE 2

SEVERITY OF OBESITY IN 101 OBESE PATIENTS

Severity	Juvenile Obese (32)				Adult Obese (69)				Totals (101)		
	M.	F.	T.	%	M.	F.	T.	%	M.	F.	T.
Mild (20%–25% overweight)	–	4	4	12	10	18	28	41	10	22	32
Moderate (25%–50% overweight)	3	8	11	35	7	14	21	30	10	22	32
Severe (more than 50% overweight)	2	15	17	53	3	17	20	29	5	32	37

Family History. Table 3 and Fig. 3 show the incidence of obesity in the families of the obese and normal groups. Obesity occurred more frequently in the near relatives of the juvenile obese group than in the adult obese group. In the normal group there was a lower incidence of obesity among all the relatives, and this was most marked in the father and spouse. Fifty per cent of the juvenile obese group had obese fathers compared with only 2% of the normal group, and 22% of the juvenile obese group were married to obese people compared with 4% of the normal group.

Influence of Pregnancy and Menopause. It is well known that women tend to become obese during pregnancy and at the menopause and that those who are already obese tend to become more obese at these times (Gurney, 1936; Greene, 1939; Sheldon, 1949; Richardson, 1952). It has also been observed (Sheldon, 1949; Richardson, 1952) that women who were overweight at marriage were more likely to gain excessive weight due to deposition of fat during pregnancy, than those whose weight was normal at marriage. It might therefore be expected that women with persistent juvenile obesity tend to become even more obese with pregnancy. The present findings do not appear to confirm this (Table 4). Only 44% of the juvenile obese group compared with 72% of the adult obese group and 53% of the normal group gained weight excessively in pregnancy, and afterwards had to wear clothes of a larger size. The numbers are small, but if the difference is real it does not necessarily conflict with the findings of Sheldon and Richardson. In a recent personal study of maternal obesity it was found that those who were overweight at marriage were prone to develop maternal obesity, but even more prone were those who had been overweight at some time before marriage and had reduced their weight. The difference was accounted for by those who had never tried to reduce their weight, among whom the incidence of maternal obesity was low. Although the exact age of onset of the obesity was not recorded, it is possible that these were cases of persistent juvenile obesity.

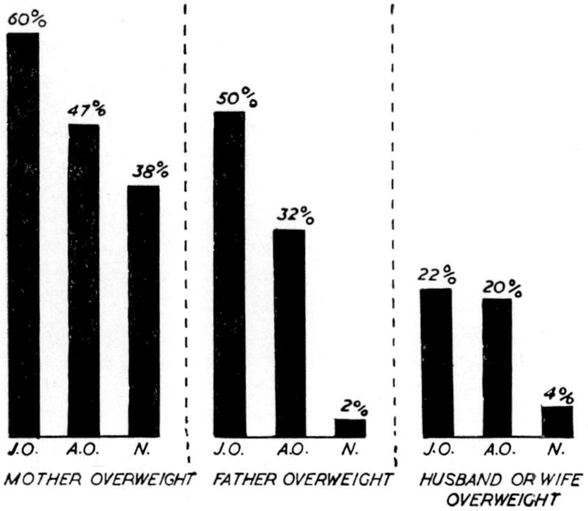

FIG. 3.—Incidence of obesity in parents and spouses of 101 obese patients and 50 patients of normal weight.
J.O.=Juvenile obese; A.O.=Adult obese; N.=Normal.

Only two women (7%) in the juvenile obese group had gained excessive weight at the menopause, compared with 12 (25%) of the adult obese group.

The figures suggest, therefore, that persistent juvenile obesity increases less during the physio-

TABLE 3

FAMILY HISTORY OF OBESITY IN 101 OBESE PATIENTS COMPARED WITH 50 PATIENTS OF NORMAL WEIGHT

Relative	Juvenile Obese (32)		Adult Obese (69)		Totals (101)		Normal Group (50)	
	No.	%	No.	%	No.	%	No.	%
Mother:								
Overweight	20	62	32	46	52	51	19	38
Normal	11	34	27	39	38	38	26	52
Father:								
Overweight	16	50	22	32	38	38	1	2
Normal	14	44	34	49	48	48	43	86
One or more sisters:								
Overweight	15	47	28	41	43	43	14	28
One or more brothers:								
Overweight	13	41	22	32	35	35	2	4
Husband or wife:								
Overweight	7	22	14	20	21	21	2	4
Normal	18	56	36	52	54	53	35	70

The apparent discrepancies in the figures are due to patients who could not remember their parents or who were not married.

TABLE 4

EXCESSIVE WEIGHT GAIN IN PREGNANCY IN 101 OBESE PATIENTS COMPARED WITH 50 PATIENTS OF NORMAL WEIGHT

	Parous Women in Groups: Juvenile Obese (18)		Adult Obese (36)		Normal (30)	
	No.	%	No.	%	No.	%
Excessive weight gain* in pregnancy	8	44	26	72	16	53
No excessive weight gain† in pregnancy	8	44	10	28	14	47
No recollection	2	12	—		—	
Weight became normal after pregnancy associated with excessive weight gain	0/8	0	2/26	8	16/16	100
Excessive weight gain at menopause	2/27	7	12/49	25	Not recorded	

* i.e. wore larger clothes after pregnancy. † i.e. wore same size of clothes after pregnancy.

logical changes of pregnancy and the menopause than other types of obesity.

Types of Appetite. Most authorities stress the alimentary cause of juvenile obesity. Østergaard (1954) found that none of his control group with large appetites gave the impression of eating urges comparable with those found in some of his obese group. Kerley and Lorenze (1941) state: 'These children are alike in possessing habitually insatiable appetites and a capacity for excessive food intake without resulting illness'. They also found that obese children had a preference for sweet and starchy foods.

In the juvenile obese group, 25 patients (78%) admitted to large appetites, and their replies were substantiated by further questions as to food intake. This compared with 28 (41%) of the adult obese group and 14 (28%) of the normal group. A preference for sweet, starchy and fried foods was common among the obese, but the normal subjects with large appetites usually ate bulky and savoury foods in preference to sweet, though they too mostly liked fried foods.

It is well recognized that psychological factors can play a large part in the aetiology of obesity. The frequency with which they are said to occur varies according to the worker, the criteria and the selection of patients. Bruch (1940), studying obese children in hospital practice, found that specific psychological factors were the most important in the production of obesity. Juel-Nielsen (1953) found psychological difficulties in nine out of 60 obese schoolchildren, and Iversen (1953) in 16 out of 40. Both these workers found that the psychological factors were less specific than in Bruch's series.

Psychiatric histories taken in the present series were no more detailed than those taken by any careful physician except that their possible connexion with appetite and food intake was carefully noted. Psychological factors that appeared to lead to increased food intake were found on the first interview in 17 (53%) of the juvenile obese group, 34 (49%) of the adult obese group and nine (18%) of the normal group. The patients were found to be of two main types:

(1) Those who normally reacted to worry and nervous tension by increase of food intake. This was by far the commonest type (Table 5). Probably most people, both normal and obese, react to stress by decrease of appetite and, if the stress is prolonged, by loss of weight. It is recognized, however, that some people react to mild and sometimes even to severe stress by increased food intake. Johnson (1947) quotes an interesting case of a thin husband and a plump wife submitted to the same psychological stress. The husband lost 13 lb. in weight and the wife gained 26 lb. before their worry ended. Freed (1947) asked 500 patients under treatment for obesity whether they ate more when nervous or worried; 370 (74%) answered 'yes'. The patients in the present series were asked the same question (Table 5). The incidence among the obese is much lower than in Freed's group, but it is nevertheless high, and is higher in the juvenile obese than in the other groups. Many patients admitted freely to this reaction and were well aware of it; others had not previously thought about it, but on being questioned they admitted that overeating was their usual reaction to stress. The overeating was usually non-specific, though in a few patients a specific craving for a particular food occurred and their descriptions of this sounded very much like the pica that is known to occur in pregnancy, and sometimes seemed to be associated with it.

TABLE 5

INFLUENCE OF WORRY AND PSYCHOLOGICAL STRESS ON APPETITE IN OBESE AND NORMAL PATIENTS

Effect of Stress on Appetite	Juvenile Obese (32)		Adult Obese (69)		Normal Group (50)	
	No.	%	No	%	No.	%
Increased	14	44	18	26	9	18
Decreased	8	25	20	29	31	62
Unaffected	10	32	31	45	10	20

M.J., aged 38 and 74% overweight, had been obese all her life and had increased markedly in weight during three pregnancies. Her father, mother, husband and daughter were all obese. Since childhood she had had a craving for milk chocolate which she tried to control. Normally she managed to restrict herself to ¼ lb. a week, but when worried or pregnant she could not pass a sweet shop without buying a bar and during these times ate at least ½ lb. every day.

It is interesting to note that the excessive eating reaction to stress was found in only 9 (18%) of the normal group.

(2) The second group were those in whom obesity developed or increased rapidly in association with a specific psychological trauma. Shorvon and Richardson (1949) described six such cases in adults. Østergaard (1954) describes obesity in children associated with a death in the family, separation of the parents or the birth of a baby. Three patients (9%) in the juvenile group and 13 (19%) in the adult group were of this type. It is probable that a

specific trauma of this kind is less likely to be recalled if it occurred in childhood than in adult life.

Results of Treatment

Bruch (1955) and Stuart (1955) found that obesity which had developed in childhood was particularly difficult to treat. The results of treatment in the obese group confirm these findings.

The criteria of success were:

(1) Poor. This group includes patients who failed to lose more than 30% of their excess weight during at least four months' treatment, and those who, within this time and before any success had been achieved, ceased to attend the clinic.

(2) Moderate. This group includes those who, during treatment lasting at least four months, lost more than 30% of their excess weight but who did not reduce their weight to within 20% of standard weight, or, in cases of mild obesity, to within 10% of standard weight.

(3) Good. This group includes all patients who reduced to within 10% of standard weight and all patients with moderate or severe obesity who reduced to within 20% of standard weight.

(4) Not yet known. This group includes all patients who had been under treatment for less than four months and who were still attending at the time of writing.

Most of the patients in groups (2) and (3) are still under treatment, and therefore it is hoped that the ultimate results will be better.

The results of treatment are shown in Table 6.

TABLE 6
RESULTS OF TREATMENT OF OBESITY

Result of Treatment	Juvenile Obese (32)		Adult Obese (69)	
	No.	%	No.	%
Poor	20	62	27	39
Moderate	8	25	17	25
Good	0	0	10	14
Not yet known	4	13	15	22

The incidence of failure is much higher in the juvenile type than in the adult type. So far, treatment has not resulted in complete success in a single case in the juvenile group. However, the fact that a quarter of them have lost more than 30% of their original excess weight is hopeful, since all these patients are still under treatment. The fact that, not only the incidence, but also the degree of success appears to be greater in the adult than in the juvenile group may be due to the higher incidence of severe obesity in the juvenile group and, therefore, the longer time necessary before complete success is achieved. Nearly all the patients in whom some success has been achieved are still attending the clinic at the time of writing.

A common difficulty in treating obesity is the appearance of new symptoms which appear to be related to the diet. Symptoms of hunger, mild depression and constipation are so common that they can be expected. *Severe reactions*, however, also occur, and, if they are not successfully treated, usually herald the failure of treatment, and the patient's failure to keep further appointments. Common among the more severe reactions are uncontrollable hunger and craving for food, severe depression, hysterical outbursts, flatulence, abdominal pain, an overwhelming preoccupation with bowel action, headaches, giddiness, faintness, nightmares and bizarre symptoms. Severe reactions occurred in nine patients (28%) of the juvenile group and in seven patients (10%) of the adult group who continued to attend the clinic (Table 7). It is probable that they were the cause of failure in some other patients to attend the clinic. When psychological complications were absent, severe reactions occurred in about a fifth of both juvenile and adult obese groups. When the complications were present, however, though severe reactions were twice as frequent in the juvenile obese, in the adult obese group they occurred only half as commonly as in the adult obese without psychological complications. The adult obese group with obvious psychological complications were more amenable to treatment than those without, whereas in the juvenile group the situation is reversed. Since these reactions often lead to failure to keep appointments, and the incidence of failure is also higher

TABLE 7
INCIDENCE OF SEVERE PSYCHOLOGICAL REACTIONS TO TREATMENT IN 101 OBESE PATIENTS

	Juvenile Obese			Adult Obese		
	No.	Reactions	%	No.	Reactions	%
All patients	32	9	28	69	7	10
With apparent psychological factors	17	6	35	34	2	6
Without apparent psychological factors	15	3	20	35	5	15

in the juvenile group, it seems likely that these reactions are an important cause of the higher incidence of failure in the treatment of the juvenile group.

Since most of these patients are still under treatment, it is probable that the ultimate incidence of severe reactions occurring among them will be higher than at present recorded.

Treated Juvenile Group. Of 21 adult patients who had been under medical care for obesity in childhood, 10 were still obese, and most of these were severely obese. Four were exceptionally tall and overweight, but not obese, and seven (five females and two males) were of normal height and within 20% of normal weight. The findings agree in the main with those of other workers (Bornhardt, 1936; Hering, 1938; Mossberg, 1948; Le Marquand, 1951; Haase and Hosenfeld, 1956).

Of the 10 patients who were still obese, four had lost weight during treatment in childhood, but none had become normal. The remaining six had not lost weight. Five of the group, as far as could be ascertained from the records, had failed to keep further appointments, presumably due to parental influence. The four patients who had grown exceptionally tall had not responded to treatment in childhood but all stated that they ceased to be obese during a later period of rapid growth, and in three of them this coincided with markedly increased activity.

Normal Juvenile Obese Group. In the 10 patients who had been under medical care for obesity in childhood and whose weight as adults was within 20% of normal weight there were several outstanding features:

(1) All these patients were at least 5% above standard weight, and none of them had ever been below it.

(2) With one exception they were all highly intelligent, compared with most other patients attending the hospital. Nine of the 10 (90%) had had a grammar school education. Among the 101 patients in the 'obese' group, only six (6%) had had a grammar school education and a large number appeared to be of very low intelligence. Only one of the 'treated juvenile obese' group who had remained obese had been to a grammar school.

Dorff (1935) found that obese children tended to be retarded. Bronstein, Wexler, Brown and Halpern (1942) found that the mean intelligence of obese children was higher than the mean of the general population, but found a tendency among them to be of either superior or retarded development. Østergaard (1954) found a normal distribution of intelligence among obese children and agreed with Bruch (1940) that serious obesity occurs less frequently under good social conditions than poor. In all the patients seen during the present investigation, there has been no case of severe obesity who had had a grammar school education, and, before the outstanding incidence of high intelligence in children who became normal was realized, a strong clinical impression was formed that the degree of success achieved in the treatment of adults was closely related to the intelligence of the patient.

(3) The mothers of these patients were intelligent and co-operative, and those who were themselves overweight (seven out of 10) made strong and successful, if sometimes intermittent, attempts to control their own weights.

(4) Weight reduction is associated with increased activity. In some cases increased activity followed weight reduction by dietary means. In others it seemed to occur spontaneously.

Discussion and Conclusion

Every case of obesity is 'exogenous' in that it is due to an intake of calories greater than the amount required for standard body weight. It can be argued that every case of obesity is 'endogenous' in that the cause for the excessive intake lies within the patient. Every case of obesity can be cured by reduction of caloric intake relative to the body's needs. Yet, in a very high proportion of cases, the condition seems untreatable by the methods in common use because the patient continues to eat in excess of the amount required for weight loss. Since this depends far more on the patient than on the doctor, a sense of hopelessness is easily induced in the minds of physicians attempting to treat the condition. Nevertheless its dangers make it important to increase our knowledge and to attempt to treat the condition whenever it is seen.

Approximately one third of all patients attending medical out-patients were found to be obese and, of these, approximately one third were found to be cases of persistent juvenile obesity. Thus more than 10% of medical out-patients had been obese from childhood. These patients did not on the whole appear to differ qualitatively from the other obese patients, but they tended to be more severely obese and a higher incidence of factors known to be associated with obesity was found among them, including large appetites, a family history of obesity and a tendency to eat more when nervous or worried.

Periods of endocrinological change, such as pregnancy and the menopause, appeared to have less influence on their weights than on those of the adult obese group.

The most marked difference between the two groups was in the results of treatment, which was much less successful in those whose obesity dated from childhood. This seemed to be at least partly due to the higher incidence of failure to keep appointments and of severe reactions to treatment in the juvenile obese group.

It is of interest that in the adult obese group treatment was more successful and the incidence of severe reactions was lower in those with obvious psychological factors complicating the obesity than in those who appeared normally adjusted. The reverse is the case in those whose obesity has been present since childhood.

In considering those patients who had suffered from juvenile obesity and who later became normal, the outstanding difference between them and those who remained obese lay in their intelligence. This finding confirmed a previous impression that intelligence is an important factor in the prevention of obesity and in the success of treatment. The present findings suggest that the usual methods of treatment are adequate for most intelligent obese children, but inadequate for the less intelligent, and it is felt that this is probably true for most adults too. The obese adult of low intelligence who has been obese since childhood or who has become addicted to food in later life is probably the most difficult of all patients to treat for obesity.

It is concluded that persistent juvenile obesity is an important cause of obesity in adult life and is, therefore, a potentially dangerous condition.

Juvenile obesity that persists into adult life tends to be more severe and more difficult to treat than obesity occurring in adult life.

Psychological factors play a larger part in persistent juvenile obesity than in adult obesity and are an important cause of failure of treatment.

The prognosis in juvenile obesity, and probably also in adult obesity, depends largely on the intelligence of the patient.

Every effort should be made to treat obesity when it first occurs.

Research should be directed particularly towards the treatment of obesity in patients of low intelligence.

I am grateful to Dr. Alexander Kahan, of St. James's Hospital, on whose patients this investigation was done. I should like to thank Dr. J. C. Burkinshaw and Mr. M. P. Curwen for information and advice, Mr. F. A. Tubbs, Librarian of St. Thomas's Hospital and his staff and Miss M. E. Charlton, Records Officer of St. James's Hospital for their assistance, Miss E. Mason for drawing the diagrams and Mrs. J. Smith for untiring secretarial assistance.

REFERENCES

Armstrong, D. B., Dublin, L. I., Wheatley, G. M. and Marks, H. H. (1951). *J. Amer. med. Ass.*, **147**, 1007.
Bornhardt, M. (1936). *Mschr. f. Kinderheilk*, **67**, 270.
Bronstein, I. P., Wexler, S., Brown, A. W. and Halpern, L. J. (1942). *Amer. J. Dis. Child.*, **63**, 238.
Bruch, H. (1939). *Amer. J. Dis. Child.*, **58**, 1001.
—— (1940). *Ibid.*, **59**, 739; **60**, 1082.
—— (1941). *J. Pediat.*, **19**, 365.
—— (1955). *Ann. N.Y. Acad. Sci.*, **63**, 68.
—— (1957). *The Importance of Overweight.* New York.
Dorff, G. B. (1935). *J. Pediat.*, **6**, 788.
Dublin, L. I. (1953). *Amer. J. publ. Hlth.*, **43**, 993.
Ellis, R. W. B. and Tallerman, K. H. (1934). *Lancet*, **2**, 615.
Evans, F. A. (1952). In Duncan, G. G. *Diseases of Metabolism*, 3rd ed. Philadelphia.
Freed, S. C. (1947). *J. Amer. med. Ass.*, **133**, 369.
Greene, J. A. (1939). *Ann. int. Med.*, **12**, 1797.
Gurney, R. (1936). *Arch. int. Med.*, **57**, 557.
Haase, K. E. and Hosenfeld, H. (1956). *Z. Kinderheilk*, **78**, 1.
Hansson, R., Brännäng, E. and Claesson, O. (1953). *Acta agric. scand.*, **3**, 61.
Hässler, —. (1935). *Mschr. f. Kinderheilk*, **63**, 404.
Hering, S. (1938). *Ibid.*, **73**, 11.
Iversen, T. (1953). *Acta Paediat.*, **42**, 8.
Johnson, W. M. (1947). *J. Amer. med. Ass.*, **133**, 1238.
Johnson, M. L., Burke, B. S. and Mayer, J. (1956). *Amer. J. clin. Nutrit.*, **4**, 37.
Jolliffe, N. (1953). *Amer. J. publ. Hlth*, **43**, 989.
Juel-Nielsen, N. (1953). *Acta Paediat.*, **42**, 130.
Kemsley, W. F. F. (1952). *Ann. Eugen. Lond.*, **16**, 316.
Kennedy, G. C. (1951). *Proc. roy. Soc. Med.*, **44**, 899.
—— (1955). *Voeding*, **16**, 40.
Kerley, C. G. and Lorenze, E. J. (1941). *J. Pediat.*, **19**, 241.
Le Marquand, H. S. (1951). *Proc. roy. Soc. Med.*, **44**, 458, 952.
McCay, C. M., Maynard, L. A., Sperling, G. and Osgood, H. S. (1941). *J. Nutr.*, **21**, 45.
Marks, H. H. (1956). *Human Biology*, **28**, 217.
Mossberg, H. O. (1948). *Acta Paediat.*, **35**, Suppl. 2.
Østergaard, L. (1954). *Ibid.*, **43**, 507.
Richardson, J. S. (1952). *Lancet*, **1**, 525.
Sheldon, J. H. (1949). *Ibid.*, **2**, 869.
Shorvon, H. J. and Richardson, J. S. (1949). *Brit. Med. J.*, **2**, 951.
Sinclair, H. M. (1954). Oxford Meeting of the British Association.
Stuart, H. C. (1955). *Quart. Rev. Pediat.*, **10**, 31.

DIABETES INSIPIDUS FOLLOWING TUBERCULOUS MENINGITIS

BY

JOHN LORBER

From the Department of Child Health, University of Sheffield

(RECEIVED FOR PUBLICATION JANUARY 27, 1958)

In tuberculous meningitis the site of the maximal infection and of the most dense exudate is the basal cisterns, particularly the cisterna chiasmatis and the cisterna ambiens. This exudate may lead to obstruction of the cerebrospinal fluid pathways, which can be readily demonstrated by pneumo-encephalograms (Lorber, 1951). Calcification of this exudate occurs in a large proportion of children who recover from the disease and can be shown two or three years after the onset of the meningitis on radiographs of the skull (Lorber, 1952; Lorber, 1958). These lesions are in close proximity to the pituitary gland and the hypothalamic nuclei. They may lead to vascular thromboses and consequently to softening of the adjacent brain substance. Furthermore, the hypothalamic nuclei may suffer as a consequence of the variable degrees of hydrocephalus produced by the obstruction of the cerebrospinal fluid.

In view of these very common developments it would be reasonable to expect endocrine sequelae to result from a disturbance of the posterior pituitary-hypothalamic mechanism. Of the endocrine disorders originating in this area diabetes insipidus is one of the best recognized examples.

Nevertheless, although by now thousands of patients must have survived tuberculous meningitis, reports of diabetes insipidus occurring as a complication during or after this illness are very few indeed (Table 1) and none of the reports furnished adequate proof of a true diabetes insipidus. All the reported cases had polyuria and polydipsia, and it is possible that full proof of diabetes insipidus was established in some of them by appropriate endocrinological tests, but these were not published. This certainly applies to the patient of Hooft and van Winckel (1957) about whom Professor Hooft kindly supplied fuller details in a personal communication which fully established the diagnosis of true pitressin-sensitive diabetes insipidus. It is possible that the 11 cases briefly summarized in Table 1 are an incomplete list. The literature on tuberculous meningitis is so vast now that mention of some cases in papers not specifically dealing with endocrine sequelae or with follow-up studies may have escaped detection. The table does not include a few cases quoted by authors without details or quoting exact references. It is noteworthy that, with one exception (Acheson and Smith, 1958), none of the reported cases was in the British or American literature.

No case of diabetes insipidus has developed among 131 surviving children who were treated in the Children's Hospital, Sheffield, and who were followed for two to 10 years after their admission. We have, however, seen and investigated a child through the courtesy of Dr. J. S. Oldham, who referred him to us because of polyuria and polydipsia, and who was proved to have true diabetes insipidus.

Case History

R. was born on February 9, 1945, and was the oldest of three children. He weighed 7 lb. He contracted tuberculous meningitis in 1948 at the age of 3½ years and was treated with intramuscular and intrathecal streptomycin. The total duration of treatment was 75 days and during this time he received 40 intrathecal injections of 50 mg. each. Following this illness he was left with severe visual and hearing defects. He was almost blind in the left eye and had poor vision in his right eye. His left ear was almost deaf and his right ear was also affected. His mental development was normal and he attended ordinary schools, as no vacancy could be found for him in a school for partially-sighted children. His headmaster reported that in spite of his physical handicaps he successfully competed with his contemporaries in academic work and he would have been above the average but for his disabilities. According to the school records his height and weight were as follows:

Date	Age (yrs.)	Height (in.)	Weight (lb.)
4.10.51	6 8/12	42¼	43½
23.11.53	8 9/12	47	51
1.6.56	11 4/12	48	56

In February, 1957, at the age of 12 years, he was struck on the head by a football. He was dizzy, but was not

TABLE 1

REPORTED CASES OF PRESUMED DIABETES INSIPIDUS FOLLOWING TUBERCULOUS MENINGITIS

Author	Number of Cases	Age (years)	Onset related to Meningitis	Other neurological Defects	Other endocrine Defects	Proof of Diabetes Insipidus	Comments
Asperger (1948) . .	1	Child	? During meningitis	Multiple	—	Clinical only	Doubtful case
Pinna (1953)	1	8	During meningitis	Died	—	Clinical and necropsy	
Conese, Colonna and La Pesa (1954) . .	1	25	Soon after recovery	No details	—	Polyuria and polydipsia urine S.G. 1,002-4	Not proven
Kissel and Arnould (1954)	1	24	11m. after recovery	+	—	Polyuria	Recovery after air encephalogram
Inglessi (1954)	1	14	3 yr. after recovery	—	Sexual infantilism	Pitressin-sensitive Polyuria and polydipsia	
Riser, Geraud, Ribaut, Gleizes, Rascol and Saint Marc (1955) . .	1	24	During treatment	—	Schizoid	Clinical	Complete recovery after 2½ yr.
Post (1955)	1	Child	After recovery	No details	—	No details	
Castel-Branco (1956) . .	2	7	During meningitis	—	—	Pitressin-sensitive	Recovery after 2 yr.
		6	3 m. after onset	—	—	Clinical	Good response to cortisone
Hooft and van Winckel (1957)	1	6	4 m. after recovery	—	—	Proved by water restriction test* Pitressin-sensitive	
Acheson and Smith (1958)	1	10	62 m. after onset	None	Atrophy of left testis (normal puberty)	Pitressin-sensitive Extreme polyuria (S.G. 1,000-6) and polydipsia	Doing well on pitressin tannate (S.G. 1,018-24)

* Personal communication.

rendered unconscious. During the following month he complained of headaches of increasing frequency and severity, but vomited only once before his admission to the Staincliffe General Hospital, Dewsbury, on March 6, 1957. On admission there he was found to have meningism and bilateral optic atrophy. The cerebrospinal fluid contained 106 white cells/ml. with 98% lymphocytes, protein 170 mg. %, chlorides 730 mg.%, and sugar 25 mg. %. Acid and alcohol fast bacilli were seen in the deposit and were repeatedly found in the cerebrospinal fluid for nine days after admission. In due course tubercle bacilli were grown on culture and were recovered from inoculated guinea-pigs. His urine was persistently acid, had a specific gravity of 1,012 on two occasions, contained a trace of albumin and there were approximately 20 leucocytes per high power field in the deposit. Acid-alcohol fast bacilli were detected in several specimens of urine up to the end of April, 1957, and tubercle bacilli were cultured and recovered from inoculated guinea-pigs. The organism was resistant to 10 μg. and sensitive both to 30 μg. of streptomycin per ml., and to 5 μg. of isoniazid per ml. A radiograph of the chest showed no lesion. A radiograph of the abdomen showed a dense calcified shadow at the level of the third lumbar vertebra, near the midline, but sometimes to the left and at another time to the right side, indicating that it was a calcified mesenteric lymph-node. A radiograph of the skull (Fig. 1) showed a dense crescentic calcification just below the posterior clinoid process of the sella at and slightly to the right of the midline.

The blood picture and blood urea were normal.

A diagnosis of a relapse of tuberculous meningitis was clinically, radiologically and bacteriologically established. An additional diagnosis of renal tuberculosis was made and this was confirmed later by an intravenous pyelogram (Fig. 2) which showed considerable right-sided hydronephrosis with a dilated and rigid right ureter. Cystoscopy was performed later and this showed inflammation around the right ureteric orifice. The orifice was depressed and was reminiscent of a 'golf hole ureter'. Catheterization of the left ureteric orifice was easy, but the catheter could not be passed into the right orifice. The urine from the left kidney gave a negative culture for tubercle bacilli.

Treatment. The treatment given was as follows: 1 g. of intramuscular streptomycin daily; 100 mg. of intrathecal streptomycin daily for 30 injections, followed by five injections in the next 11 days and followed again by daily injections for a further 16 days. (Total: eight weeks). Isoniazid was given orally in doses of 300 mg. daily from admission, and was started intrathecally in doses of 15 mg. daily a week later and continued for 18 injections. A second course of intrathecal isoniazid of 23 injections was given during the second month of treatment. In addition 5 mg. of hydrocortisone was given intrathecally daily from admission for 18 days and again during the third month from May 21 till June 10 for 21 injections. On stopping this 15 mg. of prednisolone was given by mouth daily for 17 days, 10 mg. daily for eight days and 5 mg. daily for three days.

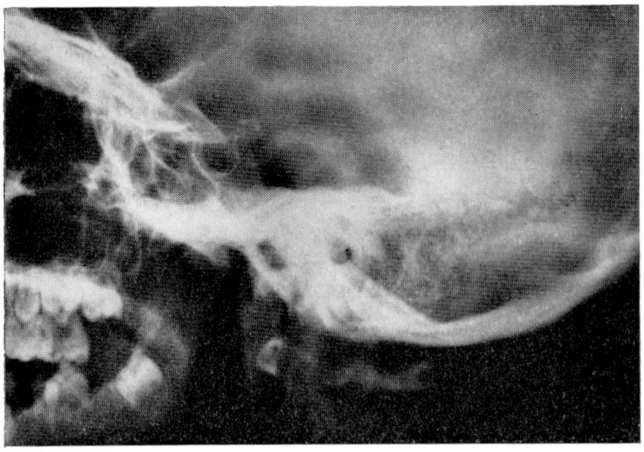

FIG. 1.—Radiograph of the skull showing calcification.

Progress. His condition slowly but steadily improved. He became more alert and lost his headaches. Occasional vomiting persisted for a few weeks but then ceased. The cerebrospinal fluid showed good improvement after the usual early fluctuations. At the end of May, 1957, it contained 11 white cells/c.mm., protein, 130 mg. % and sugar, 53 mg. %. By July 20, 1957, three and a half months after admission, the cerebrospinal fluid sugar had risen to 67 mg. % and he was thought to be well enough to go home for a holiday.

A single reading of the urinary specific gravity on July 11 had been only 1,002, and it was noted that he was drinking a great deal of water and had started to vomit water at night. He never vomited food. His urine was otherwise normal.

During his holiday at home his parents noticed increasing polydipsia and polyuria. His headaches returned and he now vomited frequently. He was readmitted to hospital on August 2, 1957, severely dehydrated. There was no deterioration in the neurological signs or in the cerebrospinal fluid, but he continued to vomit and developed a peripheral circulatory failure of such an extent that he required intravenous rehydration. During the next month he continued to drink large quantities of fluids averaging five to six pints daily and to pass even larger quantities of urine of the order of five to nine pints daily. The specific gravity was persistently very low but during a concentration test a single figure of 1,020 was obtained. At the same time the vomiting became incessant although findings in the cerebrospinal fluid remained fully satisfactory and there was no evidence of renal failure.

In view of these unfavourable developments he was transferred for further investigations to the Children's Hospital, Sheffield, on September 3, 1957. On admission his general condition was good. He was alert and interested, strikingly small for his age ($12\frac{1}{2}$ years) but not thin. His standing height was $49\frac{1}{2}$ in. (126 cm.). His other anthropometric measurements were as follows: sitting height, $29\frac{1}{2}$ in. (75 cm.); crown to umbilicus, $20\frac{1}{2}$ in. (51 cm.); umbilicus to sole, 29 in. (74 cm.); span, $51\frac{3}{4}$ in. (132 cm.). He weighed 60 lb. (27·5 kg.). Both his height and weight were below the third percentile for his age and corresponded to the 50 percentile of a boy of 7 years for height and 8 years for weight (Nelson, 1954). His penis and testicles were very small for his age and there were no secondary sexual characteristics.

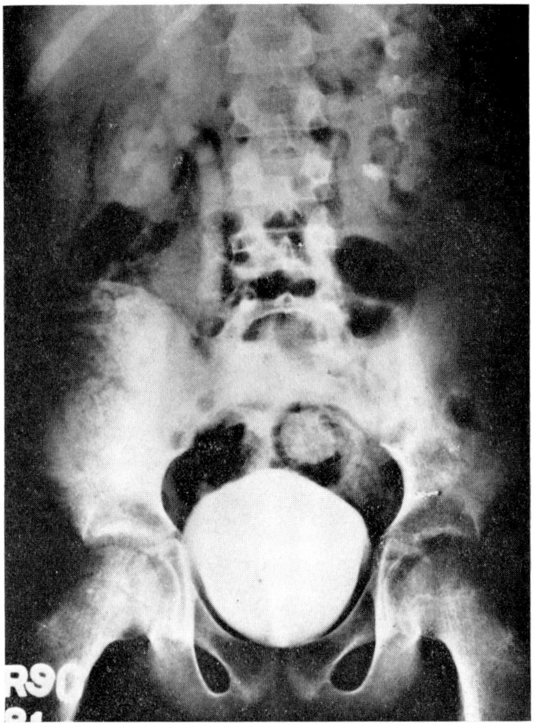

FIG. 2.—Intravenous pyelogram showing right-sided hydronephrosis.

The presence of bilateral optic atrophy and partial deafness was confirmed. Blood pressure was 120/80 mm. Hg. There was no meningism.

Investigations. The cerebrospinal fluid showed slight abnormalities consistent with recent tuberculous meningitis (43 white cells, protein 55 mg.%; sugar 41 mg.%). His urine was normal chemically and microscopically and no tubercle bacilli were seen, cultured, or recovered from inoculation of guinea-pigs. The specific gravity, however, was persistently between 1,000 and 1,005. There was no evidence of renal failure.

His visual acuity was 3/60 on the right and there was light perception only on the left. The visual fields were not constricted. Electric audiometry showed a hearing loss of 30 to 40 decibels between frequencies of 128 and 2,048 on the right ear and 75 decibels on the left ear. The resting record of the electroencephalogram was normal but over-breathing produced an abnormally big build-up with dysrhythmic changes suggesting minimal, focal residual damage.

A radiograph of the skull confirmed the presence of the suprasellar calcification. An intravenous pyelogram showed a normal kidney outline on the left, but there was no visible secretion on the right. His bone age was between 7 and 8 years.

The polydipsia, polyuria and vomiting continued. He woke several times in the night to pass large quantities of urine, but he responded well to a trial of posterior pituitary snuff. As his polyuria could not be explained on a renal basis, the test recommended by Carter and Robbins (1947) (and modified from that of Hickey and Hare (1944)) was performed on September 10, 1957. (Fig. 3).

The test was performed as follows: fluids were withheld for eight hours preceding the test and then 20 ml. of water per kg. of body weight were given by mouth over a period of one hour. Thirty minutes after the period of hydration was begun, an indwelling catheter was inserted. Urine specimens were collected in 15-minute periods and the urine flow was calculated in ml. per minute. After two control periods with an adequate urine flow, a solution of 2·5% NaCl was given intravenously at the rate of 0·25 ml. per kg. per minute for 45 minutes.

Using this test on normal individuals or in those with psychogenic polyuria there is a marked reduction of urine flow beginning after 15 minutes. In cases of diabetes insipidus there is no response.

In the case of R. the urinary output during the first two 15-minute control periods was 5 ml. and 3 ml. per minute respectively. During the intravenous infusion of 2·5% saline there was no significant reduction in the rate of urinary flow whilst at the conclusion of the infusion and immediately after the rate rose to 8 ml. per minute. The specific gravity of the urine remained very low. The test showed conclusively that this was not a case of psychogenic or habit polyuria but true diabetes insipidus. He was then given an intravenous injection of 0·1 ml. of pitressin to find out whether the diabetes was of renal or pituitary origin. There was an immediate and gross reduction in the urinary output to 0·1 ml. per minute. The volume of this sample was too small for the estimation of the specific gravity, but that of the next sample was 1,012 (Fig. 3), showing that the diabetes insipidus was pitressin-sensitive and of pituitary-hypothalamic origin.

Treatment of the Diabetes Insipidus. Treatment was begun with pituitary snuff starting at first with one capsule in the evening and after two doses was continued with one capsule morning and evening. On this regime his fluid intake and urinary output fell by about one half and varied between two and three pints per 24 hours. The specific gravity of the urine frequently rose to 1,012. This was not considered to be sufficiently good control, especially as he still woke up several times in the night, and therefore his treatment was changed to intramuscular pitressin tannate. The dose was gradually increased from 0·3 ml. on alternate days to 0·6 ml. daily. On the latter dose his fluid intake varied between 23 and 31 oz., and his urinary output between $15\frac{1}{2}$ to 20 oz. daily. The specific gravity of the urine rose to 1,020. He stopped vomiting.

He was discharged home on a maintenance dose of 0·6 ml. of pitressin tannate on alternate days.

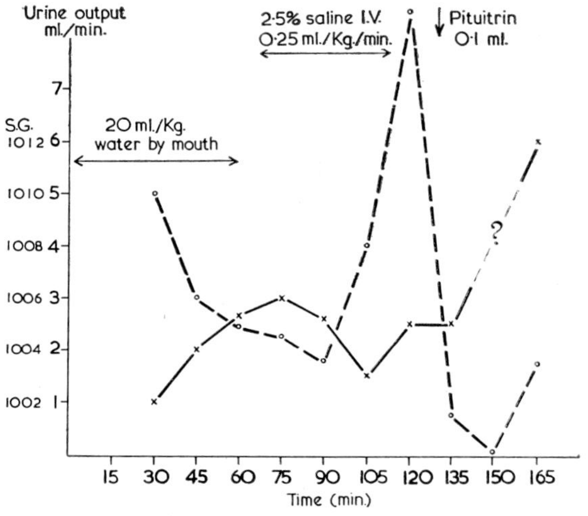

x — x = specific gravity. o — o = urine output.

FIG. 3.—Result of Carter-Robbins test in a case of tuberculous meningitis followed by diabetes insipidus (10.9.57).

Family History. As it was apparent that this boy not only had diabetes insipidus but might be a pituitary dwarf with sexual infantilism, it was necessary to go into the family history with regard to stature and sexual development.

Both his parents were small. The father was 5 ft. $6\frac{1}{2}$ in. tall (169 cm.) and his mother 4 ft. 11 in. (150 cm.). His sister who was two years younger was just taller than R. The two grandfathers were 5 ft. 5 in. (165 cm.) and 5 ft. 3 in. (160 cm.) and his grandmothers 5 ft. 4 in. (162 cm.) and 5 ft. (152 cm.) respectively. His maternal uncles and aunts were all of small build, but no measurements were available. The only available information regarding sexual development is that his mother's menarche was at 14 years and his maternal aunt's at 17 years.

Discussion

The diagnosis of diabetes insipidus of pituitary and hypothalamic origin has been established beyond doubt in our patient. He is now making good progress on pitressin treatment. It is not clear, however, whether the diabetes insipidus is a very late sequel of his first attack of meningitis which healed by meningeal calcification, or is the result of his second attack. In the earlier reported cases of diabetes insipidus the onset was either during the active phase of the meningitis or after recovery, but in none of them was it delayed by more than three years. Taking these features as guidance it seems likely that in our patient the second attack was the precipitating factor, although it is probable that the damage resulting from the first attack paved the way for the development of the disorder. That damage to the hypothalamic-pituitary mechanism did occur as a result of the first attack is undoubted, not only because of the presence of intracranial calcification immediately above the sella turcica, but more so because of the considerable retardation of the boy's growth and skeletal maturation, and by his apparent sexual infantilism. The last feature is not yet adequately proven as he is not quite 13 years old. Sexual infantilism and dwarfism was noted by Inglessi (1954) in a boy who was 14 years of age at the onset of the meningitis, and 17½ when the diabetes insipidus developed.

Another interesting feature of diabetes insipidus following tuberculous meningitis is that it is apparently capable of spontaneous recovery. Three of the reported cases recovered completely two to two and a half years after the onset, but in none of these was the diagnosis of a true diabetes insipidus adequately established.

Summary

This is a case of a boy who survived two attacks of tuberculous meningitis. The first attack occurred at the age of 3½ and he recovered with no deterioration in his good intelligence, but with grossly diminished vision and hearing. Subsequently his physical growth became very slow. At the age of 12 he had another attack of tuberculous meningitis. During the fifth month of treatment he developed the typical symptoms of diabetes insipidus. This diagnosis was established by salt and water loading tests. Treatment with pitressin led to satisfactory control of his polyuria and polydipsia. At the age of 13 he has shown no evidence of any secondary sexual characteristics.

The literature relating to diabetes insipidus following tuberculous meningitis is reviewed and its great rarity is noted.

I wish to thank Dr. J. S. Oldham for referring this patient to us, Professor C. Hooft and Dr. Honor V. Smith for details of similar cases under their care and Professor R. S. Illingworth for his criticism.

References

Acheson, R. M. and Smith, Honor V. (1958). *Quart. J. Med.*, **27**, 83.
Asperger, H. (1948). *Wien. klin. Wschr.*, **60**, 845.
Carter, A. C. and Robbins, J. (1947). *J. clin. Endocr.*, **7**, 753.
Castel-Branco, N. (1956). *Rev. ibér. Endocr.*, **3**, 422.
Conese, G., Colonna, L. and La Pesa, M. (1954). *Policlinico*, **61**, 37.
Hickey, R. C., and Hare, K. (1944). *J. clin. Invest.*, **23**, 768.
Hooft, C. and Winckel, H. van (1957). *Maandschr. Kindergeneesk*, **25**, 280.
Inglessi, E. (1954). *Arch. franç. Pédiat.*, **11**, 621.
Kissel, P. and Arnould, G. (1954). *Rev. neurol.*, **90**, 812.
Lorber, J. (1951). *Arch. Dis. Childh.*, **26**, 28.
—— (1952). *Ibid.*, **27**, 542.
—— (1958). *Amer. Rev. Tuberc.* In the Press.
Nelson, W. E. (1954). *Textbook of Pediatrics*, 6th ed. Philadelphia.
Pinna, P. (1953). *Ann. ital. Pediat.*, **6**, 365.
Post, E. (1955). *Medizinische*, **37**, 1299.
Riser, M., Geraud, J., Ribaut, L., Gleizes, L., Rascol, A. and Saint Marc. (1955). *Toulouse méd.*, **56**, 429.
Smith, H. V. Personal communication.

DIABETES MELLITUS IN A CHILD SHOWING FEATURES OF REFSUM'S SYNDROME

BY

J. B. HEYCOCK and J. WILSON

From the Sunderland Children's Hospital and the Department of Neurology and Neuro-Surgery, Royal Victoria Infirmary, Newcastle-upon-Tyne

(RECEIVED FOR PUBLICATION FEBRUARY 27, 1958)

This paper describes a diabetic child showing most of the features of a condition described by Refsum (Refsum, 1945, 1946*a* and 1946*b*, 1948, 1952; Refsum, Salomonsen and Skatvedt, 1949) under the name of heredopathia atactica polyneuritiformis. The malady is thought to be a recessive condition and is usually referred to as Refsum's syndrome. Only six other cases have so far been reported (Reese and Bareta, 1950; Clark and Critchley, 1951; Kjellson, 1953; Fleming, 1957; Olesen, 1957) and, as far as we are able to ascertain, no case has previously been described of this syndrome in association with diabetes mellitus. In view of the rarity of this association, we think that publication of this case is of interest.

Case Report

The patient, a girl, was first seen in the out-patient department in August, 1952, when she was 4½ years old. At that time she was the elder of two children, the other being a boy aged 7 months. Since then the mother has had a further child, a girl now aged 3 years. The patient had had anorexia for one month with weight loss, and also photophobia for a similar period. She had previously been quite well apart from an operation for intussusception at the age of 8 months. She was a thin girl, small in stature for her age. There was a left-sided concomitant squint and marked photophobia. Her urine was noted to contain sugar (2% Clinitest). She was admitted to the Sunderland Children's Hospital for further investigation, and particularly in order to determine whether she had diabetes mellitus. While in the ward she remained well and ate adequately. She had intermittent glycosuria, many specimens being free of sugar. During her stay in hospital she had marked photophobia and she was seen by Mr. A. Smith, consultant ophthalmic surgeon, Sunderland, who reported 'multiple epithelial erosions on both corneae'. It was thought that these could have been produced by sand when the child was playing on the beach one month previously. Her eyes were treated with 10% albucid drops and ung. atropine ½% twice daily. On this regimen the eyes became apparently normal within two weeks. A fasting blood sugar test was carried out, the result of which was 85 mg. per 100 ml.

She was discharged home but continued to lose weight and had persistent glycosuria; she was therefore readmitted to hospital in November, 1952. On this occasion her general condition was satisfactory, and her photophobia was not so obvious, but she had polyuria and persistent glycosuria. A blood sugar curve was typical of diabetes mellitus. The patient was given a 200 g. carbohydrate diet daily and soluble insulin was started in a dosage of two units twice daily. Following each injection, she became disorientated and drowsy. In view of this hypoglycaemic response an attempt was made to control her diabetes on diet alone but she continued to lose weight, and polyuria and polydipsia continued. Insulin was therefore recommenced and was now well tolerated; her diabetes appeared to be stabilized on a daily 200 g. carbohydrate diet with soluble insulin, seven units twice daily. She remained well on this regimen and, apart from a short admission to hospital for treatment of a left lower lobe pneumonia, she remained well though unusually small for her age until February, 1955.

In February, 1955, nearly three years after the start of her illness, the mother noted that the child was becoming increasingly deaf. She was seen by Mr. Rhys Evans, consultant ear, nose and throat surgeon, Sunderland, who reported that she had considerable, but not complete, bilateral hearing loss of perceptive type.

In April, 1956, nearly four years after the diabetes had been recognized, the mother noticed a progressively worsening tremor of both arms. Later titubation of the head began and in November, 1956, she began to be unsteady and to have difficulty in walking. She had to hold on to furniture to get round a room and her arms and legs became progressively weaker. She was seen by Dr. H. G. Miller, who diagnosed Refsum's syndrome and arranged admission to the Royal Victoria Infirmary, Newcastle-upon-Tyne.

On admission, aged 9 years, she was a pathetic figure, being totally deaf, dysarthric, small and underweight. She had an expressionless moon facies, and there was symmetrical wasting of the extremities of moderate degree. She had to be fed because of the severe tremor of her hands and preferred lying on pillows to sitting up. Her cardiovascular system was normal apart from a soft systolic murmur at the apex. Her skin was normal in texture and no rash or scaling was present. Abdominal palpation revealed enlargement of the liver about one and a half inches below the costal margin. Her ears showed a circular depression in the centre of both drums, possibly old healed perforations. Her intelligence was not tested formally but was probably in the low average group for her age and there was no dementia. Her neurological condition was dominated by severe deafness, gross intention tremor, dysmetria and titubation made worse by exertion or emotional disturbance. She could not walk unaided. Her speech was grossly dysarthric, slow, scanning and slurred. There was symmetrical weakness of her whole face and bilateral ptosis with slight weakness of external rectus movement and occasional rotatory nystagmus. The pupils responded sluggishly to light and accommodation. The fundi showed atypical retinitis pigmentosa with right optic atrophy. The arms and legs were symmetrically wasted both proximally and distally and there was slight wasting of the hypothenar eminences, but no fasciculation was observed and there was no muscle tenderness. All four limbs were weak and flaccid. In the arms triceps and supinator jerks could just be elicited, whilst the biceps jerks and tendon reflexes in the legs were absent. The plantar responses were flexor; the abdominal reflexes were symmetrically brisk. Intention tremor, dysmetria and dysdiadochokinesia were severe in the upper limbs and the legs were also very ataxic. It was difficult to be sure of her cooperation in the appraisal of sensation. She could recognize and differentiate between touch and prick, though in view of the docile way in which she submitted to venesection, but not to certain other procedures, we regarded pain sensation as possibly diminished. The vibration sense was impaired in the lower limbs.

Investigations. The urine showed marked glycosuria without albumen or cells. Paper chromatography confirmed the presence of glucose with normal amino-acid excretion and no evidence of indican or other indoles in the urine. Twenty-four-hour urinary 17-ketosteroid excretion was 1·7 mg.

Blood examinations showed: haemoglobin, 16·3 g./100 ml.; W.B.C. 6,250/cu. mm.; the peripheral blood film appeared normal. The erythrocyte sedimentation rate was 3 mm. in one hour. Glucose tolerance curve was typically diabetic with a fasting blood sugar of 160 mg./100 ml. Serum calcium, 9·0 mg./100 ml.; diffusible, 4·1 mg./100 ml. (Greenberg, Larson and Tufts); serum protein: total, 6·6 g./100 ml.; albumen, 4·9 g./100 ml.; globulin, 1·7 g./100 ml. (by difference); plasma phosphate, 3·4 mg. phosphorus/100 ml.; plasma iron, 127 μg/100 ml.; serum cholesterol, 260 mg./100 ml.; plasma amino acid, 3·3 mg. α amino acid nitrogen/100 ml.; plasma bilirubin, total, 0·2 mg./100 ml.—directly reacting absent; zinc sulphate turbidity, 2 units; thymol turbidity, 3 units; thymol flocculation, 0; cephalin cholesterol, +; plasma alkaline phosphatase, 6·9 units (Jenner and Kay); plasma prothrombin, 80% of normal average (one-stage Quick technique). The Wassermann reaction was negative.

Radiographs of the skull, thoraco-lumbar spine and the hands and feet revealed no abnormality. An electrocardiogram showed abnormally flat and diphasic T waves; Q-T at upper limit of normal. Audiometry showed severe inner-ear deafness (70 decibels at 1,024 cycles per second). Vestibular function was normal as judged by caloric testing at 44 degree F. Perimetry was attempted, but the patient was not sufficiently cooperative to make the result worth while. Lumbar puncture (twice): normal pressure, 1 lymphocyte per cu. mm.; protein, on the first occasion, 120 mg./100 ml., on the second, 95 mg./100 ml.

On this admission the patient's diabetes was treated by giving a free diet and increasing her soluble insulin to 20 units twice a day. Several weeks later because of several hypoglycaemic attacks insulin was reduced to 15 units twice a day. At the present time the child is at home and is walking short distances with support.

The Family History. The paternal grandmother died of diabetes mellitus. There was no history of nervous disease in the two preceding generations. The parents and two siblings were clinically normal. The optic fundi, electrocardiograms and urine of the two siblings were also normal.

Discussion

The salient features of heredopathia atactica polyneuritiformis (Refsum, 1952) are (1) Atypical retinitis pigmentosa with hemeralopia and concentric constriction of visual fields. (2) A picture of chronic polyneuritis with progressive pareses of distal parts of limbs and decreased or absent reflexes. (3) Ataxia and other cerebellar signs. (4) Increased cerebrospinal fluid protein with normal cell count. (5) In some cases abnormal electrocardiographic changes have been noted, in others neurogenic hearing loss, pupillary abnormalities and skin changes resembling ichthyosis.

The condition of the child we have described resembles Refsum's syndrome although there are several unusual characteristics, chiefly, photophobia rather than night blindness and the presence of dysarthria. We have not demonstrated parental consanguinity or a hereditary tendency, but this does not exclude recessive inheritance; on the other hand the disease may be the result of a mutation.

Differential Diagnosis. The differential diagnosis from such diseases as toxoplasmosis and neurosyphilis presents no real difficulty.

Other heredo-familial degenerations, Friedreich's disease, cerebellar ataxias, familial spastic paraplegia, bear some resemblance to the case described but features such as nerve deafness and retinitis pigmentosa are not usually present in these conditions.

Peroneal muscular atrophy (Charcot-Marie-Tooth) and hypertrophic neuritis (Dejerine and Sottas) were deemed unlikely on account of the gross ataxia and dysarthria.

As far as metabolic disorders were concerned, there was no evidence of nutritional deficiency in this child and there was no significant response to oral therapy with vitamin B complex. There was no abnormal amino aciduria; this would tend to exclude such conditions as hepatolenticular degeneration and the condition due to abnormal indole metabolism described by Baron, Dent, Harris, Hart and Jepson (1956).

In our patient the relationship between the diabetes mellitus and the degenerative condition of the central nervous system was obscure. The clinical picture was quite distinct from that of diabetic myelopathy (Garland and Taverner, 1953). Although the cerebrospinal fluid protein is elevated in both conditions, our patient's disease was insidiously progressive and quite unaffected by control of the diabetes. The family history suggests that the diabetes may have been independent.

There are many similarities between the degenerative conditions of the central nervous system in our patient and those of Friedreich's ataxia and other hereditary cerebellar ataxias and familial spastic paraplegia. It has been found that there is a higher incidence of diabetes in patients suffering from Friedreich's ataxia than in the comparable general population (Ashby and Tweedy, 1953). It now seems to be apparent that many of the heredo-degenerative diseases of the central nervous system are interrelated and that transitional cases occur. Refsum's syndrome may be another member of the hereditary ataxia group, along with Friedreich's ataxia, hereditary spastic paraplegia and peroneal muscular atrophy. It would therefore be of interest to know the incidence of diabetes mellitus in patients suffering from these degenerative conditions, and the incidence in members of affected families, as it might subsequently be possible, with adequate information, to demonstrate linkage or crossing-over between the gene or genes responsible for diabetes and those which produce the various hereditary ataxias.

Summary

A description is given of a child having many of the features of Refsum's syndrome together with diabetes mellitus.

The possible significance of the diabetes in this disease and other degenerative diseases of the central nervous system is briefly discussed.

We wish to thank Professor S. D. M. Court, Professor of Child Health, Durham University, and Dr. H. G. Miller, Department of Neurology and Neuro-surgery, Royal Victoria Infirmary, Newcastle-upon-Tyne, for their help and advice in this case and Dr. J. N. Walton for reading the manuscript.

References

Ashby, D. W. and Tweedy, P. S. (1953). *Brit. med. J.*, **1**, 1418.
Baron, D. N., Dent, C. E., Harris, H., Hart, E. W. and Jepson, J. B. (1956). *Lancet*, **2**, 421.
Clark, D. B. and Critchley, M. (1951). *Proc. roy. Soc. Med.*, **44**, 689.
Fleming, R. (1957). *Neurology*, **7**, 476.
Garland, H. and Taverner, D. (1953). *Brit. med. J.*, **1**, 1405.
Kjellson, L. (1953). *Nord. Med.*, **49**, 460.
Olesen, T. B. (1957). *Acta psychiat. neurol. scand.*, **32**, 83.
Reese, H. and Bareta, J. (1950). *J. Neuropath.*, **9**, 385.
Refsum, S. (1945). *Nord. Med.*, **28**, 2682.
—— (1946*a*). *Ibid.*, **29**, 617.
—— (1946*b*). *Acta psychiat. neurol. scand.*, Suppl. 38.
—— (1948). *Acta paediat. (Uppsala)*. Report on IXth Northern Pediatric Congress, 13.
—— (1952). *J. nerv. ment. Dis.*, **116**, 1046.
—— Salomonsen, L. and Skatvedt, M. (1949). *J. Pediat.*, **35**, 335.

THE POST-NATAL WEIGHT LOSS OF BABIES BORN TO DIABETIC AND NON-DIABETIC WOMEN

BY

JAMES W. FARQUHAR and STANLEY A. SKLAROFF

From the Departments of Child Life and Health and of Public Health and Social Medicine, University of Edinburgh, and the Simpson Memorial Maternity Pavilion, Royal Infirmary, Edinburgh

(RECEIVED FOR PUBLICATION FEBRUARY 26, 1958)

The fact that babies of diabetic women are heavier as a group than those born at the same gestational age to non-diabetic women has been attributed in part to foetal oedema. Apart from their oedematous appearance, however, such infants are said to lose more weight in the immediate newborn period than babies of healthy women, and it has been concluded that this is the result of water loss. The object of the present paper is to review the evidence for a significant difference in post-natal weight loss between the babies of diabetic and non-diabetic mothers, and to present the results of a comparative study of post-natal changes in weight with special reference to the type of 'normal' babies used as controls.

Evidence for Weight Loss

Oedema. The greater weight of babies born to diabetic women has been ascribed by White (1952) to fat, visceral enlargement and fluid retention. She considered that the babies were often oedematous, and she believed that a diuresis was responsible for the abnormal weight loss. This opinion is reflected in such well-known textbooks as those of Baird (1950), Grulee and Eley (1952), Nelson (1954), Johnstone and Kellar (1955), Ellis (1956), Price (1956) and Dunlop, Davidson and Alstead (1958). According to White the oedema may be made to pit on pressure, but Gellis (1954) described it as non-pitting. This difference of opinion is of the greatest importance because if White is correct then the diagnosis of oedema cannot be doubted. If the oedema cannot be demonstrated by pitting, however, then the diagnosis cannot be confirmed without such direct evidence as may be obtained by measurement of the body water or by careful records of body weight and fluid balance. As White and Gellis have probably shared a number of their cases and have discussed them together (Gellis, White and Pfeffer, 1949) the wide divergence of opinion between two such acknowledged authorities indicates that doubt exists about the presence of pitting oedema.

Diuresis. Although a number of papers mention the occurrence of a diuresis in such babies, no real proof of its occurrence has been provided, and no record of a fluid balance study has been found. In a previous paper Farquhar (1956) measured the 24-hour urine volumes of infants born to diabetic and to non-diabetic women. The former babies received no fluid during the first 72 hours, but each passed on average about 60 ml. more urine during the first 48 hours than the control babies who were fed from the first day of life. During the third day there was little difference between the urine volumes of the two groups. The groups were small and they were not comparable with regard to maturity or the route of delivery, but the results strongly suggested that babies of diabetic women pass rather more urine initially than normal babies. The difference in volume, however, was so small that it could not be responsible for much difference in weight loss between the groups.

Weight Loss. The studies of White (1952) and Cardell (1953) on the post-natal weight loss of infants born to diabetic mothers are well known. Although White has the larger series her analysis of the subject is less satisfactory than is that of Cardell. Her description of the amount of weight lost does not prove that this was abnormal. She did not define what she meant by weight loss and she provided no information about the control group other than that the mothers were non-diabetic women who had been delivered at the same hospital over the same time interval. She compared only the average weight loss of the two groups and even this was in terms of absolute weight and made no allowance for the greater birth weight or different maturity of the babies of diabetic women. The babies in Cardell's study were grouped first according to birth weight. He was then able to show that infants of diabetic women in his series lost significantly more weight (expressed as a percentage of birth weight) than 'control babies' of comparable birth weight. He failed to define what he meant by weight loss, although he clearly did not mean the weight loss over a fixed time interval. He gave no idea of the variability of weight loss. His control group did not match his diabetic group with regard to either maturity or the route of delivery. Neither White nor Cardell provided any detail about the technique of weighing, the environmental conditions under which their diabetic and control series were nursed or how and when they were fed.

The Problem. Because the evidence in favour of foetal oedema is inconclusive, it was decided to examine in greater detail the post-natal weight loss of babies born to diabetic and non-diabetic women.

Most of the infants in the Edinburgh series, like those delivered in the hospitals from which both White and Cardell have published their papers, have been delivered by Caesarean section. It was decided to compare the weight loss of the diabetic group not only with that of infants delivered spontaneously to non-diabetic women but also with that of babies born by Caesarean section to non-diabetic women.

The diabetic group has been subdivided into two according to the feeding history. Between the years 1948 and 1951 most of these babies were fed early because of a fear that they might suffer from hypoglycaemia. When it became recognized that this was not harmful and that inhalation occurred rather easily on the first and second days, feeding was delayed in those infants born during the years 1952 to 1955.

Consideration has been given to the comparability of the groups and also to the environmental conditions in which the infants were nursed.

Composition of Groups

A. Diabetic Mothers. The infants of diabetic mothers delivered by Caesarean section during the years 1948-55 are divided into two groups, one of which (A1) consists of 31 babies who were fed within the first 24 hours. The second group (A2) consists of 29 infants who were unfed until aged 72 hours for the reasons already given.

B. Non-Diabetic Mothers. The infants of non-diabetic mothers are divided into two groups, one of which (B1) consists of 60 babies born by Caesarean section to women who had not been in labour before operation. The second group (B2) consists of 60 babies born spontaneously by the vertex *per vaginam*. These two groups are matched with one another for maternal age and parity.

The mothers of infants in group B1 were delivered in the years 1948-49 and 1953-54. They had Caesarean sections performed because of placenta praevia in almost half the cases, because of pregnancy toxaemia in less than one sixth, and because of disproportion or previous uterine scar in the remainder. So that they might be compared in ways other than those mentioned in this paper, as many as possible of the cases were of 36 to 38 weeks' gestation.

Infants in both groups B1 and B2 were fed during the first 24 hours. Those in group B1 usually received a bottle, whereas those in group B2 were put to the breast. Infants were excluded from groups B1 and B2 if they died later during the newborn period or if they had lost blood, were pyrexial or had any congenital malformation, infection or gastro-intestinal disorder which was considered by the clinician to have a possible influence upon the weight behaviour.

Comparability of Groups

Sex, maternal age, social class (husband's occupation), parity, birth weight and maturity have all been shown to be relevant to birth weight. It was not known to what extent these would also affect weight loss, but since they were readily available they were all taken into account. It was clearly impossible to match the groups according to all these criteria, but where possible maternal age and parity were selected for matching.* These are accepted as being of fundamental importance in birth weight studies. The other characteristics are also presented for comparison.

A. Diabetic Groups. Because these groups formed the consecutive halves of a naturally occurring series no previous matching according to the above criteria was possible. The two groups are evenly balanced for foetal sex, and there is no marked difference in parity. Group A2 contains rather more babies in higher social classes than group A1 (Fig. 1). There are rather more of the heavier babies in group A1 than in A2 because of the greater variability of birth weight in A1. There is also greater variation in the maturity of infants in group A1, so that the group contains relatively larger numbers of more mature infants than does group A2. The lower birth weight and lesser maturity of infants in group A2 reflects the adoption of a more rigid policy about Caesarean section at the 36th-37th week which was adopted about 1951.

* No relationship between the infants' weight loss and maternal age or parity was found by Naish and Edwards (1952) in their study of normal babies. It was decided, however, that for the better comparison of these abnormal and normal groups these two factors should be taken into account.

B. Non-Diabetic Groups. The spontaneous deliveries (B2) were matched with the non-diabetic Caesarean deliveries (B1) for maternal age and parity (Fig. 1). The two groups are evenly balanced for foetal sex. Rather more of the infants in group B1 are of social classes IV and V. There is no marked difference in birth weight, but the babies in group B1 are distinctly less mature.

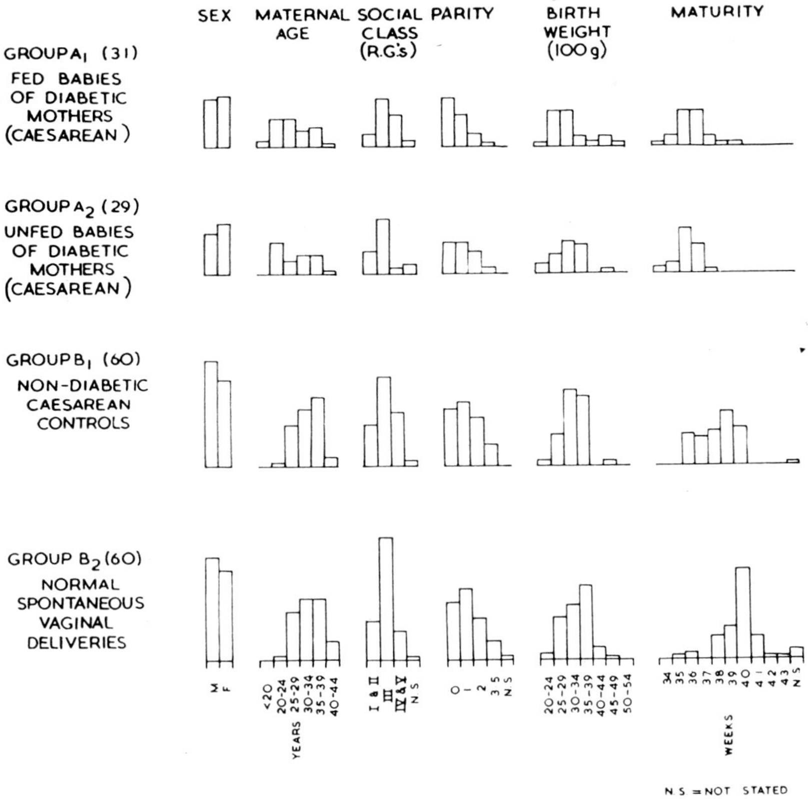

FIG. 1.—Comparison of the groups.

DIABETIC AND NON-DIABETIC GROUPS. As a result of the comparative infrequency with which Caesarean section is carried out prematurely in the non-diabetic woman, the number of babies available for inclusion in this group was rather limited, and it was found impossible to match them for maternal age and parity with either diabetic group. Older women make up a greater proportion of the non-diabetic Caesarean group (B1) than in either A1 or A2, but there is less difference in parity. Birth weight is less scattered in the non-diabetic Caesarean group (B1) but the maturity is more evenly spread over the period 36 to 40 weeks than in the diabetic groups. It may be seen from Fig. 1 that the infants of group B2 are clearly more mature than those of group B1, which in turn are more mature than those of groups A2 and A1.

Environmental Conditions During the Period of Measurement

The babies of the diabetic groups were nursed nude in premature rooms at a temperature of 80°F. Those in group A1 were moved to the main nursery after 2-3 days, and those in group A2 graduated there on the fourth or fifth day. Only a small proportion of the babies in group B1 (non-diabetic Caesarean controls) was admitted to the premature room and then usually for no longer than 24 hours. Most of them were retained in the main nursery at an environmental temperature of 70°F. and normal humidity. The babies of group B2 (spontaneous deliveries) were admitted to the main nursery from the labour ward. In the nursery all infants wore a napkin and gown. They were rolled in a cotton sheet and blanket and covered by one blanket and a light cotton coverlet.

Method of Weighing

All the babies have been weighed naked on Avery scales which are tested regularly and which are accurate to ¼ oz. (7·1 g.). They are weighed on arrival from the labour room and at the same hour each morning thereafter. The majority of babies in groups A1, A2 and B1 were born in the forenoon by elective Caesarean section. The beginning of the second day on the weight chart therefore corresponded to an age of about 22 hours. Unfortunately in group B2 the actual age at the beginning of the second day on the chart ranged from eight to about 30 hours. The retrospective nature of the study made this unavoidable. Weights were graphed on the infant charts and the plotting of the points was found to be accurate to about ½ oz. (14·2 g.) when compared with the written record. The weights of the infants in group B2 were recorded daily from birth. This applied also to the great majority of babies in group B1. In groups A1 and A2, however, the weight records during the first 48 hours were incomplete at times as some infants were nursed with the minimum of disturbance, and others were attached to experimental apparatus the efficiency of which would have been prejudiced by movement or disconnection.

Results

Criteria of Weight Changes. In defining what is meant by weight changes the features to be considered are the time interval over which the alteration occurs and the weight change in either absolute or relative terms. In this paper the relative weight loss each day is expressed as a percentage of birth weight.

Percentage Weight Loss in Relation to Birth Weight. The relationship between percentage weight loss and birth weight has been examined for several of the days after birth. No association was discovered on any of these days, and Fig. 2 illustrates this lack of

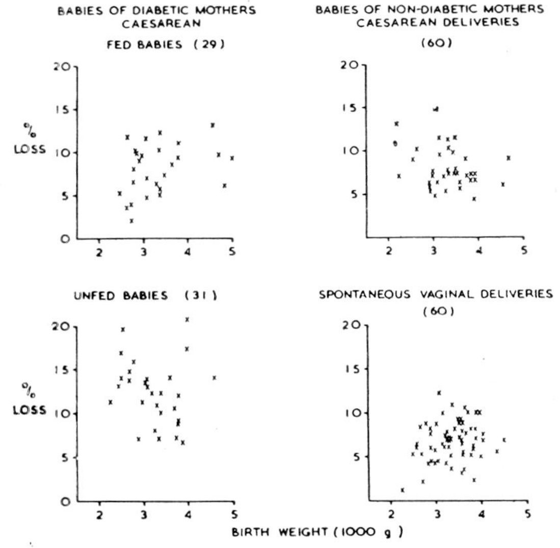

FIG. 2.—Post-natal weight loss on fourth day as a percentage of birth weight.

any relationship on the fourth day in all of the four groups. The variability of percentage weight loss changes with age. It is least at the third or fourth day after birth, and increases thereafter.

Method of Presentation. The individual weight record of each infant in the four groups has been studied and examples of the variability of individual

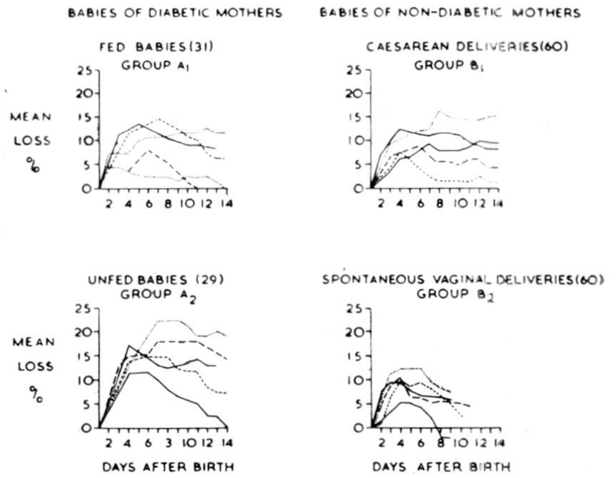

FIG. 3.—Examples of variation in post-natal weight loss in the four groups.

weight changes within each group are shown in Fig. 3. The main results, however, are presented as group averages with standard deviations (Fig. 4).

Group Differences in the Pattern of Weight Change (Fig. 4). (*a*) A significant difference in the pattern of weight change clearly exists between the two diabetic sub-groups. The unfed group (A2) loses more weight than the fed group (A1) and the rate of regain may be a little more rapid during the period up to 14 days.

(*b*) There were no significant differences in the trend of mean percentage weight changes between the fed diabetic Caesarean group (A1) and the non-diabetic Caesarean group (B1). The statistical significance of the differences between the means for each day after birth was assessed by Fisher's F test

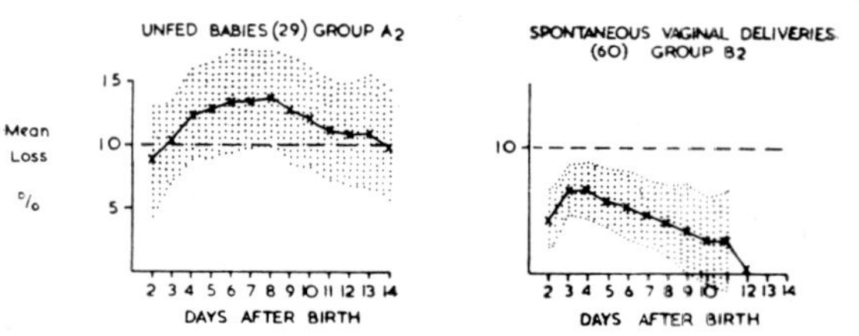

FIG. 4.—Group differences in the pattern of post-natal weight change. (Shading indicates $\pm$ one standard deviation about the mean.)

(Snedecor, 1956). In no case did the magnitude of the observed difference correspond with a probability of less than 1 in 5 ($p > \cdot 2$) of occurrence by chance in random sampling from a common population.

Although the percentage weight losses of the non-diabetic Caesarean group were slightly more variable than those of the fed diabetic group, there was no significant difference in their respective variability up to the 11th day as assessed by the F test.

(*c*) A significant difference in the pattern of weight change clearly exists between those of all the Caesarean groups (A1, A2 and B1) and that of the spontaneous group (B2). The latter loses less weight, and an earlier and more rapid regain of weight occurs.

Discussion

The newly born infant of the diabetic woman commonly has a puffy, sometimes even a bloated appearance which he loses during the first week of life. This puffiness has been attributed to oedema partly because it 'looks like oedema', partly because it changes so quickly, but mostly because pitting oedema has been demonstrated in some cases. The shedding of this fluid has been taken as the explanation of the apparent excessive post-natal weight loss. As we have stated already the babies were found by White (1952) to have pitting oedema, yet the same infants were found by Gellis (1954) to have non-pitting oedema. Neither author mentioned any exception. Oedema was accepted as the explanation of the appearance of such infants by the clinician in the Edinburgh series of over 100 cases. The baby charts appeared to show abnormal post-natal weight losses, but pitting oedema was rare and 'occult oedema' was assumed in the majority. In the second half of 1957 not one of 10 such babies showed convincing pitting oedema, although most of them were described as 'puffy' or 'flabby'. The largest of these weighed 5·0 kg. when delivered at the 36th week of gestation. He was stated by a midwife to have shown pitting oedema at birth, but when examined at three hours by one of us no evidence of it could be found. The greatest percentage weight loss of the 10 occurred in a baby who had shown no pitting oedema at birth and in whom even the characteristic puffy appearance was missing.

Direct measurement of the urine volume during the first 48 hours of life, however, showed that a group of babies born to diabetic mothers passed an average of only 60 ml. more urine than more mature infants born to non-diabetic mothers, and by the third day the urine volumes of the two groups were similar (Farquhar, 1956). Although this did in fact mean that the infants of the diabetic group passed three times as much urine on average as those of the non-diabetic group, such a difference would add comparatively little to the weight loss of infants in the diabetic group. Unless such babies lose relatively greater amounts of fluid from the skin, the lungs or the bowel, and no evidence of this has been reported, then some other explanation of their reported greater weight loss must be sought. In the first place the criteria and the consistency of weight loss should be examined.

Criteria and Consistency of Weight Loss. When it is remembered that the birth weights of infants born to diabetic women are often above average, it is clear that if their weight loss is to be compared in terms of absolute weight with that of infants born to non-diabetic women then the birth weights of the two groups must be given. This was not done by White (1952) who gave only the average absolute weight loss of the two groups. A proper comparison can be made only when the weight loss of each infant in the groups is expressed on each day as a percentage of birth weight. Although Cardell (1953) did express the weight losses of his diabetic and control groups in such relative terms he did not specify what he meant by weight loss. He probably did not take the amount of weight lost over a fixed time interval, such as from birth to the fourth day, and it may be assumed that he selected the maximum amount of weight lost irrespective of the time interval. A study of individual weight patterns in the present groups, however, has shown how difficult the selection of 'the point of maximum weight loss' may be. Quite commonly the regain of weight which follows the initial loss is interrupted by a further fall in weight which may be the result of inadequate feeding, infection or some unrecognized factor. The present paper shows the variability of individual weight patterns, but the means and standard deviations for each day and for each group have also been calculated and compared.

Comparability of Diabetic and Control Groups. The control cases recorded by both White and Cardell were born spontaneously and were usually some weeks more mature than their infants in the diabetic groups, most of which were delivered by Caesarean section. The possible influence of maternal age and parity was not considered in either. For these reasons their control cases were imperfect and it was decided that in the present investigation the diabetic groups would be compared with two groups of infants, one of which had been delivered spontaneously, and the other by Caesarean section, to non-diabetic mothers. Lack of knowledge about the exact age in hours of the present vaginal delivery group at the time of weighing probably makes very little difference to the group's general pattern of weight loss. The retrospective study of Naish and Edwards (1952) suffers from the same defect. The average weight loss increases to 6·7% of birth weight by the fourth day, and from then steady regain of weight occurs. The pattern is similar to that described by Gregory (1871), Holmes (1896), Griffith and Gittings (1907) and Kotz and Kaufman (1939) and it is quite different from that of any of the Caesarean section groups.

If the percentage of birth weight lost were to increase as birth weight increases then group comparison of relative loss would be possible only if the groups were evenly matched with regard to birth weight. For this reason the relationship of birth weight to the percentage of birth weight lost was studied for each of the present groups, and no correlation whatsoever was found. This finding opposes that of Griffiths and Gittings (1907) but confirms that of Naish and Edwards (1952) with regard to vaginal deliveries, and extends the observation to infants delivered by Caesarean section either to diabetic or non-diabetic mothers.

Delayed Feeding. The influence of delayed feeding upon the weight of the newborn baby has been studied by Griffith and Gittings (1907) and by Rott (1910). They demonstrated that the less fluid an infant receives during the first three days the more weight he will lose. The giving or withholding of extra fluid before lactation was established was believed to have been responsible for either an increase or a decrease respectively in the weight loss of infants studied by Naish and Edwards (1952) and the time of the first feed was found by Salber and Bradshaw (1954) to influence subsequent weight behaviour. The withholding of fluids until after 72 hours in group A2 was expected to influence weight loss, and the likelihood of this was increased by the high environmental temperatures in which these babies were nursed. This group did in fact lose more weight than group A1, the infants of which received fluids on the first day and were moved to a cooler nursery after 24 hours. Infants which have been dehydrated by simple water deprivation will regain weight quickly when fluids are given and this may explain why group A2 regained weight a little more rapidly than group A1.

Foetal Maturity. Although the greater weight loss and slower weight regain of group B1 when compared with group B2 is associated with the lesser maturity of group B1, the slightly greater maturity of group B1 when compared with group A2 is not associated with a similar difference in group pattern of weight loss. The small immature baby is said by Smith (1951) to lose a greater percentage of its birth weight than the mature infant, because the less mature the baby and the lower his birth weight the longer will feeding be deferred. The present study strongly suggests that deferred feeding and possibly environmental temperature exert a considerable influence on weight loss. There is no clear indication that differences in maturity alone explain the wide differences between the two non-diabetic groups, but if there is an association between maturity and the pattern of weight loss in the non-diabetic groups then this clearly does not extend to the diabetic groups.

Route of Delivery. The post-natal weight loss of infants delivered either spontaneously or by Caesarean section to non-diabetic women has been studied by Furuhjelm (1954). He subdivided his Caesarean section group into those women who had been in labour before operation and those who had not. When he compared his three groups he found that the mean weight loss of all three was equal by the third day, when it constituted about 7·2% of birth weight. This corresponds closely to the behaviour of the two non-diabetic groups in the present paper. After the third day Furuhjelm's vaginal deliveries no longer lost weight, but both Caesarean section groups continued to lose weight for two more days. The group of infants who had been born by Caesarean section to labouring women then began to gain weight parallel to the vaginal group. The group of infants who had been born by Caesarean section to non-labouring women, however, gained weight much more slowly. This also corresponds to the behaviour of the two closely matched non-diabetic groups in the present paper.

Conclusion

Had the present study been concerned only with a comparison of the post-natal weight loss of babies born by Caesarean section to diabetic women and those delivered spontaneously to non-diabetic women, then agreement would have been achieved with White and with Cardell. The conclusion that the greater weight loss of the diabetic group was the result of shedding oedema would probably have been reached. The inclusion of a non-diabetic Caesarean section group and the effort made to match this with the vaginal group and to consider the other factors previously mentioned have altered the picture completely. No evidence has been found to confirm the belief that infants born by Caesarean section to comparable groups of diabetic and non-diabetic mothers differ significantly in their post-natal weight patterns. It cannot be said therefore that the excessive weight loss of infants born to diabetic women is evidence of their having been oedematous.

No explanation is offered for the striking difference in post-natal weight between babies delivered by Caesarean section to non-labouring women and those delivered after normal labour. It is true that lactation is established more slowly in the woman delivered by Caesarean section, and during the waiting period complementary feeds may be kept small in order that the infant's hunger might act as a stimulus to the breast.

The process of labour was considered by Furuhjelm to be responsible for the differences in weight pattern between Caesarean and spontaneous groups, but the underlying condition for which Caesarean section is performed may be responsible. Furuhjelm failed to specify why the Caesarean sections were carried out on his patients, but if this were the explanation then, in the present study, diabetes mellitus would appear to have no greater influence on the post-natal weight of the foetus than placenta praevia, disproportion or previous uterine scar, which were the principal reasons for section in the control Caesarean group.

When ligature of the cord is delayed until the placenta is expelled the infant received considerably more placental blood. According to Zweifel (1878) such babies lose less weight post-natally than those whose cords were cut immediately after delivery. The cord is of course likely to be clamped more rapidly after delivery by Caesarean section than by the vagina, but Zweifel compared absolute weight losses, and his comparisons may not be valid.

Further studies will be required to explain this difference in weight behaviour, and in these the reason for Caesarean section, the nature of the labour, the time allowed to elapse before the cord is clamped, the maturity of the child and the details of feeding should be examined with greater care than has been possible in a retrospective study.

Summary

The abnormal heaviness of infants born to diabetic women has been ascribed in part to oedema.

The evidence in favour of the claims that because of this such infants lose more weight than normal babies in the post-natal period has been reviewed. Because of differences in the criteria of weight loss and in the management of the newborn, and because of the faulty construction of control groups, this evidence has been found inconclusive.

The weight loss of babies delivered by Caesarean section to diabetic women has been compared closely with that of babies similarly delivered to non-diabetic women and with babies born spontaneously to non-diabetic women.

When infants of diabetic women are subjected to prolonged fluid deprivation they lose more weight than when fluids are given early, and also lose more weight than infants of non-diabetic women by whichever route these have been delivered.

Infants of diabetic and non-diabetic women delivered by Caesarean section lose similar amounts of weight when nursed under similar conditions.

Infants delivered by Caesarean section to diabetic or non-diabetic women lose more weight over a longer period than infants delivered spontaneously to non-diabetic women. They also regain weight more slowly.

We wish to thank Professor R. W. B. Ellis for his constructive criticism of this paper, Miss A. Brown for assistance in the collection of the original data, Miss P. Johnston and Miss W. Laidlaw for computing, and Miss E. Meiklejohn for secretarial help.

References

Baird, D. (1950). *Combined Textbook of Obstetrics and Gynaecology*, 5th ed. Edinburgh.
Cardell, B. S. (1953). *J. Obstet. Gynaec. Brit. Emp.*, **60**, 834.
Dunlop, D. M., Davidson, S. and Alstead, S. (1958). *Textbook of Medical Treatment*, 7th ed. Edinburgh.
Ellis, R. W. B. (1956). *Disease in Infancy and Childhood*, 2nd ed. Edinburgh.
Farquhar, J. W. (1956). *Arch. Dis. Childh.*, **31**, 483.
Furuhjelm, U. (1954). *Études Néonatales*, **3**, 93.
Gellis, S. S. (1954). *Nelson's Textbook of Pediatrics*, 6th ed. London.
——, White, P. and Pfeffer, W. (1949). *New Engl. J. Med.*, **240**, 533.
Gregory, J. (1871). *Arch. Gynäk.*, **2**, 48.
Griffith, J. P. C. and Gittings, J. C. (1907). *Arch. Pediat.*, **24**, 321.
Grulee, C. G. and Eley, R. C. (1952). *The Child in Health and Disease*, 2nd ed. Baltimore.
Holmes, B. (1896). *Transactions of the Illinois Society for Child Study*, **2**, 201.
Johnstone, R. W. and Kellar, R. J. (1955). *A Textbook of Midwifery*, 16th ed. London.
Kotz, J. and Kaufman, M. S. (1939). *J. Amer. med. Ass.*, **113**, 2035.
Naish, F. C. and Edwards, P. W. (1952). *Arch. Dis. Childh.*, **27**, 445.
Nelson, W. E. (1954). *Textbook of Pediatrics*, 6th ed. London.
Price, F. W. (1956). *Price's Textbook of the Practice of Medicine*, 9th ed. London.
Rott, F. (1910). *Z. Kinderheilk*, **1**, 43.
Salber, E. and Bradshaw, E. (1954). *Hum. Biol.*, **26**, 156.
Smith, C. A. (1951). *The Physiology of the Newborn Infant*, 2nd ed. Oxford.
Snedecor, G. W. (1956). *Statistical Methods*, 5th ed. Ames, Iowa.
White, P. (1952). *Joslin's Treatment of Diabetes Mellitus*, 9th ed. London.
Zweifel, P. (1878). *Zbl. Gynäk.*, **2**, 1.

JAUNDICE AND INFANTILE DIARRHOEA

BY

R. G. F. PARKER

From the Bernhard Baron Institute, the London Hospital

(RECEIVED FOR PUBLICATION NOVEMBER 5, 1957)

Although it is recognized that infantile diarrhoea may sometimes be complicated by jaundice, the pathogenesis of this jaundice has not been fully elucidated. The only detailed account of the hepatic lesions in infantile diarrhoea is that of Wainwright (1950), who described in 11 of his 16 cases a form of 'hepatitis' characterized by periportal parenchymal necrosis, infiltration by polymorphonuclear leucocytes and mononuclear cells, proliferation of small bile ducts, inconstant fibrosis, periportal fatty change, distension of bile canaliculi in the centres of the lobules and congestion accompanied by varying degrees of centrilobular necrosis. In his remaining four cases there was centrilobular bile retention only. Wainwright noted a resemblance to experimental allyl formate poisoning and considered the hepatitis to be due to toxic parenchymal damage. Holland and O'Connor (1949) also attributed liver damage in infantile diarrhoea to hypothetical toxins, whilst Schlesinger, Payne and Burnard (1949) invoked nutritional deficiency.

The 13 cases which form the basis of this report came to necropsy in the Bernhard Baron Institute of the London Hospital in the years 1934 to 1954. They appear essentially similar to those described by Wainwright, although a different interpretation will be placed upon the pathogenesis of the hepatic lesions.

Description of Cases

In 9 of the 13 cases jaundice was noted during life or at necropsy. The remaining four cases were encountered unexpectedly when histological preparations were examined from 50 'control' cases of infantile diarrhoea without recorded jaundice which had come to necropsy in the years 1929 to 1956. Since in the same period there were many necropsies upon similar cases in which the liver was not examined microscopically, the true incidence of the lesions to be described could not be assessed. The hepatic lesions in the four cases without recorded jaundice were essentially similar, both qualitatively and quantitatively, to those found in cases with overt jaundice. The main features of all 13 cases are summarized in the Table.

Aetiology. The stools were examined bacteriologically in eight cases, no pathogenic organisms being found. In only the most recent case however was special search made for pathogenic strains of *Esch. coli*. The possibility of infection from a single source or of cross infection arose only in Cases 1, 2 and 8, all three of whom were in the same ward of the hospital at the same time. Two of these (Cases 1 and 8) developed both diarrhoea and jaundice whilst in hospital, having been admitted for other conditions. Case 2 was admitted with diarrhoea, jaundice appearing later. At this time there was in the same ward a child of 5 years with clinically typical virus hepatitis.

Clinical Features. It has already been noted that in four cases jaundice was not recorded during life or at necropsy. In a fifth it was present at necropsy although there was no mention of it in the clinical notes. In these five cases the duration of diarrhoea was from eight to 22 days, and in the remaining cases it was from nine to 28 days. In all but one of this latter group diarrhoea preceded jaundice by a period of seven to 16 days. In Case 12 there was vomiting for two days before jaundice was noted, but diarrhoea did not commence for another 10 days. The duration of jaundice was short (one to four days) in five cases. In the remaining three it was nine, 18 and 37 days respectively. It is clear however, from the presence of hepatic lesions without recorded jaundice and from lack of correlation between the duration of jaundice and the apparent age of the lesions as judged histologically (see Table), that jaundice was an unreliable indication of hepatic involvement in this series. The available clinical and laboratory data gave no clear indication of the nature of the jaundice, although an obstructive element was suggested in some cases. Death was not definitely attributable to hepatic failure in any case.

TABLE

CLINICAL AND PATHOLOGICAL FINDINGS IN 13 CASES OF INFANTILE DIARRHOEA WITH JAUNDICE

Case No.	Sex, Age (mths.)	Duration (Days) of Diarrhoea	Duration (Days) of Jaundice	Bile Thrombi	Proliferation of Bile Ducts	Infiltrate in Portal Tracts	Fibrosis	Fatty Change	Siderosis
1	F 5	9	2	Scanty	Slight	Scanty polymorphs	Absent	Marked	Slight
2	F 5	13	4	Scanty	Moderate	Many polymorphs	Slight	Marked	Absent
3	M 5	17	1	Scanty	Marked	Moderate polymorphs	Slight	Very marked	Absent
4	M 2½	8	Absent	Many	Slight	Slight polymorphs	Absent	Slight	Slight
5	M 4½	17	Absent	Scanty	Slight	Scanty polymorphs	Absent	Marked	Absent
6	M 8	13	Absent	Moderate	Moderate	Moderate polymorphs and lymphocytes	Slight	Marked	Absent
7	M 4½	10	P.M. only	Many	Moderate	Moderate polymorphs and lymphocytes	Slight	Moderate	Absent
8	F 8	28	18	Moderate	Probably slight	Scanty mononuclears	Moderate	Slight	Moderate
9	F 2	9	2	Many	Slight	Scanty mononuclears	Moderate	Slight	Moderate
10	F 2½	19	9	Moderate	Doubtful	Scanty mononuclears	Marked	Moderate	Slight
11	M 4	13	1	Many	Slight	Absent	Slight	Absent	Moderate
12	F 2½	27	37	Many	Absent	Absent	Absent	Absent	Marked
13	F 9	22	Absent	Moderate	Absent	Absent	Absent	Absent	Slight

Pathology. Focal ulceration of the gastro-intestinal tract was noted at necropsy in one case only. Histologically the stomach and intestines in the remainder showed only a mild or moderate non-specific acute inflammatory process, sometimes with marked oedema. Changes in organs other than the alimentary tract and liver were incidental or unimportant.

The hepatic lesions could be divided histologically into those (Cases 1 to 10, hereafter called Group I) in which there was, in addition to bile retention within the lobules, evidence of an inflammatory process in and around the portal tracts; and those (Cases 11 to 13, Group II) in which the appearances were those of obstructive jaundice without evidence of infection. This division (which is similar to that made by Wainwright, 1950) may not however be an absolute one, for, as the Table shows, there were borderline lesions (particularly in Case 4) in which biliary obstruction was marked and portal inflammation only slight.

GROUP I. In all 10 cases distended bile canaliculi at the centres of the lobules suggested obstruction to the flow of bile, slight in Cases 1, 2, 3 and 5, moderate or well-marked in the remainder (Fig. 1). In the first seven cases there was a polymorphonuclear leucocytic infiltration of the portal tracts, some of these cells being within the lumina of small bile ducts but the majority lying in the portal connective tissue or at the extreme periphery of the lobules (Fig. 2). A slight degree of periportal fibrosis was present in Cases 2 and 3 and also in Cases 6 and 7, where the presence of lymphocytes as well as polymorphonuclear leucocytes provided additional evidence of a relatively subacute inflammatory process. In Cases 8, 9 and 10 fibrosis was more pronounced, the inflammatory cell infiltrate was mild and polymorphonuclear leucocytes were virtually absent. Proliferation of small bile ducts was seen in all the more acute cases (Figs. 2 and 3), mitotic figures being usually present. Where periportal fibrosis was at all marked however it was difficult to distinguish such newly formed ducts from parenchymal trabeculae caught up in the fibrous tissue. Fatty change was present in all 10 cases, although in very varying degree. Except in the liver with most fat (Case 3) it was essentially periportal in distribution. There were no necrotic cells still *in situ* in the first nine cases. It was apparent however that, as a result of periportal inflammation, some cells had been lost from the extreme periphery of the lobules, and the presence of parenchymal mitotic figures in three cases was additional evidence of this. In Case 10 there was marked sinusoidal congestion at the centres of the lobules, and there appeared to be some loss of parenchymal cells associated with this. There was however no condensation of reticulin in the central zones, and it is probable that much of the apparent cell loss was a post-mortem artefact. Finally, slight to moderate haemosiderosis was found in five of the 10 cases, both parenchymal cells and reticulo-endothelial cells containing pigment.

GROUP II. In Cases 11, 12 and 13 inflammatory changes were absent and the most striking abnormality in the liver was moderate or pronounced

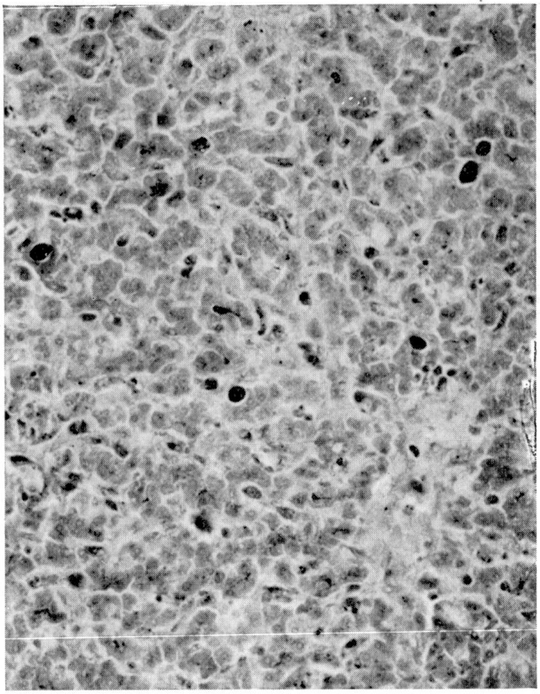

FIG. 1.—Case 4. A central vein is shown near bottom right-hand corner. There are several darkly stained bile thrombi, the majority in the centrilobular region. Haematoxylin and eosin. ×185.

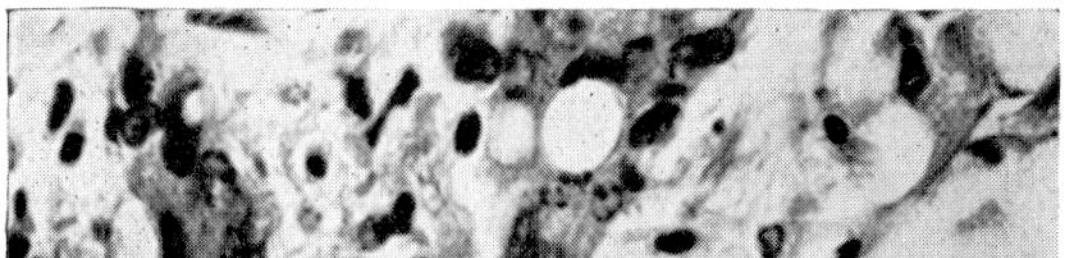

FIG. 2.—Case 2. Periportal fatty change, proliferation of small bile ducts and infiltration by polymorphonuclear neutrophils. Haematoxylin and eosin. ×490.

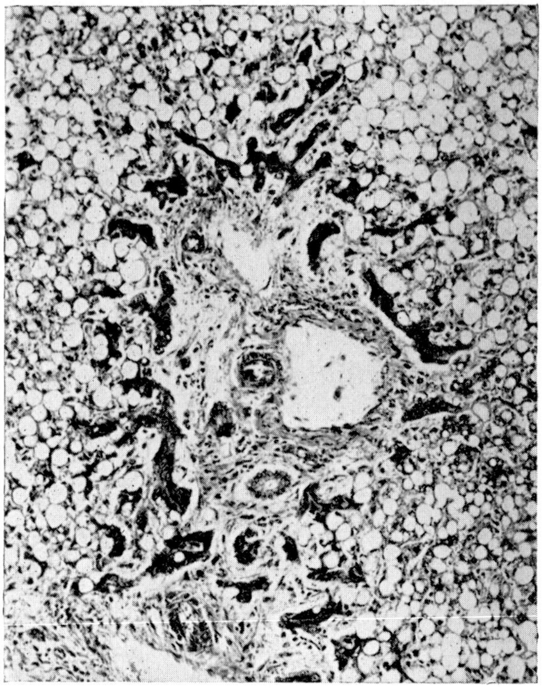

FIG. 3.—Case 6. Proliferation of small bile ducts around a portal tract and severe fatty change. Phosphotungstic acid-haematoxylin. ×120.

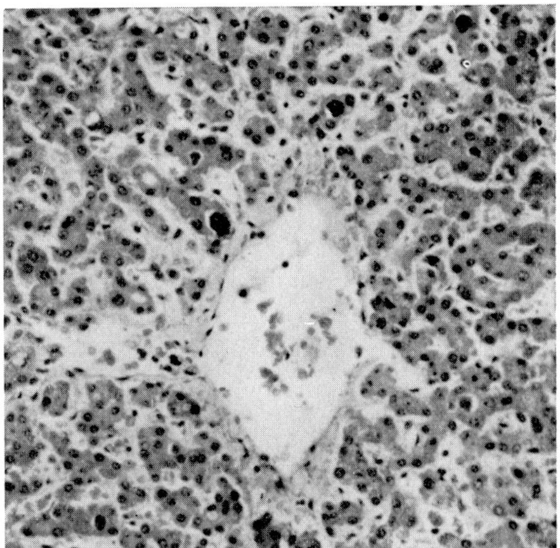

FIG. 4.—Case 11. Bile thrombi in central zone of lobule. Periodic acid-Schiff. ×185.

intralobular bile retention (Fig. 4). In Case 11 there was also slight proliferation of small bile ducts such as occurs in obstructive jaundice without accompanying inflammation, and the very slight degree of periportal fibrosis was no more than might be expected to accompany such bile duct proliferation. In Case 12 a few eosinophilic necrotic cells were present, but the appearances did not otherwise suggest virus hepatitis. Haemosiderosis was present in all three cases and occasional focal parenchymal necroses in the third.

Discussion

The pathogenesis of the hepatic lesions in these cases must be inferred very largely from the histological findings. Certain deductions of negative value may first be made. Thus although three cases (Cases 8, 9 and 11) had received blood transfusions, the microscopical features (many bile thrombi in all three, moderate periportal fibrosis in two and bile duct proliferation in the third) could hardly be attributed to haemolysis. Next, the only resemblance to neonatal hepatitis as described by Dible, Hunt, Pugh, Steingold and Wood (1954) was the presence of haemosiderosis in seven cases. A similar degree of iron pigmentation was noted in several cases of infantile diarrhoea without the hepatic lesions described above, and it was considered therefore to be a relatively non-specific finding. Nor was the picture that of virus hepatitis as seen in older subjects, the infiltration by polymorphonuclear leucocytes being particularly against this diagnosis.

Wainwright (1950) considered the essential hepatic lesion in most of his cases to be periportal parenchymal necrosis, the other changes being secondary. In all the lesions described here periportal necrosis was minimal, being readily accounted for by the inflammatory process in and around the portal tracts. It was this portal and periportal inflammation which, together perhaps with extra-hepatic biliary obstruction, appeared to be the essential hepatic abnormality in the first 10 cases in this series. Localization of the inflammation to the portal tracts might have been due to haematogenous infection, but the available evidence favoured rather an initial infection of the biliary tract, an ascending cholangitis. Thus inflammatory cells were sometimes present within the lumina of the smallest bile ducts and these same ducts showed unequivocal evidence of proliferation. Bile retention was usually in excess of what might have been expected from the amount of parenchymal damage present, and was therefore probably the result of biliary obstruction. The inflammation in and around the portal tracts probably contributed to this obstruction, but poor correlation between the intensity of the inflammation and of the bile retention suggested that the larger bile ducts may sometimes have been partly occluded. Extra-hepatic biliary obstruction was not found at necropsy in any case in this series or in that of Wainwright, and this author, whilst noting the resemblance of his lesions to cholangitis, considered the absence of demonstrable obstruction to be clear evidence that this was not their true nature. There are two objections to this conclusion. First it is doubtful whether the routine examination of the bile ducts performed at necropsy is adequate to exclude obstruction due to inflammatory swelling in the infant especially when, as the clinical evidence usually suggested in this series, the obstruction is incomplete. Secondly, whilst ascending cholangitis is very frequently associated with obstruction in adults, it would be wrong to assume that it cannot occur in the absence of obstruction in infants. Absence of inflammation in the extra-hepatic ducts would be important evidence against a non-obstructive ascending cholangitis. Wainwright failed to find such inflammation, but it is not clear how often the large bile ducts were examined in his cases. Unfortunately no sections of the extra-hepatic ducts were taken in the present series. In one section of the gall-bladder (Case 9) there was definite evidence of mild inflammation.

It is considered therefore that the hepatic lesion in the first 10 cases of this series was essentially a cholangitis associated with bile retention which may have been due in part to inflammatory obstruction of the extra-hepatic bile ducts, a true catarrhal jaundice in fact. Case 4, in which bile thrombi were numerous and inflammatory infiltration was slight, possibly bridged the gap between this group and the remaining three cases in the series (Group II) in which there was obstruction without evidence of intra-hepatic infection. Perhaps in these three cases the cholangitis had failed to reach the intra-hepatic ducts. On the other hand Case 12 was unusual clinically in that jaundice preceded the diarrhoea, and it may be therefore that a different pathological process was in operation. Virus hepatitis could not be ruled out with certainty in this case.

No pathogenic organisms were isolated in these cases and the nature of the infecting agent remained obscure. Despite a history of contact with virus hepatitis in three cases the histological evidence favoured a bacterial rather than a viral infection. On epidemiological grounds it seemed possible that at least two of these same three cases had been infected from a single source. But it would be wrong to assume from this that there exist distinct icterogenic strains among the causative organisms of infantile diarrhoea. Cholangitis is not so uncommon a complication of this condition that it would be highly unlikely to occur in three successive cases by chance. Further bacteriological and epidemiological evidence is necessary to settle this point.

Summary

Nine fatal cases of infantile diarrhoea with jaundice and four cases without recorded jaundice but with identical hepatic lesions are described.

In 10 of these cases evidence of bile retention was associated with an inflammatory process in the portal tracts which was considered to be a cholangitis. In the remaining three cases there was bile retention without inflammation.

It is suggested that all cases may represent an ascending infection of the bile ducts, sometimes stopping short of the smallest ducts and associated with varying degrees of biliary obstruction. A bacterial rather than a viral infection is favoured but the causative organism was not identified.

I wish to thank Professor D. S. Russell for her helpful criticism and Dr. K. H. Tallerman and Dr. R. H. Dobbs for permission to include cases under their care.

References

Dible, J. H., Hunt, W. E., Pugh, V. W., Steingold, L. and Wood, J. H. F. (1954). *J. Path. Bact.*, **67**, 195.
Holland, P. D. J. and O'Connor, M. H. (1949). *Irish J. med. Sci.* p. 261.
Schlesinger, B., Payne, W. W. and Burnard, E. D. (1949). *Arch. Dis. Childh.*, **24**, 15.
Wainwright, J. (1950). *Ibid.*, **25**, 286.

CONGENITAL SPHEROCYTOSIS IN INFANCY

BY

DAVID BURMAN

From the Paediatric Department, Charing Cross Hospital, London

(RECEIVED FOR PUBLICATION DECEMBER 12, 1957)

Neonatal jaundice and anaemia of infancy are both common diagnostic problems. Very rarely, both these symptoms may be due to congenital spherocytosis and, unless there is a known family history of the condition, their diagnosis may be very difficult. Difficulties in diagnosis were encountered in identical twins, whose case is reported here, and whose neonatal jaundice and subsequent anaemia were thought at first to be associated with prematurity. The unusual course of the anaemia (Fig. 1) subsequently revealed the correct diagnosis even in the absence of other affected members of the family.

The clinical features of these two cases, together with a further 41 previously reported cases occurring in the first year of life, are summarized later in Table 1. This table is analyzed in order to determine the characteristic features of congenital spherocytosis in infancy, and the management of these patients is discussed.

Case History

Female twins were born on March 22, 1956, to a multiparous woman after a 36-week normal pregnancy. Both were vertex presentations and the first weighed 4 lb. 5 oz. (1,970 g.) and the second weighed 3 lb. 12 oz.

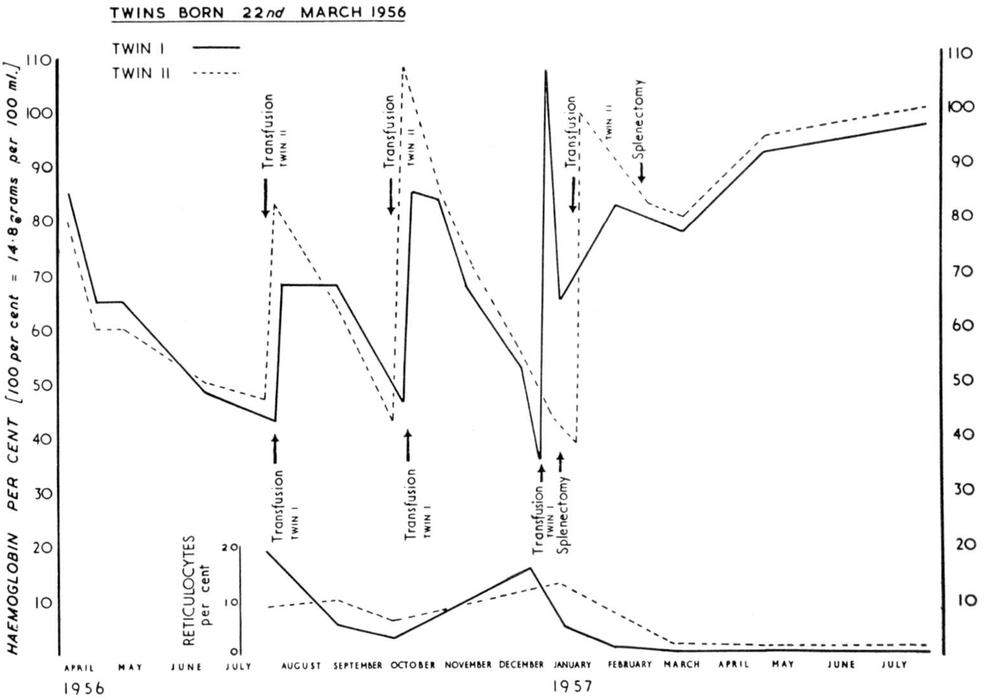

FIG. 1.—Course of anaemia in identical twins suffering from congenital spherocytosis, and progress after splenectomy.

(1,720 g.). Dissection of the placenta and membranes showed that they were monochorionic. The twins appeared identical except that there was webbing of the second and third toes on the left foot in Twin 1 only. The blood groups of both are Group O, Rh phenotype C C D ee (probable genotype CDe/CDe), M N, S+ve, P+ve, Lu−ve, K−ve, Le^a+ve, Le^b−ve, Fy^a−ve.

On March 26, both twins were noticed to be severely jaundiced and this continued until April 13. On April 5, the children appeared pale and the haemoglobin of Twin 1 was 85% (12·5 g. per 100 ml.) and of Twin 2 80% (11·8 g. per 100 ml.). By April 11 the haemoglobin had fallen to 70% (10·4 g. per 100 ml.) in both twins and on April 19 was 65% (9·6 g. per 100 ml.) and 60% (8·9 g. per 100 ml.) respectively. The twins were considered to have anaemia of prematurity associated with multiple birth. They were given ferrous sulphate from April 21, at first in doses of ¼ gr. (16 mg.) twice daily and from May 2 ½ gr. (32 mg.) was given twice daily. By June 19, Twin 1's haemoglobin had fallen to 48% (7·1 g. per 100 ml.) and Twin 2's to 50% (7·4 g. per 100 ml.) and both twins had palpable spleens. They were then given 3½ ml. of Imferon (Bengers) intramuscularly during the next month. On July 24, the twins' haemoglobin levels were 45% (6·7 g. per 100 ml.) and 42% (6·2 g. per 100 ml.) respectively.

The twins were admitted to hospital from July 24 until August 4. Investigations on Twin 1, who weighed 10 lb. 3 oz. (4,660 g.), showed haemoglobin, 43% (6·4 g. per 100 ml.); packed cell volume, 19·5%; mean corpuscular haemoglobin concentration, 32%; mean cell diameter (halometer) 6·8 microns; the red blood cells showed marked anisocytosis, poikilocytosis and polychromasia; reticulocytes, 19%; and normoblasts, 10 per 100 nucleated cells. The urine contained no bile salts and no excess urobilinogen. Two intramuscular injections of 1 ml. each of Imferon were given and on August 1 a blood transfusion of 160 ml. of whole blood. The haemoglobin on August 2 was 68% (10·1 g. per 100 ml.).

Investigations on Twin 2, who weighed 10 lb. 1 oz. (4,600 g.), showed haemoglobin, 47% (7 g. per 100 ml.); packed cell volume, 18%; mean corpuscular haemoglobin concentration, 34·4%; the red blood cells showed marked anisocytosis, poikilocytosis and polychromasia; reticulocytes, 9%; normoblasts, 10 per 100 nucleated cells; in a red cell fragility test haemolysis began at 0·48% saline and was complete at 0·32% saline; serum bilirubin was 0·5 mg. per 100 ml. The urine contained no bile salts and no excess urobilinogen. Twin 2 was given two injections of 1 ml. of Imferon and on August 1 a transfusion of 160 ml. of whole blood. On August 2, her haemoglobin was 83% (12·3 g. per 100 ml.).

On leaving hospital both twins were given ferrous sulphate gr. 1 (65 mg.) twice daily, but their spleens continued to be palpable and their haemoglobin fell progressively. They were re-admitted from October 3 to October 12. The haemoglobin level of Twin 1 was 45% (6·7 g. per 100 ml.); the red blood cells (2,530,000 per c.mm.) showed marked anisocytosis, slight poikilocytosis, slight polychromasia, some appeared macrocytic and there were a few spherocytes; the colour index was 0·88; packed cell volume, 21%; mean corpuscular haemoglobin concentration, 31%; reticulocytes, 3·1%; normoblasts, 1 per 100 nucleated cells; the direct Coombs test was negative; serum bilirubin, 1·6 mg. per 100 ml. The urine contained no excess urobilinogen; the stools contained no occult blood and the fat content was normal. On October 6, 210 ml. of whole blood were given and the haemoglobin on October 11 was 85% (12·6 g. per 100 ml.).

Re-investigation of Twin 2, who now weighed 13 lb. 2 oz. (6 kg.), showed a haemoglobin level of 43% (6·4 g. per 100 ml.); the red blood cells, 2,410,000 per c.mm., showed marked anisocytosis and poikilocytosis, moderate polychromasia and some cells appeared as polychromatic macrocytes; the colour index was 0·89; mean cell diameter, 7·0 microns; reticulocytes, 6·4%; normoblasts, 2·5 per 100 nucleated cells; a direct Coombs test was negative; serum bilirubin was 1·2 mg. per 100 ml.; the urine contained excess urobilinogen; stools contained no occult blood and the fat content was normal. On October 6, a transfusion of 220 ml. of whole blood was given and on October 11 the haemoglobin was 109% (16·1 g. per 100 ml.).

The haemoglobin fell progressively until the patients were admitted again on December 19. Both had palpable spleens and a further investigation of Twin 1, whose weight was 15 lb. 12 oz. (7·2 kg.), showed that the haemoglobin level was 53% (7·8 g. per 100 ml.); the red cells, 3,040,000 per c.mm., showed marked anisocytosis and polychromasia, moderate poikilocytosis and anisochromia and there were some spherocytes; the colour index was 0·87; reticulocytes, 16·7%; normoblasts, 1 per 100 nucleated cells; packed cell volume, 20%; mean corpuscular haemoglobin concentration, 39%; mean cell volume 66 cu. microns, mean cell diameter (halometer) 7·0 microns, and mean cell thickness 1·7 microns; no sickle cells were detected; in a red cell fragility test haemolysis commenced at 0·6% saline and was complete at 0·32% saline; a direct Coombs test was negative; serum bilirubin was 1·0 mg. per 100 ml.; no urobilinogen was detected in the urine; radiographs of the skull and long bones were normal; a test for occult blood was negative on three occasions. On December 20, Twin 1's haemoglobin was 26% (3·9 g. per 100 ml.) and she was transfused with the packed cells of 1 pint of blood. The haemoglobin rose to 108% (16 g. per 100 ml.), but fell to 65% (9·6 g. per 100 ml.) by January 8, 1957. On January 9, a splenectomy was performed by Mr. A. R. Makey under general anaesthesia. After operation the haemoglobin level gradually rose until the baby's discharge on January 25 when it was 76% (11·1 g. per 100 ml.).

The further investigation of Twin 2, who then weighed 15 lb. 3 oz. (6,940 g.), showed a haemoglobin level of 52% (7·7 g. per 100 ml.); the red cells, 2,480,000 per c.mm., showed marked anisocytosis and polychromasia, moderate anisochromia and slight poikilocytosis and there were some spherocytes present; the colour index was 0·91; reticulocytes, 15·2%; normoblasts, 1 per 200 nucleated cells; packed cell volume, 22%; mean corpuscular haemoglobin concentration, 35%, and the mean corpuscular volume 77 cμ; mean cell diameter (halometer), 7·0 microns, mean cell thickness, 2·0 microns; no sickle cells were detected; in a red cell fragility test haemolysis commenced at 0·56% saline and was complete at 0·32% saline; a direct Coombs test was negative; serum bilirubin was 0·8 mg. per 100 ml.; no urobilinogen was detected in the urine; radiographs of the skull and long bones were normal; a test for occult blood was negative on three occasions. On January 18 the haemoglobin level had fallen to 39% (5·8 g. per 100 ml.) and 300 ml. of packed blood cells were transfused prior to splenectomy. The patient developed an upper respiratory tract infection and splenectomy, together with the removal of an accessory spleen in the omentum by Mr. A. R. Makey, was postponed until February 25. Until the child's discharge from hospital the haemoglobin remained at about 80% (11·8 g. per 100 ml.).

On July 30, 1957, both twins were thriving, weighing 21 lb. 6 oz. (9,770 g.) and 20 lb. 1 oz. (9,170 g.) respectively, with a haemoglobin of 98-100% (14·5-14·8 g. per 100 ml.) and less than 1% reticulocytes. The osmotic fragility of the red cells of both twins commenced at 0·64% saline and was complete at 0·32% saline.

Pathology of Spleens. Dr. John Shore reported that the spleens of both twins were enlarged, measuring 7×4·5×3·5 cm. and 7·5×4·7×3·5 cm. respectively; with the latter specimen an accessory spleen, 0·8 cm. in diameter, was also received. The capsules were smooth and no abnormality was seen on the cut surfaces. The microscopical appearance of both spleens and of the accessory spleen were similar. The sinuses were filled with blood and appeared normal. A moderate amount of haemosiderin was present in macrophages in the pulp, most probably resulting from repeated blood transfusions. Scattered eosinophil and neutrophil polymorphonuclear leucocytes were also seen in the pulp. The malpighian follicles contained prominent germinal centres and also exhibited well-marked marginal zones of large and medium lymphocytes which lay between the lymphocytic mantle of many of the follicles and the pulp. Whilst not so prominent as those described in cases of hypersplenism by Leffler (1952), these zones were considerably wider than normal.

Family History. The family are all Irish and all the relatives in England were examined clinically and their haemoglobin and reticulocytes estimated and a film scanned for cells suggestive of spherocytes. The mother, father, second sister, a maternal aunt and a maternal uncle were all normal, but the oldest sister had an iron deficiency anaemia with a haemoglobin of 66% (9·8 g. per 100 ml.) which has since responded to oral ferrous sulphate. In October, 1957, a pair of binovular twins were born to the parents and these appeared clinically normal with normal haemoglobin, reticulocyte counts, red cell morphology and fragility.

Clinical Picture

Table 1 shows that a family history of congenital spherocytosis was present in 25 cases and absent in 15 cases. Thus, about 60% of the cases had a positive family history but this figure is probably too low, for the relatives of some of the patients in the table were not carefully investigated. This view is contrary to the earlier opinion expressed by Abt (1940) and David and Minot (1944) that a family history is rare if symptoms are present in infancy and indeed, only two cases (Cases 14 and 30) were diagnosed under the age of 3 months in the absence of such a history. The proportion of patients without a family history, however, is sufficiently high to make congenital spherocytosis preferable to hereditary spherocytosis as the name of the disease. The cases reported in this paper are the only identical twins in the table and the course of the disease in both was remarkably similar (Fig. 1). Debré, Lamy, Sée and Schrameck (1938) have reported identical twins both affected with congenital spherocytosis at the age of 4 years and Lesné, Launay and Hurez (1935) have described binovular twins both of whom were affected.

Of the 35 cases in the table whose sex is stated, 22 were boys and 13 girls, confirming the view that the disease is not sex linked.

Neonatal jaundice was present in 23 cases, but in Cases 1, 2 and 7 this could have been accounted for by prematurity. In Cases 32 and 38 jaundice was severe enough to produce kernikterus and in Cases 33, 38 and 43 it was sufficient to warrant one or more replacement transfusions. Turman, Vaughan and Shelley (1956) discovered another case with the clinical findings of kernikterus and a history of neonatal jaundice, when they investigated children attending a cerebral palsy clinic. A history of neonatal jaundice is also often obtained when cases are examined later in life (e.g. Campbell and Warner, 1926; Dawson, 1931; Bernard, Boiron and Estager, 1952). Neonatal jaundice due to congenital spherocytosis is accompanied by an erythroblastaemia and usually is present in the first few days after birth. In five cases, however, the jaundice did not appear until after the first week of life when haemolytic jaundice due to other causes is uncommon. Jaundice after the neonatal period was present in only six cases and was never a very prominent symptom. This fact supports the suggestion (Diamond, 1937) that the aphorism 'adults are more jaundiced than sick' should be revised to 'children, and particularly infants, are more sick than jaundiced' provided one excludes the neonatal period.

Anaemia was present in 38 cases of the 43 in the

SUMMARY OF PUBLISHED CASES OF CONGENITAL SPH

No.	Source	Sex	Age at Diagnosis	Family History	Neonatal Jaundice (Days)	Subsequent Ja
1	Present Cases	F	6 m.	No	4–22†	—
2	,,	F	6 m.	No	4–22†	—
3	Hawksley (1934)	F	2 d.	Yes	—	Slight from
4	Thompson (1936)	M	8 m.	—	—	Slight from
5	Diamond (1937)	F	4½ m.	No	—	Slight at 4
6	,,	M	6 m.	No	—	Slight at 5
7	Debré *et al.* (1938)	M	4 m.	Yes	Yes†	—
8	Josephs (1938)	—	5 m.	—	1–14	—
9	Abt (1940)	M	4 m.	No	—	Slight at 4
10	,,	F	1 y.	No	—	Slight at 1
11	,,	M	1 y.	No	Yes	Yes
12	Fallon (1943)	M	2 m.	Yes	—	Slight at 2
13	,,	F	4 m.	Yes	—	At 2 m.
14	,,	F	12 d.	No	From 12	—
15	David and Minot (1944)	M	4½ m.	No	—	—
16	Conrad and Schmidt (1946)	M	17 d.	Yes	From 15	—
17	Pinckney (1946)	M	6 m.	Yes	—	—
18	Macauley (1951	F	6 d.	Yes	—	—
19	Newns (1951	—	3½ m.	Yes	1–14	—
20	,,	F	7 m.	No	At 9	—
21	,,	F	1 m.	Yes	—	—
22	,,	M	1 y.	No	From 1	—
23	,,	—	1 y.	Yes	—	—
24	,,	—	10 m.	No	—	—
25	,,	—	1 y.	No	Yes	—
26	King and Shumacker (1952)	M	3 w.	Yes	Yes	—
27	,,	F	2 d.	Yes	On 2	—
28	,,	M	3 d.	Yes	From 2	—
29	,,	M	5 m.	Yes	—	—
30	,,	—	13 d.	No	From 8	—
31	Evans *et al.* (1954)	—	7 w.	Yes	—	—
32	Hindman (1954)	M	2 m.	Yes	Kernikterus 1–12	—
33	,,	F	3 d.	Yes	From 2‡	—
34	,,	—	3 d.	—	On 3	—
35	Edwards and Heaton (1955)	M	4 w	Yes	4 (w.)	—
36	Field and Tan (1955)	M	2 m.	Yes	—	—
37	,,	F	4 m.	Yes	—	—
38	Betke (1956)	M	4 d.	Yes	Kernikterus ‡ from 3	—
39	Stenstrom and Ford (1956)	M	—	Yes	Yes	—
40	,,	M	—	Yes	Yes	—
41	Robinson (1957)	M	3 m.	No	—	—
42	Shapiro *et al.* (1957)	M	2 d.	Yes	—	—
43	Smith and Franklin (1957)	M	3 d.	Yes	From 2*	—

The spleen was not palpable in Cases 19, 32, 37 and 42. * Exchange transfusions on 3rd and 4th days. † Prematu

table. In a further three, splenectomy was performed in the first 15 days, and in another at 10 weeks. The remaining case (Case 43) received two replacement transfusions on the third and fourth day of life, and did not develop anaemia in the next four months. Anaemia therefore appears to be a universal symptom of congenital spherocytosis presenting in the first year of life unless splenectomy or replacement transfusions have been performed for neonatal jaundice. Many cases, however, show no symptoms at all in infancy and Lappin (1956) reports two children of a family known to suffer from congenital spherocytosis, who have had spherocytosis and increased red cell fragility since birth but who have no enlargement of the spleen and no symptoms. The anaemia tends to be severe and many of the cases have had repeated blood transfusions in the first few months of life in a similar manner to the twins described here (Fig. 1). The anaemia may commence at any time during the first year but in the first week the haemoglobin level tended to be normal in the cases investigated, although several cases were thought to have been pale at or soon after birth.

Though the information is not included in the table itself the spleen was enlarged in 36 of the 40 cases where the state of the spleen was described. Thus in infants, as well as in later life, it is uncommon to find the spleen impalpable (Dacie, 1954a).

The characteristic features of the blood examination are reticulocytosis, which was observed in 20 cases, and the presence of spherocytes (not detailed in the table) in 26 cases. In many cases the

S DIAGNOSED DURING THE FIRST YEAR OF LIFE

emia Observed ge)	Highest Recorded Reticulocyte Level (%)	Osmotic Fragility	Splenectomy (Age)	Follow-up and Comments
w.	19·0	Increased at 9 m.	9 m.	Thriving, 19 m.
w.	16·7	Normal at 4 m.; increased at 9 m.	11 m.	Thriving, 19 m.
w.	13·4	Increased at 2 d.	—	Diagnosed by increased fragility before symptoms appeared.
m.	10·0	Increased at 8 m.	—	—
½ m.	31·0	Increased at 4½ m.	4½ m.	Thriving, 4 y. (Diamond, 1938.)
½ m.	80·0	Increased at 6 m.	—	Died before treatment.
m.	12·0	—	—	Died of otitis, 4 m.
m.	15·0	—	—	—
m.	35·0	Normal at 4 m.	-	Thriving, 14 m. without splenectomy
y.	25·0	Increased at 1 y.	15 m.	Thriving, 3 y.
m.	34·0	Normal at 1 y.	2½ y.	Thriving, 4½ y.
m.	11·0	Normal at 2 m.; increased at 2½ y.	2½ y.	—
m.	—	Increased at 4 m.	22 m.	Complete recovery.
d.	—	—	2 m.	Recovery not complete; 4 transfusions before 2 m.
m.	32·0	Normal at 4½ m.	5 m.	Thriving, 8 m.
d.	60·0	Increased at 17 d.	2½ m.	Thriving, 5 m.
m.	30·0	Increased at 6 m.	7 m.	—
d.	5·0	Increased on 6th d.	—	2 transfusions before 6 w.
w.	—	Increased	—	—
d.	—	Normal in 1st y.; increased at 8 y.	10 m.	Thriving, 7 y. after splenectomy.
w.	—	Slightly increased	2 m.	Died bronchopneumonia and suprarenal haemorrhage, 3½ m.
d.	—	Normal at birth; increased later	3½ y	—
y.	—	Increased at 1 y.	—	No symptoms.
m.	—	Increased at 10 m.	—	—
y.	—	—	—	—
w.	—	Increased at 3 w.	4 w.	Meningococcal meningitis, 12 m.
w.	—	Increased	3 w.	Meningitis, 6 m.
.	—	Increased	2 w.	Died, meningococcal septicaemia, 8½ m.
m.	—	Increased at 5 m.	6 m.	*H. influenzae* meningitis, 3½ y.
-	—	Increased	2½ m.	Died, septicaemia, 3½ m.
w.	—	—	9 w.	Meningococcal meningitis 6 m. after splenectomy.
d.	5·8	Increased at 2 m.	2 m.	At 2 y. has permanent neurological damage due to kernikterus.
.	—	—	5 d.	Thriving, 1 y.
.	—	—	3 d.	—
m.	—	Increased at 1 m.	1 m.	Thriving, 7 y.
m.	—	Increased at 2 m.	—	Unable walk at 2 y. No treatment.
m.	—	—	—	—
w.	17·0	Increased at 4 d.	—	Anaemia but no jaundice at 4 m.
h	—	Increased	16 m.	—
h	—	—	11 m.	—
w.	8·8	Normal at 4 m.; increased at 5 m.	7 m.	Pneumococcal meningitis, 9 m.
w.	13·6	Increased at 2 m.	—	Thriving, 7 m.
.	—	Increased on 3rd d.	—	Thriving. 4 m.

nge transfusion on 4th day.

reticulocytosis was marked and in the second case of Diamond (1937) it reached 80%. This was often accompanied by normoblastaemia which reached 40% of total nucleated cells in Case 5. The spherocytes can usually be identified in blood films stained with a Romanowsky dye as small deeply staining cells and the presence of larger thinner reticulocytes produces the anisocytosis and polychromasia which are frequently observed. In cases of congenital spherocytosis the mean cell diameter and the mean cell volume are smaller than usual, and the mean cell thickness is greater than normal. The changes, however, are usually not sufficiently abnormal to be of aid in substantiating the diagnosis (Young, Izzo and Platzer, 1951).

The osmotic fragility of the red blood cells was recorded in 34 cases and was normal in three cases and increased in the other 31. In five of these 31 cases the fragility was normal when first examined and increased later. In nine of the 26 cases with increased fragility on the first examination, the increase was noted in the first month of life. It is thus probably untrue that the red cell fragility may not be abnormal in infancy (David and Minot, 1944) but to demonstrate the abnormality may require a more careful technique including incubated red cell fragility, auto-haemolysis and mechanical fragility. These techniques are discussed by Young *et al.* (1951), and Robinson (1957) has found the incubated fragility increased at 4 months of age when the non-incubated fragility was within normal limits. The presence of spherocytes and an increased osmotic fragility in the neonatal period may, however, be associated with erythroblastosis foetalis due to ABO incompatibility (Crawford, Cutbush and Mollison, 1953).

The twins reported in this paper demonstrated all of the features which have been shown above to be typical of congenital spherocytosis in infancy. Although there was no family history of spherocytosis, the fact that both identical twins were affected strongly suggests that the disorder was a congenital one. They developed neonatal jaundice and subsequently a recurrent anaemia without jaundice. Their spleens were enlarged and blood examination showed the presence of spherocytes, reticulocytes and normoblasts, and the osmotic fragility of the cells was increased. Splenectomy dramatically relieved the recurring anaemia although the fragility of the red cells remained abnormal.

Management

Spencer Wells performed the first splenectomy in a case of congenital spherocytosis in 1887. Forty years later Dawson (1931) was able to make the diagnosis in retrospect by demonstrating the typical haematological picture in Spencer Wells' patient who was then completely symptom free. This demonstrates the effectiveness of the operation and today most authorities agree with Dacie (1954b) that the results of operation are so good and the mortality so low that the operation should be carried out in all patients except in the completely compensated and symptom-free cases. There are some who would go further (e.g. Young, 1955) and advise splenectomy even in the absence of symptoms.

However, recently evidence has accumulated to show that splenectomized children and infants have an increased susceptibility to infection, particularly to pneumococcal meningitis (Smith, Erlandson, Schulman and Stern, 1957). King and Shumacker (1952) thought that this association was restricted to children in the first 6 months of life, but the patients described by Smith *et al.* (1957) ranged in age from 13 months to 17 years at the time of splenectomy. Eight of the 21 children in Table 1 who had a splenectomy in the first year of life developed a serious infection post-operatively, and three of these died. Walter and Chaffin (1955) mention 10 cases of congenital spherocytosis treated in the first year of life by splenectomy and the only post-operative infection was a case of otitis media. Gofstein and Gellis (1956) discuss 17 cases of splenectomy for congenital spherocytosis under the age of 1 year and only one of their patients developed an infection, a fatal tracheo-bronchitis. By totalling from these three sources the incidence of infection following splenectomy for congenital spherocytosis in the first year of life, we find that 10, 21%, of 48 patients developed an infection and 4, 8%, died (Table 2). I have only been able to find one record of a patient developing an infection after splenectomy for this disease later in life (Gofstein and Gellis, 1956). As far as present knowledge allows any conclusion to be made, the risk of infection following splenectomy in congenital spherocytosis appears to be confined to infancy, but it must be emphasized that this age distribution is not the experience of Smith *et al.* (1957) with splenectomy performed for other conditions. Although the evidence is by no means conclusive, it is probably wise to delay splenectomy as long as possible when congenital spherocytosis occurs in infancy. The management then resolves itself into the treatment of neonatal jaundice and anaemia later in infancy.

TABLE 2

INCIDENCE OF INFECTIONS FOLLOWING SPLENECTOMY PERFORMED IN THE FIRST YEAR OF LIFE FOR CONGENITAL SPHEROCYTOSIS

Source	No. of Cases	No. of Infections	No. of Deaths due to Infection
Table 1	21	8	3
Walter and Chaffin (1955)	10	1	0
Gofstein and Gellis (1956)	17	1	1
Total	48 (100%)	10 (21%)	4 (8%)

The prevention of kernikterus is the aim of treatment in the first week of life. This is liable to occur whenever the serum bilirubin rises above 19 mg. per 100 ml. in cases of haemolytic disease of the newborn (Mollison and Cutbush, 1951). It is, therefore, usual to perform a second or subsequent replacement transfusion whenever the serum bilirubin rises above 20 mg. per 100 ml. and if this technique is carried out kernikterus can be prevented (Hsia, 1953). Replacement transfusion was performed in Cases 33, 38 and 43 in Table 1, but in Case 38 evidence of kernikterus was already present. In Case 33 splenectomy was performed soon after the replacement transfusion and produced a rapid fall in the serum bilirubin and in Case 34 splenectomy was performed on the third day to prevent neonatal jaundice rising to a dangerous level. Smith and Franklin (1957) performed a replacement transfusion on both the third and fourth days of life and at 4 months their infant was symptom-free. Repeated exchange transfusions whenever the serum bilirubin is approaching or above 20 mg. per 100 ml. appears to be the treatment of choice in the hope that splenectomy may be delayed until after infancy.

If the patient presents as anaemia in infancy, then he must be carefully observed and blood transfusion advised whenever the haemoglobin level falls too low. The indication used in treating the twins was a haemoglobin level lower than 50% (7·4 g. per 100 ml.) and this prevented the development of cardiac dilatation and impairment of growth which was noted by Bernard *et al.* (1952). In these circumstances, the risks of delaying splenectomy are the development of pigment gall stones (but this has never been found in the first year of life) and the possible occurrence of a haemolytic or aplastic crisis. If the parents are advised to return to the clinic if the patient is pyrexial or unwell in any way, then the crisis can be diagnosed early and blood transfusion is likely to be life saving (Dameshek, 1941). Repeated blood transfusions will eventually lead to transfusion siderosis and this was noticed in the histological examination of the spleens of the twins in whom three transfusions each were given and splenectomy was performed at 9 and 11 months respectively.

Summary

Identical twins suffering from congenital spherocytosis in the first year of life are described and their clinical features, together with those of another 41 cases found in the literature, are tabulated.

The majority of cases occurring in infancy are found to have a positive family history and present as neonatal jaundice or recurring anaemia with an enlarged spleen. The characteristic changes in the peripheral blood are the presence of spherocytosis, a marked reticulocytosis and an increased red cell fragility.

Because of the risk of infection, splenectomy should be postponed until after infancy. Neonatal jaundice should be treated by repeated replacement transfusions and anaemia of infancy by simple blood transfusion.

I wish to thank Dr. A. Doyne Bell and Dr. C. T. Potter for permission to publish these cases and for their helpful criticisms and advice. I also wish to thank Dr. Sydney Shaw and the staff of the Department of Clinical Pathology for most of the haematological investigations, and Dr. John Shore for the pathology report on the spleens. Figure 1 was kindly produced by Miss P. M. Turnbull of the Photographic Department.

References

Abt, A. F. (1940). *Amer. J. Dis. Child.*, **60**, 812.
Bernard, J., Boiron, M. and Estager, J. (1952). *Sem. Hôp. Paris*, **28**, 3741.
Betke, K. (1956). *Z. Kinderheilk.*, **78**, 359.
Campbell, J. M. H. and Warner, E. C. (1926). *Quart. J. Med.*, **19**, 333.
Conrad, E. and Schmidt, R. E. (1946). *Amer. J. Dis. Child.*, **72**, 731.
Crawford, H., Cutbush, M. and Mollison, P. L. (1953). *Blood*, **8**, 620.
Dacie, J. V. (1954a). *The Haemolytic Anaemias*, p. 54. London.
—— (1954b). *Ibid.*, p. 73.
Dameshek, W. (1941). *New Engl. J. Med.*, **224**, 52.
David, J. K., jr. and Minot, A. S. (1944). *Amer. J. Dis. Child.*, **68**, 327.
Dawson of Penn, Lord (1931). *Brit. med. J.*, **1**, 921.
Debré, R., Lamy, M., Sée, G. and Schrameck, G. (1938). *Amer. J. Dis. Child.*, **56**, 1189.
Diamond, L. K. (1937). *Med. Clin. N. Amer.*, **21**, 401.
—— (1938). *Amer. J. Surg.*, **39**, 400.
Edwards, W. M. and Heaton, L. D. (1955). *Amer. Practit. Dig. Treat.*, **6**, 387.
Evans, T. S., Waters, L. L. and Lowman, R. M. (1954). *Conn. med. J.*, **18**, 569.
Fallon, M. (1943). *J. Pediat.*, **23**, 721.
Field, C. E. and Tan, E. E. (1955). *Med. J. Malaya*, **10**, 60.
Gofstein, R. and Gellis, S. S. (1956). *A.M.A. Amer. J. Dis. Child.*, **91**, 566.
Hawksley, J. C. (1934). *Proc. roy. Soc. Med.*, **27**, 942.
Hindman, S. (1954). *J. Pediat.*, **44**, 213.
Hsia, D. Y. (1953). *A.M.A. Amer. J. Dis. Child.*, **86**, 484.
Josephs, H. W. (1938). *Bull. Johns Hopk. Hosp.*, **62**, 25.
King, H. and Shumacker, H. B. (1952). *Ann. Surg.*, **136**, 239.
Lappin, P. J. (1956). *R. I. med. J.*, **39**, 79.
Leffler, R. J. (1952). *Amer. J. Path.*, **28**, 303.
Lesné, E., Launay, C. and Hurez, —. (1935). *Bull. Soc. Pédiat. Paris*, **33**, 445.
Macaulay, D. (1951). *Arch. Dis. Childh.*, **26**, 241.
Mollison, P. L. and Cutbush, M. (1951). *Blood*, **6**, 777.
Newns, G. (1951). *Gt Ormond Str. J.*, **1**, 32.
Pinckney, C. (1946). *Proc. roy. Soc. Med.*, **39**, 696.
Robinson, G. C. (1957). *J. Pediat.*, **50**, 446.
Shapiro, C. M., Josephson, A. M., Rozengvaig, S. and Kauffman, A. (1957). *Ibid.*, **50**, 308.
Smith, C. H., Erlandson, M., Schulman, I. and Stern, G. (1957). *Amer. J. Med.*, **22**, 390.
Smith, I. and Franklin, A. W. (1957). *Proc. roy. Soc. Med.*, **50**, 707.
Stenstrom, J. D. and Ford, H. S. (1956). *Canad. med. Ass. J.*, **74**, 34.
Thompson, W. P. (1936). *J. Amer. med. Ass.*, **107**, 1776.
Turman, C. M., Vaughan, V. C. and Shelly, R. M. (1956). *Amer. J. Obstet. Gynec.*, **71**, 885.
Walter, L. E. and Chaffin, L. (1955). *Ann. Surg.*, **142**, 798.
Young, L. E. (1955). *Amer. J. Med.*, **18**, 486.
——, Izzo, M. J. and Platzer, R. F. (1951). *Blood*, **6**, 1073.

CONGENITAL HEART DISEASE IN ONE OF IDENTICAL TWINS

BY

H. EVERLEY JONES

From the Hallam Hospital, West Bromwich

(RECEIVED FOR PUBLICATION JANUARY 14, 1958)

As so many of the diseases afflicting children have been successfully controlled, attention has been focused increasingly on congenital abnormalities.

The developing embryo can be affected by inherited genetic factors or by the environment, and twins have been much studied to help in the differentiation of these factors. Identical twins, arising from the same ovum, have identical genetic structure, so that differences between them must arise from some difference in the environment.

Formerly, most congenital defects were thought to have a genetic basis, but recently environmental factors have come increasingly into prominence. Despite this, few cases of congenital malformation of the heart in one of a pair of monozygotic twins have been recorded. Such a case is described here with a summary of previously recorded examples.

Case History

Linda was seen at the age of 6 years because a heart murmur had been detected on examination during a mild attack of pneumonia one month previously. As she was a twin, her twin sister, Anne, was also sent for, and the two examined together.

The twins came sixth in the family, the five older siblings being singletons and quite healthy. An uncle of the mother had twins, a boy and a girl, among eight children, and an aunt of hers had girl twins beside two singletons. Whether these girls were identical twins or not is unknown.

The age of both the mother and father at the time of the birth of the twins was 37 years. Both parents were healthy, and the mother was not examined radiographically until the seventh month of pregnancy.

At birth, which was at term, Linda weighed 7 lb., and Anne 5½ lb., and the slight difference in size has been maintained since. Both twins were reared on National Dried Milk, and passed their developmental milestones together at the usual times.

Both children are liable to attacks of tonsillitis from which they suffer almost simultaneously, and both had a mild bout of pneumonia one month before the time of examination.

On examination, Linda weighed 44 lb. and measured 43 in. in height. (Anne 40½ lb. and 42 in.)

They were remarkably similar in appearance (Fig. 1),

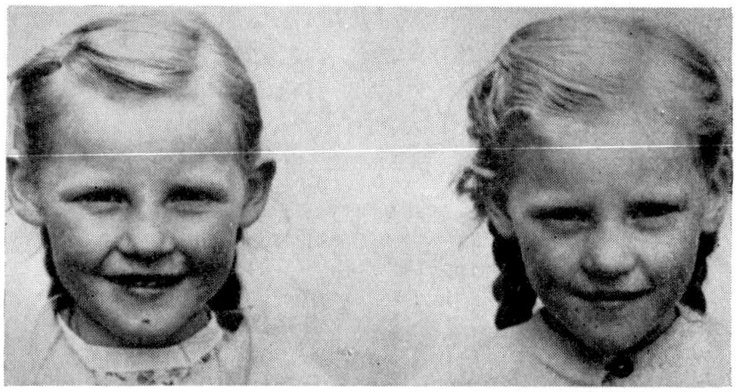

FIG. 1.—The twins—Linda on the right.

and the only differences noted were the abnormalities in Linda's cardiovascular system and the fact that Anne was left-handed while Linda was right-handed.

Examination of Linda's heart showed the apex beat to be in the fifth left interspace in the nipple line. The impulse was not remarkable. There was a harsh systolic murmur and thrill maximal in the second left interspace, and the second pulmonary sound was weak. Blood pressure was 110/70. Cardioscopy showed slight enlargement of the right ventricle and dilatation of the pulmonary artery. The lung fields appeared clear. An electrocardiogram showed right axis deviation (Fig. 2*a*). She was not cyanosed and showed no finger clubbing, and a clinical diagnosis of isolated pulmonary stenosis was made. In contradistinction the heart of Anne was normal on examination. Cardioscopy revealed a normal cardiac outline and the electrocardiogram was also normal (Fig. 2*b*).

Since first being examined, both girls have remained well apart from tonsillitis.

Evidence of Monozygosity. Unfortunately the midwife who delivered the twins has since died, and no record of the delivery has been preserved. The mother stated that there was but one afterbirth, which, though suggestive, cannot be accepted as conclusive evidence, so further corroboration was sought. Using Newman's (1940) method of similarity, the following points were noted:

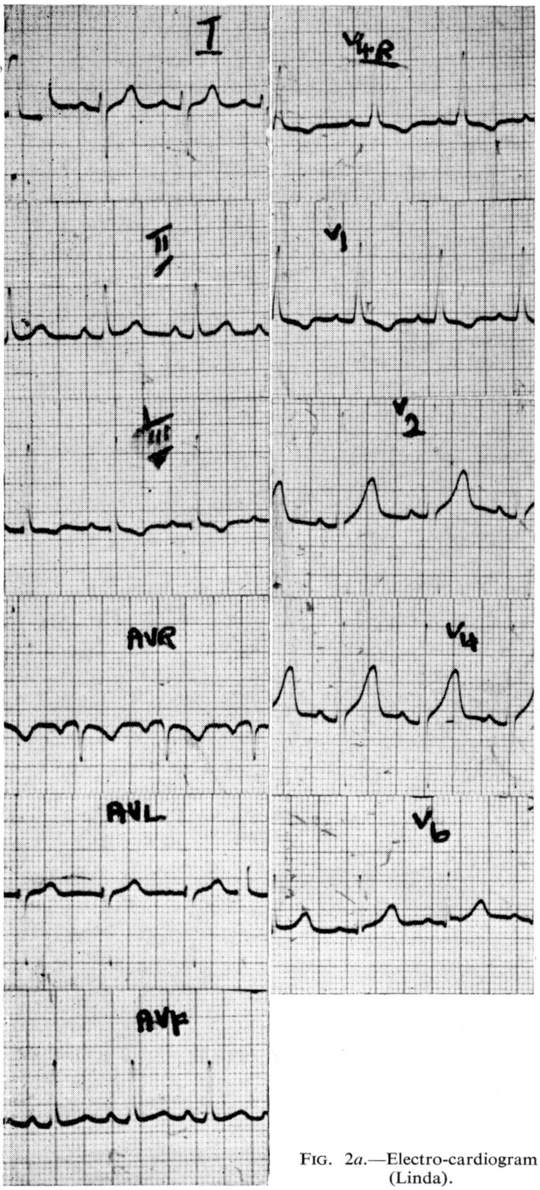

FIG. 2*a*.—Electro-cardiogram (Linda).

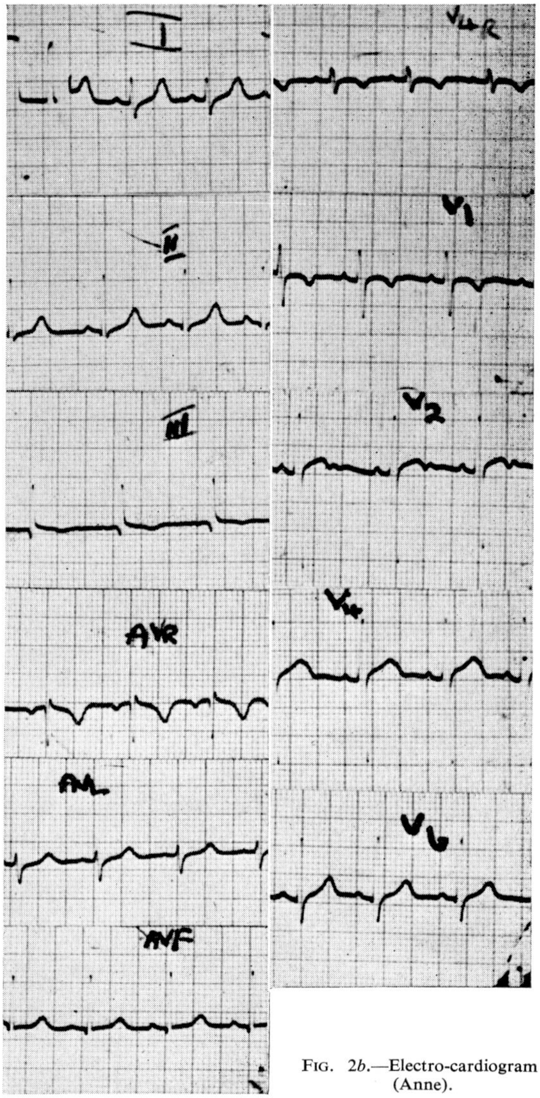

FIG. 2*b*.—Electro-cardiogram (Anne).

The features were markedly similar. The twins' hair was alike in colour, texture and whorl, as were the eyelashes. The irides were the same colour in the two girls. The lips and ears were similar. The teeth of the two were alike in appearance and time of eruption, except for one carious molar in the case of Linda.

The finger prints were interesting. The impressions of the two were remarkably similar but not identical, and the right hand of Linda resembled more closely the left hand of Anne than her own left hand.

Intelligence tests gave identical results in both girls: an intelligence quotient of 95 on Terman Merrill Form L, and a mechanical reading age (Schonell Graded Word Test) of 5·1 years.

Finally, Dr. W. Weiner, Director of the Birmingham Regional Blood Transfusion Service, kindly examined the blood of each twin, which was found to be Group AB, Rhesus negative, cdE/cde, M positive, Kell negative, in both children. He also examined the blood of the parents, siblings, two uncles, an aunt and the maternal grandmother. He concluded from these blood studies that the degree of probability of the twins being identical was 96·4%.

On this evidence there seems no doubt that the children are indeed one egg twins.

Cases in the Literature

The following instances of congenital heart disease, recorded as occurring in one egg twins, have been found in the literature:

(1) Forsyth and Uchida (1951). A pair of 6-year-old girl twins, one of whom had an auricular septal defect diagnosed clinically and by cardiac catheterization. The evidence of monozygosity was incontrovertible and better documented than in any other of the recorded instances.

(2 and 3) Wade (1952). The first was a pair of girl twins, one of whom had a patent ductus arteriosus successfully ligated. The second was a pair of girl twins, one of whom was considered to be suffering from isolated pulmonary stenosis. Evidence of monozygosity in each pair was a marked similarity in numerous features. Moreover, the finger prints of each set of twins, although not identical, were closely similar, and there were no serological differences in the blood of each pair.

(4) Goldman and Stern (1952). A pair of male twins, one of whom, when aged 10 years, was considered on clinical, radiological and electrocardiographic evidence to have an atrial septal defect. The twins were stated to have been monochorionic, and no other evidence of monozygosity was given.

(5) Jeune and Confavreux (1948). The second of male twins died at 11 weeks of age. He was cyanosed from soon after birth. Necropsy disclosed a persistent foramen Botalli, a ventricular septal defect and pulmonary infundibular stenosis. The evidence given in favour of monozygosity was that the twins were born in a single water sac, and that there was only one placenta. It is interesting that they had mirror image irregularities of the ears and palm prints (poor prints).

(6) Kean (1942). A pair of girl twins, examined when 18 years old. Both had complete situs inversus visceralis, confirmed by radiographs and electrocardiograms. One of the girls had organic heart disease as shown by a harsh thrill and systolic murmur to the right of the sternum, and an accentuated second sound on the right. This twin developed subacute bacterial endocarditis, caused by *Streptococcus viridans*, from which she subsequently died. Permission for necropsy was refused, but the author considered that she had suffered from congenital and not rheumatic heart disease. Evidence that they were a pair of one egg twins appears to be satisfactory. Although there were two placentas, this may happen when the twinning division takes place unusually early. Otherwise the similarity points described by Newman were well satisfied.

Although the evidence given in these six examples is not always complete, there seems little doubt that each pair was identical. There are, however, a few case records which, for one reason or another, cannot be definitely accepted.

(7) McClintock (1945). A female infant, the second of twins, birth weight 4½ lb., died on the fourth day. Necropsy revealed a patent ductus arteriosus and coarctation of the aorta. The other twin girl survived and was clinically normal. The only evidence of monozygosity was the presence of one placenta.

(8) Dubreuil-Chambardel (1927) described briefly a pair of twins ('identité parfaite'), one of whom had complete situs inversus visceralis, confirmed radiologically. In addition, each twin had mirror-image hare lip. Most subsequent authors have quoted this pair as an example of congenital heart disease in one of identical twins, but 'mirror imaging' in varying degree was stated by Newman to occur in about one quarter of one egg twins, although situs inversus was considered to be rare. He suggested that such a reversal might be accounted for by the twinning division occurring late in development when the two half embryos had become different in their rates of development and dominance was already present. It would seem therefore that the dextrocardia in this case was inherent in the twinning process.

(9) Reinhardt (1912) gave good evidence that a pair of twins aged 20 years, who were examined for military service, were identical. Both had dextrocardia. On clinical and radiological evidence one was regarded as having some organic cardiac lesion, type unspecified, and he was given light duties.

(10) Pezzi and Carugati (1924) described young adult twins, considered to be identical, both of whom were said to have isolated dextrocardia. The evidence is confusing (for instance the liver in one of them was stated to be palpable on the left side), but the published electrocardiograms of both twins were typical of dextrocardia. In view of Newman's writings on mirror imaging in identical twins, mentioned above, one might regard this pair as having dissimilar cardiac status.

(11) Weitz (1936) in the first edition of his book, *Die Vererbung innerer Krankheiten*, described identical twins, one of whom suffered from patent ductus arteriosus. Unfortunately I have been unable to obtain a copy of this first edition, and the second edition (1949) contains no such description.

Discussion

Reading the case records of the patients cited above, one is not always certain whether the twins were of the one or two egg variety. Newman (1940) stated that if the pair are similar in appearance, and in such points as hair texture, colour and whorl, colour of eyes, shape of lips and ears, eruption and appearance of teeth, appearance of eyebrows and eyelashes, and similarity of palm and finger prints, then it is practically certain that the pair are one egg twins. Two egg twins who are much alike always have definite differences in some of these features. The diagnosis of monozygosity by examination of the foetal membranes is not considered infallible to-day, but, if careful examination shows the presence of only one chorion, then the one egg type of twins can be assumed.

In some of the patients, the type of heart disease is not known for certain. However, it seems probable that the first six cases fulfil the requirements necessary for a diagnosis of congenital heart disease in one egg twins. Four of the remaining five are not considered completely acceptable, usually because of insufficient evidence as to the type of twinning and the kind of heart disease. The final case has not been traced.

The type of heart lesion found was varied, and these examples provide evidence of the importance of environment in the causation of congenital heart disease.

Summary

A case of congenital heart disease in one of a pair of identical twins has been described.

A brief account of other recorded examples has been given.

I am indebted to Dr. J. C. Ford, Consultant Pathologist, for help, to Dr. M. Shields for kindly performing the intelligence tests, and to Mr. D. R. Paton for the photographs.

References

Dubreuil-Chambardel, L. (1927). *Presse méd.*, **35**, 1157.
Forsyth, C. C. and Uchida, I. (1951). *Arch. Dis. Childh.*, **26**, 582.
Goldman, I. R. and Stern, N. S. (1952). *Amer. Heart J.*, **44**, 159.
Jeune, M. and Confavreux, J. (1948). *Arch. franç. Pédiat.*, **5**, 252.
Kean, B. H. (1942). *J. Hered.*, **33**, 217.
McClintock, K. (1945). *Arch. Dis. Childh.*, **20**, 47.
Newman, H. H. (1940). *Multiple Human Births.* New York.
Pezzi, C. and Carugati, L. (1924). *Cuore e Circol.*, **8**, 361.
Reinhardt (1912). *Dtsch. Milit. Z.*, **41**, 931.
Wade, G. (1952). *Brit. Heart J.*, **14**, 475.
Weitz, W. (1936). *Die Vererbung innerer Krankheiten.* Stuttgart.

THE ELECTROCARDIOGRAPHIC RECOGNITION OF VENTRICULAR HYPERTROPHY IN CONGENITAL CARDIO-VASCULAR DISEASE DURING THE FIRST YEAR OF LIFE

BY

J. S. OLDHAM

From the Children's Hospital and Dudley Road Hospital, Birmingham

(RECEIVED FOR PUBLICATION DECEMBER 9, 1957)

The value of electrocardiography in the elucidation of the diagnostic problems of congenital heart disease in infancy has been limited by lack of precise knowledge of normal features of the electrocardiogram in this age group. Battro and Mendy (1946) were the first to relate electrocardiographic patterns to age. Alimurung, Joseph, Nadas and Massell (1951) and Ziegler (1951) made detailed studies on large groups of infants and children, and their work provides standards of normality for all ages from birth to 14 years.

Publications about the electrocardiographic recognition of ventricular hypertrophy in infants are few. In these communications the existence of ventricular hypertrophy is inferred from the nature of the cardiac malformation, diagnosis being established by cardiac catheterization or contrast radiography. By these methods hypertrophy of the right ventricle may be reliably deduced, but as the techniques provide less information about the state of the left ventricle it may not be possible to distinguish between isolated right ventricular hypertrophy and combined ventricular hypertrophy.

It is the purpose of this paper to consider the value of the electrocardiogram in the determination of ventricular hypertrophy resulting from congenital cardiovascular disease in the first year of life, the type of ventricular hypertrophy and the nature of the malformation being proved by necropsy.

Investigation

Material. Forty infants were studied. Ages ranged from 2 days to 11 months at the time electrocardiograms were made. The majority of infants died within 6 months of birth. Tracings were obtained within two months of death in all cases except two, of these one child died at the age of 3 years, the other at 14 months. In 25 cases the cardiovascular lesion was one causing persistent cyanosis.

Method. In all cases standard limb leads, unipolar extremity leads and precordial leads V1, V2, V4 and V6 were used. A precordial electrode of small surface area (diameter 1·7 cm.) was employed. The recording instrument was standardized before each tracing was made.

In the interpretation of tracings the following criteria were used. The R deflection was considered abnormal if in excess of the 99·5 percentile of observed or computed maximum for age (by the standards of Ziegler (1951)). The intrinsicoid deflection in V1 was considered to be delayed if occurring 0·04 second or longer after the beginning of the QRS complex in this lead (Goodwin, 1952).

Necropsy examinations were made in all cases. Ventricular hypertrophy was invariably present. In not all cases was the heart detached from other thoracic viscera for weighing, but when this was done, heart weights ranged from 150% to 340% of that normal for age (by the standards of Potter and Adair (1940)). Cases were grouped as isolated right ventricular hypertrophy, isolated left ventricular hypertrophy, or combined ventricular hypertrophy on the basis of necropsy findings. The major cardiovascular defect in each group was as follows:

ISOLATED RIGHT VENTRICULAR HYPERTROPHY. (Total 20 cases.) Tetralogy of Fallot (6), single ventricle (3), complete transposition of the great vessels and pulmonary atresia (1), coarctation of aorta proximal to patent ductus arteriosus (2), mitral stenosis (1), isolated pulmonary stenosis (1), atrial septal defect (3), ventricular septal defect (1), congenital tricuspid incompetence (2).

ISOLATED LEFT VENTRICULAR HYPERTROPHY. (Total 3 cases.) Tricuspid atresia (2), tricuspid stenosis (1).

COMBINED VENTRICULAR HYPERTROPHY. (Total 17 cases.) Complete transposition of the great vessels (6), persistent truncus arteriosus (1), coarctation of aorta proximal to patent ductus arteriosus

TABLE 1

PATTERN OF QRS COMPLEX IN PRECORDIAL LEAD V1

Ventricular Hypertrophy	QRS Pattern									
	qR	qRS	rsR′	R	RsR′	RR′	Rs	RS	rS	Totals
Isolated right	2	1	2	11	0	0	2	2	0	20
Combined	0	0	0	0	1	1	8	6	1	17
Isolated left	0	0	0	0	0	0	0	0	3	3
Totals	2	1	2	11	1	1	10	8	4	40

(1), endocardial fibro-elastosis (2), patent ductus arteriosus (2), persistent common atrio-ventricular canal (2), ventricular septal defect (3).

Results

Ventricular Complex in V1. The types of QRS complex observed are tabulated in Table 1. In the two instances in which a qR pattern was present in V1, the complex in V2 was composed of a double peaked R and the intrinsicoid deflection was delayed in this lead. The solitary example of a qRS deflection was provided by a heart with single ventricle. In this case an rss′ pattern was present in V2.

Complexes of type R, often slurred or notched on the upstroke, were observed only in cases of isolated right ventricular hypertrophy. In 14 of 17 cases of combined ventricular hypertrophy the ventricular complex was of form Rs or RS. An rS pattern was seen only with hypertrophy of the left ventricle, whether isolated or combined.

Cases of isolated right ventricular hypertrophy could be classified in three groups on the basis of the form of the QRS complex, the amplitude of R, and the polarity of the T wave.

In the first group, of 11 cases, the intrinsicoid deflection was delayed. In 10 of these cases T was negative. In seven R was of abnormally great amplitude. This group showed incomplete right bundle branch block patterns suggesting diastolic overloading of the right ventricle (Cabrera and Monroy, 1952).

In the second group, of six cases, the ventricular complex was formed of a solitary R deflection of normal amplitude and the intrinsicoid deflection was not delayed. T was upright in four cases (abnormal in infancy except during the first 2 days of life), was isoelectric in one, and negative in one.

The third group of three cases showed features of extreme clockwise rotation of the heart, there being an initial q deflection. T was negative.

Of the 17 cases of combined ventricular hypertrophy, an incomplete right bundle branch block pattern with delay of the intrinsicoid deflection was present in 10. In four of these R was of abnormally great amplitude. Of the remaining seven cases R was abnormally tall in three.

Accepting as evidence of right ventricular hypertrophy either an amplitude of R in excess of that normal for age, or delay of the intrinsicoid deflection, the condition could be detected in 11 of 17 cases (65%) of isolated right ventricular hypertrophy (excluding from this analysis the three cases with q deflections), and in 13 of 17 cases (75%) of combined ventricular hypertrophy.

Ventricular Complex in V6. R was of amplitude in excess of that normal for age in one of three cases of isolated left ventricular hypertrophy, and in six of 17 cases of combined ventricular hypertrophy (Table 2). Delay of the intrinsicoid deflection was not of help in detecting left ventricular hypertrophy since in one case only did the intrinsicoid deflection occur after 0·04 sec., and in this case R was of abnormally great amplitude.

TABLE 2

CORRELATION OF ELECTROCARDIOGRAPHIC EVIDENCE OF VENTRICULAR HYPERTROPHY, BASED ON ABNORMAL MEASUREMENTS OF VENTRICULAR COMPLEXES IN V1 AND V6, WITH ANATOMICAL FINDINGS. (THE MEASUREMENTS WERE AMPLITUDE OF R AND TIME OF ONSET OF INTRINSICOID DEFLECTION.)

Ventricular Hypertrophy	E.C.G. Indication of Ventricular Hypertrophy				
	Right Alone	Right and Left	Left Alone	Normal Measurement	Totals
Isolated right	11	0	0	6	17*
Combined	8	5	1	3	17
Isolated left	0	0	1	2	3
Totals	19	5	2	11	37*

* 3 cases with qR or qRS patterns in VI excluded.

Ventricular Complex in VR. Extremity leads provide less direct evidence of ventricular hypertrophy than do precordial leads. VR was studied in the hope that it might provide information helpful in making distinction between isolated right ventricular hypertrophy and combined ventricular hypertrophy when the precordial electro-

TABLE 3
PATTERNS OF QRS COMPLEX IN VR

Ventricular Hypertrophy	QRS Pattern									
	QR	QRs	qR	qRs	R	rsR′	rSR′	rSrs	rS	Totals
Isolated right	4	1	3	4	2	2	2	2	0	20
Combined	0	0	5	0	0	4	4	2	2	17
Isolated left	0	0	0	0	0	0	0	0	3	3
Totals	4	1	8	4	2	6	6	4	5	40

cardiogram indicated hypertrophy of the right ventricle alone.

Patterns of the ventricular complex are analysed in Table 3. Prominent Q deflections (Q more than one third the amplitude of R), or solitary R deflections, occurred only in cases of isolated right ventricular hypertrophy. When complexes of these types were present in VR, there was usually an R or qR pattern in V1. In two cases, however, a QR in VR was associated with an Rs complex in V1; in such cases VR may be helpful in distinguishing between isolated right and combined ventricular hypertrophy.

Discussion

Goodwin (1952) was the first to suggest criteria for the electrocardiographic recognition of right ventricular hypertrophy in young children. His subjects were aged from 3 to 14 years. His criteria were based on the time of onset of the intrinsicoid deflection, and on the patterns of the QRS complex in leads V1 and aVR.

Braunwald, Donoso, Sapin and Grishman (1955) found that 11 of 45 of their cases in a similar age group did not fulfil Goodwin's criteria. They studied 51 cases of presumed isolated right ventricular hypertrophy in children aged 1 to 15 years and found that 29 (57%) exhibited an R deflection in V1 of amplitude abnormal for age, and that in 26 (51%) the pre-intrinsicoid deflection time in V1 was 0·04 sec. or longer. Accepting either of these criteria 41 (80%) could be correctly diagnosed. The authors considered that these criteria were the most satisfactory then available.

Employing these criteria only 65% of my cases of isolated right ventricular hypertrophy would be recognized, though the presence of right ventricular hypertrophy could be detected in 75% of cases of combined ventricular hypertrophy (Table 2). Numbers are too small for this disparity in results to be of statistical significance. I believe, however, that these criteria may well be of less value in the recognition of isolated right ventricular hypertrophy during the first year of life than at later periods. Certain cases revealed complexes in V1 which, though normal by measurement, were of abnormal configuration, such as qR, or R with positive T; these abnormal patterns were not shown by cases of combined ventricular hypertrophy, and were associated with types of cardiovascular malformation which usually prove fatal within a few months of birth.

Ziegler (1956) described a pattern of ventricular complex in right precordial leads which he considered to be indicative of the most advanced degree of systolic overloading of the right ventricle. This pattern consists of an R deflection single or double peaked, of near 100% amplitude of RS, followed by an upright instead of inverted T, and frequently preceded by a true initial Q wave. This type of complex was observed in five of my cases; in four of these R was of normal amplitude and the intrinsicoid deflection was not delayed; the existence of right ventricular hypertrophy thus could not be detected by measurement.

Ventricular complexes in V1 of the form qR (with negative T) were considered to be always abnormal by Goodwin (1952) and by Goldberger (1953). Goodwin (1952) and Brink and Neill (1955) regarded this pattern in V1 as indicative of right ventricular hypertrophy. No example was present in the large series of normal infants and children studied by Alimurung *et al.* (1951) but Ziegler (1951) found three examples in normal infants under 3 months of age.

The two cases showing a qR pattern in V1 in my series revealed other abnormalities in the electrocardiogram, in particular the ventricular complex in V2 was composed of a double peaked R wave, the intrinsicoid deflection being delayed, a pattern which when occurring in V1 is characteristic of right ventricular hypertrophy in this age group.

Only in a minority of cases of combined ventricular hypertrophy does direct measurement of the ventricular complexes in left precordial leads provide unequivocal evidence of hypertrophy of the left ventricle. In about 50% of cases the electrocardiogram permits the recognition of right ventricular hypertrophy alone (Table 2).

Ziegler (1956) suggested that, with QRS or T

wave evidence of right ventricular hypertrophy in right precordial leads, the occurrence of T wave inversion in leads from the left side of the precordium was strong presumptive evidence of associated left ventricular hypertrophy. In my series such T wave inversion occurred only in cases in which the R deflection in V6 was of abnormally great amplitude, itself an indication of left ventricular hypertrophy.

More helpful was the configuration of the ventricular complex in V1, since patterns of the forms R or qR were encountered only in cases of isolated right ventricular hypertrophy. The form of the complex in VR may also be of some value in making distinction between isolated right and combined ventricular hypertrophy because in the latter condition QR and R patterns were not observed.

Conclusions

It is emphasized that the material forming the basis of this study is not fully representative of congenital cardiovascular disease in infancy. The methods employed in selection were such that the series is necessarily composed of the more severe types of malformation. With this qualification the following conclusions are drawn regarding electrocardiographic findings during the first 12 months of life.

In about 90% of cases of isolated right ventricular hypertrophy the ventricular complexes in V1 are abnormal. Abnormalities are of three types: (*a*) The intrinsicoid deflection is delayed to 0·04 sec. or longer and/or R is of amplitude in excess of that normal for age. (*b*) The ventricular complex is in the form of a solitary R deflection which is followed by an upright T wave. (*c*) There is an initial q deflection.

Combined ventricular hypertrophy can be recognized in about 30% of cases from the presence in V1 of an R deflection of amplitude in excess of that normal for age and/or prolongation of the pre-intrinsicoid deflection time to 0·04 sec. or longer, together with a qR or qRs pattern in V6 in which R is of amplitude in excess of that normal for age. In about 50% of cases of combined ventricular hypertrophy the electrocardiogram reveals hypertrophy of the right ventricle alone.

When the electrocardiogram is indicative of right ventricular hypertrophy alone this is likely to be isolated if the ventricular complex in V1 is of the form qR or R, or the ventricular complex in VR is of the form QR or R.

Summary

Electrocardiograms were obtained during the first year of life from 40 infants with congenital cardiovascular disease.

The presence of isolated right ventricular hypertrophy, combined ventricular hypertrophy, or isolated left ventricular hypertrophy, was later proved by necropsy.

The value of electrocardiography in the recognition of ventricular hypertrophy, and in making distinction between isolated right ventricular hypertrophy and combined ventricular hypertrophy, is discussed.

I am grateful to physicians on the staff of the Birmingham Children's Hospital for permission to study cases admitted under their care. I am particularly indebted to Dr. C. G. Parsons for encouragement and valuable criticism, to Dr. H. S. Baar for necropsy reports, and to Miss Jean Wright who obtained most of the electrocardiograms.

References

Alimurung, M. M., Joseph, L. G., Nadas, A. S. and Massell, B. F. (1951). *Circulation*, **4**, 420.
Battro, A. and Mendy, J. C. (1946). *Arch. intern. Med.*, **78**, 31.
Braunwald, E., Donoso, E., Sapin, S. O. and Grishman, A. (1955). *Amer. Heart J.*, **50**, 591.
Brink, A. J. and Neill, C. A. (1955). *Circulation*, **12**, 604.
Cabrera, E. and Monroy, J. R. (1952). *Amer. Heart J.*, **43**, 661, 669.
Goldberger, E. (1953). *Unipolar Lead Electrocardiography and Vectorcardiography*, 3rd ed. London.
Goodwin, J. F. (1952). *Brit. Heart J.*, **14**, 173.
Potter, E. L. and Adair, F. L. (1940). *Fetal and Neonatal Death*. Chicago.
Ziegler, R. F. (1951). *Electrocardiographic Studies in Normal Infants and Children*. Springfield, Illinois.
—— (1956). *Amer. Heart J.*, **52**, 533.

THE DIFFERENTIAL DIAGNOSIS OF RHEUMATIC FEVER

BY

K. A. HALLIDIE-SMITH and E. G. L. BYWATERS

From the Rheumatism Research Unit (Medical Research Council), Canadian Red Cross Memorial Hospital, Taplow

(RECEIVED FOR PUBLICATION JANUARY 29, 1958)

Since the efficacy of continuous daily sulphonamide or penicillin administration in the prevention of attacks of rheumatic fever has now been established, and the measure recommended not only nationally but by international committees (World Health Organization, 1957), it has become increasingly important to recognize even mild cases of rheumatic fever. At the same time it is equally essential to avoid diagnosing this erroneously, since the resulting continuous daily prophylaxis is undesirable from the point of view both of the patient and of the tax-payer. We thought therefore that an account of our observations at this National Centre for Juvenile Rheumatism over the last nine years would be useful, since over this period there has accumulated considerable experience not only of rheumatic fever, but also of many conditions which masquerade as such.

Out of such prolonged experience at the House of the Good Samaritan in Boston, Duckett Jones (1944) was able to formulate a set of diagnostic criteria which have proved extremely useful in a modified form (Rheumatic Fever Committee Joint Report, 1955) for ensuring in a large therapeutic trial that cases from many different centres were of the same general type. He realized that cases of other diseases were as far as possible to be ruled out. It was realized further that many cases of genuine rheumatic fever, if first observed late in the course of the disease, or if mild, could not be fitted in and would have to be called 'probable rheumatic fever'. Furthermore, some of the criteria depend upon continuous clinical observation or laboratory tests usually possible in hospital, but only comparatively rarely made in this country in the average general practice. In this centre then, a discharge diagnosis of rheumatic fever has been made on unformulated but rather wider grounds than those of the Duckett Jones criteria, so that of 2,214 patients admitted to the unit over the nine-year period, 959 were discharged with the diagnosis of rheumatic fever. Nearly two thirds of these satisfied diagnostic criteria comparable to those of Duckett Jones, save that chorea was excluded as a major criterion and past rheumatic fever as a minor criterion. In addition, 42 cases were discharged with a diagnosis of 'possible rheumatic fever' and 202 with a diagnosis of Still's disease, the remaining 1,011 cases being various other miscellaneous disorders.

Group A. Erroneous Initial Diagnoses in Rheumatic Fever Cases

A one-in-six sample of these patients ultimately diagnosed as rheumatic fever was taken, consisting of those with surnames beginning with the initials A, B and C admitted between July, 1947, and June, 1956. In this group of 160 rheumatic fever patients, 12 were found definitely to have been initially otherwise diagnosed, though subsequently all satisfied Duckett Jones' criteria for the diagnosis of rheumatic fever. All were children between the ages of 6 and 12 years, apart from the patient initially thought to have sub-acute bacterial endocarditis, and only in that patient and the child thought to be a case of Still's disease was the ultimate diagnosis not made before transfer here. All patients have been regularly followed up since discharge, for periods between 18 months and seven years.

Poliomyelitis. These two children complained of fever and limb pains and one had neck stiffness. Normal cerebrospinal fluid was found and in both significant heart murmurs became audible subsequently.

Pneumonia. This 9-year-old girl gave a history of general malaise and limb pains. On admission to the referring hospital, she was febrile and was found to have impaired percussion note and crepitations in the right mid-zone. Following subsidence of the chest signs she developed significant heart murmurs, and later rheumatic nodules.

Meningitis. This child had a sore throat followed by limb pain and headache. Normal cerebrospinal fluid was obtained and she subsequently developed polyarthritis and heart block.

Rubella. This 7-year-old girl had a sudden onset of abdominal pain and a rubella-like rash. There was, however, a normal white count and no accompanying lymphadenopathy; she subsequently developed pericarditis and endocarditis.

Dysentery. This girl complained of abdominal pain, diarrhoea and limb pains. Stool culture was negative. She complained of limb pains after the diarrhoea settled and an organic mitral pansystolic murmur developed.

Subacute Bacterial Endocarditis. This young adult female with known rheumatic heart disease gave a five-day history of general malaise, generalized aches and pains and fever. She subsequently developed polyarthritis and a raised antistreptolysin-0 titre; repeated blood cultures were negative and there were no embolic manifestations. She responded to bed rest and salicylates.

Appendicitis. These two children both complained of abdominal pain. Normal appendices were removed, but they both subsequently developed polyarthritis and organic heart murmurs.

Suppurative Arthritis of Hip. This 9-year-old boy had a four weeks' history of pain in one hip with inguinal adenitis and fever. He subsequently developed polyarthritis and a mitral pansystolic murmur.

Still's Disease. This boy presented with a three months' history of polyarthritis, fever, rash and general malaise. It was not until after 10 weeks in this hospital that he developed heart lesions, by which time the arthritis had settled leaving no residua.

Fallen Arches. This 6-year-old boy had complained of pain in his feet for four weeks and had been treated with remedial exercises. He developed polyarthritis, and had a raised E.S.R. and A.S.O. titre.

Group B. Unsubstantiated Admission Diagnosis of Rheumatic Fever

This group consisted of all patients admitted between July, 1947, and October 31, 1956, with the presumed diagnosis of rheumatic fever, but in whom this diagnosis was not substantiated. Only those were included in whom there was fairly certain evidence from the referring letter or history on entry that they were thought to have rheumatic fever; they numbered 196.

These 196 admissions consisted of 171 children under the age of 17 years, and 25 adults. Follow-up has varied from none in a small minority to several years in some instances. There has been no evident rheumatic activity at these check-ups, and no patient has developed organic heart disease under out-patient observation. None of the patients either on long or short term follow-up has been re-admitted with rheumatic fever. They may be divided into seven broad groups which can be further subdivided as shown in Table 1. The various groups will now be considered in more detail:

TABLE 1

FINAL DIAGNOSIS OF 196 CASES REFERRED AS RHEUMATIC FEVER IN WHOM THIS DIAGNOSIS WAS NOT CONFIRMED

Functional (8):	
Physiological tachycardia	3
Hysteria	3
Neurosis and depression	2
Traumatic and Postural (11):	
Sprains	5
Slipped femoral epiphysis	2
Torn cartilage, osteochondritis dissecans, chest deformity and back ache—1 each	4
Infections (91):	
Upper respiratory tract	45
Lower respiratory tract	10
Bone and joint	10
Blood stream	4
Urinary tract	4
Pericarditis	2
Specific fevers	16
Connective Tissue Disorders (42):	
Still's and rheumatoid arthritis	24
Schonlein-Henoch purpura	8
Erythema nodosum	5
Visceral lupus erythematosus	2
Periarteritis nodosum	1
Penicillin sensitivity	1
Granuloma annulare	1
Rheumatic and Congenital Heart Disease (9):	
Congenital	2
Rheumatic	7
Blood Dyscrasias (2):	
Iron deficiency anaemia	1
Aleukaemic stem-celled leukaemia	1
Others (33):	
Arthritis	5
Arthralgia	9
Limb pains	15
Fever	3
Gout and syphilis	1
Total	196

I. Functional. This group comprised six children and two young adults. The three patients with physiological tachycardia were all children. The first had a history of recent sore throat and the referring doctor thought he had detected clinical signs of cardiac enlargement with persistent tachycardia. The second child had complained of limb pains for six weeks and was noted to have an evening temperature up to 98·8°F. and persistent tachycardia of 130-140 per minute. The third child had a recent history of cold and cough with persistent tachycardia. Nothing abnormal could be found in any of these patients, and, although the pulse rate was elevated by day, the sleeping pulse was within the normal range (Nelson, 1954).

The two young female adults complained of limb pains and general ill-health; one had had rheumatic fever as a child; she showed hysterical manifestations such as hyperventilation and no organic signs were found. The other patient also had nothing organic demonstrable, and was referred to a psychiatrist who diagnosed neurosis and depression.

The other three children all complained of pains in joints or limbs for which no organic cause was found. One had a functional wrist drop, the second hysterical gait, and the third, with an unhappy home background, admitted to exaggerating his symptoms because of desire for sympathy. All were helped by psychiatric treatment.

II. Traumatic and Postural. All the patients in this group were children, and all complained of joint pains; three patients had a history of rheumatic fever. In eight patients there was a definite history of trauma with objective signs in a single joint (knee in three cases, ankle in two, hip in two and elbow in one) with radiological evidence of slipped epiphysis in the two patients with hip involvement and of osteochondritis dissecans in the patient with elbow involvement. In the other five patients, there were normal serological findings, normal hearts and absence of other joint involvement. One patient gave a history of rheumatic fever previously, and of recent joint pains, low grade fever and suspected presystolic murmur; she was found to have a normal heart and normal temperature range, but a considerable degree of sternal deformity and scoliosis. Another girl had also had rheumatic fever and complained of pains in her back and thighs. No signs of rheumatic activity were found, but the backache was thought to be postural following her period of prolonged bedrest. The last patient gave a history of painful swelling of both knees following a sore throat. She had a normal heart and there was no evidence of rheumatic activity. Both knees tended to lock in flexion and to extend suddenly with a click, suggesting meniscus lesions. Exploration of the knee joints revealed torn cartilages, which were thought to be due to a congenital defect.

SLIPPED FEMORAL EPIPHYSIS. (i) This girl, aged 13, was referred with the following letter from her family doctor, 'Rheumatic fever 18 months ago. Now complains of pain in joints, right foot swollen. Systolic murmur at apex which has just appeared. I should be grateful if you would take her in for recurrence of rheumatic fever'. The history obtained on transfer here was of trauma to the right thigh one month previously, since when she had limped and noticed pain in the feet, knee and hip on the affected side, with recent swelling of the foot. On examination, movements of the right hip were restricted and painful and there was slight swelling of the right foot. A radiograph of the right hip showed slipped femoral epiphysis. There was evidence of mitral and aortic valve disease but this was thought to be inactive and she was transferred to an orthopaedic hospital for operation. She has now been followed up for five years and there has been no fresh rheumatic activity.

(ii) J.H., aged 14, was admitted with painful swelling of the elbow for two weeks. He had had rheumatic fever with carditis two years previously. After admission no further joints became involved and there was no evidence of recent streptococcal infection or carditis; but radiography showed osteochondritis dissecans affecting the capitellum.

III. Infections. (*a*) UPPER RESPIRATORY TRACT INFECTIONS. Of this large group, 45 (43 children and two young adults) were diagnosed as upper respiratory tract infections. The presumptive diagnosis of rheumatic fever was based on preceding upper respiratory tract infection followed by limb or joint pains, fever and general malaise in 33 patients. There were 12 patients in the whole group who did not complain of pain and in eight of them an organic systolic murmur was initially suspected, as in 16 of those who did complain of limb and joint pains. Three had had previous rheumatic fever. In all these patients, rheumatic activity was thought unlikely because of the absence of abnormal physical signs other than those of a present upper respiratory tract infection in some cases, and because of normal or rapidly settling sedimentation rate and negative evidence of streptococcal infection, except for two children (one with raised A.S.T.) whose throat swabs grew group A haemolytic streptococci.

(*b*) LOWER RESPIRATORY TRACT INFECTIONS. All these patients were children and the typical symptomatology differed from the upper respiratory tract group in that fever and cough were the presenting symptoms; pain, complained of by four children, was confined to chest or shoulder. Two children (one with primary tuberculosis and the other with bronchiectasis) had persistently elevated sedimentation rates and in four patients an organic systolic murmur was queried but not confirmed here. There was radiological proof of diagnosis in six cases (two, primary tuberculosis; one, bronchiectasis and three, lobar pneumonia). The remaining four children were diagnosed as bronchitis or resolving pneumonia in view of the chest signs on admission and the absence of cardiac involvement or streptococcal infection.

LEFT LOWER LOBE PNEUMONIA. This girl, aged 8, had had rheumatic fever and chorea five years previously. She had a sore throat one week before present admission followed by general malaise and fever. Her doctor queried precordial friction rub and thought she had had a relapse of acute rheumatism. This was not confirmed here but there were early signs of pneumonia at the left base and a subsequent radiograph showed consolidation of the left lower lobe. She responded to penicillin therapy.

(*c*) BONE AND JOINT INFECTIONS. Four of these 10 patients (nine children and a young adult male) complained of multiple joint pains and fever, but subjective and objective signs eventually became localised to one joint and diagnosis was confirmed by obtaining pus on drilling or by periosteal changes on radiographic examination. The six other patients had pain and swelling of a single joint with fever, and diagnostic proof by aspiration of purulent fluid in five cases and radiological changes in three (periostitis in two and Brodie's abscess in the third).

J.W., aged 15, was admitted to another hospital with fever and pain in the right knee. White blood cells were 8,000 per c.mm. with 80% polymorphs. Osteomyelitis was queried and she was given a short course of penicillin, but she then developed pain in other joints and was thought to have rheumatic fever. She was put on to salicylates and transferred here. She continued to run a low grade pyrexia and high E.S.R. and a bony swelling of the lower end of the right femur became apparent. White blood cells at this time were 5,000 per c.mm. with 50% polymorphs. Radiographs showed marked bony changes of osteomyelitis and the femur was subsequently drilled.

(*d*) Blood Stream Infections. Three of these cases were children and the fourth a young adult female. All complained of multiple acute painful swollen joints, fever and general malaise. In one boy an organic mitral systolic murmur was suspected. Ultimate diagnosis was based on a positive blood culture (staphylococci in two cases and streptococci in two cases), rapid response to chemotherapy and absence of cardiac involvement.

(*e*) Urinary Tract Infections. These four patients (all children) complained of limb pains and general malaise and were referred with low grade fever and a suspected organic systolic murmur in one case. All had *Esch. coli* urinary infections and one had a hydronephrosis. No other abnormal physical signs were found, and there was no evidence of carditis or of streptococcal infection.

(*f*) Pericarditis. One of these children presented with shoulder pain and fever, and the referring doctor thought that organic systolic and diastolic murmurs were present. On admission here she was found to have pericardial and pleural effusions with pericardial friction, but no evidence of endocarditis. There was no evidence of streptococcal infection. A Mantoux test at 1:1,000 was positive and radiographs showed enlarged hilar glands on one side. Symptoms and signs resolved after prolonged bed rest, and follow-up for two years showed satisfactory progress. The other child complained of general malaise and chest pain and his general practitioner found him to be febrile and thought that an organic systolic murmur was present. On admission, he had a pericardial effusion and friction rub, but no evidence of endocarditis. There was no evidence of streptococcal infection, but a Mantoux test at 1:10,000 was positive. In both these cases, the tentative diagnosis on discharge was tuberculous pericarditis, but in view of their satisfactory progress in hospital and at follow-up, in retrospect they may both have been cases of benign non-specific pericarditis.

(*g*) Specific Fevers. This group comprised 13 children and three girls aged 18-19 years. Five children had an acute episode of fever, limb pains and general malaise. This fever settled quickly after admission, no abnormal physical signs were elicited and there was no abnormal serology. They were thought to be cases of influenza, though no serological proof of diagnosis was sought.

Four patients had a discharge diagnosis of glandular fever. They all had fever and limb pains and in two of them an organic systolic murmur was questioned by the referring doctor. They were diagnosed after development of generalized lymphadenopathy and splenomegaly, abnormal mononuclear leucocytes in the peripheral blood and a positive Paul Bunnell titre in one case. No abnormal cardiac signs were noted and findings reverted to normal quite quickly.

An example of this group was a girl, aged 10. She was admitted with a history of sore throat three weeks previously and five days' fever and joint pains. On admission here she had a fever of 99°F. but no abnormal physical signs. Erythrocyte sedimentation rate was 15 mm./hr. and a white cell count was normal. Five days after admission, a white cell count showed a relative lymphocytosis of 60% and a week later 23% abnormal mononuclears were noted in a total of 15,850 W.B.C. per c.mm. Paul Bunnell titre was positive (1:224).

Six patients had acute histories with fever and muscle and joint pains in each case, but rapidly changing physical signs, finally developing features typical of measles, poliomyelitis, meningitis (no organism isolated but response to chloramphenicol therapy), infective hepatitis, erysipelas and paratyphoid fever.

The paratyphoid fever patient, an 18-year-old girl, had had rheumatic fever previously, leaving established mitral and aortic valve lesions. She gave a three-day history of fever, headache, generalized aches and pains with vomiting and diarrhoea for two days. The doctor thought she had had fresh rheumatic activity and put her on to salicylates. On admission here, vomiting and diarrhoea was a noticeable feature, and *Paratyphosus B* was isolated from blood, urine and faeces. She responded to treatment with chloramphenicol.

The patient with poliomyelitis, aged 4 years, was referred with the following letter from the general practitioner: 'History of tonsillitis two days previously. On admission she developed severe rheumatic pains in the arms and shoulders. Refuses to move the right arm because of the pain. C.N.S., all reflexes present and equal.' On admission here she was found to be febrile with slight neck stiffness and a flaccid paralysis of the right arm. The cerebrospinal fluid showed changes consistent with poliomyelitis.

The last patient in this group, a 13-year-old boy, had an acute onset of high fever, pain and weakness in one hip. There was no evidence of cardiac involvement nor of streptococcal infection and no further joints became involved; it was thought that he might have had radiculitis of virus origin.

IV. Connective Tissue Disorders. (*a*) STILL'S DISEASE AND RHEUMATOID ARTHRITIS. These 24 cases (three of whom were over 16 years of age) all presented with joint pains and the majority had had objective joint signs prior to admission; fever and general malaise were also presenting features. Eighteen had had acute symptoms and signs for over a month prior to admission here. Persistence of 'active' joints, swinging fever and in some cases lymphadenopathy or typical Still's rash, with confirmation by biopsy of synovial membrane in less classical cases, furnished the eventual diagnosis. Of these patients, five had pericarditis and in three patients a significant systolic murmur was thought to be present by the referring doctor. This latter finding was not confirmed here. It is of interest to note that while 16 of the 18 with symptoms of over one month's duration were thought to be Still's disease on entry to this hospital, all those six with histories of under one month's duration were thought to be rheumatic fever when first admitted; underlining the considerable difficulty in the early recognition of Still's disease. The following case history illustrates this point:

J.F., aged 11. Nine days before admission here he developed pains in his thighs after playing football. Next day the left ankle and right toe became swollen and painful. The general practitioner found his E.S.R. to be 72 mm./hr. and put him on salicylates. On admission here the right big toe and left ankle were hot and swollen, and the right hip painful. E.S.R. was 60 mm./hr.; heart and electrocardiogram normal. He was thought to be a case of rheumatic fever and put on cortisone. Despite high dosage, acute arthritis persisted and the left elbow also became involved. Persistent joint involvement with soft tissue thickening and raised E.S.R. with no evidence of endocarditis, favoured the alternative diagnosis of Still's disease which has been confirmed by the subsequent progress of the patient.

(*b*) SCHONLEIN-HENOCH PURPURA. Of the eight cases with Schonlein-Henoch purpura, five had polyarthritis and three had limb pains; abdominal pain was a prominent feature in four cases. In six patients there was history of preceding upper respiratory tract infection. In all cases the diagnosis was eventually clarified by the appearance of typical petechiae.

(*c*) ERYTHEMA NODOSUM. There were two adults and three children in this group. Four patients had joint pains and two had joint swelling together with fever. All developed lesions typical of erythema nodosum and the illness settled spontaneously, without an obvious cause having been discovered. Radiographs of the chest were normal and throat and nose swabs negative with no rise in antistreptolysin-O titre. The fifth patient gave a history of severe sore throat and fever treated with sulphathiazole, and he subsequently developed lesions typical of erythema nodosum. Sulphathiazole was suggested as the provocative agent after exclusion of tuberculosis.

(*g*) GENERALIZED LUPUS ERYTHEMATOSUS. Two young females were eventually diagnosed as acute lupus erythematosus. These patients both had joint pains and pericarditis. Eventual diagnosis was made in the first patient by the development of typical skin lesions with biopsy proof and L.E. cells found in peripheral blood. In the second patient proof was eventually found at autopsy. In neither was the diagnosis obvious at the time of transfer.

(*e*) PERIARTERITIS NODOSA. In this child of 11, a sore throat was followed two weeks later by polyarthritis, fever and rash of multiform type. On transfer here she had a patchy reticular erythema, pericarditis, polyarthritis and muscle pains. Skin biopsy showed changes typical of periarteritis nodosa. Subsequent follow-up has confirmed this diagnosis.

(*f*) PROBABLE PENICILLIN SENSITIVITY. This 5-year-old boy presented with pains in his knees and swelling of his face following an upper respiratory tract infection treated with penicillin. There was no evidence of arthritis, carditis or streptococcal infection on transfer, and he was thought to be sensitive to penicillin.

(*g*) GRANULOMA ANNULARE. This patient, a 6-year-old boy, gave a history of nodules on elbows, wrists, toes and neck, and pain in his knees, for six months. On admission here he had a normal E.S.R. and anti-streptolysin-O titre. Nodule biopsy resembled granuloma annulaire, though there is no record of his subsequent progress.

V. Rheumatic and Congenital Heart Disease. (*a*) CONGENITAL HEART DISEASE. These two children were referred on account of general malaise and the discovery of abnormal heart murmurs. One had signs typical of coarctation of the aorta, and the other, aged 4, was admitted with a history of a severe febrile cold following which a heart murmur had been noted. On admission here there was no evidence of rheumatic activity, but cardiovascular findings were those of patent ductus arteriosus, which was subsequently confirmed at operation two years later.

(*b*) RHEUMATIC HEART DISEASE. This group comprised six children and a 19-year-old girl, all of whom had had rheumatic fever previously with established rheumatic heart disease. The recent history was of joint or limb pains, general malaise and tachycardia. All had normal sedimentation rate, antistreptolysin-O titre and sleeping pulse, and there was no evidence of active rheumatism.

VI. Blood Dyscrasias. (*a*) Iron Deficiency Anaemia. This 14-year-old girl presented with general malaise and odd aches and pains; the referring doctor thought there was a significant heart murmur. She was found to have severe iron deficiency anaemia and an innocent basal systolic murmur. Despite full investigation, no satisfactory explanation was found other than inadequate diet.

(*b*) Aleukaemic Stem-celled Leukaemia. This 6-year-old girl was admitted from another hospital with a diagnosis of rheumatic fever. There was one month's history of general malaise with joint pains, fever, tachycardia and swelling of the left knee. E.S.R. was 32 mm./hr.; Hb., 13·8%; W.B.C., 7,000/mm^3 (polymorphs, 82%, leucocytes, 16%, monocytes, 2%). There was an unsatisfactory response to salicylates. She was thought here to be a case of rheumatic fever until, following progressive weight loss, mild generalized lymphadenopathy and anaemia, the bone marrow was examined and showed a picture of aleukaemic stem-celled leukaemia. Radiographs of the long bones showed mild generalized osteoporosis with coarse mottling.

VII. Others. This group consisted of 25 children and eight adults. In only one patient, an adult male, aged 42, could a definite diagnosis be made. He had polyarthritis and a basal diastolic murmur. These findings were confirmed here. He had a raised serum uric acid and radiological changes characteristic of gout; the Wassermann reaction was positive, accounting for the aortic incompetence. In the other 32 patients, the provisional diagnosis of rheumatic fever was not confirmed but no satisfactory alternative diagnosis could be found. Follow-up has varied from none, in a small minority, to seven years, and in no case have rheumatic fever-like episodes recurred, nor has any cardiac abnormality developed. They are grouped according to their main symptomatology as follows:

(*a*) Arthritis of Unexplained Origin. These patients, four children and one young female adult, gave a history of joint swellings but had no abnormal physical signs on admission here. No evidence of streptococcal infection was found (normal anti-streptolysin-O titre and negative nose and throat swabs) and normal E.S.R. Short term follow-up was satisfactory.

(*b*) Arthralgia. These patients gave a history of joint pains dating over several weeks or months and when examined by the family doctor there was either a slight rise in temperature, tachycardia or a suspected organic murmur. Three patients gave a history of recent upper respiratory tract infection. Clinical and serological examinations were negative in all these patients. Short term follow-up was satisfactory.

(*c*) Limb Pain. These patients all complained of limb pains, four following an upper respiratory tract infection. In four cases the referring doctor queried an organic systolic murmur; another patient had had rheumatic fever previously, and in another there was a strong family history of rheumatic fever. In other patients, low grade fever and/or tachycardia were mentioned in the referring letter. When admitted here, all investigations were negative.

(*d*) Fever. These patients were referred on account of unexplained febrile illnesses during which the general practitioner thought that an organic murmur was present. This finding was not confirmed here, and the cause of the preceding febrile episode was never established.

Observations

From the above analysis, it may be seen that many diagnoses may be confused with that of rheumatic fever. In Group B on closer study, four general categories of diagnostic errors became evident: 1. Those cases who would fulfil the Duckett Jones criteria but in whom further observation and development of fresh features provided the ultimate correct diagnosis. 2. Those who would have fulfilled the criteria if all points in the history and clinical examination could have been corroborated. 3. Those in whom there were never even questionably sufficient criteria. 4. Those in whom the diagnosis might have been rejected or the correct one established if the referring doctor had had the facilities and leisure for carrying out further investigations.

The majority in the first category are found in the connective tissue diseases, notably rheumatoid arthritis. The early acute stage of this disease closely resembles rheumatic fever, especially in children, with pericarditis, salicylate-responding pyrexia and transient joint involvement; the Rose Waaler test is usually negative. Only continued observation of the subsequent course of the disease, or the development of endocarditis, erythema marginatum or chorea provides a solution. Even chorea may be seen in acute lupus erythematosus.

The second category comprised both those in whom the referring doctor's findings were not substantiated here, or were not felt to be significant in the diagnosis of rheumatic fever, and also cases in which other points were elicited that had either been missed before or developed subsequently. In greater detail these notably concern the following:

(1) History. A careful history is an essential in the exclusion or confirmation of the less typical forms of acute rheumatism. In several instances the relationship to trauma was missed; in a large number it seemed that complaints of limb or joint pains contributed too prominently towards the proposed initial diagnosis of rheumatic fever, since they were not complained of on transfer here and did not recur. A previous history of rheumatic fever or a family history of the illness often seemed to swing the balance disproportionately in favour of a presumptive diagnosis of rheumatic fever.

(2) Fever. Temperatures of 98·8°-99·4°F. were often cited as being a significant feature. As an isolated finding in a child, this is probably of little consequence, since a normal child's temperature may often reach these levels at some time in the 24 hours.

(3) Tachycardia. This was a feature often stressed in referring letters, particularly in the group which presented primarily with limb and joint pains. Tachycardia out of proportion to the temperature has not been a common finding here, usually occurring only in those children with severe rheumatic fever or cardiac failure; in a few cases of acute rheumatism there has been a sinus bradycardia in the early stages. Even mild apprehension can cause tachycardia in a nervous child, but the sleeping pulse will be within normal range for the age group.

(4) Systolic Murmur. The presence of an organic systolic murmur was initially queried in a total of 48 patients, half of whom were in the upper respiratory tract infection group. A systolic murmur can be demonstrated in a high percentage of infants (Hallidie-Smith, unpublished work) and most normal children (Lessof and Brigden, 1957). These murmurs are usually best heard down the left sternal edge or just internal to the apex. They may be fairly localized or propagated out of the apex and up to the neck. The innocent systolic murmur never fills systole (Lessof and Brigden, 1957), and is usually maximal in early or mid systole. The character may be low pitched and musical, or rather more high pitched and blowing (Friedman, Robie and Harris, 1949). The precise aetiology of these murmurs has not been established, but they are thought to be related to flow of blood in the great vessels and are accentuated in the febrile child whose cardiac output is increased. In contrast, the organic systolic murmur is smooth and high-pitched, filling systole. It is best heard at, or just internal to, the apex, and is propagated outwards to the axilla.

The last category comprises those in whom the error of diagnosis might not have been made if the referring doctor had been able to carry out further investigations toward an alternative diagnosis, since there was often insufficient evidence for suggesting the diagnosis as it stood. The sedimentation rate is of particular value. A normal rate (less than 15 mm./hr. Westergren) at the onset of the disease, would make the diagnosis of active acute rheumatism very unlikely, although it may remain above this level for as little as two weeks. A search for evidence of a preceding streptococcal infection by isolation of the organism in throat or nose swab, or demonstration of a rise in antistreptolysin-O titre, is of some help in doubtful cases.

In other published series (McCue and Galvin, 1948; Lewy, 1952; McCue, 1954; Saslaw, Hernandez and Werblow, 1954; Wedum and Rhodes, 1955) similar points have been made about history-taking, examination and evaluation of physical signs; in each, a large proportion of cases were referred with a provisional diagnosis of rheumatic fever, which either could not be substantiated or was superseded by an alternative diagnosis, sometimes only after careful observation over a period of time. The good long-term prognosis noted in the group with upper respiratory tract infection followed by fever and limb pains is confirmed by these writers and by Kaiser (1943). In the series referred to, the overall pattern of differential diagnosis approximates to our own with certain exceptions, in part explained by the different geographical distributions of disease, e.g. sickle cell anaemia, and in part by the fact that some series only dealt with out-patient referrals. Amongst other less common diseases not listed in our series, but noted in the literature with reference to the differential diagnosis of rheumatic fever, are cat scratch fever (Lyon, 1956); meningococcaemia (Daniels, 1948); miliary tuberculosis (Freud, Weisz and Brunhofer, 1950); ascariasis (Doumer, Lorriaux and Belbenoit, 1951); juvenile hyperparathyroidism (Bogdonoff, Woods, White and Engel, 1956); Weber Christian panniculitis (Brudno, 1950); Hodgkin's disease (Paquet and Delage, 1957); berylliosis (Sprague and Hardy, 1954), sarcoidosis (Myers, Gottlieb, Mattman, Eckley and Chason, 1952); hepatitis (Martini, 1950), and irritable hip syndrome (Caravias, 1956). This last interesting entity has also been noted here. The symptoms are fever, general malaise and sudden onset of severe pain confined to the hip, all settling spontaneously and thought to be due to synovitis.

Summary

The differential diagnosis of rheumatic fever is discussed from the experience at Taplow over a nine-year-period from 1947 to 1956. The original diagnosis is reviewed in a sample of those cases ultimately diagnosed as rheumatic fever, and 12 cases are described which were originally diagnosed otherwise.

A larger series of 196 patients is described who were originally thought to have rheumatic fever, but in whom this diagnosis was eventually not substantiated. This series is subdivided into seven main diagnostic disease groups, which are discussed in detail and illustrated. The pointers in clinical investigation that led to the eventual diagnosis are listed and common erroneous interpretations of history, fever, tachycardia and systolic murmurs are discussed.

Thus the differential diagnosis of rheumatic fever still may present considerable difficulties, particularly in its milder forms. Some of these difficulties are insurmountable. Others could be overcome by more rigid adherence to diagnostic criteria, by more critical examination of the problems presenting, and by increased awareness of the significance of the physical signs elicited. Fuller investigations at an early stage in the disease, notably sedimentation rate and a search for streptococcal infection, would be helpful in the less obvious cases.

We are indebted to Dr. Wallace Brigden, Dr. Reginald Lightwood, Dr. Gerald Thomas and Dr. Paul Wood for their guidance and participation over the years.

REFERENCES

Bogdonoff, M. D., Woods, A. H., White, J. E., and Engel, F. L. (1956). *Amer. J. Med.*, **21**, 583.
Brudno, J. C. (1950). *New Engl. J. Med.*, **243**, 513.
Caravias, D. E. (1956). *Arch. Dis. Childh.*, **31**, 415.
Daniels, W. B. (1948). *Arch. intern. Med.*, **81**, 145.
Doumer, E., Lorriaux, A. and Belbenoit, C. (1951). *Bull. Soc. méd. Hôp. Paris*, **67**, 801.
Freud, P., Weisz, A. and Brunhofer, A. (1950). *Amer. J. Dis. Child.*, **79**, 676.
Friedman, S., Robie, W. A. and Harris, T. N. (1949). *Pediatrics*, **4**, 782.
Hallidie-Smith, K. A. Unpublished work.
Jones, T. Duckett (1944). *J. Amer. med. Ass.*, **126**, 481
Kaiser, A. D. (1943). *N.Y. St. J. Med.*, **43**, 1937.
Lessof, M. and Brigden, W. (1957). *Lancet*, **2**, 673.
Lewy, F. J. (1952). *Ann. intern. Med.*, **36**, 1042.
Lyon, R. (1956). *Lancet*, **2**, 555.
McCue, C. M. (1954). *J. Pediat.*, **44**, 290.
—— and Galvin, L. F. (1948). *Ibid.*, **33**, 467.
Martini, G. A. (1950). *Dtsch. med. Wschr.*, **75**, 1464.
Myers, G. B., Gottlieb, A. M., Mattman, P. E., Eckley, G. M. and Chason, J. L. (1952). *Amer. J. Med.*, **12**, 161.
Nelson, W. E. (1954). *Textbook of Pediatrics*, 6th ed., p. 854. Saunders, Philadelphia.
Paquet, E. and Delage, J. M. (1957). *Canad. med. Ass. J.*, **76**, 927.
Rheumatic Fever Committee Joint Report (1955). Rheumatic Fever Working Party of the Medical Research Council of Great Britain and the Subcommittee of Principal Investigators of the American Council on Rheumatic Fever and Congenital Heart Disease, American Heart Association. *Brit. med. J.*, **1**, 555.
Saslaw, M. S., Hernandez, F. A. and Werblow, S. C. (1954). *J. Pediat.*, **44**, 414.
Sprague, H. B. and Hardy, H. L. (1954). *Circulation (N.Y.)*, **10**, 129.
Wedum, B. G. and Rhodes, P. H. (1955). *J. Amer. med. Ass.*, **157**, 981.
World Health Organization. (1957). Report of the Committee on Rheumatic Diseases.

A SMALL OUTBREAK OF NEONATAL MENINGITIS IN A MATERNITY UNIT

BY

ERIC McKAY and JOHN SMITH

From the Royal Aberdeen Hospital for Sick Children and the Aberdeen City Hospital

(RECEIVED FOR PUBLICATION JANUARY 1, 1958)

The enterobacteriaceae are of particular importance in infancy as a cause of meningitis. Cooke and Bell (1922) postulated that certain strains of the *coli aerogenes* group might have a special tendency to invade the meninges, and suggested that full descriptions of the organisms isolated from such cases would be of value. Again, Barrett, Rammelkamp and Worcester (1942) commented on the frequent lack of sufficient detail for accurate classification of the organisms obtained in the majority of cases. Henderson (1948), in his review of Salmonella meningitis, found that a few types of salmonellae account for the majority of cases, and he also noted that three epidemics among the newborn accounted for more than one fourth of the 147 cases he had collected. A small outbreak of three cases of meningitis occurring in a maternity hospital is described, the organism being a hitherto unidentified member of the enterobacteriaceae.

Case Histories

Each of the three cases was accommodated for a few days at 'E' Maternity Hospital, Case 1 from July 2-8, 1957, and Cases 2 and 3 from August 22-28, 1957. During this period no other babies and, as far as can be ascertained, no members of staff or patients suffered from gastro-intestinal symptoms or other infections.

Case 1. K.L., a male infant of birth weight 7 lb. 8½ oz., was born by normal delivery at 'E' Maternity Hospital on July 2, 1957. He was the ninth child of healthy parents, the other children all being alive and well. The maternal membranes had ruptured immediately before the delivery, and the mother had no symptoms of urinary, gastro-intestinal or other infection. The infant was fed on evaporated milk, taking the feeds well and behaving normally until the age of 6 days when he became drowsy and refused to suck. Four hours later, when he had a brief episode of generalized twitching, the fontanelle was bulging slightly, the head was retracted, and the rectal temperature was 101°F. The baby was transferred to Aberdeen City Hospital where lumbar puncture produced a purulent, blood-stained cerebrospinal fluid. The detailed bacteriology of cerebrospinal fluid and faeces is given below. Treatment was commenced with intramuscular penicillin and streptomycin but the infant died 14 hours after admission. The positive findings at autopsy were marked congestion of the meninges, a purulent exudate over the base of the brain and bilateral adrenal haemorrhage.

Cases 2 and 3. C.F. and R.F. were twins, born five weeks prematurely at 'A' Maternity Hospital on August 18, 1957; they were transferred to 'E' Maternity Hospital on August 22 and discharged home on August 28. R.F., twin 1, was born by spontaneous vertex delivery, weighing 6 lb. 9 oz., and C.F., twin 2, by assisted breech delivery, weighing 5 lb. 12 oz. The maternal membranes ruptured only 45 minutes before delivery, and the mother had no fever or evidence of urinary or gastro-intestinal infection.

Case 2, C.F., was admitted to the Royal Aberdeen Hospital for Sick Children at the age of 12 days with a history of vomiting once 24 hours before admission with refusal to feed thereafter. On examination he was a drowsy hypotonic infant weighing 6 lb. 3½ oz., who did not appear acutely ill, but who had an intermittent slight cyanosis of the lips and peri-oral region. The rectal temperature was 98·2°F., pulse rate 146 per minute and respirations 58 per minute. A moderate degree of jaundice was present. No evidence was found of meningeal irritation or neurological abnormality and physical examination was otherwise negative. The urine contained a small amount of a reducing substance. The cerebrospinal fluid, which was under normal pressure, was greenish-yellow and turbid, containing 1,254 leucocytes (66% polymorphonuclear) per c.mm. Numerous Gram-negative bacilli could be seen on film; details of the bacteriology of cerebrospinal fluid and faeces are given below.

TREATMENT AND PROGRESS. Treatment initially was by intramuscular chloramphenicol (500 mg. daily for 29 days) and intramuscular streptomycin (120 mg. daily for 32 days). Cortisone was given by the same route in decreasing dosage for the first two weeks commencing with 100 mg. daily; this was used in view of the experience with Case 1 and also in an unsuccessful attempt to prevent the adhesions so frequently seen in coliform meningitis. Convulsions during the first few days of the illness were controlled by intramuscular paraldehyde. Continuous oxygen therapy was required for the first 11 days and parenteral fluids for 12 days. At the end of the third week exploration of the left lateral ventricle revealed thick creamy pus which was aspirated daily with instillation of 25 mg. streptomycin on each occasion for the next 10 days. The infant remained extremely ill, vomiting frequently and gradually losing weight, and for this reason the therapy was changed, chloramphenicol being replaced by sulphadiazine (0·75 g. daily for nine weeks) and streptomycin by polymyxin B (intrathecally 20,000 units twice per day for three days and once per day for a further nine days, and intramuscularly 25,000 units four-hourly for three days, then six-hourly for nine days). During his sixth week in the ward the vomiting ceased and his weight began to rise, but at the age of four months he is markedly retarded in his motor development. Ventriculography shows a gross degree of internal hydrocephalus of obstructive type, although the head measurements are not increasing rapidly.

The causative organism was not cultured from the cerebrospinal fluid after the initial specimen, but a Gram-negative organism was seen on direct film as late as the end of the polymyxin treatment.

Case 3, R.F., was admitted to the Royal Aberdeen Hospital for Sick Children two days after his twin brother. This twin had remained well until only four hours before admission, when his mother noticed intermittent peri-oral cyanosis. He refused part of a feed and whimpered frequently. Following her experience with the first twin, the mother sought immediate medical attention. Physical examination at the time of admission showed a mildly jaundiced, fairly healthy-looking baby of 6 lb. 4½ oz. No cyanosis was present, the fontanelle was not bulging, and there was no rigidity of the spine or head retraction. The tone of the legs was considered to be slightly increased, and the cry was rather shrill. The cerebrospinal fluid was turbid, greenish-yellow, containing 54,000 leucocytes (91% polymorphonuclear) per c.mm. The cerebrospinal protein was 280 mg. per 100 ml.; sugar, 15 mg. per 100 ml.; and chlorides, 710 mg. NaCl per 100 ml. Bacteriological details of cerebrospinal fluid and faeces are given below.

TREATMENT AND PROGRESS. Three short courses (14 days, 10 days, 10 days) were given of chloramphenicol and streptomycin with intervals of 14 days and eight days without antibiotics. The chloramphenicol was given intramuscularly (250 mg. twice daily) for the first course and orally (250 mg. six-hourly) for the two later courses. Streptomycin dosage was 120 mg. per day. Following these drugs oral sulphadiazine was administered for six weeks. Cortisone in decreasing dosage, commencing with 100 mg. daily, was also administered for the first 10 days. The illness of this twin ran a more benign course than in C.F. During the first few days in hospital signs of meningeal irritation developed; there were some brief episodes of twitching and also several mild cyanotic attacks, but bottle-feeding was possible throughout. The second and third courses of antibiotics were given because of recurrence of vomiting and irritability with increased numbers of pus cells in the cerebrospinal fluid although the causative organism was not cultured again. Subdural taps were negative four weeks after the onset of the illness. The present mental state of the child at the age of 4 months is difficult to assess but the general impression is unfavourable; he holds his head up with difficulty and is taking little notice of his environment.

Bacteriological Investigation

When it was found that the meningeal infection in the first case was due to an intestinal type of non-lactose fermenting organism, the faeces of the patient were examined and a similar organism was isolated. The strains obtained from the cerebrospinal fluid and from the faeces were next subjected to detailed fermentation and biochemical tests but no serological tests were carried out at this time. When the second and third cases of meningitis occurred some seven weeks later in patients from the same hospital the strains isolated from the cerebrospinal fluids and faeces were again tested for their full fermentation and biochemical activities. The reactions of the three strains isolated from the cerebrospinal fluids are given in Table 1. Similar tests applied to the strains isolated from the faeces gave the same results. The cultural and biochemical characteristics of the various strains were not identical with those usually associated with typical strains of *Esch. coli*. They differed in that they fermented adonitol, produced acid and a slight amount of gas in inositol, grew in Koser's citrate medium, produced H_2S, utilized urea after a period of delay and failed to ferment lactose. The strains from the cerebrospinal fluid and faeces of the first case were submitted to Dr. P. R. Edwards and Dr. Ewing of the

TABLE 1

BIOCHEMICAL AND FERMENTATION REACTIONS

	Cerebrospinal Fluid Strains					
	24 hours			14 days		
	KL	CF	RF	KL	CF	RF
Adonitol	AG	AG	AG	AG	AG	AG
Dulcitol	O	O	O	O	O	O
Sorbitol	AG	AG	AG	AG	AG	AG
Arabinose	AG	AG	AG	AG	AG	AG
Xylose	AG	AG	AG	AG	AG	AG
Rhamnose	AG	AG	AG	AG	AG	AG
Maltose	AG	AG	AG	AG	AG	AG
Salicin	O	O	O	AG	AG	AG
Inositol	O	SA	SA	AS/G	AS/G	AS/G
Lactose	O	O	O	O	O	O
Sucrose	O	O	O	O	O	O
Mannitol	AG	AG	AG	AG	AG	AG
Glucose	AG	AG	AG	AG	AG	AG
Indole	+++	+++	+++	—	—	—
H_2S (7 days)	+	+	+	—	—	—
Gelatin	O	O	O	O	O	O
Koser's citrate	++	++	++	+++	+++	+++
Voges-Proskauer (48 hours)	O	O	O	—	—	—
Methyl-red (48 hours)	+++	+++	+++	—	—	—
Urea agar	O	O	O	+++	+++	+++
KCN (4 days)	O	O	O	—	—	—
Motility	+++	+++	+++	—	—	—

AG = acid and gas. O = no change. SA = slight acidity.
AS/G = acid with small amount of gas. — = not tested.

TABLE 2

DETAILS OF TESTS OF THREE CEREBROSPINAL FLUID STRAINS

	Agglutination of Strains			Absorption of Sera		
	KL	CF	RF	KL	CF	RF
		'H' agglutination			*Titre after 'H' absorption*	
Serum KL 'H'	6·400	6·400	6·400	<100	<100	<100
Serum CF 'H'	12·800	12·800	12·800	<100	<100	<100
		'O' agglutination			*Titre after 'O' absorption*	
Serum KL 'O'	1·600	1·600	1·600	<100	<100	<100
Serum CF 'O'	800	800	800	<100	<100	<100

Enteric Disease Centre, Chamblee, Georgia, who reported that the organisms resembled *Esch. coli* more closely than any other type but were not related to the serological types of *Esch. coli* 1-137. They were, therefore, classified as intermediate coliforms. Since the cultural and fermentation reactions of all three cerebrospinal fluid and all three faecal strains were identical, 'H' and 'O' antigens were prepared from the K.L. and C.F. cerebrospinal fluid strains, and four rabbits were immunized. When the agglutinin titre in each animal's serum was sufficiently high, it was bled and the serum preserved with 50% glycerine. When all four sera were collected, agglutination and agglutinin absorption tests were carried out with the respective 'H' and 'O' antigens of all three strains isolated from the cerebrospinal fluid and of all three strains isolated from the faeces. The details of the tests for the three cerebrospinal fluid strains are given in Table 2 and show that they are serologically identical. As the strains obtained from the faeces gave similar serological reactions, these results are omitted.

As stated above, Ewing could find no serological relationship with any of the *Esch. coli* types 1-137. Further tests with polyvalent Salmonella and dysentery sera also failed to show any relationship with these groups of organisms. As a further confirmation of the identity of the strains isolated from the cerebrospinal fluids, their sensitivity to various antibiotics was examined. The method employed was to use the Sentest antibiotic discs prepared by Evans Medical Products, each antibiotic with the exception of bacitracin being tested in two concentrations. The results were recorded according to the approximate degree of inhibition and are given in Table 3. All three strains reacted in a more or less similar manner to 11 antibiotics, being most sensitive to chloramphenicol, neomycin and streptomycin, and less sensitive to the tetracyclines. They were insensitive to erythromycin, novobiocin, oleandomycin and penicillin.

After the second and third cases had occurred the question of the method of spread was considered. Accordingly specimens of faeces were obtained on two occasions from five nurses, four ward maids and two mothers, one being the mother of the affected twins. The nurses and maids might have had contact with the first case as well as the second and third, but the mothers could have had no contact with the first infection which occurred. None of the specimens showed the non-lactose fermenting organism so the actual source of infection was not determined. Furthermore, since the incidents occurred, all non-lactose fermenting and indole positive organisms isolated from specimens of faeces have been tested serologically with the sera prepared, but no further strains have been encountered.

Discussion

The organism isolated from the three cases was an unusual cause of meningitis. It was a non-lactose fermenting type which had fermentation and biochemical characteristics suggesting a variant of *Esch. coli*. The fact that it did not ferment lactose enabled it to be isolated from the faeces of the three cases as well as from the cerebrospinal fluids. Apparently it appears infrequently in faeces because, since the incident, some 1,500 specimens of faeces submitted for routine bacteriological investigation

TABLE 3

SENSITIVITY OF STRAINS TO TWO CONCENTRATIONS OF ANTIBIOTICS IN FORM OF SENTESTS

	Strains and Results							
	(1)				(2)			
Antibiotic	Concentration	KL	CF	RF	Concentration	KL	CF	RF
Aureomycin	10 µg.	+	+	+	100 µg.	++	++	++
Bacitracin	100 µg.	—	—	—	—			
Chloramphenicol	40 µg.	+++	+++	+++	100 µg.	+++	+++	+++
Erythromycin	1 µg.	—	—	—	10 µg.	—	—	—
Neomycin	10 µg.	+++	+++	+++	100 µg.	+++	+++	+++
Novobiocin	2 µg.	—	—	—	10 ?g.	—	—	—
Oleandomycin	2 µg.	—	—	—	20 µg.	—	—	—
Penicillin	0·5 I.U.	—	—	—	2·5 I.U.	—	—	—
Streptomycin	20 µg.	+++	+++	+++	80 µg.	+++	+++	+++
Terramycin	10 µg.	+	+	+	100 µg.	+++	+++	+++
Tetracylines	10 µg.	+	+	+	100 µg.	++	++	++

have failed to show its presence. Presumably the organism must have been distributed through the agency of a carrier, for practically a month elapsed between the occurrence of the first case and the second and third. The investigation for such a carrier, however, gave entirely negative results. Presumably also the infants ingested the infecting organism, then developed a bacteraemia, and a subsequent meningitis.

Among the many types of Salmonellae a comparatively small number have been found to be responsible for most cases of spread to the meninges. The same may well be true of other members of the enterobacteriaceae although proof of this is at present lacking. In the majority of reports of this condition the organism is recorded as *Esch. coli* or paracolon bacillus without details of fermentation or serological reactions. Complete bacteriological data should if possible be given in future reports of such cases so that an answer can be found to this problem.

Summary

Three cases are recorded of neonatal meningitis occurring in a maternity hospital and due to a previously unidentified non-lactose fermenting member of the enterobacteriaceae.

We are grateful to Professor John Craig for permission to publish these cases, to Dr. N. S. Clark for advice and criticism, and to Dr. A. Sutherland for information and laboratory specimens from the maternity unit involved.

References

Barrett, G. S., Rammelkamp, C. H. and Worcester, J. (1942). *Amer. J. Dis. Child.*, **63**, 41.
Cooke, J. V. and Bell, H. H. (1922). *Ibid.*, **24**, 387.
Henderson, L. L. (1948). *Ibid.*, **75**, 351.

NEONATAL PERFORATION OF THE COLON

BY

LEONARD HAAS

From The London Hospital

(RECEIVED FOR PUBLICATION DECEMBER 12, 1957)

Case History

Paul R., a male infant, aged 5 days, was born in hospital; his birth weight was 7 lb. 5 oz. The mother's pregnancy and the delivery were normal. Vomiting began immediately after birth and became increasingly severe. Scanty amounts of meconium were passed on the first, second and fourth days. The abdomen was said to have been protuberant as early as on the first day, and was referred to as distended on the third day of life.

The infant was seen by a paediatrician on the fifth day, who reported that he looked ill and dehydrated with balloon-like abdominal distension. Bowel sounds were present. On rectal examination a tight, narrow rectal orifice was found; there was meconium on the fingerstall. No other abnormal physical signs were detected. A radiograph of the abdomen showed that free air was present.

Progress. The child was given parenteral fluids and laparotomy was carried out. Free fluids and faeces were found in the peritoneal cavity, and there was a perforation in the transverse colon. The peritoneal cavity was cleaned out, and the transverse colon exteriorized at the site of the perforation in the form of a colostomy. The patient did not stand the operation well; he collapsed on the table and was resuscitated with difficulty. He was cold, pale and cyanosed on returning to the ward. In spite of appropriate treatment with intravenous fluids and oxygen his condition improved but little, and he died quietly 10 hours after the operation and 6 days after birth.

Necropsy confirmed the presence of a solitary perforation, 0·8 cm. in diameter, in the transverse colon, 11 cm. from the ileo-caecal valve. There was uniform dilatation of the whole of the large bowel right down to the anus. No thickened plugs of meconium were found. The peritoneum was deeply congested, with numerous scattered yellow meconium flecks. The remainder of the examination revealed no abnormality. Thus there was no evidence of meconium ileus, fibrocystic disease of the pancreas, Hirschsprung's disease or intestinal obstruction.

Discussion

Spontaneous perforation of the bowel in the newborn with peritonitis is barely mentioned in any of the standard textbooks of paediatrics. It is known to occur not only as a complication of meconium ileus and other forms of obstruction, but also in the apparent absence of any recognizable pathological lesion, when its aetiology may be quite obscure (Franklin and Hosford, 1952). Numerous factors have been implicated at different times (Thelander, 1939). Some of these have been largely of a conjectural nature, such as birth trauma, intra-uterine infection and interference with the blood supply to the bowel. Zachary (1957) in a small series of cases attributes perforation to pressure by hard plugs of meconium. In a few instances definite congenital defects of the muscle coats of the bowel have been found. Rudnew (1915) studied a case of foetal peritonitis due to perforation of the transverse colon. He found that the continuity of the muscularis mucosa was broken at frequent intervals by blood vessels and nerves surrounded by areolar tissue. The breaks in the muscularis were of considerable size, so that the mucous membrane could herniate through them. Fischer (1928) reported a case with two perforations of the colon. Examination of the areas adjacent to the perforations showed the absence of the circular and the longitudinal muscle layers. There was herniation outwards through one of the perforations of the mucosa and the muscularis mucosa. Boikan (1930) described excessive development of the lymphatic tissues and deeply penetrating crypts of Lieberkühn at the site of a neonatal colonic perforation.

Fig. 1 shows a section of the colon close to the perforation of the present case, described above. The most striking histological feature is the presence of a large number of dilated blood vessels throughout the wall of the gut. These almost replace the muscularis mucosa and interrupt at frequent intervals the circular and longitudinal muscle layers, which are scanty and ill-defined. It seems therefore that an area of weakness may have been created by this localized infiltration of the bowel wall with haemangiomatous material.

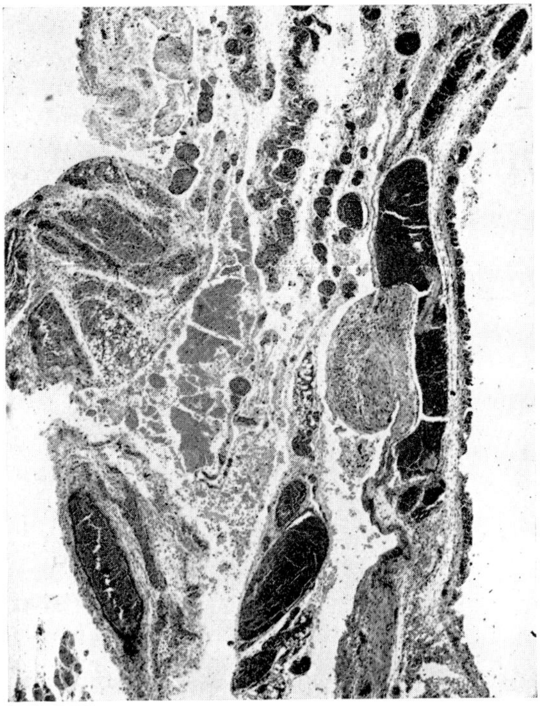

FIG. 1.—Section through colon near perforation showing haemangiomatous dilatation of vessels throughout wall.

This particular type of abnormality associated with spontaneous perforation of the intestine in the newborn does not appear to have been previously described. It is interesting, however, to compare it with the other congenital lesions reviewed above, which also weaken the muscular layers of the intestinal wall and so predispose to perforation.

Summary

A case of spontaneous perforation of the colon in a newborn infant is described.

A necropsy showed a solitary perforation and generalized peritonitis.

Histological section revealed a localized haemangiomatous abnormality at the site of the perforation, a lesion apparently not previously described.

I am indebted to Dr. K. H. Tallerman for his permission to publish this case, and for his help and encouragement. My thanks are also due to Mr. E. C. Butler, and to Dr. R. F. Parker who performed all the pathological examinations.

References

Boikan, W. S. (1930). *Arch. Path. (Chicago)*, **9**, 1164.
Fischer, A. E. (1928). *Amer. J. Dis. Child.*, **36**, 774.
Franklin, A. W. and Hosford, J. P. (1952). *Brit. med. J.*, **2**, 257.
Rudnew, W. (1915). (Quoted by Fischer, 1928). *Ueber die spontanen Darmrupturen bei Foeten und Neugeborenen.* Dissertation, Basel.
Thelander, H. E. (1939). *Amer. J. Dis. Child.*, **58**, 371.
Zachary, R. B. (1957). *Arch. Dis. Childh.*, **32**, 22.

BILATERAL PULMONARY AGENESIS

BY

ALBERT E. CLAIREAUX and H. P. FERREIRA

From the Institute of Obstetrics and Gynaecology, University of London

(RECEIVED FOR PUBLICATION DECEMBER 6, 1957)

Absence of one lung is an unusual malformation and has been the subject of an extensive review by Smart (1946) who was able to trace 33 cases of complete absence of one lung. A much more rare anomaly is complete absence of both lungs. Only three cases appear to be recorded in the literature. The first was reported by Schmit (1893) from Germany and the others by Allen and Affelbach (1925) and by Tuynman and Gardner (1952) from America. The following report appears to be the first of its kind from this country.

Case Report

The mother was a healthy primigravida aged 18 years. Apart from the usual childhood illnesses, including measles, she had been well up to the time of her pregnancy. She had no illness during pregnancy. The estimated date of delivery was May 2, 1957. When first seen on November 24, 1956, she was 18 weeks pregnant. She was Group A, Rhesus positive and the Wassermann reaction was negative. The pregnancy continued normally and labour began spontaneously at term on May 3, 1957. She was then admitted to hospital following an antepartum haemorrhage of about 100 ml. of blood. She was delivered of a male infant on May 4, 1957, following slight further blood loss.

The infant's colour was good at birth, it made several attempts at respiration and was said to have 'breathed'. A few minutes after delivery it was noted to be pale and limp. Resuscitation was attempted but was unsuccessful and heart sounds ceased 15 minutes after delivery.

Necropsy. At necropsy on May 5 the body was that of a rather small male infant weighing 2,500 g. and measuring 48 cm. in length. No congenital abnormality was found on external examination.

The falx and tentorium were intact. The brain was firm and no lesion was found on slicing.

When the thorax was opened the heart was seen to be occupying the right half of the thorax. The left side of the chest was occupied by a large thymus. Petechial haemorrhages were present in the parietal pleura and pericardium. There was no lung tissue visible and no bronchial structure was seen. The trachea was identified and was removed together with the larynx. It was noted that the trachea ended blindly (Fig. 1) and there was no

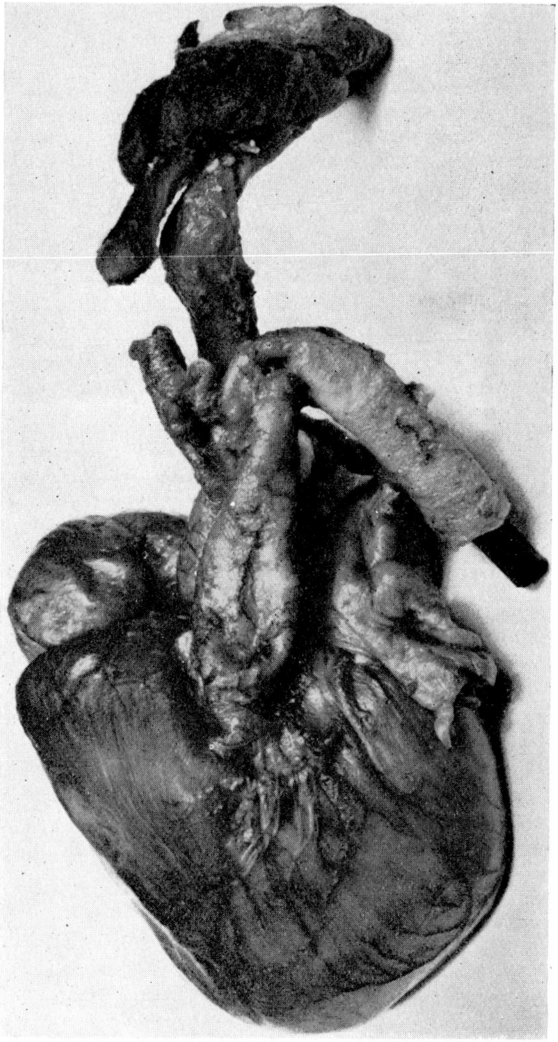

FIG. 1.—Anterior and lateral view of trachea showing rounded lower end and absence of bronchial buds. The intact oesophagus lies posteriorly. The pulmonary trunk, without branching, enters the aorta which is narrow proximally. A marker is inserted into the thoracic aorta.

evidence of an attempt at the formation of bronchial buds. The trachea measured 1·7 cm. in length and 0·5 cm. in diameter and only two poorly formed cartilagenous rings were found. It was uniform in size throughout its length and had a round end. The larynx was apparently normal. The mucosa lining the larynx and trachea was yellowish in colour.

The heart was of the expected size. There was anomalous venous drainage with a left superior vena cava opening into the left atrium (Fig. 2). The right superior vena cava and the inferior vena cava opened into the right atrium in the usual way. There was a defect in the inter-atrial septum. The tricuspid valve had a normal appearance. The pulmonary valve was also normal. The pulmonary trunk was of the usual calibre and 2·8 cm. above the pulmonary valve it joined the aorta distal to the point of origin of the left subclavian artery. There were no pulmonary arteries. The interventricular septum was intact. The aortic and mitral valves had a normal appearance. The left atrium was rather small and there were no pulmonary veins. The chamber received the left superior vena cava.

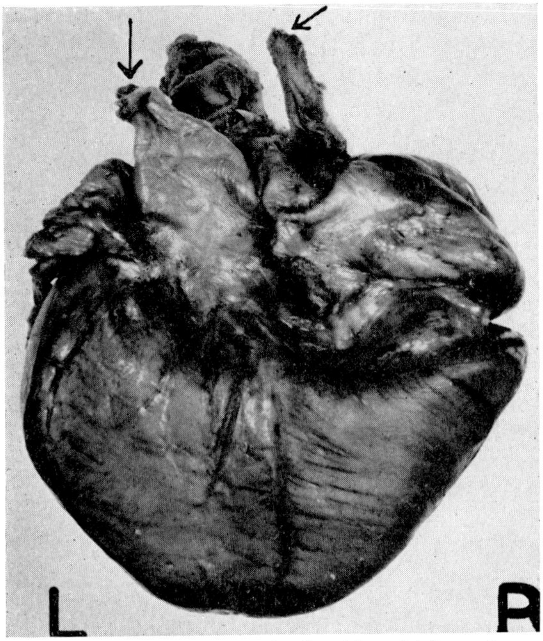

FIG. 2.—Posterior view of heart showing right and left superior vena cava (arrowed). Note absence of pulmonary veins.

The aorta arose in the usual manner and the coronary arteries had a normal appearance. The aortic arch was directed to the left and the descending thoracic aorta showed no abnormality. There were no bronchial arteries. The arch of the aorta was abnormal. Coarctation was present for a distance of 1 cm. between the origin of the innominate artery and the point where the pulmonary trunk entered. In the narrow segment of the arch the aorta was just under half the diameter of the proximal portion. The oesophagus was intact and of the usual calibre.

The peritoneum was healthy and no lesions were present in the stomach or bowel. There was no transposition of the abdominal organs. The liver was of the expected size and no lesion was found on slicing. The diaphragm reached the level of the fourth interspace on each side. The spleen and lymph nodes were normal. There was no abnormality in the genito-urinary tract.

An anatomical diagnosis of bilateral pulmonary agenesis was made. There was congenital malformation of the heart with anomalous left superior vena cava and inter-atrial septal defect; absence of the right and left pulmonary arteries (the pulmonary trunk continuing straight into the aorta); and coarctation of the aorta.

Discussion

Complete absence of both lungs is of course incompatible with life and is thus of much less clinical importance than absence of one lung. Nevertheless, it is interesting to note that an attempt at respiration was made in all cases so far reported. It thus seems certain that the initiation of respiratory movement does not depend on the presence of lung tissue. Additional malformations in our case were confined to the heart. In the case reported by Schmit (1893) the trachea was connected with the oesophagus and there was a bony abnormality in the neck. The infant described by Tuynman and Gardner (1952) had an accessory spleen. Our case also differs from that of Allen and Affelbach (1925) in that the trachea ended abruptly, but in their case and in the one reported by Tuynman and Gardner, primitive bronchial buds were present.

The cardiac malformations are also slightly different in all three cases. The pulmonary artery joined the aorta at the point where the aorta and ductus arteriosus normally meet in all the cases. The left auricle received no vessels at all in the cases of Schmit and of Allen and Affelbach. In our case an anomalous superior vena cava entered this chamber and in the case reported by Tuynman and Gardner the inferior vena cava drained into it. In their case also, the aortic arch was directed to the right, a change which was absent in the others. A patent foramen ovale was reported by Schmit and by Allen and Affelbach and in our case the inter-atrial septum was deficient. Our specimen was also unique in showing a coarctation of the aorta.

According to Arey (1940) primary bronchial budding occurs at the 4 mm. stage of the embryo, i.e. at about the fourth week of pregnancy. It would appear, therefore, that the further development of the respiratory tract was interrupted just prior to this. The abnormalities in the heart and great vessels are presumably the consequence of the failure of pulmonary development. Ellis (1917), however, has suggested that vascular anomalies may be the primary lesion. This does not appear to be likely in the present case as the development of the heart commences at about the 4 mm. stage.

Severe congenital malformations are known to follow certain virus infections in the mother, notably rubella. There was no history of any such infection in the present case. It is possible that the pulmonary and cardiovascular anomalies were genetically determined but the actual cause of the defect, as with most other congenital abnormalities, remains obscure.

Summary

A case of bilateral pulmonary agenesis in an infant born at term is reported. In addition to absence of both lungs there were a number of cardiac abnormalities, including an anomalous left superior vena cava and an inter-atrial septal defect.

We are indebted to Mr. E. Clark of the Bernhard Baron Memorial Research Laboratories, Queen Charlotte's Maternity Hospital, London, for the photographs.

References

Allen and Affelbach (1925). *Surg. Gynec. Obstet.*, **41**, 375.
Arey, L. B. (1940). *Developmental Anatomy.* 4th ed. W. B. Saunders and Co., Philadelphia. p. 233.
Ellis, A. G. (1917). *Amer. J. med. Sci.*, **154**, 33
Schmit, H. (1893). *Virchows Arch. path. Anat.*, **134**, 25.
Smart, J. (1946). *Quart. J. Med.*, **15** n.s. 125.
Tuynman, P. E. and Gardner, L. W. (1952). *A.M.A. Arch. Path.*, **54**, 306.

ATRESIA OF THE OESOPHAGUS WITH COMMON TRACHEO-OESOPHAGEAL TUBE

BY

R. G. WELCH and O. A. N. HUSAIN

From the Paediatric and Pathology Departments, Lambeth Hospital, London

(RECEIVED FOR PUBLICATION JANUARY 3, 1958)

The clinical picture and anatomical variants of oesophageal atresia are well known now that this condition can be treated surgically with fair hope of success. In about 90% of cases there is a fistula connecting the lower segment of the oesophagus to the trachea and in some 9% the atresia is present alone without a fistula. Amongst the remainder there are instances where the fistula passes from the upper pouch to the trachea, where there is a fistula connecting each segment to the trachea and where a fistula occurs without any atresia (Waterston, 1954). In the case of the infant described here, however,though in life the findings did not appear out of the ordinary, autopsy revealed a most unusual malformation and it is perhaps fortunate that the child's general condition precluded any attempt at surgical correction.

Case History

A male child, birth weight 6 lb., was born rapidly at home five weeks before term. The pregnancy had been uneventful and he was the third child of healthy parents, the mother's age being 23. Respiration could not be established and atresia of the oesophagus became apparent when a catheter could not be passed into the stomach. Intermittent gasping respiration followed mouth-to-mouth insufflation and the child was transferred to hospital where, following intra-tracheal oxygen, a more regular, but stertorous and rattling, respiration was established about two and a half hours after birth. The child remained limp and unresponsive, with intermittent cyanotic attacks and a low temperature. Numerous rales were audible all over the chest and the intestines filled with air. After some hours the intra-tracheal tube was removed but, as the child's condition and colour promptly deteriorated, it was reinserted, this time rather further than before. It was then noted that the condition remained poor until the tube was withdrawn a short way, but the significance of this was not appreciated until autopsy. After 36 hours, during which time the child never developed muscle tone or became responsive, the stertorous respirations became periodic and death followed at 48 hours.

At autopsy an oedematous and congested brain was found with blood clot around the circle of Willis and brain stem. No aneurysm or bleeding point could be identified. The right kidney and all its ureter, apart from a short distal portion, were absent. The heart was normal and there were no abnormal blood vessels apparent in the neck and chest. The oesophagus ended blindly as a pouch 1 cm. below the laryngeal entrance.

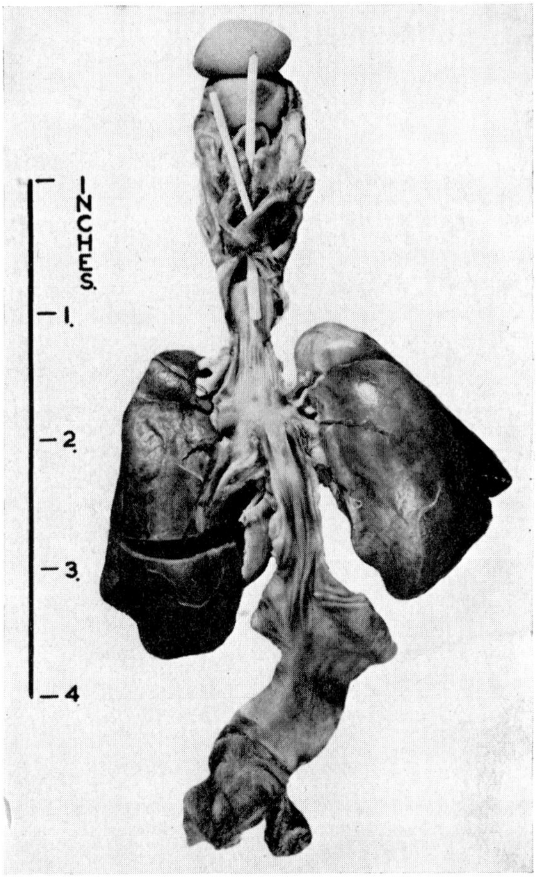

FIG. 1.—One marker lies under the oesophageal pouch and the other is passed through the larynx into the common tube.

The larynx was normal and opened wholly into a tube which appeared to be an oesophagus, but at its upper end, below the thyroid cartilage, were a normal cricoid cartilage and three poorly formed tracheal rings, all hidden behind the thyroid gland. The tube, having given off the two main bronchi in mid-thorax, passed normally through the left side of the diaphragm and into the stomach (Fig. 1). The bronchi and lobes of the lung were anatomically normal with well-formed cartilagenous rings.

Microscopy disclosed that the upper oesophageal pouch was lined by stratified squamous epithelium. There were no mucous glands and the submucosa contained a scanty muscularis mucosa. The wall was of striated muscle fibres arranged normally in outer circular and inner longitudinal coats (Fig. 2). The wall of the common tracheo-oesophageal tube contained only unstriped muscle fibres, mainly in longitudinal bundles with less well-developed outer circular fibres. The mucous glands were scattered generally throughout the submucosa, both superficial and deep, to the scanty and ill-defined muscularis mucosa, and also deep within the muscle coat. These glands had the appearance of those found in the normal trachea (Fig. 3). The epithelium gradually changed from stratified squamous above to a stratified cilated columnar form of the respiratory type near the origin of the bronchi and this passed gradually to the true respiratory mucosa in the bronchi themselves. Some of the mucosal epithelium had been stripped off by a mild inflammatory reaction and trauma (probably by the intra-tracheal tube).

The lungs were surprisingly well aerated with some scattered intra-alveolar haemorrhages.

Discussion

The interest of this case lies not only in the most unusual gross findings at autopsy but also in the histological appearance of this common tracheo-oesophageal tube which, though lacking all but the first three cartilagenous rings, had in it mucous glands of the type normally found in the trachea, as well as epithelium of both sorts. There is, of course, a wide variety of congenital anomalies involving trachea and oesophagus ranging from complete absence of the oesophagus (Wilkins, 1938) on the one hand, through absence of a segment of oesophagus (usually in association with a tracheo-oesophageal fistula), tracheal stenosis and hypoplasia (Wolman, 1941), to complete absence of trachea on the other. For two structures so intimately related in their development, it is surprising that the atresias of the oesophagus should be so much the more common. Estimates of its frequency vary, but it is probably in

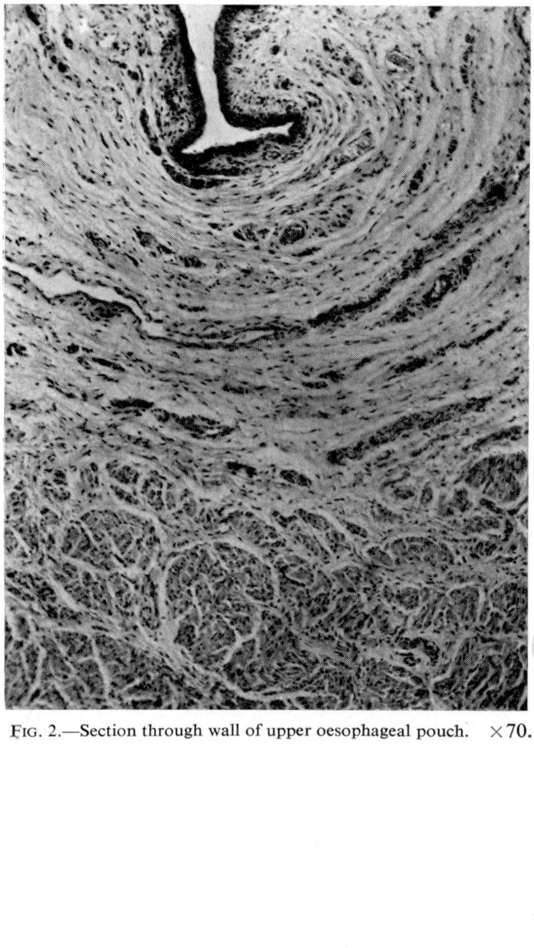

FIG. 2.—Section through wall of upper oesophageal pouch. ×70.

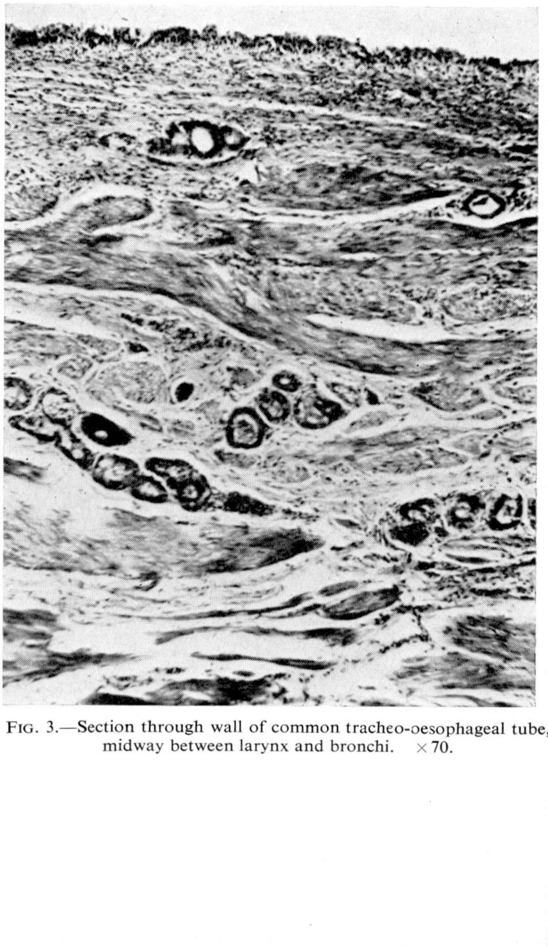

FIG. 3.—Section through wall of common tracheo-oesophageal tube, midway between larynx and bronchi. ×70.

the nature of 1 to every 1,500 births (Scott and Wilson, 1957). On the other hand, recorded examples of absence of the trachea are very rare. Fritz (1933) and Sandison (1955) have each reported a case where the bronchi opened normally into a short lower segment of trachea from the roof of which a fistula passed to a normal oesophagus. In the infants described by Kessel and Smith (1953) and Hempel (1956) the conjoined bronchi connected by a fistula to the oesophagus whilst in those recorded by Walcher (1928), Benešová and Peter (1934) and Marek (1940) the bronchi opened directly into the oesophagus. In Payne's case (1900) the main bronchi were connected to each other but to nowhere else, a state of affairs very similar to that described by Milles and Dorsey (1950). The continental authors mention a few similar cases in the earlier European literature, but the total numbers are few and in all the larynx is occluded by a sheet of cartilage or membrane with the oesophagus apparently otherwise normal, though without histological examination for the most part.

This wide range of abnormality indicates a developmental defect at a very early stage. Gruenwald (1940) has described the early stage of an oesophageal atresia and tracheo-oesophageal fistula in a 9 mm. embryo (5 to 6 weeks' ovulation age) and Ingalls and Prindle (1949) mention earlier reports of the fully developed malformation in 18·1 and 19 mm. embryos.

Normal Development. According to Frazer (1953) the first trace of the future respiratory system is apparent in the 2·9 mm. embryo (ovulation age 26 days) as a sagittal slit in the posterior part of the floor of the primitive pharynx, just cephalad to the oesophagus. This pulmonary outgrowth appears externally as a keel-like projection which soon begins to extend caudally over the ventral surface of the oesophagus, the two lung buds appearing at its lower end. By the 4 mm. stage the entodermal lung buds are projecting into a mesodermal mass continuous at its caudal end with the septum transversum which, being fixed, serves to anchor the lung buds in their subsequent development. Lateral ridges appear in the pulmonary outgrowth and fuse mesially in a caudo-cephalic direction at the same time as the oesophagus and pulmonary outgrowth are elongating rapidly, thus separating progressively the primitive main bronchi, trachea and infra-glottic part of the larynx from the oesophagus. When the pulmonary outgrowth first appears only the first two pharyngeal arches are apparent, but by the 5 mm. stage (30 days) it has come to lie between the sixth arches, just behind the hypobranchial eminence. The major (supraglottic) part of the larynx, down to and including the vocal cords and the cricoid, develops from the fourth and sixth arches and the hypobranchial eminence and is thus pharyngeal in origin, which perhaps explains why the larynx is more or less normal despite absence of the trachea beyond in the cases mentioned. In its early stages the narrow infraglottic cavity is compressed from side to side and is almost completely occluded for a short time by epithelial fusion, only small dorsal and ventral tracts leading to the patent part of the tracheal outgrowth. The larynx is well seen in the 16 mm. embryo (about the seventh week). Early in its development the cells lining the oesophagus undergo intensive proliferation but vacuoles become apparent at the end of the sixth week and, although occlusion occurs as a temporary phase in the crocodilia and reptiles (Reese, 1926), it is never complete in the human (Johns, 1952). Chondrification in the trachea becomes apparent at the 20 mm. stage.

The associated absence of kidney also helps to date development of the abnormality as the ureteric bud appears at the end of the fifth week. Rosenthal (1931), Ladd (1944) and Sandison (1955) have also recorded instances where absence of kidney is associated with tracheo-oesophageal abnormalities.

Pathogenesis. Rosenthal (1931), amongst others, has reviewed the theories of pathogenesis of oesophageal atresia, and divides them into three main groups, those based firstly upon retardation of oesophageal development at a time when it is solid (subsequently shown to be a faulty premise), secondly upon deviations and malformations of the tracheo-oesophageal septum and thirdly upon the presumed effects of changes in tension on the developing embryo (as might be exerted by an overlarge cardiac anlage, excessive flexion of the embryo or the development of blood vessels in abnormal sites).

The defect seen in this case, however, appears to be far more fundamental with the persistence of a common tube. It can best be explained on the assumption that the lateral ridges have never appeared and the pulmonary outgrowth has thus never separated from the oesophagus. The lung buds have penetrated the mesenchyme in the usual manner and with the subsequent growth of the embryo, larynx and bronchi have become widely separated. The larynx, being pharyngeal in origin, has developed normally, as have the lung buds. The existence of the dorsal oesophageal pouch behind the larynx is explained by the fact that the upper portion of the oesophagus derives partly from the pharynx (it contains striped muscle in its wall). The posterior wall of the pharynx, at the level of the pulmonary outgrowth, has formed the pouch, perhaps after the fashion of a pulsion diverticulum. Associated with this defect is a lack of chondrification of the majority of the tracheal rings.

Summary

Details are presented of an infant in whom an oesophageal atresia was found in association with a common tracheo-oesophageal tube from which arose bronchi and stomach. The pathogenesis of this and similar conditions is discussed.

Our thanks are due to Dr. B. D. R. Wilson for permission to publish details of this child and to Dr. H. Spencer and others for their help and advice.

References

Benešová, D. and Peter, P. (1934). *Čas. Lék. čes.*, **73**, 356.
Frazer, J. E. (1953). *Manual of Embryology*, 3rd ed. London.
Fritz, E. (1933). *Virchows Arch. path. Anat.*, **289**, 264.
Gruenwald, P. (1940). *Anat. Rec.*, **78**, 293.
Hempel, K. J. (1956). *Zbl. allg. Path. path. Anat.*, **95**, 226.
Ingalls, T. H. and Prindle, R. A. (1949). *New Engl. J. Med.*, **240**, 987.
Johns, B. A. E. (1952). *J. Anat. (Lond.)*, **86**, 431.
Kessel, I. and Smith, J. N. (1953). *Thorax*, **8**, 266.
Ladd, W. E. (1944). *New Engl. J. Med.*, **230**, 625.
Marek, J. J. (1940). *Ohio St. med. J.*, **36**, 1308.
Milles, G. and Dorsey, D. B. (1950). *Amer. J. Path.*, **26**, 411.
Payne, W. A. (1900). *Brooklyn med. J.*, **14**, 568.
Reese, A. M. (1926). *Amer. J. Anat.*, **37**, 195.
Rosenthal, A. H. (1931). *Arch. Path. (Chicago)*, **12**, 756.
Sandison, A. T. (1955). *Arch. Dis. Childh.*, **30**, 475.
Scott, J. S. and Wilson, J. K. (1957). *Lancet*, **2**, 569.
Walcher, K. (1928). *Dtsch. Z. ges. gerichtl. Med.*, **12**, 292.
Waterston, D. J. (1954). In *Recent Advances in Paediatrics* (edited D. Gairdner), p. 151. London.
Wilkins, S. O. (1938). *J. med. Soc. N.J.*, **35**, 737.
Wolman, I. J. (1941). *Amer. J. Dis. Child.*, **61**, 1263.

PSYCHOGENIC MEGACOLON IN CHILDREN: THE IMPLICATIONS OF BOWEL NEGATIVISM*

BY

PHILIP PINKERTON

From the Department of Psychological Medicine, University of Liverpool

(RECEIVED FOR PUBLICATION SEPTEMBER 24, 1957)

Introduction

The demonstration of a precise histopathological basis for Hirschsprung's disease (Whitehouse and Kernohan, 1948; Zuelzer and Wilson, 1948; Bodian, Stephens and Ward, 1949; Swenson, Neuhauser and Pickett, 1949; Hiatt, 1951; Lee and Bebb, 1951) has permitted a radical revision in our concepts regarding the aetiology and management of megacolon. The condition should be designated more accurately as congenital neurogenic or aganglionic megacolon. It is possible to differentiate this state from a more commonly occurring group of cases, also characterized by colonic enlargement, but in which no spastic, aganglionic segment or other organic lesion can be demonstrated. These cases have been designated as 'idiopathic' or functional megacolon (Bodian *et al.*, 1949). It is with this group that the present study is concerned.

Object of Study

Idiopathic megacolon has been attributed to a state of chronic colonic inertia (Bodian, 1952). The present investigation seeks to demonstrate, however, that megacolon can develop in children primarily on a basis of emotional factors. The condition so produced closely resembles idiopathic megacolon in clinical features and radiographic appearances. It is contended that the two entities are identical, and that, while colonic inertia forms the immediate basis of the disorder, its ultimate aetiology is psychogenic in nature.

The importance of this submission lies in the approach to treatment. It is claimed that sustained results are not procured in such cases from purely symptomatic measures of relief, and that a satisfactory long-term response is achieved only through adequate evaluation and correction of the relevant emotional factors which contribute to the condition.

Case Material

Thirty cases are presented, 19 boys and 11 girls, ranging in age from 24 months to 15 years. In all of them there was a history of functional bowel disorder varying in duration from eight months to 15 years, and presenting mainly as chronic constipation, cumulative faecal retention and overflow soiling.

The series was collected over a period of three years. The chief sources of referral were consultant paediatricians and paediatric surgeons who had previously had the cases under treatment either as out-patients or in-patients. Investigation had shown no organic basis for the disorder, and the children were referred for psychiatric opinion either because of their unsatisfactory response to standard treatment measures or because the disorder was suspected to have an emotional basis. In those of the series investigated by barium enema, radiographic appearances confirmed the presence of functional megacolon.

For comparison, a series of control cases was constructed from the record of admissions to a general paediatric hospital over the five-year period, 1950 to 1955. Examples were sought of children of equivalent age range referred with a history of constipation which warranted investigation and treatment in hospital, but in whom no organic lesion was demonstrated and who had responded satisfactorily to routine treatment procedures without subsequent relapse. Twenty-one cases, 14 boys and 7 girls, were found to fulfil these criteria.

These cases were traced and followed up independently by a senior psychiatric social worker, who conducted her assessment on each case in parallel with the model adopted for the investigation of the primary series. In this way, unbiased comparison between the two groups was made possible.

The clinical material thus comprised 51 children, 30 of whom formed the primary series under study, and the remaining 21 the control group.

* Abstracted from a thesis for the degree of M.D. awarded by the Faculty of Medicine, University of Edinburgh, 1956.

Statistical Analysis

Statistical analysis of comparable findings in these two groups is of limited value because of the small numbers involved, but, using a Chi-squared test with Yates' correction for small numbers, four significant differences between the primary and control groups are apparent. It seems reasonable to ascribe aetiological significance to each of these four factors, namely, (1) parental personality characterized by excessive rigidity and/or excessive anxiety; (2) primary coercive toilet training; (3) parental fears and prejudices relating to constipation; and (4) parental over-valuation of the child (Table I and Fig. 1).

Formulation

From the analysis of case material, compared with the findings of the control group, it is possible to construct the following formulation to explain the aetiology of psychogenic megacolon.

The primary mechanism involved, I suggest, is a state of negativism on the part of the child, expressed as persistent refusal to defaecate or, less frequently, as defiant soiling. If handled unwisely, this state may result in cumulative retention of faeces with progressive loading of the rectum and terminal colon and subsequent overflow faecal soiling. Ultimately, chronic dilatation of the distal bowel develops which is demonstrable radiographically. Confirmatory evidence of such negativistic trends in the children under study is provided in their clinical assessments.

It is significant that with one exception in the primary series, this negativistic pattern developed during the first three years of life. As such, it coincides with the period of resistance (Kanner, 1948), or the phase of defiance (Menninger, 1943), undergone by most children at the stage in their emotional development when they become aware of their independence from the mother as a separate personality. During this period, provocative and testing behaviour towards parents is common, and bowel negativism is one of the acknowledged forms which such behaviour may take.

Indeed, it is recognized as so universal a pattern that in itself it could hardly represent the entire psychogenesis of the bowel disorder. Moreover, the onset of constipation in the control group also coincided, more or less, with the period of resistance through which some of these control group children might be assumed to be passing. Yet negativism in these latter cases, where it existed, did not give rise to a degree of bowel disorder commensurate with what was found in the primary series. Clearly, therefore, additional factors must operate to bring about the differential response between the primary and control groups.

It is contended that anal negativism forms the basis of the disorder, but that it is aggravated, or intensified, by specific conditioning factors operative in the primary series to a significantly greater degree

TABLE 1

CASE FINDINGS IN PRIMARY SERIES AND CONTROL GROUP

	Primary Series (30)	Control Group (21)
Age at onset of symptoms (years):	Less than 1 12 1-3 17	8 13
Sex distribution:	Male 19 Female 11	14 7
Clinical features:	Chronic constipation 25 Pseudo-diarrhoea 5	Abdominal colic, constipation with or without vomiting: 18 Constipation: 3
Radiographic findings:	Considerable dilatation of rectum, pelvic and descending colon, often with redundancy of pelvic loops	Normal
Response to treatment with laxatives, enemata:	Of temporary benefit only	Satisfactory
Parental personality:	Perfectionist, strict or domineering: 19 Overanxious, emotionally tense: 9	Normal
History of coercive toilet training:	17	None
Parental fears of constipation:	22	1
Parental over-valuation of child:	18	2
Negativism in child:	30	5

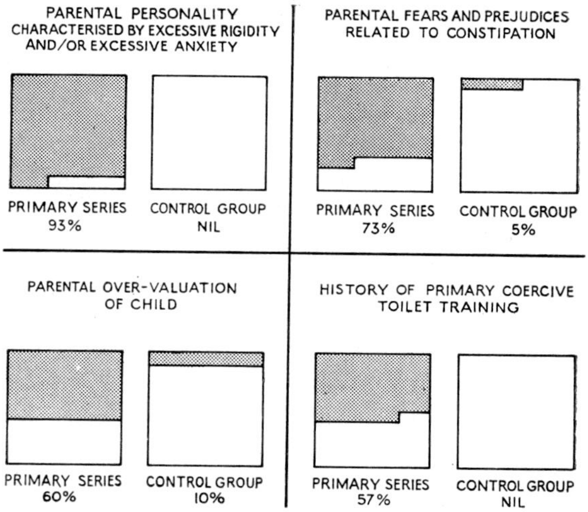

FIG. 1.—Statistically significant differences between primary and and control groups.

than they are in the control group. Given a basis of bowel negativism, it is the operation of these contributory factors, sufficiently intensely or for a long enough period, which converts the case into one of psychogenic megacolon. These factors can be classified as predisposing, precipitating and perpetuating.

Predisposing Parental Personality. The two main personality variants found among the parents of the primary series are, first, the perfectionist, rigidly obsessional parent who seeks to train the child by coercive methods to acquire bowel control at a premature stage in his development, in advance of adequate neuro-muscular maturation; and, secondly, the over-anxious, over-solicitous parent whose general attitude to the child is fraught with tension, and who closely supervises bowel evacuation because of her fears for the child's well-being.

Predisposing Parental Prejudices and Misconceptions. Linked to these emotional patterns in the parent are certain ingrained misconceptions with which the act of defaecation is still widely invested. These in turn give rise to various fears concerning the allegedly harmful effects of constipation. The over-anxious parent is specially prone to such fears.

Equally widespread is the notion of filth which invests the faeces once they are evacuated. The obsessional and fastidious type of parent is most prone to experience a sense of obnoxiousness regarding the stool, and to imbue the child with an irrational feeling of disgust or shame towards a perfectly natural product of excretion.

Thus we have the combination of personality type and parental attitude to defaecation, which accounts for much of the pressure to which these children are subjected in attempts to promote their regular bowel function.

Predisposing Environmental Factors. Particular circumstances surrounding the life situation of the child may conspire to generate excessive tension in the parents' attitude towards him and may provide the motive for excessive attention to his bodily functions. In the main, the factor involved is emotional over-valuation, which in turn contributes to excessive parental concern for the child.

Precipitating Stress Factors. Focal circumstances may provoke the immediate reaction of bowel difficulty against a background of any of the predisposing factors already discussed. There is, for example, fear of defaecation resulting from accidental fright during bowel action. While such events may induce temporary inhibition of stool, it is doubtful whether the effect ever persists and becomes chronic in the absence of predisposing factors which are already operating.

Similarly, although the disorder began as simple constipation due to intercurrent factors, in a number of the primary series it required the introduction of additional factors to elaborate the disorder into one of major bowel disturbance. It is highly significant that such a development did not take place in the control group, although each of these cases had an equivalent basis of simple constipation.

Perpetuating Factors. Excessive parental anxiety, alone or combined with excessive parental rigidity, will continue to operate if the child's initial response to treatment is unsatisfactory. In these circumstances, persisting parental tension will act as a perpetuating factor.

Continuing constipation in itself may give rise to anal spasm, secondary anal fissure, rectal prolapse or peri-anal dermatitis, any of which may perpetuate the disorder through the resulting pain on defaecation.

Yet another perpetuating factor may be the child's own reaction of anxiety and guilt in face of the persisting symptoms, or in response to parental attitudes of censure or ostracism.

It is contended that the interaction of these several contributory factors is responsible initially for evoking the child's resistance in the sphere of bowel function, and for subsequently elaborating his negativistic response to the stage at which psychogenic megacolon develops.

This hypothesis was put to the test in evolving a programme of psychotherapeutic treatment for the condition.

Treatment

Preliminary Orientation of Parental Attitude. Treatment was first directed to convincing the parents that what they had formerly regarded as a physical disorder was in fact of emotional origin, and that, in consequence, it would be necessary to substitute psychological methods of treatment for the local treatment hitherto adopted.

Parental reactions to this approach ranged from frank incredulity, through hostile resistance by obsessional parents or increased concern by over-anxious parents, to simple failure on the part of intellectually limited mothers to appreciate the relationship at all. In the latter case an authoritative approach was the only course practicable.

One of the difficulties was the implication that the parents themselves were intimately involved in the child's pattern of reaction, and that, henceforth, treatment was to be directed away from the presenting symptoms and conducted predominantly through them. In two cases, the maternal anxiety aroused by this implication proved too great for acceptance and both patients were in fact withdrawn from further attendance.

Dispersal of Parental Fears and Prejudices. In every case, acute parental concern was felt about the potential danger to the child's physical health as a result of his bowel disorder. Parents of predominantly rigid personality were as much beset by these fears as parents who were primarily over-anxious.

The task of reassurance was hindered in the majority of cases by advice or instruction about the importance of bowel regularity previously tendered by district nurses, health visitors, child welfare clinic staff, hospital medical and nursing staff or by the family doctor. Commercial advertisements about laxatives and books dealing with child care had also inadvertently helped to augment parental fears.

To overcome this attitude, and to dispel these misgivings, certain procedures proved valuable. As far as possible, for example, parents were initially interviewed in joint consultation with a paediatrician in sympathy with the psychiatric approach. At these interviews unequivocal and authoritative reassurance was given. It was necessary to repeat it until no vestige of doubt or misgiving remained in the mind of the parent. Vague or generalized advice merely served to heighten the parental anxiety. It was important to stress that no organic disease or abnormality of the bowel was present, that there would be no harmful results from persistence of the constipation, that spontaneous bowel function would be restored despite the 'stretching' of the lower bowel, that the child's rectal sensation had not been irrevocably lost and that anal fissure, rectal bleeding and rectal prolapse were only temporary sequelae. It was also necessary to explain to the parents that the child's wriggling and contortions did not represent his difficulty in expelling the faeces, but, on the contrary, indicated his determined attempt to retain them.

Although necessary, such dogmatic reassurance was of no lasting value in itself, save in the case of parents who were limited in intellectual endowment. For the majority of parents it was imperative to determine by supplementary questions how much of the initial advice had been absorbed, and to reinforce repeatedly those points which had not previously been understood or accepted adequately. Such interpretative reassurance could not be emphasized enough, reiterated too often or confirmed too insistently to ensure that it had been genuinely credited by the parents.

The limitations and dangers of excessive purgation had also to be emphasized. It was explained that, at this stage, drastic purgatives would serve no useful purpose and might, indeed, further impair bowel function. They were also likely to increase the soiling. It was equally essential that the medical advice given should be consistent, and that, therefore, laxative therapy should be discontinued, otherwise parents reasoned that if no danger were anticipated from permitting the constipation to go on untreated, why the need for maintaining laxatives.

Winnicott (1953) has referred to the need for 'symptom tolerance' in child psychiatric cases which present with physical symptoms. There is an understandable tendency among paediatricians to treat and remove presenting symptoms by direct approach as early as possible in the course of the disorder; whereas the discipline of child psychiatry advocates the frequent need for toleration of symptoms while the basic treatment is directed at the underlying causative emotional factors. This differential attitude, derived from the difference in training between the paediatrician and child psychiatrist, is exemplified in the treatment approach to the present series of cases. There was a tendency among paediatricians to continue standard treatment measures parallel with psychotherapy, either to 'make quite sure' or through a desire to resolve the disorder more rapidly by utilizing both methods of treatment together. They were intolerant of the persistence of symptoms.

Such a practice, however, is exposed to two risks. First, the parents may misinterpret it, and regard it as evidence that the medical adviser himself lacks confidence in the policy of suspending physical and medicinal measures; parental confidence is correspondingly undermined. Secondly, the maintenance of standard treatment measures may convey to the child that the emotional investment in his symptoms has not been withdrawn, and his motive for persisting in negativistic behaviour may thus be given fresh impetus.

For these two reasons, I found it advisable to suspend standard treatment procedures, apart from ensuring an adequate fluid intake.

Promotion of Parental Insight. It was just as important to avoid premature explanation to the mother of the emotional dynamics of the child's disorder in advance of her preparedness to accept such explanation. The more effective policy in practice was to withhold interpretation until the parents had disclosed their own resistances and preconceived opinions so that these could first be dealt with.

Having first assured them that there was no physical basis to the disorder, suggestions were put to them along the following lines. If there was no organic reason to prevent the child opening his bowels, why did he continue to hold back? Clearly this policy was causing him discomfort and pain and therefore, presumably, he must be deriving some compensatory gain. What might his motive be?

By such provocative suggestions, parents were stimulated to enlarge their concept of the disorder to include the possibility of emotional motivation, and to appreciate how their child's behaviour could conceivably be directed against them.

It was explained to them in general terms that young children often tried to even out the unequal balance between their own puny power, and what appeared to them to be the overwhelming authority of their mother and father. They could not defy this authority directly with impunity, but they often sought to do so indirectly by becoming obstinate and contrary in any sphere of behaviour which they sensed might upset their parents. The more concern shown over this conduct, the more the child tended to persist with it. This was emphasized as an entirely normal and almost universal pattern of behaviour. Parents must not feel therefore that they were necessarily to blame because it was adopted by their child. They had simply made the mistake, it was explained to them, of continuing to register excessive concern which the child had been quick to sense.

Modification of Parental Attitudes. At this stage, parents were sufficiently receptive to cooperate in reversing their original attitudes to the child's bowel function. They were advised to practise complete indifference towards the persistence of symptoms. No further mention must be made of the need for bowel movement, and no censure must be shown towards continued soiling. This was a difficult assignment for the mother. It meant in effect a policy of ignoring the symptoms in place of her former policy of perhaps agitated exhortation. Only confidence in the therapist, and the knowledge that she would be absolved from responsibility should anything go wrong, made it possible for her to pursue this course.

A frequent sequel, however, was the transfer of the child's negativism to some alternative sphere of conduct. Deprived of the focus of parental concern over his bowel symptoms, he might first attempt to re-establish his position by intensifying his references to bowel activity. For example, several children resorted to repeated demands to be helped in their toilet procedure. They would follow their mother around the house, insisting that she flushed the toilet for them, or unfastened their trousers, or in some similar way supervised their act of defaecation. Parents were instructed in advance to ignore all such overtures and to adhere strictly to their attitude of disinterest.

Group Therapy with Parents. In the great majority of cases, therapy was conducted predominantly through the parents and chiefly through the mother. In the course of formulating the treatment approach in the present study, a scheme was evolved for treating mothers by group therapy. Group leaders were chosen from among those mothers who had achieved the greatest depth of insight, who expressed enthusiastic support for the psychiatric view-point, and who were endowed with adequate talents for disseminating the principles which they themselves had absorbed. Four mothers emerged from the series as best suited for this purpose and as willing to co-operate. Each in turn formed the nucleus of a group of eight mothers, the membership of which changed from time to time as earlier cases acquired insight and dropped out, to be replaced by new cases. The group leadership similarly changed as a new leader came forward.

Group meetings were convened at regular weekly intervals for periods of one and a half hours under the general chairmanship of the therapist. His role was to supervise and guide the discussion but to remain as far as possible unobtrusive. He sought to promote free interchange of views between the older and more recent members, prompted by the group leader.

Considerable support was derived by new members through introduction to the group. Each in turn was relieved to find other mothers in similar straits and having to cope with identical problems. The inevitable prejudices, doubts, resistances and fears, once expressed, were more readily resolved within the group, and the acquisition of insight more readily promoted. There were repeated examples of sceptical and insecure mothers showing greater willingness to accept reassurance and advice from the group leader, or from older members of the group, than from the therapist direct. The evidence of success achieved by the psychiatric approach in earlier cases, and now placed squarely before the new case, was a potent therapeutic instrument.

Direct Therapeutic Procedures with the Child: (*a*) Admission to Hospital. In nine cases, it proved necessary to admit or re-admit the child to hospital for varying periods, under the supervision of the therapist. This step was taken with four of the children because the mother's response to reassurance had not been sustained, or because she was too limited in intellect to benefit from the guidance given without some more concrete demonstration of how to manage her child. In the remainder of this group, carping parental pressure or excessive domination of the child were most effectively curtailed by temporary removal of the patient from home.

In the absence of separate in-patient facilities, all nine cases were individually admitted to a general paediatric ward through the kind cooperation of my colleagues. The nursing staff were prompted to adopt an attitude of bland detachment towards the persistence of bowel symptoms, and equally to ignore any associated symptoms such as refusal to eat, temper tantrums, emotional withdrawal or provocative behaviour. The child was treated warmly and tolerantly but with avoidance of fuss.

In the majority of these cases no specific play therapy as such was practised with the child. Treatment essentially comprised placing the patient in a temporary residential environment, designed to counteract pre-existing influences and to achieve resolution of symptoms by engineering a suitable atmosphere. It was found that these children responded well to consistent and detached handling. In the main, they adjusted readily to ward routine, with restoration of spontaneity and regularity in bowel function after a short interval. Subsequent supportive treatment with the parents depended upon the practical example set by managing the child in hospital.

Apart from admission to hospital as a means of temporarily modifying the child's environment, direct psychotherapy was required in a further group of cases, including some who were accepted as in-patients. Such direct intervention was necessary with the child for a number of different reasons. It might be that the symptoms had become so chronic and entrenched that the child had developed an overlying bland façade which warranted definitive treatment measures. This was particularly so among the older children. Alternatively, some children were so grossly inhibited, fearful and insecure as to merit direct therapeutic help. Yet a further important indication for direct psychotherapy with the child was the unresponsive attitude of the parent, or the persistence of parental intolerance and rejection, with failure to acquire insight.

(*b*) **Play Therapy.** The aims of expressive play therapy were, first, to penetrate the child's defensive façade and establish adequate depth of contact with him; secondly, to define his fundamental problem for him through the medium of projective play techniques; thirdly, to promote the working-through of his difficulties, with associated release during play of his pent-up hostility; and, fourthly, to restore his emotional stability following the resolution of these difficulties.

Three main techniques were employed in this procedure: (*a*) the 'World Picture' technique, with portrayal of the child's own fantasy productions in a sand-tray as described by Lowenfeld (1939); (*b*) the technique of free drawing by the child on paper; (*c*) the combination of expressive drawing on paper with a device known as the aggression board. This latter technique will be described as exemplifying the treatment approach.

This apparatus was evolved by Meals and Summerskill (1951), as a technique for diverting hostility in children under treatment. It consists of a sheet of thin plywood (3 ft. by 4½ ft.), held in a thicker frame, and supported behind by a hinged brace which fits into a thick wooden base on the floor. In the plywood sheet, a square hole (8 in. by 8 in.) is cut out in the lower half. The base supports the plywood at an angle of 45°, facing the child, with the top of the board inclined away from him (Fig. 2).

In the present work, the apparatus was used by

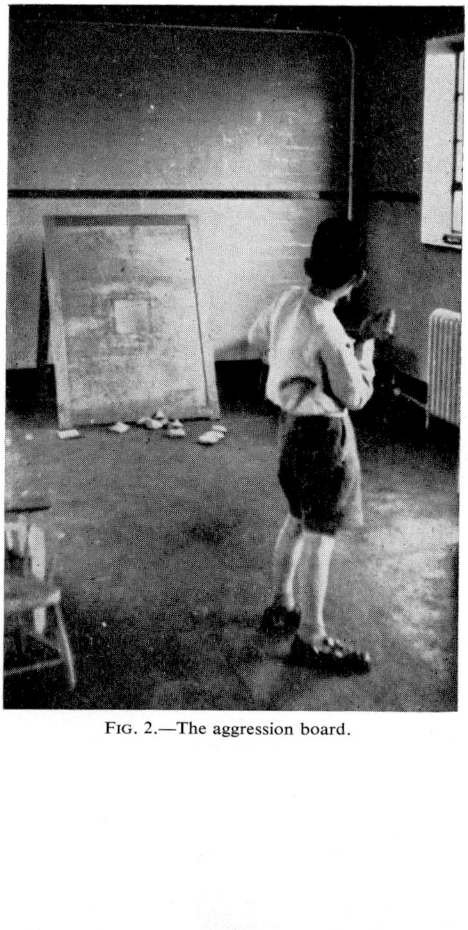

FIG. 2.—The aggression board.

inviting the child to make a drawing on a large sheet of paper of something which he particularly disliked ; no other limitation was imposed. The paper was then taped across the aperture in the plywood board so as to cover the hole. Facing the board, at a distance of four or five yards, the child was provided with 12 bean bags and encouraged to throw them, one after the other, at the picture over the opening. If he struck the target the taut paper was ripped by the impact. If he missed the drawing, the bean bag hit the surrounding plywood with a resounding noise which was obviously satisfying to the child.

The more inhibited of the children under therapy were unwilling to use the apparatus and showed fear of its aggressive potentialities. With the remaining cases, however, it proved both of diagnostic and therapeutic value. The subject matter drawn by the child as an object of his dislike provided diagnostic information, while his treatment of the drawing permitted therapeutic release of his aggressive feelings.

The following examples will suffice to indicate the type of material which emerged. Repeatedly the drawings referred to the administration of enemata by nurses as experienced by the child himself. The treatment meted out to these drawings left no doubt about the patient's hostile feelings.

Figure 3 shows a drawing undertaken by Case 9. Case 11 was more forthright in his portrayal of the same subject (Fig. 4). In this drawing, the nurse,

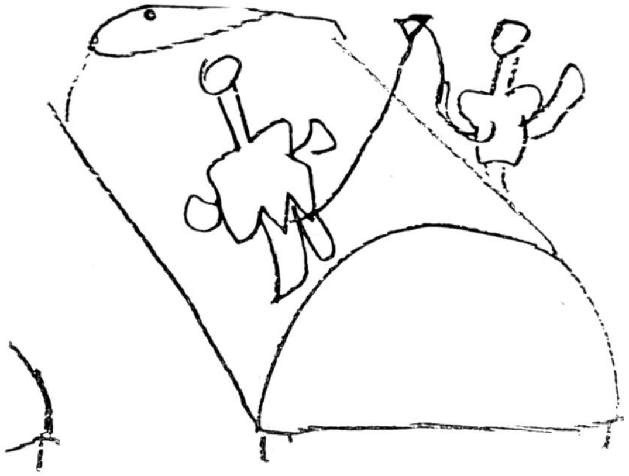

FIG. 3.—Drawing by Case 9.

menacing in appearance, is depicted as saying, 'I've never known anyone so rude, I'll give you another enema for that'. The child, though clearly sobbing, replies spiritedly, 'I'll give you an enema, you darn pest'. Treatment of this particular drawing was vigorously destructive with bean bags.

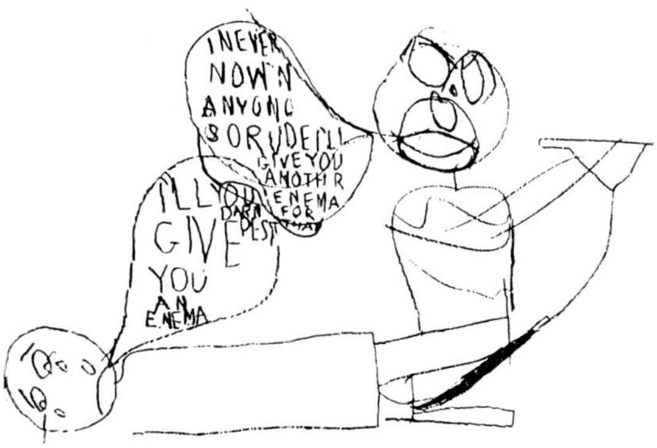

FIG. 4.—Drawing by Case 11.

Nurse: 'I've never known anyone so rude, I'll give you another enema for that.'
Child: 'I'll give you an enema, you darn pest.'

The same theme was repeated at a subsequent session, during which the child threw handfuls of wet sand violently at the plywood board when he had exhausted the supply of bean bags. The actual scene is depicted in Fig. 5.

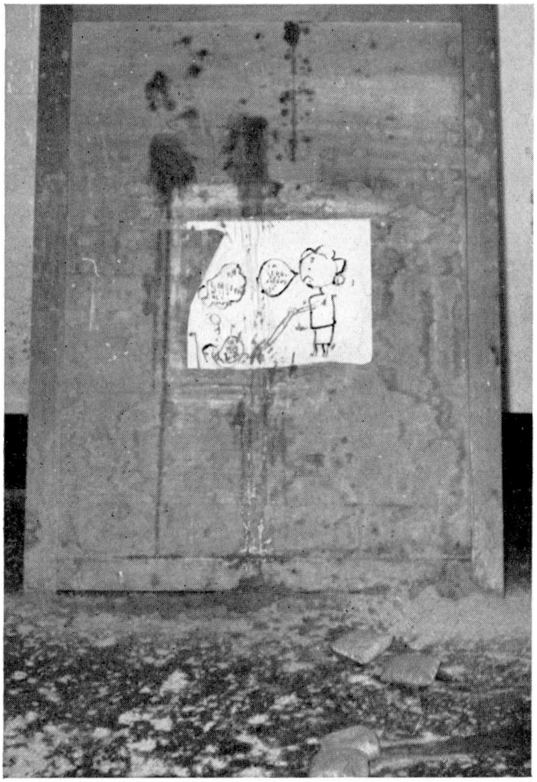

FIG. 5.—Aggression board with the drawing depicted in Fig. 6 in position.

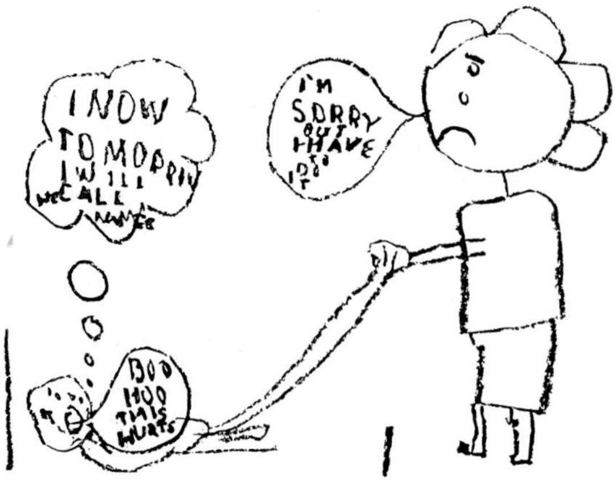

FIG. 6.
Child: 'Boo-hoo, this hurts.'
Nurse: 'I'm sorry, but I have to do it.'
Child: 'I know, tomorrow I will call you Nursie.'

Nevertheless, the verbal exchange between nurse and child in this later version is more conciliatory. The nurse, who no longer looks fierce, is saying, 'I'm sorry, but I have to do it'. The child openly concedes his discomfort ('Boo-hoo, this hurts'), but acknowledges the nurse's overture by replying, 'I know, tomorrow I will call you Nursie'. (Fig. 6.) This conciliatory trend was actually reflected in the patient's increasing stabilization and in the reduced intensity of his provocative behaviour at home.

By contrast, although the same theme was portrayed among the more inhibited and insecure children, their treatment of the subject was significantly different. For example, Fig. 7 shows a nurse administering an enema to a child behind screens in hospital. This drawing was done by a withdrawn little girl who volunteered no comment, and the picture itself seemed devoid of animation.

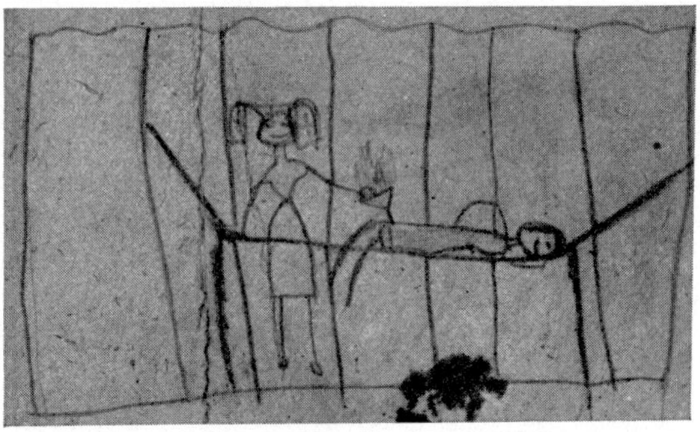

FIG. 7.

A further example of the same subject is portrayed in Fig. 8. This picture is more animated and captions have been introduced. The patient is saying, 'I'll teach you old Nursie a lesson'. The nurse, wearing a frightening expression, replies, 'No, you won't, you can't'.

It is interesting to compare this drawing with that depicted in Fig. 4, which so obviously expresses spirited defiance. In Fig. 8 the protest by the child is clearly more feeble and is emphatically overruled by the all-powerful nurse. The difference in attitude expressed in these drawings reflected the clinical difference between the first patient, a boy who was reacting with robust retaliatory behaviour, and the second patient, a girl who was much more inhibited and passive in response.

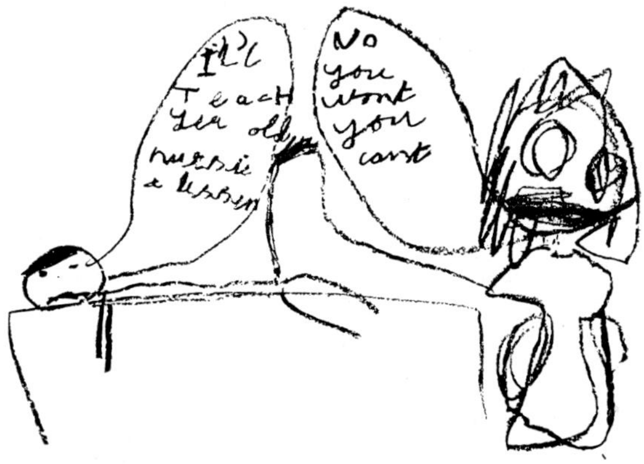

FIG. 8.
Child: 'I'll teach you old Nursie a lesson.'
Nurse: 'No you won't, you can't.'

Results of Treatment

With the kind of treatment outlined above, remission of symptoms occurred in 21 cases in the series, 17 of whom have now received no active treatment for periods up to three and a half years. Three children still continuing treatment are showing increasing symptomatic improvement. Of the remaining six cases, three failed to maintain attendance for treatment, and three have proved unamenable to psychiatric treatment (Fig. 9).

Discussion

It is noteworthy that the present series showed a preponderance of boys to girls in the ratio of almost 2 to 1 (19 boys, 11 girls). In Bodian's (1949) original group of 34 cases of idiopathic megacolon, the corresponding numbers were 25 boys and 9 girls. Bakwin (1956) has commented that resistance to bowel training and the persistence of soiling is twice as common in boys as in girls. An explanation may lie in Freud's observation that 'the little girl is as a rule less aggressive, less defiant and less self-sufficient . . . The fact that she is more easily and more quickly taught to control her excretions is very probably only the result of this docility.' (Freud, 1946.)

In several cases of the primary series, there was a manifest tendency among the mothers to overvalue their sons relative to their daughters. This might conceivably provide the motive in some cases for the excessive focus of attention on bowel regularity in the male.

The personality characteristics which were found to predominate among the parents of the children in the present study have been noted by other workers in association with difficulties over toilet performance (Lehman, 1944; Comly, 1952). The personality features of obsessional rigidity, determination and perfectionism, which were so prominent in the parents concerned, correspond to the characteristics of the 'anal character' elaborated by Freud (1916).

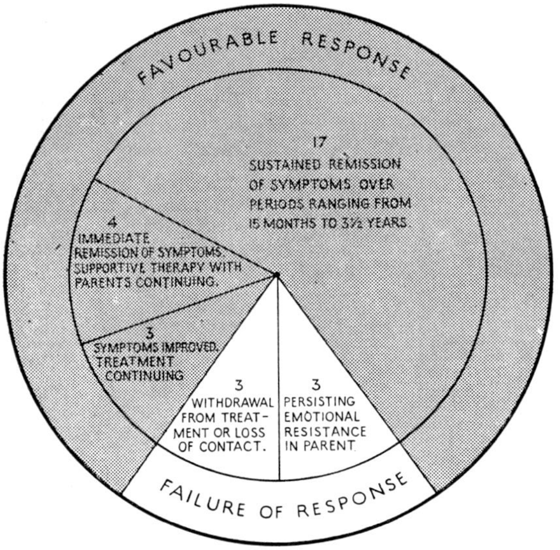

FIG. 9.—Response to treatment in the primary series.

A study of the family backgrounds of these parents yielded repeated evidence of the strict code of upbringing to which one or other parent, usually the mother, was herself subjected in her own childhood. It was significant that the parental attitude adopted toward the child was often in part determined by the parental attitude which had obtained in the previous generation.

The role of coercive toilet training in promoting bowel negativism has been stressed independently by different workers (Huschka, 1942; Swenson, 1953; Richmond *et al.*, 1954; Bakwin, 1956).

Prugh (1955) found that constipation, with or without faecal soiling, occurred twice as frequently in a group of children who had been subjected to early bowel training as in an equivalent group who had been trained at the usual time. He concluded, however, that it is not the timing or nature of bowel training which alone promotes difficulties over defaecation. In his experience, mothers who enjoy a warm and close relationship with their offspring can adopt premature or even coercive training without incurring any serious risk of subsequent bowel disorder. He adds, however, that 'if the relationship between mother and child is strained, undesirable procedures may offer a focus around which these tensions are expressed'. He therefore considers that 'the personality make-up of the mother, and her relationship to her child, are more important than her technique of toilet training'.

This view is borne out by the findings in the present series of cases, among whom 57% had been submitted to primary coercive training, whereas 93% showed evidence of parent/child tensions due to personality difficulties in the parents.

Paediatricians are alive to the fact that constipation is still widely invested by the lay public with ingrained fears and fantasies concerning its allegedly adverse effects. Accordingly, they recognize the importance of disabusing parents of such prejudices in the treatment of the child's constipation. Mac Keith (1955), Reichert (1955) and James (1955) all stress the need to emphasize to parents the wide range of normality in bowel function during infancy in order to avoid their unwarranted alarm. In the present series, the longest period of absolute constipation through resistance to defaecation was 83 days (Case 2), during which time the child, aged 3, continued to enjoy perfectly good health and remained symptom-free, eating normally and showing abundant energy throughout. Swenson (1953) reports a similar example of a child who had no bowel movement for eight months, without adverse repercussions.

In any case, some children show a constitutional tendency to infrequent bowel action, dating from the neonatal period. In the present series, there were three examples of this tendency. In each case, the mother had misinterpreted the condition as one of constipation with resulting undue concern and correspondingly rigorous treatment. Significantly, however, although the parental attitude has now been corrected and the overlying behaviour disturbance completely resolved, the child's pattern of bowel action in each case has remained unchanged, with a bowel movement occurring at three- to five-day intervals. No harm results in such cases unless the child is treated for supposed constipation.

Much depends upon the orientation of the paediatric specialist, since it is to him that the majority of cases of this kind will be referred in the first instance because of their physical presentation. Chapman and Loeb (1955) aptly comment, 'The ultimate success of referral for psychiatric opinion depends upon the referring paediatrician's skill in allaying parental guilt and anxiety about seeking such help. His ability to explain the importance of emotional factors is itself an important factor in whether parents will actually follow up the suggestion of psychiatric referral. A small amount of extra time devoted by the paediatrician in talking to parents about these gastro-intestinal problems, and how life stresses and personality factors affect the ailment, is often one of the most therapeutic things he does. It is often useful to remember that the word "doctor" derives from the Latin verb "docere" —"to teach"!'

Summary and Conclusions

Each of the 30 cases described in the current study, despite their diversity of background, had in common the factor of conflict between parent and child in the sphere of bowel function. Parental efforts to promote bowel regularity had induced a reactive state of negativism in the child, manifested as resistance to defaecation. This in turn led to chronic faecal retention, with ultimate dilatation of the rectum and terminal colon if the condition was allowed to persist for a sufficient length of time. The megacolon so produced could not be attributed to any underlying organic lesion. On the evidence presented, it is of psychogenic origin and is of common origin with the condition sometimes called idiopathic megacolon.

The conclusion drawn from the current investigation is that, while colonic inertia forms the immediate basis of the condition, its development is secondary to the state of chronic constipation which results from persistent bowel negativism.

Rational treatment of the condition should therefore be directed towards resolving the child's negativistic behaviour, since this represents the ultimate basis of the disorder. Treatment must include exploration of the emotional factors within the parent/child relationship which determine the patient's negativistic response, and appropriate re-alignment of parental attitude so that the state of conflict over bowel function is removed.

Joint consultation between paediatrician and child psychiatrist ensures that such a comprehensive approach is instituted. Parental reassurance is thereby more effectively promoted, continuity in treatment is preserved, and, although the physical symptoms are viewed with detachment, there is no risk of neglecting the local bowel disorder while pursuing the broader treatment indications. The paediatrician gains insight into the emotional dynamics of the condition and the psychiatrist gains perspective upon its physiological aspects. Each discipline reinforces the contribution of the other, and the prognosis for successful treatment is thereby enhanced.

It is a pleasure to record my thanks to Professor N. B. Capon for his unfailing interest in this work and for his kindness in providing the facilities within the Department of Child Health of the University of Liverpool which made the project possible. I would also like to thank my colleagues, Miss M. E. Gurney and Dr. W. E. Robinson, for their invaluable help with the therapeutic work; my Psychiatric Social Worker, Miss E. Ireland, for her important contribution in compiling the control group data; our Senior Clinical Psychologist, Mr. John Graham White, for his help with the statistical work; my paediatric colleagues, and in particular Dr. Hudson, Dr. Keidan, Dr. Llewellin and Dr. Todd, for their close collaboration and for their courtesy in providing access to their wards; and to my two secretaries for their industry and patience. Above all I would like to express my deep appreciation to Professor W. Mayer Gross for his support, encouragement and inspiring stimulus.

References

Bakwin, H. (1956). *Pediat. Clin. N. Amer.*, Feb., 127.
Bodian, M. (1952). *Practitioner*, **169**, 517.
——, Stephens, F. D. and Ward, B. C. H. (1949). *Lancet*, **1**, 6.
Comly, H. H. (1952). *J. Iowa St. med. Soc.*, **42**, 565.
Freud, S. (1916). *On the Transformation of Instincts, with Special Reference to Anal Erotism.* Collected Papers Vol. 2, p. 164. The International Psycho-Analytical Library, No. 8, London.
—— (1946). *The Psychology of Women*, p. 150. New Introductory Lectures on Psychoanalysis. 3rd ed. London.
Hiatt, R. B. (1951). *Ann. Surg.*, **133**, 313.
Huschka, M. (1942). *Psychosom. Med.*, **4**, 301.
James, U. (1955). *Med. Press*, **233**, 280.
Kanner, L. (1948). *Child Psychiatry*, 2nd ed., p. 39. Illinois.
Lee, C. M. and Bebb, K. C. (1951). *Surgery*, **30**, 1026.
Lehman, E. (1944). *Amer. J. Dis. Child.*, **68**, 190.
Mac Keith, R. (1955). *Guy's Hospital Gazette*, **69**, 22.
Meals, D. W. and Summerskill, J. (1951). *J. clin. Psychol.*, **7**, 376.
Menninger, W. C. (1943). *Psychoanal. Quart.*, **12**, 161.
Prugh, D. G. (1955). *Ann. N.Y. Acad. Sci.*, **58**, 35.
Reichert, J. L. (1955). *Pediat. Clin. N. Amer.*, May, 527.
Richmond, J. B., Eddy, E. J. and Garrard, S. D. (1954). *Amer. J. Orthopsychiat.*, **24**, 391.
Swenson, O. (1953). *Amer. J. Surg.*, **86**, 497.
——, Neuhauser, E. B. D. and Pickett, L. K. (1949). *Pediatrics*, **4**, 201.
Whitehouse, F. R. and Kernohan, J. W. (1948). *Arch. intern. Med.*, **82**, 75.
Winnicott, D. W. (1953). *Proc. roy. Soc. Med.*, **46**, 675.
Zuelzer, W. W. and Wilson, J. L. (1948). *Amer. J. Dis. Child.*, **75**, 40

BRITISH PAEDIATRIC ASSOCIATION

Proceedings of the Twenty-ninth Annual General Meeting

The Annual Meeting of the British Paediatric Association was held at the Old England Hotel, Windermere, from April 23 to 26, 1958.

BUSINESS PROCEEDINGS. Dr. K. H. Tallerman, M.C., took the Chair as President, and the following members were present:

F. M. B. Allen, E. C. Allibone, I. M. Anderson, J. Apley, Cécile Asher, R. Astley, H. S. Baar, T. E. D. Beavan, M. Bodian, R. E. Bonham Carter, J. V. Braithwaite, P. T. Bray, E. G. Brewis, F. S. W. Brimblecombe, R. W. Brookfield, W. A. B. Campbell, W. H. Cant, N. B. Capon, I. A. B. Cathie, N. S. Clark, T. Colver, W. R. F. Collis, Beryl Corner, S. D. M. Court, John Craig, J. O. Craig, W. S. Craig, Mildred Creak, J. Crooks, W. E. Crosbie, K. W. Cross, Mary Crosse, G. Davison, E. F. Dott, A. C. Doyne Bell, S. Doxiadis, J. L. Emery, P. R. Evans, H. L. Ellis, J. W. Farquhar, J. O. Forfar, Isabella Forshall, A. White Franklin, D. Gairdner, W. Gaisford, W. H. Galloway, R. R. Gordon, S. Graham, C. F. Harris, E. W. Hart, J. Hart-Mercer, C. C. Harvey, J. D. Hay, J. L. Henderson, W. Henderson, A. Holzel, F. P. Hudson, J. H. Hutchison, R. S. Illingworth, J. Jacobs, N. M. Jacoby, Ursula James, H. Jolly, H. Everley Jones, F. F. Kane, J. J. Kempton, G. M. Komrower, R. C. Lightwood, J. Lorber, P. MacArthur, R. A. McCance, D. MacCarthy, Agnes MacGregor, M. MacGregor, R. Mac Keith, T. P. Mann, R. Mayon-White, R. A. Miller, F. J. W. Miller, A. V. Neale, G. H. Newns, D. N. Nicholson, A. P. Norman, J. N. O'Reilly, C. G. Parsons, W. W. Payne, C. Pinckney, P. E. Polani, C. T. Potter, K. B. Rogers, A. Russell, L. Scott, R. A. Shanks, W. Sheldon, Ursula Shelley, Victoria Smallpeice, W. C. Smallwood, J. M. Smellie, J. Forest Smith, T. Stapleton, J. Thomson, M. L. Thomson, J. P. M. Tizard, R. McL. Todd, W. Walker, A. G. Watkins, Cicely Williams, Mary Wilmers, B. D. R. Wilson, D. W. Winnicott, Winifred Young, S. Yudkin.

Professor Bo Vahlquist (Windermere Lecturer) and Mr. G. J. Piller were the guests of the Association.

The following were present as guests of members of the Association:

E. Aberdeen, Charlotte Anderson, J. Baden-Daintree, R. Berg, M. F. G. Buchanan, Bera Buhrmann, Joyce Burke, E. D. Burnard, Joan M. Cashman, C. L. Chen, P. Clay, B. L. Coles, Christine Cooper, J. G. A. Davel, W. Dickson, J. H. Diggle, E. E. Doyle, D. Garrow, S. Griffin, A. D. M. Jackson, Margaret Jones, A. C. Kirby, K. M. Laurence, R. Llewelyn Davies, D. Macaulay, A. E. McCandlass, W. J. Matheson, Florence Mayer, J. Olsen, A. W. M. Page, F. Puga, A. Rigg, H. Rischbieth, S. Sjölin, Jean Smellie, F. H. Stone, G. Weston, D. Whitehouse, T. Wright.

The Annual General Meeting was held on April 24, 1958.

The Minutes of the last meeting, which had been published in the *Archives of Disease in Childhood*, were received and approved.

ELECTION OF OFFICERS. The following were elected:

PRESIDENT: Dr. J. Forest Smith.
PRESIDENT-ELECT: Dr. R. C. Lightwood.
TREASURER: Professor A. G. Watkins.
SECRETARY: Dr. P. R. Evans.

EXECUTIVE COMMITTEE, 1958-61:

Dr. J. Apley, Dr. D. V. Hubble, Dr. P. MacArthur, Dr. L. G. Scott, Dr. E. W. Hart (1958-59).

ELECTION OF MEMBERS. The following were elected:

HONORARY MEMBERS

Dr. K. H. Tallerman, Dr. H. S. Baar, Dr. Frances Braid, Professor C. Dent, Dr. A. G. Ogilvie, Dr. T. Pearse Williams.

CORRESPONDING MEMBERS

Professor S. T. Achar (Madras), Dr. R. C. Eley (Boston), Dr. A. Hartman (St. Louis), Professor D. B. Jelliffe (New Orleans), Professor E. Kerpel-Fronius (Pecs, Hungary), Dr. A. B. Sabin (Cincinnati).

ORDINARY MEMBERS

A. G. V. Aldridge, G. C. Arneil, A. D. Barlow, R. G. G. Barry, T. Bowlby, T. A. Brand, J. Coates, Christine E. Cooper, E. C. R. Couper, M. E. Disney, H. G. Farquhar, H. V. L. Finlay, B. Gans, I. H. Gosset, Gwyn R. Griffith, Sylvia K. Guthrie, T. B. Heycock, C. J. Hodson, R. Jenkins, C. W. Kesson, A. M. MacDonald, R. G. Mitchell, C. Newman, A. P. M. Page, L. J. Prosser, P. P. Rickham, T. S. Rodgers, J. M. Stansfeld, W. P. Sweetman, P. N. Swift, D. H. Wallace, H. R. E. Wallis, C. B. M. Warren, I. G. Wickes, D. A. J. Williamson, B. S. B. Wood, Barbara Woodhead.

The Treasurer's report was received and adopted and the auditors were re-appointed for a further year. The thanks of the Association were expressed to Dr. R. Lightwood at the expiry of his 11 years' work as Honorary Treasurer.

The report of the Executive Committee was received and approved and is printed below. It was agreed that next year's report should include the names of members of committees. Following a suggestion made by Dr. Beryl Corner it was agreed that the Executive Committee should arrange for more prolonged discussion on paediatric policy, either at the Annual General Meeting or at a special meeting held at another time during the year.

A proposal to alter Rule 15 to read:

'The subscription payable by ordinary members shall be fixed from time to time by the Executive Committee and reported to the members of the Association',

was referred back to the Executive Committee for further consideration.

There was considerable discussion of an offer by the Journals Committee of the British Medical Association to allow members of the Association to receive the *Archives of Disease in Childhood* at a reduced rate of subscription provided that virtually all members subscribed. On a show of hands the following resolution was passed by 42 votes to 37: 'That the Executive Committee should consider consolidating the subscription to the Association and to the *Archives of Disease in Childhood*'.

Report of the Executive Committee 1957-58

1. We note with sorrow the death of four original members, Dr. A. G. Maitland Jones, Dr. Wilkie Scott, Dr. William Brown and Dr. H. C. Cameron.

2. We congratulate Professor A. A. Moncrieff on his election to fellowship of the Royal College of Obstetricians and Gynaecologists, and Dr. C. F. Harris on his nomination as Vice-Chancellor of the University of London.

3. Reports and Committees. The report on hospital accommodation for children was published in the *Lancet* in July, 1957. The report of the Child Psychology Committee on child guidance has been submitted to the Ministry of Health. Written evidence has been submitted to the Platt Committee on the welfare of children in hospital. At the request of the Ministry of Agriculture, Fisheries and Food draft regulations on soft drinks have been studied in relation to child health and comments have been submitted. A Committee has been set up to consider paediatric care in infectious diseases hospitals and sanatoria, and another to discuss the medical care of adolescents. The Joint Committee on Prematurity has been replaced by a Standing Joint Committee of the British Paediatric Association and Royal College of Gynaecology, which will consider matters of common interest.

4. Meetings. It will be impossible to hold future meetings in Windermere and the Executive recommends that in 1959 the Annual General Meeting should be held at the Royal Hotel, Scarborough. The Canadian Paediatric Society has suggested having a joint meeting with us in Britain in 1961, and it is proposed that it shall replace our usual annual meeting in that year.

5. Diploma of Child Health. Regulations for the D.C.H. demand from clinical assistants four attendances a week. In order to encourage general practitioners to take the examination the Conjoint Board has been asked to approve less frequent attendance over a longer period and has agreed to do so.

6. Children in Adult Wards. One of the main topics for discussion during the past two years has been the question of how many children who could be nursed in children's wards are admitted to adult wards. Further information is being collected: there appears to be much regional variation.

7. Windermere Lecture. Professor Bo Vahlquist (Uppsala) delivered the Windermere Lecture entitled 'Breast milk and cow's milk in infant feeding: a clinical, serological and biochemical study in 400 children'.

Scientific Sessions

Ursula James (London). 'The Diagnosis of Urinary Infection in the Newborn.' Observations on the incidence and diagnosis of urinary infections in the newborn have been made over a period of one year in a maternity unit of 65 beds. The clinical picture and urinary investigations have been analysed, and the results compared with similar investigations in 100 normal infants. The value of actual white cell counts in the urine has been investigated, and a range of cell counts in normal infants has been compared with those found in patients with urinary infections. Suggestions are offered for making early and more certain diagnosis of infections of the urinary tract in the newborn.

W. S. Craig and M. F. Buchanan (Leeds). 'Hypocalcaemic Tetany on the Second Day of Life.' To be published in full.

F. H. Stone (Glasgow). 'Infantile Autism.' The clinical features of infantile autism (Kanner's syndrome), based on the intensive study of several cases, were described and illustrated by means of a cine-film. Aetiological factors were considered and an experimental therapeutic approach described. Suggestions were made as to future lines of research.

G. M. Komrower (Manchester). 'Sequelae of Infantile Renal Acidosis.' To be published in full.

W. Gaisford (Manchester). 'Poliomyelitis Vaccination of Newborn Infants.' Groups of newborn infants were given poliomyelitis vaccine and their titres examined to see if maternally transmitted antibodies inhibited the natural development of antibodies after vaccination and whether triple negative infants would produce reasonable titres. The effect of a booster dose seven to eight months later was also investigated.

D. Gairdner (Cambridge). 'The Fluid Shift from the Vascular Compartment Immediately after Birth.' To be published in full.

K. M. Laurence (London). 'The Natural History of Hydrocephalus.' It is generally believed that, untreated, few children with hydrocephalus survive and that those who do survive are doomed to permanent institutional care. Nearly 200 cases of untreated hydrocephalus, seen by Mr. Wylie McKissock (who rarely operates upon this condition) since 1939, have been followed up. Forty-six per cent of the series have survived with the hydrocephalus spontaneously arrested. These have been re-examined and intelligence tested. Many of those who showed evidence of spasticity and incoordination in infancy have now no 'motor trouble', and on intelligence testing 44% fall within the 'average' group (I.Q. of 85 and above). A further 20% are educable with an I.Q. of above 50, leaving only 25% requiring complete institutional care. Thirty-five per cent of the survivors are growing up as completely normal individuals, both physically and mentally. Children with acquired hydrocephalus, generally due to a basal cistern block, bore the most hopeful prognosis.

In the light of this a more hopeful approach to this condition is called for, in spite of the fact that the disease often causes some brain damage, and that mental development in many cases is temporarily delayed in the early years.

I. A. B. Cathie (London). 'On Editing the Archives.' The general functions of an editor and his responsibility to contributors and readers were briefly considered and the experience of nine years editing the *Archives of Disease in Childhood* was analysed. The types of articles submitted for publication were considered, the reasons for rejections given and the principles involved in the editing of accepted papers were discussed. Common discordances in the construction of papers and the presentation of results were outlined, as were some of the commoner grammatical extravagances. Finally, an attempt was made to indicate the type of paper most likely to give the maximum information in the minimum space and require the least amount of alteration and therefore be most acceptable.

Christine E. Cooper and S. Griffin (Newcastle). 'Oesophageal Stricture Secondary to Hiatus Hernia.' An account was given of 18 cases seen since 1952 during a study of hiatus hernia in 356 infants. The age range was 2 months to 12 years when first seen. Stricture was already present at the first visit in 15. Many had been previously treated as behaviour problems. Details of history and clinical diagnosis were presented. The importance of an experienced radiologist and careful technique during barium studies was emphasized. A preliminary account of conservative management in 15 and radical surgery in three, description of complications and emphasis on need for long-term study were given.

A. D. M. Jackson and L. Fisch (London). 'Deafness following Maternal Rubella: Results of a Prospective Survey.' Detailed clinical examinations and hearing tests (including audiograms) were carried out on a series of 57 children, whose mothers were known to have had rubella during the first 18 weeks of pregnancy. Fifty-seven controls were also examined.

The children were taken from the records of the national prospective enquiry into the effects of virus infections in pregnancy organized by the Society of Medical Officers of Health and the Ministry of Health.

A preliminary report of the findings of this investigation was presented. The results will be published in full elsewhere.

Jean Smellie (London). 'The Effect on the Infant of Large Therapeutic Doses of Vitamin D given to the Mother throughout Pregnancy.' The clinical and biochemical follow-up were described on two infants now aged 6 months and 2 years, born to a mother suffering from severe Type I renal tubular osteomalacia. She had been successfully treated with A.T. 10 for six months before the first pregnancy and received pure dihydrotachysterol throughout both pregnancies (1 mg. o.d. by mouth).

Both infants showed biochemical signs of mild vitamin D intoxication, namely a low plasma alkaline phosphatase and a slightly raised serum calcium followed by a rise of blood urea.

Lactation was suppressed in each case. In the first, the infant was fed on National Dried Milk and between 2 and 3 months became hypotonic with increased reflexes. These signs disappeared when the National Dried Milk was replaced by liquid cow's milk. The second child, fed on liquid cow's milk from birth, showed no hypotonia.

The implications of these findings were discussed, particularly in relation to the aetiology of idiopathic hypercalcaemia of infancy; for instance, that an infant may be 'sensitized' in utero to vitamin D by an excessive maternal intake of vitamin D during pregnancy in health foods and vitamin capsules.

Malcolm MacGregor (Warwick). 'Osteomyelitis Variolosa.' There is only one account in British literature, in 1887, of this interesting bone complication of smallpox, of which I had the opportunity to study 20 cases in Nigeria last year.

This short paper illustrates the condition, which is radiologically very striking, and draws some parallels with other virus affections of bone, more likely to be in the minds of members of the B.P.A.

BOOK REVIEWS

Comparative Aspects of Haemolytic Disease of the Newborn. By G. Fulton Roberts. (Pp. xi+199. 17s. 6d.) London: Heinemann. 1957.

This is an erudite little book, most amusing and interesting in its way and packed full of information. It is very rarely that the clinical, historical, pathological and comparative aspects of a disease are brought together in a single volume, but they are all here and discussed in a simple and readable style. It is not, however, by any means easy reading throughout and this is a book for the clinician who has some knowledge of the problem, or for the pathologist who does not wish to confine himself only to the finer points of serology, rather than the student.

The author has included up to date references and covers the literature fully. Some might find fault with his presentation of the case against premature induction of labour on page 138, but it would be unreasonable to make much of this.

In summary, this is a stimulating approach which might well be copied in respect to other diseases and which should remind many of us how little we know of the wider aspects of those diseases in which we are interested.

Affections Non Congénitales de l'Anus et du Rectum Chez l'Enfant. By Jean Duhamel, with Preface by Professor Robert Debré. (Pp. vii+264; 110 figures. Fr. fr. 3,600.) Paris: Masson. 1958.

This book is based on a study of 450 cases of ano-rectal disorders treated at l'Hôpital des Enfants-Malades à Paris. In the examination of such cases, the author recommends the use of an angulated frame to keep the infant in the jack-knife position. The technique of instrumentation and its dangers are set out.

The cause, clinical features, pathology and treatment of all non-congenital, ano-rectal diseases are given in detail. The solitary polyp (140 cases) and rectal prolapse (90 cases) are the two commonest conditions; anal fissure, peri-anal abscesses and fistulae are fully described. The author's view throughout the book almost completely conforms with current teaching and proctological practice. All minor operative procedures are given in detail. A few points, however, may not receive general acceptance, namely, the use of the blind external route for the sub-mucosal injection of prolapsus ani, the use of a rubber seton in treating fistulae and the injection of antibiotics, after aspiration, into peri-anal abscesses. These procedures are given only as alternatives to the more orthodox methods.

Dr. Duhamel, who was a gastro-enterologist, shows his special interest in the chapters on proctitis, anal inflammation, constipation and encopresis. More rare affections, such as multiple polyposis, malignant and venereal disease, are also included.

This book is well illustrated, mostly by clear line drawings, but a few of the photographs are of poor quality; there is a synopsis of each chapter and a useful bibliography.

The author is to be congratulated on producing this book on proctology in a special age group, for he has made available much useful information for all those called upon to treat these infant and childhood disorders. It is unfortunate that malformations and neonatal affections do not come within the scope of this book. Perhaps this omission can be remedied in a second edition.

Hydrocéphalie du Nourrison. By Marc Richard Klein. (Pp. 136; 37 figures. Fr. fr. 1,600) Paris: Masson. 1958.

This monograph of 133 pages attempts to deal with the whole problem of hydrocephalus as well as the physiology of the cerebrospinal fluid circulation. Unfortunately, it manages only to skate over the subject without giving precise data or references.

The 'classification' given merely lists tumours and lesions which may lead to hydrocephalus, and confuses rather than clarifies the problems. Investigation of such cases is dealt with in some detail, including the use of isotopes, which are, as yet, a research tool of only doubtful value. The clinical examination, however, is added as a postscript in a few lines at the end of the chapter.

Several operations are described, notably that of coagulation of the choroid plexus, which is the author's chief tool in combating the malady. Anaesthesia and post-operative problems are discussed at length.

Some of the diagrams are clear, though often irrelevant; others are confusing, while the clinical photographs are unhelpful, especially one of a hydrocephalic baby wearing a bonnet.

The impression gained from this monograph is that the author has compiled it at some speed without giving any deep thought to the problems involved.

Pseudarthrose Congenitale du Tibia et son Traitement. By M. Guilleminet and R. Ricard. (Pp. 98; 78 figures. Fr. fr. 1,800) Paris: Masson. 1958.

This is a review of the pathogenesis and treatment of congenital pseudarthrosis of the tibia, and is based upon a review of the literature and 14 personal cases of the author. Since three of these cases are too recent for assessment, and most of the others have already been reported elsewhere, it is difficult to appreciate the issue of this material in book form. The experience of the authors in the treatment of this condition lies largely in the field of inlay and sliding grafts to the tibia, with which they have had considerable success, but the bypass graft and the use of an intramedullary nail are also fully described. In such a beautifully produced book it is a pity that the bibliography is not complete, and contains minor inaccuracies.

SEVERE INFANTILE HYPERCALCAEMIA WITH SPECIAL REFERENCE TO THE FACIES

BY

M. C. JOSEPH and D. PARROTT

From the Department of Child Health, Guy's Hospital

(RECEIVED FOR PUBLICATION APRIL 30, 1958)

In 1932 Lightwood described a child aged 2 years whose illness resembled the terminal stages of severe infantile hypercalcaemia. Later Butler (1951) and Fanconi (1951) each reported similar cases and they then discussed their findings in a joint paper (Fanconi, Girardet, Schlesinger, Butler and Black, 1952). Since then there have been several reports of the severe form of this disease in this country (Creery, 1953; Dawson, Craig and Perera, 1954; Lowe, Henderson, Park and McGreal, 1954; Russell and Young, 1954; Schlesinger, Butler and Black, 1956). The incidence in America is less but recently a few cases have been reported (Sissman and Klein, 1956; Daeschner and Daeschner, 1957; Bongiovanni, Eberlein and Jones, 1957).

Lightwood and Stapleton (1953) believed that the severe type of infantile hypercalcaemia was a different syndrome from the mild type and they suggested that each should be labelled descriptively until more was known about them. They pointed out that in the mild form (Lightwood, 1952; Payne, 1952), the prognosis was good, but that in the severe form renal damage and mental retardation commonly occurred. This division into mild and severe forms is probably artificial because gradations between the two forms have emerged. We here describe three infants who were severely affected, and, in support of the conception of intermediate forms, a fourth infant who was moderately severely affected; in addition, this infant showed some of the features of infantile renal acidosis (Lightwood, 1935). We also report our observations on the facies as it is often a prominent and diagnostic feature of the disease.

Case Histories

Case 1. B.G. was the second child of healthy parents. Pregnancy and delivery were normal, and her birth weight was 7 lb. 12 oz. She was breast fed for the first three weeks, and then as lactation failed she was fed on National Dried Milk, half cream for six weeks and subsequently full cream. About 400 units of vitamin D (National Cod Liver Oil compound) were given daily.

Vomiting dated from birth, and usually occurred about half an hour after a feed; it was often bile stained. Initially she took her feeds fairly well but as her gain in weight was unsatisfactory she was admitted to a hospital at the age of 3 months; while there regurgitation occurred and a barium meal was normal; she was discharged home after four days. Her vomiting and failure to thrive continued, and at the age of 4 months one of us first saw her at an infant welfare clinic. Her weight was then 9 lb. 14 oz., and physical examination showed an apathetic infant, with a wide mouth, epicanthic folds and a concomitant squint (Fig. 1); a loud blowing systolic

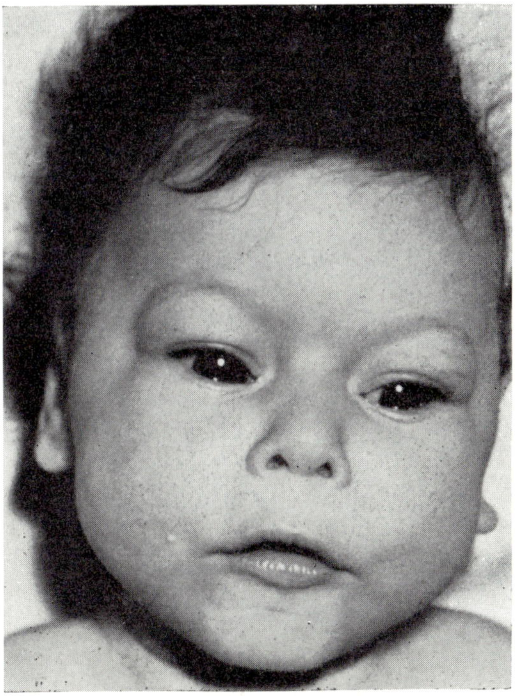

FIG. 1.—The facial appearance.

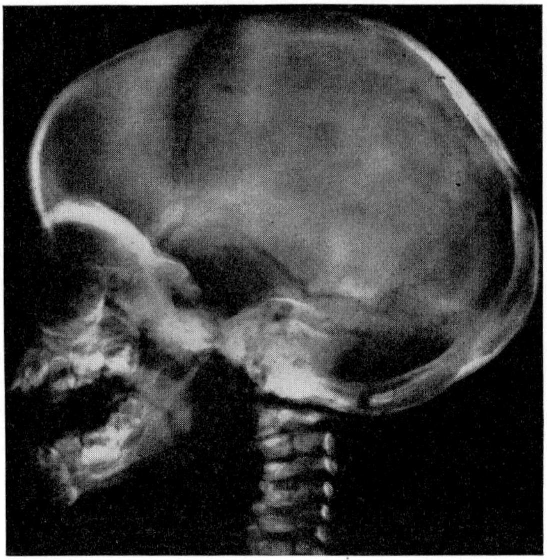

FIG. 2.—Case 1. Increased density at the base of the skull.

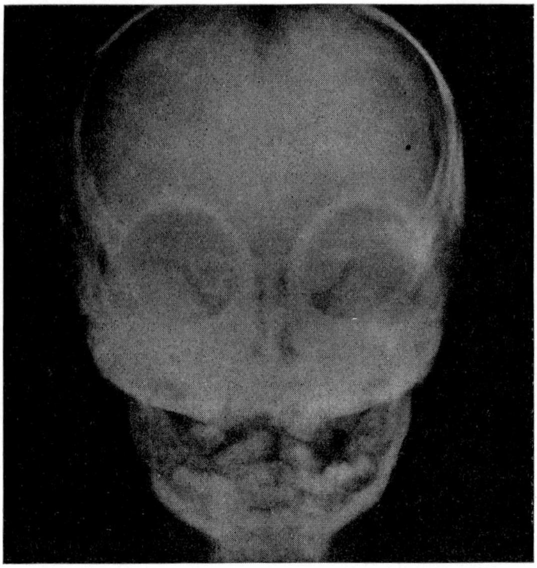

FIG. 3.—Case 1. Increased density of the periorbital bones.

murmur internal to the apex was present and the systolic blood pressure was 130 mm. Hg. A provisional diagnosis of severe infantile hypercalcaemia was made and she was admitted to Guy's Hospital for further investigation.

INVESTIGATIONS. The results of investigations on admission are shown in Table 1. The main abnormality was the raised blood urea. The serum calcium was regarded as a high normal. The serum cholesterol was normal. The electrolytes were normal. Radiographs of the skeleton showed increased density at the base of the skull (Fig. 2), of the periorbital bones (Fig. 3), at the ends of the long bones and the upper and lower borders of the vertebrae.

Serial biochemical estimations were made over the first five weeks (Table 2). Four weeks after admission the serum calcium level was unequivocally raised to 13·3 mg. %. The serum cholesterol was normal on three occasions (132 mg. %, 125 mg. %, and 117 mg. %).

TABLE 1
EARLY INVESTIGATIONS

		Blood Count		Urine				Blood Chemistry									Radiographs showing increased Density					
Case No.	Age (months)	Haemoglobin (g %)	White count (thousands/c.mm.)	pH	Albumen	White cells in deposit	Culture	Calcium (mg. %)	Phosphorus (mg. %)	Phosphatase (units K.A.)	Urea (mg. %)	Cholesterol (mg. %)	Sodium (mEq/l)	Potassium (mEq/l)	Chloride (mEq/l)	Bicarbonate (mEq/l)	Base of Skull	Periorbital Bones	Ends of Long Bones	Borders of Vertebrae	Pelvis	Ribs
1	4	11·2	10	acid	nil	±	—	11·4	4·2	13	57	132	137	4·4	101	19·8	yes	yes	yes	yes	no	no
	5							13·3	9·6	16	100	117			101	20·4						
2	5	9·5	27	4	+	+	—	13	3	6	97	160	152	3·7	102	24	yes	yes	yes	no	no	no
3	24			8	nil	—	—	12·4			133	320			97	22·5	yes	yes	yes	yes	no	no
	60			acid	nil	—	—	9·5	6·2	21	73	302					no	no		no	no	no
4	5½	10·8	12	6	nil	+++	*Esch. coli*	10·9 11·5			35			4·6	109	16						no
	7			neutral	+	++	*Proteus*	11·2			60	315			113	18·8				yes	yes	no
	12							14 9 15·8 14·6			130	200	146	4·6	113	18·8	yes	yes	yes	yes	yes	no

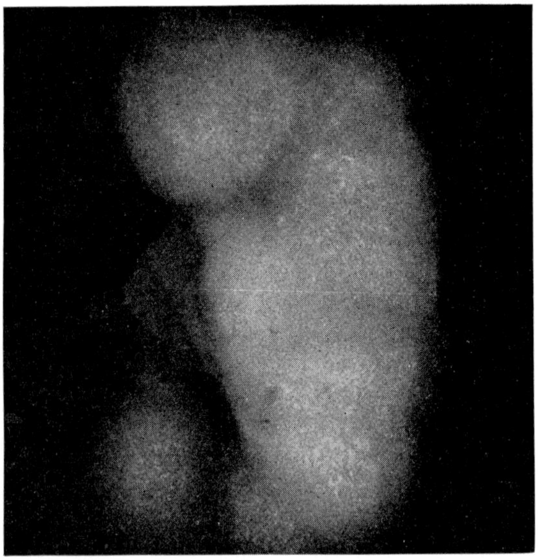

FIG. 4.—Case 1. Post mortem radiograph of kidney showing deposits in the pyramids.

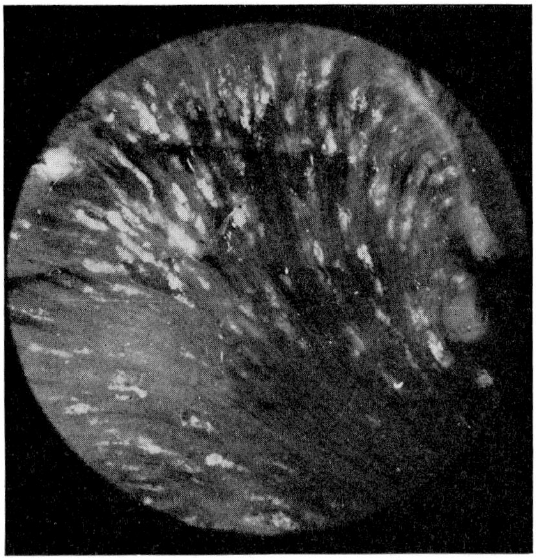

FIG. 5.—Case 1. Macrophotograph of kidney showing deposits in the pyramids (× 10).

TREATMENT AND PROGRESS. Treatment with cortisone by injection was started when she was just over 21 weeks old (Table 2); the dose varied but initially was 75 mg. daily for four days, and then 50 mg. daily. She was fed on National Dried Milk, but no added vitamin D was given. The serum calcium level dropped to 10·4 mg. % five days after starting cortisone, and apart from one raised value of 12·0 mg. % 10 days afterwards, it remained normal (Table 2). While she was on cortisone therapy a calcium balance was attempted but this was abandoned after 42 hours because she developed a severe rectal prolapse. She made slow progress, being difficult to feed, vomiting and failing to gain an adequate weight. A milk mixture which resulted in an intake of not more than 100 mg. of calcium daily was given but her anorexia became worse. At the age of 28 weeks she developed diarrhoea and the cortisone was stopped. The diarrhoea subsided, but her vomiting persisted and the serum calcium levels rose, the highest being 19 mg. % at the age of 9 months. The blood urea varied between 57 and 100 mg. %. Radiographs of the skull and the ends of the long bones showed an increase in density.

Cortisone therapy, 50 mg. daily, was started again, and she was discharged from hospital. Her symptoms persisted, however, and both her azotaemia and hypercalcaemia remained unchanged. At the age of 23 months she developed severe whooping cough; her blood urea rose to 150 mg. % and she died two days later.

NECROPSY (Dr. E. H. Bailey). The essential findings were that the kidneys weighed 15 g. (normal 45 g.). Both organs were pale. Thin streaks of calcium-like material were seen in the pyramids of both kidneys (Figs. 4 and 5). The heart weighed 75 g. (normal 55 g.). The left ventricle showed a well marked concentric hypertrophy. The right auricle was dilated and the right ventricle showed a little concentric hypertrophy. The edges of the mitral and tricuspid valves were thickened but there was no macroscopic calcification. The brain itself was normal but the right lateral sinus was completely obstructed by an ante-mortem clot. In the skull the basisphenoid and the bone forming the upper wall of the orbits were thickened. Other organs were normal.

HISTOLOGY (Dr. S. J. de Navasquez). The heart, stomach, spleen, thyroid, suprarenal glands and bone from the base of the skull were all normal. The liver showed severe passive congestion, and the lungs purulent bronchopneumonia. The intima of the aortic valve showed non-specific fibrous thickening. The cortex of the kidneys showed glomerular atrophy and periglomerular fibrosis (Fig. 6). In the medulla there were focal areas of calcium-like material which extended into and disrupted the collecting tubules in the vicinity

TABLE 2

CASE 1. BLOOD CHEMISTRY BEFORE AND DURING TREATMENT WITH CORTISONE

Age (Weeks)	Calcium	Phosphate	Phosphatase	Urea
16*	11·4	4·2	13	57
17	10·3	—	—	66
18	9·8	—	9	83
20	13·3	9·6	16	100
21	11·9	—	—	27
		Cortisone		
22	10·4	5·7	1	—
23	12·0	3·8	16	75
24½	8·8	—	—	—
25½	11·3	4·5	9	84
26	11·2	5·4	8	47
27	9·2	4·2	9	—
28	10·6	3·8	5	50

* Age on admission.

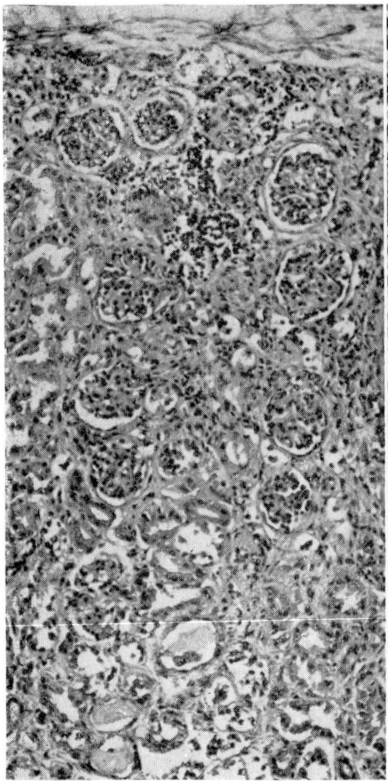

FIG. 6.—Case 1. Cortex showing glomerular atrophy and periglomerular fibrosis (H. and E. × 110).

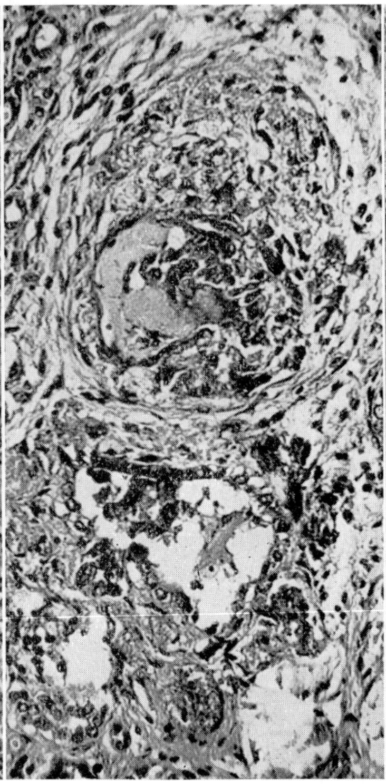

FIG. 7.—Collecting tubules showing intraluminal and subepithelial deposits of calcium-like material with disruption of the epithelium and interstitial fibrosis. (H. and E. × 175.)

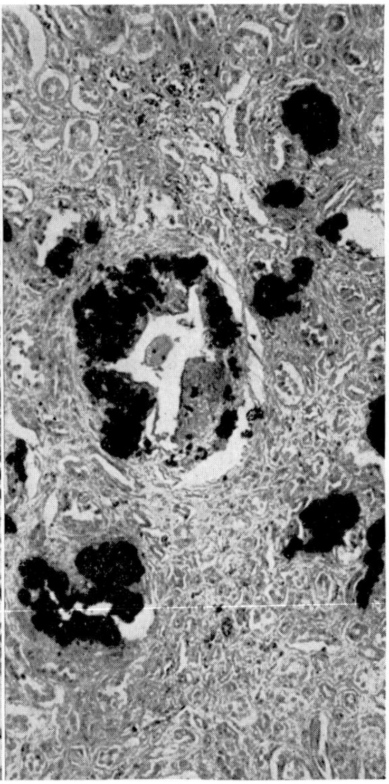

FIG. 8.—Medulla showing deposits of calcium-like material in the tubules. (von Kossa × 110.)

(Figs. 7 and 8). In addition, chronic focal pyelonephritis was present.

Case 2. B.D. was the second child of a family of three. Pregnancy was normal and her gestation period was 42 weeks; delivery was uncomplicated and her birth weight was 5 lb. 12 oz. She was breast fed for the first two weeks of life but when she was admitted to a hospital for severe conjunctivitis she was fed on half cream National milk. At this time she was noted to have an apical systolic murmur. She was in hospital two weeks and on discharge weighed 6 lb. 8 oz.

She progressed fairly well but vomited occasionally. At the age of 3 months her feeds were changed to full cream Cow and Gate milk. One month later she became listless and her vomiting became worse, and she was admitted to the Evelina Hospital. At this time she weighed 9 lb. 12 oz. Physical examination showed mild fever (100° F.), apathy, wasting, and loss of skin turgor. Her facies resembled that of Case 1, but in addition the inner third of her eyebrows was missing (Fig. 9). The pulse was regular at 130/minute and the heart was not enlarged. There was a loud systolic murmur maximal just internal to the apex. The blood pressure was 126/70 mm. Hg. There was marked hypotonia of the limb and trunk muscles. Other systems were normal.

INVESTIGATIONS. The results of investigations on admission are shown in Table 1. The urine contained albumen and an excess number of white cells; the serum calcium and blood urea were both raised. Radiographs showed increased density at the base of the skull, of the periorbital bones and at the ends of the long bones.

TREATMENT AND PROGRESS. Various feeds were tried, but her vomiting and anorexia persisted. She gained only 2 lb. in weight over a period of six months. A diet containing not more than 150 mg. of calcium daily was given for two months, but although her serum calcium levels became normal after six weeks, her symptoms persisted. Two weeks later, she was given normal milk feeds and this coincided with a gain in weight, which continued until her discharge four months later at the age of 19 months; at this time she weighed 16 lb. 14 oz., her hypotonia was less and she was able to sit up unaided. Her facies was unchanged. The serum calcium was 11·6 mg. % and the blood urea 40 mg. %.

She continued to progress very slowly, her weight at 2 years being 18 lb. 2 oz. Six months later she was readmitted weighing 19 lb. At this time she was beginning to say a few words and was walking with help; her squint was worse but the systolic murmur was now blowing and the systolic blood pressure was 110 mm. Hg.

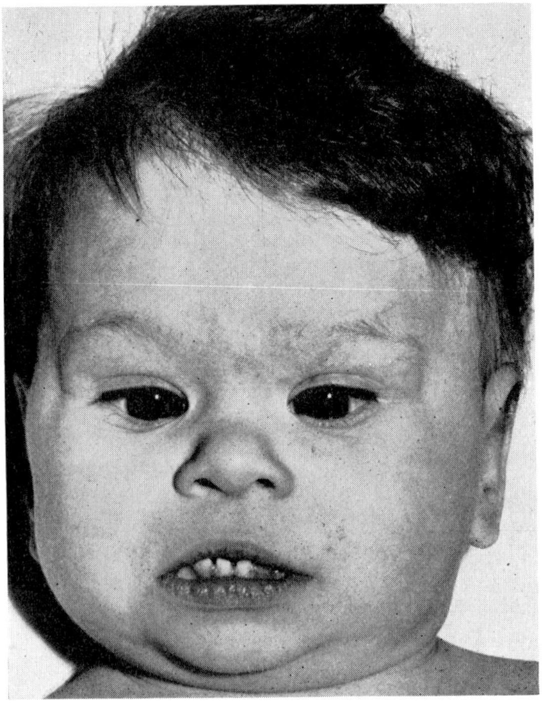

FIG. 9.—Case 2. The facial appearance; note loss of inner third of eyebrows.

The haemoglobin was 9 g. %, serum calcium 12·6 mg. %, phosphorus 4 mg. %, alkaline phosphatase 9 units (King Armstrong) and urea 65 mg. %. Radiographs of the skull and ends of the long bones showed a decrease in density.

A calcium balance was done when she was $2\frac{3}{4}$ years old and, following this, cortisone 15 mg. b.d. was given by injection. She became brighter, her appetite increased and she put on weight rapidly and consistently; the serum calcium fell to 7·8 mg. % but the blood urea remained elevated at 48 mg. % (Fig. 10).

Two months later the systolic murmur was less loud. The calcium balance was repeated while she was taking cortisone. She was discharged at the age of 3 years taking cortisone 25 mg. daily by mouth; this was continued for seven months. At the age of 4 years she weighed 24 lb. and was about 22 inches tall; her facies was unchanged but the systolic murmur was barely audible; the serum calcium was 9·8 mg. % and the blood urea 43 mg. %. Radiographs of her skeleton still showed some increase in density. Her I.Q. was 40.

Case 3. The clinical features of this patient have been already described (Schlesinger *et al.*, 1956). Briefly, vomiting and anorexia began when he was 11 months old. He was investigated but no firm diagnosis was made until the age of 2 years when he was seen by Dr. Philip Evans who observed the facies, physical and mental retardation and a loud systolic murmur. The

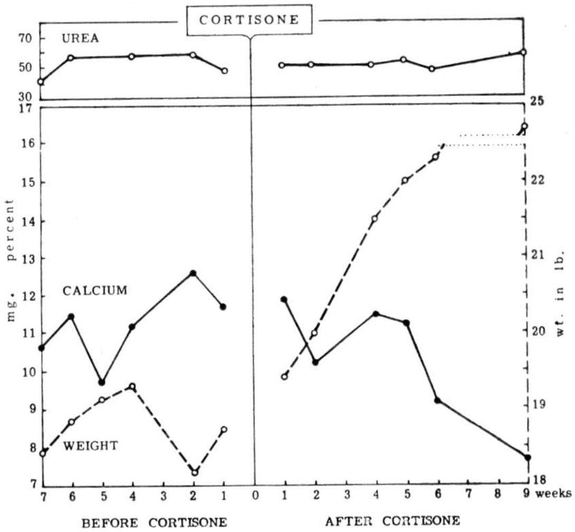

Fig. 10.—Case 2. Response to cortisone.

main investigations are shown in Table 1. The blood urea was 133 mg. %, serum calcium 12·4 mg. % and blood cholesterol 320 mg. %. The base of the skull and periorbital bones showed moderate increase in density.

Over the course of the next few months he began to improve slowly, the vomiting and anorexia became less and he began gaining weight. He was seen again at the age of 5 years, because of attacks of abdominal pain. He was a mentally retarded child whose behaviour resembled that of a 2-year-old; the facies and the squint were unchanged. No systolic murmur was present. Serum calcium, phosphorus and phosphatase were normal, but the blood urea was 73 mg. % and the blood cholesterol 302 mg. %; the urine, radiograph of the skull and intravenous pyelogram were normal and the bone age corresponded with the chronological age.

Case 4. P.B. was a second child; pregnancy and delivery were normal. His birth weight was 7 lb. 3 oz. As his mother had a history of tuberculosis he was never breast fed. For the first four months he was fed on half cream milk and subsequently on full cream milk. At the age of 4 months he began to vomit and the National Cod Liver Oil Compound (800 units of vitamin D), which he had been taking, was omitted. He continued to vomit and lose weight and at the age of $5\frac{1}{2}$ months he was admitted to a hospital. Examination then showed a fairly fit-looking infant with a normal facies; his forehead was prominent, and his temples were narrow. No physical signs were present except those of mild dehydration. His weight was 14 lb.

INVESTIGATIONS. The results of investigations are shown in Table 1. The urine was infected with *Esch. coli*; the serum calcium and blood urea were normal, but the plasma chloride was raised and the bicarbonate lowered.

TREATMENT AND PROGRESS. Subsequent examination of the urine did not confirm the presence of an infection.

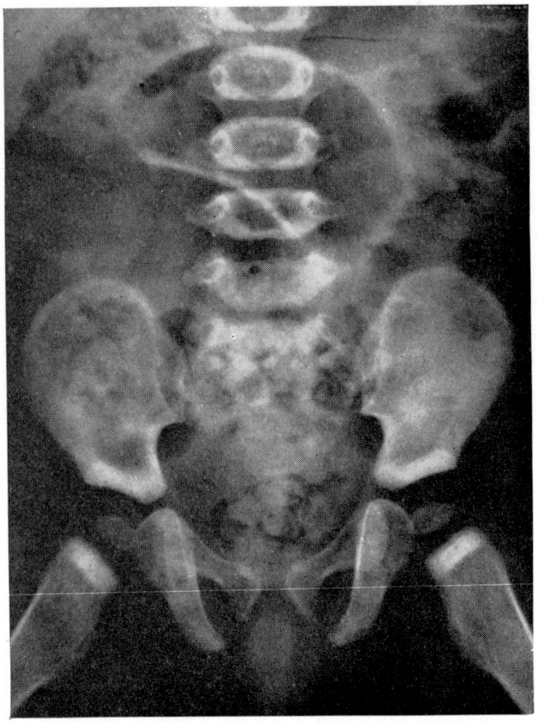

FIG. 11.—Case 4. Increased density adjacent to hip joints, of the iliac crests and of the superior and inferior borders of the lumbar vertebrae.

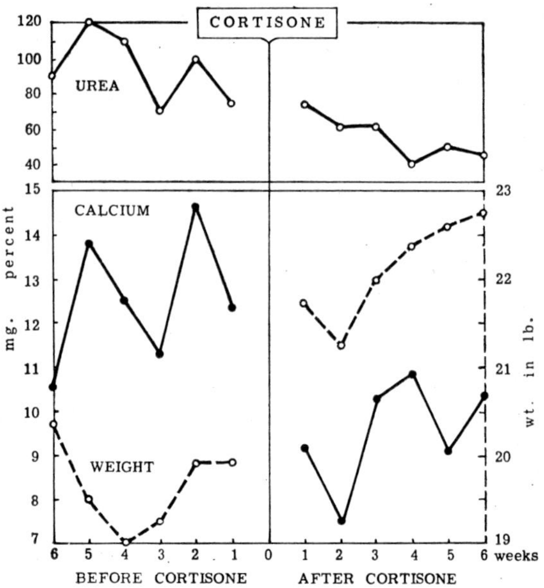

FIG. 12.—Case 4. Response to cortisone.

While in hospital he developed a series of upper respiratory infections. He vomited when he was fed on full cream milk, but when this was changed to half cream no vomiting occurred. He was discharged symptomless taking half cream milk. No firm diagnosis was made.

He progressed slowly until the age of 7 months when vomiting recurred and he developed severe constipation. He was admitted to Guy's Hospital. On examination there were no physical signs except those of constipation. The results of investigations are shown in Table 1.

In view of the previous and present findings, it was thought likely that he had infantile renal acidosis with hypercalcaemia and he was treated with a mixture of 10 gr. sodium citrate and 2·5 gr. of citric acid four times daily. He began gaining weight and the plasma bicarbonate rose to 26 mEq/l. and the plasma chloride fell to 104·6 mEq/l. When the alkali was discontinued the plasma bicarbonate fell to 16·2 mEq/l. and the chloride rose to 111 mEq/l. Treatment with alkali was reintroduced and he responded well, gaining 12 oz. in the first week.

Two months later he developed severe bronchitis and was readmitted. Examination at this time showed no physical signs additional to those of bronchitis; the systolic blood pressure was 110 mm. Hg; the blood urea was 130 mg. % and the serum calcium 9 mg. %. The α_2 and β globulins were increased. Radiographs of the skull, long bones, vertebrae and pelvis showed increased density (Fig. 11). Subsequent serum calcium levels remained high, rising to 15·8 mg. % and 14·6 mg. % on two occasions. He vomited periodically and gained weight slowly. A milk containing not more than 100 mg. of calcium daily was given for two months without appreciable effect clinically or biochemically. A calcium balance was performed at this stage, and following this he was given cortisone by injection, 25 mg. b.d. He responded well both clinically and biochemically; his serum calcium fell to 7·6 mg. % later rising to within normal limits (Fig. 12). He was discharged taking the same dose of cortisone by mouth. Three months later the calcium balance was repeated while he was taking cortisone.

His subsequent progress was good and he gained weight satisfactorily. The cortisone was stopped after 10 months. He continued to do well and at the age of 4¾ years he weighed 38 lb.; the blood pressure was 110/70 mm. Hg and no physical signs were present; there was no evidence of mental retardation. The urine was acid and normal. The blood urea was 44 mg. %, serum calcium 11 mg. % and phosphate 3·7 mg. %.

Radiologically the long bones were normal but the base of the skull and periorbital bones still showed some increase in density.

Calcium Balance Studies

Balance Methods. The patient was equilibrated on a constant calcium intake for three days and thereafter stools and urine were collected between stool carmine markers over a period of four days. The type of feed and calculated intake of vitamin D are indicated in Table 3. A metabolic bed was used, and the stools were collected into cellophane-lined containers. In girls the urine was collected through a vulval mould and in boys through Paul's tubing. All receptacles for stools and urine were previously rinsed with distilled sterile water. Duplicate aliquots of stools, urine and a homogenate of a duplicate diet were digested with fuming nitric and perchloric acids. The digest was made up to volume and insoluble fatty acids were filtered off. After adjustment of pH, calcium was precipitated with excess oxalate and estimated by titration with standard potassium permanganate solution.

Table 3 shows the results of the balances. Cases 2 and 4 each had two balances, before and after cortisone therapy. Balances were attempted in Cases 1 and 2 in the early stages of their illness but were not completed as they were badly tolerated. Case 1 had a short balance lasting 42 hours while she was on cortisone, and although the results have been recorded, interpretation must be especially cautious. However, the figure of 38% retention is similar to that reported by Forfar, Balf, Maxwell and Tompsett (1956) and Morgan, Mitchell, Stowers and Thomson (1956) in affected infants of the same age while taking cortisone. The daily retention of calcium in Case 2 was 30% which is between one and a half and three times more than normal at this age (Daniels, 1941; Watson, McGuire, Meyer and Hathaway, 1945; McLean, Lewis, Jensen, Hathaway, Breiter and Holmes, 1946; Irving, 1950). The daily retention in Case 4 was about normal when expressed as a percentage of intake but in absolute figures (137 mg. and 248 mg.), both children retained between one and a half and three times normal (Shohl, 1939; Holmes, 1945; Mitchell, Hamilton, Steggerda and Bean, 1945). Schlesinger, Butler and Black (1952) and Forfar *et al.* (1956) in affected children of similar age reported daily retentions of 74 mg. and 126 mg. of calcium (7·7% and 16% of intake).

Effect of Cortisone. The effect of cortisone on calcium retention is shown in Table 3. In Case 2 calcium retention increased from 30% to 37% and in Case 4 from 20% to 33%. The total intake varied in our children, but Watson *et al.* (1945) found that similar variations of intake did not influence the percentage retentions in normal children. The effect of cortisone on calcium retention which we observed was similar to that found by Fletcher (1957) in a boy of 3 years in whom the faecal calcium decreased when he was given 15 mg. of cortisone daily. However, although others (Bonham Carter, Dent, Fowler and Harper, 1955; Forfar *et al.*, 1956; Morgan *et al.*, 1956) have found that cortisone increases the faecal calcium and therefore reduces calcium retention, their studies were on younger patients in whom cortisone therapy had been of shorter duration. Nevertheless, we cannot satisfactorily account for the difference in these findings, especially as cortisone was so effective in reducing the serum calcium levels (Figs. 10 and 12).

The Facies

The unusual facial appearance was recognized by Butler (1951) and Fanconi (1951), and it has been used to help distinguish the severe from the mild type. How soon after birth it develops is unknown. The mother of B.G. told us that she thought the face was 'queer looking' at birth, and it was sufficiently characteristic at 4 months of age for the clinical diagnosis to be made (Joseph, 1956).

The facies in this disease has received less attention than some of the other features, but since it usually indicates severity, it is both an important diagnostic and prognostic sign.

There have been too few examples observed for all the facial variations and combinations to be known, and for a great many generalizations to be made, and the following notes are no more than an attempt to focus attention on some of the changes. One of the difficulties we have encountered is our ignorance of the range of normal, if any face can be called normal. The facial appearance in this disease is due to the presence of a combination of features, but we do not know which particular

TABLE 3
CALCIUM BALANCES IN CASES 1, 2 AND 4

Case	Age (yr.)	Diet	Daily Vit. D Intake (units)	Calcium (mg. %)	Urea (mg.)	Daily Cortisone (mg.)	Calcium (mg. daily) Intake	Faeces	Urine	Retention	%
1 B.G.	½	Milk	700	11·2	84, 47	50	1,255	700	72	473	38
2 B.D.	3¼	Mixed	12	11·7	31		455	255	63	137	30
,,	3½	Mixed	44	9·2	47	50	1,066	512	119	373	37
4 P.B.	2	Milk, egg	66	11 13	93, 73		1,208	890	70	248	20
,,	2¼	Mixed	78	12·1 14·1	80, 60	50	702	342	123	237	33

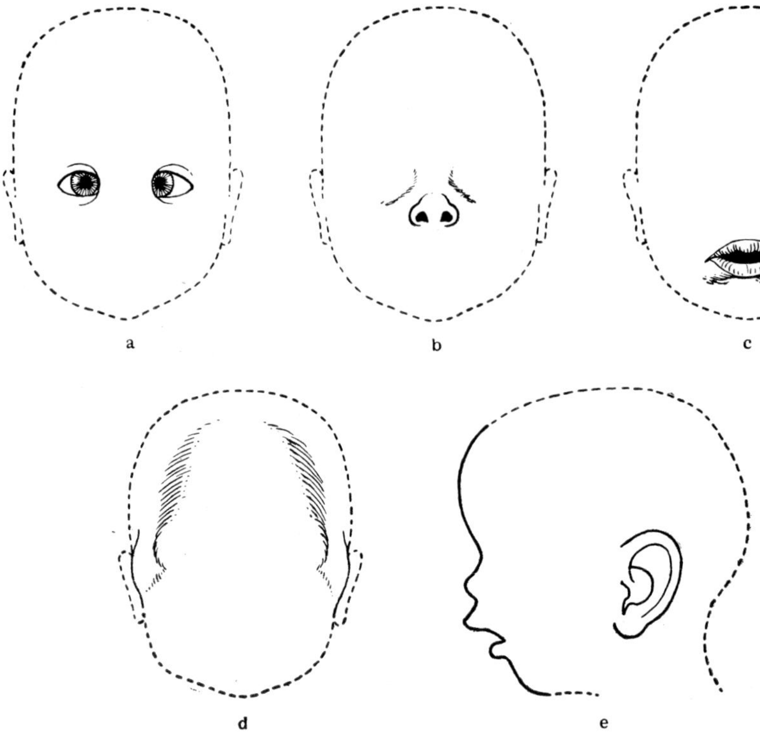

FIG. 13.—Components of the facies.

combination is necessary to produce the facies; indeed it is likely that different combinations will affect the facies, and this is probably what occurs.

Lowe *et al.* (1954) have described the facies as elfin-like; although we agree that this applies to the general shape of their face, it disregards their expression of misery and irritability. Surely elves have a sprightly air:

> 'Couronnés de thym et de marjolaine
> Les Elfes joyeux dansent sur la plaine.'
> *Leconte de Lisle*

The Individual Facial Features. Epicanthic folds and commonly a concomitant squint are present (Fig. 13a). The nose is pinched and retroussé, with the nostrils pointing forwards (Fig. 13b); because there is some filling in at the sides of and across the nose, the appearance has been likened to that of a pekinese dog (*British Medical Journal*, 1954). The upper lip is prominent and appears loose (Fig. 13e); it lacks the usual bow and the pars villosa may persist (Fig. 13c). The mouth is sometimes asymmetrical and is generally kept open, the lower lip hanging slackly. The temples are narrow (Fig. 13d). The profile is affected by the receding chin and by the rounded and sometimes prominent forehead (Fig. 13e). The ears may be large but are normally placed (Fig. 13e).

The ears have been described as being low set (Butler, 1951; Schlesinger *et al.*, 1952) but we think they appear so because these children frequently adopt a 'chin-up' position (Fig. 14). This deception is added to if the ramus of the mandible is short or if its angle with the body of the mandible is more acute than normal. The ear may also appear low if the vertex of the skull is deep; this was well illustrated when the father of an affected boy said he thought that his son's head was high rather than that his ears were low. Finally, a relative increase in the amount of the pinna below the meatus will make the ear appear low in the same way as a large ear may.

The profile of these infants runs downwards and backwards and therefore the Frankfurt line does not form even an approximate right angle with the profile. Although the ear appears low the external auditory meatus maintains a normal relationship with the base of the skull (Fig. 15).

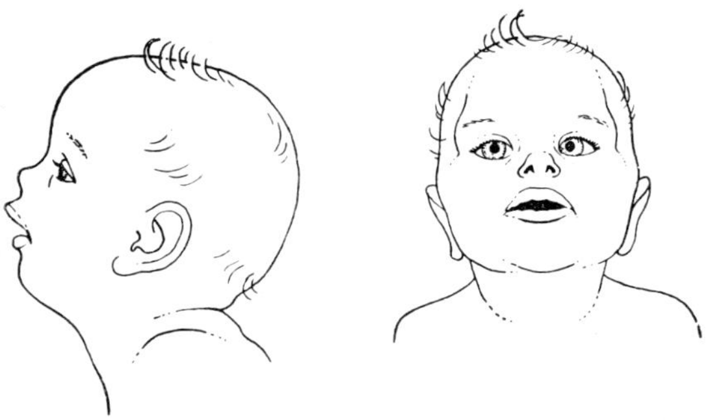

FIG. 14.—The ears appear low because the head is held extended

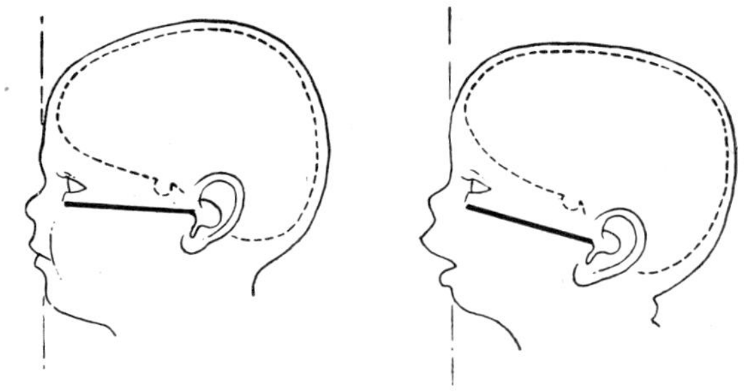

FIG. 15.—The Frankfurt line has been drawn and shows that the external auditory meatus has a normal relationship to the base of the skull.

The cause of the facies is unknown. Russell and Young (1954) have suggested that it is due to abnormal growth of the basisphenoid. Schlesinger *et al.* (1956) reviewed 10 cases of the severe type and all had both the characteristic facies and radiological changes in the skull. Our Cases 1, 2 and 3 were similar in these respects. Case 4 showed changes in the skull but except for a prominent forehead the facies was not characteristic. Of more than a score of infants with the less severe form of hypercalcaemia (Lightwood, 1952; Lowe *et al.*, 1954; Bonham Carter *et al.*, 1955; MacDonald and Stapleton, 1955; Forfar *et al.*, 1956; Morgan *et al.*, 1956; Rhaney and Mitchell, 1956; Kendall, 1957), none had radiological changes in the skull; in three the facial appearance was described as normal and in the remainder there was no comment. These observations suggest that the bone changes in the skull are responsible for the facies, but because some of the facial features seem to be due to alterations in the contours of the soft tissues, it is possible that the bone changes only play some part in the facial appearance.

Types of Idiopathic Hypercalcaemia

Stapleton and Lightwood (1953) suggested that certain clinical and radiological features served to distinguish cases of simple idiopathic hypercalcaemia with failure to thrive from those with general retardation and osteosclerosis. Lowe *et al.* (1954) have elaborated the differences. The former type is transient and relatively benign, without significant bone changes, systolic murmurs, hypertension or mental retardation. The latter type is sustained and severe, has bone changes, significant systolic murmurs, hypertension, characteristic facies, mental retardation and often a raised blood cholesterol. During the past few years, there have been many reports of infants with hypercalcaemia, and some have had features which have made it difficult to place them in one or other category. We are uncertain which criteria are valid in order to classify the affected infant. Transient and benign is no help as three infants who conformed to this type came to necropsy (Rhaney and Mitchell, 1956; Morgan *et al.*, 1956). Systolic murmurs may be present in both types; they were recorded in the simple type by Lowe *et al.* (1954), Creery and Neill (1954) and MacDonald and Stapleton (1955), but were absent in some of the severe cases collected by Schlesinger *et al.* (1956). Hypertension is also unreliable; MacDonald and Stapleton (1955) reported its presence in a simple case, while Creery (1953) and Lowe *et al.* (1954) found normal readings in two severe cases. Radiological changes in the bones are not absolute but increased density of the base of the skull has only been described in the severe forms, although it was not present in three patients who died (Rhaney and Mitchell, 1956). The characteristic facies has been described as only occurring in the severe form but Rhaney and Mitchell (1956) reported its absence in their three fatal cases. It is probably too early to evaluate the incidence of mental retardation, but in general the survivors in the simple group have developed normally whereas the few survivors of the severe form have been grossly retarded. The facies and bone changes in the skull usually occur together and indicate severity, with renal impairment and possible mental retardation. Cases 1, 2 and 3 had these changes and Case 1 died and Cases 2 and 3 are both grossly retarded (I.Q. 40). But absence of skull changes and of the facies does not necessarily indicate a good prognosis, as shown by the deaths reported by Rhaney and Mitchell (1956) and Morgan *et al.* (1956).

Creery (1953) has suggested that all grades of idiopathic hypercalcaemia occur and later others have supported this conception (Russell and Young, 1954; Lightwood, 1955). Case 4 was an example of an intermediate grade. He resembled the simple type by the presence of a raised α_2 globulin, and the absence of abnormal facies, of hypertension, of a systolic murmur and of mental retardation. On the other hand, he resembled the severe type by the presence of bone changes in the skull, vertebrae and pelvis, by a raised serum cholesterol and by his slow recovery. Additionally he had some of the changes seen in renal acidosis. Lightwood (1952) and Payne (1952) reported that an associated renal acidosis was occasionally present in simple hypercalcaemia and Lightwood (1955) found this in six of 50 cases. In none of these patients, however, were there bone changes such as those found in Case 4.

As it is now recognized that the prognosis is not always good in the simple or so-called benign cases, it is suggested that the term 'benign' should no longer be used.

Necropsy Findings

The findings at necropsy and the histological changes have been described and discussed fully by Dawson *et al.* (1954), Lowe *et al.* (1954) and Schlesinger *et al.* (1956). Darmady and Stranack (1957, 1958) have microdissected a number of these kidneys and consider that the focal areas of deposit are probably a phosphate protein complex, and should at the moment be referred to as 'calcium-like'.

The changes in the kidneys found in Case 1 were similar to those previously reported. Although nephrocalcinosis was not diagnosed before death, calcium-like material was clearly seen in the cut surface of the kidney macroscopically and radiologically (Figs. 4 and 5). Darmady and Stranack (1958) have fully described their findings on microdissection of the kidney in Case 1 and we are grateful to them for allowing us to use their report and microphotograph. Briefly, they found focal areas of calcium-like material adherent to the basement membrane and projecting laterally from the proximal tubule wall. Similar areas were seen in the distal and collecting tubules (Fig. 16).

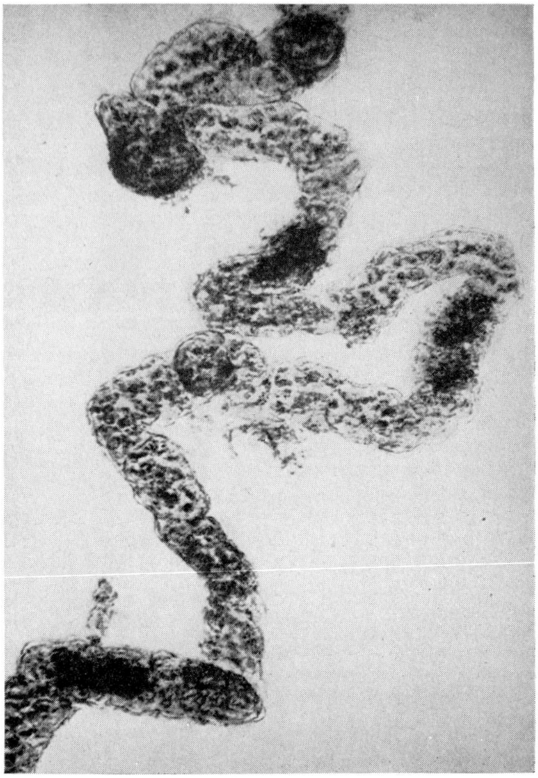

FIG. 16.—A portion of proximal tubule shows a plaque of calcium-like material adherent to the basement membrane and further areas are seen lower in the nephron. At the bottom left hand corner of the picture an albuminous case is seen lying in the lumen of the tubule. The architecture of the proximal tubule is normal. (× 280.)

Conclusion

The cause of infantile hypercalcaemia and an explanation of many of its clinical features remain unanswered. The exact incidence of the condition is unknown but Morgan *et al.* (1956) have pointed out that in Dundee between 1953 and 1955 it accounted for 4·6% of all medical admissions of children aged 6 to 12 months, ranking fourth in frequency after respiratory infections, feeding difficulties and otitis media. We do not know whether its incidence is diminishing, but if sensitivity to vitamin D (*Lancet*, 1954) is an important contributory factor, then the recent recommendation (Her Majesty's Stationery Office, 1957) that the vitamin D content of National Dried Milks and Cod Liver Oil Compound should be halved is likely to reduce the incidence of a disease which may cause physical and mental retardation, and sometimes death.

Summary

The clinical, radiological and biochemical features of four patients with severe infantile hypercalcaemia are described. In addition, one of the patients had renal acidosis.

Three patients were treated with cortisone, and in two the response was good; the third died and the results of necropsy are discussed. Balance studies on these three patients reveal an increased retention of calcium, and cortisone was found to augment this retention.

The individual features of the facies are illustrated

and discussed. It is suggested that patients having the characteristic facies are usually severely affected and are likely to have sequelae of mental retardation and renal insufficiency.

The types of infantile hypercalcaemia are discussed and it is suggested that the mild and severe types should not be considered separate syndromes.

Cases 1, 2 and 3 were under the care of Dr. P. R. Evans and Case 4 was under the care of Dr. R. C. Mac Keith. We thank Dr. W. H. H. Merivale for help with the calcium balances, and Dr. J. Dow for help with the interpretation of the radiographs. Miss S. Treadgold of the Medical Illustration Department contributed much to the section on the facies, and we thank her for her help and for the drawings. The remaining illustrations were made by the Photographic Department to whom we are indebted.

References

Bongiovanni, A. M., Eberlein, W. R. and Jones, I. T. (1957). *New Engl. J. Med.*, **257**, 951.
Bonham Carter, R. E., Dent, C. E., Fowler, D. I. and Harper, C. M. (1955). *Arch. Dis. Childh.*, **32**, 399.
British Medical Journal (1954). Leading article, **2**, 1155.
Butler, N. R. (1951). *Proc. roy. Soc. Med.*, **44**, 296.
Creery, R. D. G. (1953). *Lancet*, **2**, 17.
—— and Neill, D. W. (1954). *Ibid.*, **2**, 110.
Daeschner, G. L. and Daeschner, C. W. (1957). *Pediatrics*, **19**, 362.
Daniels, A. L. (1941). *Amer. J. Dis. Child.*, **62**, 279.
Darmady, E. M. and Stranack, F. (1957). *Brit. med. Bull.*, **13**, 21.
——, —— (1958). In the press.
Dawson, I. M. P., Craig, W. S. and Perera, F. J. C. (1954). *Arch. Dis. Childh.*, **29**, 475.
Fanconi, G. (1951). *Schweiz. med. Wschr.*, **81**, 908.
——, Girardet, P., Schlesinger, B. E., Butler, N. R. and Black, J. A. (1952). *Helv. paediat. Acta*, **7**, 314 and 335.
Fletcher, R. F. (1957). *Arch. Dis. Childh.*, **32**, 245.
Forfar, J. O., Balf, C. L., Maxwell, G. M. and Tompsett, S. L. (1956). *Lancet*, **1**, 981.
Her Majesty's Stationery Office (1957). Report of the Joint Sub-Committee on Welfare Foods.
Holmes, J. O. (1945). *Nutr. Abstr. Rev.*, **14**, 597.
Irving, J. T. (1950). *S. Afr. med. J.*, **24**, 601.
Joseph, M. C. (1956). *Brit. med. J.*, **1**, 1112.
Kendall, A. C. (1957). *Ibid.*, **2**, 682.
Lancet (1954). Leading article, **2**, 127.
Leconte de Lisle, C. M. R. (1925). *Oxford Book of French Verse*, p. 442. St. John Lucas.
Lightwood, R. (1932). *Arch. Dis. Childh.*, **7**, 193.
—— (1935). *Ibid.*, **10**, 205.
—— (1952). *Ibid.*, **27**, 302.
—— (1955). *Rev. port. Pediát.*, **18**, 335.
—— and Stapleton, T. (1953). *Lancet*, **2**, 255.
Lowe, K. G., Henderson, J. L., Park, W. W. and McGreal, D. A. (1954). *Lancet*, **2**, 101.
MacDonald, W. B. and Stapleton, T. (1955). *Acta Paediat. (Uppsala)*, **44**, 559.
McLean, D. S., Lewis, G. K., Jensen, E., Hathaway, M., Breiter, H. and Holmes, J. O. (1946). *J. Nutr.*, **31**, 127.
Morgan, H. G., Mitchell, R. G., Stowers, J. M. and Thomson, J. (1956). *Lancet*, **1**, 925.
Mitchell, H. H., Hamilton, T. S., Steggerda, F. R. and Bean, H. W. (1945). *J. biol. Chem.*, **158**, 625.
Payne, W. W. (1952). *Arch. Dis. Childh.*, **27**, 302.
Rhaney, K. and Mitchell, R. G. (1956). *Lancet*, **1**, 1028.
Russell, A. and Young, W. F. (1954). *Proc. roy. Soc. Med.*, **47**, 1036.
Schlesinger, B., Butler, N. and Black, J. (1952). *Helv. paediat. Acta*, **7**, 335.
——, ——, —— (1956). *Brit. med. J.*, **1**, 127.
Shohl, A. T. (1939). *Mineral Metabolism*, p. 50. New York.
Sissman, N. J. and Klein, R. (1956). *Clin. Res. Proc.*, **4**, 36.
Stapleton, T. and Lightwood, R. (1953). *Lancet*, **2**, 255.
Watson, E. K., McGuire, E. W., Meyer, F. L. and Hathaway, M. L (1945). *J. Nutr.*, **30**, 259.

CONGENITAL ABSENCE OF THE INTRAHEPATIC BILE DUCTS

BY

LEONARD HAAS and RICHARD H. DOBBS
From the Children's Department, The London Hospital

(RECEIVED FOR PUBLICATION MARCH 24, 1958)

Routine histological examination of the liver during the acute stages of neonatal obstructive jaundice, whether of biopsy or of autopsy specimens, reveals a variety of different pathological conditions.

Congenital absence of the intrahepatic bile ducts appears to be a rare cause of obstructive jaundice in the newborn. The purpose of this paper is to draw attention to the condition by reporting two cases, and by discussing its main clinical and pathological features in the light of these two and eight other cases that have been found in the medical literature. One of the present cases was previously shown at a clinical meeting (Smythe and Dobbs, 1949) as a case of xanthomatosis, and later included in a monograph on this subject by Ahrens, Harris and MacMahon (1951) who considered the underlying pathology to be intrahepatic biliary atresia.

Neonatal obstructive jaundice with pale stools and dark urine has been common to all described cases, and in no way differed from that found in, for instance, congenital extrahepatic obstruction of the bile ducts or neonatal hepatitis. But, though the diagnosis was arrived at histologically in seven out of the 10 cases only after the age of 2 years, certain features common to the post-neonatal course of all of them appear to make the condition a recognizable clinical entity at least before the end of the first year of life.

Case Descriptions

Case 1. E.H., female, died aged 2 years 9 months. (Previously reported by Smythe and Dobbs, 1949; Ahrens *et al.*, 1951). She was the second child of healthy parents. The mother suffered from toxaemia in both pregnancies. The first child is alive and well. The birth was normal, the infant weighed $6\frac{1}{2}$ lb. and was apparently healthy. Jaundice was noted on the second day of life and rapidly deepened. The serum bilirubin was not estimated at this stage. The stools became clay coloured and remained so for the first two months, after which they became yellow and sometimes brown. The urine is alleged not to have contained bile pigments during the neonatal phase of the disease though from the age of 5 months onwards tests for bilirubin were always positive. Pruritus was a troublesome symptom from the first few days of life: persistent scratching often led to excoriations and bleeding, and the child was always unhappy and fretful. Nevertheless feeds were taken well and she gained weight slowly. At the age of 20 months widespread deposits of yellow material appeared in the skin. At the same time pruritus became more marked and scratching was mainly aimed at these deposits which frequently bled freely.

The child's condition remained stationary and in September, 1948, at $2\frac{1}{2}$ years of age, she was admitted to The London Hospital for investigation. She was then found to be a thin, undersized and unhappy child, 21 lb. in weight and 32 inches in height. There was moderate generalized jaundice of the skin and the conjunctivae. The body was covered with innumerable yellow, raised xanthomatous deposits, especially marked over the hands, elbows, ankles and legs (Figs. 1 and 2). Miliary xanthomata were found on the palms and soles and longitudinal yellow streaks in the creases of the skin and along the gum margins. Both liver and spleen were enlarged and palpable 1 inch below the costal margin, the liver edge

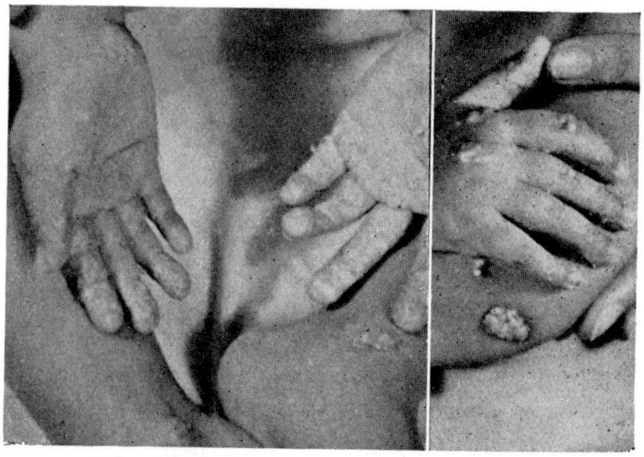

FIGS. 1 AND 2.—Case 1. Skin xanthomata.

being firm and smooth. A systolic murmur was audible over the praecordium.

The relevant investigations at this time were as follows: liver function tests: serum bilirubin, 4·5 mg. per 100 ml.; alkaline phosphatase, 36 units; serum proteins, 6·3 g. per 100 ml. (albumin, 4·1; globulin, 2·2); thymol turbidity, 2·5 units; cephalin and colloidal gold tests were negative. Apart from the raised serum bilirubin these tests were compatible with normal hepatic function. Serum cholesterol was 1,200 mg. per 100 ml. Urobilin and urobilinogen as well as a trace of bile were present in the urine. Stercobilin was present in the stools. A skin biopsy confirmed that the deposits in the subcutis were cholesterol.

No change in the clinical picture was observed during her stay in hospital. She was considered to be suffering from an incomplete or partial obstructive jaundice associated with generalized xanthomatosis. This was believed to be the primary abnormality and as such she was presented at the Royal Society of Medicine (Smythe and Dobbs, 1949).

The child died three months after discharge from hospital at the age of 2 years and 9 months. Just before death she became deeply jaundiced with a bilirubin of 13·6 mg. per 100 ml. Autopsy revealed a bilateral acute pyelonephritis as the immediate cause of death*. Xanthomatous deposits were found in the endocardium and the subintima of the great vessels, as well as on the posterior surface of the epiglottis and the epiglottic folds. The liver was enlarged and jaundiced. The gall bladder contained a moderate amount of brownish bile which could be easily expressed along the main cystic and hepatic ducts which appeared to be patent. The spleen was enlarged and firm but showed no definite abnormality.

The microscopy of the liver has been described in detail by Ahrens *et al.* (1951), and will be discussed later.

Case 2. S.P., female, was 5 years old in May, 1958. She was born of a healthy mother after a normal pregnancy and there have been no other siblings (1958). The father is not known. The child was delivered by forceps, weighed 6 lb. 2 oz. and was apparently healthy. Jaundice was noted on the fourth day of life and this rapidly increased in severity. The stools became pale and the urine dark. A congenital obstruction to the flow of bile was suspected, and a laparotomy was performed on the sixteenth day of life. At operation the gall bladder was found to be empty and deeply buried in the fissure. The cystic duct was traced to where the common bile duct should have been, but the latter could not be identified with certainty. There was no extrahepatic distension of the bile ducts and aspiration of the liver did not locate any collection of bile. An unfavourable prognosis was given. However, though the child remained thin and jaundiced her general condition did not deteriorate.

She was re-examined at the age of 8 months when her complexion was described as pale olive. Her serum bilirubin was 1·5 mg. per 100 ml., and stercobilin was identified in the stools. Since then there has been no increase in the degree of clinical jaundice and her general health has also remained relatively good.

She was admitted to The London Hospital in June, 1956, at the age of 3 years 1 month. She was then a stunted child, 27 lb. in weight and 30 inches in height. There was very slight generalized jaundice. The liver was enlarged, its edge was smooth, firm and palpable three and three-quarter inches below the costal margin. The tip of the spleen was just palpable. There was a systolic cardiac murmur audible over the praecordium.

The relevant investigations at this time were as follows: liver function tests: serum bilirubin, 4·5 mg. per 100 ml.; alkaline phosphatase, 54 units; thymol turbidity, 0·8 units; thymol flocculation, 0; zinc sulphate test, 3·5 units; serum proteins, 7 mg. per 100 ml. (albumin, 5·1; globulin, 1·9). Apart from the raised serum bilirubin and the slightly raised alkaline phosphatase these tests were compatible with normal hepatic function. Cholesterol was 1,600 mg. per 100 ml.; total lipids, 3,800 mg. per 100 ml.; and lipo-proteins, 1,300 mg. per 100 ml. The urine contained bilirubin, and urobilinogen within normal limits. Stercobilin was present in normal quantities in the stools. The bone age was within normal limits.

The child's general health remained good. She was cheerful and happy in spite of continued pruritus which caused a great deal of scratching. A sparse papular eruption first noted one month after admission was soon followed by the appearance of numerous yellow shiny xanthomatous deposits in the skin flexures and over the buttocks (Fig. 3). No skin biopsy was done. She grew two and a half inches within the course of nine months but failed to gain any significant amount of weight.

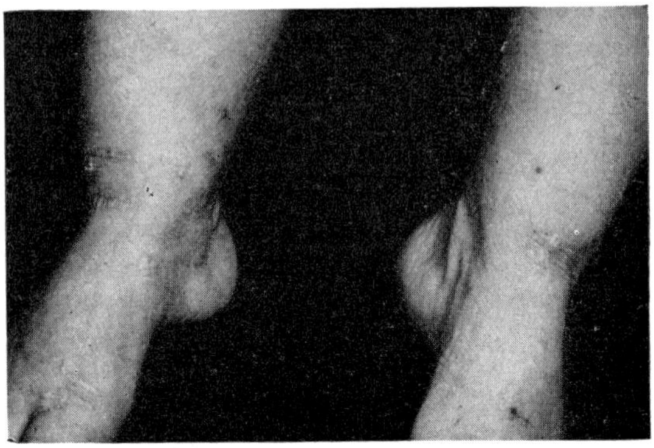

FIG. 3. Case 2. Skin xanthomata.

This clinical picture reminded us of Case 1, and of the histological description by Ahrens, to whom autopsy material had been sent. A tentative diagnosis of intrahepatic biliary atresia was made, and a drill biopsy of the liver was performed. This showed a histological pattern almost identical with that of Case 1, for a description of which the monograph by Ahrens and his colleagues should be consulted (Ahrens *et al.*, 1951)

* (Autopsy no. 5/42. General Hospital, Southend, Essex.)

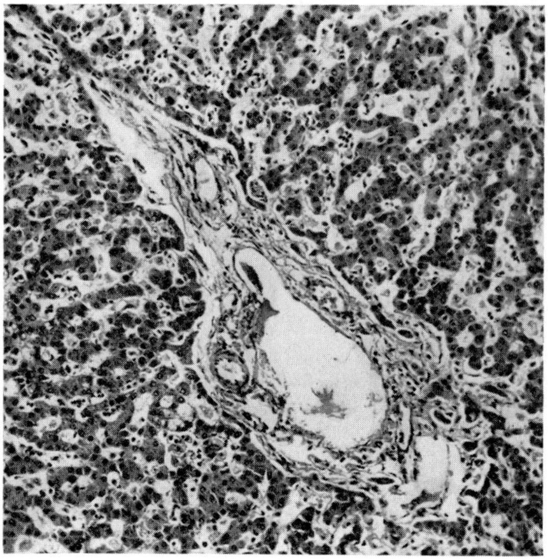

FIG. 4.—Case 1. Section of liver showing portal tract containing portal vein and hepatic artery but no bile duct. H. and E. × 110.

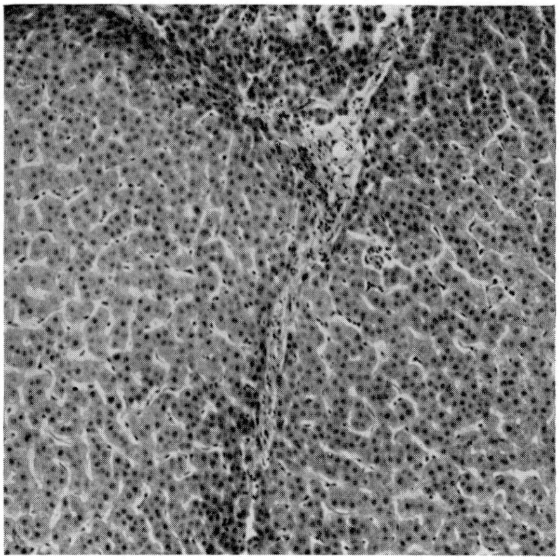

FIG. 5.—Case 2. Section of liver from biopsy specimen showing single thin fibrous band in otherwise normal parenchyma. H. and E. × 105.

(Figs. 4, 5 and 6). Briefly the most important and apparently essential abnormality in both cases was found in the portal tracts: portal veins and normal hepatic arteries were present but the accompanying bile ducts were absent. In contrast the intralobular canaliculi were present in both cases, and contained inspissated bile casts in Case 1 but not in Case 2. The portal tracts were infiltrated with small round cells in both cases, more marked in Case 1, in which a slight excess of extralobular fibrous tissue was also present. The liver cells looked normal. The Kupffer cells in Case 1 were large and contained lipoid material. The architecture of the lobules was still normal and there was no evidence of cirrhosis.

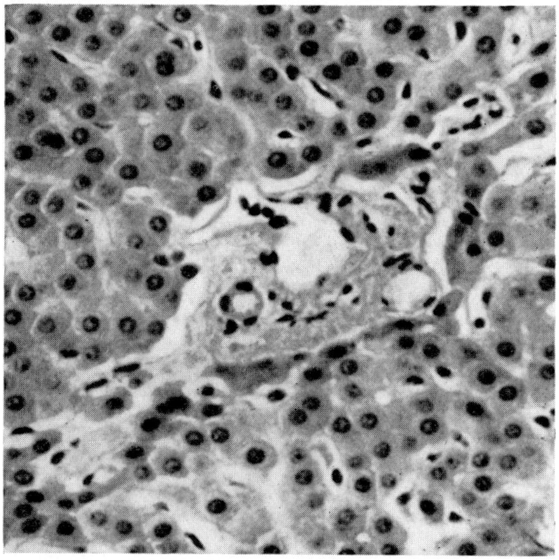

FIG. 6.—High power view of same section as Fig. 5 showing portal tract with absent bile duct. H. and E. × 325.

Discussion

Ahrens *et al.* (1951) were the first to describe this condition in detail. They reported two cases of their own as well as two others, one of which was Case 1 above. They also collected nine further cases from the literature which they thought comparable, though in seven of these the clinical and pathological details appear to us insufficient to be sure that they belong to the same group. The two remaining cases, however, Case 2 reported by Dahl-Iversen and Gormsen (1944), and the one reported by Sacrez, Fruhling and Rohmer (1946), are clearly the same condition on clinical as well as histological grounds. We have been able to find three more cases which have been fully described since then (MacMahon and Thannhauser, 1952; Moyson, Gillet and Richard, 1953; Sass-Kortsak, Bowden and Brown, 1956) and brief references to three others in which clinical details are not given (MacMahon and Thannhauser, 1952; Redo, 1954; Kiesewetter, Koop and Farquahr, 1955).

There are, therefore, now 10 well-documented cases of this condition, two male and eight female.

The important features of these 10 cases are summarized in Table 1. Four of the children, including Case 2 of this report, were alive and relatively well at the time of reporting. Two of them, the only two boys in the series, are known to have reached the ages of 10 and 12 respectively (MacMahon and Thannhauser, 1952; Harris, 1957). Apart from the infant who died at birth all these children have certain features in common: (1) They suffered from obstructive jaundice in the first week of life. As they lived on, their jaundice became less intense and bile pigment reappeared in the faeces. (2) The extrahepatic biliary system, either at laparotomy or at autopsy, was found to be patent in nine of the 10 patients. In one (Ahrens *et al.*, 1951: Case 3), although the gall-bladder was found to contain bile at autopsy, the cystic duct was patent for only 1 cm. and then became a thick fibrous cord which extended to the ampulla of Vater. The hepatic ducts in this case were not identified. (3) Elevation of the serum lipids was found in all seven cases in which this estimation was carried out. The serum cholesterol levels were often very high and well above 500 mg. per 100 ml. except in one case in which the readings varied between 212 and 300 mg. per 100 ml. between the ages of 7 weeks and 3 months at which age she died (Sass-Kortsak *et al.*, 1956). (4) Xanthomatous cutaneous deposits were present in all but four cases. The youngest recorded appearance of these was at the age of 1 year 3 months (Ahrens *et al.*, 1951: Case 3), and the oldest at approximately the age of 6 (McMahon and Thannhauser, 1952). In all these cases pruritus preceded the appearance of xanthomata by several months. (5) The microscopical changes of the liver in all cases showed essentially the same abnormalities as described above. These consisted of absence of the bile ducts in the portal tracts, slight infiltration of portal tracts with lymphocytes, plasma cells and polymorphs, normal looking liver cells and absence of any distortion of lobular architecture or significant increase of fibrous tissue in the portal tracts even in late stages of the disease.

The more frequent causes of neonatal obstructive jaundice differ both clinically and pathologically from this syndrome. In extrahepatic biliary atresia in which the site of obstruction may be anywhere between the portal tracts and the ampulla of Vater, the jaundice persists until the infant dies. During the neonatal period there is marked proliferation of perilobular bile ducts with gross dilatation in places of the larger bile ducts in the portal tracts and many of them are plugged by inspissated bile. Even in the early stages there is increase of fibrous tissue in the portal tracts which becomes very marked in those infants surviving more than a few months. The liver cells are often swollen and contain bile pigment. In the course of time true cirrhosis may ensue (Figs. 7 and 8).

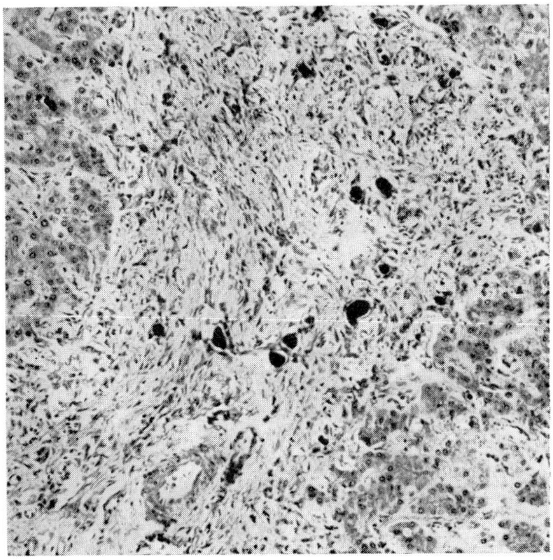

FIG. 7.—Section of post-mortem specimen of liver from patient with extrahepatic biliary atresia, showing wide fibrous tissue bands in portal region. Numerous portal bile ducts with inspissated bile casts. H. and E. × 105.

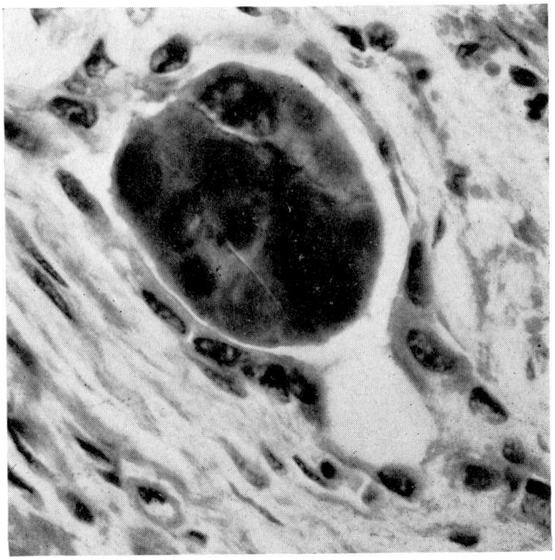

FIG. 8.—High power view of same case showing presence of portal bile duct surrounding inspissated bile cast. H. and E. × 830.

In neonatal hepatitis the jaundice may persist for a number of weeks but is followed in the majority

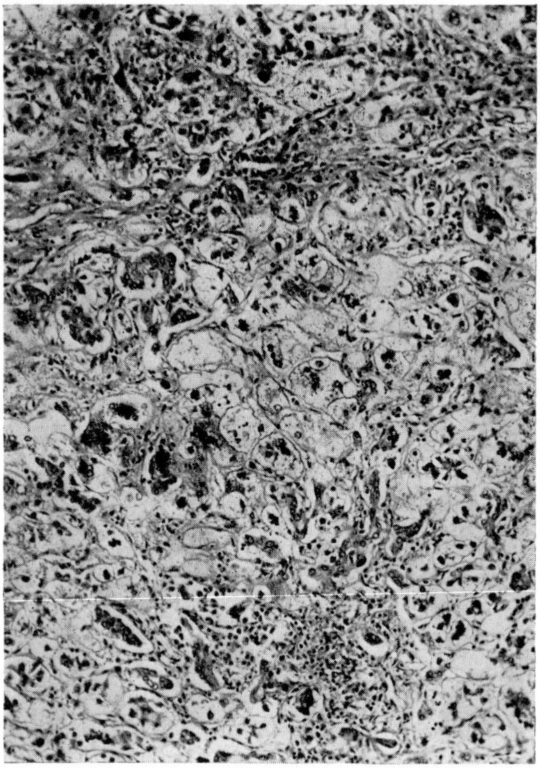

FIG. 9.—Section of post-mortem specimen of liver from child with neonatal hepatitis, showing large multinucleate parenchymal cells.

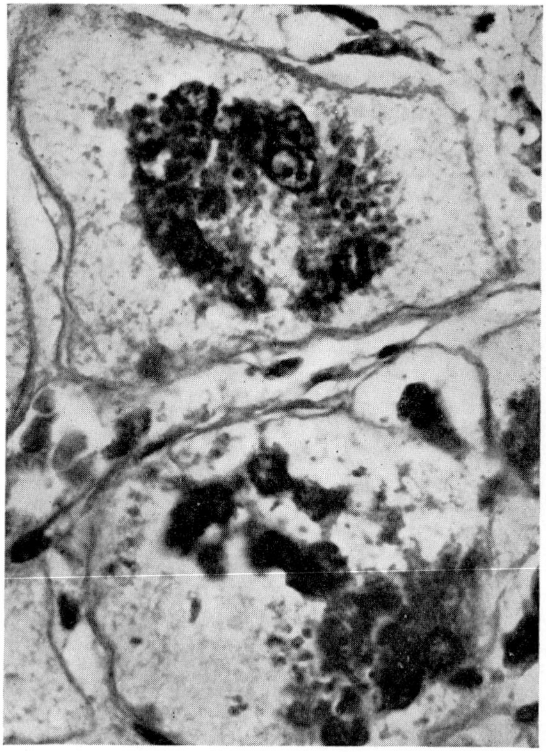

FIG. 10.—High power of same section.

of cases by a complete recovery. There is, however, a mortality rate of 20% and a further 10% of patients develop cirrhosis of the liver (Gellis, Craig and Hsia, 1954). The microscopical picture during the neonatal stage shows marked variation in the size of the liver cells, with distorted multinucleated giant cells scattered throughout the liver substance (Craig and Landing, 1952; Bodian and Newns, 1953). In

Author	Dahl-Iversen and Gormsen (1944)	Sacrez *et al.* (1946)	Case 1	Cas
Age of reported onset of jaundice	Birth	8 d.	1 w.	2 d.
Age of appearance of xanthomata	—	—	1 yr. 9 mth.	3½ yr.
Age of first reported hyperlipaemia	—	—	1 yr.	3 yr. 9
Highest and lowest recorded serum cholesterol levels in mg./100 ml.	—	—	1,816 149	1,0 6
Age of onset of pruritus	—	—	1½ yr.	3 yr.
Age of reporting	Birth	2 yr. 7 mth.	3½ yr.	6½ yr.
Age of liver histology	Birth	2 yr. 7 mth.	1 yr. 1 mth.	3 yr. 9
Age of death	Birth	2 yr. 7 mth.	3 yr. 6 mth.	–
Cause of death	'Lethargy'	Meningitis	Liver failure	–
Extrahepatic biliary system	Normal	Normal	Normal	Norma

the chronic stage of the disease the lobular architecture is distorted by fibrous tissue and a true cirrhosis may follow (Figs. 9 and 10) (Bodian and Newns, 1953; Dible, Hunt, Pugh, Steingold and Wood, 1954).

In the bile-inspissation syndrome of Lightwood and Bodian (1946) prolonged haemolytic jaundice due to Rhesus incompatibility became complicated by biliary obstruction; this they showed histologically to be associated with inspissation of bile in the canaliculi.

A variety of other conditions occasionally cause liver damage associated with jaundice, pale stools and dark urine in the newborn. Inclusion-body disease was reviewed by France (1951); umbilical sepsis with generalized septicaemia, toxoplasmosis, congenital syphilis and herpes simplex, by Sherlock (1955). The clinical course of all these diseases is short and acute and totally unlike the condition under discussion.

It seems that in no other neonatal condition, particularly not in the later stages of either extrahepatic bile duct atresia or neonatal hepatitis, do hypercholesterolaemia or xanthomatosis occur. The association of liver disease with chronic jaundice and deposits in the skin has been known for more than a century (Addison and Gull, 1851). More recently Ahrens and others (Ahrens and Kunkel, 1949; MacMahon and Thannhauser, 1949; Ahrens, Payne, Kunkel, Eisenmenger and Blondheim, 1950), in their comprehensive monographs have fully discussed this relationship; briefly, elevation of the serum lipids is found in chronic biliary obstruction from any cause of sufficient duration provided liver cell function remains normal. When the serum cholesterol remains above a level of about 1,800 mg. per 100 ml. for longer than a few months, xanthomatous deposits begin to appear in the skin.

Aetiology and Treatment

Ahrens *et al.* (1951) consider the absence of the intrahepatic bile ducts to be a developmental anomaly and, indeed, the typical histological picture was seen in one newborn infant as well as in another 3 months of age. At present treatment is entirely symptomatic. Pruritus may be relieved by the administration of methyl testosterone (Lloyd-Thomas and Sherlock, 1952) and, in Case 2, stenediol, 10 mg. on alternate days, was tried with good effect. An attempt was made to lower the circulating lipids by giving a diet devoid of all animal and saturated vegetable fats (Bronte-Stewart, Antonis, Eales and Brock, 1956) for two periods of two months each and one of one month, with intervening periods of a month. The result was disappointing, there being neither appreciable reduction of the serum lipid levels nor any regression of the xanthomata.

Summary

Two cases of congenital absence of intrahepatic bile ducts are described.

Together with eight other similar cases from the literature, their clinical and pathological features are discussed and are contrasted with those of other causes of neonatal obstructive jaundice.

Though some of these other conditions appear very similar during the neonatal period, the clinical course of intrahepatic atresia is sufficiently characteristic during the next nine to 12 months for a diagnosis

(1951) Case 3	MacMahon and Thannhauser (1952)	Moyson *et al.* (1953)	Sass-Kortsak *et al.* (1956)	Present paper Case 1†	Case 2
	8 d.	3 mth.	3 d.	2 d.	4 d.
nth.	6 yr.	—	—	1 yr. 8 mth.	3 yr. 2 mth.
—	12 yr.	9 mth.	7 w.	2 yr. 6 mth.	3 yr. 1 mth.
—	1,686	300 212	922 362	1,200 1,081	1,600 500
mth.	Uncertain	—	—	5 mth.	3 yr. 1 mth.
	10 yr.	$11\frac{1}{4}$ mth.	7 w.	$2\frac{1}{2}$ yr.	3 yr. 1 mth.
mth.	10 yr.	$11\frac{1}{2}$ mth.	$3\frac{1}{2}$ mth.	2 yr. 9 mth.	3 yr. 3 mth.
nth.	—	—	3 yr. 6 mth.	2 yr. 9 mth.	—
itis, liver failure	—	—	Staphylococcal pneumonia	Pyelonephritis	—
cystic and common ducts	Normal	Normal	Normal	Normal	? Normal

rens *et al.* (1951).

to be made, whilst probably at any time a liver biopsy will be pathognomonic.

We would like to express our thanks to Dr. Kenneth Tallerman for permission to allow us to report our second case, to Dr. Preedy for performing the liver biopsy and also to Dr. Weinbren for his histological reports.

REFERENCES

Addison, T. and Gull, W. (1851). *Guy's Hosp. Rep.*, **7**, 265.
Ahrens, E. H. Jr., Harris, R. C. and MacMahon, H. E. (1951). *Pediatrics*, **8**, 628.
—— and Kunkel, H. G. (1949). *J. clin. Invest.*, **28**, 1565.
——, Payne, M. A., Kunkel, H. G., Eisenmenger, W. J. and Blondheim, S. H. (1950). *Medicine (Baltimore)*, **29**, 299.
Bodian, M. and Newns, G. H. (1953). *Arch. franç. Pédiat.*, **10**, 169.
Bronte-Stewart, B., Antonis, A., Eales, L. and Brock, J. F. (1956). *Lancet*, **1**, 521.
Craig, J. M. and Landing, B. H. (1952). *Arch. Path. (Chicago)*, **54**, 321.
Dahl-Iversen, E. and Gormsen, H. (1944). *Acta chir. scand.*, **89**, 333.
Dible, J. H., Hunt, W. E., Pugh, V. W., Steingold, L. and Wood, J. H. F. (1954). *J. Path. Bact.*, **67**, 195.
France, N. E. (1951). *Arch. Dis. Childh.*, **26**, 588.
Gellis, S. S., Craig, J. M. and Hsia, D. Y. Y. (1954). *Amer. J. Dis Child.*, **88**, 285.
Harris, R. C. (1957). Personal Communication.
Kiesewetter, W. B., Koop, C. E. and Farquahr, J. D. (1955). *Pediatrics* **15**, 149.
Lightwood, R. and Bodian, M. (1946). *Arch. Dis. Childh.*, **21**, 209.
Lloyd-Thomas, H. G. L. and Sherlock, S. (1952). *Brit. med. J.*, **2**, 1289.
MacMahon, H. E. and Thannhauser, S. J. (1949). *Ann. intern. Med.*, **30**, 121.
——, —— (1952). *Gastroenterology*, **21**, 488.
Moyson, F., Gillet, P. and Richard, J. (1953). *Helv. paediat. Acta*, **8**, 281.
Redo, S. F., (1954). *Arch. Surg. (Chicago)*, **69**, 886.
Sacrez, R., Fruhling, L. and Rohmer, J. A. (1946). *Arch. franç. Pédiat.*, **3**, 78.
Sass-Kortsak, A., Bowden, D. H. and Brown, R. J. K. (1956). *Pediatrics*, **17**, 383.
Sherlock, S. (1955). *Diseases of the Liver and Biliary System.* Oxford.
Smythe, P. M. and Dobbs, R. H. (1949). *Proc. roy. Soc. Med.*, **42**, 86.

REPLACEMENT TRANSFUSION AS A MEANS OF PREVENTING KERNIKTERUS OF PREMATURITY

BY

V. MARY CROSSE, PATRICIA G. WALLIS and ANNA M. WALSH
From Sorrento Maternity Hospital, Birmingham

(RECEIVED FOR PUBLICATION FEBRUARY 25, 1958)

The possibility of premature babies developing kernikterus from jaundice not due to haemolytic disease is now generally recognized (Aidin, Corner and Tovey, 1950; Zuelzer and Mudgett, 1950; Hsia, Allen, Diamond and Gellis, 1953; Billing, Cole and Lathe, 1954; Crosse, Meyer and Gerrard, 1955; Meyer, 1956).

In haemolytic disease kernikterus has been practically eliminated by the use of repeat replacement transfusion to wash out the excess of bilirubin, and this form of treatment therefore seems to be indicated for the prevention of kernikterus due to prematurity.

Since the beginning of July, 1955, bilirubin levels have been estimated each morning (and when necessary in the evening also) in all premature babies showing definite clinical jaundice during the first eight days of life; and replacement transfusion has been performed in each case in which the level reached 18-20 mg.% during this period or was rising so rapidly that it would probably have reached this level before the next morning. Haemolytic disease has been proved or disproved in each case by full examination of the blood of both mother and baby. The transfused babies have been followed up carefully to assess any damage (however small) which might have resulted from the jaundice or from the transfusion.

Material

The 1,320 babies studied were the total number of admissions to the three premature baby units under our care during the two-year period from July 1, 1955, to June 30, 1957.

The degree of jaundice was roughly estimated by blanching the skin, either by stretching or by pressure. If examined by daylight it soon became possible to decide whether the level of bilirubin had reached approximately 10 mg.% or not. If it appeared to have reached this level, blood was taken for bilirubin estimation and to exclude haemolytic disease. In two of the units blood was taken by femoral puncture, and in one by multiple heel prick.

Results

Number of Babies who Required Transfusion. Table 1 shows all premature babies admitted to the three premature baby units during the two years under investigation, and the number who required replacement transfusion for hyperbilirubinaemia not due to haemolytic disease. The 1,320 babies are divided into three birthweight groups: group A includes all babies up to 1,500 g. at birth, group B babies from 1,500-2,000 g., and group C babies from 2,000-2,500 g.

With the exception of group A, the percentage of babies requiring transfusion diminished as the birthweight increased. Because many babies weighing less than 1,500 g. die before they can develop hyperbilirubinaemia, the transfused babies are also given as a percentage of the babies at risk (babies alive at 48 hours) but even when this is done group A still shows the smallest percentage of babies transfused. The reason for this is difficult to understand unless it was due to the small numbers involved. It is of interest that this discrepancy was not present among the babies treated in Sorrento premature baby unit which deals with the highest proportion of small babies. In Sorrento during the past two and a half years, eight out of 207 babies weighing less than 1,500 g. at birth (group A) were transfused (3·9%). If only the 99 babies at risk (alive at 48 hours) are considered, 8·1% were transfused. For comparison, 8·5% of the babies at risk were transfused in group B, and 7·5% in group C. If by chance, one more baby in group A had been transfused, this would have raised the percentage in this group to 9·1%.

Of the total 1,320 premature babies admitted, 92 (8·4%) required replacement transfusion for hyperbilirubinaemia not due to haemolytic disease. It is of interest to find that the five cases of kernikterus which occurred during this series were all in group B.

Number of Babies who Required more than One Transfusion. If, after the first transfusion, the level of bilirubin rose again to dangerous levels, the same

TABLE 1
BABIES REQUIRING REPLACEMENT TRANSFUSIONS

Birth Weight	Total Admissions	Babies at Risk (alive at 48 hr.)	Babies Transfused		
			No.	% of total	% of babies at risk
Group A (Up to 1,500 g.) ..	262	137	8	3·1	5·8
Group B (1,500–2,000 g.) ..	564	499	49	8·7	9·8
Group C (2,000–2,500 g.) ..	494	464	35	7·1	7·5
Total	1,320	1,100	92	7·0	8·4

criteria as before were used as indications for a repeat transfusion.

Table 2 shows the number of transfusions required by each affected baby in each of the three birthweight groups. The proportions of transfused babies requiring more than one transfusion show the same variations as in Table 1 but of course the numbers concerned are extremely small.

Of all transfused babies, 19·6% required more than one transfusion to keep the bilirubin below a dangerous level.

All five babies who later showed signs suggestive of kernikterus required more than one replacement (one baby required four, one required three and the remaining three babies two each).

Mortality Due to Transfusion. There were two deaths among the transfused babies but only one was due to transfusion. This baby weighed 3 lb. 4 oz. at birth. The transfusion was technically easy and 250 ml. were exchanged but unfortunately no deficit was left. The baby collapsed and died five minutes after the completion of the transfusion. An autopsy showed that death was due to heart failure. Since this occurrence a deficit of 20-40 ml. has always been left.

The second death occurred in a baby which weighed 4 lb. 11 oz. at birth. This baby's mother had severe pre-eclampsia. The condition of the baby was extremely poor at birth and continued so. Jaundice developed rapidly and on the third day a replacement transfusion became necessary. The baby improved slightly after the transfusion but 12 hours later collapsed suddenly and died. An autopsy showed that death was due to gross atelectasis and the transfusion was not believed to have contributed to the death.

Babies in whom a Satisfactory Replacement was not Obtained. A replacement was called unsatisfactory if less than 80 ml./lb. (176 ml./Kg.) were exchanged.

Among the 92 first transfusions there was a failure to obtain a satisfactory replacement in three cases: this was due to spasm of the umbilical vein in two cases and failure to cannulate the umbilical vein in one.

There were also three failures among the 18 repeat transfusions. In each case the umbilical vein had been ligated after the first transfusion, and re-cannulation of the umbilical vein was impossible. In two of the three cases, the saphenous route was not attempted; in the third it was attempted but failed.

One baby comes into both these groups because the first transfusion was incomplete and the repeat transfusion failed. Five babies are therefore concerned, and two of these five babies developed kernikterus.

All six unsatisfactory replacements occurred during the early part of the period under review, and with our present technique failure should be rare. When spasm of the umbilical vein occurs, the replacement is now abandoned for one or two hours, after which time the spasm has usually relaxed. If it has not done so after this time the saphenous route is used. Repeat transfusions are now made easier by

TABLE 2
NUMBER OF TRANSFUSIONS REQUIRED

Birth weight	Babies Transfused	Transfused Babies				%Requiring more than one Transfusion
		No. of transfusions				
		One	Two	Three	Four	
Group A (Up to 1,500 g.) ..	8	7	1	—	—	12·5
Group B (1,500–2,000 g.) ..	49	38	9	1	1	22·4
Group C (2,000–2,500 g.) ..	35	29	4	2	—	17·1
Total	92	74 (80·4%)	14 (15·2%)	3 (3·3%)	1 (1·1%)	19·6

leaving the catheter *in situ* for several days in case a further transfusion should become necessary.

Age at First Transfusion. Fig. 1 shows the age at first transfusion for each of the three birthweight groups separately, and also for all cases together.

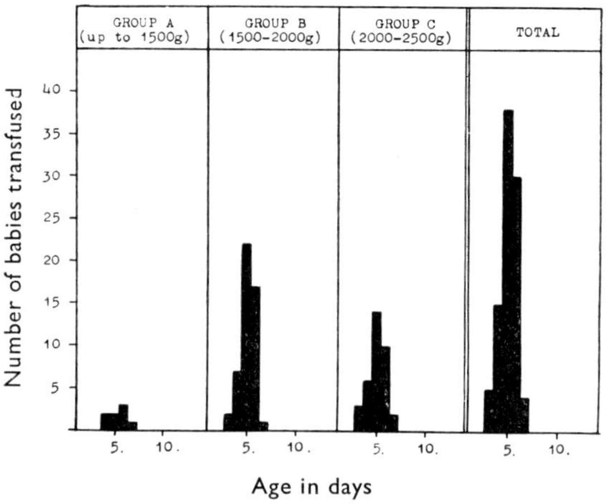

FIG. 1.—Age at first transfusion (92 babies).

In group A the first transfusion was performed between the ages of 3 days and 7 days, with the maximum incidence during the sixth day of life. In group B and C the first transfusion was performed between the ages of 2 days and 7 days and the maximum incidence was during the fifth day of life.

Of all 92 transfusions, five (5·4%) were undertaken on the third day of life, 15 (16·3%) on the fourth day, 38 (41·3%) on the fifth day, 30 (32·6%) on the sixth day, and four (4·4%) on the seventh day.

Of the five babies who developed kernikterus, the first transfusion was done on the third day in one case, on the fourth day in two cases, and on the fifth day in two cases.

Levels of bilirubin at which the decision was made to replace. (115 transfusions.) Fig. 2 shows these levels for each of the three birthweight groups separately, and for all cases together.

For 53 transfusions (46·1%) the decision was taken when the level of bilirubin was between 17 and 20 mg.%. In three of the four cases (3·5%) in which the decisions were made at lower levels, the jaundice was increasing so rapidly that it was not considered safe to leave the babies until the following morning; and in one case the reported level was believed to be incorrect because of the clinical severity of the jaundice.

For 58 transfusions (50·4%) the decision was made at levels over 20 mg.%. In the light of present knowledge this was too late because in all five babies who developed kernikterus, the decision to transfuse was made at levels over 20 mg.%. The decision to transfuse was made at levels over 20 mg.% for three out of nine transfusions (33·3%) in group A, for 32 out of 63 transfusions (50·1%) in group B, and for 23 out of 43 transfusions (53·5%) in group C.

When the decision to transfuse was taken at levels higher than 20 mg.%, this was usually due to lack of experience in judging the depth of jaundice. In some

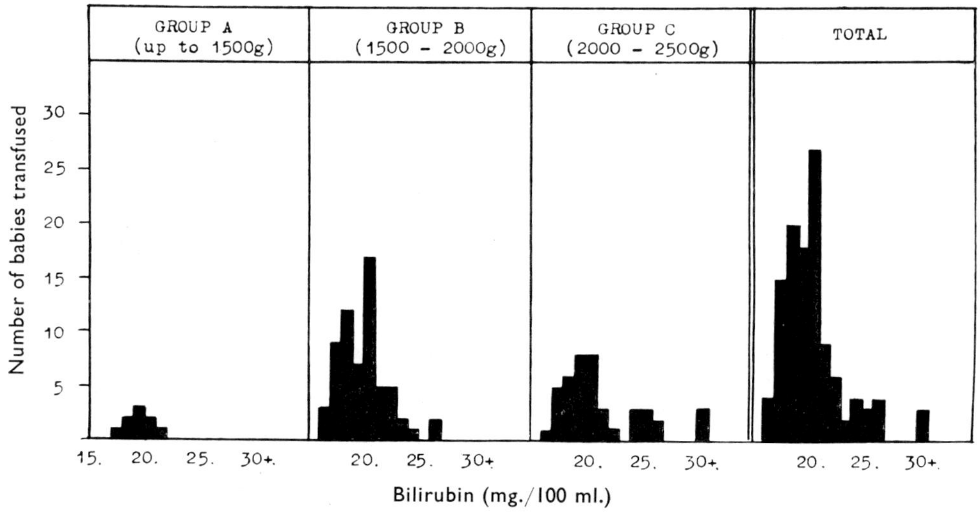

FIG. 2.—Level of serum bilirubin at which decision was taken to transfuse (115 transfusions).

cases the bilirubin level was first estimated when the critical level had already been reached; and in others the rate of increase in the depth of jaundice was not appreciated. It has been found that, with experience, the serum bilirubin level can be assessed clinically up to about 10-12 mg.%, but above that level it is impossible to judge the levels at all accurately clinically, and bilirubin estimations are now made much more frequently.

In the early months of the investigation different serum bilirubin results were frequently obtained by the various laboratories on the same blood. It was felt that the indications must be definite before embarking on what seemed a major operation, but as confidence in the safety of replacement transfusion was gained, and as the laboratory technique became more standardized, there was less hesitation in deciding to replace at lower and safer levels.

Highest Serum Bilirubin Levels Reached by Babies. Fig. 3 shows the highest bilirubin levels reached by babies in each of the three birthweight groups separately, and by all babies together.

In 29 (31·5%) of the 92 transfused babies the bilirubin level was kept below 20 mg.%; in 39 (42·4%) it rose to 20-22 mg.%, in 21 (22·8%) it rose to 22-27 mg.% and in three (3·3%) it rose above 30 mg.%. A rise to levels between 20 mg.% and 27 mg.% could be explained in each case by lack of experience either in judging the degree of the jaundice or in appreciating the rate of increase.

As regards the three babies in whom the bilirubin level rose to 30 mg.% or more, the following remarks may be of interest:

Baby R. (5 lb. 6 oz.) The bilirubin level reached 20 mg.% by the fourth day, but due to some misunderstanding the baby was not transfused. The level on the fifth day had risen to 30 mg.% and replacement transfusion was undertaken immediately. Luckily this child showed no signs of kernikterus and has developed normally.

Baby B. (4 lb. 1 oz.) This baby developed kernikterus and particulars are given in the section on the follow-up of all transfused babies.

Baby S. (5 lb.) This baby was slightly jaundiced on the first day and by the second day the bilirubin level had reached 14·6 mg.%. The level was not estimated that evening because the jaundice was not believed to have deepened. However the next morning the level was reported as 30 mg.% and an immediate replacement was performed. The child showed no signs of kernikterus and has developed normally.

These three babies were born during the first six months of the period under review. Bilirubin levels are now taken more frequently and such high levels are avoided.

The five babies who developed kernikterus were all in group B, and in each case the bilirubin level rose to 22 mg.% or more (two rose to 22 mg.%, two to 23 mg.% and one to more than 30 mg.%).

It is of interest that none of the 68 babies with levels below 22 mg.% developed kernikterus, while four of the 21 (19·2%) with levels of 22-27 mg.%, and one of the three (33·3%) with levels over 30 mg.% developed this complication.

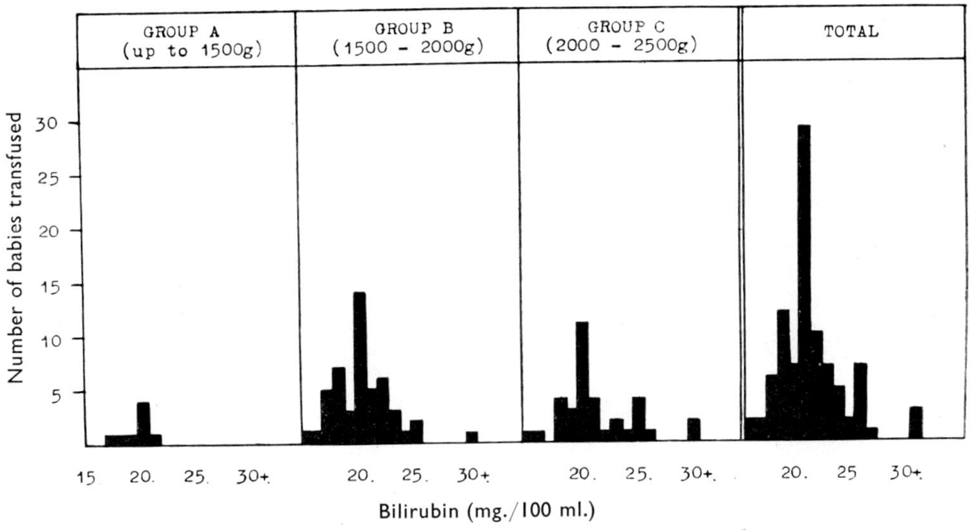

Fig. 3.—Highest serum bilirubin levels reached (92 babies).

No baby over 2,000 g. developed kernikterus. When babies under 2,000 g. are considered by themselves, four out of the 12 (33·3%) with bilirubin levels of 22-27 mg.% and the only one with a bilirubin level over 30 mg.% developed kernikterus. This was in spite of the fact that these high bilirubin levels were present for a relatively short time, except in the case of baby B.

Reduction in Bilirubin Level Achieved by Transfusion. It is impossible to give complete figures for this because technical difficulties often prevented the collection of all the required samples of blood. However, in cases in which the necessary samples were obtained, the reduction in the bilirubin level during transfusion usually varied from 45%-65%.

Follow-up of Transfused Babies. A great effort has been made to follow-up the 92 transfused babies. This has been difficult owing to the wide geographical area from which the units draw their cases. It was intended that each baby should be seen at three-monthly intervals until the age of at least 1 year. Actually 83 of the 90 surviving transfused babies have been followed to the age of 1 year, and one to the age of 9 months. The remaining six have moved to unknown addresses and all efforts to trace them have failed. There is, however, no reason to believe that any of these six babies are abnormal; when last seen by the doctor or health visitor they were considered normal.

The following five babies have developed signs which are probably due to kernikterus:

Baby G. (3 lb. 7 oz.) On the fourth day the bilirubin level rose from 16 mg.% in the morning to 20 mg.% in the evening; then unfortunately there was a delay of five hours before the baby was transfused. By this time the jaundice had increased (bilirubin 22 mg.%) and early signs of kernikterus had developed, i.e. head retraction, eye rolling and periods of apnoea during which cyanosis developed. This child is now spastic and possibly retarded, but is not deaf.

Baby K. (4 lb.) A transfusion was given on the fifth day when the bilirubin level was 21 mg.%, but a complete exchange was not achieved due to spasm of the umbilical vein after 100 ml. had been exchanged. The catheter was removed and the vein ligated. The following day the bilirubin level rose to 23 mg.%, but the umbilical vein could not be cannulated and the femoral route was not attempted. The bilirubin level began to fall the next day. No head retraction or other signs of kernikterus were seen and there were also no signs of birth injury or asphyxia during early life. The child is now mildly spastic, very emotional and probably slightly retarded, but is not deaf. In spite of the apparent absence of signs of kernikterus in the early days, this baby must be included because of the history of hyperbilirubinaemia.

Baby B. (4 lb. 1 oz.) This child was transfused on the third day (bilirubin 20 mg.%) and again on the sixth day (bilirubin 22 mg.%), but this time the umbilical vein went into spasm after 60 ml. had been exchanged. No further attempt was made because it was felt (wrongly) that the level of bilirubin would probably fall after this age. In fact the baby became more deeply jaundiced and signs of kernikterus developed on the ninth day when the bilirubin level was found to have reached 38 mg.%. This child is now definitely spastic and retarded, is having convulsions and probably has a hearing defect.

Baby C. (3 lb. 8 oz.) This child was transfused on the third day (bilirubin 18 mg.%). By the fourth day the bilirubin level had risen again to 20 mg.% but the baby was not transfused until six hours later when the bilirubin level had reached 22 mg.%. A third transfusion was carried out on the fifth day (bilirubin 20 mg.%). On the sixth day the bilirubin level had risen again to 18·4 mg.% but transfusion was not performed. By the seventh morning the baby had developed head retraction and the bilirubin level was again 22 mg.%. In spite of the head retraction a fourth transfusion was undertaken (with the hope of limiting the degree of brain damage) and after this the level of bilirubin fell steadily. This child now shows no spasticity but has been late in reaching all his mile-stones. There is a tendency to athetosis and there also appears to be some hearing defect.

Baby H. (3 lb. 15 oz.) This child was in a poor condition from birth. He had marked atelectasis and an enlarged liver, he also showed signs of cerebral irritation; he was not expected to survive. The first transfusion was undertaken on the fourth day (bilirubin 21 mg.%), a second on the fifth day (bilirubin 23 mg.%) and a third on the seventh day (bilirubin 20 mg.%). After this the level of bilirubin gradually fell. There were no definite signs of kernikterus at any time, but the general condition was very poor throughout the first week of life. This child is now spastic and probably retarded, but is not deaf. It is possible that this child's disability was the result of birth asphyxia, but he is included as a probable case of kernikterus because the bilirubin was allowed to rise to 23 mg.% on the fifth day.

From a study of these cases, it appears that all five were preventable, and much has been learnt from these failures.

A better realization of the rapidity of the rise in the level of the bilirubin by more frequent estimations during the critical period, thus enabling transfusions to be undertaken at lower levels, would have been helpful in all five cases.

The realization that the bilirubin could still rise to dangerous levels after the sixth day of life would have helped Baby B.

A reduction in the time between taking the actual blood sample and starting the transfusion might have saved babies S and C.

Better technique to avoid incomplete exchanges might have helped babies K and B, i.e. a period of rest to allow venous spasm to relax, leaving the catheter *in situ* in case further transfusions become necessary, and the use of the saphenous route if the umbilical route fails.

Discussion

In order to assess the value of replacement transfusion in hyperbilirubinaemia not due to haemolytic disease, it is necessary to know what proportion of the premature babies admitted to our units would have developed kernikterus without such preventive treatment.

During the two years 1953 and 1954, the excessive use of vitamin K increased the number of cases of kernikterus occurring in our units (Crosse *et al.*, 1955), but before this unhappy episode, i.e. during the eight-year period 1945-1952, 1·08% of all admissions developed kernikterus, and approximately 70% of these babies died.

If this incidence (1·08%) is applied to the 1,320 admissions during the two years under review the expected number of cases of kernikterus would be 14. Of these, nine or 10 would have died, and four or five would have survived but suffered cerebral palsy. Instead, one baby has died (from transfusion) and five babies have developed cerebral palsy, two of whom are only slightly affected. If certain failures in diagnosis and technique had not occurred, these five cases might have been prevented. (Unfortunately the bilirubin level was allowed to rise above 22 mg.% in each case.)

Until some better method of preventing this important and dangerous complication of prematurity becomes available (e.g. conversion of the lethal indirect-acting into the harmless direct-acting bilirubin; or reduction of the rate of breakdown of the red blood cells so that the immature liver can cope with the reduced amount of bilirubin) replacement transfusion appears to be the only way of coping with the situation.

To avoid failures such as those described it is obviously necessary to keep the bilirubin level below 20-22 mg.% at all times, and this entails an exacting regime. In all hospitals where premature babies are treated, it is necessary to have a sufficient number of experienced nurses and doctors who can decide when the bilirubin level is approaching 10-12 mg.% and promptly take blood samples for laboratory estimation. Accurate estimations must be made on these samples, and the bilirubin level promptly reported. If the level is over 18 mg.% replacement should be performed with as little delay as possible. If the bilirubin level is rising rapidly a decision to replace may be made at a lower level, especially if the decision has to be made in the evening, with a long night ahead and the difficulty of assessing the degree of jaundice in artificial light and the reduction of laboratory facilities. In order to have some idea of the rate of rise in the level of bilirubin, the first estimation should not be left too late.

Full cooperation with the blood transfusion service is necessary to avoid undue delay between deciding to transfuse and performing the transfusion.

Medical staff with experience in replacement transfusion must be available at all hours of the day and night, and two assistants (nurses or medical students) should also be available.

Summary

The development of jaundice has been carefully observed in 1,320 premature babies admitted to three premature baby units during a period of two years, and exchange transfusions have been undertaken in 92 babies (8·4%) who developed hyperbilirubinaemia not due to haemolytic disease.

Of the transfused babies, 19·6% required more than one transfusion.

There were two deaths among the 92 babies transfused (115 transfusions), but one of these deaths could not be attributed either to the transfusion or to kernikterus.

The highest bilirubin level reached was less than 20 mg.% in 31·5%, 20-22 mg.% in 42·4%, 22-27 mg.% in 22·8%, and over 30 mg.% in 3·3%. No baby with a bilirubin level below 22 mg.% developed kernikterus, but 19·1% of those with levels of 22-27 mg.%, and 33·3% of those with levels over 30 mg.% developed this complication.

Of the 92 transfused babies five later showed signs which were probably due to kernikterus.

Until some better way has been found to prevent or treat hyperbilirubinaemia not due to haemolytic disease, it seems that replacement transfusion is the best way of preventing kernikterus.

We are very grateful to Dr. T. C. Meyer, Dr. Joan Angus, Dr. Frances Thompson and Dr. Daphne Hall, who performed many of the transfusions; to Dr. A. H. Henley for technical advice; to the laboratory staffs of Little Bromwich General Hospital, Sorrento Maternity Hospital and Marston Green Maternity Hospital; to Dr. W. Weiner and the staff of the Blood Transfusion Service; to Dr. H. S. Baar and Dr. F. E. D. Griffiths for the two autopsies; and to the Sisters and nursing staff of the three premature baby units without whose help this work could not have been undertaken.

References

Aidin, R., Corner, B. and Tovey, G. (1950). *Lancet*, **1**, 1153.
Billing, B. H., Cole, P. G. and Lathe, G. H. (1954). *Brit. med. J.*, **2**, 1263.
Crosse, V. M., Meyer, T. C. and Gerrard, J. W. (1955). *Arch. Dis. Childh.*, **30**, 501.
Hsia, Y. H., Allen, F. H., Diamond, L. K. and Gellis, S. S. (1953), *J. Pediat.*, **42**, 277.
Meyer, T. C. (1956). *Arch. Dis. Childh.*, **31**, 75.
Zuelzer, W. W. and Mudgett, R. T. (1950). *Pediatrics*, **6**, 452.

SERUM TRANSAMINASE VARIATIONS IN CHILDHOOD

BY

PAOLO TOLENTINO and MARCELLA ROSSI

From the Departments of Infectious Diseases and Paediatrics, University of Genoa

(RECEIVED FOR PUBLICATION MARCH 10, 1958)

The study of serum transaminases has recently entered clinical practice. In December, 1954, Wróblewsky and La Due demonstrated an increase of glutamic-oxalacetic (GOT) transaminase in the serum of patients suffering from various liver diseases and in carbon tetrachloride intoxication. In 1955, de Ritis, Coltorti and Giusti demonstrated an increase of both aspartic-ketoglutaric (GOT) and alanine-ketoglutaric (GPT) transaminases in the serum of patients with infectious hepatitis. This increase was accompanied by a remarkable inversion of the ratio between aspartic-ketoglutaric (GOT) and alanine-ketoglutaric activity (GPT), ($\frac{GOT}{GPT}$,) which stands above unity in healthy people and notably below in infectious hepatitis. While the increase of serum transaminase is generally ascribed to extensive necrosis of the hepatic cells and the consequent passage into the blood of cellular enzymes, the inversion of the ratio has not yet been satisfactorily explained.

A series of clinical and experimental observations made during the last two years has enabled us to reach some interesting conclusions. Our clinical researches concerned about 100 cases of acute infectious diseases, including infectious hepatitis, rheumatic fever, measles, scarlet fever, whooping cough, chickenpox, infectious mononucleosis, mumps and poliomyelitis. In some of the above-mentioned diseases multiplication of the causal agent in the liver during the incubation stage takes place, and liver damage is frequently observed at needle-biopsy.

In estimating the serum transaminases we used the method of Tonhazy, White and Umbreit (1950) reading with Pulfrich's photometer, filter S 53. The results are set out in Figs. 1, 2 and 3, the values being expressed in micromoles of pyruvic acid.

These figures show that only in infectious hepatitis, from virus A or B, is there a definite increase of both transaminases accompanied by the characteristic inversion of the ratio. This specific finding is probably related to the extensive liver

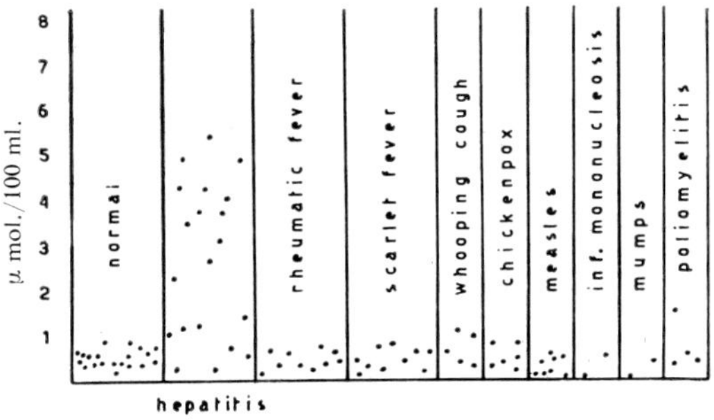

FIG. 1.—Serum aspartic-ketoglutaric (GOT) transaminase.

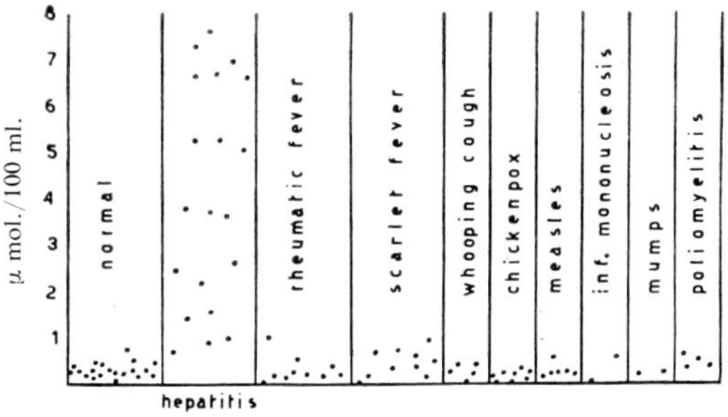

FIG. 2.—Serum alanine-ketoglutaric (GPT) transaminase.

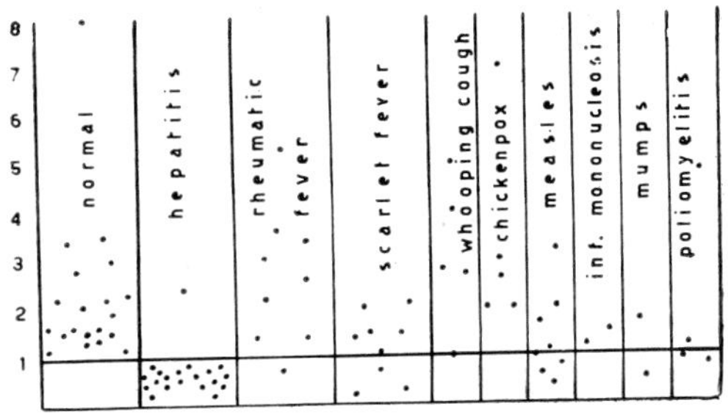

FIG. 3. $\frac{GOT}{GPT}$ ratio in some infectious diseases.

4

necrosis that is present only in this disease. However, we found the ratio inverted without a considerable increase of transaminase in a certain percentage of cases in other infectious diseases; we never found inversion in healthy subjects (Tolentino and Rossi, 1957a).

In numerous cases of hepatitis we estimated the serum transaminases throughout the course of the disease and observed that the values decreased with clinical improvement and rose again during relapses. The last pathological finding to disappear was the inversion of the GOT/GPT ratio.

In some cases we were also fortunate enough to be able to show that the increase in serum transaminases occurred very early, appearing about a month before the clinical manifestations. We observed this in children from a school, who were in contact with hepatitis patients. Fig. 4 charts the course of one such case and demonstrates that the

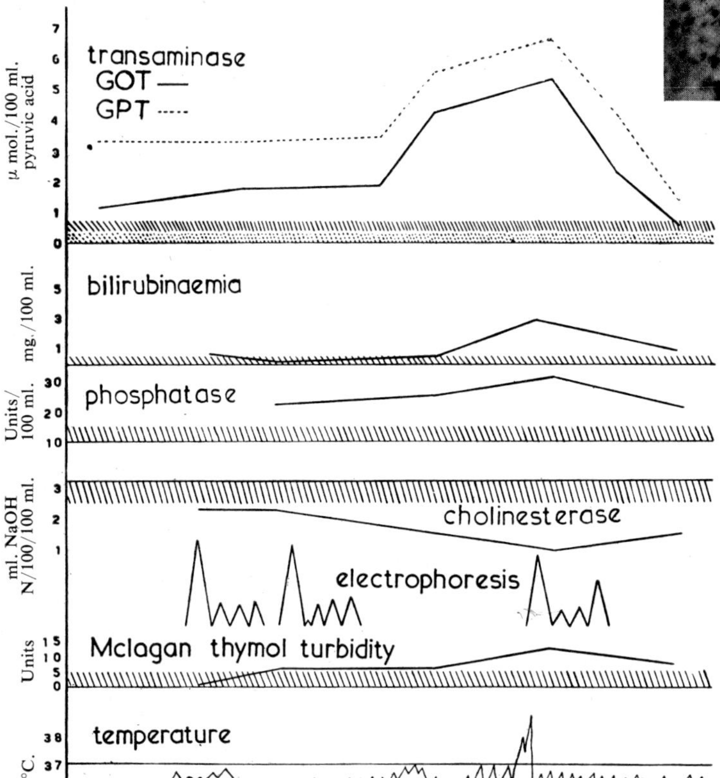

FIG. 4.—Clinical course and laboratory data during the incubation period and acute phase of a case of infectious hepatitis. Shading=normal values.

Methods: *Transaminase:* Tonhazy-White-Umbreit. *Bilirubinaemia:* Jendrassik Czike. *Phosphatase:* King-Armstrong. *Cholinesterase:* Stedman-Lucas. Electrophoresis on paper.

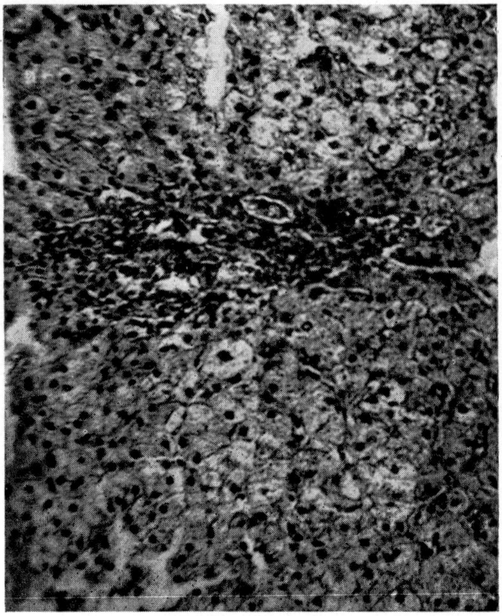

FIG. 5.—Needle-biopsy 30 days before jaundice (infectious hepatitis). Hydropic swelling of liver cells and inflammatory portal inflammation. H. and E. × 130.

pathological increase of transaminases, with inversion of the ratio, appeared as early as 36 days before fever and jaundice. The estimation of transaminases is, therefore, a valuable aid in detecting cases of hepatitis just at the beginning of the incubation period, with obvious prophylactic advantages. Thus it should be used routinely in blood donors in order to eliminate those with pathological values (Tolentino and Rossi, 1957b).

Since at the beginning of the incubation period there is sufficient necrotic damage of the hepatic cells to induce an increase of transaminases, and to be manifest at biopsy (as demonstrated in one case in Fig. 5), it seems that even at this early stage the virus is exerting its injurious action upon the liver. The unusually long duration of the incubation stage could be due to a peculiar slowness of virus multiplication, and clinical signs would appear only when a sufficient portion of tissue had been destroyed.

As has been mentioned above a dissociation exists in some clinical cases between increase of the transaminases and inversion of the ratio: on the one hand some infectious diseases show an inversion of the GOT/GPT ratio without an increase of values, while on the other hand obstructive (as opposed to infective) jaundice demonstrates increased values without inversion (cases of obstructive jaundice of the newborn) (Kove, Goldstein and Wróblewski, 1957; some cases of ours). We sought an explanation of these phenomena in animal experiments.

This research gave the following results:

(1) In guinea pigs bile-duct ligature produced after only one hour a very quick and remarkable increase (about 10 times) of aspartic-ketoglutaric (GOT) transaminase and a smaller increase of alanine-ketoglutaric (GPT) transaminase; the normal ratio (Fig. 6) was therefore maintained.

(2) In mice infected with mouse hepatitis by virus MHV_3 there was an increase of serum transaminases just as in human infectious hepatitis (Fig. 7), and this increase was preceded by a similar inversion of the ratio in the mitochondria of the damaged liver (Tolentino, Nordio and Rossi, 1957).

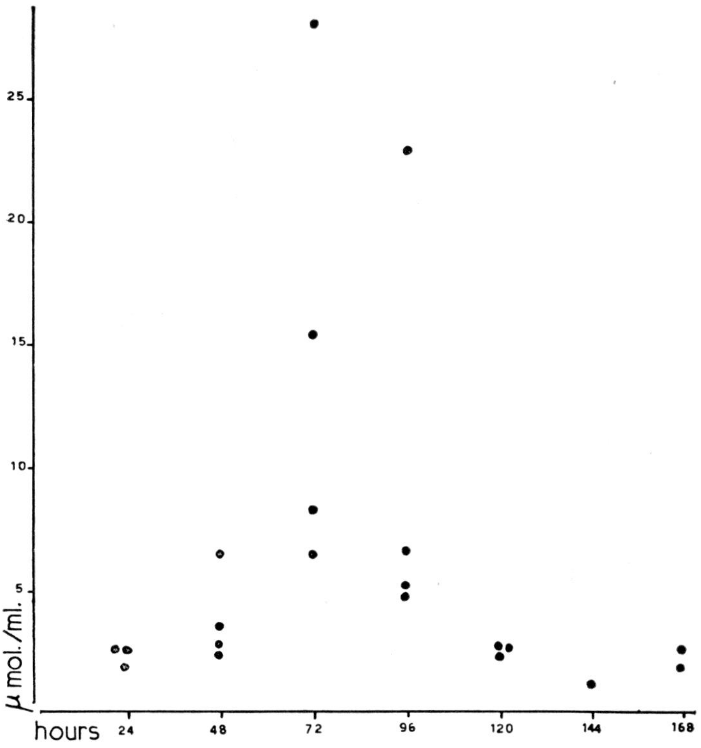

FIG. 7.—Serum transaminase (aspartic-ketoglutaric (GOT)) in mice inoculated with sub-lethal doses of mouse hepatitis virus (MHV_3).

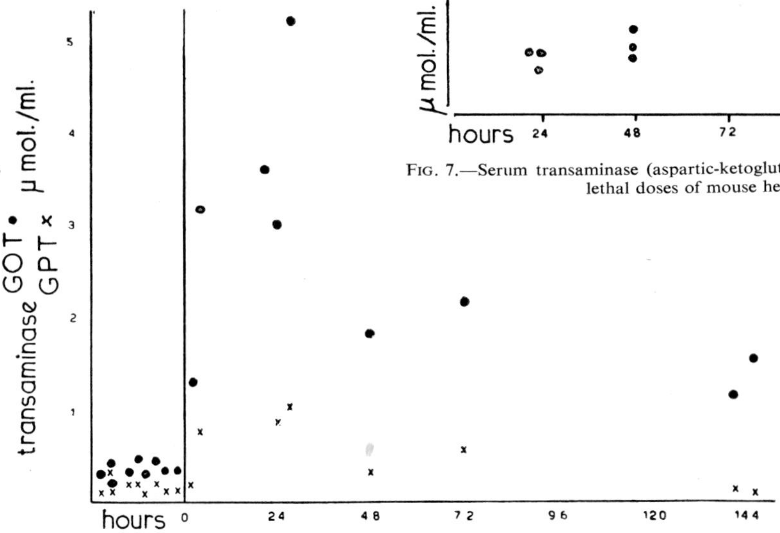

FIG. 6.—Serum transaminases in guinea pigs before and after ligature of the bile duct.

TABLE 1

VALUES OF LIVER TRANSAMINASES IN NORMAL AND IN TYPHOID-VACCINATED GUINEA-PIGS

Transaminase Activity	Normal			Vaccinated		
	GOT	GPT	Ratio GOT/GPT	GOT	GPT	Ratio GOT/GPT
Liver homogenate (µmol./100 mg.) ..	44·14	6·85	6.85	51·30	13·26	4.27
Mitochondria (µmol./mg. N) ..	9·78	1·14	8.48	9·00	3·66	2.90
Supernatant phase (µmol./mg. N.) ..	7·96	1·29	9.47	7·55	2·14	4.26

(3) In guinea-pigs immunized by typhoid vaccine an increase of alanine-ketoglutaric (GPT) transaminase in the mitochondria and in the supernatant fluid occurred with an alteration of the GOT/GPT ratio in favour of alanine-ketoglutaric (GPT) transaminase (Table 1) (Tolentino, 1957).

Previous research in our department had demonstrated that antigenic stimulation, such as provided by vaccination or infectious diseases, produces a hydropic swelling of the hepatic cells related to their increased function. The simultaneous internal displacement of transaminases in the cell may be responsible for the inversion of the serum transaminases (without a significant increase) in some infectious diseases. In infectious hepatitis the phases succeed each other: there is first, hydropic swelling with internal displacement of enzymes, followed by cellular necrosis and a consequent passage of cellular enzymes into the blood. In obstructive necrosis, produced by bile duct ligature, on the contrary, the first phase, the internal displacement of the enzymes, is absent and therefore there is no inversion of the ratio in the blood.

REFERENCES

Kove, S., Goldstein, S. and Wróblewski, F. (1957). *Pediatrics*, **20**, 590.
Ritis, F. de, Coltorti, M. and Giusti, G. (1955). *Minerva Med.* (*Torino*), **46**, 1207.
Tolentino, P. (1957). Intern. Conference of Hepatol. Perugia.
——, Nordio, S. and Rossi, M. (1956). *Boll. Soc. ital. Biol. sper.*, **32**, 780.
—— and Rossi, M. (1957a). *Minerva pediat.* (*Torino*), **9**, 377.
——, —— (1957b). *G. Mal. infett.*, **9**, 552.
Tonhazy, N. E., White, N. G. and Umbreit, W. W. (1950). *Arch. Biochem.*, **28**, 36.
Wróblewski, F. and La Due, J. S. (1954). *J Lab. clin. Med.*, **44**, 958.

A TEST FOR COELIAC DISEASE

BY

W. W. PAYNE and V. JENKINSON

From The Hospital for Sick Children, Great Ormond Street, London

(RECEIVED FOR PUBLICATION APRIL 28, 1958)

The relationship between wheat flour in the diet and the development of symptoms in children with coeliac disease observed by Dicke (1950) has been established. Subsequent investigations indicated that the injurious factor occurs principally in the gliadin fraction (van de Kamer, Weijers and Dicke, 1953). Weijers and van de Kamer (1955) used gliadin in a method of testing wheat sensitivity hoping that the test would be helpful in the diagnosis of coeliac disease.

In order to determine the value of this gliadin tolerance test, it was performed on a series of children with coeliac disease and on controls. The children with coeliac disease were patients of Dr. Wilfrid Sheldon and attended his clinic regularly. The diagnostic criteria used were those given by May (in Garrod, Batten and Thursfield, 1947). The diagnosis was confirmed by a favourable response to a diet free of wheat and rye gluten. The beneficial effect of the diet is manifested by an improvement in appetite and temperament, disappearance of steatorrhoea and an increase in growth. Growth is carefully followed by height and weight charts (Sheldon and Lawson, 1952).

Material

Thirty-three cases of coeliac disease were studied. The diagnosis was made according to the criteria stated in 25 cases. In eight cases the diagnosis was based on clinical data associated with the response to a gluten-free diet, and relevant biochemical investigations were not made.

The children were in all stages of the disease and treatment. Two of the children were in the active phase. Treatment had not been instituted when they were tested. Eight children had been on a gluten-free diet for periods of a few days to one month before their gliadin tolerance test. These children have since shown a satisfactory response to the therapeutic diet. The rest of the cases had been treated for some years, having had periods on a gluten-free diet and on a normal diet. Some children, who had been treated for more than four years, still deteriorated when returned to a normal diet. A few patients had apparently recovered after prolonged treatment; they had shown no recurrence of symptoms when returned to a normal diet and growth continued at the expected rate. Six children in this series were either undiagnosed or untreated for a long time after the onset of symptoms.

Control cases were selected from convalescent patients who had had diseases with no alimentary tract involvement, with the exception of one child, who was a normal healthy unlike twin of one of the coeliac patients. Four children who were convalescent from disorders of the alimentary tract from causes other than coeliac disease formed a second control group. A summary of the details of these cases is tabulated:

Case	Sex	Age (Yr.)	Diagnosis
A.H.	♀	2½	Dyschezia
N.H.	♂	7½	Malabsorption syndrome with abnormal pattern of second part of duodenum.
S.T.	♀	11	Chronic constipation with faecal incontinence. Congenital anal stenosis. Operation: division of fibrosed anal ring. Faecal incontinence continued. Vaginal septum.
M.K.	♀	11	Chronic watery diarrhoea. Giardia cysts found. Congenital atrial septal defect.

Gliadin was prepared according to the procedure recommended by van de Kamer (personal communication). The patient to be tested fasted, usually, for 12 hours; the period of fast was sometimes reduced to eight hours when the condition of the patient made it advisable, e.g. in the case of a young ailing child. A sample of blood was taken by fingerprick from a fasting subject into a heparinized tube. A dose of gliadin (350 mg./Kg. body weight) in water was fed to the patient, and hourly samples of blood were taken for five consecutive hours.

The plasma glutamine was estimated in each sample as glutamic acid (Prestcott and Waelsch, 1946, 1947). Free glutamic acid was removed by adsorption on acid alumina. The filtrate was hydrolyzed in acid medium for one hour. The glutamic acid set free was separated on acid alumina and estimated. A glutamic acid standard was used in place of the solution recommended by Prestcott and Waelsch (1946). A series of standard curves were made and found to be linear over a range of 0-25 γ glutamic acid. A standard sample was estimated in parallel with test samples and all readings were related to it. The average difference between repeat estimations of 50 test samples drawn at random from our results was 0·7 mg./100 ml. Duplicate estimations were done when possible. It has been assumed that the glutamic acid liberated by short acid hydrolysis of the filtrate was entirely derived from the plasma glutamine; since other glutamine-containing compounds may contribute the measured substance is known as 'apparent' plasma glutamine (Prestcott and Waelsch, 1947).

Recording of Results

The maximum increase of apparent plasma glutamine occurred at variable times. The greatest increase, irrespective of time of occurrence, is recorded as a percentage of the fasting value, which is the form adopted by Weijers and van de Kamer (1955). There is no reason to suppose that there is any relation between the fasting plasma glutamine and the absolute increase after gliadin; therefore, the absolute increase in mg./100 ml. is also recorded. The results are given in the following tables.

Table 1 shows that the mean maximum increment of apparent plasma glutamine of these children with coeliac disease is significantly greater than that of normal children. A few children who had recently recovered from dysfunction of the alimentary tract show a mean percentage rise which is intermediate between that of normal children and coeliac children. The mean percentage in this group is not significantly different from children with no recent gastro-intestinal disturbance, nor from coeliac children. The absolute rise is the same as that of coeliac children.

Tables 2a and b show that there is no relation between age and magnitude of increase of apparent plasma glutamine in this series of controls and coeliac patients. The numbers of control children in different age groups are insufficient for a complete analysis, but there is no indication of an age relationship (Table 2a). Age can be disregarded when grouping the coeliac patients according to a clinical assessment (Table 2b).

Table 3 shows that the mean rise of apparent plasma glutamine of children treated for less than two years is significantly greater than that of normal children. Children who remained intolerant of gluten even after four years of treatment show a similar difference. There is no correlation in this series between magnitude of rise of apparent plasma glutamine and phase of the disease, whether symptoms are active or controlled by treatment.

The number of children who, after prolonged treatment, no longer appeared intolerant of gluten, was small. The mean rise of plasma glutamine did not differ significantly from normal children, but this may be the result of the limited size of the sample.

The six patients who remained undiagnosed or untreated for some time after the appearance of the disease were grouped together, but they do not form a homogeneous group. It is not surprising that their response to gliadin is variable.

TABLE 1

	No. of Estimations	Maximum Increment of Apparent Plasma Glutamine: As % of fasting value		mg./100 ml.	
		Mean	S.D.	Mean	S.D.
Controls:					
Group 1	13	22·62	21·53	1·04	1·10
Group 2 .. .. Children with recent alimentary dysfunction	5	40·80	17·55	2·42	1·21
Coeliac patients ..	38	51·24	37·32	2·42	1·38

Significance of difference between means of:

Control groups 1 and 2:	$P>0·05$	$P>0·05$
Control group 1 and coeliac group:	$P<0·01$	$P<0·01$
Control group 2 and coeliac group:	$P>0·05$	$P>0·05$

Using Cochran's approximation.

TABLE 2A

Control Children recovered from Diseases with no Alimentary Tract Involvement	No. of Estimations	Maximum Increment of Apparent Plasma Glutamine: As % of fasting value		mg./100 ml.	
		Mean	S.D.	Mean	S.D.
0-4 yr. ..	2	11		0·75	
5-9 yr. ..	6	30·67	20·62	1·42	1·06
10-14 yr. ..	5	12·4	22·01	0·70	1·18

TABLE 2B

Coeliac Patients	No. of Estimations	Maximum Increment of Apparent Plasma Glutamine: As % of fasting value		mg./100 ml.	
		Mean	S.D.	Mean	S.D.
0-4 yr. ..	13	54·23	40·91	2·24	1·39
5-9 yr. ..	19	55·37	38·76	2·71	1·46
10-14 yr.	6	31·67	18·34	1·88	1·01

Significance of difference between means of:

0-4 yr. and 5-9 yr.	$P>0·05$	$P>0·05$
0-4 yr. and 10-14 yr.	$P>0·05$	$P>0·05$
5-9 yr. and 10-14 yr.	$P>0·05$	$P>0·05$

Using Cochran's approximation.

TABLE 3

Independent Clinical Assessment of Children Tested	No. of Estimations	Maximum Increment of Apparent Plasma Glutamine: As % of fasting value		mg./100 ml.	
		Mean	S.D.	Mean	S.D.
Controls:					
Group I	13	22·62	21·53	1·04	1·10
Group 2 .. .. Children with alimentary dysfunction	5	40·80	17·55	2·42	1·81
Coeliac Patients:					
All cases treated less than 2 yr.	14	51·57	40·57	2·19	1·36
Intolerant of gluten after more than 4 yr. treatment	14	52·07	31·26	2·65	1·05
Recovered after long treatment	4	45·50	35·24	2·38	1·96
Treatment commenced late after onset of symptoms	6	52·33	52·14	2·48	1·92

Significance of difference between means of:
Control and coeliac patients:
(*a*) Treated for less than 2 yr. $P<0\cdot05$ $P<0\cdot05$
(*b*) Intolerant of gluten after more than 4 yr. treatment. $P<0\cdot05$ $P<0\cdot01$
(*c*) Recovered after long treatment. $P>0\cdot05$ $P>0\cdot05$
(*d*) Treatment commenced late after onset of symptoms. $P>0\cdot05$ $P>0\cdot05$
Using Cochran's approximation.

Comparison of the mean rise of apparent plasma glutamine as a percentage of the fasting value of children who remained intolerant of gluten even after prolonged treatment and that of normal controls shows that the probability of the difference between the two results being due to chance, lies between 1 in 20 and 1 in 100. When the increase in mg./100 ml. is used instead, the probability is less than 1 in 100. The explanation of the difference lies in the fact that the fasting level of plasma glutamine tended to increase with age in these coeliac children. There are indications that the same trend may occur in normal children over a lower range, but in this case the trend was not significant. Further estimations are necessary to substantiate the indications of a rise of fasting level with age.

Table 4 shows that five children, who were tested while on a gluten-free diet and while on a normal diet, demonstrated no relationship between diet and rise of plasma glutamine.

In Table 5 the coeliac children were grouped according to the diet at the time of the test. The similarity of the mean rise in the two groups supports the conclusion that diet has no influence on the test.

None of the children with coeliac disease showed aggravation or recurrence of symptoms after the dose of gliadin used in the test.

TABLE 4

Effect of Diet on Increase of Apparent Plasma Glutamine

Patient	Age (yr.)	Gliadin Tolerance Test 1: Diet	Period of Diet (mth.)	Maximum Increment of Plasma Glutamine %	mg./100 ml.	Gliadin Tolerance Test 2: Diet	Period of Diet (mth.)	Maximum Increment of Plasma Glutamine %	mg./100 ml.
C.I. ..	14	G.F.D.	28	9	0·6	Normal	6	26	2·0
M. McC. ..	8	G.F.D.	30	45	1·7	Normal	4	41	3·6
C.M. ..	3	G.F.D.	15	77	4·3	Normal	5	13	1·2
L.P. ..	7	Normal	33	38	3·1	G.F.D.	8	79	4·2
J.A. ..	7	Normal	18	98	5·3	G.F.D.	4	23	1·1

G.F.D. = Gluten free diet.

Discussion

These results confirm the observations of Weijers and van de Kamer (1955), who found a greater increase of plasma glutamine in coeliac children than in normal children after ingestion of gliadin. The increase in our series of coeliac patients is not as great as that found by Weijers and van de Kamer. Alvey, Anderson and Freeman (1957), also found after a test dose of gluten an increase in blood glutamine which was greater in four coeliac children

TABLE 5

Diet	No. of Estimations on Coeliac Children	Maximum Increment of Apparent Plasma Glutamine: As % of fasting value		mg./100 ml.	
		Mean	S.D.	Mean	S.D.
Gluten free	28	51·18	35·85	2·29	1·29
Normal	10	51·40	43·24	2·67	1·74

than in four normal children, but the increment was again of a lesser degree than that reported by Weijers and van de Kamer.

The intermediate position of children convalescent from gastro-intestinal disorders other than gluten-induced coeliac disease suggests that the abnormal increase of plasma glutamine may be a non-specific effect common to other gastro-intestinal disturbances. The number of these children tested was too small to show conclusive evidence.

The increase of plasma glutamine measured in five children tested while on a gluten-free diet and on a normal gluten-containing diet showed no correlation with the prevailing diet. The results from these children exhibit considerable variation between two tests in the same child. A very wide standard deviation is evident in this series indicating an overlap in the range of results from the various groups. The variance found in the results from the coeliac group is significantly greater than that in the control group of children with no recent gastro-intestinal dysfunction (Table 1). This probably reflects the unreliability of a test dependent on rate of absorption in children where absorption is disturbed (Alvey, *et al.*, 1957). We would conclude in accordance with other workers that the test in its present form is unreliable in individual cases.

Later experiments by van de Kamer and Weijers (1955) showed that it was glutamine bound in protein, as it occurs in gliadin, which probably caused the abnormal increase of apparent plasma glutamine in children with coeliac disease and was the injurious factor. Frazer (1956) reported the presence of abnormally large amounts of a glutamine-containing peptide in the blood of one patient fed with a peptide fraction obtained from a tryptic digest of wheat gluten. The toxicity of this fraction was eliminated after digestion by an extract of pig's intestinal mucosa. The work of Alvey *et al.* (1957) substantiates the evidence indicating that the toxic factor in gluten is probably a peptide. They were able to show that the smaller peptides of gluten caused an increase of fat excretion in a patient with mild clinical symptoms.

The difference between normal children and children with coeliac disease is sufficiently pronounced to encourage further investigation of the amino-acid and peptide pattern of the blood after ingestion of gliadin or fractions of this protein.

Summary

A gliadin tolerance test was performed on control children and children with coeliac disease.

The increase of apparent plasma glutamine after a test dose of gliadin is significantly greater in children with coeliac disease than in control children convalescent from diseases with no gastro-intestinal involvement. A small group of children convalescent from gastro-intestinal dysfunction from causes other than coeliac diseases showed an increase intermediate between normal controls and coeliac children.

There is no quantitative relation between increase of plasma glutamine and phase of the disease, whether acute or non-symptomatic through withdrawal of wheat and rye gluten from the diet.

Diet appears to have no influence on the degree of increase of plasma glutamine.

The overlap of range of results from controls and coeliac patients is considerable and does not recommend the test as a diagnostic one.

We wish to thank Dr. Wilfrid Sheldon and other members of the staff for allowing us access to their patients. We are grateful to Dr. Sheldon for his help and interest in the study and to Dr. C. O. Carter for his tuition and advice on methods of statistical analysis. We are also indebted to Mr. A. Whitfield for his skilled assistance in the laboratory.

This investigation was done under the auspices of the Research Committee, The Hospital for Sick Children, Great Ormond Street.

References

Alvey, C., Anderson, C. M. and Freeman, M. (1957). *Arch. Dis. Childh.*, **32**, 434.
Dicke, W. K. (1950). *Coeliakie.* M.D. Thesis. Utrecht.
Frazer, A. C. (1956). *Proc. roy. Soc. Med.*, **49**, 1009.
Garrod, A. E., Batten, F. E. and Thursfield, H. (1947). *Diseases of Children.* 4th ed. Edited by Paterson, D. and Moncrieff, A. A., **1**, 343. London.
Kamer, J. H. van de. Personal communication.
—— and Weijers, H. A. (1955). *Acta paediat.* (*Uppsala*), **44**, 465.
——, —— and Dicke, W. K. (1953). *Ibid.*, **42**, 223.
Prestcott, B. A. and Waelsch, H. (1946). *J. biol. Chem.*, **164**, 331.
——, —— (1947). *Ibid.*, **167**, 855.
Sheldon, W. and Lawson, D. (1952). *Lancet*, **2**, 902.
Weijers, H. A. and Kamer, J. H. van de (1955). *Acta paediat.* (*Uppsala*), **44**, 536.

A LONGITUDINAL STUDY OF THE GROWTH AND DEVELOPMENT OF PREMATURELY AND MATURELY BORN CHILDREN

PART I. INTRODUCTION

BY

CECIL MARY DRILLIEN

From the Department of Child Life and Health, Edinburgh

(RECEIVED FOR PUBLICATION DECEMBER 16, 1957

Over the past 40 years many studies of the later growth and development of premature infants have been reported in the literature with widely varying conclusions (for example: Ylppö, 1920; Capper, 1928; Hess, Mohr and Bartelme, 1934; Blegen, 1952; Alm, 1953). In a comprehensive review of the early literature Benton (1940) puts forward four reasons for its contradictory nature. These are: the substitution of 'clinical impression' for standardized tests; the lack of attention paid to socio-economic factors; inadequate numbers and unsatisfactory controls; and the biased nature of the samples.

The longitudinal developmental study which is described in this paper has been designed to take into account these important points.

The chief difficulty in planning a long-term study of this type is to obtain the co-operation of parents representing a cross section of the general population, and having gained co-operation to maintain it over a period of years. This is well illustrated by reference to some current long-term studies. For the longitudinal research in child development being carried out from the Child Study Centre, London (Moore, Hindley and Falkner, 1954), the parents of 18·4% of the 272 children originally selected, declined to participate in the study at the beginning. In a similar study from the Centre International de l'Enfance, Paris, 16% of the 515 children were never seen. In addition it was reported (Pernot, 1955) that not more than 15% attended all seven of the examinations arranged during the first two years.

Present Study

During the period 1953 to 1955, over 1,000 mothers delivered in two large Edinburgh maternity hospitals took part in an investigation into the social factors affecting premature birth (Drillien, 1957). Every surviving premature infant and every pair of twins was selected for the developmental study, the only stipulation being that the family be resident in Edinburgh and likely to be so for the next six months. Illegitimate infants were only excluded if adoption was proposed. The sample so obtained was heavily weighted by the larger premature babies between 4½ and 5½ lb. at birth. It was therefore decided to include all babies of 4 lb. or less, who were resident in the surrounding counties.

The control group of infants who were mature at birth, on a weight basis, was selected by taking the next mature birth from the hospital record list occurring after every alternate premature birth. This method of obtaining a control sample has been chosen in preference to the commonly used matching technique (e.g., Douglas and Mogford, 1953) which is based on the assumption that social and economic differences between two groups will be removed by matching for certain broad categories such as social class, sex, age of parents, place in family and locality. This method has not been employed in the present study as it was felt that many more diverse influences affect the later growth and development of the child than can be covered by taking into account a few broad groupings. It has, in fact, been noticed on many occasions that two neighbouring families matched closely by such factors may show widely differing standards of child care and household management.

The mothers were not asked initially to co-operate in a long-term survey, but were asked to allow a visit and examination when their baby was 6 months old. At this time every mother agreed to co-operate, although later two withdrew their consent. Table 1 gives the total numbers of children originally recruited, by sex and birth weight. Tables 2 and 3 give the numbers of twin pairs and the birth weight distribution of individual twins by sex. It was hoped that after the first visit at 6 months of age, the mothers would be sufficiently interested to continue co-operation and this has, in fact, been the case. Losses from the sample have been minimal and have been due mainly to emigration, or removal to a considerable distance (i.e., more than 30 or 40 miles). Children who were grossly mentally defective were removed from the sample after one year if the diagnosis had been established. Two children were lost from the sample in the first two years for this reason. Table 4 gives the number

TABLE 1

TOTAL NUMBER OF SINGLETONS ORIGINALLY RECRUITED BY BIRTH WEIGHT AND SEX

Birth Weight (lb. oz.)	M.	F.	Total
3·0 and under	10	4	14
3·1–3·8	13	15	28
3·9–4·0	14	12	26
4·1–4·8	18	20	38
4·9–5·0	30	25	55
5·1–5·8	37	53	90
5·9–6·8	6	14	20
6·9–7·8	22	27	49
7·9–8·8	21	14	35
8·9 and over	9	6	15
Total	180	190	370

TABLE 2

TOTAL TWIN PAIRS ORIGINALLY RECRUITED

Twin Pairs of Unlike Sex:		
Both over 5½ lb.	14	
Both under 5½ lb.	22	
Male over 5½ lb., female under 5½ lb.	7	
Female over 5½ lb., male under 5½ lb.	6	
Total	49	
Twin Pairs of Like Sex, Identical:	F.	M.
Both over 5½ lb.	1	2
Both under 5½ lb.	11	7
One over 5½ lb., one under 5½ lb.	1	5
Total	13	14
Twin Pairs of Like Sex, not Identical:	F.	M.
Both over 5½ lb.	7	7
Both under 5½ lb.	3	5
One over 5½ lb., one under 5½ lb.	7	5
Total	17	17
Surviving Twin of Like Sex, Other Twin Stillborn or Died Before Discharge	F.	M.
Over 5½ lb.	1	1
Under 5½ lb.	2	1
Total	3	2
Total no. of twin pairs	110	
Total no. of twin pairs one only surviving	5	
Total no. of infants	225	

TABLE 3

BIRTH WEIGHT DISTRIBUTION OF TWINS RECORDED SEPARATELY BY SEX

Birth Weight (lb. oz.)	M.	F.	Total
3·0 and under	2	6	8
3·1–3·8	1	3	4
3·9–4·0	12	7	19
4·1–4·8	15	13	28
4·9–5·0	11	17	28
5·1–5·8	22	21	43
5·9–6·8	30	22	52
6·9–7·8	15	18	33
7·9–8·8	5	5	10
Total	113	112	225

TABLE 4

LOSSES FROM SAMPLE

Age (months)	Total	Examination Completed	Examination not Completed	Lost from Sample*
6	595	572	13	10
12	585	564	3	18
18	567	548	5	14
24	553	538	6	9

*Total 51: death (9); refused to co-operate (7); moved or emigrated (33); removed from sample because of gross mental defect (2).

of examinations completed at 6, 12, 18 and 24 months of age, the number of examinations missed and losses from the sample. Out of the original 595 children recruited, 544 (91·4%) remained in the survey at 2 years.

Although at the time these children were born about 75% of all Edinburgh births took place in hospital, it seemed possible that a sample of children selected from hospital deliveries only might be biased, particularly as regards social background and parity of the mother. All births in Edinburgh are notified to the Public Health Department of the Corporation as being under or over 5½ lb. at birth, and access to these records was allowed. It was therefore decided to obtain some comparative information about all births in Edinburgh during the 12-month period October, 1953, to October, 1954 (Drillien and Richmond, 1956). Every premature birth together with one in 10 of all mature births was investigated and the following information recorded about each: birth weight, legitimacy, age of mother, parity and occupation of the father.

The survey sample can therefore be compared with the general infant population to see how far the two are alike and in drawing any general conclusions from the sample cognisance can be taken of the differences observed.

Tables 5 and 6 give the parity and social class distribution of the survey sample as compared with the general population, for premature infants of

TABLE 5

PARITY DISTRIBUTION, EXPRESSED AS PERCENTAGE, OF SURVEY SAMPLE COMPARED WITH ALL INFANTS BORN IN EDINBURGH, 1953 TO 1954

Birth Weight (lb. oz.)	Parity											
	0		1		2		3		4		5 and over	
	Survey	Edin.	Survey	Edin.	Survey	Edin.	Survey	Edin.	Survey	Edin.	Survey	Edin.
>5·8	58·9	36·6	21·0	27·9	15·1	15·5	3·4	8·0	0·8	8·0	0·8	6·0
4·1 to 5·8	56·8	48·9	20·8	22·6	10·4	14·7	6·6	5·1	6·6	5·1	2·7	4·6
<4·1	47·1	51·0	19·1	14·9	19·2	12·8	11·8	12·8	11·8	12·8	—	8·5

TABLE 6

SOCIAL CLASS DISTRIBUTION, EXPRESSED AS PERCENTAGE, OF SURVEY SAMPLE COMPARED WITH ALL INFANTS BORN IN EDINBURGH, 1953 TO 1954

Birth Weight (lb. oz.)	Social Class					
	1 and 2		3		4 and 5	
	Survey	Edin.	Survey	Edin.	Survey	Edin.
>5·8	21·8	26·9	55·5	53·6	22·7	19·5
4·1 to 5·8	15·3	12·5	51·4	57·1	33·3	30·4
<4·1	14·7	19·1	66·2	55·4	19·1	25·5

4 lb. or less at birth, those between 4 lb. 1 oz. and 5 lb. 8 oz., and those mature at birth.

The social class distribution of the survey sample and the Edinburgh infants is very close and appropriate statistical tests show that there is no reason to suppose that the survey sample is biased in any way with respect to social class distribution.

Parity distribution in the premature groups is also sufficiently close to be free from bias, but in the mature control group there is an excess of first births in the survey sample, which must be taken into account in drawing general conclusions about the effect on the child of place in family.

As nearly all twin pregnancies are delivered in hospital, it has been assumed that the sample of twins will be representative of twins in the general population.

Procedure and Methods

Hospital Interview. All mothers were interviewed in the maternity hospital and consent to the initial visit obtained. At the same time particulars were noted of the mother's social background both before marriage and since, and any complication of the pregnancy or delivery.

First Home Visit at Six Months. At the initial home visit a special effort was made to establish a good relationship with the mother and to secure her continuing interest in the survey.

Full particulars were taken of housing and certain information was obtained about other children in the family. Details of feeding, vitamin supplements, and protective immunization were noted. At this and every subsequent interview a record was made of any illness necessitating medical attention or hospital admission.

A brief clinical examination was carried out and the children graded as to general nutrition and health, and a note made of any minor abnormalities which had not received medical attention. The children were weighed in light, indoor clothing, an appropriate deduction being made for the clothes worn, and, from the age of 2 years, crown-heel and crown-rump lengths were taken recumbent on a portable measuring board.

The developmental level was estimated on the response to the Gesell developmental tests.

Subsequent Examinations. The children are seen every six months (± 7 days) up to the age of 18 months and at 2 years old (± 14 days) and thereafter they are seen once yearly (± 14 days). It was originally anticipated that after the initial visit a proportion of the mothers would be willing to bring their babies for examination to a central clinic, thus saving much time and providing standard conditions for examination and testing. In practice it has been found that the number of mothers who are willing to do this is very small. Even the best-intentioned find it difficult to attend regularly at a set time especially if there are other children in the family. Mothers from the two extremes of the social scale are the most reluctant to attend a clinic, and insistence on such attendance inevitably introduces bias in the social composition of the sample. In many cases the mother has become pregnant again during the course of the survey, and this is an added deterrent to further clinic attendance.

Mental testing may be difficult, especially after the first year, in the presence of other members of the family and absence of adequate table and floor space. Nevertheless as the children are seen at regular intervals an incomplete testing at one visit can be confirmed and completed on the next occasion.

Some authorities hold strongly to the view that developmental testing can not be considered valid unless carried out under standard conditions. This would be more convincing if the subjects for testing came from a standard environment. It may be argued that the child's own house approximates more nearly to a standard setting than an impersonal clinic room to which children from different types of homes react in a different way. In practice it has been found that the children who have been tested both at home and in the clinic are more responsive in their own homes.

Table 7 gives the proportion of children seen within the pre-arranged period. Up to 18 months quite a large percentage were examined more than seven days after the set age. In some cases, this was due to illness of mother or child, or absence on holiday, but in the majority it was due to a change of address and the inevitable lapse of time before the family could be traced and a fresh appointment made. One hundred and ninety-five changes of address have been recorded. This is 35% of total families and does not include those who have been lost to the survey by removal. Nearly all were seen within 14 days, and it will be noticed that at 2 years old (± 14 days) only a small percentage were not seen within this period. A suitable adjustment has been made for measurements and estimated developmental levels if the child was seen within four weeks of the pre-arranged date. Measurements for children seen later than four weeks have not been included in the subsequent analyses.

Although much of the information collected is necessarily subjective in character, an attempt has been made to adhere to certain standards throughout. Some of these are now described.

TABLE 7

PERCENTAGE OF CHILDREN SEEN LATER THAN PRE-ARRANGED DATE

Age (mths.)	%
6 ± 7 days	14
12 7 days	10
18 7 days	11
24 ±14 days	5

Housing

The following criteria were employed in grading housing accommodation:

(1) A separate living room not used for sleeping. (2) Sufficient bedrooms for the child in question to sleep apart from the parents after the age of 1 year and with not more than two other children of the same sex, or one adult. (3) Adequate furnishings, in particular that the child should be able to occupy a separate cot or bed. (4) Modern cooking facilities (gas or electric cooker), and a kitchen sink. (5) A supply of hot water. (6) A bathroom. (7) An inside W.C. (8) Easy access to a garden or green. (9) A reasonable standard of cleanliness and structural repair.

The following classification was adopted according to the number of points satisfied:

1=Very good	9
2=Good	7 to 8
3=Fairly good	5 to 6
4=Fair	3 to 4
5=Poor	1 to 2
6=Very poor	0

The majority of municipally owned houses were classified as very good, although some come in the next category as they failed to satisfy points 3 and 9. The majority of privately owned houses belonging to parents in social classes 1 and 2, also were graded as being very good. Privately owned houses belonging to families in social class 3, were usually graded as good, or fairly good, overcrowding being the commonest problem here.

Many rented houses occupied by families in social classes 3, 4 and 5 were graded as fair or poor, these most often being of the room and kitchen type, without a bathroom or hot water, and often with a shared toilet on the landing.

Houses graded as very poor possessed none of the facilities mentioned above and in addition were kept in a state of squalor and filth.

A house which might have been considered good or fairly good when the child was under 1 year old, and the only child in the family, might drop to a lower category at a later age and when other children were born.

Fig. 1 gives the percentage of singletons in the survey living in these grades of accommodation at 6 months by social class.

As would be expected there is a marked social gradient in the standard of accommodation. In social classes 1 and 2, 91% were occupying houses graded as good or very good, compared with 27% in social classes 4 and 5. Of the total population studied 54% were living in good or very good accommodaton and 27% in poor or very poor houses. By the age of 2 years the situation had improved a little, 58% now living in good accommodation and 20% in poor. In 16% of the total, the housing had improved due mainly to rehousing by the municipal authority and in 4% the housing had deteriorated.

Social Class

The social class of the child's father has been

recorded, the classification used being based on that given by the Registrar General (1951) in the Classification of Occupations, 1950, with certain minor modifications (Drillien, 1957) principally the addition of a social class 6 to cover homes in which the mother was widowed, divorced or separated from her husband, or where the child was illegitimate.

In addition to the social class classification, working class mothers and fathers, if seen, have been graded as being superior working class, average or poor.

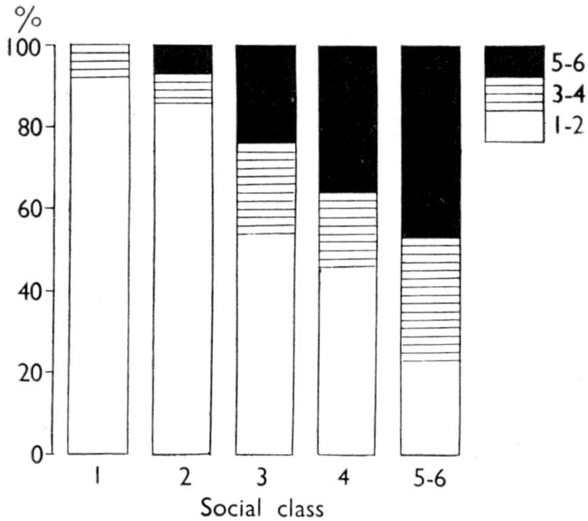

FIG. 1.—Standard of housing by social class.

Maternal Efficiency

The following points were noted when considering the efficiency of the mother: (1) Cleanliness of the house, the child and his clothes. (2) Feeding habits and diet. (3) Advantage taken of welfare facilities, such as vitamin supplements, protective immunization and infant clinics. (4) Management of training problems such as weaning, sleeping and toilet training. (5) The relationship of the mother with the child, other children in the family, and the father. (6) Maternal health.

Maternal efficiency was graded as being: very good, good, fair and poor. This grading was necessarily a purely subjective assessment, but is considered valid as all examinations were carried out by the same person and the same standards adopted throughout. In some cases the grading of efficiency changed as the child grew older. The mother who could deal adequately with a baby might prove less capable of coping with a toddler. The standards of others though satisfactory with the first child became less satisfactory as succeeding pregnancies entailed more work and responsibility.

Some mothers, especially those in the higher social groups, with an only child, though giving every material care and much affection, yet were over-anxious and fussy in their handling. A separate note has been made of this and it appears to have some bearing on the genesis of behaviour problems, which will be dealt with in a separate paper.

Fig. 2 gives the grading of maternal efficiency by social class at the initial home visit. In the total sample, maternal care was graded as good, or very good, in 84% of homes. This comes very close to the findings in the Newcastle 1,000-family survey (Spence, Walton, Miller and Court, 1954) in which at least 85% of the families were regarded as receiving a good standard of child care.

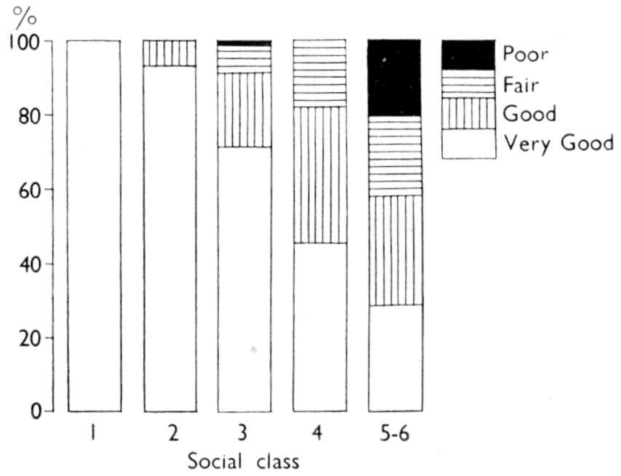

FIG. 2.—Efficiency of the mother by social class.

Again there is a marked social gradient. In social classes 1 and 2, maternal efficiency was considered good or very good in 100% of cases, compared with less than 60% in social class 5. In one-fifth of homes in this latter group, maternal efficiency was considered poor. The children were found to be dirty, inadequately clothed and fed, subject to a disproportionate amount of illness, and in many cases lacking in security and affection.

At 2 years of age the percentage of maternal efficiency graded as fair or poor had risen from 16% to 20%, mainly due to deterioration in standards with succeeding pregnancies in social class 5.

All children in the survey have now reached the age of 2 years and subsequent papers will present the data collected for this age period under the following headings: (1) Physical growth in relation to birth weight, height of parents, nutrition, early illness and social class. (2) Mental development in relation to birth weight, gestation time and social class. (3) Morbidity in relation to nutrition, maternal efficiency, place in family, housing and social class. (4) Patterns of maternal care.

REFERENCES

Alm, I. (1953). *Acta paediat. (Uppsala)*, **42**, Suppl. 94.
Benton, A. L. (1940). *Amer. J. Orthopsychiat.*, **10**, 719.
Blegen, S. D. (1952). *Acta paediat. (Uppsala)*, **41**, Suppl. 88.
Capper, A. (1928). *Amer. J. Dis. Child.*, **35**, 262.
Douglas, J. W. B. and Mogford, C. (1953). *Brit. med. J.*, **1**, 748.
Drillien, C. M. and Richmond, F. (1956). *Arch. Dis. Childh.*, **31**, 390.
—— (1957). *J. Obstet. Gynaec. Brit. Emp.*, **64**, 161.
Hess, J. H., Mohr, G. J. and Bartelme, P. F. (1934). *The Physical and Mental Growth of Prematurely Born Children.* Chicago.
Moore, T., Hindley, C. B. and Falkner, F. (1954). *Brit. med. J.*, **2**, 1132.
Pernot, M. P. (1955). *Études sur la Croissance Somatique et le Développement Psychique de l'Enfant.* Paris.
Registrar General (1951). Classification of Occupations, 1950. London.
Spence, J., Walton, W. S., Miller, F. J. W. and Court, S. D. M. (1954). *A Thousand Families in Newcastle Upon Tyne.* London.
Ylppö, A. (1920). *Z. Kinderheilk.*, **24**, 1

A LONGITUDINAL STUDY OF THE GROWTH AND DEVELOPMENT OF PREMATURELY AND MATURELY BORN CHILDREN

PART II.—PHYSICAL DEVELOPMENT

BY

CECIL MARY DRILLIEN

From the Department of Child Life and Health, Edinburgh

(RECEIVED FOR PUBLICATION DECEMBER 16, 1957)

This paper is the second in a series presenting findings in a long-term study of growth and development in a representative sample of nearly 600 premature and maturely born children, delivered in two Edinburgh maternity hospitals in the years 1953 to 1955. The sample, the method of selection, the procedures carried out and the social standards employed have already been described in Part I (Drillien, 1958).

All children in the survey have reached the age of 2 years, and results are now given of the analysis of weight and height measurements, in the first 2 years of life for different birth weight groups in relation to certain genetic and environmental factors. The children were examined at 6, 12, 18 and 24 months of age. At 6 months, infants were weighed on baby scales recording accurately to 1 oz. Thereafter they were weighed on a spring balance type of scale incorporating a seat. These scales are calibrated in ounces up to a weight of 50 lb., but are only considered to be accurate to the nearest 4 oz. Both scales were checked periodically against standard weights. The children were weighed in light indoor clothes, without shoes, and an appropriate deduction made for the clothes still worn. At 2 years old recumbent length without shoes was recorded on a portable measuring board calibrated in centimetres.

Mean Measurements of Weight and Height

Tables 1 to 4 give mean weights, weight increments and standard deviation of these means, at ages 6, 12, 18 and 24 months, for four birth weight groups, of male and female singletons and twins. At each age, mean weight is related to birth weight, the prematurely born showing little tendency to reduce their initial weight handicap. At 2 years the total weight increment since birth for singletons is highest in the smallest birth weight group. The difference between means of the group $4\frac{1}{2}$ lb. or less at birth, and that over $7\frac{1}{2}$ lb. at birth is 14 oz. for males and 13 oz. for females. The appropriate statistical test shows that a difference of this magnitude is not significant at the 5% point.

In the case of multiple births, the differences in mean weight at 2 years are greater than the differences in mean birth weight, both male and female twins showing smaller weight increments in the lower birth weight groups. Again these differences are not statistically significant.

Table 5 gives mean heights and height increments at 2 years for the same birth weight groups. Here again those who were largest at birth maintain their superiority in height at 2 years, but the height increments for both male and female singletons and twins are greater for those smallest at birth. Here the difference in height increment is statistically significant. There appears to be a definite tendency for those smallest at birth to reduce their height handicap significantly by 2 years of age.

Among singletons, boys show a bigger weight increment than girls at 2 years, amounting to just over 1 lb. both for those premature and mature at birth. In the twin groups the boys again show a bigger weight increment of $\frac{1}{2}$ lb. for those $5\frac{1}{2}$ lb. or less at birth, and $1\frac{1}{2}$ lb. for those above that birth weight. There is very little difference between the sexes in height increment either for single or multiple births.

These results are similar to those given by Lowe and Gibson (1953) who found that mean weight was closely related to birth weight, but that there was

TABLE 1

MALE SINGLETONS. MEAN WEIGHTS AND WEIGHT INCREMENTS FOR DIFFERENT BIRTH WEIGHT GROUPS

Age (mth.)	Birth Weight (lb. oz.)	Weight (oz.)	S.D.	Weight Increment (oz.)	S.D.	No.
6	4·8 and under	219	4·1	159	3·7	46
	4·9 to 5·8	250	4·1	169	3·9	60
	5·9 to 7·8	281	6·8	171	6·8	28
	7·9 and over	297	4·5	160	3·9	30
12	4·8 and under	308	6·4	251	6·1	53
	4·9 to 5·8	336	4·5	254	4·5	62
	5·9 to 7·8	366	8·3	255	8·6	26
	7·9 and over	383	6·7	246	6·6	30
18	4·8 and under	353	6·5	297	6·0	51
	4·9 to 5·8	374	4·4	292	4·3	64
	5·9 to 7·8	413	9·3	302	9·6	26
	7·9 and over	428	8·4	291	8·0	29
24	4·8 and under	394	6·6	335	6·5	53
	4·9 to 5·8	408	4·8	327	5·1	62
	5·9 to 7·8	439	8·5	328	8·3	26
	7·9 and over	457	8·9	321	8·7	30

TABLE 2

FEMALE SINGLETONS. MEAN WEIGHTS AND WEIGHT INCREMENTS FOR DIFFERENT BIRTH WEIGHT GROUPS

Age (mth.)	Birth Weight (lb. oz.)	Weight (oz.)	S.D.	Weight Increment (oz.)	S.D.	No.
6	4·8 and under	216	7·3	155	4·1	47
	4·9 to 5·8	227	3·9	152	6·9	75
	5·9 to 7·8	260	8·7	152	3·8	40
	7·9 and over	271	6·1	139	6·5	20
12	4·8 and under	307	6·7	248	3·6	41
	4·9 to 5·8	320	6·5	243	4·8	77
	5·9 to 7·8	339	6·5	231	6·1	39
	7·9 and over	367	9·9	239	11·5	20
18	4·8 and under	352	6·3	294	6·0	43
	4·9 to 5·8	359	5·1	277	5·0	75
	5·9 to 7·8	380	6·2	266	5·3	37
	7·9 and over	407	9·7	271	8·4	19
24	4·8 and under	390	6·8	324	11·0	42
	4·9 to 5·8	395	5·9	314	5·5	75
	5·9 to 7·8	414	5·5	306	6·4	38
	7·9 and over	440	10·4	309	9·9	19

TABLE 3

MALE TWINS. MEAN WEIGHTS AND WEIGHT INCREMENTS FOR DIFFERENT BIRTH WEIGHT GROUPS

Age (mth.)	Birth Weight (lb. oz.)	Weight (oz.)	S.D.	Weight Increment (oz.)	S.D.	No.
6	4·8 and under	222	6·5	158	5·8	28
	4·9 to 5·8	241	5·3	158	5·3	31
	5·9 to 7·8	272	4·6	171	4·8	42
	7·9 and over	298	4·8	174	6·2	5
12	4·8 and under	296	7·2	235	7·9	25
	4·9 to 5·8	327	9·0	248	9·6	28
	5·9 to 7·8	362	5·8	257	5·7	39
	7·9 and over	365	8·9	240	9·4	6
18	4·8 and under	353	7·6	285	7·8	27
	4·9 to 5·8	378	7·5	294	7·3	29
	5·9 to 7·8	402	6·9	300	6·8	37
	7·9 and over	409	12·2	285	13·0	6
24	4·8 and under	376	8·4	312	8·5	27
	4·9 to 5·8	410	7·1	327	7·2	28
	5·9 to 7·8	442	7·4	343	7·8	39
	7·9 and over	450	17·8	325	18·8	5

TABLE 4

FEMALE TWINS. MEAN WEIGHTS AND WEIGHT INCREMENTS FOR DIFFERENT BIRTH WEIGHT GROUPS

Age (mth.)	Birth Weight (lb. oz.)	Weight (oz.)	S.D.	Weight Increment (oz.)	S.D.	No.
6	4·8 and under	204	5·8	144	4·6	30
	4·9 to 5·8	239	5·1	157	5·1	34
	5·9 to 7·8	263	6·6	158	6·4	34
	7·9 and over	283	12·8	152	10·5	4
12	4·8 and under	290	7·5	230	7·4	30
	4·9 to 5·8	320	12·9	242	7·6	32
	5·9 to 7·8	342	6·4	241	6·5	36
	7·9 and over	379	11·2	250	9·2	5
18	4·8 and under	338	9·8	277	9·0	29
	4·9 to 5·8	367	7·5	288	7·4	32
	5·9 to 7·8	387	6·4	284	6·0	34
	7·9 and over	427	18·7	322	29·0	4
24	4·8 and under	373	8·0	310	7·7	30
	4·9 to 5·8	390	10·1	310	10·1	28
	5·9 to 7·8	415	5·9	313	5·7	33
	7·9 and over	466	6·6	340	5·7	5

TABLE 5

MEAN HEIGHTS AND HEIGHT INCREMENTS AT TWO YEARS FOR DIFFERENT BIRTH WEIGHT GROUPS

	Birth Weight (lb. oz.)	Height (cm.)	S.D.	Height Increment (cm.)	S.D.	No.
Male Singletons	4·8 and under	81·1	1·7	38·9	·9	52
	4·9 to 5·8	84·0	·37	37·9	·47	63
	5·9 to 7·8	86·8	1·47	36·5	·91	26
	7·9 and over	87·4	·58	35·4	·63	29
Male Twins	4·8 and under	82·3	·85	38·6	·71	24
	4·9 to 5·8	83·8	·61	37·0	·77	28
	5·9 to 7·8	86·3	·53	36·9	·63	38
	7·9 and over	84·8	·80	33·4	1·07	5
Female Singletons	4·8 and under	82·7	·65	39·5	·64	42
	4·9 to 5·8	83·2	·43	36·8	·45	74
	5·9 to 7·8	85·2	·53	38·0	·72	37
	7·9 and over	86·4	·68	34·9	·66	19
Female Twins	4·8 and under	80·7	·65	38·1	·67	28
	4·9 to 5·8	82·3	·71	36·3	·79	28
	5·9 to 7·8	84·4	·63	34·9	·77	32
	7·9 and over	87·5	·37	36·9	·94	5

little correlation between weight increment and birth weight. At 3 years the average male increment was 1 lb. greater than that for females. Similarly Falkner (1958) found that the mean weight increment from birth to 2 years was 1½ lb. greater for boys, but there was no difference in mean recumbent length increment for boys and girls between 4 weeks and 2 years of age. He also states that birth weight and early length differences are maintained up to the age of 3 years.

The Effect on Height and Weight of Certain Environmental Factors

It is known that prematurely born children tend to come from an inferior socio-economic background, which may account in part for their failure to catch up in weight and height with those mature at birth. Information was collected about the environmental background of each case, including the standard of maternal efficiency, frequency of illness and adequacy of the diet.

Maternal efficiency has been graded as: (1) Very good, (2) Good, (3) Fair and (4) Poor. Diet has been graded as: (1) Good, (2) Fair and (3) Poor. Frequency of illness has been graded according to the number of medical conditions requiring attention from the family doctor or hospital admission as follows: (1) No illness. (2) A few minor disorders, e.g., head colds, mild digestive disturbances or mild attacks of specific fevers. (3) One to three more serious infections, e.g., bronchitis, tonsillitis, otitis media or one hospital admission. (4) Four or more infections as above and one hospital admission. (5) Four or more infections and two hospital admissions. (6) Four or more infections and three or four hospital admissions. (7) Four or more infections and five or more hospital admissions. Hospital admissions for surgical conditions such as hernia or pyloric stenosis have not been included.

Table 6 gives mean weight and height increments at 2 years, for three birth weight groups, by four grades of maternal efficiency. Weight and height increments are substantially higher when maternal efficiency is very good, the effect of maternal efficiency being most marked in those who were premature at birth. Table 7 gives similar means by frequency of medical illness, here graded as: A, no serious illness (1 and 2), B, some illness (3), and C, frequent illness (4, 5, 6 and 7). Again the prematurely born with little or no illness show a marked increase in weight and height increments especially in those smallest at birth. Analyses of weight and height increment by grade of diet are given in Table 8 and show a similar result. Tables 9, 10 and 11 give the proportion of children in the three birth weight groups, by the different efficiency, illness and diet grades.

In the premature groups there is a striking excess of inefficient mothers, frequent illness and poor diet, especially in those who were $4\frac{1}{2}$ lb. or less at birth. To get some idea of the extent to which prematurely born children might catch up in weight and height if they were reared in the most favourable environ-

TABLE 6

MEAN WEIGHT AND HEIGHT INCREMENTS AT TWO YEARS BY EFFICIENCY GRADE OF MOTHER

	Male			Female		
Birthweight (lb. oz.)	4·8 and under	4·9 to 5·8	5·9 and over	4·8 and under	4·9 to 5·8	5·9 and over
			Weight Increment (oz.)			
Efficiency						
1	347·4	339·0	326·2	328·2	342·2	316·4
2	316·7	311·4	345·1	312·3	311·5	300·0
3	329·3	326·4	346·4	306·1	300·1	304·8
4	295·0	320·7	321·5	281·7	266·8	287·6
Difference between 1 and 4	52·4	18·3	4·7	46·5	75·4	28·8
			Height Increment (cm.)			
Efficiency						
1	39·1	39·3	36·4	39·9	37·2	36·1
2	39·1	36·9	36·4	38·1	36·5	35·4
3	39·3	35·8	36·0	38·8	36·8	33·4
4	33·8	34·6	33·0	36·1	31·7	34·1
Difference between 1 and 4	5·3	4·7	3·4	3·8	5·5	2·0

TABLE 7

MEAN WEIGHT AND HEIGHT INCREMENTS AT TWO YEARS BY FREQUENCY OF ILLNESS

	Male			Female		
Birthweight (lb. oz.)	4·8 and under	4·9 to 5·8	5·9 and over	4·8 and under	4·9 to 5·8	5·9 and over
			Weight Increment (oz.)			
Illness						
A	352·7	334·9	333·5	355·0	327·7	315·3
B	315·1	322·2	328·8	311·0	310·5	308·1
C	309·8	318·8	332·7	290·9	284·9	302·9
Difference between A and C	42·9	16·1	0·8	64·1	42·8	12·4
			Height Increment (cm.)			
Illness						
A	40·9	38·7	37·1	40·1	37·6	35·3
B	39·7	37·7	35·1	41·6	35·8	36·4
C	37·6	34·9	35·8	36·7	35·4	34·4
Difference between A and C	3·3	3·8	1·3	3·4	2·2	0·9

TABLE 8

MEAN WEIGHT AND HEIGHT INCREMENTS AT TWO YEARS BY GRADE OF DIET

	Male			Female		
Birth Weight (lb. oz.)	4·8 and under	4·9 to 5·8	5·9 and over	4·8 and under	4·9 to 5·8	5·9 and over
			Weight Increment (oz.)			
Diet						
1	337	330	331	334	326	316
2	322	321	328	295	305	275
3	310	315	347	285	268	287
Difference between 1 and 3	27	15	−16	49	58	29
			Height Increment (cm.)			
Diet						
1	39·5	38·6	36·4	39·6	37·2	36·2
2	41·0	36·7	35·5	38·1	36·5	33·3
3	37·1	35·1	34·1	37·8	34·8	34·3
Difference between 1 and 3	2·4	3·5	2·3	1·8	2·4	1·9

TABLE 9

EFFICIENCY OF MOTHER BY BIRTH WEIGHT OF BABY

	Male			Female		
Birth Weight (lb. oz.)	4·8 and under	4·9 to 5·8	5·9 and over	4·8 and under	4·9 to 5·8	5·9 and over
Efficiency						
1	38·[illegible]	46·8	65·0	55·6	53·4	65·3
2	32·5	29·9	19·0	23·6	27·2	13·7
3	15·0	15·6	10·0	11·1	14·6	15·8
4	13·8	7·8	6·0	9·7	4·9	5·3
Total	100·0	100·0	100·0	100·0	100·0	100·0

TABLE 10

FREQUENCY OF ILLNESS BY BIRTH WEIGHT OF BABY

	Male			Female		
Birth Weight (lb. oz.)	4·8 and under	4·9 to 5·8	5·9 and over	4·8 and under	4·9 to 5·8	5·9 and over
Illness						
A	39·7	37·0	48·5	45·6	54·0	51·6
B	26·9	35·9	35·4	30·9	26·0	28·4
C	33·3	27·2	16·2	23·5	20·0	20·0
Total	100·0	100·0	100·0	100·0	100·0	100·0

TABLE 11

GRADE OF DIET BY BIRTH WEIGHT OF BABY

	Male			Female		
Birth Weight (lb. oz.)	4·8 and under	4·9 to 5·8	5·9 and over	4·8 and under	4·9 to 5·8	5·9 and over
Diet						
1	52·5	56·7	76·0	62·5	59·2	71·1
2	27·5	33·3	20·0	22·2	33·0	22·7
3	20·0	10·0	4·0	15·3	7·8	6·2
Total	100·0	100·0	100·0	100·0	100·0	100·0

mental conditions, a selected group has been extracted from the total premature sample, consisting of those who had a minimum of illness, a good diet and very good maternal care. No difference was found in mean weights when these selected prematures were further divided by social class of father, although as would be expected there was a predominance of children with fathers in social classes 1 and 2.

Fig. 1 shows the mean weights, from birth to 2 years, of selected premature infants who were $4\frac{1}{2}$ lb. or less at birth, those who were between $4\frac{1}{2}$ and $5\frac{1}{2}$ lb. at birth, and the total control group of maturely born infants. By the age of 2 years the smallest singleton premature infants, both male and female, are only 14 oz. below the mean weight of

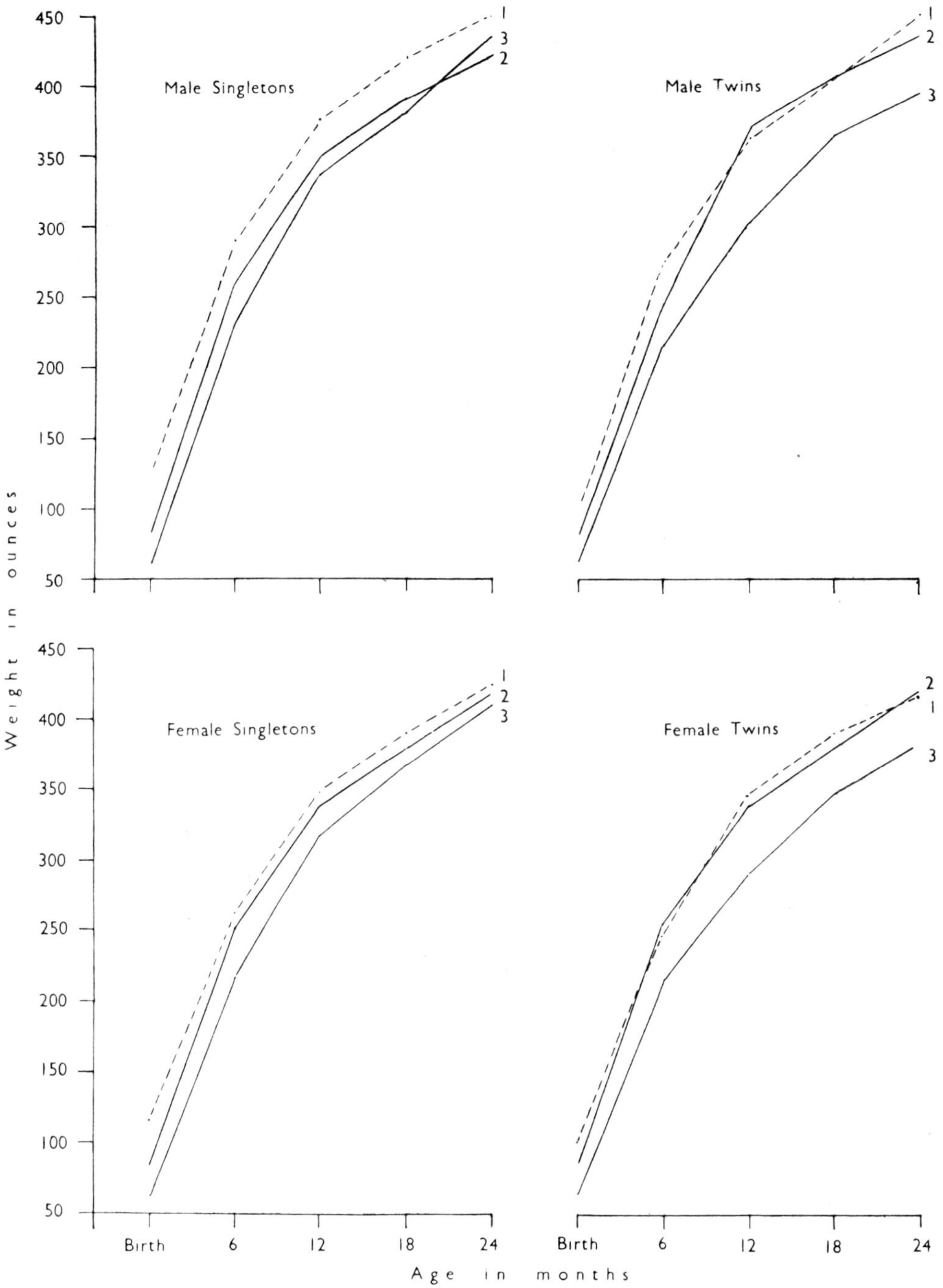

FIG. 1.—Mean weights of selected prematurely born children and mature controls. 1. Mature controls. 2. Premature: birth weight 4 lb. 9 oz. to 5 lb. 8 oz. 3. Premature: birth weight 4 lb. 8 oz. or less.

the mature controls, the differences at birth being 65 oz. for males and 55 oz. for females. However, in twin births those who were smallest at birth, even when given the best environmental conditions, are still substantially behind the control group who were over 5½ lb. at birth, although those with a birth weight between 4½ and 5½ lb. have caught up with the control group.

In height, the selected prematurely born are very little behind the control group at 2 years except for twins who were less than 4½ lb. at birth, who show little reduction in their initial height handicap.

No significant correlation was found between length of gestation and 2-year weight increment. It might be expected that small babies born at term, often to mothers of small stature, would show a smaller weight gain after birth, but this was not obvious at 2 years. Douglas and Mogford (1953) also found no relationship between weight gain and gestation time.

In addition to the social factors already considered, one would expect growth to be influenced by genetic factors. In each case the height of the parents was recorded and those data included in the subsequent analysis.

Correlation and Regression Analysis

Tables 12 and 13 give the first order correlation coefficients between weight and height increments at 2 years and the following factors: mother's height, father's height, frequency of illness, the seven grades of illness frequency being used in this analysis, diet, maternal efficiency and social class of father. Two factors (mother's height and father's height) are presumably mainly genetic, and four (illness, diet, maternal efficiency and social class) are primarily environmental. The separation is not absolute. Heights of the parents will depend to some extent on diets in their own youth, and so will be partly socially conditioned. It was shown in a previous study, including these same women (Drillien, 1957), that mothers of premature babies are, on the whole, significantly shorter than mothers of mature controls and that average height was related to the woman's environment during childhood. The correlations will be reduced by imperfections in the assessment or measurement of the factor concerned. This is likely to affect in particular the social factors of diet and maternal efficiency which could only be approximately specified. The heights of mothers were recorded accurately during their stay in hospital, but a record of father's height was obtained by enquiry and is therefore less reliable. The correlation coefficients found may therefore be regarded as minimal and the true values, if they could be observed, would in general

TABLE 12

FIRST ORDER CORRELATION COEFFICIENTS BETWEEN WEIGHT INCREMENT AT TWO YEARS AND VARIOUS FACTORS

	Premature Singleton		Twins		Mature Singleton	
	Male	Female	Male	Female	Male	Female
No. of Cases	111	103	99	92	55	49
Weight Increment and:						
Mother's height	·1837	·4416	·2801	·3840	−·0162	·2966
Father's height	·2456	·3692	·2732	·3769	·3138	·2055
Illness	−·2368	−·3114	−·2830	−·3654	−·1446	−·2325
Diet	−·1482	−·3952	−·1974	−·3072	−·0771	−·2233
Mother's efficiency	−·1526	−·2905	−·2755	−·2942	·0790	−·1725
Father's social class	−·2011	−·2279	−·1234	−·2255	−·1601	−·2708
Baby's birth weight	−·1089	−·1064	·1408	·1572	−·0092	·1238
Minimum value for significance at 5% point	·1867	·1939	·1978	·2053	·2656	·2815

TABLE 13

FIRST ORDER CORRELATION COEFFICIENTS BETWEEN LENGTH INCREMENT AT TWO YEARS AND VARIOUS FACTORS

	Premature Singleton		Twins		Mature Singleton	
	Male	Female	Male	Female	Male	Female
No. of Cases	109	102	98	90	54	48
Length Increment and:						
Mother's height	·2890	·3777	·3082	·1702	·5020	·4504
Father's height	·3045	·3423	·1567	·2350	·3106	·3229
Illnesss	−·2345	−·1549	−·2215	−·2272	−·3439	·0592
Diet	−·1414	−·2336	−·2132	−·0708	−·0533	−·3196
Mother's efficiency	−·2354	−·1941	−·2999	−·2097	−·1764	−·1959
Father's social class	−·2045	−·1361	−·1621	−·2404	−·2537	−·1233
Baby's birth weight	−·2616	−·2816	−·3335	−·1890	−·1983	−·1118
Minimum value for significance at 5% point	·1884	·1949	·1988	·2706	·2680	·2845

be higher. Tables 12 and 13 indicate that the correlations between weight and length increments, and the genetic factors are comparable in magnitude to those with the social factors. In the premature and twin groups there is good concordance, the differences observed being within the expected range of random fluctuation. Not all the individual coefficients are statistically significant, but joint tests combining the four groups of male and female prematures and twins, show that the overall significance is beyond question for each of the separate genetic and social factors. As noted previously, the prematurely born singletons show a negative correlation between birth weight and weight increment, whilst the twins show a positive correlation indicating that there is a tendency for the singleton prematures to reduce their initial weight handicap by 2 years, though in the case of twins the reverse applies. However, in no case is the correlation coefficient significant at the 5% point. When height increment is considered, a negative correlation between length at birth and height at 2 years is found for all groups of singletons and twins, and taken together these findings are statistically significant. In the mature groups numbers are smaller and the significance of results thereby lowered.

In general, social factors appear to be relatively less important and genetic factors more so in those mature at birth. Of the social factors studied, frequency of illness gives the highest and most consistent correlations in the premature and twin groups. This is no doubt due to the fact that greater accuracy was possible in recording these data than for the other social factors, except for social class which *per se* seems of least importance in determining rate of growth. The various social and genetic criteria are not independent of one another. To disentangle the relative contributions of the different factors, extensive use has been made of the techniques of multiple correlation and regression analysis. For this it was necessary first to find the correlation of each of the factors employed with all the others. Table 14 gives these correlations and levels of significance.

Mother's height is quite highly correlated with father's height in each group, indicating a fairly high degree of assortative mating. Parental heights are also correlated significantly with all the social factors excepting frequency of illness. Frequency of illness is correlated with diet, social class and maternal efficiency, the last correlation, about ·5, being very high. Diet is correlated highly with social class and very highly with maternal efficiency, the values being about ·45 and ·75. Many multiple regressions were computed relating weight and length increment to various combinations of the genetic and social factors listed in Tables 12 and 13. In general, a combination consisting of mother's height (M), father's height (F) and one or two of the social factors will give significant, or near significant, regression coefficients for all factors included, but the most significant social factor varies in the different groups of infants. This is not surprising, for, as Table 14 shows, all social factors are quite highly intercorrelated among themselves. Each one is a more or less adequate partial measure of the others. The social factor which most often gave

TABLE 14

CORRELATION COEFFICIENTS BETWEEN THE VARIOUS GENETIC AND SOCIAL FACTORS EMPLOYED IN THE ANALYSIS

	Premature Singletons		Twins		Mature Singletons	
	Male	Female	Male	Female	Male	Female
No. of Cases	111	103	99	92	55	49
Mother's Height and:						
Father's height	·2581	·5093	·4392	·3809	·2321	·4958
Illness	—·0404	—·1390	—·1303	—·1930	—·0384	—·0633
Diet	—·2070	—·2236	—·2713	—·3595	—·0554	—·2399
Mother's efficiency	—·1718	—·2888	—·2991	—·3175	—·2510	—·2048
Father's social class	—·2079	—·2232	—·1760	—·2740	—·2218	—·1107
Father's Height and:						
Illness	—·0350	—·0857	—·1783	—·2693	—·0402	—·3512
Diet	—·2008	—·2036	—·4063	—·3670	—·1472	—·2260
Mother's efficiency	—·1610	—·1968	—·3466	—·4195	—·1122	—·2983
Father's social class	—·1867	—·2006	—·3504	—·2447	—·1337	—·2722
Illness and:						
Diet	·2405	·4263	·3894	·4656	·4500	·5404
Mother's efficiency	·5335	·4962	·5204	·4414	·4483	·4962
Father's social class	·2657	·2837	·3136	·1251	·3305	·5275
Diet and:						
Mother's efficiency	·7676	·7210	·7805	·8362	·7464	·7201
Father's social class	·5291	·3745	·4603	·4673	·3965	·4188
Mother's efficiency and:						
Father's social class	·5369	·4142	·5275	·5342	·4432	·5344
Minimum value for significance at 5% point	·1867	·1939	·1978	·2053	·2656	·2815

the highest regression coefficient, in combination with parental heights, was frequency of illness (I). The regression coefficient for the combination of three factors, M, F and I, is shown in Table 15. Column 1 shows the regression coefficients when all variates are scaled so that the standard deviations are unity. These are strictly comparable with the correlation coefficients set out in Tables 12 and 13, and indicate what the correlation between weight or length increment and the particular factor would be if the other factors were held constant. Column 2 gives the F tests of significance for these coefficients. A figure of 4 or more indicates significance at the 5% level. Column 3 gives regression coefficients in terms of the actual measurement. These figures give the average excess weight increment in ounces, or height increment in centimetres, per inch extra height in mother or father, and per unit decrease in the grading scale for illness. In weight one would expect an increased increment of about 4 oz. for every extra inch in mother's height, 3 oz. for each extra inch in father's height and ½ lb. decrease in weight increment for each increase in illness frequency grading from one to seven.

The standard deviation for maternal height is about 2·4 inches and for paternal height about 2·9 inches, the range of mother's height being 10 inches, and 12 inches for fathers (i.e., 95% of the heights are included in the range mean height ± 2 S.D.). Therefore one would expect a difference in weight increment at 2 years of about 40 oz. between children of the shortest and tallest mothers, rather less between the children of the shortest and tallest fathers, and 3½ lb. between those in the lowest and highest illness frequency grades. Similarly in height, one would expect an increased increment of about ·7 cm. for every extra inch in mother's height, ·4 cm. for every extra inch in father's height, and 1 cm. decrease in height increment for each increase in illness grade.

In spite of the inevitable fortuitous variation between the comparable coefficients there is a consistent picture. Whether for weight or height increment the primarily genetic factors (M and F) and the representative environmental factor (I) have a significant influence when the other type of factor has been fully taken into account. Perhaps the best way of expressing this is to work out the partial multiple correlation coefficients as shown in Table 16. These give the multiple correlations between weight or length increment and (1) Mothers' and fathers' heights, when all social factors are held constant. (2) Social factors (illness, diet and maternal efficiency), when parental heights are held constant.

It is evident that these partial coefficients are comparable in magnitude, with the genetic coefficients on the whole rather higher. Considering that parental heights themselves contain a social component and that the correlations with social factors are more likely to be attenuated by unavoid-

TABLE 16

PARTIAL MULTIPLE CORRELATION COEFFICIENTS

	Singleton Premature		Twins	
	Male	Female	Male	Female
Weight Increment and:				
Parental heights*	·2601	·4359	·2683	·3665
Social factors†	·2484	·3846	·2584	·2811
Length Increment and:				
Parental heights*	·3697	·3792	·2500	·1896
Social factors†	·2581	·1602	·2530	·2990

* Parental heights held constant † Social factors held constant.

TABLE 15

COEFFICIENTS FOR MULTIPLE REGRESSION OF WEIGHT OR LENGTH INCREMENT ON PARENTAL HEIGHT AND FREQUENCY OF ILLNESS

	1 Regression Coefficients in Standard Measure (partial Correlations)			2 F Values for Regression Coefficients			3 Regression Coefficients in Units of Measurement (Increment per inch height)		3 (Increment per illness grade)
	M	F	I	M	F	I	M	F	I
				Weight Increment at 2 Years (oz.)					
Premature Singletons:									
Males	·1214	·2065	-·2247	1·682	4·868	6·166	2·2333	3·1556	-8·6743
Females	·3099	·1898	-·2520	9·731	3·695	8·626	5·4279	2·9282	-11·7322
Twins:									
Males	·1834	·1513	-·2321	3·053	2·047	5·866	3·1632	2·5719	-8·7757
Females	·2538	·2102	-·2598	6·584	4·352	7·487	4·0116	2·8555	-8·6260
				Length Increment at 2 Years (cm.)					
Premature Singletons:									
Males	·2271	·2452	-·2253	6·330	7·379	6·604	·7055	·6272	-1·4576
Females	·2608	·2004	-·0994	5·942	3·558	1·159	·8629	·5806	-·8702
Twins:									
Males	·2868	-·0013	-·1885	7·179	·0002	3·718	·9597	-·0043	-1·3884
Females	·0764	·1581	-·1637	·469	1·916	2·269	·2394	·4264	-1·0809

able inaccuracy of the assessments, it may be fairly concluded that in the groups studied genetic and environmental factors are of approximately equal importance in their influence on growth, whether measured by weight or by length increment during the first 2 years.

In few studies of the growth of prematurely born children has attention been paid to social background. Hess, Mohr and Bartelme (1934), using a control group of siblings, found that prematurely born boys had caught up in weight and height by 3 years, and girls somewhat earlier, except for those who were less than $3\frac{1}{4}$ lb. at birth. They point out that these children were all specially supervised from birth unlike the control group. Thirty per cent of their premature sample were first born and had no controls. Douglas and Mogford (1953) found that their premature group were lighter and shorter than their controls at 4 years. The mothers of those prematures who caught up or surpassed the controls by 4 years were taller and heavier than the mothers of those who failed to catch up. They conclude that the height of the mother gives the best indication of the likely growth pattern of her premature baby and that the small size of certain prematurely born children is genetically determined.

Summary

A statistical analysis is presented of a study of physical growth, in the first 2 years of life, in a group of 600 premature and maturely born children, including 200 twin births. The following conclusions were reached:

Throughout the 2-year period mean weights are closely related to mean birth weight. The smallest prematurely born singletons show a small increase in weight increment at 2 years. The smallest twins show a smaller weight increment, but neither finding is statistically significant.

In height, those largest at birth maintain their height superiority at 2 years, but there is a significant excess height increment in those smallest at birth.

Boys show a greater weight increment at 2 years than girls. There is little difference between the sexes in height increment.

Rate of growth whether measured by weight or height increment is affected by certain environmental factors. Substantially higher increments are recorded when maternal efficiency and diet are considered to be good, and frequency of illness is minimal. Environmental factors appear to exert a more marked influence on growth in the prematurely born than in the mature controls. In all premature groups there is a striking excess of inefficient mothers, poor diet and frequent illness.

Prematurely born singletons reared in the most favourable environmental conditions have very nearly caught up with the mature group in both weight and height by 2 years. This applies also to twins who were over $4\frac{1}{2}$ lb. at birth, the smaller twins still being substantially behind the control group.

Genetic factors as deduced from parental heights also have an influence on rate of growth. Genetic and environmental factors were intercorrelated to quite a high degree. Using the technique of correlation and regression analysis it was found that genetic and environmental factors are of approximately equal importance in their influence on growth whether measured by weight or height increment at 2 years.

It is a pleasure to thank my secretary and research assistant, Miss A. E. Moore, Dr. Barnet Woolf who gave advice on the statistical analysis and Professor R. W. B. Ellis for his interest and encouragement throughout.

This research programme is being supported by a grant from the Scottish Hospital Endowments Research Trust.

References

Douglas, J. W. B. and Mogford, C. (1953). *Arch. Dis. Childh.*, **28**, 436.

Drillien, C. M. (1957). *J. Obstet. Gynaec. Brit. Emp.*, **64**, 161.

—— (1958). *Arch. Dis. Childh.*, **33**, 417.

Falkner, F. (1958). *Ibid.*, **33**, 1.

Hess, J. H., Mohr, G. J. and Bartelme, P. F. (1934). *The Physical and Mental Growth of Prematurely Born Children.* Chicago.

Lowe, C. R. and Gibson, J. R. (1953). *Brit. J. prev. soc. Med.*, **7**, 78.

PANCREATITIS IN YOUNG CHILDREN

BY

J. COLLINS

From the Roan Antelope Copper Mines, Luanshya, N. Rhodesia

(RECEIVED FOR PUBLICATION FEBRUARY 7, 1958)

Pancreatitis is rare in very young children and the medical literature contains comparatively few accounts of the associated pathology. The purpose of this paper is to describe the findings in the pancreas in four cases in which disease of this gland was discovered at autopsy and to discuss the pathogenesis of the condition. Three of the children concerned were Bantu of N. Rhodesia and were the only ones found to have pancreatitis in the routine examination of material from 100 consecutive autopsies on African children. The fourth child, included for comparison, was an Edinburgh girl and the only case of pancreatitis in the records of 1,812 consecutive post-mortem examinations conducted during the five years 1952-56 by the staff of the Pathology Department of the Royal Hospital for Sick Children, Edinburgh.

Case Histories

Case 1. A female Bantu child, aged 18 months and weighing 13 lb. 4 oz., was admitted to the African Hospital, Luanshya, where she was found to have bronchopneumonia, diarrhoea and vomiting (of several days' duration) with marked dehydration and kwashiorkor of moderate severity. She responded well to treatment but relapsed on the eighth day with further vomiting and diarrhoea for which she again required parenteral fluids. Soon after resuming oral feeding she suddenly collapsed and died in less than three hours. At necropsy the typical appearance of an acute haemorrhagic pancreatitis was found with haemorrhage extending for a considerable distance in the retro-peritoneal tissues both proximally and distally to the pancreas. Fat necrosis was not obvious and no abnormality was present in gall bladder, bile ducts or the terminal portion of the main pancreatic duct. On microscopical examination of the pancreas, the most striking changes were in the interlobular ducts most of which were dilated, some to a remarkable extent, while many contained eosinophilic material which had completely occluded the lumen. This material had often a distinctly laminated appearance and was sufficiently soft to be readily cut by the microtome knife, although tearing of the tissues in the immediate vicinity had occurred in some instances (Fig. 1). The epithelium lining some of these occluded ducts was unusually tall and columnar, and was occasionally more than one cell layer in thickness, but squamous metaplasia was not present in any of numerous sections examined.

In a few ducts rupture of the wall had occurred with herniation of the contents and in these situations there was a varying degree of round cell infiltration, many of the cells being polymorphs, but elsewhere the dilated and occluded ducts did not appear to have excited any significant reaction, only a very few lymphocytes being found in their walls and immediate surroundings. The main pancreatic duct was normal.

Haemorrhage, although widespread, was confined

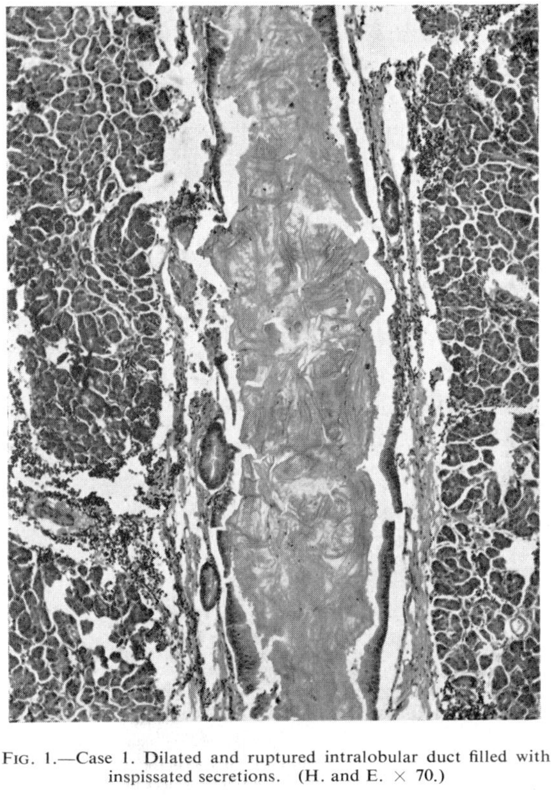

FIG. 1.—Case 1. Dilated and ruptured intralobular duct filled with inspissated secretions. (H. and E. × 70.)

mainly to the interlobular septa and the external pancreatic surface, where too the early changes of fat necrosis were present. The walls of a few vessels close to ruptured ducts showed the partial necrosis described by Rich and Duff (1936).

Apart from a few small foci of necrosis near ruptured ducts, the gland parenchyma and islets of Langerhans showed no abnormality except in one area where there had been former destruction and healing by fibrosis was occurring (Fig. 2) and in which the remains of ducts and eosinophilic material could, with difficulty, be distinguished.

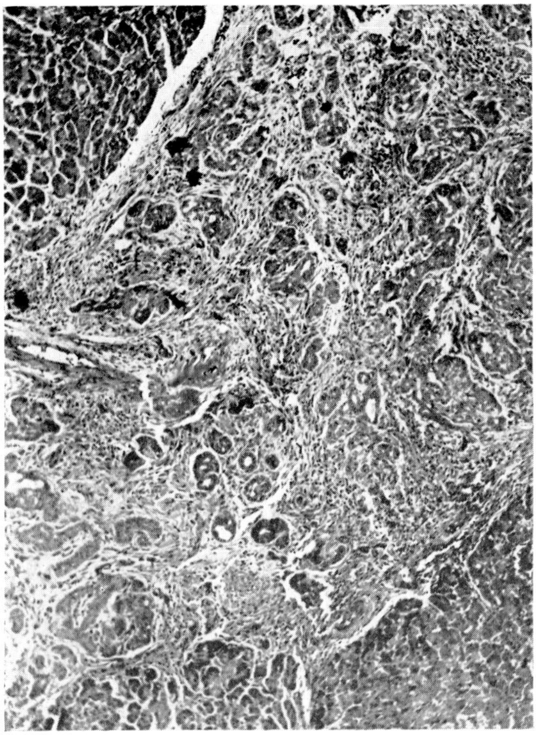

FIG. 2.—Case 1. Healing by fibrosis of an area of former destruction (H. and E. × 70.)

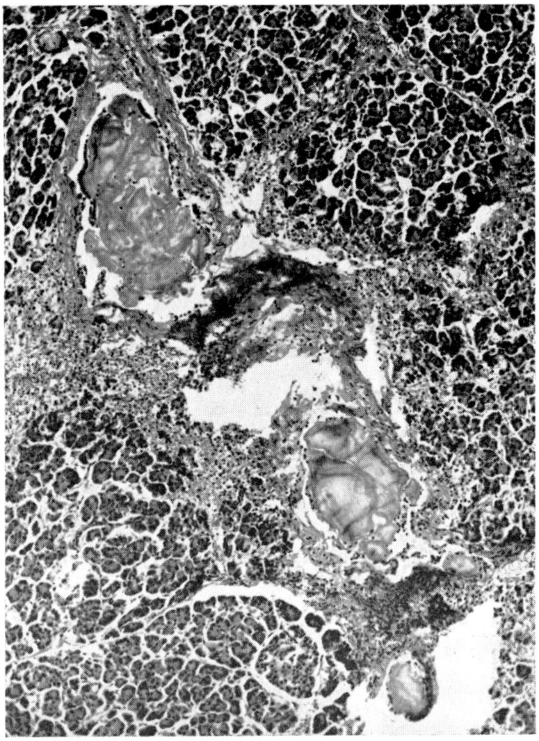

FIG. 3.—Case 2. Dilated and ruptured intralobular duct filled with inspissated secretions. (H. and E. × 70.)

Case 2. (71/53. Edinburgh). She was aged 2 years 9 months, and was under treatment for scalds involving 30% of the body surface. After some initial difficulty she had responded satisfactorily for 10 days; she then suddenly developed abdominal distension and vomiting, became shocked and collapsed, and, in spite of all attempts to improve her condition, died in 48 hours. Her previous history included hospitalization at 6, 9 and 14 months of age for persistent vomiting for which no cause was discovered. At autopsy an extensive pneumonia was present and some excess of free fluid in the abdomen. The pancreas appeared normal, but microscopic examination revealed an acute haemorrhagic pancreatitis, very similar in appearance to that of Case 1, but with less haemorrhage. The interlobular ducts were dilated and occluded by eosinophilic, laminated material (Fig. 3) and some had ruptured, but the duct epithelium showed neither hyperplasia nor metaplasia.

Case 3. A Bantu girl, aged 2 years and weighing 14 lb. 4 oz., was admitted to hospital at Luanshya with a history of convulsions for 24 hours and diarrhoea and vomiting for six or seven days. She was unconscious, very dehydrated, had a severe pneumonia with marked respiratory distress and died shortly after admission. At autopsy a confluent bronchopneumonia was found with numerous pin-head-size abscesses, subsequently shown to be staphylococcal in origin. There was no meningitis. The pancreas appeared unduly pink, but no actual haemorrhage was noted and no abnormality of the gall bladder, bile ducts or the terminal portion of the main pancreatic duct. Microscopically sections from the body of the pancreas showed many dilated interlobular ducts occluded by eosinophilic material similar in all respects to that already described. Some of these ducts had ruptured with partial herniation of contents, and in these areas round cell infiltration was evident (Fig. 4). The duct epithelium was of normal appearance as was the main pancreatic duct. In a few areas some dilatation of pancreatic acini and ducts was present without duct occlusion being found.

Case 4. A Bantu girl, aged 2 years and weighing 18 lb., was admitted to the African Hospital, Luanshya, with bronchopneumonia, moderately advanced kwashiorkor with oedema of the feet and legs and some areas of skin exfoliation, and also severe gastro-enteritis. After initial improvement she developed thrombocytopenic purpura and rapidly succumbed to intestinal haemorrhage.

At autopsy the presence of bronchopneumonia, purpura and intestinal haemorrhage was confirmed, but the pancreas appeared to be normal. Microscopically sections of the lungs showed a giant-cell pneumonia. Sections of the body of the pancreas showed a small, completely disorganized area, with foci of necrosis surrounded by dilated and partly necrotic acini. Early fibroblastic proliferation was present and a patchy round cell infiltration. A few severely damaged ducts were recognizable and seemed to be occluded by eosinophilic material. Staining with P.A.S. simplified recognition of these ducts and one is shown in Fig. 5.

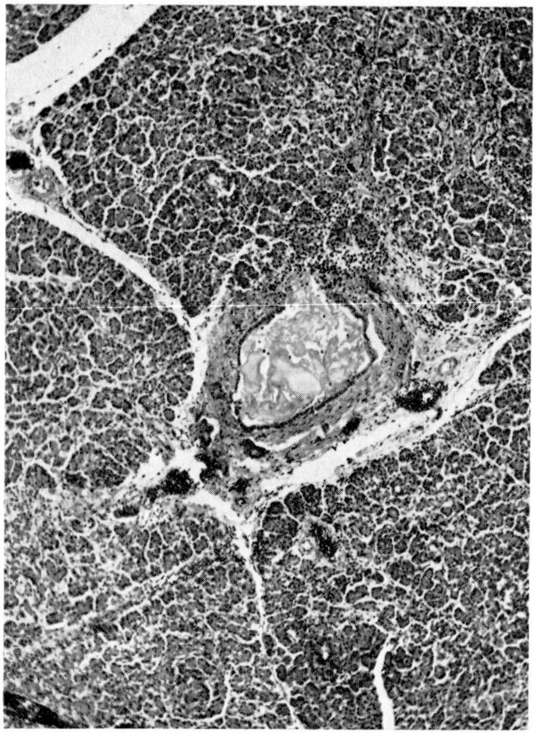

FIG. 4.—Case 3. Dilated and ruptured intralobular duct filled with inspissated secretions. (H. and E. × 70.)

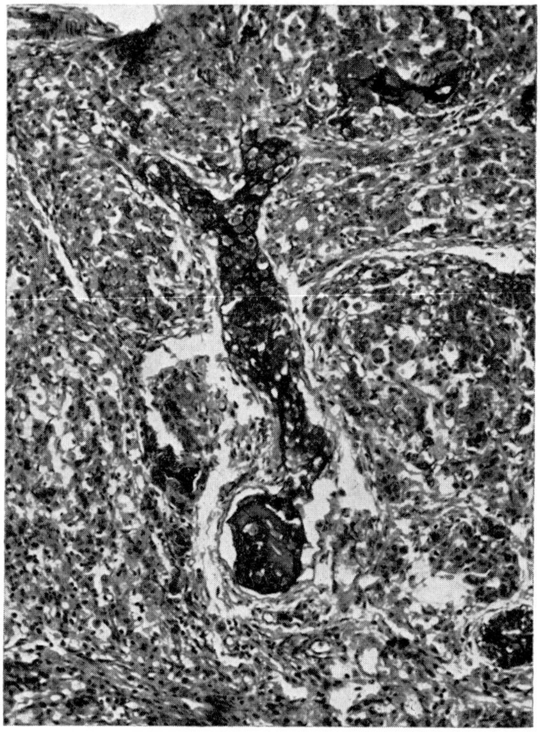

FIG. 5.—Case 4. Severely damaged duct, filled with inspissated secretion, in area of destruction. (P.A.S. × 120.)

Comment

The pathology in Cases 1 and 2 was that of a typical acute haemorrhagic pancreatitis, while that in Case 3 was of lesser severity. In the pancreas of Case 1, however, there was also a small scarred area from a previous incident, not yet completely healed, and Case 4 showed the picture of a similar area at a much earlier stage.

In the first two cases, death was due to the pancreatic condition and this too may have contributed to the fatal outcome in the third, although the pneumonia alone was sufficient to have caused the death of the child. The very small focus of healing pancreatic damage found in Case 4 cannot be regarded as other than an incidental finding.

Discussion

Our knowledge of the pathogenesis of acute haemorrhagic pancreatitis was considerably extended by the work of Rich and Duff (1936) and since that date many others have stressed the importance of the mechanical factor in the initiation of this condition. In Rich and Duff's series of cases this factor was duct occlusion caused by epithelial hyperplasia and metaplasia, but they also mention three cases in which inspissated secretions, staining irregularly with eosin, were present and which were sometimes associated with inflammatory signs in the walls of the affected ducts.

More recently, Wainwright (1951) found, in the routine examination of material from 2,500 autopsies on persons over 25 years of age, four instances in which inspissated material alone was present in pancreatic interlobular ducts and 81 others in which it was associated with duct epithelial hyperplasia; he suggested that the presence of this material could contribute to duct obstruction. As there can be little doubt that the intraductal material in the four cases presented here did in fact cause duct obstruction it seems worthwhile to discuss the nature and probable cause of these eosinophilic plugs.

In these four cases, the absence of any significant tissue reaction in the vicinity of affected ducts, except where rupture has occurred, and the general similarity of the appearance of the intraductal material to that found in cases of fibrocystic disease of the pancreas, seems to confirm that these eosinophilic plugs are in fact inspissated secretions; moreover their somewhat laminated appearance points to formation over a period of time with enlargement occurring at intervals.

Andersen (1938), referring to similar material, believed that its formation was due to a disturbance of the autonomous nervous stimulation of glandular pancreatic secretion and Baggenstoss (1948) thought that such inspissation could be caused by vagal stimulation, dehydration and possibly malnutrition, especially protein deficiency.

That vagal stimulation does result in the formation of an unnaturally thick and viscid pancreatic juice, rich in enzymes, is a known physiological fact but that protein deficiency can exert a similar effect must be regarded as doubtful, for in kwashiorkor, a disease of protein deficiency the pathology of which has been extensively studied, inspissated pancreatic secretions are very infrequently found (Trowell, Davies and Dean, 1954) and the main pancreatic lesion is a loss of zymogen granules and collapse of the acinar cells (Davies, 1948), a condition hardly compatible with the production of viscid secretion.

The formation of these plugs may be connected with dehydration as the presence of slightly dilated ducts filled with eosinophilic secretions is a common finding in children and others dying in a dehydrated state (Bodian, 1952). Fig. 6 shows a portion of pancreas from such a case and it is possible that in certain circumstances such pools of secretion may become inspissated and form pancreatic ductal obstructions.

In Central Africa, dehydration in children is most often the result of diarrhoea and vomiting which, at certain seasons of the year, is so widespread that most young African children are affected and many at such frequent intervals that the weights recorded for Cases 1, 3 and 4 are by no means unusual. Since vomiting and diarrhoea may be expected to give rise to vagal stimulation as well as dehydration, the combination of these factors should result in the formation of an abnormally viscid pancreatic secretion. Furthermore, children suffering severely from diarrhoea and vomiting usually refuse all food, and few African mothers in such circumstances would make any effort to coax them to take anything other than perhaps a little water, thereby removing any stimulus for the pancreas to commence the production of more normal secretions to wash out the unnaturally thick and viscid material present in the ducts.

It seems reasonable to assume that if such a state of affairs continued over a period of days, as it

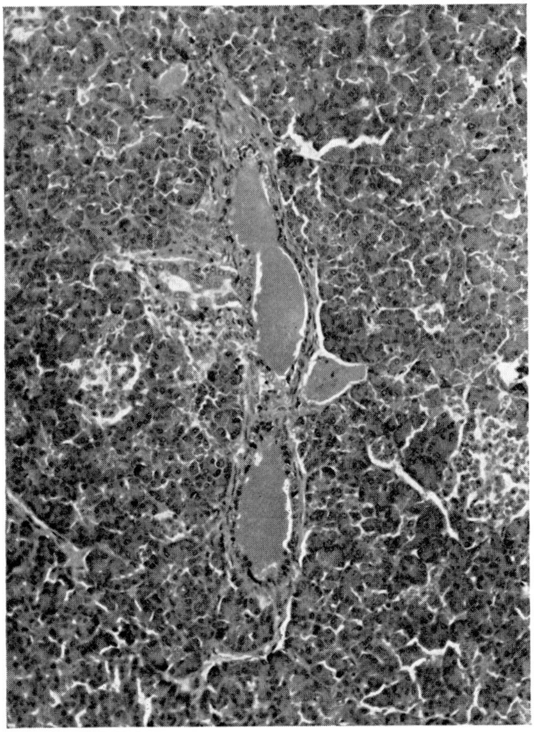

FIG. 6.—Pooled secretions in intralobular duct of a child dying from gastro-enteritis and dehydration. (H. and E. × 120.)

frequently does, inspissation would occur and the seed be sown for future pancreatic damage.

Once inspissation is present it is probable that further deposition would follow, as occurs for example in the case of renal calculi, particularly on any fresh occurrence of similar circumstances, so giving rise to the laminated appearance of the deposit as well as the dilatation and finally obstruction of the affected ducts.

Such a mechanism could account for the occluded ducts found in all three Bantu cases and probably too for those in the Edinburgh child, whose early history contains episodes of persistent vomiting requiring admission to hospital on three occasions. It is also probable that in the latter case her scalds gave rise to some degree of dehydration, as well as vagal stimulation, which may have added to inspissations already present.

Once duct obstruction has occurred rupture is probably inevitable sooner or later, but that the resulting pancreatitis can be confined to a very small area is illustrated in Cases 1 and 4 and the detection of such minute lesions on naked eye examination may be impossible.

If this theory of the cause of these intraductal obstructions is correct then, apart from the normal procedures to remedy dehydration, other measures to overcome vagal stimulation (where this is present) and to encourage normal pancreatic secretions are indicated in all very young sick children.

Summary

The pathology in four cases of pancreatitis in children is described and illustrated.

In each instance inspissated secretions had caused the dilatation, obstruction and subsequent rupture of intralobular ducts and in two cases the resulting pancreatitis had been confined to a very small area and was undergoing healing by fibrosis.

It is suggested that this inspissation is brought about by a combination of vagal stimulation, dehydration and the absence of normal pancreatic secretions over a period of time probably measured in days.

My thanks are due to Dr. A. C. Fisher, O.B.E., Chief Medical Officer of the Roan Antelope Copper Mines Ltd., for permission to publish this paper; Dr. Agnes R. Macgregor, Consulting Pathologist to the Royal Hospital for Sick Children, Edinburgh, for access to her records and the material for Case 2; Dr. R. F. Ogilvie, Consulting Pathologist, Royal Infirmary, Edinburgh, for much helpful advice and to Mr. T. C. Dodds, of the Medical Photographic Unit, University of Edinburgh, for the photographs.

REFERENCES

Andersen, D. H. (1938). *Amer. J. Dis. Child.*, **56**, 344.
Baggenstoss, A. H. (1948). *Arch. Path. (Chicago)*, **45**, 463.
Bodian, M. (1952). *Fibrocystic Disease of the Pancreas*. London.
Davies, J. N. P. (1948). *Lancet*, **1**, 317.
Rich, A. R. and Duff, G. L. (1936). *Bull. Johns Hopk. Hosp.*, **58**, 212.
Trowell, H. C., Davies, J. N. P. and Dean, R. F. A. (1954). *Kwashiorkor*, p. 148. London.
Wainwright, C. W. (1951). *New Engl. J. Med.*, **244**, 161.

HERPES ZOSTER OPHTHALMICUS IN CHILDREN

BY

S. M. TUCKER*

From St. Andrew's Hospital, Bow, London

(RECEIVED FOR PUBLICATION JANUARY 30, 1958)

Herpes zoster ophthalmicus, first described fully by Jonathan Hutchinson in 1866, is very rare in children, being predominantly an adult affection (Doggart, 1933; Björk, 1950; Duke-Elder, 1952). Koch (1939), in reporting a case in a child of 5½ years of age, states that only one other child, aged 12, developed zoster ophthalmicus at the Mayo Clinic before 1938. In a fairly exhaustive analysis of the literature by Poulsen (1955) only 17 cases had been reported in children, three of whom had the disease within the first year of life. Poulsen adds his own contribution, that of a boy of 15 months. Several standard text books (Mitchell Nelson, 1954; Cecil and Loeb, 1951; Price, 1956) make little or no mention of herpes zoster ophthalmicus in infants and children.

Edgerton (1945), in a detailed analysis of herpes zoster ophthalmicus, found about 2,250 cases in the world literature. The average age of these cases was 43 years. He could only find 44 cases under 13 years of age, but did not attempt to differentiate between the epidemic or symptomatic forms. He does, however, state that in the vast majority of cases of ophthalmic zoster, the disease was secondary or symptomatic.

In view of the great deal of evidence which has accumulated recently linking the virus of herpes with that of chickenpox (Bokay, 1909; Brain, 1933; Amies 1934; Weller, 1953; Simpson, 1954; Blank and Rake, 1955) it is surprising to find so few authenticated cases of herpes zoster in children, while chickenpox is such a common and highly infectious exanthema. Chickenpox has its maximum incidence in childhood, whereas herpes is more commonly observed from the ages of 20 to 65 years. Edgerton (1945), on the other hand, quotes Evans and Fox (1905) as saying that herpes zoster ophthalmicus was common in the young. They state that one half of their patients were under 14 years of age. Cases of ophthalmic zoster in children have been reported by other authors as well, but few detailed descriptions can be found in the British literature. Roll (1920), presenting the case of a child of 3 years, commented on the unusually early age for such a condition.

The following typical case appears to be one of the few documented cases in the British literature of epidemic herpes zoster ophthalmicus affecting the first division of the trigeminal nerve in a child.

Case History

D.T., a boy aged 6 years, admitted on July 17, 1956, was the fourth child of healthy parents. He had a normal infancy except for frequent bouts of tonsillitis from the age of 2 years which usually improved without treatment. Tonsillectomy was finally resorted to during June, 1955. He also had a bout of diarrhoea earlier in 1955 but this was very mild. He had mumps, measles and whooping cough during infancy and chickenpox in 1952. Three of the other four children had all had chickenpox many years previously and none of them had had herpes zoster at any time. There was no recent history of having been in contact with herpes or chickenpox.

The boy's present illness began four days before admission to hospital, when his main complaints were of abdominal pain and headache. He was kept in bed and observed.

Three days before admission, he began to complain of pain over his left eye associated with mild photophobia. For the following three days he was pyrexial with a temperature range of 99°-100°F., vomited on a few occasions and still complained of abdominal pain and headaches. The pain over his left eye had now become more acute and the child was subsequently admitted for investigation.

On examination his general condition was good but the temperature was raised to 99°F. He was reluctant to eat and vomited up what was offered to him. His frontal headache was most painful at this stage but again there were no abnormal findings in any of the other systems. Careful daily examination did not reveal any rash or other abnormal physical findings but on the child's fourth day in hospital a mild conjunctivitis of the left eye was noted with some erythema around the eye. No oedema was present. There was no evidence of any vesicle formation.

On July 21, 1956, a classical cutaneous zoster affecting the ophthalmic branch of the left trigeminal nerve was observed which included the nasociliary branch on that

* Present address, Middlesex Hospital, London.

side (Fig. 1). The vesicles extended only to the midline and involved the left side of the forehead, both upper and lower eyelids, the left eyebrow, and the root of the nose on the left together with the bridge and the tip. Many of the vesicles had broken down. The left eye was now inflamed and swollen and the upper lid overrode the lower as the eye became closed. Conjunctivitis and iritis were also present. The pupil was inactive but the fundi and discs were normal. The vessels appeared engorged. Diffuse corneal oedema was also present with some impairment of sensation. The tension of the eye appeared normal. Two other vesicles were seen elsewhere on the trunk.

On July 22 the herpetic dermatitis had become infected and left keratitis was noted. Atropine 1% eye drops were instilled into the affected eye and aureomycin 1% ointment applied to the infected vesicles. The temperature had now risen to 103°F. and the child was extremely ill. Left pre-auricular adenopathy was present. The temperature remained high until July 25, when the ophthalmologist reported that iridocyclitis with punctate keratitis was present. It was decided to continue with atropine, and cortisone drops were added four-hourly.

Within a few days the temperature subsided to normal and the child appeared much happier. He began taking food adequately for the first time since the onset of his illness. The cutaneous herpes had improved considerably but it was noted that the hair on the left side of the head, at the upper limit of the ophthalmic division, had thinned considerably. The right eye remained normal throughout.

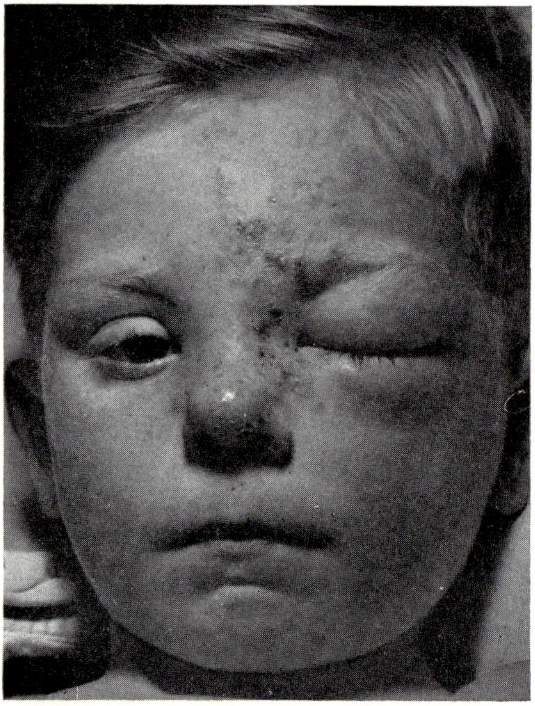

FIG. 1.

Progress continued and on August 1 the left eye was still mildly inflamed but the chemosis was distinctly less; there was marked ciliary injection and the cornea was very hazy. Typical deep spots were seen in the corneal stroma. Considerable punctate keratitis was present. The pupil was small and was not fully dilated on atropine.

On August 10 keratitis was still present. The eye had become whiter and the pupil was still not fully dilated. The corneal ulcers no longer stained up on fluoroscopy, but characteristic deep white spots were seen in the corneal stroma. Photophobia remained intense.

On August 14 the eye was a little improved, the pupil was wider and there were extensive central nebulae. No corneal sensation was detected. The chemosis and swelling had by this time completely resolved but the herpetiform scars were still evident. The hair was sparse on top but the rash had cleared up.

On September 26, about five weeks later, the cornea showed a ground glass appearance with a few deep residual corneal spots. One month later this had cleared and the corneal haze was noted to be gradually disappearing. No posterior synechiae were present.

In November, 1956, residual corneal dot opacities were still present. Vision in the left eye was only 6/60. The left pupil had now become eccentric. The hair on the forehead had begun to grow again but was still not normal.

Vision improved as the months went by and was found to be 6/36 in the left eye by February, 1957.

He was last seen in June, 1957, one year after the initial infection, when he was found to have supraorbital scarring, normal hair growth of the left forehead, and an eccentric left pupil. Vision had now improved to 6/9. He had been very well in himself for the past few months and had resumed schooling. Sensation in the left eye had returned to normal.

Discussion

Herpes zoster ophthalmicus usually follows a mild course in children, and it is the rule that all traces of the infection clear up with little residual damage. Ocular complications are usually mild and the children do not appear unduly perturbed by the disease. Post-herpetic neuralgia, so common in affected adults, rarely troubles the child (Björk, 1950).

This case differs from the general observations in some essential points. The child was extremely ill and toxic once the herpes became evident, most unlike many of the cases reported (Poulsen, 1955). Loss of hair in the ophthalmic division was very noticeable and this finding does not appear to have been commented upon much previously. Normal vision had not completely returned one year after the original illness, although improvement has been maintained.

Aetiologically, two types of herpes zoster ophthalmicus are described (Duke-Elder, 1952): (1) The epidemic form which is caused by a specific virus and produces a lesion in every way comparable with herpes zoster elsewhere. This form is usually of sudden onset with severe constitutional disturbances such as fever, prostration and vomiting and these general signs often precede the neuralgic pain of the herpes. (2) The symptomatic form due to the involvement of the ganglion secondarily in infective, neoplastic or traumatic disturbances, e.g. syphilis, tuberculous meningitis or a pontine tumour. It may also be caused by drugs, e.g. arsenic or carbon monoxide poisoning. This form cannot be definitely diagnosed as such unless the patient shows other evidence of the causal agent, which may not appear until months or years later. Many of the cases reported in children may well be this symptomatic form with the evidence or cause of the trouble as yet not manifest.

The case described falls into the first group. Duke-Elder states that herpes zoster ophthalmicus of the epidemic type almost always affects adults and the aged; it runs a fairly similar course in all cases from onset to subsidence.

Doggart (1933) lists three principal features in the diagnosis of epidemic herpes zoster: (1) Pain along the course of distribution of the first division of the fifth cranial nerve; (2) A skin rash appearing about three days later on a portion of the corresponding area of the face or head; (3) Limitation of the rash to one side.

Ocular complications usually occur in about 50% of adults affected, the main ones being keratitis, iritis, scleritis, ocular muscle palsies and optic neuritis. If the naso-ciliary branch of the ophthalmic division of the trigeminal nerve is involved by a lesion of the tip of the nose, the eye will very often be involved as well (Hutchinson, 1866). This case illustrates the rule quite convincingly.

Relation of Herpes Zoster to Varicella. The virus causing herpes zoster is now believed to be identical with the virus of varicella and there is a large amount of clinical and experimental evidence for the association (Bokay, 1909; McEwen, 1920; Jacobi, 1921; Simpson, 1954; Blank and Rake, 1955).

Minor antigenic differences may be present but the two viruses appear to be very closely related. They may differ perhaps in the mode of attack by the virus: in herpes zoster spread is by the lymphatics, whereas in chickenpox it is usually via the blood stream (Low, 1919). There remains the possibility of the occurrence of two forms of epidemic herpes zoster, one allied to chickenpox and one allied to herpes. Most evidence, however, supports the monistic theory that zoster and chickenpox are different manifestations of infection by the same virus, zoster being usually a reawakening of the latent infection of chickenpox (Blank and Rake, 1955).

Simpson (1954) after studying an epidemic on the Shetland Island of Yell of ordinary varicella and also of varicella caught from a shingles contact on the same island, could find no distinction in the clinical manifestations, in the mean reproductive cycles, in the infectiousness of the disease or in the solidity of the protection conferred by a previous attack against varicella of the same or of the alternative origin, i.e. complete cross immunity, and concluded that the varicella caught from shingles is due to the same virus as ordinary chickenpox. He also showed that people infected with chickenpox derived from a case of zoster were subsequently immune for a few years to ordinary chickenpox infection; and similarly, people who had previously had chickenpox were not infected when exposed to the virus derived from a case of zoster.

Experimental evidence of Kundratitz (1925) and Bruusgaard (1932) as early as 1925 is in line with the views expressed by Simpson (1954) and they offer laboratory evidence of close similarities between the two aetiological agents.

Summary

Herpes zoster ophthalmicus is a rare form of herpes infection in children, being primarily an adult affection. A case of a boy of 6 years is presented who showed the classical unilateral eruption together with some other unusual features. The association of the herpes zoster virus with varicella is discussed.

I am indebted to Dr. B. D. R. Wilson under whose care the child was admitted for helpful advice and criticism and to Mr. L. M. Green for ophthalmological comments.

REFERENCES

Amies, C. R. (1934). *Brit. J. exp. Path.*, **15**, 314.
Björk, A. (1950). *Acta derm.-venereol. (Stockh.)*, **30**, 34.
Blank, H. and Rake, G. (1955). *Viral and Rickettsial Diseases of Skin, Eyes and Mucous Membranes of Man.* Boston.
Bokay, J. von. (1909). *Wien. klin. Wschr.*, **22**, 1323.
Brain, R. T. (1933). *Brit. J. exp. Path.*, **14**, 67.
Bruusgaard, E. (1932). *Brit. J. Derm.*, **44**, 1.
Cecil, R. L. and Loeb, R. F. (1951). *Textbook of Medicine.* London and Philadelphia.
Doggart, J. H. (1933). *Brit. J. Ophthal.*, **17**, 513.
Duke-Elder, S. (1952). In *Textbook of Ophthalmology.* Vols. II and V. London.
Edgerton, A. E. (1945). *Arch. Ophthal. (Chicago)*, **34**, 40, 114.
Evans and Fox. (1905). *Brit. J. Derm.*, **17**, 199.
Hutchinson, J. (1866). *Ophth. Hosp. Rep.* **3**, 72; **5**, 191.
Jacobi, O. (1921). *Z. Kinderheilk.*, **29**, 368.
Koch, F. L. P. (1939). *Arch. Ophthal. (Chicago)*, **21**, 118.
Kundratitz, K. (1925). *Wien. klin. Wschr.*, **38**, 502.
Low, R. C. (1919). *Brit. med. J.*, **1**, 91.
McEwen, E. L. (1920). *Arch. Derm. Syph.*, **2**, 205.
Nelson, W. E. (1954). In *Textbook of Paediatrics*, 6th ed. London and Philadelphia.
Poulsen, P. A. (1955). *Acta med. scand.*, **151**, 131.
Price, F. W. (1956). In *Textbook of Medicine*, 9th ed., London.
Roll, G. W. (1920). *Proc. roy. Soc. Med.*, **13**, 81.
Simpson, R. E. H. (1954). *Lancet*, **2**, 1299.
Weller, T. H. (1953). *Proc. Soc. exp. Biol. (N.Y.)*, **83**, 340.

OBSERVATIONS ON THE BROMIDE PARTITION TEST IN THE DIAGNOSIS OF NON-PURULENT MENINGITIS

BY

V. S. NICOL and H. T. FAWNS

From the Paediatric Unit and Department of Pathology, Worcester Royal Infirmary

(RECEIVED FOR PUBLICATION FEBRUARY 10, 1958)

The Bromide Partition Test

In its earliest stages when treatment will produce the most favourable results, tuberculous meningitis may be difficult to diagnose clinically, since other infective non-bacterial conditions of the central nervous system may present a similar clinical picture at their onset.

Since the bromide partition test and its use in the diagnosis of tuberculous meningitis were described (Taylor, Smith and Hunter, 1954) we have found it a useful aid to diagnosis in six cases of tuberculous meningitis and 20 cases of non-tuberculous meningitis (Fig. 1).

Normally after oral or intravenous administration of sodium bromide, the ratio of serum bromide/cerebrospinal fluid bromide is above 1·65 (usual range 2-3). In cases of tuberculous meningitis the integrity of the blood cerebrospinal fluid barrier is affected and there is an early fall in the ratio below 1·65 towards unity, with a return to normal when the infection is brought under control. In other types of non-purulent meningitis a fall in the ratio does not occur. In cases of purulent meningitis this fall may, or may not, occur. In five cases of purulent meningitis described by Cheek (1956) there was a low ratio in two cases, in the other three the ratio was normal. Owing to the different clinical course of purulent meningitis, this type of test should not be necessary, and no cases of purulent meningitis are included in our series.

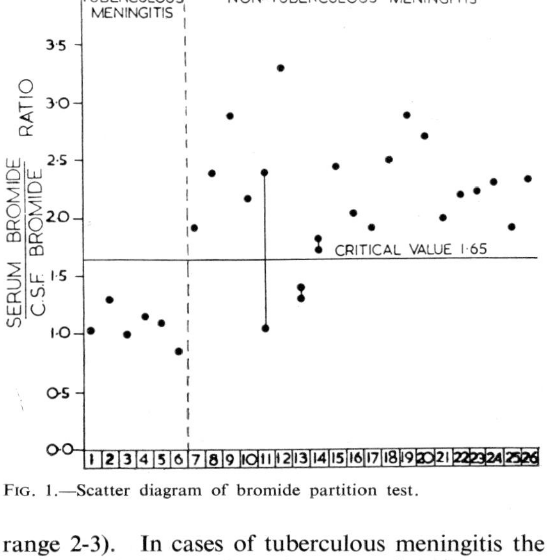

FIG. 1.—Scatter diagram of bromide partition test.

The method used is that described by Taylor, Smith and Hunter (1954). Sodium bromide is given orally, 0·25-1 g. t.d.s., for three days, or as a single intravenous injection of 2-8 g. (the solution contains 8 g. in 30 ml.). Venous blood, 5 ml., and lumbar cerebrospinal fluid, 8 ml., are collected 24 hours after intravenous, and 48 hours after oral administration, for bromide estimation. The authors of the original paper stress the importance of collecting lumbar cerebrospinal fluid as fluid obtained by cisternal or ventricular puncture yields different values.

Analytical Method

Bromide was estimated by the method of Hunter (1953) which is the technique of choice for this test as it enables the relatively small serum and cerebrospinal fluid levels to be estimated with greater accuracy than by other methods (Hunter, Smith and Taylor, 1954). This method is a quantitative application of the Van der Meulen reaction, whereby bromide is oxidized to bromate by hypochlorite. The excess hypochlorite is removed with sodium formate, after which the bromate liberates a corresponding amount of iodine from potassium iodide, which is titrated with N/200 sodium thiosulphate, using a starch indicator. The end point is sharp and satisfactory.

One ml. of serum or cerebrospinal fluid is required for each estimation.

In the majority of cases estimations were carried out in duplicate and the mean value reported. In a few cases, however, shortage of material made this impossible. It is essential to carry out a 'reagent blank' with each test, as there is a somewhat large and variable blank value arising from reagents, which must be deducted

TABLE 1

FIGURES FOR THE FIRST 10 DUPLICATED ANALYSES OF SERUM AND OF CEREBROSPINAL FLUID, SHOWING THE MEAN VALUES REPORTED AND THE DEGREE OF ACCURACY*

Specimen No.	Serum				Cerebrospinal Fluid			
	I	II	Mean	Accuracy (%)	I	II	Mean	Accuracy (%)
1	35·6	36·2	35·9	±0·84	13·0	13·4	13·2	±1·52
2	61·0	61·2	61·1	±0·16	65·0	63·0	64·0	±1·56
3	35·6	34·1	34·8	±2·21	32·0	29·6	30·8	±3·90
4	131·0	129·0	130·0	±0·77	5·8	5·8	5·8	±0·00
5	92·8	91·2	92·0	±0·87	26·4	27·4	26·9	±1·86
6	17·6	19·2	18·4	±4·30	18·5	19·5	19·0	±2·63
7	14·2	13·4	13·8	±2·90	24·7	24·7	24·7	±0·00
8	56·0	57·0	56·5	±0·89	27·7	25·7	26·7	±3·72
9	24·5	24·5	24·5	±0·00	5·7	3·8	4·75	†±20·0
10	19·7	19·5	19·6	±0·51	27·0	27·0	27·0	±0·00
	Accuracy: average ±1·35% (Range: 0·00–4·30%)				Accuracy: average ±1·69% (Range: 0·00–3·90%)			

* Results are expressed as bromine mg. %.

† Not included in calculating the average and range for this series. This much larger error is due to the difficulty in estimating the very small amount of bromine present.

from the serum and cerebrospinal values. Initially, the method involves ashing protein-free alcoholic extracts of serum and cerebrospinal fluid in nickel crucibles, but apart from these no special apparatus is required other than what is normally available in a clinical laboratory. The original method suggests that 4 ml. of alcoholic supernatant fluid be used for the estimation after protein precipitation. This is satisfactory for cerebrospinal fluid but in the case of sera we frequently found it difficult to realize this volume. As a routine, we therefore employed 3·5 ml. and corrected the calculation accordingly. The accuracy of the method appears satisfactory. From the point of view of a busy clinical laboratory, one might perhaps make the criticism that it is somewhat time-consuming.

Results are expressed as mg. % of bromine, and Table 1 gives the figures for the first 10 duplicated analyses, for serum and cerebrospinal fluid respectively. Some of these figures refer to adult cases of meningitis and are not dealt with in this paper. The accuracy is expressed as the percentage difference between the individual analyses and the mean value reported. Hunter (1953) claims an accuracy of approximately ± 1% for the method, and the majority of our own analyses agree with this. At the outset of this work, recovery tests were carried out with sodium bromide added to serum at a concentration of 10 mg. %, expressed as bromine. The recovery range was 97% to 104%, but it was possible to improve on this standard of accuracy with the higher concentrations encountered in the test specimens.

TABLE 2

Case No.	Serum Bromide (mg. %)	C.S.F. Bromide (mg. %)	Serum CSF Ratio	Mantoux 1·1000	Culture C. Guinea Pig G.	Cerebrospinal Fluid Findings: Cells (per c.mm.)	Protein (mg. %)	Glucose (mg. %)	T.B. Family History	Diagnosis
1	19·2	18·4	1·04	—	CG+	424	240	21	—	
2	38·2	27·6	1·38	+	G+	62	120	43	— (milk)	
3	27·0	27·0	1·00	+	C—	350	260	15	—	Tuberculous meningitis
4	30·8	25·9	1·19	+	C—G—	244	180	20	+	
5	20·2	18·4	1·10	+	C—	230			+	
6	24·2	28·1	0·86	+	C—G+	128	128	40	—	
7	33·0	17·2	1·92	—	C—G—	1,340	80	45	—	Non-specific meningitis
8	13·9	5·8	2·40	—	G—	176	30	49	—	Non-specific meningitis
9	13·8	4·75	2·90	—	C—	266	55	60	+	Poliomyelitis
10	28·3	13·2	2·18	+	C—	3	80	62	—	Tuberculoma of cerebellum
11	27·3 } 38·0	25·0 } 15·6	1·09 } 2·40	—	G—	260	150	55		Non-specific meningitis
12	45·0	13·5	3·35	—	C—	454	30	46	—	Non-specific meningitis
13	33·4 } 47·5	24·0 } 35·0	1·40 } 1·36	—	C—	828	30	40	—	Non-specific meningitis
14	42·0 } 48·0	24·5 } 26·3	1·72 } 1·82	—	C—	324	58	52	+	Mumps. Encephalitis
15	13·8	5·6	2·45	—	C—	62	40	90	+	Non-specific meningitis
16	14·9	7·2	2·05	—		800	48	55	—	Non-specific meningitis
17	37·3 } 59·4	19·4 } 30·6	1·93 } 1·93	+	C+ (from foot)	94	35	43	—	Miliary tuberculosis
18	14·2	5·7	2·50	—	C—	20	54	40	—	Mumps. Encephalitis
19	38·4	13·4	2·90	—	C—G—	432	30	37	—	Mumps. Encephalitis
20	23·8	8·6	2·76	—		90	70	70	+	Non-specific meningitis
21	30·4	15·2	2·00	—		3	32	78	—	Non-specific meningitis
22	25·0	11·4	2·20	+ (BCG)	C—	140	60	59	+	Poliomyelitis
23	27·5	12·3	2·24	—	C—G—	216	70	46	+	Non-specific meningitis
24	51·5	22·8	2·25	—	C—	202	40	67		Poliomyelitis
25	18·1	9·5	1·92	—		90	20	80	—	Mumps. Encephalitis
26	51·5	21·9	2·36	—	C—	48	35	54	+	Poliomyelitis

Material and Results

In the six cases of tuberculous meningitis (Table 2) the bromide ratio was depressed in all cases. In Cases 3 and 5 the test was useful in confirming the clinical diagnosis. Case 1 presented the typical features of tuberculous meningitis but the Mantoux reaction was negative on admission. A bromide ratio of 1·04 was useful additional evidence in favour of the diagnosis. Cases 2, 4 and 6 presented diagnostic problems as the clinical picture was not typical, and, as they illustrate the practical value of the test, they are presented more fully.

Case 2. A girl, aged 5 years, was well until the day of admission when she was suddenly unable to speak, did not recognize her mother and looked vacant for a few minutes. She vomited at the end of the attack. There was nothing relevant in her previous or family history, but the milk supply was from a doubtful source. The child was well on admission and physical examination was negative. Investigations included: haemoglobin 81%, white blood cells 8,000 per c.mm., 62% polymorphs. The urine was normal and there were no pathogens in the stool. A Mantoux test was 1:1,000 positive. Radiographs of the skull and chest were normal, while that of the abdomen showed calcified mesenteric glands. She was well for 10 days when she had a further minor convulsion lasting a few seconds. Three days later she was less well and vomited several times. Physical examination remained negative. Lumbar puncture showed 62 cells per c.mm., protein 120 mg. %, glucose 43 mg. %. She was thought possibly to be suffering from early tuberculous meningitis and was started on streptomycin, isoniazid and P.A.S. while a bromide partition test was done, the ratio being 1·38 which was in favour of the diagnosis. A guinea pig inoculated with the original cerebrospinal fluid showed evidence of tuberculosis. She made an excellent recovery.

Case 4. A boy, aged 2 years, whose father had recently been admitted to a sanatorium with pulmonary tuberculosis, was found to have an early primary complex just discernible on his contact film. Unfortunately, the family did not attend for their Chest Clinic appointment and shortly afterwards this child was admitted following a convulsion with a history of vomiting and irritability of one week's duration. On examination he was unconscious and twitching. There was no meningism, or localizing signs in the central nervous system. He had an acute right otitis media requiring paracentesis, otherwise physical examination was negative. Investigations included haemoglobin 68%, white blood cells 11,000 per c.mm., 50% polymorphs. A radiograph of the skull was normal, that of the chest showed a right primary complex. Pus from the right ear was sterile and *M. tuberculosis* was not isolated. Cerebrospinal fluid cells were 244 per c.mm., 91% lymphocytes, protein 180 mg. %, glucose 20 mg. %. A Mantoux test was 1:1,000 positive. The child was thought to be suffering from tuberculous meningitis and was started on treatment with streptomycin, isoniazid and P.A.S. A bromide ratio of 1·19 confirmed this diagnosis and was useful in ruling out the possibility that he was suffering from an intracranial complication of his ear disease.

Case 6. A girl, aged 6 years, was admitted as a 'pyrexia of unknown origin' with a five days' history of headache, abdominal pain and vomiting. Physical examination was negative. Routine investigations included haemoglobin 72%, white blood cells 14,000 per c.mm. A radiograph of the chest was normal. The urine contained a trace of albumen. Agglutinations to *Salmonella* and *Brucella* groups were negative. A blood culture was sterile and there were no pathogens in the stool. A Mantoux test was 1:1,000 positive. Cerebrospinal fluid cells were 128 per c.mm., protein 128 mg. %, glucose 40 mg. %. Bromide ratio 0·86.

During the investigations apart from a pyrexia she remained relatively well and there were no clinical signs of tuberculous meningitis until the diagnosis had been made and she was on treatment with streptomycin, isoniazid and P.A.S.

In the above six cases presenting as tuberculous meningitis, proof of the diagnosis was obtained in five. Three were confirmed by guinea pig inoculation (Cases 1, 2, 6) and two others developed choroidal tubercles (Cases 4, 5). In the remaining case the subsequent course of the disease was typical of tuberculous meningitis, and there is little doubt about the final diagnosis. Treatment with anti-tuberculous drugs does not affect the bromide ratio in the early stages. Cases 1, 2, 4, 5 and 6 were started on treatment a few days before or during the bromide partition test. Case 3 had been on treatment for 17 days when the test was done. This is particularly useful as treatment may be started at once in uncertain cases without affecting the result, and, conversely, the patient need not be committed to a full course of treatment in the event of a negative result.

Case 14 illustrates the latter point. A child, aged 15 months, whose father had had a recent pulmonary tuberculosis, was admitted following a convulsion. Ten days previously his brother had developed mumps and he had had transient facial swelling. Physical examination was normal. Relevant investigations included a Mantoux test 1:1,000, and 100 negative. Radiographs of the chest and abdomen were normal. Cerebrospinal fluid cells were 324 per c.mm., 89% lymphocytes, protein 58 mg. %, glucose 52 mg. %. The fluid was taken on admission at night and a technician reported acid-fast bacilli in the smear. In view of this he was started on treatment with streptomycin, I.N.A.H. and P.A.S. The bromide ratio was 1·72 and a repeat ratio 1·82. In view of the history, clinical course and high bromide ratio he was thought to be probably suffering from mumps encephalitis and he did not have a full course of anti-tuberculous drugs.

The bromide ratio is said to rise when infection is brought under control (Taylor, Smith and Hunter, 1954). In three of our cases repeat bromide partition tests were done during treatment (Fig. 2). Clinical improvement was accompanied by a rising ratio in each case. In Case 6 when the response to treatment was initially poor, the bromide ratio remained low, rising later when the clinical condition was also improving.

In the 20 cases of non-tuberculous meningitis the bromide ratio was normal in 18 of the cases. It was particularly helpful in six of these children (Cases 9, 15, 20, 22, 23, 26) who presented with early non-purulent meningitis and in whose case there was a family history of tuberculosis. Further, when poliomyelitis has been prevalent, or when there has been a history of contact with a disease such as mumps when encephalitis may occur, the bromide partition test has been a useful aid in eliminating tuberculous meningitis which must always come into the differential diagnosis.

Three of the cases with normal bromide ratios had positive Mantoux reactions. One had had B.C.G. The other two, one of interest, are presented more fully.

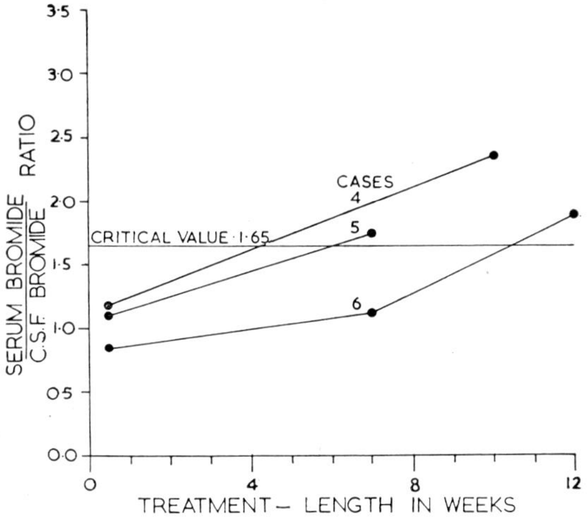

FIG. 2.—Alterations in the $\frac{\text{serum bromide}}{\text{C.S.F. bromide}}$ in tuberculous meningitis cases treated with P.A.S., I.N.A.H. and I.M. streptomycin.

Case 10. A girl, aged 9 years, was admitted with a history of general ill health, poor appetite, loss of weight and a noticeable falling off in her school work, of one year's duration. In the five days before admission she had had six attacks of headache, nausea and vomiting followed by unconsciousness for one minute. Physical examination was normal apart from a systolic murmur in her heart (pulse 86 per minute, blood pressure 95/50) and early papilloedema. Investigations included haemoglobin 78%, white blood cells 7,000 per c.mm., 74% polymorphs. The E.S.R. was 60 mm. in one hour. Blood urea was 38 mg. %. Blood chemistry was normal. There was a trace of albumen in the urine. Radiographs of the chest and abdomen were normal. A radiograph of the skull showed increased digital markings. Lumbar puncture showed fluid at increased pressure, cells 3 per c.mm. mononuclear, protein 80 mg. %, sugar 62 mg. %, Lange 5,554,310,000. The Wassermann reaction was negative, a Mantoux test positive. In view of her positive Mantoux, raised E.S.R. and changes in the cerebrospinal fluid, a bromide ratio was done, which at 2·18 was against a diagnosis of tuberculous meningitis.

She developed increasing papilloedema and ataxia and was transferred to a neuro-surgical unit where craniotomy was performed. A tuberculoma of the cerebellum was found and successfully removed. The normal bromide ratio in this case was both helpful and interesting.

Case 17. A girl, aged 2½ years, was admitted with a history of a minor injury to her right foot a few days previously: an indurated swelling had developed at the site of the injury. On the day of admission she vomited and had a series of generalized convulsions. On examination she was convulsed and neck stiffness was present. There was a fluctuant swelling on the dorsum of her right foot and her right knee was swollen. There were no other abnormal signs. Investigations included haemoglobin 71%, white blood count 11,300 per c.mm.. 80% polymorphs. There were no pathogens in the stool, A radiograph of the skull was normal, that of the chest showed increased shadowing at the right hilum. A Mantoux test was 1:1,000 positive. Urine protein was 700 mg. %, with two pus cells per high power field in uncentrifuged urine. Blood urea was 34 mg. %. An E.S.R. was 21 mm. in one hour. Cerebrospinal fluid cells were 94 per c.mm., 19% polymorphs, 81% lymphocytes, protein 35 mg. %, glucose 43 mg. %. Pus from the swelling of the foot contained tubercle bacilli. The bromide ratio was 1·93.

She was thought to be suffering from miliary tuberculosis and was started on treatment with streptomycin, isoniazid and P.A.S.

The normal bromide ratio, which was confirmed on a repeat test, is interesting. Cheek (1956) quotes Taylor, Smith and Hunter as saying that in miliary tuberculosis not involving the central nervous system the bromide ratio remains normal. In this case the meningeal signs and cerebrospinal fluid changes occurred during the period of invasion and she did not develop a true tuberculous meningitis.

In two of the cases the bromide ratio was low, giving false positive results.

Case 11. A girl, aged 11 years, was admitted as a surgical emergency with abdominal pain which rapidly improved, but she developed a pyrexia and persistent headache. Relevant investigations included a Mantoux test, 1:1,000 negative. Cerebrospinal fluid cells were 260 per c.mm., 94% lymphocytes, protein 150 mg. %, glucose 55 mg. %. She was kept under observation and put on no treatment while a bromide ratio was done, the ratio being 1·09. By then she was quite well and the cerebrospinal fluid was returning to normal. A repeat ratio was 2·40.

Case 13. A boy, aged 4 months, who had had signs of a cerebral injury in the neonatal period was admitted following a convulsion. Physical examination was normal. Relevant investigations included a Mantoux test, 1:1,000 negative. Cerebrospinal fluid cells were 828 per c.mm., 94% lymphocytes, protein 30 mg. %, glucose 40 mg. %. The bromide ratio was 1·40. The child remained well and, as the cerebrospinal fluid was also improving, he was given no treatment and continued to improve. A repeat ratio was 1·36. He made an uneventful recovery.

These results agree with those of Taylor, Smith and Hunter (1954) who reported 7% false positive results in their series.

Summary

The serum/cerebrospinal fluid bromide ratio ('bromide partition test') of Taylor, Smith and Hunter (1954) has been applied in 26 cases of non-purulent meningitis of which six were tuberculous and 20 non-tuberculous.

In the tuberculous cases the accuracy was 100%, no false negatives being obtained. In three of the tuberculous cases, the ratio was determined at intervals during treatment and clinical improvement was accompanied by a rising ratio.

In the non-tuberculous cases, the accuracy was 90%, two out of 20 cases giving false positive results (Cases 11 and 13). Similar findings have been reported by Taylor, Smith and Hunter who found a low ratio in 7% of 66 cases of non-tuberculous meningitis.

Taken in conjunction with the clinical findings, the bromide partition test appears to be a valuable adjunct in the early diagnosis of tuberculous meningitis and may prove also to be a useful criterion for following the course of clinical improvement.

We are grateful to Dr. P. Kidd for first drawing our attention to this diagnostic technique and to Dr. A. G. V. Aldridge for his interest in the work and for permission to publish material relating to his cases. Mr. F. Hughes kindly prepared Figs. 1 and 2 for us.

References

Cheek, D. B. (1956). *Pediatrics*, **18**, 218.
Hunter, G. (1953). *Biochem. J.*, **54**, 42.
——, Smith, H. V. and Taylor, L. M. (1954). *Ibid.*, **56**, 588.
Taylor, L. M., Smith, H. V. and Hunter, G. (1954). *Lancet*, **1**, 700.

PNEUMATOSIS INTESTINALIS IN CHINESE CHILDREN

BY

C. S. MUIR

From the Department of Pathology, University of Malaya

(RECEIVED FOR PUBLICATION MARCH 5, 1958)

Pneumatosis cystoides intestinorum hominis is a rare condition. Although about 250 cases have been described to date only seven of these have come from the Orient: five Chinese adults (Tung and Ngai, 1933; Yin, 1937; Ling, Ku and Su, 1948), and two Indian adults (Tribedi, 1941; Davies, 1941). This paper records five cases occurring in Singapore, one in an adult, the remainder in children.

The lesion consists of gas-containing cysts of varying size, either sessile or pedunculated, within the wall of the intestinal tract. There may, in addition, be similar cysts on the surface of other abdominal organs and on the parietal peritoneum.

Case Histories

Case 1. C.J.M., a 3-month-old male Cantonese child, was admitted to the General Hospital, Singapore, on August 20, 1953, and died five minutes after reaching the ward. The child's mother stated that he had had diarrhoea for the past two days. Over a similar period of time she had noticed increasing breathlessness. The child's temperature was 104° F. Dyspnoea was extreme and numerous crepitations were heard on auscultation of the lung bases.

Dr. E. B. La'Brooy, who performed an autopsy, reported that the body was that of a thin, male Chinese infant, height 2 ft. 4 in., weight 1 st. 1 lb. The heart appeared normal. The respiratory passages were partially blocked by mucopurulent exudate, and the lungs showed patchy areas of consolidation with areas of collapse posteriorly. The liver showed gross fatty change. Hyperaemia of the mucosa was present in the small intestine. Two lymph follicles showed superficial necrosis and bile staining of sloughing tissue. The large intestine showed several irregular ulcers of lymph follicles. There were numerous bubbles of gas in the mucosa of the ileum. The stools were not cultured.

HISTOLOGY. A section of colon showed well-marked pneumatosis. The majority of gas spaces had no lining endothelium (Fig. 1, top left). Several of these unlined spaces had giant cells in the wall and an occasional macrophage round about. Another space showed an incipient lining, which appeared to be formed by condensation of surrounding tissue. In this wall (Fig. 2), three giant cells were seen (cf. Fig. 30: Wright, 1930). Moderate numbers of macrophages were present in the neighbourhood.

Case 2. A.B.H., aged 1 month, a male Chinese infant, was admitted to the General Hospital, Singapore, in a dehydrated condition, with a three-day history of diarrhoea and vomiting after feeds. No pathogenic organisms were grown from the stools. The child died.

Dr. Ng Chiau Gian found a patent foramen ovale on autopsy. There was a thin layer of sero-purulent fluid inside the peritoneal cavity, and small mucosal ulcers in the lower part of the ileum and colon. In a portion of the ileal wall, which showed no signs of inflammation, there were numerous blebs of gas, possibly post-mortem in origin.

HISTOLOGY. Sections of colon showed a very well-developed pneumatosis. The gas spaces were lined by a low endothelium. Towards the centre of the section an abscess containing mononuclears, polymorphs and much debris was present. This extended from the mucosa to the muscle layers and was of the 'collar-stud' type (Fig. 3). Just below this abscess, within the muscle layers, an amoeba was seen (Fig. 4).

Case 3. G.H.J., a 1-month-old male Hokkien child, was admitted to the General Hospital, Singapore, on December 1, 1956, with a complaint of persistent regurgitation of feeds of several days' duration. A diagnosis of duodenal stenosis was made and on December 15 laparotomy was performed. A volvulus of mid-ileum was reduced and numerous adhesions divided. The child died on January 2, 1957, after a short period of vomiting.

At autopsy the body was that of a thin, male Chinese infant. The abdomen was rather bloated, and there was a well-healed transverse lower abdominal surgical scar. The heart appeared normal. The lung parenchyma showed early bronchopneumonic change. The normal anatomy of the gut was deranged by multiple adhesions: a major portion of caecum was tacked down to the liver and the appendix was adherent to the small bowel. The loops of small bowel were adherent to each other, showing numerous kinks although no definite obstruction

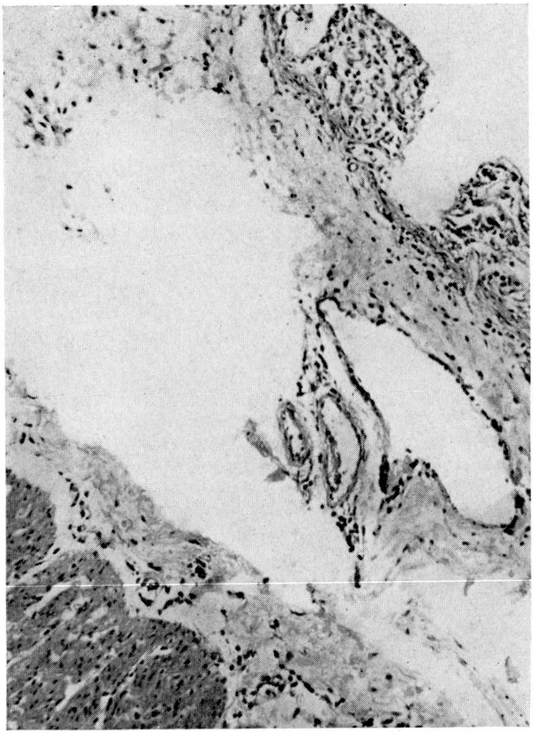

FIG. 1.—P.M. 1492/53. Section of intestinal wall showing, at middle right, a gas space with an incipient lining. On either side is unlined gas space. H. and E. × 135.

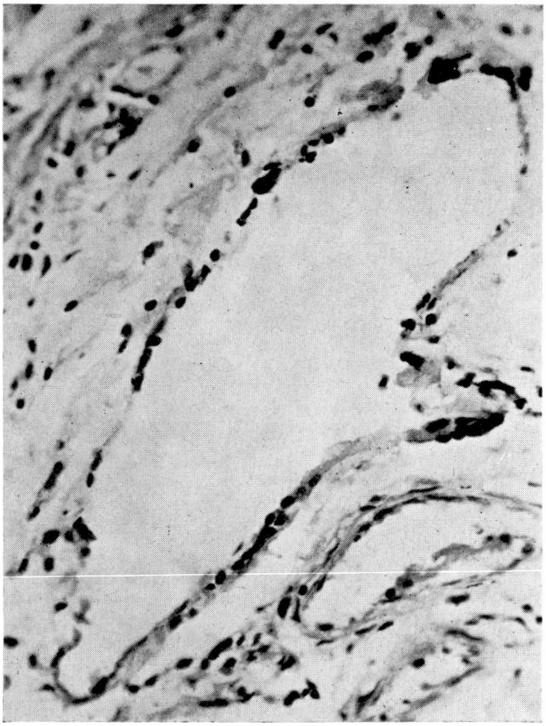

FIG. 2.—P.M. 1492/53. Higher magnification of the gas space above shows it to be partially lined by a condensation of surrounding tissue. In the wall three giant cells are seen. Moderate numbers of macrophages are present in the surrounding tissue. H. and E. × 336.

could be detected. One portion of jejunum was tacked down between the liver and the diaphragm. The gut was generally dilated, red in colour and in places showed desquamation of the mucosal epithelium.

HISTOLOGY. Section of the ileum showed pneumatosis (Figs. 5, 6 and 7). Nearly all the gas spaces had an endothelial lining although this was not well marked in places. Macrophages were moderately plentiful; the cytoplasm was less bulky than in other sections. Moderate numbers of giant cells were seen (Fig. 8).

Case 4. O.B.C., a 63-year-old Henghwa male, was admitted to the General Hospital, Singapore, on April 25, 1957, with a complaint of four months' increasing abdominal swelling. A firm nodular mass was palpated in the upper abdomen and the liver was grossly enlarged. He was considered to be suffering from gastric carcinoma.

Dr. A. O. Aaron's autopsy report stated that the heart appeared to be normal. The lungs were the seat of numerous small circumscribed tumour nodules. The liver weighed 4,300 g., being largely replaced by secondary tumour. There was no evidence of cirrhosis. There was a large circular carcinomatous ulcer 5 cm. in diameter on the lesser curvature of the stomach close to the pylorus. The submucosa of the ileum and colon showed pneumatosis.

HISTOLOGY. Section of the colon showed moderately well-developed pneumatosis. All the gas spaces were lined by a low endothelium. Very few giant cells or macrophages were seen.

Case 5. N.P.M., a 12-year-old Hokkien girl, was admitted to the General Hospital, Singapore, on December 26, 1957, and died one hour later. She gave a history of two days' abdominal pain associated with vomiting. She had passed numerous stools on the day prior to admission.

At autopsy the heart appeared normal. The lungs showed changes, possibly early bronchopneumonic. The entire gut from mid-jejunum to descending colon was inflamed and showed areas of patchy superficial necrosis. The necrotic areas were deeply bile stained. In the mid-jejunum and upper ileum several small areas, each about 5 cm. long, were seen which showed air bubbles in the gut wall. This was probably early pneumatosis.

HISTOLOGY. Section of the lower jejunum (Fig. 9), showed a moderate degree of disruption of the tissues of the sub-mucosa. This was presumably caused by gas. Around these areas macrophages and eosinophils were prominent (Figs. 10 and 11; cf. Fig. 25: Wright, 1930). These macrophages had a prominent ovaloid nucleus and a bulky homogeneous pink cytoplasm.

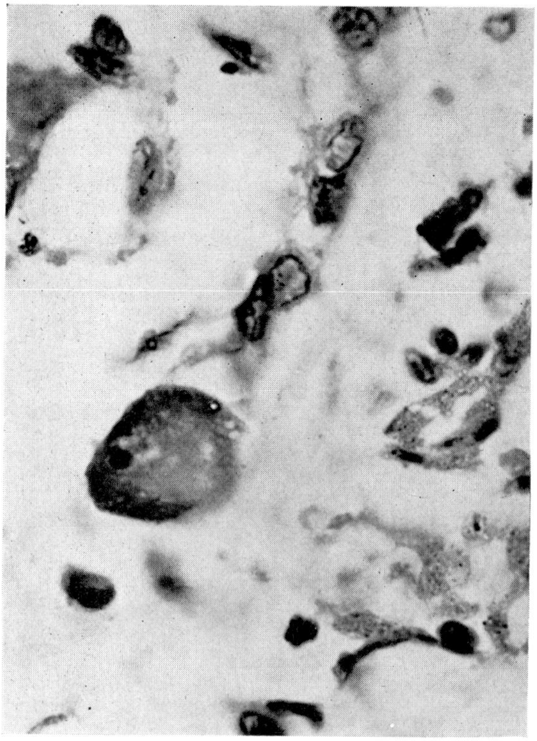

FIG. 3.—P.M. 1167/57. Amoebic abscess of ascending colon superimposed on pneumatosis. H. and E. × 135.

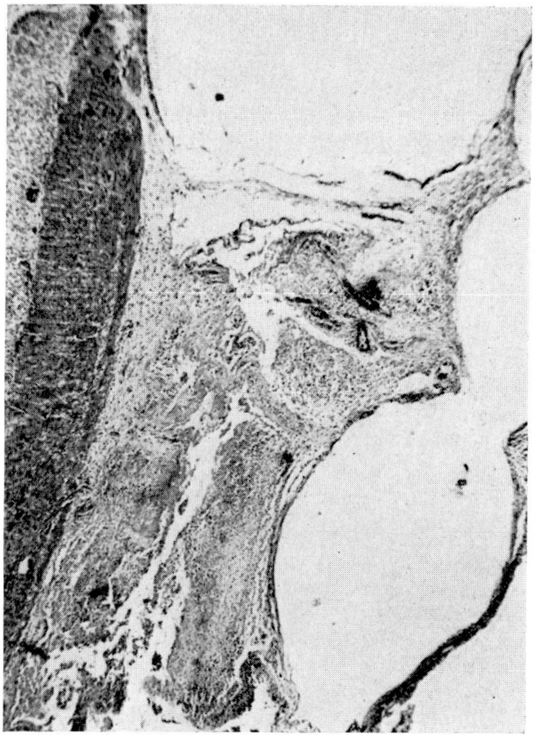

FIG. 4.—P.M. 1167/57. An amoeba within the muscle coats. H. and E. × 1,200.

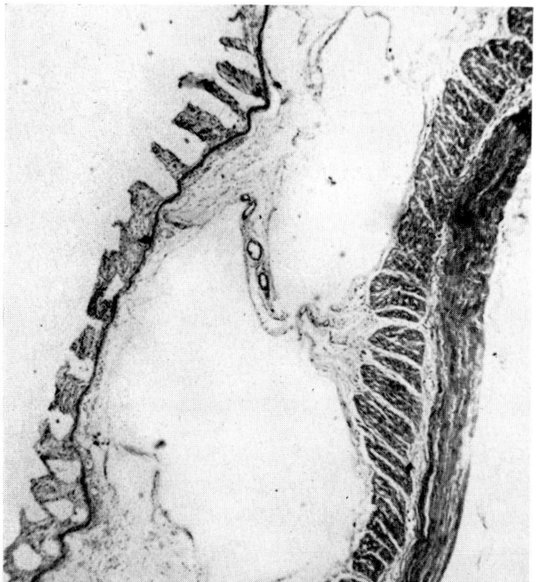

FIG. 5.—P.M. 7/57. Section showing submucosal pneumatosis.

Elsewhere in the section several lined gas spaces were seen. One of these (Fig. 12), was lined for about three-quarters of its circumference by a low endothelium, the remainder by a condensation of surrounding tissue. Around this space moderate numbers of macrophages were present.

Aetiology

The exact cause of pneumatosis is unknown. Several theories have each, from time to time, attracted some support.

First in the field was the neoplastic hypothesis. Bang (1876) described the first well-documented case and considered the cysts to be the product of a new growth, which, taking its origin from giant cells in the lymphatic vessels, spread, elaborating a gas as it did so. Mair (1907) believed that the lesion was a true neoplasm whose cells produced gas. Finney (1908) who reported the first American case subscribed to this viewpoint.

The bacterial theory attracted workers who considered that the cysts were the work of gas-producing organisms. Dupraz (1897) did, indeed, isolate a variety of organisms which he termed *Bacterium*

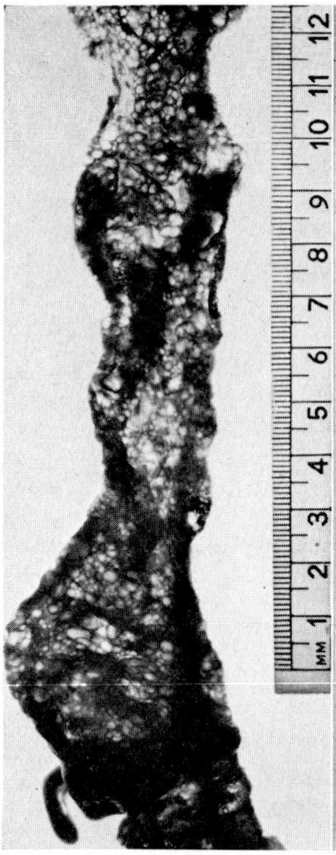

FIG. 6.—P.M. 7/57. Macroscopic appearance of caecum by incident light.

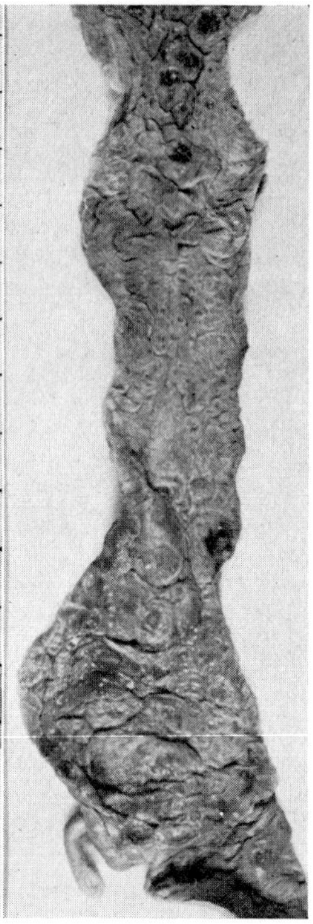

FIG. 7.—Same portion of gut as in Fig. 6. By transmitted light the extent of involvement is much more readily appreciated.

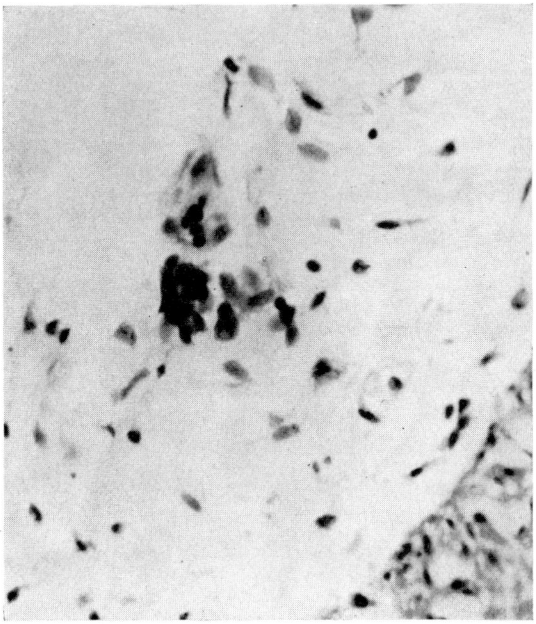

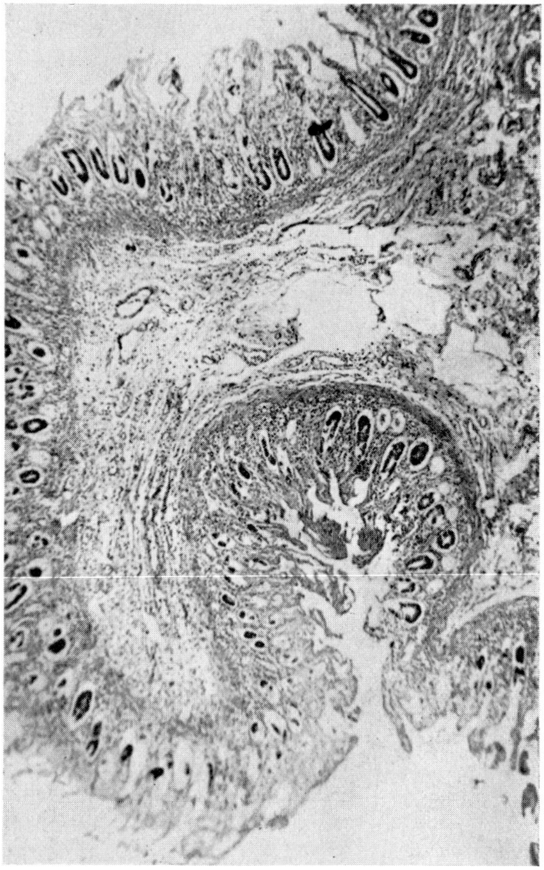

FIG. 9.—P.M. 2609/57. The lower jejunum shows a moderate degree of disruption of the sub-mucosal tissues. H. and E. × 37.

coli lymphaticum aerogenes which, if given orally to animals, reproduced the lesions. All his animals died, however, within 48 hours. Naeslund (1924) cultured from gas cysts in the intestinal wall of swine a variant of *Esch. coli* which he termed *Bacillus pneumatosis*. He obtained weakly positive serological reactions between a suspension of these organisms and the sera of positive swine. Healthy animals, i.e., those without gas cysts of the intestines, did not show this reaction. Injection of these bacteria failed to reproduce the lesions.

The biochemical theory is favoured by those who draw an analogy between the lesions in man and those occurring in the pig. Swine suffer from the condition quite frequently, a fact known since Mayer (1825) described the condition in an otherwise healthy hog. Known as swine emphysema it is

FIG. 8.—P.M. 7/57. A giant cell in the wall of a partially lined gas space. H. and E. × 336.

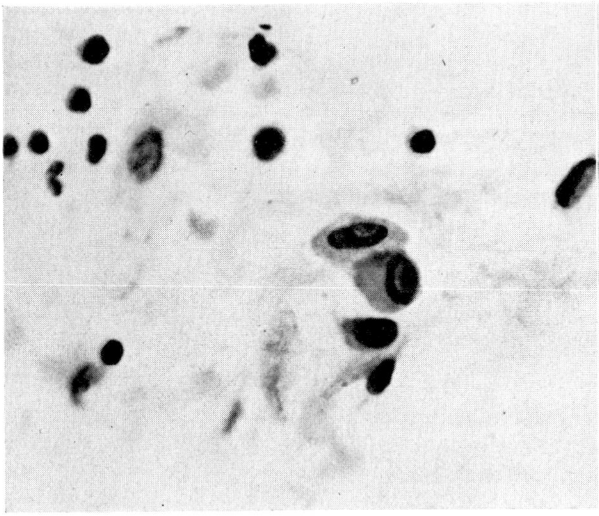

FIG. 10.—P.M. 2609/57. Macrophages around the gas spaces in the intestinal wall. H. and E. × 880.

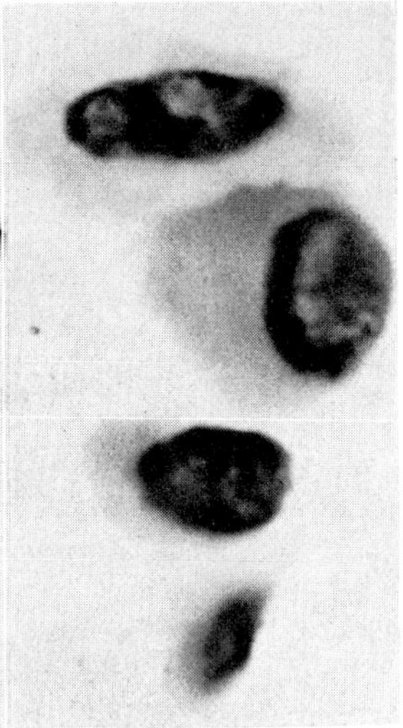

FIG. 11.—P.M. 2609/57. The macrophages in Fig. 10 at a higher magnification. H. and E. × 2,200.

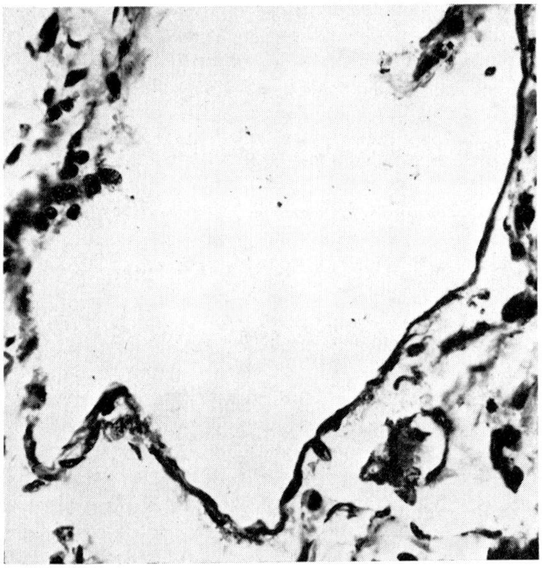

FIG. 12.—P.M. 2609/57. A low endothelium partially lines this gas space on the bottom and right sides, blending gradually at the top left into a condensation of the surrounding tissues. Moderate numbers of macrophages are present. H. and E. × 350.

related in some way to diet, as the disease can be readily reproduced on feeding a diet of polished rice (Biester, Eveleth and Yamoshiro, 1936). Such a relationship is not apparent in man. Pneumatosis has also been observed in sheep (Mills, 1925) and in chickens (Naeslund, 1924).

At present the mechanical theory seems to attract the most adherents. If air be injected directly into the gut wall it follows the lymphatics to the mesentery and within a few days is gradually absorbed. Masson (1925) concluded that lymph stagnation is the basis of the phenomenon. This occurs in tortuous or obstructed lymph vessels, carbon dioxide and lactic acid being absorbed into the obstructed segment. Carbon dioxide is liberated and nitrogen, oxygen and methane diffuse in, the relative proportions of the gases being governed by their partial pressures.

Tung and Ngai (1933) expended considerable effort in trying to reproduce pneumatosis in the dog. They attempted to mimic as closely as possible the conditions obtaining in their patients, both of whom had, in addition to pneumatosis, stenosing peptic ulcers. They reproduced such a stenosing ulcer in one of their dogs and filled the stomach with air and salt solution. Air bubbles appeared, both inside and outside the lymphatics, which moved distally with each peristaltic movement. The animals were allowed to recover from anaesthesia. On the second day after operation the dogs vomited, refused to eat, and appeared quite sick. On reopening the abdomen air bubbles were seen in the lymphatics of the gastric serosa and in those of the omental attachments. Straus (1954) attempted to do the same in the large intestine of the dog. He found that gas cysts did form slowly if air were injected into the lumen of a segment of bowel which had been obstructed both distally and proximally. It seems, therefore, that obstruction favours the formation of these cysts, although it cannot be the whole answer as one would expect to see them more frequently in association with, say, obstructing carcinomata of the colon.

Pathology

The ileum, followed by the colon, are the most frequently affected portions of the gut; both may be involved at once (MacKenzie, 1951). The stomach and gall bladder (Mills, 1925) and the falciform ligament of the liver (Pybus, 1934) have been reported as affected. The amount of gut involved varies. It is often confined to a loop constricted by adhesions or volvulus, sometimes to a loop containing intestinal parasites, usually nematodes (Tung and Ngai, 1933). In the adult the gas cysts are found mainly in the serosa. In children the cysts tend to be submucosal, cysts in the muscle coats being rare. The average cyst is 4-5 mm. in diameter. Koss (1952) reports one cyst 3·5 cm. in diameter in the distal caecum. The gas is a mixture of 70-90% nitrogen, 3-20% oxygen, and 0-15% carbon dioxide. Traces of methane have been detected (Urban, 1910).

In children the cysts appear microscopically as thin-walled sacs lined entirely, or in part, by a single layer of flat endothelium. This lining may not be present. In adults as a rule giant cells are present; in the child they may not be so conspicuous. Wright (1930) has shown that air acts as a foreign body evoking a giant cell response. These giant cells are in many instances mere aggregations of nuclei some 10 to 50 in number and are found near the gas-filled space (Fig. 8). Tung and Ngai (1933) describe in their adult cases a second type of cyst lined by a dense fibrous tissue. In their Fig. 6 they show giant cells in the lumen of one example of this type of cyst, which they regard as being older than the thin-walled variety. They made serial sections of their specimens and found that the endothelium lined spaces communicated with lymphatic vessels, whereas the fibrous variety did not. Koss (1952), examining serial sections, was unable to demonstrate a breach of the continuity of mucosa in the region affected by gas cysts or to demonstrate a definite transition between a cyst and a lymphatic vessel. It seems, therefore, that in time the thin-walled cysts become fibrosed and obliterated. The photomicrographs in his paper show a similar disposition of the giant cells in thick-walled cysts.

Clinical Features

In the infant the most common presenting symptom is diarrhoea (Botsford and Krakower, 1938; Judge, Cassidy and Rice, 1949; MacKenzie, 1951). In the adult pyloric obstruction following peptic ulcer is found in about 60% of cases (Nitch and Shattock, 1919). Pyloric lesions tend to be associated with pneumatosis of the small gut, while obstructive signs are found more commonly with large gut lesions (Kreeger and Littmann, 1954).

Intestinal obstruction is, particularly in the adult, the most likely complication. This may be precipitated by volvulus induced by the cyst mass, by the adhesions which seem to arise as a result of the cysts, or by mechanical blockage of the bowel lumen. Koss (1952) quotes a case in which pneumatosis caused intussusception. Haemorrhage from the bowel may occur (Matthews, 1954; Kreeger and Littmann, 1954; Pontius, 1954). Pneumoperitoneum will result if a sufficient number of cysts burst.

Diagnosis. Diagnosis is usually made on the operating table or at autopsy.

A straight radiograph of the abdomen may be helpful, particularly so if there should be a pneumoperitoneum. Pneumoperitoneum may be simulated by the gas from the mesenteric cysts passing retroperitoneally and accumulating between the parietal peritoneum and the diaphragm. The so-called Chilaiditi sign (the interposition of a loop of bowel between liver and diaphragm) is often positive. Barium meal or enema will show filling defects. The condition has been diagnosed on sigmoidoscopy (Matthews, 1954) and on sigmoidoscopic biopsy (Kreeger and Littmann, 1954).

Treatment. Incidental discovery calls for no active measure. Koss (1952) has observed that the disease is self-limiting. Should obstruction occur the offending segment of gut may be removed. There appears to be no agreement as to how the lesion should be treated in childhood.

Discussion

Apart from the submucosal situation of the cysts, Case 4 is typical of pneumatosis in the adult. The rest show features common to nearly all others described in infants. Diarrhoea was the presenting symptom. A volvulus with intestinal obstruction and adhesions were found in Case 3. This latter case shows the Chilaiditi sign, a not infrequent occurrence in pneumatosis with small bowel involvement. Koss (1952) would exclude many of the cases reported in children, preferring to class them as intestinal emphysema. He observes that in many of these cases on microscopy, the cyst wall is devoid of epithelial lining, and cites the cases of Botsford and Krakower (1938) and Judge *et al.* (1949). He states, 'The cases in which there is evidence of cyst lining are accepted, and the others are considered as cases of emphysema, possibly a terminal event, with intestinal gas penetrating into the intestinal wall generally and not selectively into the lymphatics.'

While one must respect the views of the author of a careful and exhaustive review, he and many others have failed to appreciate the significance of the work of Wright (1930). Wright injected, under aseptic conditions, various gases into the subcutaneous tissues of guinea pigs. He found that nitrogen remained in the tissues for three days after injection and at the end of this time the crepitation typical of surgical emphysema could still be elicited. With oxygen, a gas which diffuses much more readily, crepitation could be detected at the end of 24 hours.

A study of the cellular response to these gases showed that while the response varied quantitatively with each gas used, qualitatively it was much the same. Within two days of the introduction of gas into the subcutaneous tissues, tissues which are surely not so different from those of the sub-mucosa or sub-serosa, there appeared round the gas spaces epithelioid type cells, derived, he felt, from the monocytes, by virtue of their appearance when stained supravitally. By the tenth day numerous giant cells derived from these epithelioid-like cells were present, some being 15-40μ in diameter. By the fourth day portions of the walls of the gas spaces were lined by flat cells, which morphologically resembled an endothelioid or serous lining. Although he thought that the possibility that these cells arose from capillary or lymphatic endothelium could not be ruled out, he could find no evidence that they did so and concluded that this lining arose from the epithelioid cells. By the end of two months the walls of these gas spaces were thickened and the lumina contained many giant cells, a picture closely resembling the 'older' cysts of Tung and Ngai (1933).

Although the author has been unable to identify the epithelioid nature of the cells described by Wright (1930), nearly all the sections examined from the cases of pneumatosis described showed a characteristic cell which has been described as a macrophage in the text. This cell, with an oval or round nucleus and a homogeneous dusky pink cytoplasm, is found in great numbers around early lesions and to a lesser extent around the more advanced ones. This cell may be the intestinal counterpart of Wright's epithelioid cell, and, indeed, cells which are described as mononuclears in Fig. 25 of his paper look identical with the author's macrophages.

The sequence of events would thus seem to be:

(*a*) The intestinal gases gain entrance to the sub-mucosal tissues, disrupting them to form gas spaces (Fig. 9) around which a macrophage response is evoked (Fig. 10).

(*b*) The tissues surrounding these spaces condense to form a lining, which gradually becomes altered to an endothelium (Figs. 2 and 12). In these walls typical giant cells, probably derived from the macrophages, are found (Figs. 2 and 8).

(*c*) As the gas space, now a lined gas cyst, becomes older, it may either dilate as in Figs. 5 and 6 or sclerose as in the cases of Tung and Ngai (1933).

This histological interpretation is open to criticism. It does not explain the mode of formation of sub-serosal gas cysts, nor the mode of entry of the gases when there is apparently no breach in the gut wall. It may be that there are two mechanisms of genesis for pneumatosis, a lymphatic one, and the more mechanical one outlined above. It is felt that the exclusion of certain cases by Koss (1952) is, on the basis of the evidence presented above, unwarranted. The immunological approach of Naeslund (1924) is worth repeating.

It is not without interest to note that even in the fresh specimen I could not elicit the crepitation which is so characteristic of subcutaneous emphysema. Although this absence of crepitus has not been commented on before, no reference to its presence could be found in other cases.

Summary

Five cases of pneumatosis occurring in persons of Chinese race are reported. The literature is briefly reviewed. Special reference is made to the differences of opinion which exist on the classification of gas cysts of the intestine in children, and a theory of pathogenesis for the condition is promulgated.

I wish to thank Professor Kirk for kind help and criticism; Mr. V. Nalpon for sections and photomicrographs and my wife for secretarial assistance.

References

Bang, B. L. F. (1876). *Nord. med. Ark.*, **8**, 1. (Cited by Finney (1908). *Loc. cit.*)
Biester, H. E., Eveleth, D. F. and Yamashiro, Y. (1936). *J. Amer. vet. med. Ass.*, **88**, 714.
Botsford, T. W. and Krakower, C. (1938). *J. Pediat.*, **13**, 185.
Davies, S. T. (1941). *Indian med. Gaz.*, **76**, 94.
Dupraz, A. L. (1897). *Arch. Méd. exp.*, **9**, 282.
Finney, J. M. T. (1908). *J. Amer. med. Ass.*, **51**, 1291.
Judge, D. J., Cassidy, J. E. and Rice, E. C. (1949). *Arch. Path. (Chicago)*, **48**, 206.
Koss, L. G. (1952). *A.M.A. Arch. Path.*, **53**, 523.
Kreeger, N. and Littman, L. (1954). *New Engl. J. Med.*, **251**, 779.
Ling, C. Y., Koo, S. N. and Su, Y. H. (1948). *Chin. med. J.*, **66**, 435.
MacKenzie, E. P. (1951). *Pediatrics*, **7**, 537.
Mair, W. (1908). *Med. Chron.*, **47**, 422.
Masson, P. (1925). *Ann. Anat. path.*, **2**, 541.
Matthews, F. J. C. (1954). *Brit. med. J.*, **1**, 851.
Mayer, J. (1825). Quoted by Koss (1952). *Loc. cit.*
Mills, H. W. (1925). *Surg. Gynec. Obstet.*, **40**, 387.
Naeslund, J. (1924). Zur Kenntnis der Pneumotosis cystoides intestinorum. Thesis. Uppsala, Stockholm.
Nitch, C. A. R. and Shattock, S. G. (1919). *Proc. roy. Soc. Med.*, Sect. of Path., **12**, 46.
Olson, J. D. (1954). *A.M.A. Arch. Surg.*, **68**, 899.
Pontius, G. V. (1954). In discussion on paper by Olson (1954). *Loc. cit.*
Pybus, F. C. (1934). *Brit. J. Surg.*, **21**, 539.
Straus, F. H. (1954). In discussion on paper by Olson (1954). *Loc. cit.*
Tribedi, B. P. (1941). *Calcutta med. J.*, **38**, 285.
Tung, P. C. and Ngai, S. K. (1933). *Chinese med. J.*, **47**, 1.
Urban, K. (1910). *Wein. med. Wschr.*, **60**, 1750.
Wright, A. W. (1930). *Amer. J. Path.*, **6**, 87.
Yin, Y. C. (1937). *Chinese med. J.*, **51**, 541.

PHYSICAL DEVELOPMENT OF SCHOOLGIRLS IN UPPER BURMA

BY

C. V. FOLL

From the Burma Oil Company (1954) Ltd., Rangoon

(RECEIVED FOR PUBLICATION MARCH 17, 1958)

It is still popularly believed that the onset of menstruation occurs earlier in tropical climates than in temperate ones. Ellis (1950) studied puberty in Nigeria and found, in his second series, that the median age of the menarche was 14·4 years. This was significantly later than Wilson and Sutherland's (1949) figure of 13·6 for Oxford schoolgirls, the same authors' (1950) figure of 13·49 for Dorset, Oxford and Essex schoolgirls, and Provis and Ellis's (1955) figure of 13·35 for Edinburgh schoolgirls. Wilson and Sutherland (1950) also recorded some observations from Ceylon, and showed a distinct urban-rural difference in the mean age of the menarche; the respective ages being 12·84 and 14·39 years. Such urban-rural differences were not found in their English series.

In this paper it is hoped to confirm Ellis's Nigerian findings and also to provide some information about schoolgirl growth and development in Burma.

Social Factors, Nutrition and Environment

During December, 1957, 702 schoolgirls, aged 10 to 18 years, were interviewed in Chauk, a town of some 25,000 inhabitants in Upper Burma. The girls were predominantly Burmese, the remaining few being Chinese, Indian or Anglo-Indian. Chauk is a relatively wealthy town and food is plentiful, the basic diet being vegetable (occasionally meat) curry and rice. Some fish and fresh vegetables would commonly be included in most diets. Malnutrition is rarely seen in the town.

Chauk is about 1,470 miles north of the Equator, and in the hot weather the temperature reaches about 112° F. There are approximately 24 inches of rain each year. There is no malaria and the 'dry zone' in which it lies is one of the healthiest parts of Burma.

The schoolgirls were asked their age and whether or not they had started menstruating. Unlike many tropical peoples where age estimation is largely guess-work, the Burman has an accurate knowledge of his children's ages for several reasons. It is customary for almost all Burmans to have a horoscope made; this is based on an absolutely accurate time and date of birth. Many important decisions are made only after consulting the horoscope, and propitious days are sought for weddings, going into hospital for operations or deliveries, opening new cinemas and other business undertakings. A Burmese year consists of 12 lunar months, alternately 29 days and 30 days long. During the course of every third year there is an extra month. Each full moon is treated as a Sabbath day and many are times of special celebration.

The schoolgirls' heights and weights were also recorded. Weighing was done with the girls clad in angyis (nylon or cotton blouses) and longyis (type of long, usually cotton, skirt). The total weight of clothes would be less than 2 lb. Their height was recorded with the girls barefooted.

Age of Menarche

From the results obtained, it was possible to calculate graphically by probit analysis the 'median' age of the menarche, that age at which half the girls have started their periods; this was found to be 14·4 years. Table 1 shows a comparison between this figure and those obtained by Ellis (1950) and by Wilson and Sutherland (1950).

TABLE 1

COMPARATIVE AGE OF MENARCHE IN VARIOUS GROUPS

Series		Median Age of Menarche
Wilson and Sutherland	(1949)	13·6
(England)	(1950)	13·6
Ellis and Provis	(1955)	13·35
(Scotland)		
Ellis	(1950) 1st series	14·22
(Nigeria)	2nd ,,	14·40
Wilson and Sutherland	(1950) Urban	12·10
(Ceylon)	Rural	14·5
This Series	(1957)	14·40
(Burma)		

From the table it may be seen that the Chauk results confirm Ellis's findings in Nigeria, and also Wilson and Sutherland's rural results in Ceylon.

Height and Weight

Table 2 shows the mean heights and weights arranged in age groups before and after the menarche.

TABLE 2

NUMBERS, MEAN HEIGHTS AND WEIGHTS OF CHILDREN IN PRESENT SERIES

Age	Before Menarche			After Menarche		
	No.	Height (in.)	Weight (lb.)	No.	Height (in.)	Weight (lb.)
10	72	48·37	53·85			
11	91	49·97	57·22	1*	53·00	84·00
12	85	52·48	66·09	8*	57·56	77·88
13	58	53·65	73·26	49	54·83	84·43
14	20	55·50	82·50	71	55·46	88·07
15	3*	56·50	84·00	100	55·24	91·33
16	1*	54·00	82·00	74	55·36	93·86
17	2*	54·30	88·00	47	54·23	93·59
18				20	54·88	90·70

* Numbers too small to be of significance.

It may be seen that there is considerable increase in height from year to year until the age of 14 is reached, after which height remains almost constant. There is a similar increase in weight. The cessation of growth in height at the age of 14 is earlier than in the English series and it appears from these results that growth may take place earlier in children in the tropics. For instance, the average height and weight for a Scottish girl aged 11½ years (Provis and Ellis, 1955) is 55·7 in. and 74·5 lb. (nude weight). In this series, for a Burman 11½ years old, the height was 50 in. and weight 57 lb., a difference of 5·7 in. and 17·5 lb. This is considerably less than differences in height and weight of the older children as will be shown later.

Another factor that must be considered is that there is a substantial drop in the heights of the 17-year-old group, i.e. those girls born in 1940-41. These children would have suffered during their infancy from the various privations that were common during the Japanese invasion and occupation. A further series taken in 5 years' time would no doubt throw further light on this. Generally speaking children stay at school until older in Burma than in England.

The height difference between the pre-menarche group aged 13 and 14 is 1·85 in.; this group is largely composed of girls who will start menstruating the following year. This pre-menarchial growth spurt has been reported on by Simmons and Greulich (1943).

Comparison between 13- and 14-year-olds before and after the menarche shows a very slight difference in height but a marked difference in weight. This might be taken to confirm the view of Wilson and Sutherland (1950) that increase in height at this age is unaffected by sexual development, though it could also mean that the pre-menarchial spurt of growth has already occurred by the age of 14.

Body Build

The measure used is the height (in inches) divided by the cube root of the weight (in pounds); the means of height and weight for each group were used (Table 3).

TABLE 3

BODY-BUILD (MEAN HEIGHT IN IN. DIVIDED BY CUBE ROOT OF MEAN WEIGHT IN LB.)

Age	Body-build	
	Before Menarche	After Menarche
10	12·80	
11	12·96	*
12	12·98	*
13	12·82	12·49
14	12·75	12·47
15	*	12·21
16	*	12·18
17	*	11·94
18		12·21

* Fewer than 10 measurements, value omitted.

In the pre-menarche group it may be seen that height and weight increase in the same proportions. but the post-menarche group shows that girls become heavier for their height.

This study also shows that the Burmese girl is considerably smaller than her English counterpart. For instance the average weight and height (from Wilson and Sutherland's, 1950, series) of a 13½-year-old English girl who has not menstruated is 95·8 lb. and 60·8 in.; her Burmese contemporary weighs 73·3 lb. and is 53·6 in. tall. Similarly the English figures for a post-menarche 14½-year-old are 119·9 lb. and 62·5 in. compared with the Burmese 88·1 lb. and 55·5 in. In other words, the Burmese girl of 13-14 years onwards is some 7 in. shorter and 20-30 lb. lighter than the English girl. That they are smaller from birth has been reported on in an earlier study in Chauk, where the average birth weight for some 200 consecutive single deliveries in 1957 was found to be 6 lb. 7 oz. for boys and 6 lb. 3 oz. for girls (Foll, in press).

The average figures for Scottish newborns (full term by dates, but not all weighing more than 5½ lb.) were 7 lb. 9 oz. (boys) and 7 lb. 5 oz. (girls).

Summary

A study has been made of 702 predominantly Burmese schoolgirls in Chauk, Upper Burma.

The median age of the menarche is found to be 14·4 years, thus confirming Ellis's (1950) view that the onset of menstruation takes place later in tropical climates and not earlier as is often believed.

The study of height and weight confirms Wilson and Sutherland's (1950) suggestion that in adolescent girls growth is of two superimposed types: physical growth dependent on age and sexual growth dependent on sexual development.

It is suggested that growth starts earlier in the tropics and that little growth in height takes place after the age of 14.

Early nutritional deprivation may well have an effect on subsequent growth.

The Burmese girl is shown to be lighter and shorter than her English and Scottish contemporary.

I am indebted to Professor R. W. B. Ellis for his advice and helpful criticism in the preparation of this paper; also to the Management of the Burma Oil Co. (1954) Ltd. for facilities granted to me, to the headmasters of the various schools who so willingly co-operated, and especially to Dr. Onmar Khin who interviewed the children.

REFERENCES

Ellis, R. W. B. (1950). *Brit. med. J.*, **1**, 85.
Foll, C. V. (1958). In press. *J. Trop. Pediat.*
Provis, H. S. and Ellis, R. W. B. (1955). *Arch. Dis. Childh.*, **30**, 328.
Simmons, K. and Greulich, W. W. (1943). *J. Pediat.*, **22**, 518.
Wilson, D. C. and Sutherland, I. (1949). *Brit. med. J.*, **2**, 130.
——, —— (1950). *Ibid.*, **2**, 862.

THE PREVALENCE OF DENTAL CARIES IN RELATION TO MATURITY

BY

J. N. MANSBRIDGE

From the Department of Public Health and Social Medicine, University of Edinburgh

(RECEIVED FOR PUBLICATION MARCH 27, 1958)

This study constitutes part of an investigation of the epidemiology of dental caries in 4,034 Edinburgh children in the age range 5-17 years. Of this total sample, 1,730 children were examined as part of a joint investigation with H. S. Provis and R. W. B. Ellis, who were making an anthropometric study of the children (Provis and Ellis, 1955). Therefore for this group of children data relating to certain anthropometric measurements were available in addition to the dental findings.

As socio-economic factors often influence growth, it was decided that a proportion of this sample of children should derive from private, fee-paying schools. Because of the influence of these factors on growth, it seemed not unreasonable to suppose that they could also influence dental health. When the dental state of children from fee-paying schools was compared with that of an otherwise comparable group of children from non-fee-paying schools differences in dental caries experience were found to exist. Thus, in the deciduous dentition, prevalence of dental caries was found to be lower among the fee-paying than amongst the non-fee-paying group, while in the permanent dentition the reverse was observed ; that is, dental caries was now found to be more prevalent among the fee-paying than among the non-fee-paying children. Furthermore, it was also found that the proportions of the various tooth surfaces attacked by caries differed between these two classes of children.

Analysis of the data suggested that independent aetiological factors operate in differing degree in the two contrasting social groups and these findings, supported by evidence from the literature, suggest the view that these effects reflect poorer structural quality of the teeth in the lower social class and a more caries-provoking diet of children from a higher social class environment.

Thus, by selection, the children compared were in the main divided into those belonging predominantly to Social Class I, while the remainder (the non-fee-paying children) represented Social Classes III, IV and V (Registrar General, 1931). This division of the sample distinguished unmistakably two distinct groups of differing social environments. The information available relating to the occupation of the child's father was in most instances insufficiently precise to discriminate between the various social levels of which the non-fee-paying children were comprised. For this reason these children constituted a socially heterogeneous group.

It is well recognized that differences in both stature and weight of children vary according to socio-economic level and, since such variation is probably related to standards of diet and nutrition, the possibility existed that physical differences within the non-fee-paying group of children might discriminate between the various social strata of which the group was composed, in terms of diet and nutrition.

Clements (1953) examined data relating to heights and weights of British children over the past 70 years. These data show clearly the differences that exist in height and weight between children drawn from upper, middle and lower income groups, and also indicate that children are growing more quickly now than they were some years ago. Furthermore, while these changes have taken place in all social groups, the greatest increases have occurred in the lower income groups, with the result that the disparity between children from upper and lower income groups has now been greatly reduced. Of considerable interest is the fact that during both world wars this upward trend was interrupted, to be continued again after World War I during the inter-war period. This effect of both world wars is interesting for Sognnaes (1948) showed that during both wars there was a considerable reduction in the prevalence of dental caries in those countries involved. This reduction in caries was considered to be related to dietary changes, particularly those in regard to sugar consumption. He also showed that at the end of the wars after a delay of some years the prevalence of dental caries began to increase and continued towards the pre-war level.

Since, for this sample of Edinburgh school children, there were available data relating to lying height, nude weight and a clinical assessment of sexual maturity, it was decided that a comparison of dental caries experience with certain physical measurements of non-fee-paying children should be undertaken in order to see whether the differences in dental caries found between fee-paying and non-fee-paying children would be repeated between children of differing physique.

The literature revealed only two investigations in which the relationship between physique and dental caries was studied. Cunningham (1934), in an investigation of the relation of dental caries to disease, menstrual experience and physical measurements in 11,117 young women aged 15 to 19 years, found some evidence that the tall women showed a higher prevalence of dental caries than those of medium or short stature. This difference was found to be statistically significant.

Discussing these findings, she expresses the view that many of the women of 15-18 years may not yet have attained full stature, and since dental caries increases with age, it was possible that the taller women were also among the oldest in the sample. It is unfortunate that no attempt was made to study the age distribution of these women.

Hurme (1936), in a study of 54 case histories of first-year students, in which prevalence of caries, height and health records were compared, found that when the number of D.M.F. teeth (decayed, missing and filled) was compared with height, the relationship, although not well marked, showed the number of D.M.F. teeth to be slightly less in the shorter half of the group. However, when the extremes of the distribution were compared, the short individuals had fewer D.M.F. teeth than the tall. Furthermore, since most of the tall individuals happened to belong to the youngest age group, the difference between the tall and the short was obviously not a function of chronological age in this instance.

The discrepancy between chronological and developmental age in individual children can be considerable and in consequence differences can exist between the number of teeth erupted at any given age. Therefore differences in total dental caries experience in children at the same age may be due in part to this. Also, even when all teeth have erupted, some individuals will have had their teeth exposed in the mouth to risk of attack for a longer period than others of the same chronological age.

Boas (1933) presented data to show that in a homogeneous social group, development of the dentition and general physical development as measured by height are associated. Talmers (1952) also observed that children of both sexes who had erupted their second molars early, were usually advanced in both height and weight for their age. Conversely, those children who were late in eruption of the second molars were below average in height and weight. It was also noticed that the relationship between body size and eruption was more marked among the boys than among the girls.

Clearly, then, any association found between prevalence of dental caries and physique might also be explained by differences in the rate of development, rather than by absolute differences in physique.

Methods

The Sample. This has been described previously (Provis and Ellis, 1955).

Measurement of Dental Caries. The children were examined in the schools during school hours. The dental examinations were conducted using plane mouth mirrors and Ash No. 54 probes, and illumination was obtained by the use throughout of a portable lamp, using a 60-watt bulb. The dental findings were dictated to an assistant who recorded them on a standard dental chart.

The D.M.F. index (Klein, Palmer and Knutson, 1938) has been used to measure the prevalence of dental caries of the permanent teeth in these children. Using this index, the dental caries experience of an individual is expressed in the sum of all decayed, missing and filled permanent teeth, thus past experience of the disease in terms of treatment, i.e. extractions and fillings, is included with present untreated carious teeth to give the total caries experience of the individual at the time of examination.

Analysis. As a preliminary step in order to see whether or not any relationship existed between the incidence of dental caries and height and weight, the children were ranked in order of the greatest to least height and similarly for weight, for each age and for both sexes separately. Each yearly age group was then divided into thirds and comparison of dental caries experience was made between the greatest third and the least third for height and weight separately.

Results. It was found that up to and including the age of 11 years in both sexes the differences in dental caries experience between the tallest and shortest and between the heaviest and the lightest were quite insignificant and inconsistent. However, from 12 to 17 years of age for both sexes the taller children showed a consistently greater number of D.M.F. teeth per child than those who were shorter at the same age, with one exception only; that was in girls aged 17 years, where the shortest girls showed an appreciably greater average number of D.M.F. teeth per girl than the tallest.

When weight and dental caries experience were compared, the heaviest girls showed a consistently higher average number of D.M.F. teeth from 12 to 17 years than the lightest girls, but in boys the data showed less consistency and at 12, 13 and 17 years the lightest boys showed a higher average dental caries experience, but at 14, 15 and 16 showed the same trend as the girls, that is, the heaviest had the greatest D.M.F.

Figures 1 and 2 illustrate the differences in D.M.F. between these two groups and the numerical data are presented in Appendix Tables 1 and 2.

It was found that these differences could not be explained entirely on the basis of the numbers of teeth erupted, for the average number of D.M.F. teeth per 100 teeth erupted clearly indicated a higher incidence of caries in the taller and heavier children relative to the number of teeth erupted, compared with the shorter and lighter. Also, the differences in mean age of the children seemed inadequate to explain the differences shown in dental caries experience. As mentioned earlier, it was observed that under 12 years of age the differences in dental caries between the tallest and shortest and between the heaviest and lightest were both insignificant and inconsistent. This contrast and the age at which notable differences began to appear suggested the possibility that sexual maturation may exert some influence in the incidence of dental caries and be responsible for the differences in caries between groups of contrasting physiques.

The data relating to dental caries prevalence in the total sample of Edinburgh children indicated that the greatest increase in the annual increment of caries was found to occur in girls between the ages of 13 and 14 years and in boys between 15 and 16 years of age, a difference of two years (Appendix Table 3).

Provis and Ellis (1955), in a study of the same Edinburgh children, found that boys began to show evidence of sexual maturation on the average two years later than girls. The median age of pubescence in boys was 13·45 years and in girls 11·30 years, while the median age of adolescence was for boys 15·35 years and for girls 13·35 years.

It is apparent that the peak increase in dental caries and the onset of adolescence correspond in time for both sexes. The suggestion is strong, therefore, that these two events may be related in some way.

For these children a clinical assessment of sexual maturity, made by H. S. Provis, was available. Three grades of maturity were recognized, 'non-

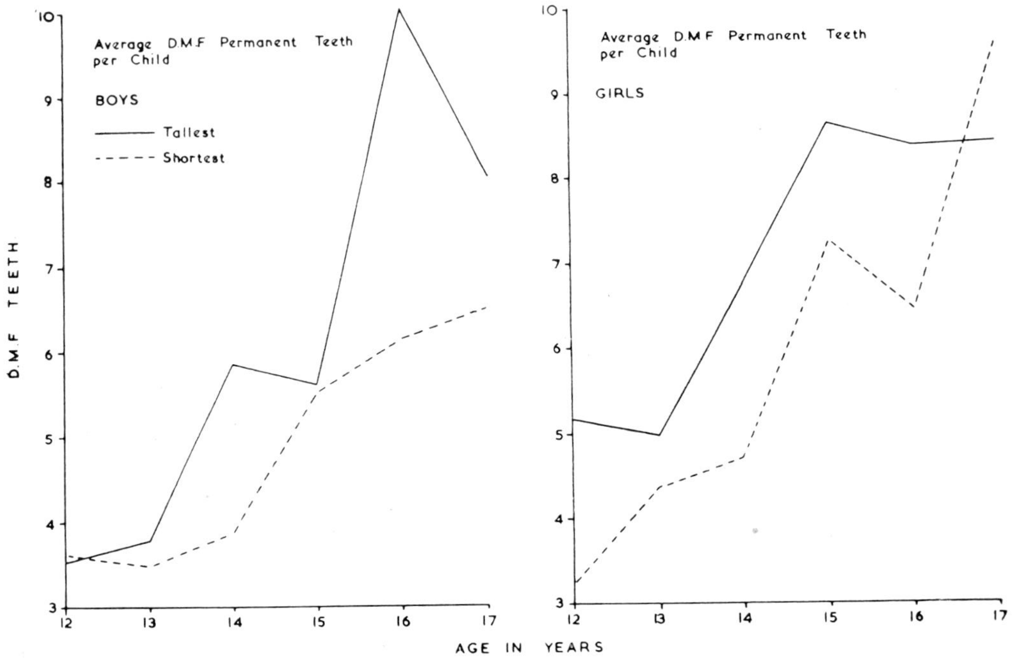

FIG. 1.—D.M.F. for tallest and shortest third of age group.

pubescent', with no evidence of sexual development, 'adolescent' as an advanced stage of maturity, while the 'pubescent' grade was intermediate. The assessment of maturity in boys was determined by the distribution of pubic and axillary hair, together with degree of development of the genitalia, according to the criteria of Ellis (1946). In girls, the beginning of pubescence was defined by breast enlargement, while the onset of menstruation was taken as the commencement of adolescence.

Therefore for each yearly group in the upper and lower thirds for height and weight, the data relating to degree of maturation were examined. These data are presented in Table 1 as combined totals for all age groups and are also given in greater detail in Appendix Tables 4 and 5.

It can be seen from these data that a very much larger proportion of the children in the upper thirds for both height and weight are in a more advanced stage of sexual maturation than those children who happen to be in the lower thirds.

To determine whether an association existed between sexual maturation and the incidence of dental caries, a comparison of dental caries experience was made between children of the same age but at different levels of maturation. For this purpose all the children for whom maturation data were available were taken as the sample.

TABLE 1

NUMBER OF CHILDREN IN THE DIFFERENT STAGES OF SEXUAL MATURATION

	Boys			Girls		
	NP	PB	AD	NP	PB	AD
Tallest	15	51	49	—	34	77
Shortest	58	39	18	13	38	60
Heaviest	14	53	48	—	29	82
Lightest	72	32	11	17	40	64

NP = Non-pubescent. PB = Pubescent. AD = Adolescent.

A preliminary examination of the data had revealed differences in dental caries between pubescent and adolescent children at the same age. However, differences were also observed in the number of teeth erupted in the different maturity groups even at the same age (Appendix Table 6). These differences were not large and it was clear that they contributed in part only to the differences in dental caries. For this reason it was decided that comparison between the different maturity grades would be confined to those children who had erupted all permanent second molars. In this way comparison would be made between children of the same age and sex and in approximately an equal stage of dental development to examine the relationship, if any, between sexual maturation and the incidence of dental caries.

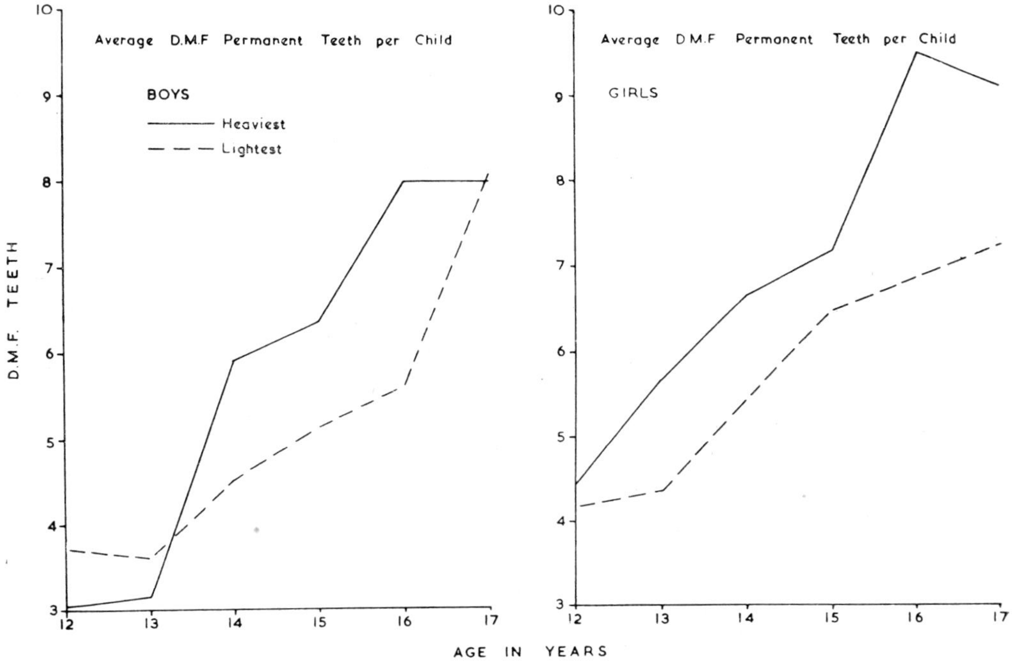

FIG. 2.—D.M.F. for heaviest and lightest third of age group.

When these requirements had been met, the distribution of children by age in each of the three maturity gradings was such that only two comparisons could usefully be made:

(1) Between 31 pubescent and 35 adolescent girls, aged 13 years, and

(2) Between 28 pubescent and 28 adolescent boys, aged 15 years.

The number of children in the non-pubescent group who had erupted all four second molars was, at any age, too small to justify comparison with a pubescent group of equivalent age.

It is generally recognized that attack of the teeth by dental caries is in part a function of the length of time that they are exposed in the mouth after eruption (Palmer, Klein and Kramer, 1938). Clements, Davies-Thomas and Pickett (1953) suggest that eruption of the second permanent molar and puberty are approximately coincident. It was considered possible, therefore, that differences in dental caries between children of the same age, who differed only in degree of maturation, might prove to be merely a reflection of the differences in time of eruption of the second molar. For example, it can be expected that the second molars of those children who are adolescent have been erupted in the mouth for a longer period than is the case of those children who are only pubescent at the same age. A second comparison was therefore made between the adolescent and pubescent children of both sexes in which the second molars were excluded from consideration. The results of these comparisons are presented in Tables 2, 3, 4 and 5.

It can be seen that those children who are less advanced in maturity have a smaller number of decayed, missing and filled teeth than those who are more mature at the same age. Furthermore, the adolescent children have an average number of D.M.F. teeth which more closely approximate that for the total Edinburgh sample at their age, while the pubescent children have an average more appropriate to a younger age.

The influence of the second molar upon the average number of D.M.F. teeth is considerable, but even when these teeth are excluded, a difference between the two maturity groups remains, which is in the same direction as before.

An examination of the distribution of dental caries of the individual teeth revealed no significant differences in distribution, that is, the pattern of attack in the two groups was substantially the same. The only difference observed was in amount of caries as indicated by the D.M.F. values in Tables 2 and 3. To test the possibility that differences in degree of dental caries might exist between the two maturity groups, the data were arranged to present dental caries measured in terms of affected tooth surfaces. The results indicated, however, that dental caries measured in this way shows differences between the groups equivalent to those observed when using the D.M.F. index. For these data then, the D.M.F. index provides a good measure of dental caries experience.

Thus far the evidence clearly suggests that degree of sexual maturation is associated in some way with the dental caries experience of the child. It was appreciated, however, that the number of children between whom comparison was made was of necessity small and, taking into account the high variability of dental caries in individuals, it was manifestly desirable that some measure of this possible association be obtained and tested. The comparison of dental caries experience between children in the greatest and least thirds of height and weight had shown that the difference in dental caries

TABLE 2

MEAN NUMBER OF DECAYED, MISSING AND FILLED TEETH IN 13-YEAR-OLD GIRLS

Maturity Grading	No.	Mean No. Teeth Erupted	Mean D.M.F. Teeth
Pubescent	31	27·42	4·81
Adolescent	35	27·28	5·40
Ungraded Total Edinburgh Sample	151	26·92	5·58

TABLE 3

MEAN NUMBER OF DECAYED, MISSING AND FILLED TEETH IN 15-YEAR-OLD BOYS

Maturity Grading	No.	Mean No. Teeth Erupted	Mean D.M.F. Teeth
Pubescent	28	27·68	5·68
Adolescent	28	27·53	6·54
Ungraded Total Edinburgh Sample	111	27·55	6·25

TABLE 4

MEAN NUMBER OF DECAYED, MISSING AND FILLED TEETH, SECOND MOLARS EXCLUDED, 13-YEAR-OLD GIRLS

Maturity Grading	No.	Mean D.M.F. Teeth
Pubescent	31	3·42
Adolescent	35	4·17

TABLE 5

MEAN NUMBER OF DECAYED, MISSING AND FILLED TEETH, SECOND MOLARS EXCLUDED, 15-YEAR-OLD BOYS

Maturity Grading	No.	Mean D.M.F. Teeth
Pubescent	28	4·36
Adolescent	28	4·79

in these children might also have been influenced to some extent by differences in both the number of teeth erupted and chronological age. The inter-relationship of these possible factors presented a complicated situation and therefore, in an attempt to disentangle the effects of these various factors, multiple regression equations were calculated separately for boys and girls, in which the number of D.M.F. teeth was used as the dependent variate and some or all of the following in differing combinations were taken as independent variates:

Height	Maturity
Weight	with stages: Non-pubescent
Age	Pubescent
Number of teeth erupted	Adolescent

For this purpose, within the age range 11-17 years the entire sample for which these data were available was used and consisted of 629 boys and 581 girls. As might be expected, the number of D.M.F. teeth increased with age and with the total teeth erupted, these two indices being, of course, themselves highly correlated. When the effect of these was discounted, a marked difference appeared between the sexes. Among boys there was a highly significant increase of D.M.F. teeth with maturity, but there was no such effect with girls.

To investigate this further, the regressions were done in another way. In each year of age D.M.F. teeth were used as a dependent variate and the first and second stages of maturation (pubescent and adolescent) as independent variates. From the sums of squares and cross-products of these a pooled regression was done for boys and another for girls. The effect of this is to give a measure of the difference, over the range of ages studied, in number of D.M.F. teeth between children of like age according to which stage of maturation they had reached.

These regressions for both sexes showed that the number of teeth erupted was significantly associated with the stage of pubescence, but not with adolescence.

Discussion

It has been shown that differences in dental caries exist between those children who are tallest and heaviest and those who are shortest and lightest in the same yearly age group. However, these differences in physique could not be ascribed only to differences in standards of nutrition, if at all, and in consequence the original objective of this comparison, which was to discover whether differences in physique might discriminate between differing social levels, has not been achieved. It can be seen from the data presented in Appendix Tables 1 and 2 that the tallest and heaviest children were on average fractionally older and had a greater number of teeth erupted. In addition, it was found that the great majority of the tallest and heaviest children had reached a more advanced stage of maturity than those who were shortest and lightest.

With regard to the differences in dental caries between these children, it was appreciated that these differences could be due either to the greater number of teeth erupted, or to the slightly greater age of the tallest and heaviest children, or to both of these factors. However, neither of these seemed adequate to explain fully the observed differences in dental caries, although it was recognized that they could contribute in part. There remained, therefore, the generally more advanced maturity of the taller and heavier children as a possible factor in their greater prevalence of dental caries. It had also been observed that no consistent differences in caries experience existed between these two groups of children of contrasting physique up to 11 years of age, but that major differences were only found in the age group 12-17 years, during the period from puberty to adolescence. Furthermore, the data relating to the incidence of dental caries in the larger total sample of Edinburgh children indicated that the greatest annual increment of caries corresponded in time with the onset of adolescence in both sexes.

These facts therefore suggested that sexual maturation and susceptibility to caries may be associated in some way. A comparison between adolescent and pubescent children of the same chronological age, who had erupted all their second molars, revealed differences in dental caries for both sexes that seemed only attributable to differences in degree of sexual maturation, and further indicated that these differences involved the whole dentition, not only the more recently erupted second molars.

However, Parfitt and Parfitt (1954), in a study of the caries experience of a number of individuals from childhood to middle age, as derived from the records of private practice, presented data which showed no change in the caries incidence rate between the ages of 6-21 years, and commented that, while it has been suggested that puberty may have some influence on caries incidence rate, the data examined by them in their study did not show any such change. Of the 60 cases studied in this age range, 20 showed no change in caries incidence rate, but the remaining 40 individuals showed variations in the caries rate during this period, as many showing a decrease as an increase. They concluded, therefore, that puberty did not affect the caries incidence rate measurably.

The data provided by this study of Edinburgh children are insufficient to show what the mechanism involved in this phenomenon may be, but the findings, together with evidence from other studies, suggest a possible explanation.

Boas (1933) presented data showing that in a homogeneous social group, development of the dentition and general physical development as measured by height are associated. He demonstrated that early dentition was related to early increase in stature.

Talmers (1952) also observed that children of both sexes who had erupted their second molars early were usually advanced in both height and weight for their age. Conversely, she found that those children who were late in eruption of the second molars were below average in height and weight.

Clements *et al.* (1953) found that there was a trend towards the earlier eruption of the lower C, PM_1 and M_2 teeth in those children who showed physical signs of puberty compared with those who showed no signs of puberty.

The data for Edinburgh children indicated that the tallest (and heaviest) children had a consistently greater number of teeth erupted than the smallest (and lightest) at approximately the same age, and are therefore in agreement with these other three studies. Also, the data given in Appendix Table 6, showing the average number of teeth found at various stages of physical maturation in both boys and girls, appear to confirm the view that tooth eruption and general physical development are closely related.

Of particular interest are the findings of Ellis (1946) in a study of height and weight in relation to onset of puberty in boys aged 11-16 years. He found that not only were boys of a higher maturity group heavier and taller than boys of the same age in a lower maturity group, but that difference between the growth curves could be demonstrated as far back as the sixth year. There is thus good evidence that general physical development and eruption of teeth are associated, and further, that those children who mature early have been early in general physical development from a much earlier age, while those in whom the onset of puberty is late, have been late in general physical development throughout their early years.

It seems possible to suggest, therefore, that in terms of dental development, those who mature late (e.g. in this study, boys who at 15 are classed as pubescent) may have been late in eruption of their teeth throughout their whole period of dental development. In consequence their teeth would have been exposed to risk of attack by dental caries for a shorter period than in the case of those children who have erupted their teeth at the usual times or earlier.

While the differences in decayed, missing and filled teeth between pubescent and adolescent children of the same age could be explained in terms of differences in times of dental development, the possibility exists that these differences in caries experience may be dietary in origin. The period of sexual maturity is accompanied by a rapid acceleration in growth and in consequence nutritional needs are increased, together with corresponding increase in appetite. Widdowson (1947) presents data from which it is apparent that caloric intake reaches a peak for boys at 15 years of age and for girls at 14 years.

Her data relating to total sugar consumption of children are also of some interest, showing that in boys, the highest average intake was 37·7 oz. per week at 15 years of age, and in girls 26·0 oz. per week at the age of 14 years. Total sugar consumption included sugar taken as such, sweets including chocolate, jams, cakes, biscuits, sugar in puddings and in cooked fruit. It was also found that up to the age of 8, differences in sugar consumption between the sexes were negligible, but from 9 years upwards boys consumed more than girls and at 15 they were eating nearly twice as much. Between 15 and 18 years boys ate more than twice as much as girls of similar age.

A finding of considerable importance was the very great variation in food consumption of children at the same age and the fact that these extreme variations were compatible with normal physical development. Ellis (1951), commenting upon this observation regarding variations in food consumption in individual children of the same age, poses the question as to whether maturity grading of children in such a study might not reveal less variation in caloric intake in relation to stage of maturity reached than was observed when the children were grouped by chronological age.

Since an increased intake of refined carbohydrate, especially sugar in sticky form between meals, has been shown to be associated with an increase in susceptibility to dental caries (Gustafsson, Quensel, Lanke, Lundqvist, Grahnén, Bonow and Krasse, 1954), the high consumption of these items of diet by children in the 13-15 years old age group suggests another possible explanation of the differences in dental caries found between pubescent and adolescent children of the same age. That is, those who mature physically early may then have subsisted for a longer period upon a diet containing a high level of refined carbohydrates than those of the same age who matured later. Gustafsson *et al.* (1954) clearly demonstrated the rapidity with which susceptibility to dental caries could be altered by increasing or decreasing the intake of sugars in certain forms, even in adults. These writers also pointed out that similar dietary changes in children might be expected to produce even more marked differences in susceptibility.

Although two quite different possible explanations may be offered to account for the differences in dental caries experience found in this study between pubescent and adolescent children, these explanations are not mutually exclusive. It is therefore possible that both differences in time of development of the dentition and differences in susceptibility due to dietary changes may both play their part in producing the results described in this study.

From the multiple regression analysis confirmation of previous findings in this study was obtained that, for boys, sexual maturity and dental caries incidence are associated and, more precisely, that this association is related to adolescence but not to pubescence. Furthermore, the differences in D.M.F. teeth between adolescent and pubescent boys of the same chronological age attributable to maturity alone was 1·8 teeth. For girls, however, the differences in dental caries experience between those who are adolescent and those who are pubescent at the same age were not found to be significantly associated with stage of maturity. It is of some interest that Talmers (1952) noted that the relationship between body size and eruption of second molars was less marked in girls than in boys.

This difference between the sexes was not expected since the previous evidence suggested that, if in fact sexual maturity and dental caries incidence were associated, it would have been so for both sexes inasmuch as:

(1) For the total Edinburgh sample the greatest increment of dental caries was found to correspond in time with the onset of adolescence in both sexes, i.e., between 13 and 14 years in girls and 15 and 16 in boys. It was seen, however, that the increase in D.M.F. teeth in boys between 15 and 16 was greater than the increase in girls between 13 and 14 years.

(2) The tallest and heaviest thirds of each yearly age group showed a significantly greater proportion of children in more advanced stages of maturity than those in the least thirds. This was true for both sexes.

(3) The comparison between pubescent and adolescent children of the same chronological age, who had also erupted all their second permanent molars indicated that there was a higher incidence of caries in the adolescent children of both sexes and that this difference in caries affected the dentition as a whole, not *only* the second molars.

It is recognized that individual variations in dental caries incidence are considerable and result in large standard deviations. Consequently because of this variability any difference in D.M.F. rates between groups of individuals must be large to be statistically significant. Taking all the evidence into account, the possibility exists that the difference in dental caries experience observed between girls at different stages of maturation may, in fact, be associated with maturity in much the same way as boys, even if not of such magnitude as to show a statistically significant relationship.

It is concluded, therefore, from the evidence obtained that adolescence in boys is associated with a higher dental caries incidence than is found in pubescent boys of the same age.

It is suggested that this may be due either to a longer total exposure of the teeth in the mouth or to dietary factors associated with adolescence, or to a combination of both factors together.

Finally, the regressions for both sexes provided statistical evidence that the number of teeth erupted was associated with pubescence. This confirms the observations made from the data presented in Appendix Table 6, and also those of Clements *et al.* (1953).

Summary and Conclusions

Data are presented which show a relationship between dental caries experience and stage of sexual maturation in children.

When children of the same chronological age and at an equal stage of dental development were compared, it was found that children further advanced in maturation showed a higher dental caries experience than those who were less advanced. Also this difference in dental caries appeared to influence the dentition as a whole.

Possible reasons for this are discussed.

From the evidence obtained in this investigation it is concluded that earlier sexual maturation is associated with an increased prevalence of dental caries in boys.

For girls no statistically significant evidence was obtained to indicate that a similar relationship exists, although other evidence suggests that this may be so.

Finally, it was also found that for both sexes those children who reach the stage of pubescence early have a greater number of permanent teeth erupted than non-pubescent children of the same chronological age.

I wish to thank Professor J. H. F. Brotherston and Professor R. W. B. Ellis for their most helpful advice and criticism. I am also indebted to Dr. H. S. Provis for his co-operation in this study, to Dr. W. N. Boog Watson, Chief School Medical Officer and Mr. G. Moody, Chief Dental Officer, of the City of Edinburgh, for their most helpful co-operation in the collection of the original data.

My sincere thanks are due to Dr. Barnet Woolf for his valuable statistical advice and to Miss M. Brown for her assistance in the computation of the raw data.

REFERENCES

Boas, F (1933). *Hum. Biol.*, **5**, 429.
Clements, E. M. B. (1953). *Brit. med. J.*, **2**, 897.
— —, Davies-Thomas, E. and Pickett, K. G. (1953). *Ibid.*, **1**, 1421.

Cunningham, R. L. (1934). *J. dent. Res.*, **14**, 439.
Ellis, R. W. B. (1946). *Arch. Dis. Childh.*, **21**, 181.
—— (1951). *Brit. J. Nutr.*, **5**, 151.
Gustafsson, B. E., Quensel, C. E., Lanke, L. S., Lundqvist, C., Grahnén, H., Bonow, B. E. and Krasse, B. (1954). *Acta odont. scand.*, **11**, 232.
Hurme, V. O. (1936). *J. dent. Res.*, **15**, 395.
Klein, H., Palmer, C. E. and Knutson, J. W. (1938). *Publ. Hlth. Rep. (Wash.)*, **53**, 751.
Palmer, C. E., Klein, H. and Kramer, M. (1938). *Growth*, **2**, 149.
Parfitt, G. J. and Parfitt, J. B. (1954). *Brit. dent. J.*, **96**, 183.
Provis, H. S. and Ellis, R. W. B. (1955). *Arch. Dis. Childh.*, **30**, 328.
Registrar General (1931). Classification of Occupations. H.M.S.O., London.
Sognnaes, R. F. (1948). *Amer. J. Dis. Child.*, **75**, 792.
Talmers, D. A. (1952). *N.Y. St. dent. J.*, **18**, 314.
Widdowson, E. M. (1947). *Spec. Rep. Ser. Med. Res. Coun. (Lond.)*, No. 257.

APPENDIX

TABLE 1

DENTAL CARIES IN RELATION TO HEIGHT

No.	Tallest Third				Shortest Third			
	Mean Age (yr.)	Mean No. Teeth Erupted	Mean No. D.M.F. Teeth per Child	D.M.F per 100 Teeth Erupted	Mean Age (yr.)	Mean No. Teeth Erupted	Mean No. D.M.F. Teeth per Child	D.M.F. per 100 Teeth Erupted
Boys								
23	12·6	25·7	3·5	13·7	12·5	23·8	3·4	14·2
24	13·5	26·5	3·8	14·3	13·2	25·2	3·5	13·9
24	14·5	27·6	5·9	21·3	14·5	26·4	3·9	14·7
21	15·4	27·8	5·6	20·2	15·2	27·2	5·4	19·7
13	16·6	28·5	10·1	35·3	16·4	27·7	6·1	22·2
10	17·5	28·6	8·1	28·3	17·4	28·7	6·5	22·6
Girls								
26	12·7	26·2	5·2	19·8	12·5	25·1	3·2	12·9
26	13·6	26·8	5·0	18·7	13·4	26·2	4·4	16·7
17	14·6	27·6	6·8	24·5	14·4	26·8	4·8	17·8
19	15·5	28·1	8·6	30·7	15·3	27·7	7·3	26·2
14	16·5	28·9	8·4	29·0	16·4	28·1	6·4	22·9
9	17·5	28·0	8·4	30·2	17·5	27·8	9·5	34·4

TABLE 2

DENTAL CARIES IN RELATION TO WEIGHT

No.	Heaviest Third				Lightest Third			
	Mean Age (yr.)	Mean No. Teeth Erupted	Mean No. D.M.F. Teeth per Child	D.M.F. per 100 Teeth Erupted	Mean Age (yr.)	Mean No. Teeth Erupted	Mean No. D.M.F. Teeth per Child	D.M.F. per 100 Teeth Erupted
Boys								
23	12·6	25·3	3·0	12·0	12·5	23·3	3·7	15·9
24	13·6	26·6	3·2	11·9	13·4	24·8	3·6	14·6
24	14·5	27·7	5·9	21·4	14·5	26·6	4·5	17·1
21	15·4	27·6	6·4	23·1	15·2	27·3	5·1	18·8
13	16·6	28·1	8·0	28·4	16·4	27·8	5·6	20·2
10	17·4	28·8	8·0	27·8	17·4	28·6	8·1	28·3
Girls								
26	12·6	26·2	4·4	16·9	12·5	25·2	4·2	16·8
26	13·6	27·1	5·6	20·8	13·3	26·1	4·3	16·6
17	14·5	27·3	6·6	24·3	14·4	26·8	5·5	20·6
19	15·5	28·1	7·2	25·5	15·3	27·6	6·5	23·7
14	16·6	28·6	9·5	33·2	16·4	28·2	6·9	24·3
9	17·6	28·3	9·1	32·2	17·4	27·8	7·2	26·0

TABLE 3

DENTAL CARIES PREVALENCE BY AGE AND SEX IN A SAMPLE OF 4,034 EDINBURGH CHILDREN

Age (yr.)	Boys			Girls		
	No.	Mean D.M.F. Teeth per Child	Annual Increment in Mean D.M.F. Teeth	No.	Mean D.M.F. Teeth per Child	Annual Increment in Mean D.M.F. Teeth
5	135	0·12	0·00	144	0·19	0·00
6	200	0·65	0·53	170	0·70	0·51
7	170	1·69	1·04	171	2·13	1·43
8	204	1·83	0·14	202	2·31	0·18
9	192	2·20	0·37	193	2·64	0·33
10	183	2·64	0·44	204	3·12	0·48
11	207	3·41	0·77	218	4·17	1·05
12	199	4·10	0·69	205	4·71	0·54
13	123	4·47	0·37	151	5·58	0·87
14	117	5·15	0·68	133	7·11	1·53
15	111	6·23	1·08	119	7·73	0·62
16	69	7·97	1·74	90	8·63	0·90
17	62	8·11	0·14	62	9·11	0·48

TABLE 4
THE NUMBER AND PERCENTAGE OF BOYS IN THE VARIOUS STAGES OF SEXUAL MATURATION

Age Group	Number						Percentage					
	NP	PB	AD	NP	PB	AD	NP	PB	AD	NP	PB	AD
	Tallest			Shortest			Tallest			Shortest		
12	11	12	—	22	1	—	48	52	—	96	4	—
13	4	19	1	21	3	—	17	79	4	87	13	—
14	—	18	6	13	10	1	—	75	25	54	42	4
15	—	2	19	2	16	3	—	9	91	9	77	14
16	—	—	13	—	8	5	—	—	100	—	62	38
17	—	—	10	—	1	9	—	—	100	—	10	90
Total	15	51	49	58	39	18	13	44	43	50	34	16
	Heaviest			Lightest			Heaviest			Lightest		
12	10	13	—	23	—	—	43	57	—	100	—	—
13	4	19	1	22	2	—	17	79	4	92	8	—
14	—	17	7	16	8	—	—	71	29	67	33	—
15	—	4	17	3	16	2	—	19	81	14	77	9
16	—	—	13	—	8	5	—	—	100	—	62	38
17	—	—	10	—	1	9	—	—	100	—	10	90
Total	14	53	48	64	35	16	12	46	42	56	30	14

NP = Non-pubescent. PB = Pubescent. AD = Adolescent.

TABLE 5
THE NUMBER AND PERCENTAGE OF GIRLS IN THE VARIOUS STAGES OF SEXUAL MATURATION

Age Group	Number						Percen age					
	NP	PB	AD	NP	PB	AD	NP	PB	AD	NP	PB	AD
	Tallest			Shortest			Tallest			Shortest		
12	—	21	5	9	17	—	—	81	19	35	65	—
13	—	9	17	3	16	7	—	35	65	12	61	27
14	—	3	14	1	4	12	—	18	82	6	24	70
15	—	1	18	—	1	18	—	5	95	—	5	95
16	—	—	14	—	—	14	—	—	100	—	—	100
17	—	—	9	—	—	9	—	—	100	—	—	100
Total	—	34	77	13	38	60	—	31	69	12	34	54
	Heaviest			Lightest			Heaviest			Lightest		
12	—	22	4	13	11	2	—	85	15	50	42	8
13	—	5	21	3	20	3	—	19	81	12	76	12
14	—	2	15	1	6	10	—	12	88	6	35	59
15	—	—	19	—	3	16	—	—	100	—	16	84
16	—	—	14	—	—	14	—	—	100	—	—	100
17	—	—	9	—	—	9	—	—	100	—	—	100
Total	—	29	82	17	40	54	—	26	74	15	36	49

NP = Non-pubescent. PB = Pubescent. AD = Adolescent.

TABLE 6
MEAN NUMBER OF TEETH ERUPTED PER CHILD AND ASSESSMENT OF SEXUAL MATURATION

Age (yr.)	Assessment of Sexual Maturity	Boys		Girls	
		No.	Mean No. of Teeth Erupted	No.	Mean No. of Teeth Erupted
11	Non-pubescent	—	—	29	21·69
	Pubescent	—	—	34	24·09
12	Non-pubescent	70	24·14	13	25·69
	Pubescent	21	25·90	67	25·60
	Adolescent	—	—	7	26·71
13	Non-pubescent	42	25·55	—	—
	Pubescent	43	25·98	39	26·79
	Adolescent	—	—	46	27·04
14	Non-pubescent	19	26·58	—	—
	Pubescent	53	27·28	13	26·54
	Adolescent	15	27·47	54	27·46
15	Pubescent	35	27·34	—	—
	Adolescent	52	27·69	—	—

FAMILIAL DYSAUTONOMIA

BY

T. McKENDRICK

From the Paediatric Unit, Hillingdon Hospital, Middlesex

(RECEIVED FOR PUBLICATION APRIL 11, 1958)

Familial dysautonomia is a rare syndrome of childhood affecting the nervous system. As the name suggests, dysfunction of the autonomic system is a prominent feature. It was first recognized as a separate entity by Riley, Day, Greeley and Langford (1949), the first large series being described by Riley (1952). So far, about 70 patients have been recorded. Though the fully developed syndrome is unmistakable, not all its features can be elicited in infancy and it is likely that some patients have died undiagnosed. Some of the constituent features may suggest other commoner diseases such as fibrocystic disease of the pancreas, cerebral palsy or childhood schizophrenia. There may therefore be further patients as yet unrecognized in long stay hospitals or mental deficiency institutions, or attending psychiatric clinics. These unfortunate children and their families can be helped (Riley, 1957) so that early recognition is important.

With the exception of one from Vienna (Tyndel, 1955), all the cases so far recorded have been from America or Canada (Forster and Tyndel, 1956). The following example is unusual in that the diagnosis was certain at the age of 8 months despite the absence of a family history of this condition.

Case Report

B.A. is the third child of Jewish parents. When she was born her father was aged 41 and her mother 39. Both had been healthy and there was no history of consanguinity. Their first child, a boy of 16, and their second, a girl of 10½, were healthy and had both been breast fed for about nine months. B.A. was born at term by uncomplicated breech delivery following moderately severe maternal pre-eclampsia in the last month of pregnancy. Her birth weight was 6 lb. 4½ oz. She showed mild asphyxia at birth, but the only other abnormality noted then was that the fourth toe of each foot tended to cross medially under the third. Breast feeding was not established as the baby never sucked properly.

Advice was sought when she was 8 months old because of the following symptoms:

(1) Coldness of the extremities since the first few days of life and always present irrespective of clothing, room temperature or weather. Her hands and feet were frequently blue with cold, and sometimes swollen.

(2) Profuse sweating from her head and body since coming home from the maternity hospital. She invariably needed a complete change of dress and bed clothes each morning.

(3) Feeding difficulty had been present since birth and appeared to be due to dysphagia. Since the age of 1 month she began to put her thumb into her mouth after each mouthful of feed, apparently to assist swallowing. As a result, each feed took an hour or more and many were never finished. She frequently spat out or refused feeds, and never seemed hungry. Solids were consistently refused.

(4) Breath-holding attacks. These began at the age of 5 months and had increased in frequency from one or two to three or four daily. Either without warning or whilst crying, she would hold her breath, become cyanotic and lose consciousness for a few seconds. No sequelae had been noted.

(5) Emotional instability. She was easily and unpredictably upset, and to a much more profound degree than were her siblings at the same age. Sometimes she could not be consoled.

In spite of her discomfort and frustration, however, she had never produced any tears. There had been no vomiting, no excessive dribbling and her bowel actions were normal. There was no history of intercurrent illness, and she had never apparently been febrile. Her weight gain, though slow, had been fairly constant. She did not smile until 4 months old. Shortly after this she began to try to hold her head up, but at 7 months she was not sitting and made little attempt to play with toys.

Examination. B.A. was miserable but lusty. In spite of loud cries of misery and fear, there were no tears, though her conjunctivae were moist. Her hands were constantly active, but the movements were those of a child of 4 or 5 months of age. Throughout the examination she frequently interrupted her wailing by pushing her left thumb in her mouth to suck it only a few times before resuming her cries. There was mild plagiocephaly and slight asymmetry of the ears. The pulse was regular at 164 per minute. The heart was clinically normal, a quiet, short, blowing, apical mid-systolic murmur being considered physiological. Blood pressure: (whilst awake, by flush method) systolic 120 mm. mercury in arm, 90 mm. in leg; (whilst asleep, by auscultation) 106/60 mm. in arm, 80/50 mm. in leg. Though the hands and feet were abnormally cold and blue, the radial and tibial pulses were easily palpable. The trunk and limbs showed cutis marmorata but her scalp and neck were wet with perspiration. No abnormality was found in the chest, abdomen, genitalia, ears, or nose and no enlarged glands were felt. The limbs showed full ranges of movement.

An examination of the nervous system showed that the fundi and pupillary reactions were normal. There was absence of corneal reflexes, associated with hypo- or anaesthesia of the corneae; some sensation was present in the rest of the area supplied by the trigeminal nerve, but the child did not resent a swab soaked in ammonia being held under her nose, nor did this produce any tears. The movement of the eyes and face was normal. There was a brisk gag reflex. Abnormal swallowing mechanism was noticed: a bolus of food when placed on the back of the tongue would be swallowed with an effort in two to three seconds; elsewhere in the mouth it was rejected. The limb movements were immature and there were no tendon reflexes present in arms or legs.

Developmental Assessment. (Gesell.) Made at 35 weeks by Dr. E. P. G. Michell. "The developmental profile was uneven and showed retardation in all areas. Gross motor performance was particularly affected; fine motor adaptive, less so. Predominantly, test behaviour was at the 20-24 week level."

Investigations. There were no cells, casts, albumen or organisms in the urine. A pooled specimen over several days showed no abnormal amount of pressor amines. Haemoglobin was 80%; white cells, 18,700 per c.mm., polymorphs, 39%; lymphocytes, 56%; monocytes 4%; eosinophils, 1%. Blood urea, 29 mg. per 100 ml.; blood cholesterol 105 mg. per 100 ml.; serum calcium, 9·6 mg. per 100 ml.; serum alkaline phosphatase 24·8 K-A units per 100 ml.; serum sodium, potassium, chloride and bicarbonate levels normal; plasma electrophoretic pattern within normal limits. The Wassermann reaction was negative; a Mantoux test 1 in 1,000 was negative. Electrocardiogram rate 165 per minute; sinus rhythm; P.R. 0·11 second; Q.R.S. 0·04 second; electrical axis vertical; there was less evidence of right ventricular preponderance than is usual at this age; ST segments and T waves were within normal limits. Radiographs of the chest and abdomen were normal. Bone development was compatible with age. A barium swallow was normal. Cerebrospinal fluid was clear and colourless; sugar, chlorides and protein were all within normal limits; there was no excess of globulin. Lange showed no reaction. An electroencephalogram showed no evidence of any paroxysmal disturbance or unilateral cerebral lesion. Subcutaneous injection of 0·125 mg. neostigmine bromide produced a few tears (Kroop, 1956).

Progress. During her 10-day stay in the ward she was kept in a cubicle of average temperature 70° F. The extremities became pink and warm. The rectal temperature varied irregularly between 97·0 and 100·2°F. When she was asleep the pulse was usually 120 per minute but when she was awake it was contantly raised to 160 per minute. She had three short breath-holding attacks, all related to examination or handling by nursing staff. Feeds continued to take an hour or more and many were left unfinished. Her weight remained about $14\frac{3}{4}$ lb.

She was discharged receiving phenobarbitone gr. $\frac{1}{4}$ twice daily. Subsequently there were only about six breath-holding attacks during the following 10 weeks. The blood pressure has once been as high as 146/86 mm. of mercury. One attack of bronchitis lasting three weeks occurred at the age of 9 months. At the age of 1 year she was less miserable than before admission. Developmental assessment (Gesell) at 53 weeks by Dr. E. P. G. Michell showed a similar pattern to that at 35 weeks. Her performance was on the whole at the 28-32 week level, but one test was performed at the 40-week level. At this time she began to show indifference to painful stimuli.

Discussion

This child shows many of the features of the syndrome as described in the literature. Other common but not essential features are not present and some cannot be assessed. Table 1 summarizes these.

TABLE 1

Feature	Present	Not Present	Not Fully Assessed
Hereditary factors	Jewish parents	Occurrence in siblings Consanguinity of parents	
Autonomic dysfunction	Absence of tears Excessive sweating Paroxysmal hypertension Poor control of peripheral circulation Abnormal swallowing mechanism	Skin blotches Bowel upsets Excessive dribbling Attacks of high fever	Postural hypotension
Voluntary motor-disturbance	Poor co-ordination Absent tendon reflexes	Orthopaedic deformity	Dysarthria
Sensory disturbance	Corneal anaesthesia		Indifference to pain Dysaesthesia Proprioceptive disturbance
Psychological features	Breath-holding attacks Emotional lability Retarded development	Vomiting attacks	
Other features	Retarded growth	Frequent respiratory infections Corneal ulceration	Tendency to accidental injury

She also had the typical facial expression, difficult to describe adequately, but apparently compounded of suspicion, fear and misery.

Of this diverse collection of symptoms, some are present so frequently as to be considered essential to the diagnosis. These are: (1) Jewish ancestry. (2) Reduced tear secretion. (3) Excessive sweating. (4) Feeding difficulty. (5) Cold hands and feet. (6) Postural hypotension. (7) Poor motor co-ordination. (8) Corneal anaesthesia. (9) Relative indifference to pain, and (10) Emotional lability.

A variable number of the other features in the table may be present. Also occasionally reported have been persistent leucocytosis, neonatal flaccidity and persistent thumb sucking. The predominating features tend to vary with age. Thus feeding difficulty is commonly the earliest symptom; absence of tears is not noteworthy before 2 months of age; motor inco-ordination is seldom appreciated before 6 months. After the age of 6 months breath-holding attacks begin, and parents may focus attention on apparent mental retardation or on excessive dribbling. Vomiting attacks usually predominate in those aged 2 to 5 years. Sensory disturbance and postural hypotension can be evaluated only after infancy.

The diagnosis in extreme infancy is not easily made, and usually doubt remains throughout the first year of life. Riley (1957) suggests that in the neonatal period at least the following should be present: (1) Family history. (2) Pronounced feeding difficulty and (3) Lack of deep tendon reflexes.

Family history, however, can never be more than suggestive, and has been found in only about a third of all cases so far reported. Feeding difficulty is common in newborn infants but in this condition it is marked and frequently shows no sign of ameliorating for several months. Though swallowing is more commonly reported to be abnormal, difficulty in sucking has also been noted. Tendon reflexes are not always absent in older cases. In some they vary from time to time, and it may be that they disappear as the child grows.

Moloshok and Reuben (1954) were able to gather the neonatal histories of 14 of their patients. They found that apart from feeding difficulty there was a high incidence of apnoeic or cyanotic attacks simulating atelectasis, hypothermia, attacks of high fever, excessive oral secretion, vomiting and failure to thrive. The present case suggests that profuse sweating and poor circulatory control may also occur in the neonatal period.

Differential Diagnosis. Provided that it is considered, familial dysautonomia is unlikely to be confused with other conditions. There are, however, points of similarity with several commoner diseases in infancy. Thus the vasomotor instability, sweating, hyporeflexia and misery occur also in pink disease. This condition, however, rarely affects children under the age of 6 months, whereas dysautonomic children are abnormal from birth. Photophobia, severe skin irritation and increased urinary excretion of pressor amines (Farquhar, Crawford and Law, 1956) often found in pink disease, have not been described in dysautonomia. In the latter, feeding difficulty as opposed to anorexia is typical.

Because of frequent lower respiratory infections, poor nutritional state, sweating, hypotonia and febrile episodes, fibrocystic disease of the pancreas may be suspected. Suspicion may be heightened by radiographic demonstration of areas of consolidation, atelectasis or emphysema. These are usually attributed to aspiration of food or vomitus as a result of inco-ordinated swallowing. Moloshok and Moseley (1956) have suggested that increased bronchial secretion may be responsible, much as the changes in fibrocystic disease are related to the unduly viscid secretion throughout the respiratory tree. Though the duodenal juice may be viscid and scanty in dysautonomia, pancreatic function is normal (Shwachman, Leubner and Catzel, 1955).

Cerebral palsy may show similar motor defects but sensory and vascular disturbances are not marked. Rarely, absence of tears may be due to congenital absence of the lachrymal glands, sometimes associated with other congenital defects in the face, skull or cranial nerve nuclei (Sjögren and Eriksen, 1950).

Later in childhood several other conditions require differentiation. The attacks of fever, vomiting, abdominal pain, headache and sweating may simulate the periodic syndrome. In this condition and in migraine, however, there are usually no physical signs.

Less easy to disprove is the presence of a phaeochromocytoma. Smid and DuShane (1955) could find fewer than a dozen under the age of 10 recorded in the literature. Both a phaeochromocytoma and dysautonomia may produce paroxysms of headache, pallor, sweating, abdominal pain, peripheral vasoconstriction and hypertension. Phaeochromocytoma, however, is not accompanied by nervous abnormalities and the attacks respond well, if temporarily, to adrenolytic agents such as phentolamine or piperoxane; there is also a great increase in urinary excretion of pressor amines.

Many of the psychological features of dysautonomia may superficially resemble those of schizophrenia. Exaggerated response to emotional stress, withdrawal from surroundings in vomiting attacks, often with repetitive or self-injurious behaviour and apparent inability to concentrate, may all be seen in both conditions. Schizophrenic children may also show poor vasomotor control, muscle inco-ordination, and apparently retarded development. Examination, however, shows that dysautonomic children are not psychotic, nor is there any history suggesting precocious development followed by regression.

Finally some children with congenital indifference to pain have been described with absent tendon reflexes and retarded development, but there the similarity to dysautonomia ends.

Prognosis. The outlook as regards survival is uncertain. About a fifth of all the recorded cases have died, some in the first year of life, others in childhood. Most of the deaths seem to have been due to respiratory infection, with or without hyperpyrexia. At least one has been attributed to renal damage, and one child died following a haematemesis.

Of the survivors, the pattern of early development is becoming fairly well defined. Affected children remain below average height and weight. Their lives are punctuated by frequent illness and injury. The latter may begin with teething: by a combination of habitual rubbing of the tongue or cheek on teeth and indifference to pain, severe ulceration may result. Besides respiratory infection, corneal ulceration due to defective lachrymation is common. Motor performance is severely handicapped by inco-ordination and development is therefore retarded. Adaptation to these disabilities is poor.

No less a handicap is the psychological abnormality. The cycle of personality traits and their reactions in the family are described by Freedman, Helme, Havel, Eustis, Riley and Langford (1957). In infancy the situation is relatively simple. The affected infant is likely to be miserable and to show exaggeration of infantile reaction to stress. The case described here suggests that this is not entirely resistant to sedative therapy, but little information on the subject is available.

Later in childhood a more complicated situation develops. These children, realizing that they have unique and incurable physical handicaps, make many demands on their parents and become tyrannical. Yet they lack initiative and remain over-dependent on others. They tend to become very attached to adults other than their parents, especially women, and are rarely friendly to other children. The parents, even when the diagnosis is known to them, tend to feel afraid of their child's symptoms and to resent them. Some parents even feel guilty. Most try to gratify the child's inordinate demands. Such appeasement, especially when variable, reduces the child's sense of security. To the difficulty of controlling the "milieu interieur" is added that of trying to compensate for a changing social environment, and the whole cycle is enhanced. Partial or complete rejection by one or both parents may result.

The long term outlook is not known. The oldest patient so far recorded was 23 years old in 1957 (Riley, 1957). She had not fully compensated for her disabilities. Other patients are thought to be developing renal damage due to hypertension. Adult cases have never been described. It is not inherently impossible that adaptation, both physical and psychological, can eventually take place.

Summary

The clinical findings in a Jewish girl, aged 8 months, with familial dysautonomia are reported. The diagnosis was suggested by absence of tears, excessive sweating, paroxysmal hypertension, poor peripheral circulatory control and dysphagia. Poor muscle co-ordination, absence of tendon reflexes and corneal anaesthesia indicated that there was also disturbance of motor and sensory systems. Breath-holding attacks, emotional lability, retardation of development and relative failure to thrive were also present. Diagnosis is on clinical grounds alone.

The differential diagnosis in infancy includes pink disease, fibrocystic disease of the pancreas, cerebral palsy and congenital absence of lachrymal glands and in older children the periodic syndrome, schizophrenia and phaeochromocytoma.

Dysautonomia is not necessarily fatal, but the physical difficulties and psychological disturbances in child and family make the rearing of the child difficult.

I am grateful to Dr. H. V. L. Finlay for his permission to publish this account and also for much helpful advice and criticism. My thanks are also due to Dr. E. P. G. Michell for the developmental assessment.

REFERENCES

Farquhar, J. W., Crawford, T. B. B. and Law, W. (1956). *Brit. med. J.*, **2**, 276.
Forster, W. and Tyndel, M. (1956). *J. ment. Sci.*, **102**, 345.
Freedman, A. M., Helme, W., Havel, J., Eustis, M. J., Riley, C. M. and Langford, W. S. (1957). *Amer. J. Orthopsychiat.*, **27**, 96.
Kroop, I. G. (1956). *J. Pediat.*, **48**, 328.
Moloshok, R. E. and Moseley, J. E. (1956). *Pediatrics*, **17**, 327.
—— and Reuben, R. N. (1954). *J. Mt Sinai Hosp.*, **21**, 137.
Riley, C. M. (1952). *J. Amer. med. Ass.*, **149**, 1532.
—— (1957). *Advanc. Pediat.*, **9**, 157.
——, Day, R. L., Greeley, D. M. and Langford, W. S. (1949). *Pediatrics*, **3**, 468.
Shwachman, H., Leubner, H. and Catzel, P. (1955). *Advanc. Pediat.*, **7**, 257.
Sjögren, H. and Eriksen, A. (1950). *Brit. J. Ophthal.*, **34**, 691.
Smid, A. C. and DuShane, J. W. (1955). *Amer. J. Dis. Child.*, **90**, 81.
Tyndel, M. (1955). *Wien. med. Wschr.*, **105**, 189.

AUTOPSY FINDINGS IN A CASE OF PITUITARY DWARFISM

BY

A. T. SANDISON

From the Departments of Pathology, the University and Western Infirmary, Glasgow

(RECEIVED FOR PUBLICATION MARCH 20, 1958)

Although the condition of pituitary dwarfism has been recognized for some considerable time, there is still a relative lack of published autopsy findings and the following case is reported briefly for this reason.

Lack of hypophysial growth hormone (almost certainly elaborated in the alpha cells of the pars anterior) during infancy or childhood results in varying degrees of under-development which may range from obvious dwarfism to slight degrees of lack of normal stature. In some cases, so-called primordial dwarfs may be small at birth and grow at a much reduced rate, while in others the child may grow normally for a varying period of time.

The term *infantilism*, sometimes used synonymously with dwarfism, may more strictly be applied to individuals in whom there is impairment of growth, sexual development and intellect while *nanism* implies restriction of growth in stature only. Infantilism is often referred to as the Levi-Lorain syndrome, the condition having been described by Lorain (1871) and by Levi (1908). Post-mortem studies are infrequent since the uncomplicated condition is not incompatible with good health. In childhood the patient is perfectly formed but somatic growth is slow. Development of the primary and secondary sexual phenomena does not occur at puberty and the genitalia usually remain infantile. This is not invariable, however, and some limited degree of sexual development may occur. Epiphyseal closure may be delayed but the ultimate stature attained is considerably below normal due to lack of growth hormone. Purely intellectual development may be satisfactory but emotional and behaviour patterns may be immature. These patients are slender with graceful limbs, ankles and wrists, and they often have fine, smooth skin and soft silky hair (Price, 1946).

Hypophysial dwarfs are usually born of normal parents, and some cases are recorded of hypophysial dwarfs producing normal offspring. They show good body symmetry, the physique being that of early childhood in which the lower measurements are relatively short. Most are thin and obesity is rather uncommon. The genitalia are generally under-developed and the secondary sexual characteristics may be absent or retarded. There may be amenorrhoea in the female and azoospermia in the male. Nevertheless, as indicated above, hypophysial dwarfs may occasionally be fertile. The skeletal framework is smaller and more fragile than normal and epiphyseal closure tends to be delayed. The appetite may be small and the basal metabolic rate low. There is not the profound impairment of the central nervous system noted in cretins, nor does one see the myxoedematous infiltration of subcutaneous or submucous tissues present in juvenile myxoedema. The metabolic consequences of adrenal hypoplasia are much less conspicuous than in Addison's disease. Glucose tolerance is sometimes increased. Occasionally radiography may show a small sella turcica but this is not common; indeed the sella may be enlarged due to adenoma or craniopharyngioma. It has been suggested that the term *ateleiosis* might well be used for the generality of dwarfism until the true extent of hypopituitarism in the causation of these cases is established (Cecil and Loeb, 1955).

For full consideration of types of dwarfism reference may be made to Wilkins (1950). Many of the points made above are confirmed and some further suggestions are put forward. Wilkins points out that androgen deficiency may be shown by low levels of 17-ketosteroids and by the relative absence of body hair. Often the testes and ovaries are immature and there is a low level of follicle-stimulating hormone. The facies is childish and immature but with attainment of the fourth decade a peculiar 'oldish-young' look may appear due to atrophy and wrinkling of the skin.

The pathology of this condition was first discussed by Erdheim (1916, 1925) who introduced the term 'nanosomia pituitaria'. Reference may be made also to Kraus (1926). Brief discussions are given in the textbooks of Cappell (1951) and Anderson (1953). Among the commoner causes of pituitary nanosomia are intra- or extra-cellular cranio-pharyngioma which may show marked retrogression. Other conditions described are fibrosis of the pars anterior (possibly ischaemic in origin), colloid-cystic degeneration, congenital syphilis, chronic hydro-cephalus and hypophysial malformation. Russfield and Reiner (1957) have described three cases of dwarfism without mechanical destruction of the pituitary and postulate possible failure of production of growth hormone by so-called 'amphophil' cells. The thyroid gland may be atrophic but the parathyroids, which are probably not under hypophysial control, are unaffected. The adrenals may be small and occasionally diabetes mellitus or even diabetes insipidus has been described. The latter condition would suggest possible hypothalamic damage; hypothalamic damage may undoubtedly be responsible for obesity when this is present. It seems probable that lack of alpha cells leads to growth impairment while beta cell insufficiency is responsible for genital dystrophy. Cappell has pointed out that in the Lawrence-Moon-Biedl syndrome there is evidence of a hereditary influence, the dwarfism here being associated with retinitis pigmentosa and polydactyly.

In the case now to be described a 15-year-old girl died from malignant astrocytoma. An associated dwarfism was the result of pituitary hypoplasia and of the presence of chromophobe adenoma and developmental cyst in the small pars anterior.

Case History

The patient, a 15-year-old girl, was admitted to the wards of Dr. J. A. W. McCluskie at the Western Infirmary, Glasgow. She was the fifth child of normal parents, the siblings being normal, alive and well. Parturition was two months premature and the patient then weighed 1·6 Kg. Mental and physical growth was from the first retarded and all the landmarks of development were delayed in appearance. At the age of 22 months she weighed only 6·0 Kg. instead of the expected 11·0 Kg. At this time she was seen by Professor Stanley Graham at the Royal Hospital for Sick Children, Glasgow, and was then noted to be mentally backward. Her height was 65 cm. (normal 80 cm.) and the circumference of the head was 39 cm. (normal 47 cm.). The cranial sutures were well united. At this time a course of antuitrin G was given without obvious effect.

By the age of 30 months she could walk without aid but intelligible and coherent sentences were not formulated until the age of 7 years. During the four years before admission there had been little or no somatic growth but the patient was able to undertake simple domestic tasks. At the age of 13 years, for a period of three months only she menstruated, apparently normally, but thereafter amenorrhoea was invariable. There was, however, some development of secondary sexual characteristics.

Some five weeks before admission the patient fell heavily and was dazed for a short time. Two weeks later her behaviour suggested gross visual defect and she became inactive. Aphasia and incontinence then developed although after a time some capacity for speech returned.

On examination, the patient proved to be imbecile and uncooperative. The hands and feet were small, the maximum circumference of the head was 44 cm. and the distance from the anterior superior iliac spine to the internal malleolus was 55 cm. There was bilateral webbing of the second and third toes. The teeth were of primary dentition and in poor condition. The palate was normal, as were the ear drums. The left pupil was larger than the right; neither reacted to light and both lenses were rather opaque. The tendon reflexes were difficult to elicit but the plantar responses were flexor.

The erythrocyte sedimentation rate was 6 mm. in the first hour. The Wassermann reaction was negative. The white blood count was 16 500/c.mm. with a polymorphonuclear leucocytosis. A radiograph of the chest was negative: the skull was small but showed no abnormality; the bones of the forearm were normally ossified. Lumbar puncture showed an opalescent fluid under pressure. Cells were 650 polymorphs per c.mm. Sugar was 68·0 mg. %; protein, 160 mg. %; chlorides, 708 mg. %. There was no growth on culture and tubercle bacilli were not demonstrated. Despite intrathecal penicillin and oral sulphadimidine the condition of the patient deteriorated and she died 10 days after admission.

Post-Mortem Examination (Dr. J. M. Johnstone). The body length was about 120 cm., the mean for a girl of this age being 161 cm. The head, hands and feet were small but well-formed and the limbs in proportion to the trunk. The fingers were of 'spindle' type. The facial appearance was older than the stated age suggested. The trunk was rather obese and the breasts were low hemispheres with poorly developed nipples and areolae. On dissection they proved to be largely fatty. The pubic hair was normal but axillary hair was scanty.

The heart (110 g.) showed no congenital defects and the lungs (left, 120 g.; right, 95 g.) were normal. The alimentary tract, liver (440 g.), spleen (40 g.) and kidneys (each 30 g.) showed no evidence of acquired disease. The uterus was infantile and the ovaries small without obvious follicle or corpus luteum formation. The adrenals and thyroid were small. No parathyroid adenoma was discovered.

The brain was congested and the convolutions were flattened. There was bulging of the left frontal lobe; this proved to be due to a haemorrhagic, necrotic tumour with central cystic degeneration which occupied the whole frontal lobe, extended back to the left caudate nucleus and crossed into the right frontal lobe for a little way

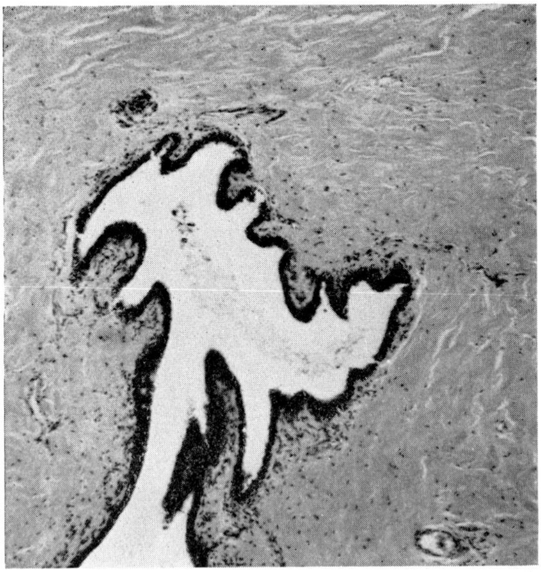

FIG. 1.—Section of breast to show simple duct system without evidence of lobule formation. Haemalum and eosin. × 75.

via the anterior commissure. The optic nerves and chiasma appeared normal. The pituitary was small.

Histological Examination (A. T. Sandison). The heart, lungs, liver, spleen and kidneys showed no significant change. The pancreatic islets appeared normal. The thyroid acini contained abundant well-stained colloid and were lined by cuboidal epithelium. Parathyroid and adrenals showed no structural abnormality. The breasts were largely fatty but in the fibrous strands there were ducts of simple immature type without evidence of lobule formation (Fig. 1). The ovarian cortical stroma was only moderately cellular; a few small ripening follicles of immature appearance were seen. The cervix uteri was normal and the endometrium appeared inactive with some dilatation of the glands.

The cerebral neoplasm was a highly cellular, vascular and necrotic astrocytoma producing little or no glia. The cells varied from spheroidal to spindle-cell type but mitotic activity was not great.

PITUITARY. This was hypoplastic, the mid-level horizontal cross-sectional area being about two-thirds of that of some glands from females of similar age. The pars anterior was greatly congested with prominent vascular spaces. One lateral lobe was occupied by a rather haemorrhagic, trabeculated, small-cell chromophobe adenoma with protein-containing fluid between the trabeculae (Fig. 2). The chromophobe cells present

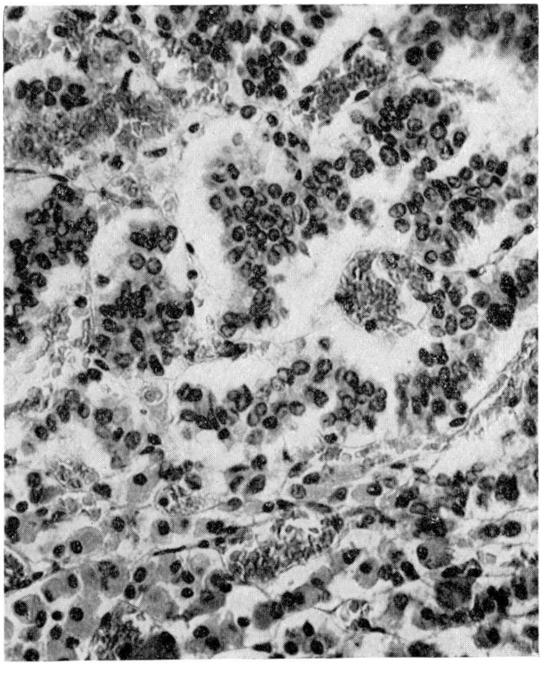

FIG. 2.—Chromophobe adenoma of pituitary with normal chromophil cells of pars anterior at the bottom. Picromallory stain. × 420.

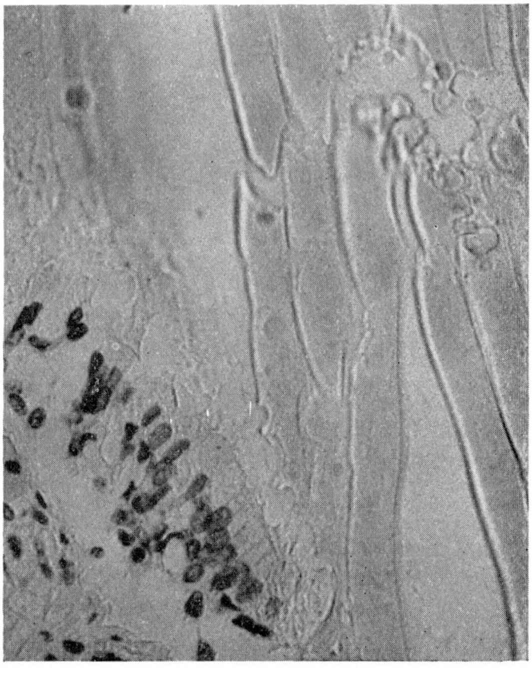

FIG. 3.—Developmental cyst of pars anterior containing colloid-like substance and lined by ciliated epithelium. Heidenhain's iron haematoxylin. × 420.

contained no granules stainable by the periodic-acid Schiff method. The opposite lateral area was largely occupied by a colloid-containing cyst which was lined partly by cubical and partly by tall columnar ciliated epithelium (Fig. 3). The remaining parenchyma contained well-granulated alpha and beta cells which were arranged rather haphazardly. The nature of these cells was confirmed by staining with the Mallory, phosphotungstic-acid haematoxylin, eosin-methylene blue and McLetchie and Pearse methods.

Discussion

The cause of death in this child was a malignant astrocytoma of the left frontal region which had produced obvious clinical effects for a period of six to seven weeks only. The patient, however, had been small at birth and had failed to grow normally; no increase in stature had been noticed in the four years before death. Mental development had also been retarded considerably although she could carry out simple domestic tasks. It is interesting to recall that the patient had menstruated three times at the age of 13 years but that this had not again occurred. Pubic hair developed despite the infantile genitalia but the breasts, although at first sight normal, were largely fatty. The normal developing breast at this age is a fibrous cone enveloped at the periphery by fat. Furthermore, the breast parenchyma was immature on histological examination.

The dwarfism here was of proportionate type and associated with mental retardation and poor development of sexual characteristics. This picture is not inconsistent with pituitary insufficiency and this was substantiated by histological examination. The pituitary in this instance was hypoplastic. Furthermore, a considerable bulk of the gland was occupied by a simple chromophobe adenoma and by a cyst of developmental Rathke type as shown by the ciliated lining. These abnormalities must have further reduced the volume of functional pars anterior. Undoubted alpha and beta cells were demonstrated in rather haphazard arrangement but these must have been inadequate for the production of sufficient growth hormone and gonadotrophins.

Summary

A 15-year-old girl who died of malignant astrocytoma was a dwarf of proportionate type from birth. There was also retarded mental development and poor sexual development. This dwarfism was the result of hypoplasia of the pituitary gland, the pars anterior of which was largely occupied by a simple chromophobe adenoma and a developmental cyst.

My thanks are due to Dr. J. A. W. McCluskie for permission to publish this case and to Dr. J. M. Johnstone for allowing me to quote from his autopsy records. I am also grateful to Mr. N. L. Russell for technical assistance and to Mr. W. Mason for the photographs.

References

Anderson, W. A. D. (1953). *Pathology*, 2nd ed. London.
Cappell, D. F. (1951). Muir's *Textbook of Pathology*, 6th ed. London.
Cecil, R. L. and Loeb, R. F. (1955). *Textbook of Medicine*, 9th ed. Philadelphia and London.
Erdheim, J. (1916). *Beitr. path. Anat.*, **62**, 302.
—— (1925). *Ergebn. allg. Path. path. Anat.*, **21**, 482.
Kraus, E. J. (1926). In Henke and Lubarsch *Handbuch der Spezielle Pathologischen Anatomie und Histologie*, **8**, 899.
Levi, E. (1908). *Nouv. Inconogr. Salpêt.*, **21**, 297, 421.
Lorain (1871). Lettre préfacée à la thèse de Faneau de la Cour. *Du féminisme et de l'infantilisme chez les tuberculeux*. Paris.
Price, F. W. (1946). *A Textbook of the Practice of Medicine*, 7th ed. London.
Russfield, A. B. and Reiner, L. (1957). *Lab. Invest.*, **6**, 334.
Wilkins, L. (1950). *The Diagnosis and Treatment of Endocrine Disorders in Childhood and Adolescence*. Springfield, Illinois.

INSUFFICIENT GLUCURONIDE FORMATION IN THE NEWBORN AND ITS RELATIONSHIP TO THE PATHOGENESIS OF ICTERUS NEONATORUM

BY

M. VEST

From the Children's Hospital, University of Basel, Switzerland

(RECEIVED FOR PUBLICATION FEBRUARY 24, 1958)

In the last few years the pathogenesis of icterus neonatorum and kernikterus has aroused renewed interest (Napp and Plotz, 1949; Obrinsky, Allen and Anderson, 1954; Billing, Cole and Lathe, 1954; Meyer, 1956). The discovery by Schmid (1956) and Billing, Cole and Lathe (1957) that bilirubin is excreted in the bile as a glucuronide now makes it possible to reinvestigate this problem more specifically. The accumulation of bilirubin in the blood after birth suggests that the excretory capacity of the liver is inadequate. Such an inadequacy has been demonstrated only indirectly, either by the diminished ability of newborn and premature infants to excrete bromsulphalein dye (Mollison and Cutbush, 1949; Yudkin and Gellis, 1949; Obrinsky, Denley and Brauer, 1952; Perl, 1957) or by the fact that an inverse relationship exists between the amount of bile pigment in the meconium and the subsequent rise of the bilirubin in the serum (Ross, Waugh and Malloy, 1937; Fashena, 1948; Napp and Plotz, 1949; Vest, 1958).

It therefore seemed promising to investigate the glucuronic acid conjugating ability of the liver in newborn and premature infants. Storey and Dutton (1955) have demonstrated that the conjugation of substances like p-aminophenol, menthol and others with glucuronic acid is catalyzed by an enzyme system in the microsomes of the liver and requires uridine diphosphate glucuronic acid (UDPGA) as the glucuronide donor. The enzymatic formation of bilirubin glucuronyl seems to involve the same system (Schmid, Hammaker and Axelrod, 1957).

A diminished glucuronide synthesis in young animals as compared with adult animals was demonstrated *in vitro* with liver tissue from mice (Karunairatnam, Kerr and Levvy, 1949), rabbits (Hartiala and Pulkkinen, 1955) and rats (Vest, 1958). The purpose of this paper is to report the results of an investigation into the capacity of the liver of full term and premature infants to form glucuronides.

Method

We chose the substance acetanilide (Antifebrin) to assess glucuronide formation. After oral administration this compound is excreted to 80% as N-acetyl-p-aminophenol-glucuronide, very little (about 4%) appears as free N-acetyl-p-aminophenol, and an insignificant part is de-acetylized in the body to aniline (Brodie and Axelrod, 1948a). This can give rise to the formation of methaemoglobin if an overdose is given. In the adult some 80% of the given amount of acetanilide is excreted in the urine within 24 hours. The dosage administered was 10 mg./kg. body weight, an amount which does not produce any toxic effects. The acetanilide was given in milk or by stomach tube. The urine was collected for a period of 48 hours, but separately for each 24-hour period. Before and several hours after the administration of the acetanilide the methaemoglobin level in the blood was examined by the method of Evelyn and Malloy (1938). P-aminophenol (free and total conjugated) was determined by the method of Brodie and Axelrod (1948b). It was found necessary, however, to repeat the extraction with ether-isoamyl-alcohol as we were unable to recover all the p-aminophenol from urine in one step. Moreover, normal colour development with phenol and sodium hypobromite occurs only if the solution is distinctly alkaline. Therefore a surplus of sodium carbonate has to be added to the bromine water.

The method of Jendrassik and Gróf (1938) was used in the micro modification of With (1943) for the determination of bilirubin in the serum. The subjects investigated were 94 premature, full term infants and older children at the Children's Hospital, Basel.

Results

Fig. 1 shows the amount of p-aminophenol in the 24-hour urine expressed as a percentage of a given dose of acetanilide in relation to the age of the children. The graph includes the regression line for full term and premature infants. It can be seen

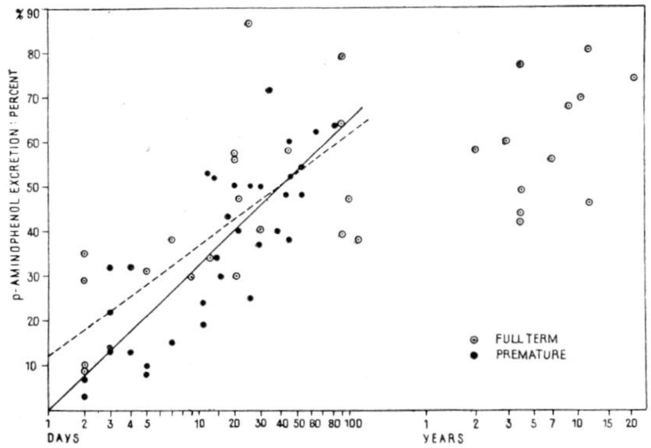

FIG. 1.—Excretion of p-aminophenol as glucuronide in 24 hours expressed as percentage of a given dose of acetanilide in relation to the age of the children.

that the excretion is much lower in newborn infants than in infancy and childhood and that premature infants have a still lower capacity to excrete a given amount of acetanilide. At the age of about 3 months the average excretion is not much below that of older children or of young adults and the difference between full term and premature infants can no longer be demonstrated. Free p-aminophenol was traceable in the urine of only a few cases and was generally well below 5% of the ingested acetanilide. Fig. 2 demonstrates how the ability to excrete acetanilide as glucuronide develops in the various premature and full term infants in the first 3 months of life. In almost every case this ability

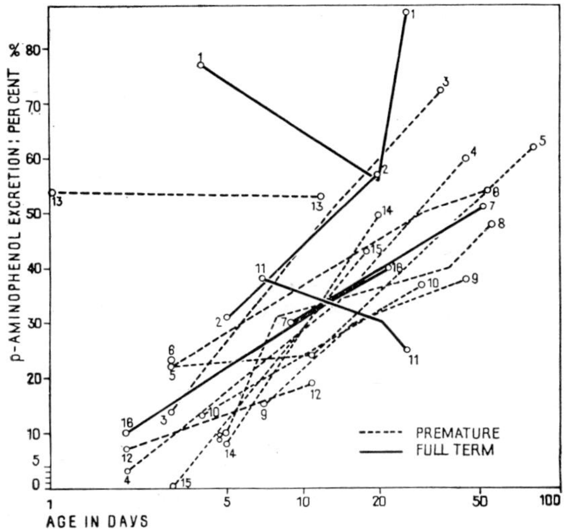

FIG. 2.—Increasing capacity of p-aminophenol-glucuronide excretion in individual premature and full term infants during the first 3 months of life.

is very low in the beginning, but rises conspicuously within 10 to 20 days after birth. This ability immediately after birth is satisfactory only in a few infants (Cases 1 and 13). Figs. 3 and 4 are examples of the relationship which exists between the capacity of the newborn to eliminate Antifebrin as p-aminophenol-glucuronide and the height of the serum bilirubin concentration. An inverse relationship can be clearly demonstrated: with the increasing ability to form and excrete p-aminophenol-glucuronide the bilirubin level decreases to normal. Because of a rising bilirubin concentration in one infant an exchange transfusion was performed (Fig. 4) in order to remove bilirubin from the circulation, but with only temporary success. However, with increasing ability to conjugate glucuronic acid the bilirubin level falls steeply. One fact remains to be mentioned: Figs. 3 and 4 show two examples of the

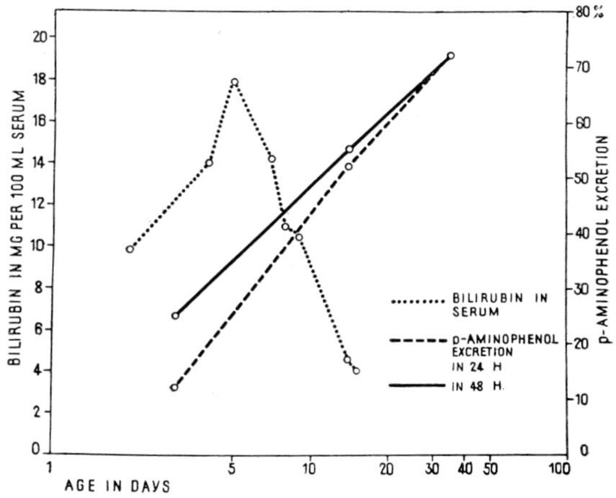

FIG. 3.

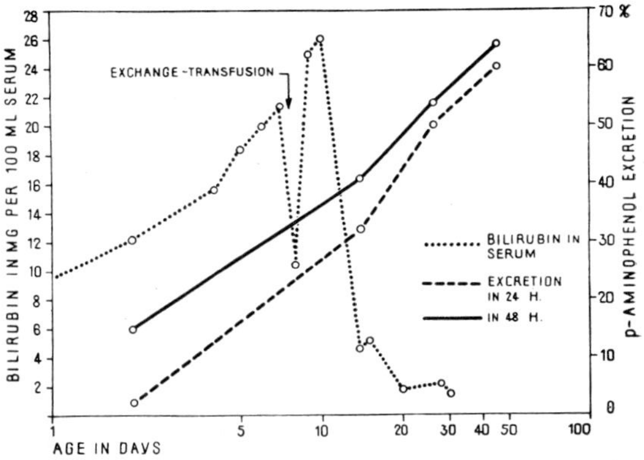

FIG. 4.

FIGS. 3 and 4.—Premature infants. Examples of the relationship between the capacity to excrete acetanilide as p-aminophenol-glucuronide and the height of the serum bilirubin concentration.

amount of p-aminophenol excreted in 24 hours as well as the cumulative excretion in 48 hours. It is noteworthy that in infants tested in the first days after birth the excretion in the first 24 hours amounts to half or less of the 48-hour value. On the other hand, in infants aged over 15 to 30 days the difference between the 24-hour excretion and the cumulative excretion in 48 hours is small. Therefore in the first few days of life the excretion is not only diminished but also much delayed. Later in infancy and childhood, no p-aminophenol can generally be demonstrated in the second urine portion because all has already been eliminated in the first 24 or even 12 hours.

Discussion

The results shown demonstrate that the ability to excrete a given amount of acetanilide is greatly diminished in the newborn and premature infant and that the normal function develops within 3 months after birth. In the first few days after birth the excretion is also very much delayed.

There are two possibilities with regard to the underlying cause of this diminished excretion in the newborn. First, the excretory capacity of the kidneys might be insufficient or secondly, the liver might not be able to conjugate glucuronic acid. A simple calculation will demonstrate that the kidney is not at fault. Assuming a low absolute p-aminohippuric acid (PAH) clearance of 20 ml./min. in a newborn baby and a PAH blood level of 2·5 mg. per 100 ml., the kidney would eliminate 0·5 mg. PAH per minute from the plasma, i.e. 30 mg. in one hour. These figures are chosen deliberately on the low side of actual measurements and in most cases the kidney is able to clear two or three times as much. Since the molecular weights of PAH and p-aminophenol-glucuronide are not very different, it is reasonable to assume that the kidney should be able to excrete at least 720 mg. of p-aminophenol-glucuronide in 24 hours. We have seen that the newborn baby is unable to excrete a dose of only 10 mg. acetanilide per 1 kg. body weight within this length of time. There can be no doubt that the excretory power of the kidney in the newborn would be adequate to meet this demand. One must conclude, therefore, that the liver of the newborn infant is unable to conjugate a sufficient amount of p-aminophenol with glucuronic acid. It must be remembered that this conjugation is necessary in order to make it possible for the kidney to excrete p-aminophenol. The same enzyme system is responsible for the conjugation of bilirubin to bilirubin glucuronide. Therefore the investigations described in this paper gave a direct indication of the cause of increased bilirubin accumulation in the newborn and of the pathogenesis of icterus neonatorum. Generally the bilirubin concentration in premature infants is high after birth. Concurrently these infants have also the lowest p-aminophenol excretion. This corresponds well with the fact that premature infants have the lowest content of bile pigment in meconium (Ylppö, 1913; Vest, 1958). As we have briefly mentioned, other functions of the liver are poorly developed in the newborn as well, e.g. the ability to excrete bromsulphalein or to conjugate benzoic acid with glycin or the formation of prothrombin and proconvertin (Loeliger and Koller, 1952; van Creveld, Paullsen, Ens, van der Meij, Versteegh and Versteegh, 1954; Vest and Meier, 1957).

In contrast with the congenital familial non-haemolytic icterus (Crigler and Najjar, 1952) in which an isolated defect of the glucuronic acid conjugating system exists (Schmid, Axelrod, Hammaker and Rosenthal, 1957) there is a deficiency in more than one metabolic liver function in the newborn baby. One of these, the insufficiency of the glucuronic acid conjugating system, accounts for the hyperbilirubinemia and gives rise to icterus of the newborn.

Summary

The capacity of the liver to form glucuronides was tested in full term and premature infants by administration of acetanilide in a dosage of 10 mg./kg. body weight and by measurement of the amount of p-aminophenol-glucuronide in the urine. Adults and older children are able to excrete about 80% of this value in 24 hours or less, whereas newborn and especially premature infants only eliminate a few % in 24 hours. Even in 48 hours the total excretion in newborn infants amounts to only about 10% or less. Within the first weeks of life the power to conjugate glucuronic acid steadily increases and by the age of 3 months normal function is generally reached.

There exists an inverse relationship between the ability to form glucuronides and the height of the bilirubin concentration in the serum. As the capacity of the liver to form glucuronides increases the serum bilirubin level begins to fall. It is concluded that this insufficiency in the formation of glucuronides by the liver might be regarded as the underlying cause of icterus neonatorum.

References

Billing, B. H., Cole, P. G. and Lathe, G. H. (1954). *Brit. med. J.* **2**, 1263.
——, ——, —— (1957). *Biochem. J.*, **65**, 774.
Brodie, B. B. and Axelrod, J. (1948a). *J. Pharmacol.*, **94**, 29.
——, —— (1948b). *Ibid.*, **94**, 22.
Creveld, S. van, Paullsen, M. M. P., Ens, J. C., van der Meij, C. A. M., Versteegh, P. and Versteegh, E. T. B. (1954). *Et néo-natal.*, **3**, 53.
Crigler, J. F. and Najjar, V. A. (1952). *Pediatrics*, **10**, 169.
Evelyn, K. A. and Malloy, H. T. (1938). *J. biol. Chem.*, **126**, 655.
Fashena, G. J. (1948). *Amer. J. Dis. Child.*, **76**, 196.

Hartiala, K. J. V. and Pulkkinen, M. (1955). *Ann. Med. exp. Biol. Fenn.*, **33**, 246.
Jendrassik, L. and Gróf, P. (1938). *Biochem. Z.*, **297**, 81.
Karunairatnam, M. C., Kerr, L. M. H. and Levvy, G. A. (1949). *Biochem. J.*, **45**, 496.
Loeliger, A. and Koller, F. (1952). *Acta haemat.* (*Basel*), **7**, 157.
Meyer, T. C. (1956). *Arch. Dis. Childh.*, **31**, 75.
Mollison, P. L. and Cutbush, M. (1949). *Ibid.*, **24**, 7.
Napp, J. H. and Plotz, J. (1949). *Arch. Gynäk.*, **176**, 781.
Obrinsky, W., Allen, E. L. and Anderson, E. E. (1954). *Amer. J. Dis. Child.*, **87**, 305.
——, Denley, M. L. and Brauer, R. W. (1952). *Pediatrics*, **9**, 421.
Perl, E. (1957). *Schweiz. med. Wschr.*, **87**, 334.
Ross, S. G., Waugh, T. R. and Malloy, H. T. (1937). *J. Pediat.*, **11**, 397.
Schmid, R. (1956). *Science*, **124**, 76.
——, Hammaker, L. and Axelrod, J. (1957). *Arch. Biochem.*, **70**, 285.
——, Axelrod, J., Hammaker, L. and Rosenthal, I. M. (1957). *J. clin. Invest.*, **36**, 927.
Storey, I. D. E. and Dutton, G. J. (1955). *Biochem. J.*, **59**, 279.
Vest, M. (1958). *Physiologie und Pathologie des Neugeborenenicterus*, In press. S. Karger. Basel and New York.
—— and Meier, W. (1957). *Ann. paediat.* (*Basel*), **189**, 282.
With, T. K. (1943). *Hoppe-Seyl. Z. physiol. Chem.*, **278**, 120.
Ylppö, A. (1913). *Z. Kinderheilk.*, **9**, 208.
Yudkin, S. and Gellis, S. S. (1949). *Arch. Dis. Childh.*, **24**, 12.

THE FIRST ARCH SYNDROME

BY

J. McKENZIE

From the Department of Anatomy, University of Aberdeen

(RECEIVED FOR PUBLICATION FEBRUARY 17, 1958)

Although disfiguring abnormalities of the face have been a problem to the plastic surgeon for many years and the accompanying embarrassment and morbidity have equally exercised the ingenuity of the psychiatrist, there is yet neither satisfactory treatment nor an adequate mask to shield the sufferer. Accordingly, the search for the cause and possible means of prevention has been intensively pursued for many years.

From an examination of the clinical features, anatomy and embryology of the following anomalies of the head and neck, it is clear that all arise from abnormal development of the first visceral arch and should be regarded as comprising a 'first arch syndrome': (*a*) The Treacher Collins syndrome or mandibulofacial dysostosis; (*b*) Pierre Robin syndrome (hypoplasia of the mandible with glossoptosis); (*c*) mandibular dysostosis; (*d*) deformities of the external and middle ear; (*e*) congenital deaf-mutism; (*f*) cleft lip and cleft palate; (*g*) hypertelorism; (*h*) a recently described syndrome exhibiting congenital deafness and hypertelorism.

Treacher Collins Syndrome. Berry (1889) and Treacher Collins (1900) each described patients showing a small notch at the junction of the outer third and inner two thirds of each lower eyelid, associated with 'an unusual want of prominence of the malar bones'. Subsequent writers, de Lima and Montiero (1923), Isakowitz (1927), Lockhart (1929), Waardenburg (1932), Herman (1936), van Linnt and Hennebert (1936), McEnery and Brennemann (1937), Debusmann (1940) and Mann (1943), added to the syndrome agenesis of the mandible, poorly developed eyelashes in the medial part of the lower lid, abnormalities of the external and middle ear, deafness, drooping of the outer canthus giving an anti-mongoloid obliquity of the palpebral fissures, microphthalmos and a marked hereditary trait. Franceschetti and Klein (1949) recognized the association of those features, proposed the term mandibulofacial dysostosis and attributed the condition to 'an inhibitory process occurring towards the seventh week of embryonic life and affecting the facial bones deriving from the first visceral arch. . . . The syndrome is of genic origin and is transmitted in an irregular mode . . . dealing with an unstable gene of occasional pleotropic, polyphaenic effect'. Hövels (1953*a*) also reviewed the subject and (1953*b*) claimed that these first arch anomalies resulted from maldevelopment of the head neural crest.

Pierre Robin Syndrome. In the newborn, hypoplasia of the mandible associated with a tendency for the tongue to block the pharynx (glossoptosis) has attracted attention because of the attendant feeding difficulties, choking fits and emaciation. Apart from their occurrence in the Treacher Collins syndrome, these features may be present alone, comprising the Pierre Robin syndrome. As described by Lenstrup (1925), Ely and Farber (1930), Davis and Dunn (1933), Robin (1934) and Lapage (1937), the condition shows a remarkable tendency to spontaneous improvement; this, and the fact that the symphysis menti is nearly vertical and the angle of the mandible nearly a right angle (Walker, 1956), have diverted attention from the purely teratogenic theory of origin to that expressed by Llewellyn and Biggs (1943), viz., that the micrognathia is purely a mechanical effect produced by the pressure of the chin against the sternum in the vertex position of the foetus; these authors went even further: they claimed that the frequent complication of cleft palate may be the result of the tongue being pushed back into the mouth and preventing the fusion of the palatal processes.

Mandibular Dysostosis. Obviously, micrognathia may occur in varying degrees, some so slight as to be unnoticed, and it is probably only in cases with a disproportionately large tongue interfering with respiration and feeding that the condition calls for attention. Nager and Reynier (1948) did not mention glossoptosis when they described mandibular hypoplasia in association with defects of the ear; they called this syndrome mandibular dysostosis.

Deformities of the External and Middle Ear. These require no description here. Wilson (1955) in his classification observes that the more severe the defect of the auricle the more likely the involvement of the meatus, that accessory auricles and pre-auricular fistulae tend to be hereditary and that in anomalies involving the external and middle ear the most frequently involved ossicles are the malleus and the incus.

Congenital Deafmutism. Dealing with abnormalities of the inner ear, Wilson (1955) states that they are 'inextricably mixed up with deafmutism', while Altmann (1950) describes the pathological changes found in the cochlea of two deaf mutes; there appears to be great difficulty in differentiating pathological from congenital abnormal alterations. McKenzie (1958) has shown, from audiometric examination of five cases of congenital deafmutism, that the condition is caused by an abnormality of the middle ear. On this account, and because of its association with congenital anomalies of the first visceral arch, the probability is that congenital deafmutism, also, arises from the same initial developmental fault.

Cleft Lip and Cleft Palate. Here the most likely cause is a failure or disturbance in the development of either the maxillary or frontonasal process, usually the maxillary, causing sufficient inhibition of growth to prevent approximation of these processes at the scheduled time. In cleft lip it is worth noting how the ala or alae and dorsum of the nose succeed, by dint of appreciable flattening or 'spreading', in bridging the difficult gap between the nasal process and the maxilla. Accompanying congenital lesions include anomalies of the ear, deafness, microphthalmos and asymmetry of the mandible.

Hypertelorism. Ocular hypertelorism is a term coined by Grieg (1924) to describe the unusually wide interval between the medial canthi in two cases which he was fortunate to dissect. The following features may be seen in his illustrations: there is a wide nasal aperture, its roof formed of greatly expanded nasal bones with a small sutural bone between them; the maxillae are slender and seem stretched to their utmost to fulfil their duty of bounding the nasal aperture and, even allowing for the absence of teeth and consequent bone resorption, they are undoubtedly hypoplastic; the angle between the axes of the orbits is increased, hence the patient's difficulty when looking at near objects stereoscopically; the zygomatic bones may not be quite up to the mark developmentally but at least they have the distinction of being able to support the skull (less the mandible) when it is set on the table; in the base of the skull the unusual feature is the great width of the cribriform plates of the ethmoid and of the body of the sphenoid including the hypophyseal fossa, with persistence of the craniopharyngeal canal, the original track of Rathke's diverticulum; the greater wing of the sphenoid is narrow and no greater in size than the lesser wing, the deficiency in the temporal region resulting from this anomaly and from the rather poor development of the temporal squama being compensated for by sutural bones. Greig believed that the developmental fault lay in that portion of the cartilaginous base of the skull which gives rise to the ethmoid and the body, lesser wings and medial half of the greater wings of the sphenoid.

Deafmutism with Hypertelorism. Fisch andRenwick (1956) drew attention to the combination of these conditions when they appealed for help in tracing cases characterized by the following features: (*a*) lateral displacement of the inner angles of the eyes, (*b*) a broad nose root, (*c*) different colours of the right and left eyes, (*d*) white forelock and (*e*) congenital deafness.

Case Histories

The cases described below illustrate conditions comprising the first arch syndrome.

Case 1. A.R. (Figs. 1 and 2) was described and discussed by McKenzie and Craig (1955), the essential points being the receding chin with a large tongue held towards the back of the mouth, the palpebral fissures slanting downwards at the outer ends, the lower eyelid bent at the junction of the inner two thirds and outer third, eyelashes scanty in the medial two thirds, hypoplasia of the malar bones and low set ears. The child died at the age of 10 weeks from feeding difficulties and cyanotic attacks. The trunk was normal at autopsy; dissection of the head revealed absence of the zygomatic bone and the zygomatic process of the temporal bone, the maxilla completing the orbital margin and providing attachment for the masseter (Fig. 3); the squamous temporal was very small, the deficiency made up by surrounding bones and by an extra bony plaque. In the mandible the body was foreshortened, the coronoid process everted and the head elongated anteroposteriorly; the articular eminence was absent. In the ear, the incus and stapes were normal. There was no parotid gland but the facial musculature was

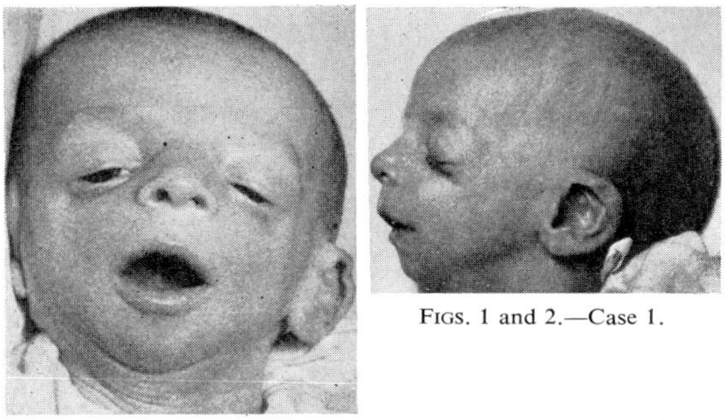

FIGS. 1 and 2.—Case 1.

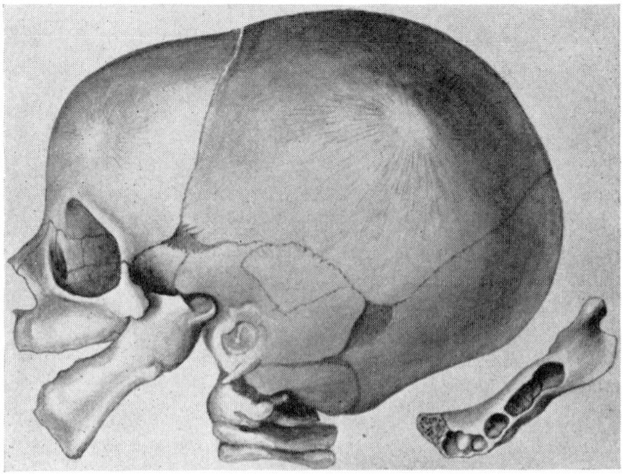

FIG. 3.—Case 1. Lateral view of skull.

well developed. The maxillary artery supplied inferior dental, posterior superior dental and middle meningeal branches but petered out before it reached the pterygo-maxillary fissure; the lower surface of the palate was supplied by the posterior superior dental artery while the nose received blood from a vessel which arose from the maxillary artery near the inferior dental artery, ran along the lower head of the lateral pterygoid muscle, entered the pterygopalatine fossa from behind and finally ran up to and through the sphenopalatine foramen into the nose. The infra-orbital artery was a branch of the ophthalmic artery.

Case 2. In G.A., aged 17 (Fig. 4), the only obvious anomaly of the head is the markedly receding mandible which reveals on the lateral radiograph (Fig. 5) an infantile appearance, namely short anteroposteriorly, an unusually wide angle, a short ascending ramus and a body lacking in depth and comprising chiefly alveolar bone; the maxilla, also, would be unusually small without its alveolar part. In the occipitomental view (Fig. 6), there is a bony deficiency in both zygomatic arches. At the age of 3, he began to complain of pain about his knees on exercise and within a year or so it was noticed that he was becoming knock-kneed. By the age of 7, radiographic examination showed anterior bowing of the femoral shafts with haziness of the bone structure around their lower epiphyses suggesting a slight degree of rickets. Two years later there was an equally marked but opposite curvature of the upper ends of the tibiae. The lower ends of the forearm bones were also curved due to abnormal epiphyseal growth. Osteotomies in the lower limbs at the age of 15 to correct the deformities have been complicated by non-union. Renal rickets and other metabolic disorders have all been excluded. He has one sister 21 years older than himself.

Case 3. M.N., aged 9 (Figs. 7 and 8), presents marked asymmetry of the face due to absence of the ascending ramus of the mandible on the left side and absence of the left zygomatic bone with a poorly developed maxilla; the left auricle is represented by several small tubercles lying further forward than normal and the left external auditory meatus is absent. Hearing is good but probably only with the right ear. A moderate degree of hypertelorism is present, the frontonasal angle flattened, the tongue musculature poor on the left side and the palatal

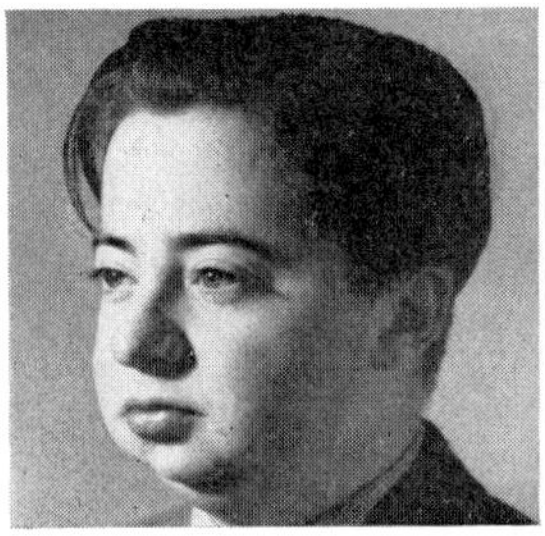

FIG. 4.—Case 2.

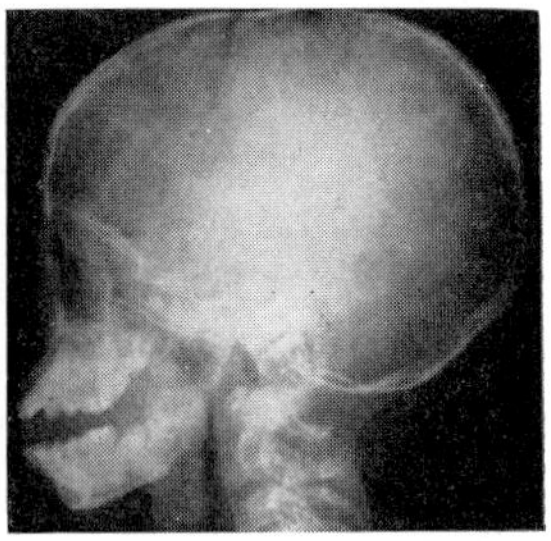

FIG. 5.—Case 2. Lateral radiograph.

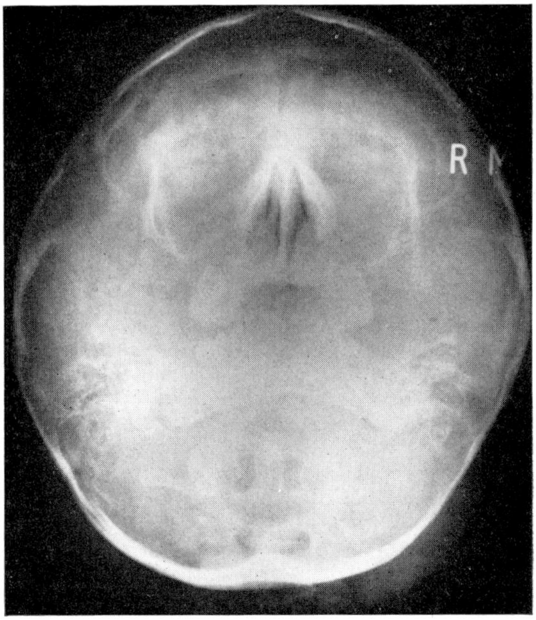

FIG. 6.—Case 2. Occipitomental radiograph.

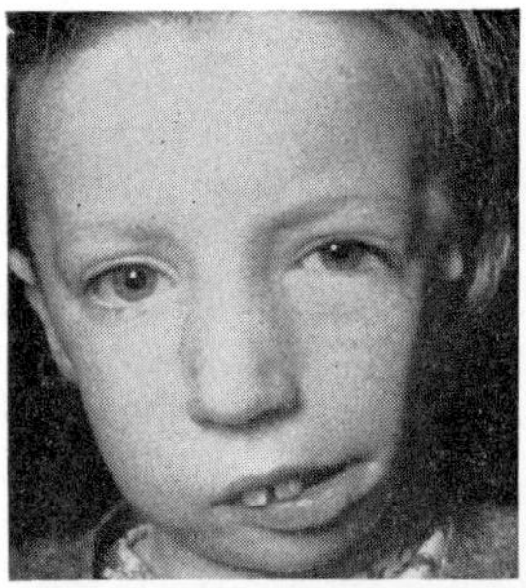
FIG. 7.—Case 3.

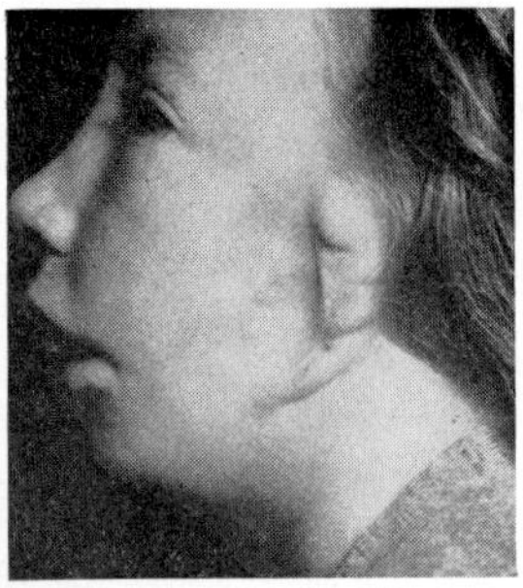
FIG. 8.—Case 3.

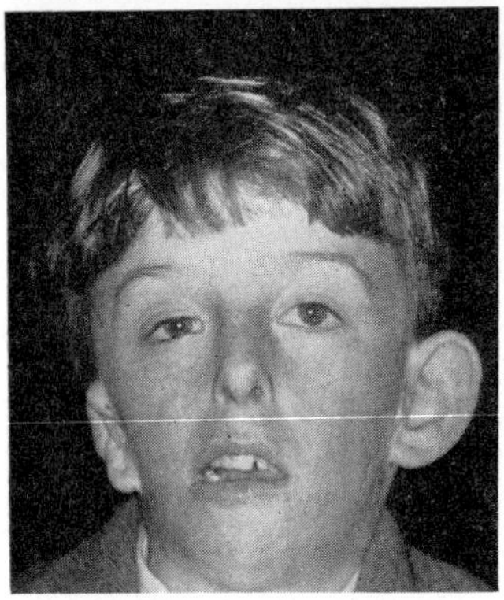
FIG. 9.—Case 4.

arch high but intact.

Case 4. A.G., aged 10 (Fig. 9), shows hemiatrophy but no bony deficiency of the jaw on the right side, irregularity of the oral mucocutaneous junction and hypoplasia of the right cheek with drooping of the outer canthus.

Case 5. A.A.M., aged 1 year, was recognized at birth as a very feeble, hypotonic, listless child with depressed bridge of nose, widely set eyes, simple low-set ears, flattened left forehead and flattening of the back of the skull on the opposite side; the soft palate was cleft and there was an obvious twist of the mandible, the tip of the chin being pushed over to the right side (Fig. 10). There has been considerable improvement since then; now it is difficult to identify the deformity of the mandible (Fig. 11) but the depressed, excessively wide bridge of the nose is still present with flattening of the bony orbital margin. Her weight as well as mental and physical development are all poor, feeding difficulties not entirely due to cleft palate restricting her progress.

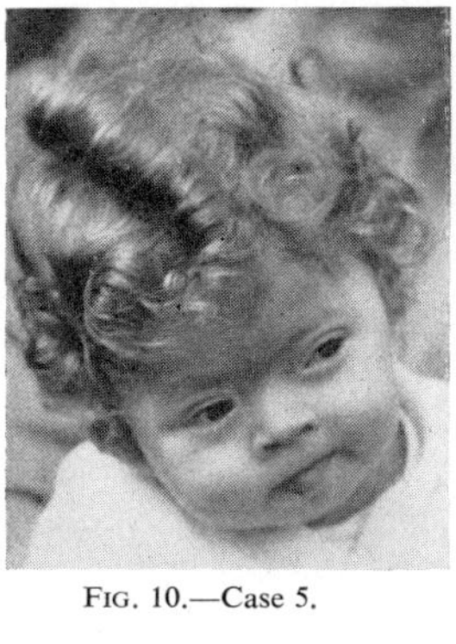
FIG. 10.—Case 5.

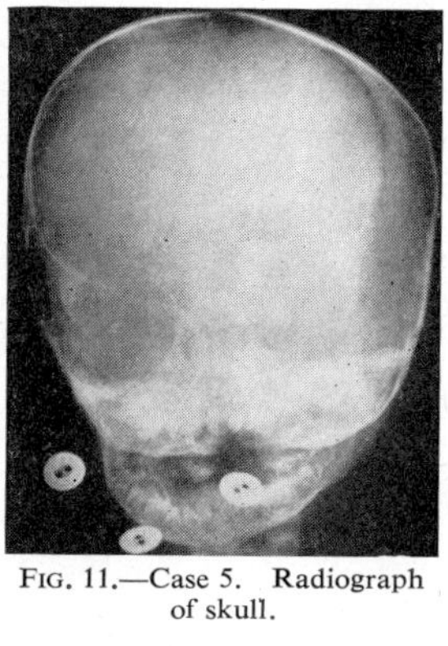
FIG. 11.—Case 5. Radiograph of skull.

Case 6. In A.M. (Fig. 12), much of the conjunctiva is exposed by the S-shaped lower lids which are atrophic and without eyelashes in their medial two thirds. The bilateral defect of the zygomatic bone is visible as well as palpable and a broadening of the interval between the medial canthi is present. The grandfather of this child, but no other member of the family, shows flattening over the zygomatic bones without eyelid defect but with deformities of the external ear and external auditory meatus.

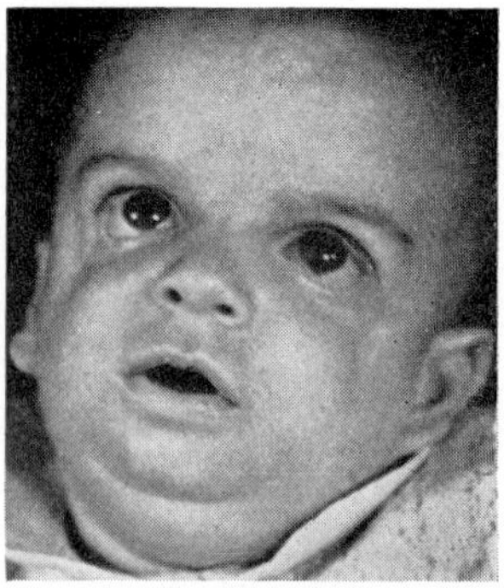
FIG. 12.—Case 6.

Case 7. R.F., aged 28, is the only member of his family showing a congenital abnormality; from birth there have been mere nodules of skin and cartilage representing the auricles; both external auditory meati are absent. Although there is considerable deafness he can carry on a reasonable conversation with the help of lip-reading and can understand what is being said on the radio. Apart from his deafness he is normal,

Case 8. B.R., aged 11, shows malformation of his right ear, deformity of the helix, antihelix and lobule with absence of the tragus and external auditory meatus. At an exploratory and reconstructive operation in 1951, it was reported that the anterior and inferior walls of the external auditory canal were missing, also the tympanic ring; the incus was the only middle-ear structure that could be identified.

Case 9. In R.A., aged 14, the left ear shows absence of the tragus and microtia, and there are two tiny accessory auricles; the right ear was markedly deformed at birth with absence of the auditory canal; hearing is diminished, more so on the right side where a conversational voice is heard at 6-8 ft. in contrast to 16-18 ft. on the left.

Case 10. E.M., aged 4 (Figs. 13 and 14), is a deafmute; the striking features in his appearance are the very wide

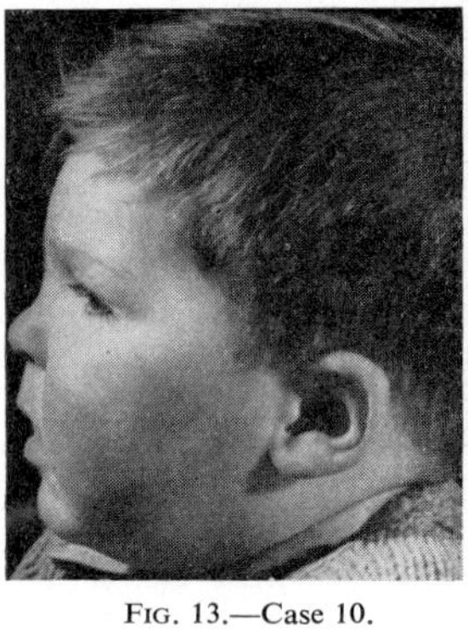
FIG. 13.—Case 10.

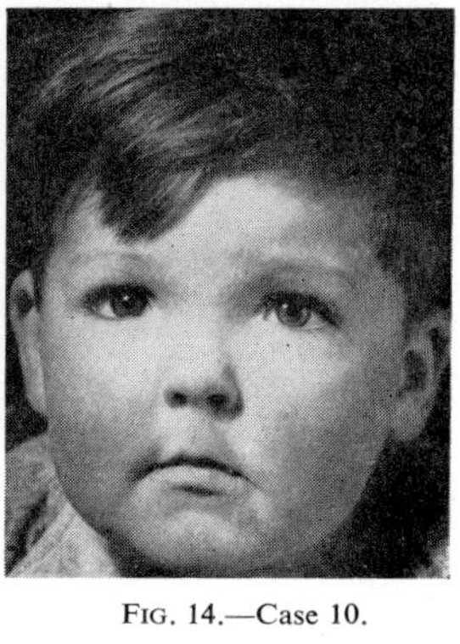
FIG. 14.—Case 10.

nasal bridge, the different colour of the irises, one blue and the other brown, a narrow palatal arch rising very steeply on either side but showing no cleft and a narrowness or 'pinching' of the nostrils and upper lip region. In the middle of the hair line over the forehead are a few white hairs; this white forelock, like the congenital deafness, is a marked feature in his ancestry; his mother, who declined to be photographed, is congenitally deaf and also had a white forelock when younger but her hair is now all white; she shows no hypertelorism but the frontonasal angle is nearly a straight line. The pedigree chart (Fig. 15) reveals that two brothers of the mother each have a white forelock and congenital deafness and that her father, although not deaf, had the characteristic forelock. No details are available regarding the cause of the 'wasting' in the three brothers and one sister of the mother who all died during their first year. The child's father is only partially deaf probably as a result of middle-ear disease in childhood.

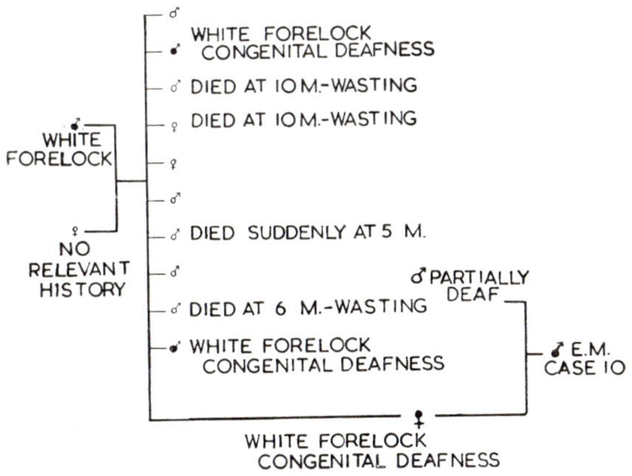

FIG. 15. Pedigree chart of case 10.

Case 11. D.S., aged $5\frac{1}{2}$ (Fig. 16) is also deaf-mute and is suspected of being mentally backward. There is an anti-mongoloid obliquity of the palpebral fissures and his mother volunteers the information that he 'does not weep with his left eye'. This can be due only to hypoplasia of the lacrimal gland on that side. There is no family history of deafness or congenital abnormality.

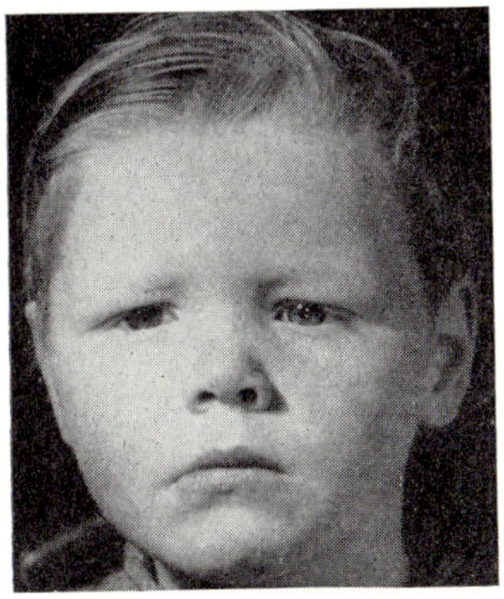

FIG. 16.—Case 11.

Embryology of the First Visceral Arch

Figure 17 shows the contributions to the face of the first (mandibular) arch and its maxillary process

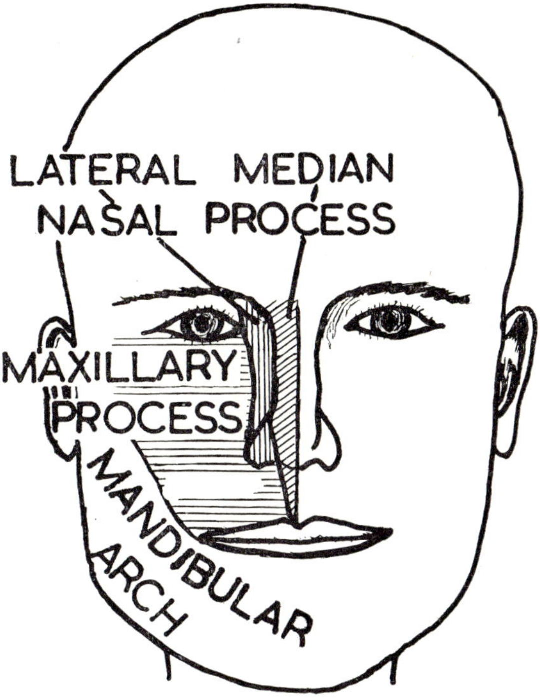

FIG. 17.—Contribution of mandibular arch to structure of face.

and of the frontonasal process. The external auditory meatus is the persistence of the posterior end of the first ectodermal groove while the middle ear and the auditory (Eustachian) tube represent the first, and possibly part of the second, endodermal pouch. Of the pinna, only the tragus and the area immediately around it derive from the first arch, the remainder from the second arch (Wood-Jones and I-Chuan, 1934). The dorsal ends of the first (Meckel's) and second (Reichert's) cartilages provide the ear ossicles, the incus and malleus from the first, the stapes from the second. Although the pterygo-quadrate cartilage (part of Meckel's cartilage seen in lower vertebrates) cannot be identified in the human embryo, two cartilaginous masses adjoining the primitive base of the skull are believed to be derivatives, namely the cartilaginous models and later the centres of ossification for the greater and lesser wings of the sphenoid bone. That for the greater wing is supplemented at a later stage by an intramembranous centre of ossification and the same is probably true for the lesser wing. Tandler (1902) and Padget (1948) have described the development of the vascular supply to the first visceral arch and its environs: after the disappearance of the first and second aortic arches, the blood supply of this region is left to small mandibular arteries arising on either side from the dorsal aorta (the future internal carotid artery). The mandibular artery confines its activities to the maxillary process (the primitive maxillary artery); the hyoid artery supplies the second visceral arch tissues; the mandibular arch proper receives blood from the ramifications of a newly formed vessel, the ventral pharyngeal artery running forwards from the truncus arteriosus. From the hyoid artery, a newly formed vessel turns forwards through the mesodermal condensation representing the stapes and (as the stapedial artery) grows to a far greater size than its parent vessel; it then advances on the mandibular arch, thereafter dividing into two branches, one, the supra-orbital division proceeding dorsally and cranially, the other, the maxillomandibular division ventrally and medially towards the maxillary process and mandibular arch. The former division passes at first lateral to the trigeminal ganglion and then accompanies the ophthalmic artery to the orbit. The maxillomandibular vessel replaces the now dwindling primitive maxillary artery by sending one branch (the infra-orbital ramus) into the maxillary process while a second branch joins the distal end of the ventral pharyngeal artery to form the mandibular artery (the inferior dental of the adult). Ventrally, the external carotid is already growing towards the mandible and distributing on the way its more proximal branches like the lingual and the facial. Finally it joins the bifurcation of the maxillomandibular artery, takes over its two branches now called inferior dental and maxillary arteries, reverses the flow of blood in the proximal part of the maxillomandibular vessel transforming it into the proximal part of the middle meningeal artery, the distal and main part of which is derived from the supra-orbital division of the stapedial. At the point where it arises from the hyoid, the trunk of the stapedial begins to narrow becoming the superior tympanic branch of the middle meningeal artery. The original hyoid artery persists as the tiny carotico-tympanic artery. In his article Padget (1948) provided an explanation of why there should sometimes be a branch from the anterior division of the middle meningeal artery anastomosing with the ophthalmic artery or even giving origin to the lacrimal and other orbital branches; an ophthalmic branch can be traced to the eye from the supra-orbital division of the stapedial to assist in the supply of the eye and orbit; later the terminal part of the vessel is annexed by the future definitive artery and used as its lacrimal or other orbital branches.

The Etiology of the First Arch Syndrome

The detailed anatomy of Case 1 showed marked vascular anomalies and, in spite of a well-known range of 'normal' variation in such vessels, these findings are enough to incriminate the arterial system in the production of hypoplasia of the zygomatic bone, if not as the original cause then at least as an important intermediary. Only one reference can be traced in the literature to a defect of the first visceral arch region associated with a vascular anomaly: Tomes (1872) described a mandible showing marked hypoplasia of the left body and ramus with no inferior dental foramen and consequently no mental foramen on that side, 'the vascular supply of this side of the jaw was derived from several small vessels entering the front of the jaw on its inner and outer aspects'. Tomes compared his with a similar specimen described by his father 11 years before; there the canal for the inferior dental artery 'was very small and did not emerge at a mental foramen but was lost in the bone'.

From the description given above of the normal blood supply of the first arch it is clear that, in the interval (third to fifth week) between the disappearance of the first aortic arch and the full development of the external carotid artery, the first visceral arch has a hazardous existence, dependent during that time on the relay of three successive vessels, the remains of the first aortic arch, the stapedial artery with its branches and the external carotid artery and on some split-second timing on their part as one relinquishes and the next adopts the supply of that region. Before considering the numerous mishaps which may occur at this time, it is as well to recall the effect of obliteration of any large artery during adult life; provided the patient is young and healthy, arterial anastomoses with adjacent vessels can compensate for the injured artery and within a relatively short time the tissues are receiving adequate nourishment for their needs at rest but they may have to wait an appreciable period before full activity is possible. Compensatory anastomoses will be as active during embryonic life and survival will be as easily assured. These tissues, however, are not at rest; they are seething with an activity less obvious than muscular contraction but far more vital to themselves, namely growth and differentiation which are known to have a high utilization of oxygen and other nutriments.

Far too many hitches may occur in the three weeks so critical to the first visceral arch region for each to receive adequate discussion here, and only a few with their consequences will be mentioned. The stapedial artery which, after all, is a phylogenetically labile vessel and therefore likely to vary, may be very poorly developed; this implies a late start, an inadequate flow of blood and possibly an early involution and if no vessel contemporary with it or its branches seeks to help, the maxillary process would find itself without blood after degeneration of the primitive maxillary artery; the mandible would be inhibited in its growth when the time came for the ventral pharyngeal artery to disappear; the supra-orbital ramus of the stapedial artery struggling to supply the tissues of the side of the head may be unable to assist the primitive ophthalmic vessel with the normally profuse circulation to the eye and the orbit; poor development of either branch of the maxillomandibular division may be sufficient to prevent death of the tissues in the maxillary process and the mandibular arch but barely enough to allow normal growth, while, unless the external carotid artery reaches this region before the stapedial degenerates, the same results may follow as from an inadequate supply by that artery.

All the compensatory anastomoses may develop in response to such a serious defect as a poorly developed stapedial artery and consequently no evidence of any abnormality may be apparent in later life. On the other hand a dilatory response by one of the neighbouring vessels may result in a relatively short but nevertheless crucial period of malnutrition in a region normally supplied by the stapedial. Juggle with these possibilities and it becomes perfectly clear how failure of one vessel (the stapedial) to play its full part in normal development may result in complete chaos in the subsequent development of the first visceral arch and its derivatives, or perhaps only focal derangements such as inhibition of growth in the maxilla, mandible or ear, or, if conditions at the time happen to be particularly favourable, no perceptible abnormality.

Objections to this explanation may be raised on the grounds that these abnormal events take place between the third and fifth weeks, an appreciable time before any sign of an ossification centre appears in the mandible or maxilla (sixth week) or before the appearance of the hillocks representing the pinna (also sixth week). To cause an upset in initial bone formation, however, a lapse in the maintenance of an adequate blood supply need not occur at, or immediately before, the stipulated time of appearance of the ossification centre; the latter phenomenon is merely a phase in a series of reactions which began some time previously and interference with the blood supply to the region at an earlier date may give rise to an abnormality which is only apparent later.

Genetics of the First Arch Syndrome

There are too many instances recorded of transmission through several generations for the syndrome to be explained in any other way than by hereditary factors: Debusmann (1940) found 10 members in three generations of one family, Straith and Lewis (1949) described the variations in the syndrome occurring in a mother and her four children, the father having normal features; affected brothers were reported by de Lima and Montiero (1923); a mother and daughter by Berry (1889) and a father and two daughters by Isakowitz (1927); the father of Case 1 described here has a hare lip; Case 10 reflects the features presented by his grandfather and the cases of deafmutism in one family reported by McKenzie (1958) have prototypes in their mother, father and four paternal uncles. Franceschetti and Klein (1949) concluded from their review that mandibulofacial dysostosis was hereditary.

Whether the gene responsible for the syndrome is recessive or dominant may be judged from the incidence of the syndrome; having no relationship to sex or to consanguinity, it must be regarded as dominant although there, too, modifying factors exist, such as the lapse of the syndrome in the second generation followed by its re-appearance in the third, and the many different guises it assumes in its history. These characteristics depend on the expressivity, penetrance and the specificity of the gene concerned. Expressivity is (*a*) the activity of the gene itself which depends on the quantity of some substance produced by it in initiating the reaction for which it is responsible as well as (*b*) its activity in relation to the rest of the genes and to the environment (Waddington, 1939). 'Different genes vary greatly in their response to particular environmental changes' (Gates, 1946). Penetrance is a measure of the frequency with which the characteristic features of a gene appear in the carrier while its specificity refers to the kind of effect rather than to the amount.

In this syndrome there is the unique opportunity not only of displaying the morphological sequences which lead to the anomalies in the child but also of explaining the variable expressivity and specificity and moderate penetrance of the gene. The gene, we must presume, is responsible for the maldevelopment or even suppression of the stapedial artery while the compensatory processes (anastomoses) will provide the degrees of penetrance, although other factors must be sought to explain the variability of the compensatory reactions. The results of experimental teratology can, at least partially, solve this problem. Since the time of Saint-Hilaire (1826) it has been well known that anomalies may be produced in chicks by abnormal environment such as shaking the eggs or covering them with varnish. Dareste (1891) and Féré (1899) furthered these experiments while Stockard (1909) and Spemann (1938) exploited the possibilities in the amphibian, but it was not until Hale (1935) showed that anophthalmos and cleft palate occurred in pig embryos when the sows were fed on vitamin-A-deficient diets that the production of congenital anomalies in mammals became a common experimental procedure. Many teratogenic agents have since been used, e.g., riboflavin deficiency (Gilman, Perry and Hill, 1952; Nelson, Baird, Wright and Evans, 1956), folic acid deficiency (Thiersch, 1952; Nelson, Asling and Evans, 1952), pantothenic acid deficiency (Giroud, Lefebres, Prost and Dupuis, 1955) and ionizing radiations (Wilson and Karr, 1951; Wilson, Jordan and Brent, 1953). Ingall's (1952) remarks concerning the multiplicity of these experiments adequately sum up the present position: 'From the welter of investigations has come an ever-growing list of teratogenic agents . . . As the number rises, however, the question of specificity seems to become less important than dosage and timing of the agent used. The very diversity of teratogenic stresses and agents suggests that any substance that can kill can induce abnormal growth when acting in critical dosage at an appropriate moment of development'.

One of the most vulnerable regions for congenital abnormalities in these experimental animals is that of the first visceral arch, e.g., micrognathus, cleft lip, cleft palate, microphthalmos and anophthalmos, while the only histological investigation after deficient diets in pregnancy was carried out by Giroud, Lefebres, Prost and Dupuis (1955) on deformed limbs; they reported that 'arrest of the blood circulation in the dilated marginal veins (of the limbs) had occurred. The vascular endothelium had then disappeared and the coagulated blood had come in direct contact with the tissues'. Not only is it possible then to produce a condition like the first arch syndrome but it also appears from experimental procedures as well as anatomical findings that teratogenic effects are mediated through the vessels of the part concerned and, since the blood vessels of the first visceral arch normally provide it with a rather hazardous existence at one period, it is not surprising that this region is among the most vulnerable.

It is not suggested from such findings that the first arch syndrome is caused by dietary deficiency or conditions akin to the experimental procedures, for these were extreme and unlikely to occur naturally. It is enough to postulate a gene or genes as the initial factor inhibiting or even preventing the development of the stapedial artery, but the compensatory anastomoses of the surrounding vessels in such an emergency call for unusually large supplies of nourishment; the normal or minimal amount for normal development is unlikely to allow for compensatory reactions. The result, then, will be inhibition of growth in the area supplied by the faulty stapedial artery and its branches. The penetrance of the gene causing the first arch syndrome therefore depends on the nutritional state and diet of the mother during the first few weeks of pregnancy, even if the diet is minimal or 'adequate' the child may be abnormal because only an excellent nutritional state can successfully prevent the appearance of the anomaly. The expressivity and specificity of the gene, on the other hand, depend on the details and timing of the maladjustments occurring among the vessels concerned.

Discussion

The inherent tendency for improvement in the shape and development of the mandible seen in Case 5 and in children with the Pierre Robin syndrome requires further explanation. Throughout the normal development, which comprises not only an orderly progression of morphological changes but also a similarly regulated sequence of chemical reactions, there is a precise interval of time allotted to each item of growth or differentiation and all are closely interwoven. The growth and differentiation of an organ or tissue postponed beyond its normal period of activity will be proceeding under the stresses of an inimical environment, and the later the attempt is made the more it is likely to be suppressed entirely. Genetic influences or environmental factors, as we have seen, may inhibit any developmental process and prevent its completion or even its commencement within the specified time, and this initial setback will be perpetuated in successive stages of development in the organ or tissue in spite of attempts to make up the leeway. The growth of an organ or part of the body like the mandible may be compared with the journey of a long-distance express train after it has been delayed in the early part of its trip; the normal schedule provides it with immediate clearance at all junctions and signals but, if it be late, then it must contend with the demands of other trains which are on time and must take precedence over it. The delay is thus maintained if not aggravated, but the train will eventually reach its destination after facing the hazards of an unscheduled journey.

In Case 5 and in the Pierre Robin syndrome an early upset in the nutrition of the mandible and possibly of the other parts of the face was sufficient to retard growth but not to cause irreparable damage or prevent recovery; during the last few weeks of pregnancy the normal intra-uterine pressure was enough to distort this under-developed bone struggling under adverse conditions to make up its leeway. Only after birth (during the first year or two of life) does the mandible have the freedom to complete its development, correct the deformity and assume its genetically determined shape. The same explanation will suffice for deformities such as club-foot, but several bones are involved in these cases and structural adaptation of unaffected tissues usually occurs before birth.

In Case 2 where an infantile mandible and defective zygomatic arches were associated with unexplained anomalies of the limb bones, there had been, during the third to fifth week of intra-uterine life, a nutritional disturbance influencing the first visceral arch, already affected by an abnormal stapedial artery, and leaving in its wake the characteristic features of the syndrome. This superimposed nutritional upset, however, also interfered with the initial capillary growth in the limb buds, inhibiting their development without altering the structural pattern. Whether there had been a distortion of the limbs caused by intra-uterine pressure and visible at birth is unknown but there is normally a distinct curvature in the legs of the newborn infant. Although during normal postnatal development, the bones are adequate to withstand the weight of the child, in this case the epiphyses and their newly formed bone were prematurely subjected to strenuous activity which was not favourable to processes striving to make up lost ground; the metaphyseal region, then, like the mandible in Case 5 before birth, yielded to the forces applied to it, forces which would not have affected normally growing bone. It should be noted also that not only are the bones of the lower limbs more distorted than those of the upper limb because of weight-bearing but also that the regions showing the curvatures are at the more actively growing ends of the bones, namely around the knee and at the wrist joint. In all likelihood, if the activities and weight of the child had been restricted up to, say the age of 8 or 10 (there are obvious difficulties and objections to such a course), these aspects of the child's development would have been in step with the growth of the limb bones and no deformity would have resulted. This is borne out by the history that the curvatures of the limbs did not increase markedly, if at all, in his teens.

Superficially, the cause of hypertelorism seems remote from the first visceral arch; closer examination, however, shows that the presenting feature, the wide interocular distance, is really a compensatory effect for poor development of the maxillary process, an effect seen also in cases of cleft lip and palate. Greig's first case showed poorly developed maxillae, unusually small squamous temporals and greater wings of sphenoid (all in first arch territory). In Case 10, the frontonasal process had spent itself in spreading or expanding laterally at the expense of its downward development and thereby provided an extremely high, slot-like palatal arch; no cleft had occurred because the palatal processes of the maxillae had succeeded in joining the nasal septum before being drawn upwards by the delayed growth of the over-taxed frontonasal process. The pinched appearance around the nostrils and upper lip arose from the same cause. A straining of the nutrition in the frontonasal process in such cases may account for the white forelock immediately above it, while variations in the blood supply to the two eyes could easily be the cause of their being different colours.

Fisch and Renwick (1956) and McKenzie (1958) showed that congenital deafmutism may occur in association with first arch deformities and the latter author demonstrated the middle ear origin of the condition. On clinical examination there is no evidence of any defect within the middle ear, hence the presumed normality of the ossicles; but the incus may be at fault because of its origin from the first arch (Meckel's) cartilage while the stapes, although a remnant of the second (Reichert's) cartilage, has the stapedial artery traversing it in the early stages of its development. The exact site of the abnormality, however, will have to await confirmation, although Wilson (1955) states that the ossicles are seldom abnormal in an otherwise normal ear but, if so, it is usually the stapes which is at fault.

Summary

Eleven cases illustrating the clinical features of eight different types of congenital anomaly or syndrome affecting the head and neck are described along with the relevant literature on each.

From a consideration of the clinical features, the anatomy described in several cases, the embryology of the first visceral arch and its environs, especially the development of the blood vessels, and, from an examination of the hereditary features, it is claimed that all the anomalies mentioned comprise one hereditary syndrome (the 'first arch syndrome') caused by a dominant gene or group of dominant genes with variable specificity and expressivity and with only a moderate degree of penetrance.

I am indebted to Professor R. D. Lockhart for his advice, help and interest during the preparation of this paper; and to the following for allowing me access to their case notes: Dr. George Swapp, Aberdeen (Case 2); Mr. A. B. Wallace, Royal Hospital for Sick Children, Edinburgh (Cases 3, 4 and 6); Dr. P. MacArthur, Royal Northern Infirmary, Inverness (Case 5); Mr. I. S. D. Thomson, Royal Aberdeen Hospital for Sick Children (Cases 8 and 9); and Dr. Dorothy Younie, Senior Assistant M.O.H., Aberdeen (Case 10).

REFERENCES

Altmann, F. (1950). *Arch. Otolaryng. (Chicago)*, **51**, 852.
Berry, G. A. (1889). *Roy. Lond. ophthal. Hosp. Rep.*, **12**, 255.
Collins, E. Treacher (1900). *Trans. ophthal. Soc. U.K.*, **20**, 190.

Dareste, C. (1891). *Recherches sur la Production Artificielle des Monstruosités*, 2nd ed. Paris.
Davis, A. D. and Dunn, R. (1933). *Amer. J. Dis. Child.*, **45**, 799.
Debusmann. (1940). *Arch. Kinderheilk.*, **120**, 133.
Ely, R. C. and Farber, S. (1930). *Amer. J. Dis. Child.*, **39**, 1167.
Féré. (1899). *Cinquantenaire de la Société de Biologie*, Vol. Jubilaire, p. 360.
Fisch, L. and Renwick, T. K. (1956). *The Teacher of the Deaf*, **54**, 150.
Franceschetti, A. and Klein, D. (1949). *Acta ophthal.* (*Kbh.*), **27**, 143.
Gates, R. R. (1946). *Human Genetics*, Vol. 1. New York.
Gilman, J. P. W., Perry, F. A. and Hill, D. C. (1952). *Canad. J. med. Sci.*, **30**, 383.
Giroud, A., Lefebres, J., Prost, H. and Dupuis, R. (1955). *J. Embryol. exp. Morph.*, **3**, 1.
Greig, D. M. (1924). *Edinb. med. J.*, **31**, n.s., 560.
Hale, F. (1935). *Amer. J. Ophthal.*, **18**, 1087.
Herman. (1936). *Bull. Soc. belge Ophtal.*, **73**, 60.
Hövels, O. (1953*a*). *Z. Kinderheilk.*, **73**, 532.
—— (1953*b*). *Ibid.*, **73**, 568.
Ingalls, T. H. (1952). Conference on Prematurity, Congenital Anomalies and Birth Injuries, New York Academy of Medicine, June, 1952.
Isakowitz, J. (1927). *Klin. Mbl. Augenheilk.*, **78**, 509.
Lapage, C. P. (1937). *Lancet*, **1**, 323.
Lenstrup, E. (1925). *Acta paediat.* (*Stockh.*), **5**, 154.
Lima, J. A. Pires de, and Montiero, H. B. (1923). *Arch. Anat. Antrop.* (*Lisboa*), **8**, 185.
Linnt, A. van, and Hennebert, P. (1936). *Bull. Soc. belge Ophtal.*, **73**, 57.
Llewellyn, J. S. and Biggs, A. D. (1943). *Amer. J. Dis. Child.*, **65**, 440.
Lockhart, R. D. (1929). *J. Anat.* (*Lond.*), **63**, 233.
McEnery, E. J. and Brennemann, J. (1937). *J. Pediat.*, **11**, 468.
McKenzie, J. (1958). *Brit. med. J.* In press.
—— and Craig, J. (1955). *Arch. Dis. Childh.*, **30**, 391.
Mann, I. (1943). *Brit. J. Ophthal.*, **27**, 13.
Nager, F. R. and de Reynier, J. P. (1948). *Practica otorhinolaryngologica*, Suppl. 2, Vol. 10.
Nelson, M. M., Asling, C. W. and Evans, H. M. (1952). *J. Nutr.*, **48**, 61.
——, Baird, C. D. C., Wright, H. V. and Evans, H. M. (1956). *Ibid.*, **58**, 125.
Padget, D. H. (1948). *Contr. Embryol. Carneg. Instn.*, **32**, 205.
Robin, P. (1934). *Amer. J. Dis. Child.*, **48**, 541.
Saint-Hilaire, E. G. (1826). *Journ. Comp. du dict. de sc. Med.*, **24**, 256.
Spemann, H. (1938). *Embryonic Development and Induction.* London.
Stockard, C. R. (1909). *J. exp. Zool.*, **6**, 285.
Straith, C. L. and Lewis, J. R. (1949). *Plast. reconstr. Surg.*, **4**, 204.
Tandler, J. (1902). *Morph. Jb.*, **30**, 275.
Thiersch, J. B. (1952). *Amer. J. Obstet. Gynec.*, **63**, 1298.
Tomes, C. S. (1872). *Trans. odont. Soc. G.B.*, **4**, 130.
Waardenburg, P. J. (1932). *Das menschliche Auge und seine Erbanlagen.* Haag.
Waddington, C. H. (1939). *An Introduction to Modern Genetics.* London.
Walker, D. G. (1956). Unpublished M.D. Thesis. Dublin.
Wilson, T. G. (1955). *Diseases of the Ear, Nose and Throat in Children.* London.
Wilson, J. G., Jordan, H. C. and Brent, R. L. (1953). *Amer. J. Anat.*, **92**, 153.
—— and Karr, J. W. (1951). *Ibid.*, **88**, 1.
Wood-Jones, F. and I-Chuan, W. (1934). *J. Anat.* (*Lond.*), **68**, 525.

BOOK REVIEWS

Pediatric Gynecology, 4th ed. By GOODRICH C. SCHAUFFLER. (Pp. 349; 84 figures. 57s.) London: Interscience Publishers. Chicago: Year Book Publishers. 1958.

The fourth edition of this useful book has been slightly enlarged and contains many fresh illustrations. A seven-page section on female pseudohermaphroditism has been added and 'masturbation is, at last, given a monographic consideration'; no less than 17 pages! Here and there the author seems, perhaps, unduly concerned over the upbringing and *mores* of the American teenager, and his ideas on such going's-on as teenage pregnancy, masturbation, female circumcision and even clitoridectomy in that surprising country leave the (English) reviewer confused and somewhat breathless. The section, however, on the truly pathological disorders of the female child's genital and urinary systems are straightforward, clearly if wordily expressed and useful, and the appropriate aspects of endocrinology, chemo- and antibiotic therapy and treatment with steroids are all clear and up to date.

The subject is certainly worth a book to itself and this volume more than adequately fulfils its purposes.

The Compleat Pediatrician. By W. C. DAVISON and JEANA DAVISON LEVINTHAL. (Pp. vi + 257. 35s.) London: Staples Press. 1958.

The fact that seven editions have been published in America is evidence of the popularity of this book in its land of origin. Further editions have been or are in process of being published in Japan, Spain and Italy. An English edition has been considered essential and *The Compleat Pediatrician* is now published for the first time in Great Britain. The reviewer is uncertain as to what exactly is implied by the use of the term 'English edition'. The spelling employed in the title shows no departure from American practice.

There is none who can but admire the immense industry devoted to bringing this book up to date without sacrifice of its unique character. It is small wonder that Professor Davison has felt the need for assistance and he is to be congratulated on enlisting the services of his daughter, herself a paediatrician, as co-author. The original format of the book has been retained. Those conversant with earlier editions will find no difficulty in recognizing amendments and additions made in the light of recent advances in modern paediatrics. Greater use is made of practical footnotes than formerly. This is to be commended as is the introduction of a few carefully selected references.

There can be no questioning the value of this book if judiciously used as a discriminating guide to the collection of clinical facts relevant to the individual case. The volume is not to be regarded as a short cut to diagnosis or treatment. On the contrary it is an aid to memory and thoroughness. As the authors themselves emphasize, training and experience are essential to reliable evaluation of clinical facts no matter how meticulously amassed. Recognition of this fact is essential if the maximum help is to be derived from this admirable publication.

The Management of Childhood Asthma. By FREDERIC SPEER. (Pp. xii + 116; 13 figures. 36s.) London: Blackwell Scientific Publications; Springfield, Illinois: Charles C. Thomas. 1958.

Any doctor, except an allergist, will read this primer with mounting impatience at the lopsided view given of children with asthma. Calm will return when he realizes that the book deals with the treatment of childhood asthma and not of asthmatic children, and that the text concerns only asthma due to specific allergens in the United States. Within these boundaries here is an excellent account of history taking, skin testing, elimination diets for food allergens, orthodox drug treatment and hyposensitization methods.

Of 315 cases studied in the mould and pollen laden atmosphere of Kansas City and its environs the recorded sensitivities were to alternaria (67·6%), ragweed (42·9%), housedust (38·1%), helminthosporium (22·5%) and grass (17·8%). All the rest rate low (cat, 4·1%; dog, 2·2%). Between the lines Dr. Speer reveals himself as a shrewd and doubtless highly effective physician, with more in his management than pure allergy, but as director of a paediatric allergy clinic he has to be loyal to the unitarian view that asthma is always due to specific allergens if we are clever enough to find them. He recognizes (and treats) 'unusual psychic stress' as a contributing factor. From the only alternative conception mentioned, that of a psychogenic origin, he dissents like most physicians and most psychiatrists. How sad that asthma and allergy clinics have to nail some special colour to the mast. The truth could be that asthma is a symptom and not a disease *sui generis* and that each case has to be studied afresh and in the broadest possible terms, although a few are purely allergic and a few neurotic. Dr. Speer recognizes that there may be widespread symptoms even outside the respiratory tract, but these are 'evidence of systemic allergy'. We close the book hearing a faint echo of the Preacher: 'Allergy, allergy, all is allergy'.

Technique Chirurgicale Infantile. By BERNARD DUHAMEL in collaboration with SIMONE SEGAUX. (Pp. 354; 289 figures. Fr. fr. 2,800.) Paris: Masson. 1957.

This book makes interesting reading because it is the work of a thoughtful surgeon with an original mind. He gives reasons for his preferred methods, and the factual statement of his experience and results in several chapters is a welcome feature in this class of book. The work covers abdominal surgery, the neck, harelip and cleft palate but excludes thoracic lesions (except oesophageal atresia and hiatus hernia), neurosurgery (except spina bifida) and orthopaedics.

Some of the methods, however, may seem over-ingenious to the British reader: a technique for combined herniotomy and appendicectomy would seem of very limited value. Readers will also probably desire a larger and more detailed series of results before preferring his operation for Hirschsprung's disease to the well-tried Swenson type. Bodian is mentioned in the text on several occasions though no specific reference is given. The reviewer feels sure that the opinions attributed to him, e.g., that rectosigmoidectomy should only be considered 'dans les formes graves, rebelles au traitement classique', are quite unlike Bodian's present opinions.

The book will be interesting reading for paediatric surgeons but it could not be recommended as a text for one unfamiliar with the field.

Aktuelle Problem der Kindertuberkulose. By H. WISSLER. (Pp. viii + 71; 17 figures. D/M 12.80.) Stuttgart: Georg Thieme. 1958.

In this monograph Professor Wissler, late physician-in-chief of the Children's Sanatorium pro Juventute in Davos, Switzerland, discusses current problems of tuberculosis in childhood. Fully aware of the geographical variation in importance of such problems, he nevertheless succeeds in selecting for consideration questions of universal interest. He deals in lucid and precise language with topics ranging from recent advances in bacteriology and epidemiology to the oscillations in B.C.G. policy.

However, the therapeutic aspects of primary tuberculosis, mediastinal and cervical adenitis, tuberculous meningitis, as well as bone and joint tuberculosis, have not been overlooked. The place of the steroids in the treatment of the various clinical manifestations has been critically assessed on the basis of reports available in the literature but also on personal experience.

Each chapter is followed by a short but well-selected bibliography. The x-ray reproductions are generally good and the diagrams clear with the exception of one on page 39 (reproduced from Dubois) comparing mortality from tuberculous meningitis in cases treated with streptomycin alone with those having streptomycin + I.N.H.

The monograph is particularly useful for those who have not had the opportunity or the time to follow the vast literature on childhood tuberculosis but nevertheless have to treat tuberculous children in their day-to-day practice. It provides a succinctly and pleasantly written guide.

Children Under Five. By J. W. B. DOUGLAS and J. M. BLOMFIELD. (Pp. 177; 8 figures. 21s.) London: Allen and Unwin. 1958.

In 1946 a joint committee of the Population Investigation Committee and the Royal College of Obstetricians and Gynaecologists, wanting information on the maternity services and the cost of childbearing, investigated the circumstances of all confinements that took place in Great Britain during the first week in March of that year, and later published its results. At the end of the investigation there remained available a representative sample of children drawn from all types of homes in the country, and, with a certain amount of luck, the enthusiasm of a small group of workers and the financial help of various interested bodies, this sample has been and is still being followed as it grows up. Periodically during the intervening years a series of papers and monographs have appeared giving the results of various studies in this group. The latest of these, the book under review, embodies the analysis of the answer to a questionnaire sent in 1950 to the parents of a somewhat curtailed remnant of the original group of infants who were by then 4 years old. The questions related to the social class, education of parents, home arrangements and the care of children in the home, growth and illness of the infants, separation from the mother, accidents, broken homes, toilet training and some special information regarding the prematures.

The information is set out, for the most part, in tabular and statistical form, and the conclusions, 75 of them, are usefully summarized in the final chapter.

It is not easy to be sure how valuable all this information is and certainly many of the conclusions will not be news to anyone working with small children. We all agree, for instance, with conclusion no. 7 that 'a large proportion of children shared their beds particularly in Scotland and in both countries many slept either in the same bed or in the same room as their parents'; and it will come at least as useful ammunition to turn to the relevant tables and find that the figure for the 4-year-old children of England and Wales is 26% and for Scotland 51%. Again many of us suspecting that admission to hospital is usually only a minor psychological trauma, will breath a sigh of relief to read that 'a preliminary examination suggested that short periods of separation were not important, and we therefore matched (with controls) only those children who were separated for four weeks or more'. Moreover, though in the latter group there was a higher incidence of nightmares, thumb sucking, nail biting and bed wetting, there did not appear to be greater emotional instability, and this was also true of the 178 children living in homes broken by death, divorce or separation. It should be fascinating to watch the whole survey group as it grows up.

THE FLUID SHIFT FROM THE VASCULAR COMPARTMENT IMMEDIATELY AFTER BIRTH

BY

DOUGLAS GAIRDNER, JOHN MARKS, JANET D. ROSCOE and R. O. BRETTELL
From the Cambridge Maternity Hospital

(RECEIVED FOR PUBLICATION MAY 20, 1958)

In an earlier paper (Gairdner, Marks and Roscoe, 1952) we drew attention to the fact that the haemoglobin (Hb) level during the first day of life is generally much higher than at birth. We questioned the adequacy of the current explanation, that any rise in the Hb level after birth is the result of transfer of placental blood, and suggested that the effect merited study. We now present further observations comparing the composition of cord blood at birth with venous blood taken from a few minutes to a few hours after birth. Hb, packed cell volume, (PCV), plasma protein and plasma sodium have been measured. From these comparisons we conclude that after birth there is usually a shift of fluid, mainly whole plasma, from the circulation. The volume of the plasma shift may be large, amounting to an appreciable fraction of the initial plasma volume, and the effect may consequently prove to be of some clinical importance.

Material

Ninety-two infants were studied, of whom 73 were delivered vaginally and 19 by caesarean section. The mother's permission for blood sampling was obtained. Most of the subjects were normal, but a few of the mothers had toxaemia or diabetes; the results in these were similar to those of the normals and have not been separately analysed.

Methods

The cord was always clamped as soon as conveniently possible, both in vaginal and caesarean deliveries. A blood sample was taken by puncture of the umbilical vein between placenta and clamp. Subsequent specimens were taken from an external jugular, internal jugular or femoral vein, or from the ductus venosus (i.e. the continuation of the umbilical vein). The ductus venosus was used particularly for samples within a few minutes of birth. We have found that the ductus venosus can often be catheterized conveniently by inserting a wide-bore trocar into the terminal part of the umbilical vein in the cord, and threading a polythene catheter through it. Samples were taken into heparinized tubes. Hb and PCV were estimated as described previously (Marks, Gairdner and Roscoe, 1955), Hb being estimated in duplicate in most cases. Plasma protein was estimated by the biuret method, using 0·2 ml. plasma. Plasma sodium was estimated by flame photometer. These four estimations required about 2·5 ml. of blood.

Results

(i) **Change in Hb Level a Few Hours After Birth.** In 92 infants samples were taken one to eight hours after birth and compared with cord blood. These included 19 caesarean deliveries, all but two of which were elective, and thus performed before the onset of labour. Results are shown in Fig. 1. Twenty-two cases showed a negligible change (less than $\pm$ 5%) in Hb level after birth; in two cases there was a fall exceeding 5%, while the remaining 68 (74% of the sample) showed a rise exceeding 5%. This rise amounted to 6-15% in 24 cases, to 16-25% in 23 cases, and to 26% or over in 21 cases. In five cases the rise exceeded 40%, the most extreme example being that of an infant born with an abnormally low haemoglobin level of 10·5 g./100 ml. which six hours after birth had risen to 17·0 g., a rise of 63%. For the series as a whole the mean Hb levels were 16·6 g./100 ml. (S.D. 1·96) for cord blood and 19·1 g./100 ml. (S.D. 2·36) at one to eight hours, giving a mean postnatal rise of 16%. The figure of 16·6 g. for cord blood Hb is not significantly different from 16·9 g., the value found in our earlier series (Marks *et al.*, 1955).

Since the means of the Hb rise (see Fig. 1) are as great at three hours as later (four to six hours), it seems that when the Hb level rises after birth the effect tends to be complete within three hours of birth, and perhaps in much less than this, judging from the few values available for one and two hours.

It will be seen from Fig. 1 that infants delivered by elective caesarean section showed the same order

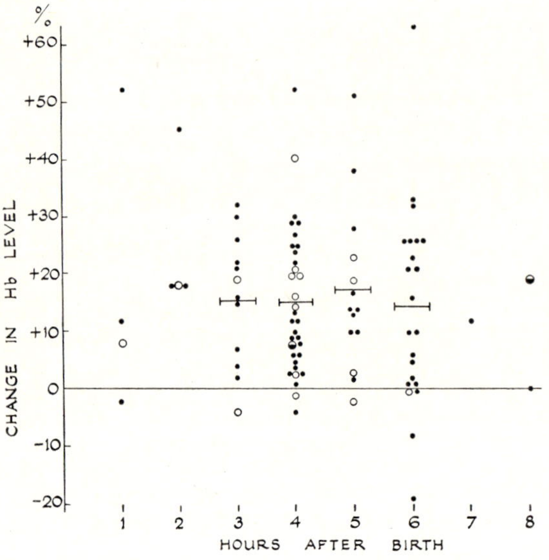

FIG. 1.—Change in Hb level in first few hours after birth.
● 73 infants delivered vaginally.
○ 17 infants delivered by elective caesarean section.
◓ 2 infants delivered by non-elective caesarean section.
Averages are shown for 3, 4, 5 and 6 hours.

of postnatal rise in Hb levels as did vaginally delivered infants, a crucial fact which bears on the part played by placental blood transfer in the postnatal Hb rise, to be discussed later.

(ii) **Change in the Hb Level a Few Minutes After Birth.** In order to determine how soon after birth the rise in Hb level begins, in 15 cases one or more venous samples were taken a few minutes after birth, either by means of a catheter introduced into the ductus venosus, or by puncture of another vein. Results are shown in Fig. 2. In seven cases the change in Hb level did not exceed ± 5%; in one case there was a fall of 6·5%; in the remaining seven cases there were rises of from 7% to 19%. It will be noted that in both vaginal and elective caesarean deliveries the Hb level often showed a significant rise within a few minutes of birth. The rises within the first few minutes thus may approach those seen at a few hours and demonstrate that the changes can occur very rapidly after birth.

(iii) **Uniformity of Samples from Different Veins.** At this stage it was felt imperative to establish that the changes were real and did not merely reflect some difference in the composition of blood in different veins. In five infants, the youngest aged 20 minutes, samples were taken from more than one vein. Results (Table 1) show that in no subject did the Hb level vary by more than 0·3 g./100 ml. in different veins, a maximum variation of 1·5%.

(iv) **Change in Packed Cell Volume.** In 39 cases the PCV was estimated in addition to the Hb level,

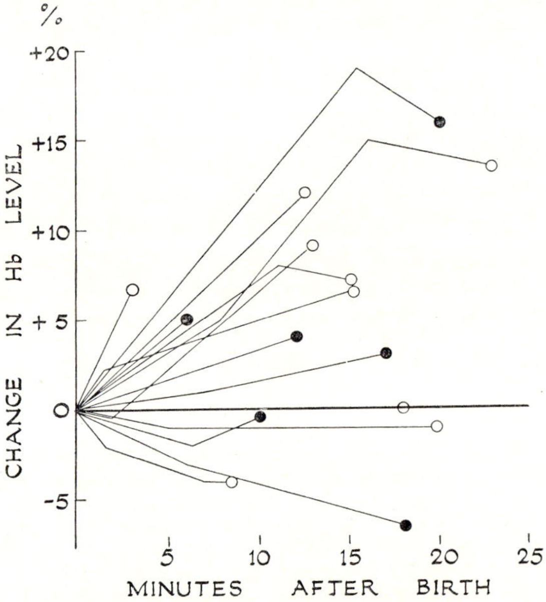

FIG. 2.—Change in Hb level in the first few minutes after birth.
● 6 infants delivered vaginally.
○ 9 infants delivered by elective caesarean section.

TABLE 1

UNIFORMITY OF BLOOD SAMPLES FROM DIFFERENT VEINS

Case	Age	Hb (g./100 ml.) Jugular Vein Int.	Jugular Vein Ext.	Femoral vein	Sagittal sinus	Ductus venosus	Difference
1. Normal	20 min.			17·6		17·6	0
2. Mild haemolytic disease	3 hr.	16·3				16·2	0·1
3. Normal	6 hr.	15·2		15·1			0·1
4. Mongol	27 hr.	20·0		20·0	20·2		0·2
5. Mongol	9 days		L. 20·8				
			R. 20·5		20·5		0·3

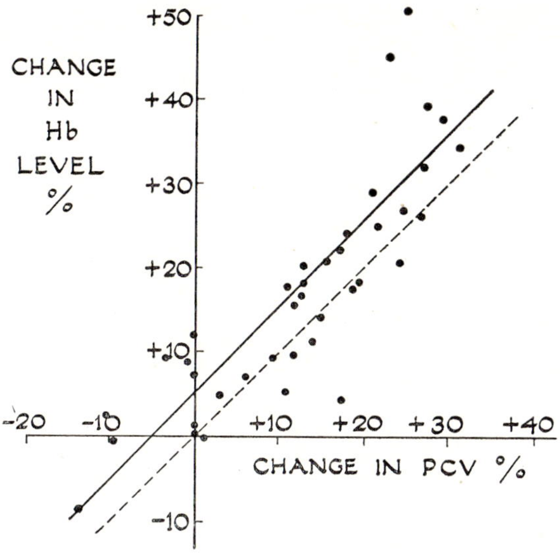

FIG. 3.—Relation of change in Hb level 1-8 hours after birth, to change in PCV, 39 cases. The broken line bisects the axes. Note that the change in Hb tends to exceed the change in PCV

and in Fig. 3 the percentage change in PCV is compared with the percentage change in Hb level. If the Hb and PCV had moved strictly in parallel, the points would have been grouped around the broken line shown; in fact the majority fall well above this line, i.e. the rise in Hb level is usually proportionately greater than the rise in PCV level. The calculated regression line is shown. In order to test the significance of this trend the percentage change in PCV was compared with the percentage change in Hb by the χ^2 test. The difference was highly significant ($\chi^2 = 215\cdot9$, d. of f. $= 38$, $p =< 0\cdot001$).

Since the ratio $\frac{\text{Hb concentration}}{\text{PCV}}$ defines the mean corpuscular Hb concentration (MCHC), these results are equivalent to stating that after birth there is a significant rise in MCHC. In a series of 21 cases* the mean MCHC of cord blood was 32·3 and in blood at one to eight hours 33·6, an increase of 4·0%.

* It was discovered that one of the centrifuges used had been running at less than the prescribed 3,000 r.p.m. leading to incomplete packing of red cells and to incorrectly high PCV values. Therefore the 18 cases involved were excluded when calculating MCHC values, leaving the 21 cases quoted.

These 18 cases have not been excluded from the data for Fig. 3 for the following reason. Since the effect of incomplete packing is relatively greater in blood samples having a high PCV, the percentage increase in PCV after birth would tend to have been *over*-estimated. The point we have sought to demonstrate in Fig. 3 is that when, after birth, the Hb rises, the PCV tends to rise relatively *less*. The error under consideration would therefore tend to shift results in a direction opposite to that of the trend we are demonstrating.

(v) **Change in Plasma Protein Concentration a Few Hours After Birth.** Plasma protein was measured in 17 cases, care being taken to reject any sample showing haemolysis, to which blood samples in the early days of life are annoyingly prone. The protein concentration showed either a negligible change of less than $\pm$ 5% (six cases) or a small postnatal rise of from 6% to 20% (11 cases). The mean value for cord blood was 6·5 g./100 ml. and at one to eight hours was 7·0 g., a mean postnatal rise of 7·7%.

(vi) **Change in Plasma Sodium Concentration.** This was measured in 14 cases. The mean value for cord blood was 145 mEq./1 and at one to eight hours was 146 mEq./1, a non-significant difference.

Discussion

To summarize the main findings, within a few hours of birth, there is frequently:

(1) A substantial rise in the Hb level, which reaches its maximum within three hours. In many cases this rise exceeds 25%, and it may reach 50% or more. In some cases the rise exceeds 10% within 15 minutes of birth.

(2) A rise in MCHC, averaging 4·0%.

(3) A rise in plasma protein concentration of up to 20%.

(4) No change in plasma sodium concentration.

Before considering the possible mechanisms responsible for these changes, it is essential to define certain terms used throughout the discussion and to relate them to each other.

In order to estimate the relative proportion of red cells in a sample of blood, we have centrifuged it in a Wintrobe tube for 30 minutes. The proportion of red cells thus determined is the *packed cell volume* (PCV). The PCV does not in fact represent the true volume of the red cells in the blood, since there is a small amount of trapped plasma in the red cell layer. Within the ranges of haematocrit and centrifugation applicable to this study, this can be allowed for by utilizing a factor of 0·95 (Chaplin and Mollison, 1952). The PCV thus corrected is the *venous haematocrit*. Thus,

$$\text{venous haematocrit} = 0\cdot95 \times \text{PCV}.$$

Blood in small vessels contains a greater proportion of plasma than does that in large vessels. Consequently the haematocrit of blood from a vessel such as a vein (venous haematocrit) is higher than the true *body haematocrit*. The ratio

$$\frac{\text{body haematocrit}}{\text{venous haematocrit}}$$

has been found to have a value of 0·91 in adults (Chaplin, Mollison and Vetter, 1953) and of 0·87 in newborn infants a few hours old (Mollison, Veall and Cutbush, 1950). Thus for an infant after birth,

$$\text{body haematocrit} = 0{\cdot}87 \text{ venous haematocrit}$$
$$= 0{\cdot}87 \times 0{\cdot}95 \times \text{PCV}$$
$$= 0{\cdot}83 \times \text{PCV}.$$

The postnatal rise in the haemoglobin level might be brought about by one of three possible mechanisms:

(1) A redistribution of plasma within the vascular compartment.

(2) An addition to the red cell volume.

(3) A loss of plasma fluid.

(1) **Redistribution of Plasma Within the Vascular Compartment.** As has already been stated, the ratio $\frac{\text{body haematocrit}}{\text{venous haematocrit}}$ in newborn infants a few hours old has the value of 0·87. In the foetus before birth there is no direct evidence of such a difference between the haematocrit in different parts of the circulation. If we choose to suppose that in the foetus the distribution of red cells and plasma is uniform, after birth a redistribution of plasma would take place, with some of the plasma in effect pooling in the smaller vessels. Then, considering an infant where *at birth* the venous haematocrit is h_1, this will be identical with the body haematocrit, while *after birth* the venous haematocrit h_2 will be given by

$$h_2 = \frac{\text{body haematocrit}}{0{\cdot}87} = \frac{h_1}{0{\cdot}87},$$

from which the percentage rise in haematocrit after birth $100\left(\frac{h_2 - h_1}{h_1}\right)$ can be calculated as 15%.

Since PCV is proportional to venous haematocrit this figure of 15% would also be the percentage increase in PCV after birth.

Under these hypothetical conditions, then, redistribution of plasma within the vascular compartment could in theory cause the PCV to rise by as much as 15%, but not more. However, rises greater than 15% are often observed (see Fig. 3).

While, therefore, we have no reason to believe that in foetal life the small vessels do contain less plasma relative to large vessels than is the case in the infant after birth, we cannot exclude this possibility. But if after birth some redistribution of plasma within the vascular compartment does occur, then it is clear on quantitative grounds that this can do no more than make some contribution to the large rise in PCV which is often observed.

(2) **Addition to the Red Cell Volume.** It will be convenient first to define the approximate size of the increase in red cell volume which would be necessary to produce the observed effect. This can be calculated in terms of the change in PCV for an average infant as follows.

We may take as a typical instance an infant of 3·4 kg., with a PCV at birth of 53%, rising by 15% after birth to 61%, corresponding therefore to a body haematocrit of 44% at birth and 50·6% after birth. With a PCV of 61% the blood volume after birth, obtained from the data of Mollison, Veall and Cutbush (1950) can be estimated to be 90 ml./kg. or 306 ml. If it be assumed that (*a*) the plasma volume remains the same after birth as before birth, then the composition of the circulating blood will be as shown in Fig. 4 (a), while if (*b*) the blood volume be assumed to remain constant, then the state of affairs after birth will be as in Fig. 4 (b).

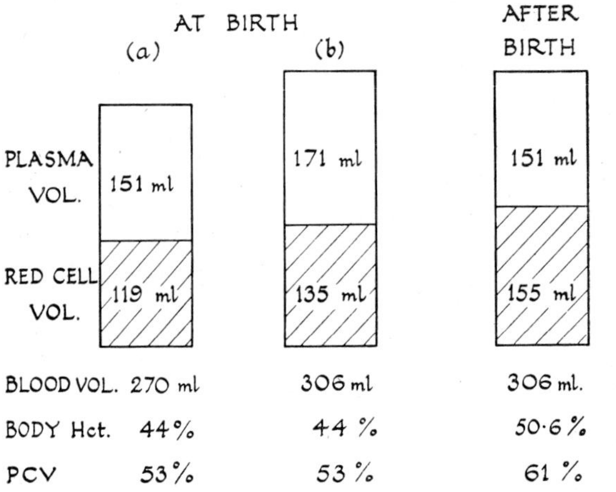

FIG. 4.—Calculated changes in red cell volume after birth, to account for an observed change in PCV from 53% at birth to 61% after birth: (*a*) assuming *plasma* volume unchanged, (*b*) assuming *blood* volume unchanged.

It will be seen that the calculated gain in red cell volume after birth is either (*a*) 155-119 = 36 ml., which is 23% of the initial red cell volume, or (*b*) 155-135 = 20 ml. which is 15% of the initial red cell volume, depending on which of the two assumptions is made.

This calculation gives an idea of the order of magnitude of the gain in red cell volume, i.e. 20 to 36 ml., which would be necessary to account for a postnatal rise of 15% in PCV such as is observed in a typical infant. With these figures in mind we may proceed to consider three possible sources of red cells which might be added to the circulation after birth. (It should be appreciated that many infants show a much greater postnatal rise in PCV than 15% (see Fig. 3) and would consequently require even larger red cell supplements.)

(*a*) Red Cells Derived from Transfer of Placental Blood. In the past it has often been observed that the mean Hb concentration is higher on the first day of life than in cord blood, and where attention has been paid to this difference it has usually been assumed that the postnatal rise in Hb level is the result of placental blood transfer. This view received weighty support from the work of DeMarsh, Windle and Alt (1942, 1948) who compared the Hb and haematocrit of cord blood with that of blood from the sagittal sinus at a few hours after birth. The latter gave Hb and haematocrit values on an average some 12-15% higher, but only if the cord clamping had been delayed, no such difference being seen in infants whose cord had been clamped at once. These authors' findings are thus completely at variance with our own, since throughout our series the cord has been clamped as soon as conveniently possible, yet a significant postnatal rise in Hb level has been observed in the majority of infants.

We have sought without success to find an explanation for this difference in results. Thus DeMarsh and co-workers took their blood samples from the sagittal sinus, a source we have not used in this series. However, a number of our samples were taken from the internal jugular vein, which, as the direct continuation of the sagittal sinus, is most unlikely to contain blood of different composition. Furthermore, reference to Table 1 shows that in two subjects investigated the Hb level of sagittal sinus blood was the same as in other veins.

The possibility exists that significant amounts of placental blood might be rapidly transferred to the baby during the terminal stages of delivery. In order to establish the fact that the postnatal rise in Hb level occurs independently of placental blood transfer, the effect was studied in 17 infants delivered by elective caesarean section, before the onset of labour. In these cases, too, the cord was clamped as soon as possible, so that it seems certain that no appreciable amount of placental blood could have been transferred to the infant. Nevertheless a postnatal rise in Hb level took place in much the same proportion of these subjects as in those delivered vaginally (Fig. 1), and this rise often exceeded 20%.

We must conclude that the postnatal rise in Hb level occurs independently of placental blood transfer (although it is, of course, likely to be augmented by any placental blood transfer that is allowed to take place).

(*b*) Red Cells Derived from Reservoir Sources. The spleen which weighs only about 10 g. at birth is clearly incapable of providing any significant addition to the red cell volume.

The only other viscus which requires consideration is the liver. This highly vascular organ weighs about 150 g. at birth, but even so it seems hardly conceivable that it could be capable of releasing as much as 20 ml. of red cells, or 13% of its weight.

(*c*) New Red Cells Derived from Haemopoietic Centres. According to Seip (1953) red cells delivered from haemopoietic tissue into the circulation are all reticulated and persist as reticulocytes for about one day. A large addition of new red cells would thus result in a correspondingly large rise in the number of circulating reticulocytes. Therefore, in the present context, where an average rise of the order of 15% in the red cell volume is being considered, the proportion of reticulocytes would be expected to rise from a normal level at birth of 3-4%, to nearly 20%. It may be said at once that no rise of this magnitude occurs. Wegelius (1948) found a slight transient rise in the reticulocyte level from 2·8% at birth to 3·7% at two hours. Seip (1955) also found that the level rose slightly, e.g. from 4·1% at birth to 4·5% after birth, but pointed out that this is what would be expected from the fact that new reticulocytes are added to a smaller volume of blood after elimination of the placental circuit. Our own data (Gairdner *et al.*, 1952) have given similar results, the reticulocytes numbering between 3% and 4% both in cord blood and in blood taken during the first day. These results therefore show that red cells from haemopoietic centres cannot be the source of the postnatal rise in haemoglobin level.

Thus we may conclude that addition to the red cell volume does not play a significant part in the haemoglobin rise that we have observed in infants after early clamping of the umbilical cord.

(3) **Loss of Plasma Fluid.** By exclusion of the other possible mechanisms we must conclude, then, that the postnatal rise in Hb level must be mainly due to haemoconcentration from a shift of fluid from the vascular compartment.

Two other simultaneous changes support the idea of fluid shift:

(i) A rise in the concentration of plasma protein.

(ii) A rise in the MCHC of the red cells.

The increase in the MCHC implies that there is usually some contraction of the red cells from shift of intracellular fluid into the plasma, at the same time as fluid is extruded from the vascular compartment.

If the blood volume after birth is v, the red cell

and plasma volumes at birth, and a few hours after birth, can be defined in terms of the Hb level and the PCV *at birth* (Hb_1, PCV_1) and *after birth* (Hb_2, PCV_2) as shown in Fig. 5.

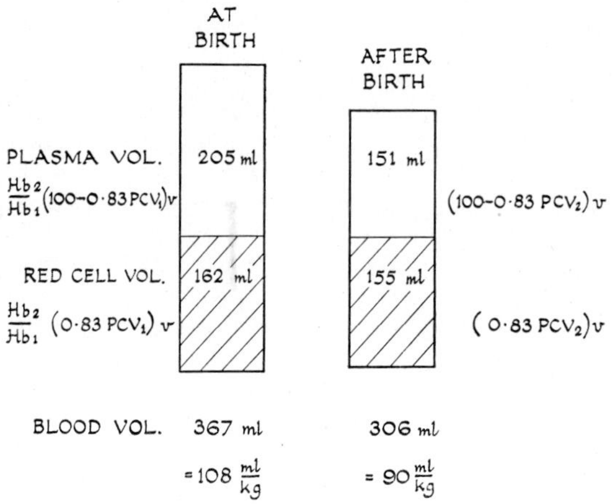

FIG. 5.—Method of calculating red cell and plasma volumes at birth and after birth, in terms of blood volume after birth (v). Numerical values for a typical infant (see text) are shown.

Using this general scheme it is simple to calculate the volume of the plasma fluid shift corresponding to any observed change in Hb level and PCV. As an example we have taken a typical case of a 3·4 kg. infant where the Hb after birth rises by 20% from 16·9 to 20·3 g./100 ml. and the PCV by 15% from 53 to 61%. The blood volume after birth, corresponding to a PCV of 61%, is 90 ml./kg. (Mollison *et al.*, 1950), and from this values for the plasma and red cell volumes at birth and after birth have been calculated (Fig. 5).

According to this calculation it will be seen that in a typical case such as that quoted the volume of fluid extruded from the vascular compartment will be 367-306 = 61 ml., while the plasma volume will diminish by 205-151 = 54 ml. The difference between these figures is accounted for by the 7 ml. of fluid that has shifted from the red cells, equivalent to a contraction of about 4% in the red cell volume. The 54 ml. of plasma fluid lost from the vascular compartment out of an initial plasma volume of 205 ml. represents 26% of the initial plasma volume.

The Composition of the Fluid Lost from the Vascular Compartment

Plasma being composed of electrolytes, protein and water, the question next to be answered is whether all these constituents are lost in the same proportions in which they exist in the plasma.

The percentage increase in the concentration of a solute when the volume of a solution diminishes from V_1 to V_2 is given by $100\,\frac{(1/V_2 - 1/V_1)}{1/V_1}$ which reduces to $100\left(\frac{V_1}{V_2} - 1\right)$. If the terms V_1 and V_2 are replaced in this expression by the values for the plasma volume at birth and after birth as given in Fig. 5, this expression becomes

$$100\left(\frac{Hb_2}{Hb_1} \cdot \frac{100-0\cdot 83\ PCV_1}{100-0\cdot 83\ PCV_2} - 1\right)$$

If now the fluid lost from the vascular compartment were protein-free, then the above expression would give the percentage increase in plasma protein concentration in terms of the changes in Hb level and PCV after birth. If, on the other hand, the fluid lost were whole plasma, there would be no change in the concentration of plasma protein. In Fig. 6 the percentage change in the plasma protein concentration, calculated on the supposition that

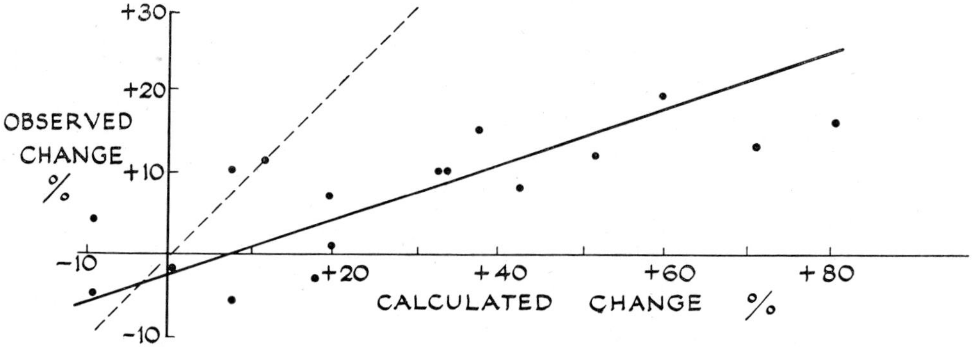

FIG. 6.—Observed change in plasma protein concentration one to eight hours after birth (17 cases), related to change calculated on the supposition that the fluid lost from the vascular compartment after birth is protein-free. Regression (continuous) line shows that observed change is about one quarter as great as calculated change.

the fluid lost is protein-free, is plotted against the observed change. It will be seen that the points mainly fall far below the broken line representing a 1:1 ratio between the calculated and the observed changes in protein concentration. The position of the regression line shows that the observed change in protein concentration is on the average only about one quarter of the calculated value, and from this fact we may infer that the protein content of the fluid which leaves the vascular compartment is roughly three-quarters that of the plasma.

In the same way, the fact that the plasma sodium shows no postnatal rise implies that any fluid lost from the vascular compartment contains about the same concentration of sodium as does plasma.

In brief, therefore, we may conclude that the fluid lost is largely whole plasma, although the small increase in plasma protein concentration indicates that some additional protein-free fluid also leaves the vascular space.

The Fluid Shift from the Red Cells. We have seen that there is generally a rise in the MCHC in the first few hours after birth, averaging 4·0%. The fact that the MCHC is appreciably higher after birth than at birth is evident also when studying the data provided by other authors who have examined both cord blood and blood taken after birth on Day 1; their results are set out in Table 2. For the four series quoted the average postnatal increase in MCHC is about 3%.

An increase of 3% in the MCHC implies a contraction in the volume of the red cell by about the same amount. We have not made direct observations to check whether in individual cases the mean corpuscular volume (MCV) decreases in parallel with the MCHC increase after birth, and in view of the inaccuracy of red cell counts it would be a laborious task to attempt. However, there is some evidence from the literature that the MCV after birth on Day 1 is, on the average, some 3% lower than at birth (Table 2).

There is thus good evidence that after birth there is a contraction in the volume of the red cells which, on the average, amounts to about 3%. This rapid decrease in volume must be largely caused by a shift of fluid from the cells.

The cause of the fluid shift from the red cells is undecided. Our data show no correlation between the increase in MCHC and the increase in Hb level after birth so that, for example, the MCHC may increase in cases where there is no postnatal Hb rise. It therefore seems that the shift of fluid from the red cells on the one hand and from the plasma compartment on the other, may prove to be independent effects.

Certainly our data do not suggest that the contraction of the red cells is a response to alteration in the osmotic pressure of the plasma, for the plasma sodium, which (with the chloride) makes the major contribution to the osmotic pressure of the plasma, shows no consistent rise after birth. The small increase noted in plasma protein concentration after birth would have only an insignificant effect on the total osmolarity of the plasma.

It is, however, known (Jacobs and Parpart, 1931) that red cells contract under the following three conditions: a rise in O_2 tension; a fall in CO_2 tension; or a shift of the *p*H towards the alkaline side; and it is possibly a combination of these three effects which causes the haematocrit of arterial blood to be about 1% lower than that of venous blood (Henderson, 1928; Hope and Verel, 1955). After birth, as soon as air-breathing begins, all three effects operate, the blood *p*H (which has the largest effect on red cell size) shifting from 7·33 to 7·43, according to Graham and Wilson (1954). It must be stressed that the gas tensions in a sample of blood examined by ordinary haematological techniques can bear little relation to those in the body. Nevertheless changes in O_2 and CO_2 tensions provide an attractive theory to explain the postnatal contraction of red cells and this possibility requires further study.

TABLE 2

CHANGE IN COMPOSITION (MCHC) AND SIZE (MCV) OF RED CELLS AFTER BIRTH

Author	Number of Cases	(1) Birth (Cord Blood)	(2) After Birth (Day 1)	Difference (1)—(2)
		Mean Corpuscular Hb Concentration (%)		
Present series	21	32·3	33·6	+4·0%
Waugh *et al.*, 1939	45	30·0	31·5†	+5·0%
Vahlquist, 1941	24	32·2	32·4	+0·6%
Guest and Brown, 1957	59	32·6	33·5	+2·7%*
		Mean Corpuscular Volume (c. μ.)		
Vahlquist, 1941	24	116·2	113·2	−3·0%
Guest and Brown, 1957	59	113	110	−2·7%*

* Differences statistically significant. † Day 2.

The Mechanism of the Postnatal Shift of Plasma. We have inferred that in a typical newborn infant birth is quickly followed by the shift of an appreciable fraction of the plasma volume, amounting in an average case to some 54 ml. of plasma. At present we can do no more than speculate about the mechanism of this substantial shift of plasma, which often begins within a few minutes of birth and appears to be complete within an hour or two.

From animal and human studies it is known that plasma fluid with varying amounts of protein is continuously flowing out of capillaries. Some of this fluid is reabsorbed on the venous side of the capillary, while the remainder, including practically all the protein, is recovered by the lymphatics and eventually returned to the circulation. It is less well known how considerable is the amount of protein which thus leaves the circulation, giving rise to a regular extravascular circulation of plasma protein via the lymphatic system, the lymph having a concentration of protein of about half that in plasma itself. In the dog it has been estimated that 50-100% of the total plasma protein leaves the circulation each day (Yoffey and Courtice, 1956).

Under physiological conditions the main variable factor determining the amount of plasma fluid leaving a capillary is the hydrostatic pressure within the vessel. The cause of the postnatal plasma shift may well therefore be sought in the drastically changed haemodynamics of the infant following birth. The re-routing of the blood stream which takes place must presumably lead to a greatly increased blood flow at some sites. At no site is such a change better defined than in the lungs. This subject is discussed by Dawes (1958) who has shown that (in the lamb) birth is followed by (i) a large fall in pulmonary arterial pressure and (ii) a large increase (perhaps threefold) in pulmonary blood flow. The very large decrease in the pulmonary vascular resistance, which these two facts together imply, points to the probability of a large rise in the pressure within the smaller pulmonary vessels. This pressure has not as yet been susceptible to measurement.

It is suggested, then, that the loss of protein-rich fluid takes place from capillaries subjected to an increased pressure following circulatory rearrangements at birth, and that the pulmonary circulation is one site where conditions are such as to favour this.

Blood Volume at Birth. Determinations of the blood volume of the newborn infant have in practice been made when the infant was a few hours old, by which time we must assume from our data that the postnatal change in plasma volume will have already taken place. This conclusion is supported by inspection of the data given by Mollison *et al.* (1950) in their paper on blood volume in newborn infants, where the (corrected) haematocrit of the normal infants studied is, with a few exceptions, well above the normal mean value of 50% for cord blood, averaging about 60%. It follows that the blood volume of the infant at birth is appreciably larger than is currently accepted. Referring, for example, to the situation represented in Fig. 5, it will be seen that the inferred blood volume *at birth* was 108 ml./kg., compared with 90 ml./kg. after birth. In this case, therefore, the blood volume at birth was 20% larger than after birth, 18% being accounted for by a larger plasma volume, and 2% by a larger red cell volume.

The Hydraemic State of the Foetus. It is clear therefore that, compared with the infant after birth, the foetus tends to be in a state of hydraemia, i.e. to have a larger plasma volume.*

The question arises as to how far the wide range over which the normal Hb level in the cord blood varies is partly a function of the degree of hydraemia. In Fig. 7 the postnatal rise in Hb level has been plotted against the cord Hb level. The regression line is shown and this is highly significant ($r = 0{\cdot}352$, $p = <0{\cdot}01$). It can be seen that there is a tendency for the largest postnatal rises in Hb level to occur amongst those infants that have a low initial level.

This is an interesting finding, because it throws some light on a fact which has puzzled us, the remarkably wide range of the normal cord Hb level, the 95% range being 13·7-20·1 g. (Marks *et al.*, 1955), with occasional values observed as low as 10·4 g. and as high as 22·0 g. The findings shown in Fig. 7 strongly suggest that the lower Hb values are the result of haemodilution. For instance, while 18 out of 92 infants were born with a cord Hb below 15 g., a few hours after birth only two infants showed so low a level.

As we have inferred that immediately after birth the plasma volume may decrease appreciably, it is of interest that there is some evidence of a similar lability of the plasma volume in the foetus before birth. Born, Dawes and Mott (1956) observed that in the foetal lamb subjected to hypoxia, as by decreasing the oxygen content of the air inspired by the ewe, there was a rise averaging 11% in the oxygen capacity (i.e. the Hb concentration) of the foetal blood, the oxygen capacity tending to return

* In contrast to this use of the term *hydraemia* in its strict sense, the term has sometimes been loosely applied to the foetus, and equally to the newborn infant, in the sense that the water and salt content of the body is high (Gans and Thompson, 1957).

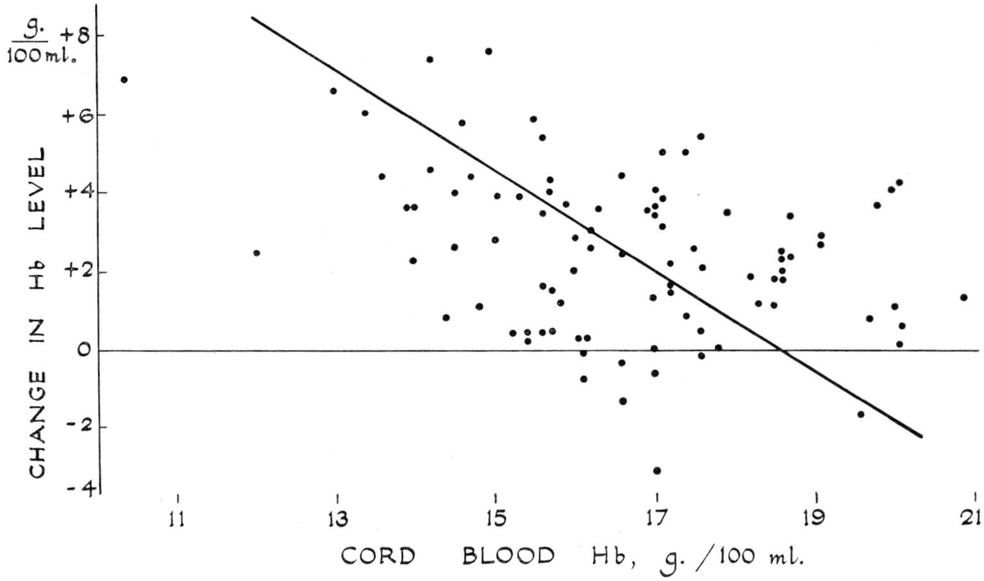

FIG. 7.—Change in Hb level one to eight hours after birth related to cord blood Hb level (92 cases). The regression line shows that the lower the cord blood Hb level, the larger the postnatal haemoconcentration effect.

to its original level after oxygenation was restored. This effect was shown not to be due to placental blood transfer and would be most readily explained on the basis of the readiness of the foetus to lose plasma from the circulation. The same explanation may account for the observation of Cook, Brodie and Allen (1957) that the mean cord blood Hb level of infants born with evidence of pre-natal hypoxia (meconium staining of nails, skin and cord) was 19·2 g./100 ml., significantly higher than the level of 17 g. in normal infants, and attributed by these authors to haemoconcentration. A similar conclusion was reached by Sjöstedt, Engelson and Rooth (1958) who found that infants showing meconium staining of the skin tended to have an abnormally low oxygen saturation of umbilical vein blood, and an abnormally high mean Hb level, 17·0 g. against the normal 16·1.

The Premature Infant and Plasma Shift. Only a few of the infants studied in this series were premature. In these few the usual tendency for the Hb level to rise strikingly after birth has been observed and it seems likely that in premature as in normal infants, birth is often followed by a shift of plasma from the circulation. A fluid shift which is evidently a physiological process in the normal infant might, however, prove an important handicap to an immature infant. The conspicuous tendency for the premature infant to develop generalized subcutaneous oedema within a few hours of birth comes to mind in this connexion, since it implies that immediately after birth there is a substantial shift of fluid from an undetermined source into the interstitial spaces. Moreover, there is some evidence to suggest that this fluid has a high content of protein, since Baar (1956) has been able at necropsy to collect oedema fluid from the leg in some premature infants. He found the protein content of this fluid to be near to that of plasma, with a concentration of from 3 to 7 g. %, and an electrophoretic pattern similar to that of plasma, save that the proportion of albumen was rather higher.

More important from the point of view of the vital functions is the part played by oedema in the pulmonary failure which is the main cause of death in the premature. From the standpoint of morbid anatomy there are two facets to these cases: resorption atelectasis, and intra-alveolar 'hyaline membrane'. The latter is only seen in infants that have survived several hours (Potter, 1952) and is probably formed from a transudate of plasma protein. We have already given reasons why the lungs are likely to be one of the sites where plasma is extruded postnatally. It is suggested that in the premature infant the normal mechanism by which the lymphatic system recovers protein leaving the circulation is overwhelmed, and that pulmonary oedema follows, with some of the protein-rich oedema fluid exuding into the alveolar space. In the average infant at birth the lungs weigh about 60 g., compared with a volume of fluid entering the extravascular space which we have estimated in a typical case to amount to about 61 ml. Thus even a small part of this fluid, if it remained in the lungs, might be of functional significance in the immature infant.

This reasoning leads then to the view that pulmonary oedema may be the primary disturbance in the pulmonary failure which so often overtakes the premature baby within a few hours of birth, and that one factor in the pathogenesis of the oedema may be the postnatal shift of plasma from the circulation.

Summary

Immediately after birth there is a rise in concentration of Hb and in PCV in the majority of infants. The rise may be discernible within a few minutes of birth and is probably completed within an hour or two. It occurs in the absence of any transfer of placental blood.

The possible causes are considered in detail and it is concluded that the effect is brought about by a shift of fluid from the vascular compartment.

This fluid is mainly whole plasma, and its volume may amount to a large fraction of the circulating plasma at birth, a quarter or more.

In addition, there is a shift of fluid from the red cells, the volume of red cells contracting after birth by an average of 3%.

The cause of these fluid shifts is discussed and it is suggested that the plasma loss may be a consequence of the re-routing of the circulation after birth.

These results imply that the foetus *in utero* is hydraemic, i.e. has a large plasma volume.

Haemodilution is thus in part responsible for the wide range of the normal cord Hb level.

Possible clinical implications are mentioned, particularly in relation to the pulmonary failure of the premature infant.

We gratefully acknowledge biochemical help given us by Professor R. A. McCance, F.R.S., Dr. R. S. Lawrie and Mr. S. H. H. Davison, and haematological facilities granted us by Dr. D. G. Chalmers.

References

Baar, H. S. (1956). Quoted by Crosse, V. M. (1957). *Ann. paediat. Fenn.*, **3**, 153.
Born, G. V. R., Dawes, G. S. and Mott, J. C. (1956). *J. physiol.*, **134**, 149.
Chaplin, H. and Mollison, P. L. (1952). *Blood*, **7**, 1227.
——, —— and Vetter, H. (1953). *J. clin. Invest.*, **32**, 1309.
Cook, C. D., Brodie, H. R. and Allen, D. W. (1957). *Pediatrics*, **20**, 272.
Dawes, G. S. (1958). In *Recent Advances in Paediatrics*, ed. D. Gairdner, 2nd ed. Churchill, London.
DeMarsh, Q. B., Windle, W. F. and Alt, H. L. (1952). *Amer. J. Dis. Child.*, **63**, 1123.
——, Alt, H. L. and Windle, W. F. (1948). *Ibid.*, **75**, 860.
Gairdner, D., Marks, J. and Roscoe, J. D. (1952). *Arch. Dis. Childh.*, **27**, 214.
Gans, B. and Thompson, J. C. (1957). *Proc. roy. Soc. Med.*, **50**, 929.
Graham, B. D. and Wilson, J. L. (1954). *A.M.A. Amer. J. Dis. Child.*, **87**, 287.
Henderson, L. J. (1928). *Blood, a Study in General Physiology*, chap. 7. Yale University Press, New Haven.
Hope, A. and Verel, D. (1955). *Clin. Sci.*, **14**, 501.
Jacobs, M. H. and Parpart, A. K. (1931). *Biol. Bull.*, **60**, 95.
Marks, J., Gairdner, D. and Roscoe, J. D. (1955). *Arch. Dis. Childh.*, **30**, 117.
Mollison, P. L., Veall, N. and Cutbush, M. (1950). *Ibid.*, **25**, 242.
Potter, E. L. (1952). *Pathology of the Fetus and the Newborn.* Year Book Publishers, Chicago.
Seip, M. (1953). *Acta med. scand.*, Suppl. 282.
—— (1955). *Acta paediat.*, **44**, 355.
Sjöstedt, S., Engelson, G. and Rooth, G. (1958). *Arch. Dis. Childh.*, **58**, 123.
Wegelius, R. (1948). *Acta paediat.*, **35**, Suppl. 4.
Yoffey, J. M. and Courtice, F. C. (1956). *Lymphatics Lymph and Lymphoid Tissue*, 2nd ed., chap. 2. Arnold, London.

THE PLASMA AMINO ACIDS IN MALNUTRITION:

PRELIMINARY OBSERVATIONS*

BY

ROLAND G. WESTALL,† ELLEN ROITMAN, CARMEN DE LA PEÑA, HOWARD RASMUSSEN, JOAQUIN CRAVIOTO, FEDERICO GÓMEZ and L. EMMETT HOLT, JR.

From the Department of Pediatrics, New York University College of Medicine and the Group for Research in Infant Malnutrition, Hospital Infantil, Mexico

(RECEIVED FOR PUBLICATION MAY 20, 1958)

It is generally appreciated that malnutrition is the world's foremost paediatric problem. Directly or indirectly it makes the major contribution to child mortality. Nevertheless, it remains an entity which is not well defined, or, more accurately, a combination of entities only some of which are well defined. We recognize the effects of certain specific food factors, the accessory food factors or vitamins, and we have some knowledge of changes brought about by deficits of the inorganic components of diet. The effects of caloric deficits, of protein deficits and of possible deficits of specific amino acids have, however, been difficult to separate. Protein and caloric deficits are commonly associated and the existence of syndromes of specific amino acid deficiency has not been definitely established although there is some evidence that they exist.

It appears that the more exact definition of this area of deficiency will depend on chemical studies. We already know that plasma protein levels fall in protein deficiency, particularly the albumin fraction, and that blood urea is also reduced. We know that certain protein enzymes in the blood and the liver (Waterlow and Patrick, 1954; Burch, Arroyave, Schwartz, Padilla, Béhar, Viteri and Scrimshaw, 1957) are diminished. It has seemed to us that observations on the free amino acids of the plasma might be of help in delineating specific entities within this area. The free amino acid level of the plasma might prove to be a more significant index of protein adequacy than other criteria that have been applied and the plasma free amino acid pattern, even if it could not be correlated with symptoms of specific amino acid deficiency, might yet be of considerable value in pointing to limiting amino acids and thus providing a sounder basis for dietary supplementation than has hitherto been available. Preliminary studies of urinary amino acids in kwashiorkor by members of our group (Cheung, Fowler, Norton, Snyderman and Holt, 1955), by Maggioni (1957) and by Hansen (1957) had shown abnormal amino acid excretion patterns, but since these might have been of renal origin it seemed preferable to explore the blood patterns rather than to extend the observation of urinary amino acids.

The observations reported here were made on four children admitted to the nutrition ward of the Hospital Infantil, Mexico City, with severe clinical evidences of malnutrition. There was no clinical evidence of vitamin deficiencies. They were all thought to be suffering from caloric deficiency as well as from protein deficiency, but the severity of the protein deficiency was much more marked in one of these subjects (M.M.C.) than in the other three. Only this patient exhibited the oedema and skin pigmentary changes typical of kwashiorkor. The serum of these four patients was studied initially and at intervals during the phase of recovery by the technique of column chromatography. Individual case histories are given below.

Case Histories

Case 1. R.A.M. (231195), a boy aged 1 year 11 months, was admitted to the Hospital Infantil on June 11, 1957, suffering from diarrhoea. No reliable information was obtainable about his past history or present illness. He was grossly undernourished, though not dehydrated, and the panniculus adiposus was minimal. His weight was 6·7 kg., height 71 cm. The skin showed somewhat deeper pigmentation on the dorsal surfaces of the hands and feet than elsewhere, but there were no discrete lesions. The liver was palpable 2 cm. below the costal margin in the mammary line. No evidence of infection was discovered, and the tuberculin reaction was negative. The bone age corresponded to that of a child of 6 months, according to Todd's Atlas (1937).

* This study was supported in large part by a grant from E. I. du Pont de Nemours and Co., Wilmington, Del.

† Present address: Medical Unit, University College Hospital Medical School, London.

The diarrhoea proved not to be severe, only five to six stools a day being passed. No pathogens were isolated on culture, but a microscopic examination revealed ova of *Hymenolepsis nana* and cysts of *Giardia lamblia*. The appetite was good and the patient took increasing amounts of the regular ward diet which consisted of whole cow's milk with supplements of bread, rice, banana, liver, lean beef and beans.

The samples of blood serum for amino acid assay were taken on the dates shown in Table 1.

During the period in hospital there was a gradual improvement in the child's general appearance. During the first four days he lost some weight, but after this there was a steady gain which reached 8·7 kg. on August 7, the day of discharge. Evidence of the 'recovery syndrome' (Gómez, Ramos Galván and Cravioto Muñoz, 1952) was first noted on June 20. The abdomen was enlarged with signs of free fluid in the abdominal cavity and prominent superficial abdominal veins. The liver edge at this time was felt 4 cm. below the costal margin. A blood examination at this time showed:

R.B.C. 3·3 millions, haematocrit 28%, haemoglobin 6·8 g., W.B.C. 18,000 (P. 57%, E.4%, L. 35%, M. 4%). The urine was normal. The stools at this time showed only *Giardia* cysts. Total plasma proteins 7·43 g. %; albumin 3·82 g., total globulin 3·61 g. ($\alpha = 0{\cdot}7$, $\beta = 1{\cdot}59$, $\gamma = 1{\cdot}32$).

By July 7, hepatomegaly and ascites had further increased as had the prominence of the abdominal vein, and examination of the blood showed the following:

R.B.C. 3·1 millions, haematocrit 26%, haemoglobin 7·3 g., W.B.C. 8,000 (P. 46%, E. 3%, B. 1%, L. 48%, M. 2%). Total protein 7·60 g., albumin 3·63 g., total globulin 3·97 g. ($\alpha = 1{\cdot}55$, $\beta = 1{\cdot}15$, $\gamma = 1{\cdot}27$).

Between July 7 and August 7 evidence of the recovery syndrome diminished markedly, but did not altogether disappear, and a blood study on July 25 showed:

R.B.C. 3·4 millions, haematocrit 29%, haemoglobin 7·3 g., W.B.C. 6,500 (P. 23%, E. 5%, L. 69%, M. 3%).

Case 2. E.F.A. (231172), a boy of 2½ years, was admitted to the Hospital Infantil on June 10, 1957, with malnutrition which had developed since weaning at 2 months of age. For a time he had been fed on a mixture of dilute cow's milk and tea, but on this he had not thrived and had suffered attacks of diarrhoea associated with fever and loss of weight. These attacks had recurred at intervals up to the time of admission. After the age of 1 year he had received almost no milk, his diet consisting of corn meal, beans, bread and noodle soup.

On admission the patient was found to be markedly undernourished. His weight was 5·7 kg., height 71 cm. The anterior fontanelle was still open (2 × 2 cm.). The skin showed no oedema, but there was a striking loss of subcutaneous fat. There was some excessive diffuse pigmentation, particularly on the extremities, but no discrete lesions. The liver edge was not palpable. Bone age corresponded to that of a child of 6 months (Todd, 1937).

The patient was given the regular ward diet. For the first two days some weight was lost but thereafter there was a steady gain, reaching 6·3 kg. on June 21, 6·8 kg. on July 10 and 7·1 kg. on August 7, the day of discharge. He had improved steadily up to June 25 when he developed bronchopneumonia which necessitated the use of antibiotics and oxygen. This attack was, however, brief and did not interrupt his weight gain. By June 28 the pulmonary signs had virtually disappeared. Evidence of the recovery syndrome was noted on July 8: the abdominal veins were engorged and the liver was now palpable 1½ cm. below the xyphoid. By August 1 these signs were receding.

Routine studies of the blood morphology and of the plasma proteins were made on three occasions:

On June 21: R.B.C. 3·6 millions, haematocrit 31%, haemoglobin 8·9 g., W.B.C. 12,000 (P. 63%, E. 2%, L. 30%, M. 5%). Total plasma proteins 6·9 g. %, albumin 3·31 g., total globulins 3·59 g. ($\alpha = 0{\cdot}44$, $\beta = 1{\cdot}99$, $\gamma = 1{\cdot}11$). Urine was normal. Stools showed cysts of *Giardia lamblia*.

On July 8: R.B.C. 3·1 millions, haematocrit 26%, haemoglobin 8·2 g., W.B.C. 6,000 (P. 36%, B. 8%, L. 54%, M.2%). Total protein 6·35 g. %, albumin 3·63 g., globulin 2·72 g. ($\alpha = 0{\cdot}73$, $\beta = 0{\cdot}72$, $\gamma = 1{\cdot}57$).

On August 2: R.B.C. 4·7 millions, haematocrit 40%, haemoglobin 12 g., W.B.C. 9,700 (P. 56%, E. 4%, L. 38%, M. 2%). Total plasma protein 6·07 g. %, albumin 3·09, total globulin 2·98 ($\alpha = 1{\cdot}54$, $\beta = 0{\cdot}36$, $\gamma = 1{\cdot}08$).

Case 3. F.C.G. (231194), a boy of 3 years, was admitted to the Hospital Infantil on June 11, 1957, with a history of bouts of diarrhoea since the age of 8 months. The attack for which he was admitted had lasted 15 days, and was precipitated by measles. The diarrhoea was not severe, only five to six stools a day being passed.

On admission the patient was markedly wasted, his weight being 8·0 kg., height 80 cm. The skin showed general pigmentation but no discrete lesions. There was no oedema. The liver was not palpable. Laboratory examinations on admission showed a normal urine. No pathogenic bacteria were cultivated from the stools, but cysts of *Giardia lamblia* were present. The blood showed: R.B.C. 3·6 millions, haematocrit 31%, haemoglobin 10·3 g., W.B.C. 2,000 (P. 38%, L. 60%, M. 2%). Total protein 5·35 g. %, albumin 3·12, globulin 2·23 ($\alpha = 0{\cdot}64$, $\beta = 0{\cdot}32$, $\gamma = 1{\cdot}27$).

For the first five days in hospital the patient was given a diet of corn meal and fish flour; for a second five-day period he was fed with corn and beans supplemented with glycine; after this he received the regular ward diet, similar to that given to the two patients previously described. Loss of weight was confined to the first 24 hours after admission. After this he gained steadily, reaching a weight of 9·6 kg. on August 6, the day of discharge. The diarrhoea proved to be mild, subsiding after the first few days, and the general appearance improved steadily.

The signs of the recovery syndrome, enlargement of the abdomen with hepatomegaly and engorgement of the superficial abdominal veins, were first noted on

July 8. The liver edge was felt 5 cm. below the costal margin and there was some evidence of free fluid in the abdominal cavity. On August 1 these signs, though still detectable, were definitely on the wane.

A routine blood examination on July 5 showed the following: R.B.C. 3·8 millions, haematocrit 32%, haemoglobin 9·1 g., W.B.C. 6,700 (P. 44%, E. 1%, L. 53%, M. 2%). Total proteins 7·02 g. %, albumin 3·94, total globulin 3·08 ($\alpha = 0·91$, $\beta = 0·52$, $\gamma = 1·65$).

Case 4. M.M.C. (231196), a girl of 1 year 7 months, was admitted to the Hospital Infantil on June 11, 1957, with a history of diarrhoea and vomiting for two months. For the preceding two weeks she had been weak and apathetic, and there was loss of appetite and oedema of the legs. Her diet had consisted largely of beans and noodle soup, but some milk had been given two to three times a week, possibly as much as 10 oz. on the days it was given. She was markedly undernourished, weight being 7·4 kg., height 77 cm. Discrete skin lesions, hyperpigmented and scaly, and typical of kwashiorkor, were present on the arms and legs and to some extent on the trunk. The hair was dry and relatively depigmented; it was easy to pull out. The tongue was red with hypertrophy of the fungiform and atrophy of the filiform papillae. There was tremor of the arms and a definite carpopedal spasm.

The patient was given calcium intravenously with prompt disappearance of the tetanic symptoms. The routine ward feeding was given from the start. Diarrhoea and vomiting were not observed in the hospital, and no parasites were found in the stools. The appetite and general well-being improved steadily. Weight was lost during the first two weeks in hospital as the oedema disappeared, the lowest point, 6·6 kg., being reached on June 25. After this the weight steadily increased to 8·6 kg. on August 9, the day of discharge. On June 27 it had increased and engorgement of the abdominal veins was observed. There was evidence of free fluid in the abdominal cavity on July 8. Defervescence of all these manifestations was clearly evident during the first days of August.

Routine blood studies were made on four occasions with the following results :

1% picric acid following precisely the details described by Moore and Stein (1954) for deproteinizing the plasma and removing the excess picric acid. The conditions used for the column chromatographic analyses again followed closely those described by Stein and Moore (1954) except that Dowex 50 × 5% cross-linked resin was used instead of a blend of the 4 and 5% cross-linked resin recommended by the above authors.

Results

The plasma amino acid concentrations in mg./100 ml. of plasma of the four patients, initially and during recovery, are given in Table 1. A range of normal values is also included. These normal values are derived partly from an analysis of plasma amino acids of normal children of similar age, which we have performed in the Pediatric Department of Bellevue Hospital, New York, and partly from the few figures available from published reports (Huisman, 1954; Stein and Moore, 1954; Iber, Rosen, Levenson and Chalmers, 1957). Throughout we were unable to detect any tryptophan in the plasma of the four children in this study nor was this amino acid found in the plasma of our normal children of this age group. We found it in older children and Stein and Moore reported a well-defined peak in their diagram of adult plasma. However, the latter authors reported that some loss of tryptophan can occur during the analytical procedure. We can only assume, therefore, that in children of 1 to 3 years the plasma concentration of tryptophan is so low that its presence is masked by the small losses inherent in the method.

The figures for ammonia and urea are also given since these are also determined by this method. The ammonia figure does not represent true ammonia present in plasma at the time of sampling since it is well known that ammonia is liberated and the concentration builds up during the deproteinization procedure. The figure for total amino acids

Date	R.B.C. (millions)	Hct. (%)	Hb (g.)	W.B.C.	Polys. (%)	Total Protein (g.%)	A/G	Globulins α	Globulins β	Globulins γ
June 12	3·2	—	9·1	6,200		3·76	1·56/2·20	0·69	0·68	0·83
,, 24	3·3		9·5	15,600	83	5·03	2·34/2·69	0·71	0·14	1·24
July 4						6·75	3·75/3·00	1·03	1·17	0·80
,, 31	4·5	38	11·2	15,600	28					

Experimental Procedure

Blood samples were taken at four different times from each patient, the first soon after admission, another sample about eight to nine days later, a further sample at the 25-30 day period and a final sample at eight to nine weeks. Approximately 20 ml. of blood, taken at least three hours after the last meal, was drawn with a heparinized syringe from the jugular vein. The sample was centrifuged and 10 ml. was shaken with 50 ml. of

represents the sum of the amino acids which were determined individually.

The changes observed in the plasma of the three patients who showed neither oedema nor appreciable skin changes were fairly consistent. They were least conspicuous in R.A.M. who showed the least reduction in weight and who during treatment failed to increase his total amino acid concentration

TABLE 1

AMINO ACID CONCENTRATION (MG./100 ML. BLOOD PLASMA)

Amino Acid	F.A.E. (2½ yr.) ♂				F.G.C. (3 yr.) ♂				R.A.M. (1 yr. 11 m.) ♂				M.M.C. (1 yr. 3 m.) ♀				Normal Range
	Day 1	11	30	60	Day 1	9	25	55	Day 1	8	25	55	Day 1	9	26	55	
Alanine	0·3	3·7	1·9	1·3	1·6	10·0	6·2	3·6	3·3	2·3	2·1	2·4	0·7	5·4	2·5	3·3	3·0–4·8
Aspartic acid	0·03	0·0	0·07	0·20	0·02	0·0	0·20	1·0	0·1	0·0	0·4	0·1	0·04	0·0	0·2	0·5	0·1–0·2
Asparagine + glutamine	2·1	4·0	2·8	1·5	2·6	5·0	3·2	3·0	3·9	3·9	1·5	4·0	2·0	7·7	1·7	2·3	3·0–5·0
α-aminobutyric acid	0·05	0·1	0·1	0·2	0·08	0·0	0·0	0·4	0·0	0·0	0·0	0·0	0·0	0·1	0·1	0·4	0·2–0·4
Arginine	0·4	0·9	0·4	—	0·4	0·8	0·5	0·4	0·4	0·6	0·6	0·4	—	0·5	0·7	0·9	0·8–1·4
Cystine	0·6	0·7	0·8	0·6	0·6	0·6	1·5	0·4	1·0	0·7	4·0	0·4	0·1	0·2	1·6	0·4	1·0–1·5
Glutamic acid	1·3	1·3	0·8	1·8	0·8	0·7	0·1	1·8	0·9	0·7	0·1	1·9	0·6	1·7	1·7	2·0	1·0–1·5
Glycine	2·2	3·0	1·3	1·2	1·9	0·6	0·7	2·1	1·9	1·7	0·6	1·8	0·8	1·3	1·8	1·5	1·0–2·0
Histidine	0·8	0·8	1·0	—	1·0	0·9	1·0	1·5	0·7	0·0	1·2	1·2	1·2	1·7	1·4	1·2	1·0–1·7
Isoleucine	0·5	1·0	0·7	1·0	0·7	0·8	1·2	0·9	0·7	0·7	0·7	0·9	0·8	0·7	0·7	1·5	0·8–1·5
Leucine	0·7	1·7	1·1	1·1	0·4	1·3	2·2	1·5	1·0	1·3	1·1	1·7	0·4	1·2	1·3	2·0	1·5–2·9
Lysine	0·9	2·3	1·0	—	0·9	2·7	1·4	2·1	0·7	1·7	2·3	1·9	0·6	3·6	2·6	2·4	1·5–2·4
Methionine	0·1	0·3	0·1	0·1	0·15	0·5	0·4	0·4	0·4	0·2	0·2	0·4	0·2	0·2	0·3	0·1	0·3–0·6
Ornithine	0·3	0·8	0·3	—	0·3	0·6	0·4	0·5	0·3	0·4	0·0	0·6	0·1	0·8	1·1	1·1	0·6–0·8
Proline	0·8	2·4	1·3	1·1	1·6	2·2	1·7	2·4	2·2	1·4	2·1	2·4	0·7	3·1	1·8	3·1	1·5–3·0
Phenylalanine	0·7	1·3	0·7	—	0·7	1·2	2·3	1·4	1·2	1·5	1·3	0·9	0·3	0·5	0·7	1·9	1·0–1·7
Serine	0·7	1·5	1·1	1·1	1·2	4·6	1·9	1·2	1·4	1·4	1·3	1·4	0·6	2·2	1·2	1·6	1·3–2·2
Taurine	1·3	0·2	0·4	0·6	0·6	1·5	0·8	0·3	0·3	0·9	0·5	0·3	0·2	0·5	2·1	0·9	0·9–1·8
Threonine	0·3	1·0	0·6	1·0	0·4	1·4	1·4	0·9	0·5	0·5	1·1	0·9	0·2	1·5	1·2	1·6	1·2–1·6
Tyrosine	0·7	1·3	0·9	—	0·6	0·6	1·4	1·7	1·3	1·1	1·0	1·5	0·1	0·2	0·7	1·9	1·5–2·3
Valine	1·2	3·0	1·7	2·1	0·8	1·6	3·3	1·9	1·7	1·7	2·9	1·7	0·2	1·7	2·0	2·7	2·0–3·0
Total	15·98	31·30	19·07	14·9*	17·35	37·60	31·80	29·40	23·9	22·5	25·0	26·8	9·84	34·7	27·4	33·3	28–33
Ammonia	0·23	0·22	0·05	—	0·26	0·20	0·30	0·4	0·18	0·3	0·3	0·5	0·28	0·38	0·07	0·20	
Urea	17·5	13·3	11·2	2·5	9·33	13·1	11·6	1·5	7·3	14·1	2·7	1·4	0·7	4·5	28·6	15·0	20–30

in the plasma. The general findings were as follows:

R.A.M., the least affected of the group, showed only a slight reduction in total amino acids although the urea concentration was low. Some of the amino acids were just within normal range, but significant reductions were present in the concentrations of threonine, taurine, lysine, leucine, ornithine and arginine. The eight-day specimen showed approximately the same picture except that aspartic acid was absent. In the two later specimens a fall in urea was noted, a phenomenon seen in the other subjects in association with the recovery syndrome.

F.A.E. and F.C.G. showed the same changes as R.A.M. and, in addition, several others. Their total amino acid concentrations were substantially reduced and several other individual amino acids were distinctly low in the initial specimen: alanine, aspartic acid, isoleucine, methionine, phenylalanine, tyrosine and valine. In the second specimen, the total amino acids had returned to normal as had the individual amino acids with the exception of aspartic acid and tyrosine. The tyrosine was slow in returning to normal and aspartic acid was absent in the eight-day specimen but returned later. Again the later specimens showed a reduction in urea.

M.M.C., the one who exhibited oedema and the typical kwashiorkor skin changes, showed the most profound changes in the plasma amino acids. The blood urea was extremely low and the total free amino acids were roughly one third of the normal value. Virtually all the amino acids were reduced to some extent with the exception of glycine, histidine and isoleucine. The most striking reductions were observed in the case of tyrosine, valine and cystine (to one tenth or less of the normal level). Substantial reductions (to one third or less of the normal level) were noted also in the concentrations of ornithine, threonine, taurine, leucine, alanine and phenylalanine. The levels of the remaining amino acids were reduced but less spectacularly so. The specimen taken nine days later showed a marked rise in the total amino acid figure to a level somewhat above normal. The increase was largely brought about by an abnormally high concentration of alanine and serine but at the same time the levels of the majority of the amino acids, which had been low, had returned to normal. Exceptions were phenylalanine and cystine and, most markedly, tyrosine. The subsequent specimens remained normal in respect of the amino acid concentration but tyrosine was particularly slow in reaching a normal level. Again, blood urea was low in the final specimen.

Discussion

A definite interpretation of these preliminary findings must await confirmative studies. At the most, the present data can be regarded only as suggestive. As regards the most limiting amino acid in the indigent Mexican diet, as far as it can be judged from these results which do not permit an evaluation of tryptophan in this respect, arginine, ornithine and threonine would seem to be consistently affected even in mild cases, and leucine, valine, lysine and tyrosine thereafter. Urea is also consistently low. Methionine, phenylalanine and alanine, although not so affected in the milder cases, were markedly affected in the more severe case with typical kwashiorkor symptoms. Here also, the cystine and tyrosine concentrations were particularly low. From the above data it would be difficult to incriminate any one particular amino acid as being limiting in the Mexican diet.

With regard to imbalance of amino acids in the plasma of these patients, it follows that some imbalance must exist since the levels of some amino acids are more affected than others. However, there was certainly no abnormally high concentration of any one amino acid and the only general comment is that the glycine concentration was consistently higher than the alanine level in the initial samples whereas the reverse ratio applies in all normal plasmas.

We are, however, impressed with the possibility that the low protein diet, particularly in the case of the severely affected patient, M.M.C., interfered with the development and activity of enzymes concerned with the metabolism of amino acids. The low concentrations of arginine and ornithine suggest some interference with the urea cycle. The low concentration of cystine seen in M.M.C. suggests a deficiency in its synthesis from methionine. Even more striking in this patient is the reduced level of tyrosine as compared with phenylalanine which supports the suggestion previously made on excretion data (Cheung *et al.*, 1955) that there is this condition, a deficiency of the enzyme which converts phenylalanine into tyrosine, phenylalanine hydroxylase.* A deficiency of this enzyme had been postulated by an increased excretion of phenylalanine in the urine, a phenomenon also noted by Maggioni (1957). The slow recovery of the blood tyrosine level of our patient is also worthy of comment. It may be that assays of this enzyme will prove useful in characterizing protein deficiencies.

The marked drop in the plasma urea concentration two months after treatment began puzzled us greatly, coinciding as it appeared to do with the presence of the recovery syndrome (Gómez *et al.*, 1952). Conceivably this might be due to impaired deamination. It might also be due to some re-utilization of urea although why this should occur so late is not easy to understand. A more likely explanation would be that the recovery growth spurt causes an extremely high utilization of protein and consequently little nitrogen is available for excretion. This argument can be supported to some extent by the low level of plasma taurine in the three patients with low blood urea at this time. Dent (personal communication) points out that in a number of disease states where the utilization of protein is poor and the subject is also in negative nitrogen balance owing to excessive enzymic breakdown of body protein, the excretion of taurine, which is derived from cystine or cysteine, is high. He believes also that the converse is true and that with high utilization of protein there is little wastage of cystine and consequently a low excretion of taurine. Unfortunately, in this series of cases we were unable to cope with equivalent analyses of urine but it is now obvious that in subsequent studies it would be desirable to carry out amino acid analyses on the urine as well as the plasma.

In considering the levels of the various amino acids in the initial samples of plasma we can say without doubt that they are, in general, much below normal. To go beyond that we find ourselves at a loss as to what further inferences can be drawn as we lack the basic knowledge. For instance, in the absence of an adequate protein intake at what level of plasma amino acid concentration does the body call upon endogenous proteins to reinforce the plasma amino acids? Further, once the endogenous protein available is used up how far can the plasma amino acid level fall before the vital organs are affected? It is difficult to see how this knowledge can be adequately answered by work on experimental animals, particularly as in kwashiorkor we are dealing with children in a narrow age group. An extensive study of kwashiorkor patients, including those with the mildest and the severest forms, would, in time, give us the answer to these questions.

Summary

A study is reported of the free amino acids of blood plasma in four patients suffering from severe malnutrition. Three of these showed no specific clinical symptoms of protein deficiency, whereas the fourth exhibited oedema and skin lesions typical of kwashiorkor, and can hence be regarded as a well defined type of protein deficiency.

A tendency to aminoacidopenia was found in all four patients, involving certain essential as well as certain unessential amino acids. It is suggested that

* Since this paper was written we have had the opportunity of studying the blood of three other patients with the frank kwashiorkor syndrome, one from French West Africa and two from Nigeria. The findings, which will be reported elsewhere, showed certain differences from those reported here, but the exceptionally low tyrosine value was consistently found.

these changes are best interpreted on the basis of defective enzyme systems.

Particular attention is called to evidence pointing to a deficiency of the enzyme phenylalanine hydroxylase in the frank kwashiorkor syndrome.

REFERENCES

Burch, H. B., Arroyave, G., Schwartz, R., Padilla, A. M., Béhar, M., Viteri, F. and Scrimshaw, N. S. (1957). *J. clin. Invest.*, **36**, 1579.

Cheung, M. W., Fowler, D. L., Norton, P. M., Snyderman, S. E. and Holt, L. E. (1955). *J. trop. Pediat.*, **1**, 141.

Dent, C. E. Personal communication.

Gómez, F., Ramos Galván, R. and Cravioto Muñoz, J. (1952). *Pediatrics*, **10**, 513.

Hansen, J. D. L. (1957). Proceedings of Conference held at Princeton, 1955. Josiah Macy Jr. Foundation, p. 42.

Huisman, T. H. J. (1954). *Pediatrics*, **14**, 245.

Iber, F. L., Rosen, H., Levenson, S. M. and Chalmers, T. C. (1957). *J. Lab. clin. Med.*, **50**, 417.

Maggioni, G. (1957). *Moderne Probleme der Pädiatrie*, II, 161. Karger, Basel.

Moore, S. and Stein, W. H. (1954). *J. biol. Chem.*, **211**, 893.

Stein, W. H. and Moore, S. (1954). *Ibid.*, **211**, 915.

Todd, T. W. (1937). *An Atlas of Skeletal Maturation.* 1. The Hand. C. V. Mosby, St. Louis, Mo.

Waterlow, J. C. and Patrick, S. J. (1954). *Ann. N.Y. Acad. Sci.*, **57**, 750.

HYPOCALCAEMIC TETANY DEVELOPING WITHIN 36 HOURS OF BIRTH*

BY

W. S. CRAIG and M. F. G. BUCHANAN

From the Department of Paediatrics and Child Health, University of Leeds

(RECEIVED FOR PUBLICATION MAY 16, 1958)

Introduction

Paediatric literature contains many brief references to the occurrence of neonatal tetany. Clinical signs developed in the first week of life in only a small proportion of the recorded cases. The number of infants reported as showing signs of hypocalcaemic tetany within a few hours of birth is extremely small. Willi (1939) described eight and Bakwin (1937) four babies in whom tetany developed on the first day of life. In a more recent comprehensive study of the causes of tetany in infancy and childhood Gribetz (1957) uses the term 'first day tetany' when referring to the biochemical imvestigations of Gittleman and his co-workers. Gittleman, Pincus, Schmerzler and Saito (1956) made a special study of calcium levels on the first day of life and found low serum calcium levels with significant frequency in premature infants and in babies born at term to mothers with a history of abnormal pregnancy and/or labour.

In October, 1956, the occurrence of violent neuromuscular hyperexcitability in the day-old baby of a diabetic mother in the Leeds Maternity Hospital aroused suspicions of tetany. The baby's serum calcium was 6·2 mg. per 100 ml. Within a period of one month similar findings were encountered in the newly born babies of two other mothers with diabetes mellitus. A detailed clinical study of babies newly born to diabetic mothers was commenced. As the study proceeded a resemblance was noted between the movement pattern in these babies and that seen in a number of newly born premature infants of healthy mothers. The resemblance was one of quality rather than severity. Low serum calcium levels were obtained in a high proportion of the premature babies with neuromuscular hyperactivity. A decision was therefore made to extend the investigation to include all babies manifesting neuromuscular hyperexcitability shortly after birth.

The primary purpose of this article is to present the findings in connexion with 26 babies in whom hypocalcaemic tetany developed within 40 minutes to 36 hours of birth. As a corollary to the main study findings are also given in infants who in the first 36 hours of life either (*a*) showed clinical signs suggestive of tetany in the absence of a low serum calcium level (seven infants), or (*b*) presented no abnormal clinical features despite the presence of a low serum calcium level (two infants).

Clinical Material

Of the 35 babies included in the total study, 30 were born in the Leeds Maternity Hospital, three in St. Mary's Hospital, Leeds, and two at home prior to admission to Leeds Maternity Hospital. For the purposes of the study tetany was considered to be present if exaggerated neuromuscular hyperactivity was associated with a total serum calcium level of 8 mg. per 100 ml. or less. Total serum calcium determinations were obtained by the permanganate titration method. Ultrafilterable calcium levels were estimated in a limited number of cases. The method employed was the one described by Lavietes (1937) and used by Hopkins, Howard and Eisenberg (1952). The decision to regard a total serum calcium of 8 mg. (and less) per 100 ml. as low takes account of the recorded opinions of other workers. Bakwin (1937), Willi (1939) and Kendig (1942) consider that a serum calcium level below 8 mg. per 100 ml. provides confirmatory evidence of a clinical diagnosis of tetany. In their comprehensive laboratory study Gittleman *et al.* (1956) regarded total serum calcium levels under 8 mg. per 100 ml. as low. Studying a series of 55 healthy newborn babies Mitchell and Stevenson (1932) found a serum calcium level of under 8 mg. per 100 ml. in only one infant. In another control series of 48 healthy newborn babies investigated by Dodd and Rapoport (1949) the serum calcium level was above 8 mg. per 100 ml. in every instance.

* Based upon a paper given at the Annual Meeting of the British Paediatric Association, 1958, and illustrated by a cinematograph film.

Clinical Observations

I. Hypocalcaemic Tetany (26)

(1) **The Clinical Picture.** Neuromuscular hyperactivity associated with hypocalcaemia was noted in 26 infants. All infants were under observation while being nursed in incubators. Details concerning these babies are given in Table 1. In each case signs were first noted within 36 hours of birth. The severity of the clinical picture varied, being violent in seven, pronounced in 14 and mild in five babies.

TABLE 1

HYPOCALCAEMIC TETANY WITHIN 36 HOURS OF BIRTH

Neuromuscular Excitability			Total Serum Calcium* (mg./100 ml.)	
Degree	Age at Onset (hr.)	Duration (hr.)	On 2nd day of life	Lowest estimate in 1st 72 hr. of life
Violent (7)	22	108	2·6	2·6
	10	120	5·1†	5·1
	1	130	6·0	6·0
	24	32	6·2	6·2
	10	62	7·1	6·8
	8	30	7·3	6·8
	1	21	8·0	8·0
Pronounced (14)	19	36	6·1	5·7
	4	77	6·4	6·4
	7	72	6·7	4·6
	36	24	6·8	6·8
	17	52	6·8	6·8
	24	36	7·2	6·8
	6	18	7·3	7·3
	22	48	7·3	6·5
	22	60	7·4	7·4
	14	72	7·6	7·6
	18	32	7·8	7·8
	13	90	7·9†	7·9
	6½	130	8·0	8·0
	24	48	8·0	8·0
Mild (5)	33	24	5·6	5·6
	17	24	7·0	7·0
	24	36	7·1	7·1
	4	40	7·8	7·3
	22	24	7·9	7·3

* The concentration of calcium in the cord blood was estimated in 21 cases. The lowest level obtained was 9·9 mg., the average being 10·5 mg. per 100 ml.

† Given exchange transfusion on account of haemolytic disease.

A detailed description of the signs in certain of the infants included in this series has already been recorded (Craig, 1958). Clinical signs were characterized by an abnormal movement pattern consisting of alternating phases of generalized hyperactivity and silent, exhausted immobility. Hyperactivity took the form of coarse waving movements of the limbs, agitated vibrations of the hands and fine persistent tremors of the fingers. The toes were splayed out. In severe cases the cry was squeaky and hollow and the expression one of distress. In all babies there were periods of apnoea and during phases of severe agitation the entire body acquired a grey cyanotic tinge. Cyanotic apnoea not due to aspiration of fluid was particularly liable to occur at the time of feeds.

Other features noticed in a proportion of cases were tachypnoea, tachycardia, repetitive blinking of partially closed eyelids, and the ejection of minute meconium stools. Trousseau's and Chvostek's signs were not present but in four babies a position simulating pedal spasm was assumed following local pressure on the lower limbs. Laryngeal stridor was a feature in two babies. Phases of neuromuscular hyperexcitability occurred spontaneously, and as a result of stimulus by touch, noise, vibration and light. Repeated stimuli resulted in temporary diminution of response. Spontaneous phases recurred at short intervals over varying periods of 12 hours to six days. There were convulsions in four infants. Details of the abnormal movement pattern in these 26 babies are summarized in Table 2.

TABLE 2

CLINICAL FEATURES OF HYPOCALCAEMIC TETANY WITHIN 36 HOURS OF BIRTH

26 INFANTS

Generalized neuromuscular hyperexcitability	26
Convulsions	4
Simulation of carpo-pedal spasm	4
Spontaneous attacks of apnoea and/or cyanosis	13
Apnoea stimulated by feeding	13
Frequent regurgitation	10
Hollow or squeaky cry	13
Stridor	2
Tachycardia	4
Tachypnoea	5
Complete disappearance of abnormal clinical features	26
Total serum calcium level of 10 mg. or more per 100 ml. on or before seventh day of life	26

None of the babies was given cow's milk or alkaline therapy prior to the onset of tetany and at no time did any suffer from vomiting, diarrhoea or excessive fluid loss.

(2) **The Biochemical Picture.** Biochemical findings in the 26 examples of hypocalcaemic tetany are given in Table 3.

(3) **The Influence of Calcium Therapy.** Calcium was given to five babies with clinically violent tetany. The results were not uniformly conclusive. Rapid improvement followed oral administration in one infant, and intramuscular administration in another. In the remaining three babies the impression was gained that combined intramuscular and oral therapy may have accelerated the disappearance of clinical signs of tetany.

(4) **The Obstetric Background.** Details are summarized in Table 4. There were two cases of placenta praevia, one being associated with toxaemia. Delivery was spontaneous in 15 cases and by caesarean section in 11 cases.

TABLE 3

BIOCHEMICAL FINDINGS DURING FIRST 4 DAYS OF LIFE IN HYPOCALCAEMIC TETANY: 26 INFANTS

Baby	Day	Total Ser. Ca. (mg./100 ml.)	Ultrafilt. Ca. (mg./100 ml.)	Phosphorus (mg./100 ml.)	Alk. Phosph. (Units*/100 ml.)	Blood Urea (mg./100 ml.)
(A) Violent Hyperexcitability (7)						
Ma	2	6·2	—	—	—	—
	4	10·0	—	3·0	23	68
T	2	2·6	—	5·7	36	176
	4	8·1	—	8·4	—	92
G	1½	8·0	—	—	—	—
	2	6·0	—	5·6	—	—
H	2	6·8	—	—	21	48
	3	7·1	3·1	7·0	—	—
	4	8·6	—	—	—	42
Mo	2	6·8	—	5·0	24	30
	3	7·3	3·5	—	28	22
R	½	5·1	—	—	—	—
	3	—	—	5·3	—	83
G	1	8·0	—	5·6	—	—
(B) Pronounced Hyperexcitability (14)						
S	2	4·6	—	6·8	18	44
	3	6·7	3·6	—	—	—
L	1	7·3	3·6	—	—	46
	2	7·8	2·9	—	—	—
W	½	8·3	—	4·5	—	46
	1½	6·8	—	—	—	—
	2¼	7·2	4·9	—	—	—
D	1¼	6·4	—	5·0	—	32
	2	8·0	4·9	—	—	—
N	1½	6·5	—	—	—	—
	2½	7·4	4·5	3·0	20	35
N	1½	7·3	4·1	—	—	—
	2½	—	—	—	—	31
T	1¾	6·1	3·2	—	—	35
T	2	8·0	—	7·1	26	62
W	1½	6·8	—	4·5	—	46
	2½	7·2	4·9	—	—	—
F	2	7·6	—	—	—	—
S	1	5·7	—	—	—	35
	2	6·1	3·2	—	—	—
Wm	1½	6·8	—	—	—	—
	2½	—	—	—	—	—
W	¾	8·1	—	5·4	—	—
	1¾	7·9	—	5·0	—	—
McG	1¼	9·0	—	—	—	46
	2	8·0	—	—	—	—
	3¼	9·8	—	—	—	—
(C) Mild Hyperexcitability (5)						
I	1¼	7·0	3·5	—	—	—
S	1	7·8	—	5·8	9	53
	2	7·3	—	—	—	—
M	2	5·6	2·8	—	—	—
	3	7·0	—	7·4	—	34
S	1¼	7·9	—	—	—	—
Mac	1½	7·1	—	—	20	35
	2	7·5	3·9	—	—	—

* King Armstrong units.

TABLE 4

OBSTETRIC BACKGROUND IN HYPOCALCAEMIC TETANY WITHIN 36 HOURS OF BIRTH: 26 INFANTS

A. *Born at Term* (38 weeks and over)			
	Healthy mother:	spontaneous delivery: breech	1
		caesarean section: prolonged labour	1
		caesarean section: placenta praevia	1
		elective caesarean section: disproportion	1
B. *Short Gestation Period* (less than 38 weeks)			
	Healthy mother:	spontaneous delivery: vertex	4
		,, breech	2
		both infants of a twin pregnancy	2
		one infant of twin pregnancies	2
	Diabetic mother:	spontaneous delivery: vertex	3
		elective caesarean section	7
	Pre-diabetic mother:	spontaneous delivery: vertex	1
	Eclampsia and placenta praevia:	caesarean section	1

II. Neuromuscular Activity in the Absence of Hypocalcaemia

A tentative diagnosis of tetany based on clinical observations was made on the second day of life in seven infants in whom the total serum calcium level was above 8 mg. per 100 ml. The clinical picture was pronounced in six and mild in one. All seven babies were delivered spontaneously, presentation being by the vertex in five cases and by the breech in two. The estimated gestation period was 37 weeks or less in the case of five babies: and 40 and 41 weeks in the remaining two. In no case was there a history of maternal toxaemia. Two of the premature infants were the firstborn of twin pregnancies (see IV (2) below). The onset of neuromuscular hyperexcitability took place three, 16, 20, 23 and 29 hours after birth and persisted for 12, 30, 72, 24 and 72 hours respectively in five babies. The corresponding percentages of serum calcium on the second day of life were 8·5, 9·3, 8·8, 11·6 and 8·7 mg.

In two instances neuromuscular hyperexcitability in the absence of hypocalcaemia occurred in babies given exchange transfusions.

III. Hypocalcaemia without Associated Neuromuscular Hyperexcitability

Two examples were encountered of hypocalcaemia not associated with neuromuscular hyperexcitability. Both occurred in infants newly born to diabetic mothers. In each case the estimated gestation period was 36 weeks, delivery was spontaneous, and the serum calcium level on the second day of life was 7·3 mg. per 100 ml.

IV. Some Special Groups

The 35 infants reported in this study include a high proportion of infants born prematurely, a number of babies born to diabetic mothers, several infants of twin pregnancies and four babies given replacement transfusions on account of haemolytic disease.

(1) **Premature Infants.** The estimated gestation period of 29 babies was less than 38 weeks, ranged from 31 to 37 weeks and averaged 36 weeks. Ten of the infants were born to diabetic mothers, the average birth weight being 7 lb. 7 oz. The birth weight of one baby born to a pre-diabetic mother was 6 lb. 12 oz. The average birth weight of the remaining 18 premature infants was 4 lb. Of the 29 premature babies hypocalcaemia was a feature of 24, being associated with violent, pronounced and mild hyperexcitability in five, 13 and four cases respectively. In two babies there was no hyperexcitability despite the presence of hypocalcaemia; and hyperexcitability was present in five infants in whom the serum calcium was above 8 mg. per 100 ml.

(2) **Twin Pregnancies.** Hypocalcaemic tetany was found in the babies of four twin pregnancies. In one such pregnancy both babies were involved; and in another both infants showed clinical signs of pronounced neuromuscular hyperexcitability but only one infant had a total serum calcium level under 8 mg. per 100 ml. In each of two other pregnancies one infant showed evidence of hyperexcitability and was the only infant with hypocalcaemia. A feature of each of the four twin pregnancies was that the total serum calcium level was lower in the second than the first live-born infant. Details are given in Table 5.

TABLE 5

SERUM CALCIUM LEVELS IN FOUR TWIN PREGNANCIES

Baby	Hyper-excitability	Total Serum Calcium (mg./100 ml.)	Birth Weight (lb.	oz.)	Maturity (weeks)
N 1	Pronounced	7·4	4	6	35
N 2	Pronounced	7·3	5	7	35
T 1	Nil	8·6	5	4	36
T 2	Pronounced	5·7	3	14	36
S 1	Pronounced	8·8	3	9	34
S 2	Pronounced	7·8	3	6	34
Mc 1	Nil	8·3	3	10	33
Mc 2	Mild	7·1	3	13	33

One of the infants with pronounced neuromuscular agitation in the absence of hypocalcaemia was a twin, the other product of the pregnancy being a macerated foetus.

None of these babies was born to a diabetic mother.

(3) **Infants Born to Diabetic Mothers.** Ten babies with clinical tetany were born to mothers with diabetes mellitus and one to an obese mother with a pre-diabetic type of glucose tolerance curve. All 11 infants were premature and all were singletons. Of the 11 babies, 10 gave total serum calcium levels below 8·0 mg. per 100 ml., the values ranging from 2·6 to 7·5 mg. %. In the remaining baby the corresponding figure was 8·0 mg. per 100 ml. Two infants (see section III) with low serum calcium levels showed no clinical evidence of abnormal neuromuscular instability. They were unique in this respect among all babies included in this investigation. In babies born to diabetic mothers neuromuscular hyperexcitability was violent in four, pronounced in four and mild in two infants. Clinical signs of tetany in the baby of the pre-diabetic mother were violent.

During the period of this investigation only three babies who had been newly born to diabetic mothers were found to show neither neuromuscular hyperexcitability nor hypocalcaemia.

(4) **Exchange Transfusions.** Pronounced or violent neuromuscular hyperexcitability was encountered in four babies given exchange transfusions on account of haemolytic disease. A total serum calcium level below 8 mg. per 100 ml. was obtained in two cases. In the interval between the commencement and completion of transfusion a fall of 3 mg. per 100 ml. was recorded in one baby, and a fall of 2 mg. per 100 ml. in another. Potassium levels were not estimated. Blood used for the exchange transfusions was citrated and had been stored for a period not exceeding five days. No calcium preparations were given during the transfusions.

Discussion

Biochemical Considerations. It is known that the serum calcium level falls transitorily during the first few days of life (Editorial, 1950). Gittleman *et al.* (1956) noted that in a number of newborn infants the concentration of calcium in the serum was less than 8 mg. per 100 ml. on the first day of life. They found that the incidence of hypocalcaemia was greater in infants delivered by caesarean section and in premature infants than in babies delivered spontaneously at term. Respiratory embarrassment, a tendency to regurgitate, convulsions, tremors and twitching of the extremities were seen in a number of the premature babies, and infants delivered by caesarean section (Gittleman, 1957). Zetterström and Arnhold (1958) stress the frequent occurrence of hypocalcaemia in the newly born babies of diabetic mothers. The occurrence of 'first-day hypocalcaemia' is referred to by Gribetz (1957) and has been demonstrated by Bruck and Weintraub (1955).

Clinical Approach. The investigations carried out by Gittleman *et al.* (1956) and Bruck (1955) were concerned primarily with biochemical findings. By way of contrast the present study is based primarily upon clinical observations. Admittedly the study is of only limited scale. It can be said, however, that despite its contrasting approach the results are in many respects in keeping with those of the two American investigations. The present series provides confirmatory evidence of a noteworthy incidence of hypocalcaemia in the early hours of life more especially among premature infants, babies born to diabetic mothers, and infants delivered by caesarean section. It is of interest too that while five of the 20 premature infants with hypocalcaemia in the present series were the products of twin pregnancies the premature infants in Gittleman's series included a number of twins. Our findings further resemble those of Gittleman (1957) in that the serum calcium levels in twins of the same pregnancy were usually different.

A more important result of the present study is evidence of the presence on the first or second day of life of a characteristic clinical picture of neuromuscular excitability in a large proportion of infants in whom there is 'first-day hypocalcaemia'. The association of neuromuscular hyperexcitability with hypocalcaemia warrants use of the term tetany, and is in accordance with views expressed by Bakwin (1937, 1939), Shannon (1934), Willi (1939), Bass (1942) and Kendig (1942).

Correlation of Clinical and Biochemical Findings. In their investigation of clinical tetany appearing between the first and thirteenth day of life Dodd and Rapoport (1949) found an approximate parallelism between the severity of symptoms and the depression of calcium levels. They record that the serum calcium varied between 6 and 9 mg. per 100 ml. in the infants with clinical tetany, although in a few babies with 'mild to moderate signs' levels of above 9 mg. were obtained.

The findings in our series of infants in whom clinical signs of tetany developed within 36 hours of birth do not reveal any rigid parallelism between the severity of clinical signs and the depression of calcium concentrations. It is probably significant, however, that in clinically violent cases the total serum calcium level averaged 6 mg. per 100 ml. while the corresponding figure for all other cases with manifest signs was 7 mg. per 100 ml. This may be an over-simplification. To some extent the physical tone and strength of an infant determine the severity of general systemic reactions to underlying trauma, infection or biochemical disturbance. This is evident in the subdued nature of the convulsions which are seen in small premature infants with severe intracranial trauma, meningitis or pyelonephritis. In the present series of infants an approximate relationship existed between birth weight and the clinical picture: the average birth weight of infants with violent, pronounced and moderate clinical tetany was 6 lb. 12 oz., 5 lb. 15 oz. and 4 lb. 10 oz. respectively. This in turn may be related to the positive correlation between birth weight of the premature infant and the concentration of calcium in the plasma noted by Gittleman and Pincus (1951).

A further point of interest is that Dodd regarded a total serum calcium level of less than 9 mg. % as evidence of hypocalcaemia in the newborn. Had this standard been applied in the present series six of the seven infants we have regarded as examples of neuromuscular hyperactivity in the absence of hypocalcaemia (section II) would have been included among babies with hypocalcaemic tetany (section I). Another consideration is the interval of time between the onset of clinical signs of tetany and the taking of specimens for calcium estimations. As already emphasized clinical signs appeared within 36 hours of birth in every baby. An endeavour was made to obtain serum on the second day of life as a routine. The need to minimize disturbance of the babies ruled out any question of subsequent daily estimates. Almost certainly therefore the lowest concentration of calcium in the serum was not determined in every case. This is of importance because we gained the impression that although an approximate parallelism existed in the individual case between the trend of the clinical pattern and that of the serum calcium level, clinical signs of tetany tended to precede the appearance of pronounced hypocalcaemia, and the gradual disappearance of clinical signs tended to lag behind elevation of the serum calcium to a normal level.

The absolute level to which the serum calcium falls may not be the only factor of significance. Severe clinical tetany developed during exchange blood transfusions in two cases in which the serum level did not fall below 8 mg. per 100 ml. The fall in level in each of these cases, however, was considerable and occurred within one and a half hours (section IV (4)). It is possible, therefore, that separately or jointly the speed and magnitude of the depression of calcium concentration may be of importance. Farquhar and Smith (1958) have investigated the disturbance of electrolyte balance which occurs during exchange transfusion. They found that the serum potassium level frequently increases and the calcium ion falls irrespective of the total serum calcium, creating conditions favouring the development of neuromuscular hyperexcitability. Estimates of serum potassium levels were not made in our study. In this study four infants given exchange transfusions, including the two referred to above, developed neuromuscular hyperexcitability in association with hypocalcaemia, and it is of interest that in three of the infants the first evidence of irritability was present before transfusion was commenced.

Differentiation of Abnormal from Normal. There is no arbitrary level of serum calcium which serves to distinguish an abnormally low from a normal concentration of calcium in the serum of the newborn infant. This applies especially to infants aged only 1 or 2 days in view of the temporary physiological fall in serum calcium level which occurs at this time. Midwives with prolonged experience of the care of premature infants are agreed that 'jumpiness', or 'preminess' as some term it, is a feature in the first few days of life of many of the smallest infants for whom they are responsible. In the present study neuromuscular hyperexcitability was noted in 27 premature babies (section IV (1)). It is probable that these examples of clinical tetany represent an intensified form of the clinical 'ditheriness' characteristic of a significant proportion of small premature babies in general. If this postulate is correct it can be argued with justification that just as no clear line of demarcation exists between physiological and pathological hypocalcaemia, so there is no definable clinical feature differentiating normal from abnormal neuromuscular excitability. This does not invalidate application of the term tetany to cases in which neuromuscular excitability and hypocalcaemia are found in association. It does, however, suggest that hypocalcaemic tetany *per se* occurring within 36 hours (say) of birth should be regarded as an exaggeration of a normal physiological state rather than as a distinct abnormal clinico-biochemical entity. The fact that unusual clinical and biochemical features disappear spontaneously gives support to this view.

It has been said that 'the concurrence of clinical tetany and hypocalcaemia [in the newborn] may suggest a causal relationship but this has not been clearly established' (Editorial, 1950). Observations made in this study do not clarify the continuing uncertainty in this connexion. They do, however, afford evidence that the occurrence of clinical tetany within 36 hours of life is probably favoured by a number of those factors which Gittleman *et al.* (1956) found contributed to hypocalcaemia on the first day of life. These factors include premature birth, delivery by caesarean section and maternal diabetes. It is possible that multiple pregnancy may be another factor.

Summary

Hypocalcaemic tetany is defined as abnormal neuromuscular hyperexcitability associated with a total serum calcium level of 8 mg. per 100 ml. or less.

The occurrence of hypocalcaemic tetany within 40 minutes to 36 hours of birth in 26 babies is described.

'Recovery' was complete in all cases.

Details of the clinical and biochemical findings are given.

The significance of the data presented is discussed.

Generous assistance was received from many colleagues including the consultant obstetrical, resident medical and midwifery staffs of the Leeds Maternity Hospital and St. Mary's Hospital, Leeds. Particularly valuable help was given by Miss M. Pattullo, S.R.N., S.C.M., and Dr. M. Sturges. Routine laboratory examinations were undertaken by Mr. R. K. Martindale of the Leeds Maternity Hospital. Confirmatory estimates were kindly carried out under the direction of Dr. W. Goldie at St. James's Hospital, Leeds, or of Dr. W. W. Payne and Dr. R. H. Wilkinson at The Hospital for Sick Children, London. Estimates of ultrafilterable serum calcium were made at the last-named hospital. Valuable assistance in obtaining references was given by the Librarian, The Royal College of Physicians, Edinburgh.

References

Bakwin, H. (1937). *Amer. J. Dis. Child.*, **54**, 1211.
—— (1939). *J. Pediat.*, **14**, 1.
Bass, M. H. (1942). *J. Mt Sinai Hosp.*, **9**, 314.
Bruck, E. and Weintraub, D. H. (1955). *A.M.A. Amer. J. Dis. Child.*, **90**, 653.
Craig, W. S. (1958). *Pediatrics*, **22**, 297.
Dodd, K. and Rapoport, S. (1949). *Amer. J. Dis. Child.*, **78**, 537.
Editorial (1950). *Quart. Rev. Pediat.*, **5**, 271.
Farquhar, J. W. and Smith, H. (1958). *Arch. Dis. Childh.*, **33**, 142.
Gittleman, I. F. (1957). Personal communication.
—— and Pincus, J. B. (1951). *Pediatrics*, **8**, 778.
——, ——, Schmerzler, E. and Saito, M. (1956). *Ibid.*, **18**, 721.
Gribetz, D. (1957). *A.M.A. J. Dis. Child.*, **94**, 301.
Hopkins, T., Howard, J. E. and Eisenberg, H. (1952). *Bull. Johns Hopk. Hosp.*, **91**, 1.
Kendig, E. L., (1942). *J. Pediat.*, **21**, 510.
Lavietes, P. H. (1937). *J. biol. Chem.*, **120**, 267.
Mitchell, A. G. and Stevenson, F. E. (1932). *J. Amer. med. Ass.*, **99**, 1502.
Shannon, W. R. (1934). *Arch. Pediat.*, **51**, 23.
Willi, H. (1939). *Mschr. Kinderheilk.*, **80**, 309.
Zetterstrom, R. and Arnhold, R. G. (1958). *Acta paediat. (Uppsala)*, **47**, 107.

CELLULAR IMMUNITY AT BIRTH

THE MECHANISM AND NATURE OF THE PHAGOCYTIC RESPONSE

BY

M. S. EDWARDS, L. L. GRIFFITHS and P. N. SWIFT

From Farnborough Hospital, Kent

(RECEIVED FOR PUBLICATION JUNE 27, 1958)

Immunity in the infant has been extensively studied in the past and numerous investigations have been made into the development of specific immunity, the production of antibody and the passive transfer of antibody from the mother. On the other hand comparatively little work has been devoted to elucidating the complexities of the cellular response since Tunnicliff (1910) observed that phagocytosis by infants' leucocytes of streptococci, staphylococci and pneumococci was less active than in adults until the age of about 2 years. Subsequently it was demonstrated that the efficiency of phagocytosis was to a large extent determined by factors in the serum. In this connexion the studies of Mudd, Lucké, McCutcheon and Strumia (1929) were particularly important since they clarified our understanding of mechanisms by which serum enhances phagocytosis in the immunized animal and the role of antibody therein. Ward and Enders (1933) were able to elaborate upon these observations and correlated the effects of complement and antibody. They concluded that complement acts merely in the role of a catalyst which accelerates the effect of antibody. A similar view put forward by Topley and Wilson (1929) was that 'in normal serum the low concentration of specific antibodies necessitates the adjuvant action of a considerable amount of complement before its presence can be detected so that the complementary action appears to dominate the picture, while the high concentration of specific antibody in an immune serum reduces the complementary effect to a mere enhancement of an effect which takes place in its absence'.

Ward and Enders (1933), in one of the few reports dealing with infants, found that the titre of complement in infants under the age of 1 year was as high as that in adults. It seemed probable, therefore, that the inferiority of phagocytosis in infancy might be due to substances other than complement.

The findings of Gluck and Silverman (1957) are thus consistent with earlier work in that they showed that a phagocytosis-promoting factor was located in the α_1, α_2 and β-globulin fractions of the serum protein.

Matoth (1952) produced evidence which suggested that infants' leucocytes were inherently less active than those of adults and considered that the effect of serum was unimportant in spite of the fact that he noted infant serum to be less potent than adult serum in promoting phagocytosis.

The picture of cellular immunity in early infancy is thus incomplete and as much of the earlier work was carried out with immune sera and virulent micro-organisms their conclusions and results cannot be applied without due criticism to the explanation of the newborn infant's vulnerability to infections by bacteria of low pathogenicity.

The present investigation was designed in the light of previous work to study the processes involved in normal phagocytosis by the leucocytes of cord blood and the functional interdependence of leucocyte and serum in the infant at birth.

Method

The procedure for measuring phagocytosis which we adopted was a modification of that originally described by Wright (1921) for the determination of the opsonic index. The efficiency of phagocytosis is expressed as the number of leucocytes in a total count of 100 leucocytes which have ingested one or more yeast cells, as described by Hamburger (1927), and similar to the procedure employed by Mudd *et al.* (1929). We found this more reliable in practice than Wright's method in which the number of particles in each leucocyte was counted. The present method also has the advantage that when yeast cells are employed there is less difficulty in differentiating between particles within the cells and those on its surface.

Materials. Maternal blood (10 ml.) obtained by venepuncture within half an hour after delivery and 10 ml. of infants' blood from the umbilical vein was collected and 5 ml. of each placed in a dry bottle and

5 ml. into a bottle containing 50 i.u. heparin. Ten millilitres of blood from a normal adult was collected into a dry bottle for use as control.

Preparation of Sera. The serum obtained from the blood in each dry bottle after clotting and centrifugation was divided between two tubes, one of which was heated to 56° C. for 30 minutes to inactivate complement. Both were then kept at 4° C. until used, within 24 hours.

Preparation of Cell Suspensions. The plasma from 3 ml. of the heparinized maternal or infant's blood was withdrawn after centrifugation. The packed cells were then washed three times with 10 times their volume of modified Hanks' solution and the supernatant fluid withdrawn. Deposit, 0·5 ml., was aspirated from the bottom of the tube with a Pasteur pipette to effect some concentration of the leucocytes in the upper layers. The resultant leucocyte-rich deposit was kept at 4° C. until used.

Yeast Cell Suspension. Yeast cells were finally chosen since experiments with carbon particles and starch granules had proved unsatisfactory because of the difficulties and inaccuracies in counting the ingested particles. Yeast cells possess the advantage of uniform size suitable for counting and yet not so large as to cause gross distortion of the leucocyte. As Hanks (1940) demonstrated a relationship between the degree of phagocytosis and the number of micro-organisms in suspension, it has been necessary to determine the optimal concentration of yeast cells to ensure uniformity. The proportion of leucocytes exhibiting phagocytosis of yeast cells was found to increase in proportion to the number of yeast cells in suspension, until a concentration of 75,000 yeast cells per c.mm. was reached. Suspensions containing greater numbers of cells produced little further increase in the number of actively phagocytic leucocytes although the number of ingested particles per leucocyte (i.e. the phagocytic index) continued to increase. In the present experiments, therefore, a concentration of 100,000 yeast cells per c.mm. was chosen, since minor variations were found to produce no significant effect. On the other hand in estimating phagocytosis by means of the phagocytic index, variations in the number of yeast cells caused relatively large variations in the number of particles ingested. For this reason the phagocytic index was considered less reliable for studies involving numerical comparisons, though it has been estimated in the present series on the majority of specimens and shows a close correlation with the total number of active leucocytes (Fig. 1).

Preparation of Suspension of Yeast Cells. Yeast strain CN 1845 was propagated on nutrient agar and subcultured in nutrient broth for three to four days. After centrifugation and washing three times in 10 ml. normal saline the cells were suspended in normal saline at a concentration of 100,000 cells per c.mm. The selected concentration was obtained by serial dilution and counting in a Neubauer chamber. The cells in suspension were then killed by heating to 65° C. in a sealed tube for 15 minutes.

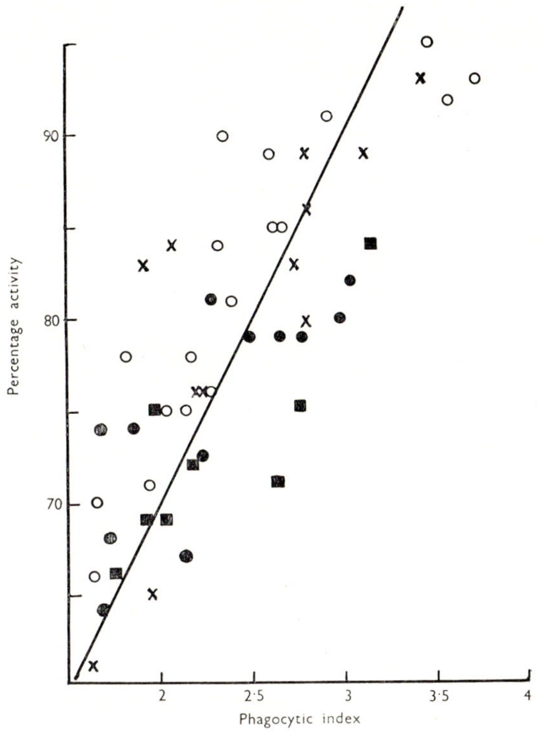

FIG. 1.—Relation of percentage activity of maternal and infant leucocytes to phagocytic index.

Demonstration of Phagocytosis. A suspension of leucocytes (0·1 ml.) of each mother or child was placed in each of six tubes containing equal volumes of serum and yeast cells, as follows:

Tube 1	Leucocytes + killed yeast cells	+ fresh adult serum
,, 2	,, ,, ,, ,,	+ heated adult serum
,, 3	,, ,, ,, ,,	+ fresh infant serum
,, 4	,, ,, ,, ,,	+ heated infant serum
,, 5	,, ,, ,, ,,	+ fresh maternal serum
,, 6	,, ,, ,, ,,	+ heated maternal serum

In each experiment the leucocytes of the mother and those of her own infant were prepared and tested simultaneously. After thorough mixing by shaking, the 12 tubes were placed in a water bath at 37° C. for 30 minutes and agitated every five minutes. After 30 minutes phagocytosis was inhibited by cooling in cold water, and films were made from each tube, fixed with methyl alcohol, and stained with Leishmann's stain.

Cell Counts. A total of 200 polymorphs was counted and the number which ingested one or more yeast cell noted. The number of leucocytes showing phagocytosis was expressed as percentage activity.

Twenty pairs of cell preparations in the various sera were made by this method. The mean error of the method was determined in a pilot experiment, and found to be ± 2% in counts of 200 cells.

Results

In Table 1 are tabulated the percentage numbers of leucocytes exhibiting phagocytosis of yeast cells when suspended in adult, infant and maternal sera. Comparison of the total number of active cells or the mean number of cells in each category can be made and the validity of any difference referred to Student's *t* distribution.

Comparison of the activity of the cells in their own unheated sera (columns 3 and 5A), which is the nearest approximation *in vitro* to the conditions of postnatal life, shows a small difference in mean activity between infant and maternal cells. It is not possible to make a statistical comparison under these conditions, but it is felt that the difference (79·6%-72%) may reflect somewhat greater activity on the part of maternal cells, which would be in accord with the findings of previous investigators.

The Effect of Unheated Serum on Phagocytosis. In 20 experiments the activity of infants' leucocytes has been assessed in their own unheated serum, in that of their own mother and in that of a seemingly normal adult. Likewise the activity of maternal leucocytes has been assessed in their own unheated serum, in that of their own infant and in that of an adult. The mean activity of infants' leucocytes, columns 1, 3 and 5, and maternal leucocytes columns 1A, 3A and 5A, is about the same with each of the three sera (Table 1).

Infant cells seem to be more active in maternal serum, and maternal cells more active in the sera of infants and adults, but these differences are statistically insignificant.

The Effect of Heated Serum on Phagocytosis. The influence of heated serum on phagocytosis is assessed by comparing the activity of leucocytes from an infant or mother in unheated and heated serum. The comparison has been made in their own serum, in that of their own mother or infant and in adults' serum. A highly significant difference between the number of leucocytes of infant and maternal origin showing phagocytosis in fresh and the number showing phagocytosis in heated sera is apparent (Table 1).

The influence of heated serum on phagocytosis is assessed by comparing the activity of leucocytes from the same infant or from the same mother in maternal, infant and adult sera (Table 2a, b). In each of the 20 experiments, the infants' leucocytes have been tested in their own, in their mothers' and in adults' heated serum. The maternal leucocytes have been tested in their own, their own infants' and normal adult serum.

The number of infant and maternal leucocytes exhibiting phagocytosis is significantly greater in heated maternal serum (and to a less extent heated adult serum) than in infant serum.

TABLE 1
THE NUMBER OF LEUCOCYTES % EXHIBITING PHAGOCYTOSIS

Pair No.	Infant Leucocytes						Maternal Leucocytes					
	Adult		Cord Serum		Maternal		Adult		Cord Serum		Maternal	
	1 unheated	2 heated	3 unheated	4 heated	5 unheated	6 heated	1A unheated	2A heated	3A unheated	4A heated	5A unheated	6A heated
1	58	23	62	5	60	17	65	9	64	5	70	9
2	82	30	80	6	94	65	91	24	80	10	57	15
3	68	5	57	6	75	9	88	4	86	6	86	5
4	73	19	74	4	80	10	93	10	90	6	93	10
5	73	12	66	15	69	36	80	8	77	10	82	14
6	77	8	71	7	80	9	86	12	85	8	89	12
7	87	15	80	16	81	15	89	8	87	8	92	11
8	65	10	64	11	71	23	76	12	74	5	74	10
9	64	11	66	6	64	32	68	9	71	3	65	13
10	76	14	78	8	79	19	89	4	85	9	76	11
11	75	12	76	16	68	15	85	5	92	7	81	17
12	80	22	79	15	81	40	80	12	89	5	86	11
13	82	14	84	12	82	18	83	17	91	10	83	20
14	80	4	72	3	79	9	94	8	93	7	93	7
15	73	4	69	3	67	4	70	4	75	2	61	3
16	70	14	69	14	75	21	88	14	81	10	76	14
17	69	7	66	6	70	13	74	7	75	7	84	14
18	73	19	78	15	74	18	94	13	90	9	83	13
19	84	9	75	4	79	8	90	7	95	6	89	5
20	73	10	75	5	74	7	82	5	84	4	72	9
Mean	74·1	13·1	72·05	8·85	75·1	19·4	83·25	9·6	83·2	6·85	79·6	11·15

(The numbers are the mean of two counts of 100 cells.)
In each pair the mother's leucocytes and her own infant's leucocytes are tested in their own, or the other's serum. Adult serum was obtained from a normal adult.

TABLE 2a

DIFFERENCES BETWEEN THE NUMBERS OF ACTIVE INFANT LEUCOCYTES IN THE HEATED SERA OF MOTHERS, ADULTS AND INFANTS

Heated Serum	Infant Leucocytes (% activity)	Difference (N = 20)
Infant ..	8·85	t = 2·38 (significant)
Adult ..	13·1	p ≏ 0·05
Infant ..	8·85	t = 2·99 (highly significant)
Maternal ..	19·4	p = 0·01
Adult ..	13·1	t = 1·72 (not significant)
Maternal ..	19·4	p = 0·1

TABLE 2b

DIFFERENCES BETWEEN THE NUMBERS OF ACTIVE MATERNAL LEUCOCYTES IN THE HEATED SERA OF MOTHERS, ADULTS AND INFANTS

Heated Serum	Maternal Leucocytes (% activity)	Difference (N = 20)
Infant ..	6·85	t = 2·0 (significant)
Adult ..	9·6	p = 0·05
Infant ..	6·85	t = 3·45 (highly significant)
Maternal ..	11·15	p ≏ 0·001
Adult ..	9·6	t = 1·25 (not significant)
Maternal ..	11·15	p ≏ 0·2

Inherent Activity. The intrinsic activity of infants' and mothers' leucocytes was assessed by comparing their activity when suspended in an identical serum. The results are shown in Table 3, and show that mothers' leucocytes are more active to a highly significant degree than infants' leucocytes in both infants' and adults' serum. When suspended in maternal serum on the other hand, infants' leucocytes show the same activity as those of their mothers.

Comparison of the activity of mothers' and infants' leucocytes in the same heated sera is shown in Table 4. In the heated serum of infants and adults no significant difference in their activities is demonstrable, but in heated maternal serum the infants' leucocytes show significantly more phagocytosis than their mothers' leucocytes.

Relation of Phagocytosis to Maturity of the Leucocyte. The average number of nuclear lobes per leucocyte was estimated for each infant and mother in counts of 100 cells.

In infants' leucocytes the average number of lobes was found to be 2·41 and in the mothers' leucocytes 2·86, but no relation can be demonstrated, in either unheated or heated serum, between the average number of lobes of the leucocytes and number of phagocytosing cells on the same film.

Relation of Phagocytosis to Birth Weight. The weights of the infants in the present series ranged from 6 lb. 5 oz. (2·85 Kg.) to 8 lb. 11 oz. (4·03 Kg.) at birth. All infants were delivered at full term.

No significant correlation was apparent in the weight of the infants and the activity of their leucocytes. Our findings are thus in accordance with those of Gluck and Silverman (1957).

Discussion

Previous studies on phagocytosis in infancy have established that leucocytes are less active at this age than in later childhood and adult life. Matoth (1952), who employed starch granules, concluded that the leucocytes were themselves relatively inactive and considered that the influence of substances in the serum was small. Gluck and Silverman (1957), however, have demonstrated that the addition of adult serum to the blood of babies of birth weight below 2,000 g. brings about a significant increase in the proportion of effective phagocytes.

It seems probable in view of these reports that the inherent activity of the cells and the enhancing effects of serum may both contribute to the inferiority of infant leucocytes.

The results of the present investigation confirm the existence of significant differences between the phagocytic activity of cord and mothers' leucocytes under certain conditions.

The Phagocytosis-promoting Factors in Serum. Although infants' and mothers' leucocytes appear (Table 3) to be less active in their own unheated serum than in heterogeneous serum the difference is small and may well have occurred by chance. The figures therefore indicate that phagocytosis occurs with similar frequency in both unheated sera and no significant difference between the effects on phagocytosis by infants' and mothers' serum can be assumed.

TABLE 3

DIFFERENCES BETWEEN THE ACTIVITIES OF INFANT AND MATERNAL LEUCOCYTES IN UNHEATED SERA

Serum	Infant Leucocytes (% activity)	Maternal Leucocytes (% activity)	Difference (N = 20)
Infant ..	72·05	83·2	t = 4·8 (highly significant)
Adult ..	74·1	83·2	t = 2·9 (highly significant)
Maternal	75·1	79·6	t = 1·0 (not significant)

TABLE 4

DIFFERENCES BETWEEN THE ACTIVITIES OF INFANT AND MATERNAL LEUCOCYTES IN HEATED SERA

Serum	Infant Leucocytes (% activity)	Maternal Leucocytes (% activity)	Differences (N = 20)
Infant ..	8·85	6·85	t = 1·5 (not significant)
Adult ..	13·1	9·6	t = 1·9 (not significant)
Maternal	19·4	11·15	t = 2·4 (significant)

For this reason the seeming superiority of maternal over infant leucocytes, albeit small, cannot simply be attributed to differences in whole serum on the strength of these findings.

Phagocytosis by infant and maternal leucocytes of particles sensitized by heated serum is much less efficient than that of particles sensitized by unheated serum. As a result of the greater loss in the activity of mothers' leucocytes in heated serum, the activity of infants' cells is equal to or greater than that of their mothers. We have no evidence that this is due to a greater capacity for spontaneous phagocytosis on the part of infant leucocytes.

The influence of the different sera on phagocytosis has been studied in order to determine whether this finding might be explained by differences in the sera.

In contrast to the constancy with which ingestion occurs in unheated sera, well-marked and significant variations are observed in heated sera (Table 2a, b). In the heated serum of infants, phagocytosis by infants' or mothers' leucocytes is less than that in heated adult serum and less to a highly significant degree than that in heated maternal serum. These observations imply that serum factors determine activity in the absence of complement, and they suggest, moreover, that the heat-stable enhancing factor is of importance in determining the ultimate activity of the phagocyte. We may assume that the heat stable fraction of serum which enhances phagocytosis is present with greatest effect in maternal serum and least effect in infant serum. Whether this is due to quantitative or qualitative differences in the active constituents of the heat-stable fraction is not known, though the findings of Gluck and Silverman (1957) and our own studies on the serum globulin are compatible with the view that they may be due to qualitative changes. In the present investigation the Popper reaction, which depends on the amount of α and β globulins, was higher in heated serum of most infants (mean 3·85 compared with 2·65 in unheated serum) and of all mothers (mean 4·3 compared with 2·3 in unheated serum). The Kunkel reaction, which depends principally upon the γ-globulin fraction, was reduced in all heated sera and especially in maternal sera (mean 1·25 compared with 4·3 in unheated serum). In order to confirm these changes electrophoretic separation (Griffiths, 1952, 1953; Griffiths and Brews, 1953) was performed on seven paired sera and it demonstrated that a small increase in the amount of α_2-globulin and a small reduction in the γ-globulin occurs as a result of heating maternal serum.

The influence of the heat-labile fraction of serum may be estimated by finding the numerical difference between activity in unheated and in heated serum. The figure thus obtained is a measure of the number of leucocytes which owe their activity to the heat-labile fraction. It offers a convenient means of measuring quantitatively the phagocytosis-promoting effect of heat-labile fraction or complement.

When this figure is plotted graphically against the number of active cells in unheated serum (Fig. 2a, b) a close correlation with the overall activity of

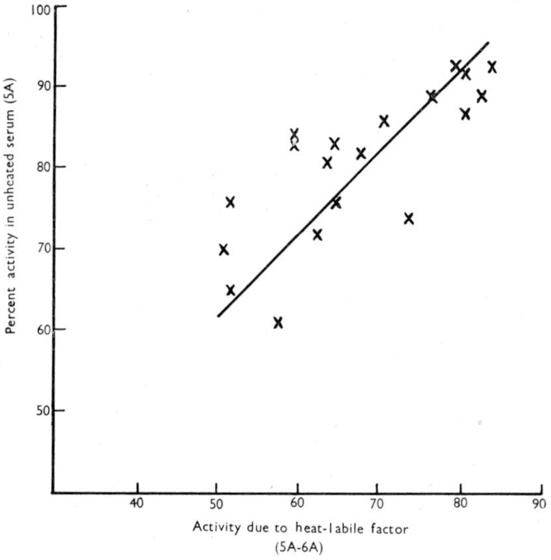

FIG. 2a.—Relation of activity of maternal leucocytes in unheated maternal serum (5A) to activity due to heat-labile factor (5A-6A).

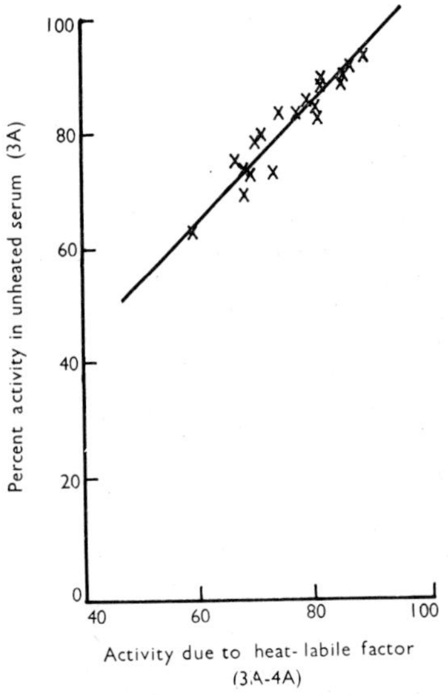

FIG. 2b.—Relation of activity of maternal leucocytes in unheated infant serum (3A) to activity due to heat-labile factor (3A-4A).

maternal leucocytes is demonstrated, which indicates that phagocytosis is directly related to the opsonic effect of the heat-labile fraction of serum.

This finding is in accordance with present views on the role of complement as the dominant influence on normal phagocytosis.

Since the correlation of total phagocytosis by maternal leucocytes and heat-labile fraction is the same in both infant and maternal serum it may be inferred that complement is present in infant serum to the same extent as in maternal serum, as found by Ward and Enders (1933). Since we have been unable to demonstrate any lack of effective complement in infant serum, differences in phagocytic activity between infant and maternal leucocytes cannot be explained by postulating differences in complement. In so far as it is possible to separate the functions of leucocyte and serum it appears that the heat-stable fraction of infant serum in some way as yet undetermined is deficient in a phagocytosis-promoting factor. Of the substances in serum which are not destroyed at 56° C. specific antibodies are known to influence phagocytosis. We have attempted by employing a non-pathogenic strain of yeast throughout these experiments to avoid interference by specific immunity and we consider such interference most improbable.

Hormonal status particularly in respect of oestrogens and corticosteroids influences phagocytosis, but the concentration of these substances in the blood of mother and infant is similar at birth, and differences in phagocytosis would not be expected unless their leucocytes differ in sensitivity to the effects of hormones.

The Response of the Leucocyte. From the foregoing discussion upon the phagocytosis-promoting effects of serum it is apparent that the paucity of an active heat-stable factor in infant serum accounts at least in part for the relative inactivity of infant leucocytes. This conclusion is not inconsistent with the conclusions of Gluck and Silverman (1957) that the activating component may be in the α and β fractions of the serum protein, though proof that the factor observed by us is identical with that of Gluck and Silverman is not within the scope of the present investigation.

The observation that the infants' leucocyte is relatively more dependent upon a heat-stable factor than upon complement suggests that there may be a difference in the cells' response to sensitized particles. In this connexion it is interesting to note that the heat-stable phagocytosis-promoting factor in maternal serum does not exert an effect of similar magnitude on the leucocytes of the mother herself (Table 4) which seems to be affected mainly by complement (Fig. 2).

Evidence of the nature of the differences between the responses of maternal and infant leucocytes can be obtained by further analysis of their behaviour under certain conditions.

It has already been shown that phagocytosis by maternal leucocytes in unheated serum bears a close quantitative relationship to activity due to complement and is thus presumed to be determined by complement (Fig. 2). The activity of infant leucocytes bears some but not such a close relation to complement in their own serum, and in maternal serum no relation that can be demonstrated (Fig. 3a, b, c).

Since it has already been shown that the opsonic effect of complement is similar in both sera it is concluded that the avidity of infants' leucocytes for particles sensitized in the presence of complement is less than that of their mothers'.

In maternal serum, in spite of a striking absence of any quantitative relationship to complement, the total activity of infant cells is greater. The knowledge that maternal serum is comparatively rich in a heat-stable enhancing factor combined with the knowledge that the activity of infants' leucocytes is not quantitatively dependent on complement provides evidence that their activity is more dependent on a heat-stable factor in serum. The fact that the mothers' leucocytes retain their dependence upon complement excludes the possibility that this is a non-specific effect of maternal serum and serves to confirm that there is an inherent difference in cellular response. Likewise our findings are not compatible with the view that this is an effect of antibody passively transferred from the mother.

The difference in response is characterized by a marked avidity of infants' leucocytes for particles sensitized by the heat-stable fraction of maternal serum. In nature, however, there are no opportunities after birth for micro-organisms invading the infant to be sensitized by maternal serum and thus for the infant to receive any protection which this mechanism might provide. If it does play a role in defence against infection in life it must do so while the foetus is *in utero* and the placenta intact, for only in these circumstances are conditions such that invading micro-organisms will have been sensitized by contact with maternal serum. As there is no significant difference between the activity of mothers' and infants' leucocytes when there has been sensitization by unheated maternal serum (Table 3), it is probable that, *in utero*, the foetal leucocytes are as efficient as those of their mothers.

The present investigation has shown that the

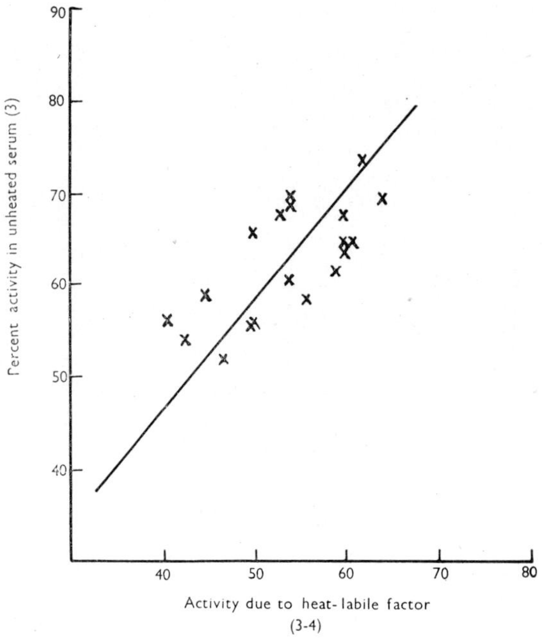

FIG. 3a.—Relation of activity of infant leucocytes in unheated infant serum (3) to activity due to heat-labile factor (3-4).

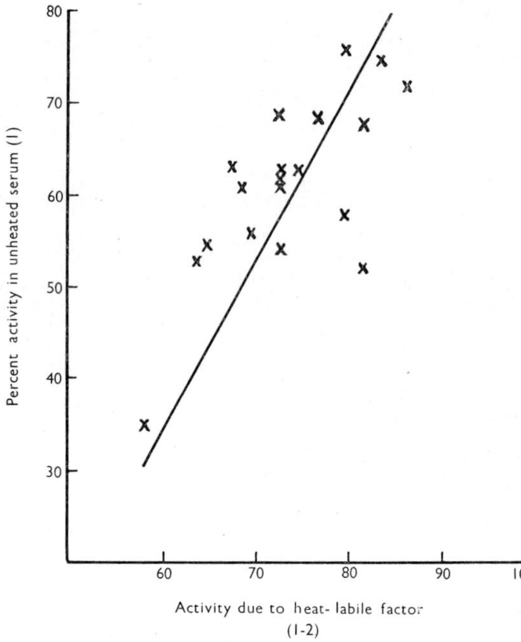

FIG. 3b.—Relation of activity of infant leucocytes in unheated adult serum (1) to activity due to heat-labile factor (1-2).

cellular response in the normal non-immune infant at birth resembles the response in the immune adult, in which antibody appears to be relatively more important than complement. The evidence suggests that this altered or perhaps more primitive response is due to an inherent difference in the leucocyte at this age. It differs from that in the mother by virtue of differences in their serum which is relatively deficient in a heat-stable enhancing factor and by virtue of differences in the leucocytes which appear to be more avid for yeast cells sensitized by the heat-stable fraction of maternal serum and less to the effects of complement.

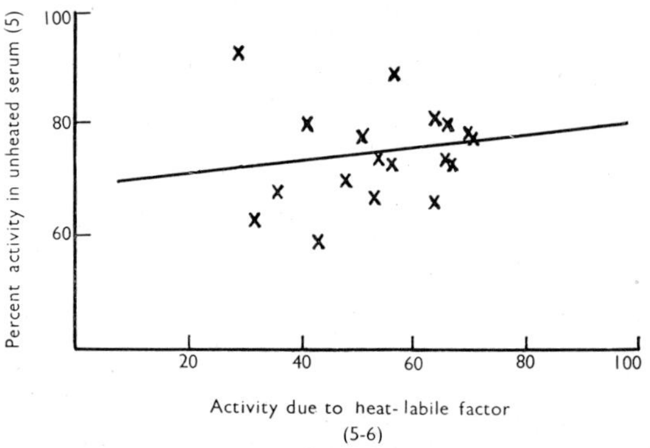

FIG. 3c.—Relation of activity of infant leucocytes in unheated maternal serum (5) to activity due to heat-labile factor (5-6).

Conclusion

The results of the present investigation provide evidence of differences between the mechanisms controlling phagocytosis in cord blood and those in maternal blood. Normal phagocytosis by maternal leucocytes is determined primarily by the heat-labile fraction of serum. Normal phagocytosis by leucocytes of cord blood, on the other hand, is less responsive to the effect of heat-labile factors and more to the effect of heat-stable factors in serum. Although observations on the nature of the heat-stable factor have been made, its identification is outside the scope of the present investigation.

This heat-stable factor is found in cord, adult and maternal sera, but to greatest effect in maternal serum, and to least effect in cord serum. The leucocytes of cord blood have a relatively greater avidity for particles sensitized by maternal serum.

While it is possible that these phenomena may have some protective role in the foetus, it is difficult to visualize how they might benefit the infant after birth. The withdrawal of protection afforded by maternal serum and the readjustment of the cellular response to one dominated by complement may well play a part in the infant's vulnerability to infection.

Our findings are not compatible with views which attempt to explain the infant's susceptibility on the basis of simple and separate defects in its leucocytes or serum. The functions of leucocytes and serum are closely interdependent and in the infant at birth both show significant differences from those of the mother.

Summary

The phagocytic activity of leucocytes has been measured by finding the percentage which ingest killed yeast cells. Activity as estimated by this method bears a close correlation to the phagocytic index.

The activity of the leucocytes of cord blood and of the leucocytes of the mother have been measured in unheated cord, maternal and normal adult serum and in heated cord, maternal and adult serum.

The efficiency of phagocytosis by cord and mothers' leucocytes in different sera can be compared to demonstrate the influence of serum and leucocytes on phagocytosis.

Unheated cord and maternal serum are equally effective in promoting phagocytosis.

Heated cord serum is significantly less effective than heated maternal serum in promoting phagocytosis.

Heated sera are much less effective than unheated sera in promoting phagocytosis.

Mothers' leucocytes are more active than those of their infants except in mothers' unheated serum when activity is equal.

In heated sera, infants' leucocytes are as active as those of their mothers except in mothers' heated serum where they are more active.

The activity of maternal leucocytes is closely correlated with the heat-labile fraction of serum which is present in both infants' and mothers' sera. The activity of infants' leucocytes is less closely dependent on the heat-labile factor of serum and especially of mothers' serum.

It is concluded that cord serum is relatively deficient in a heat-stable factor capable of enhancing phagocytosis and that the leucocytes of cord blood are less dependent upon the heat-labile factors in serum than are maternal leucocytes. The heat-stable fraction of maternal serum most effectively enhances phagocytosis by cord leucocytes.

To Dr. S. R. M. Bushby we are indebted for his assistance in selecting the test organism and for supplies of yeast strain CN 1845. We wish to thank both Dr. Bushby and Professor George Brownlee for their advice and helpful criticisms at all stages of the work. The study was made possible by a financial grant received from the South-east Metropolitan Regional Hospital Board.

REFERENCES

Gluck, L. and Silverman, W. A. (1957). *Pediatrics*, **20**, 951.
Griffiths, L. L. (1952). *J. clin. Path.*, **5**, 294.
—— (1953) *J. Lab. clin. Med.*, **41**, 188.
—— and Brews, V. A. L. (1953). *J. clin. Path.* **6**, 187.
Hamburger, H. J. (1927). In *Handbuch der biologischen Arbeitsmethoden*, ed. E. Abderhalden. Abt. 4, teil 4, p. 953. Urban and Schwarzenberg, Berlin.
Hanks, J. H. (1940). *J. Immunol*, **38**, 159.
Matoth, Y. (1952). *Pediatrics*, **9**, 748.
Mudd, S., Lucké, B., McCutcheon, M. and Strumia, M. (1929). *J. exp. Med.*, **49**, 779.
Topley, W. W. C. and Wilson, G. S. (1929). *The Principles of Bacteriology and Immunity*, Vol. 1, p. 176. Arnold, London.
Tunnicliff, R. (1910). *J. infect. Dis.*, **7**, 698.
Ward, H. K. and Enders, J. F. (1933). *J. exp. Med.*, **57**, 527.
Wright, A. E. (1921). *Technique of the Teat and Capillary Glass Tube*. Constable, London.

THROMBOTIC MICROANGIOPATHIC HAEMOLYTIC ANAEMIA

BY

M. J. ROBINSON, N. P. ORCHARD and A. R. EDEN
From the Austin Hospital, Heidelberg, Melbourne

(RECEIVED FOR PUBLICATION JUNE 9, 1958)

Introduction

The syndrome of thrombotic microangiopathic haemolytic anaemia is rare and almost all the cases reported have been in adults. Very few cases occurring in childhood have been reported and the youngest recorded case was 22 months old (Craig and Gitlin, 1957).

We report the clinical and pathological details and the response to treatment of a child aged 21 months, who was seen at the Austin Hospital, Melbourne.

Case Report

J.L., a male child aged 21 months, was admitted to the Austin Hospital, Melbourne, with a week's history of malaise, anorexia, fever and a suggestion of pain, tenderness and mild swelling of both wrists and ankles. Six days before admission a red, blotchy urticarial rash was noted over the diaper area but this faded after three days.

He had had similar but milder symptoms following immunization with triple antigen, also following a course of sulphonamide, and one mild attack appeared spontaneously. These early episodes lasted only a few days. There were no significant past illnesses and the family history was not relevant.

On physical examination he was flushed and unco-operative. The temperature was 103° F., the pulse 164 and respirations 28 per minute. A fine purpuric rash diffusely involved the face and both upper extremities. Both wrists were swollen and tender and movement was restricted by pain; in addition, there was mild swelling of both knees and ankles. A mild tonsillitis and an otitis media were present. A provisional diagnosis of anaphylactoid purpura of the Schönlein type was made and he was treated with aspirin.

During the first week in hospital his temperature ranged between 99° F. and 103° F. (Fig. 1). The blood examination showed the haemoglobin to be 9 g. % (60%), the white cell count 20,000 per c.mm., with 70% neutrophils (showing a marked shift to the left), 25% lymphocytes and 5% monocytes; the red cells and platelets were normal, and no lupus erythematosus cells (repeated examinations), glandular fever cells or malarial parasites were seen; the reticulocyte count was less than 1%. Examination of the sternal marrow revealed no abnormality. The clotting and prothrombin times were normal but clot retraction was poor. The Paul-Bunnell and Coombs tests were negative. Repeated blood cultures and agglutination tests, the Mantoux and Casoni tests and the Wassermann and Kahn reactions were all

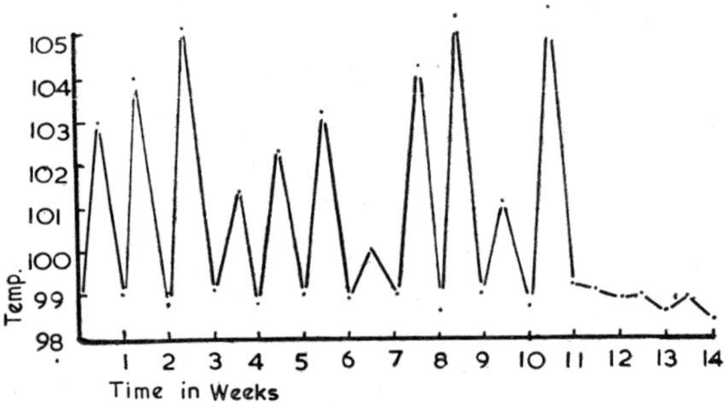

FIG. 1.—Temperature range during first admission.

negative. Liver function tests, the blood urea and the serum proteins and electrophoresis were normal. The cerebrospinal fluid was normal as were radiographs of the chest and long bones. The throat swab grew a β haemolytic streptococcus.

The rash reappeared during the second week and the temperature, malaise and irritability persisted. A four-week course of aureomycin did not affect the temperature.

One month after admission the spleen became palpable and there was a mild generalized lymphadenopathy. At this stage the white blood count rose to 32,400 per c.mm. but the haemoglobin did not fall. After three months of hospitalization his temperature subsided spontaneously and being quite well he was allowed to go home. He remained well for the next six months when he developed a rash, resembling erythema marginata, on his arms and chest. Six weeks later the swinging temperature recurred and on one day his joints became painful. Similar episodes recurred weekly until he was readmitted three weeks later because of persistent pyrexia, irritability and a disclination to move his limbs.

Examination at this stage revealed a fine generalized red papular rash, slight generalized lymphadenopathy and a temperature of 103° F. (Fig. 2.) The haemoglobin was

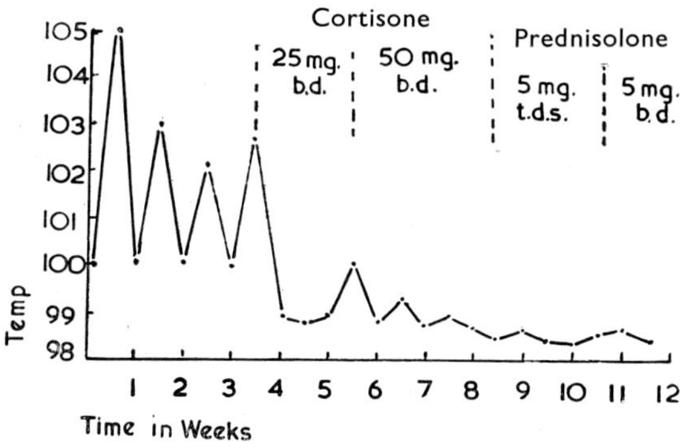

FIG. 2.—Temperature range during second admission.

11 g. % (74%); white cell count 24,600 per c.mm. with 60% neutrophils, 4% eosinophils, 33% lymphocytes and 3% monocytes; reticulocytes 12%. The platelets were 100,000 per c.mm.; this was the lowest figure obtained, and the count the next day was normal. In addition the red cell fragility in hypotonic saline was slightly increased and spherocytes were observed for the first time. The serum bilirubin was 3·2 mg./100 ml. and urinary urobilinogen was markedly increased and the faecal urobilinogen excretion per day was 300 mg.

The white blood count gradually rose to 56,000 per c.mm. in the next four weeks; the marked shift to the left and the presence of 8% myelocytes rendered the blood picture leukaemoid. The haemoglobin level waxed and waned in association with a fall and rise in the reticulocyte count, which reached 15% at one stage. The spherocytes increased in number and became a permanent feature.

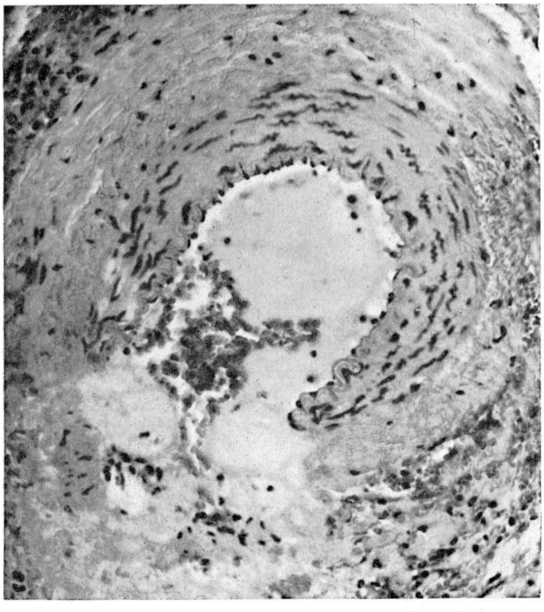

FIG. 3.—Section of the arteriole in the pericapsular region of the lymph node, showing a hyaline thrombus, rupture of the vessel wall and haemorrhage into the surrounding tissues. Haematoxylin and eosin. × 700.

The possibility of thrombotic microangiopathic haemolytic anaemia was suggested by one of us (N.P.O.) and a combined axillary lymph node and pectoral muscle biopsy was taken. Sections of the muscle showed no abnormality. Sections of the lymph node revealed reactive hyperplasia only, but striking changes were observed in the small calibre vessels in the pericapsular region (Fig. 3.) One vessel was almost completely occluded by a mass of hyaline material. There was a breach in the vessel wall with resulting haemorrhage into the perivascular tissues. There was no perivascular reaction whatsoever. Other vessels were occluded and in the thrombi could be seen endothelial cells, fibroblasts and the clefts of recanalization. Some vessels showed endothelial hyperplasia and others subendothelial accumulation of hyaline material. These histological findings confirmed the diagnosis. Sections were stained by Weigert's, Mallory's P.T.A.H., Biebrich scarlet-aniline blue and Pearse's P.A.S.-orange G-haematoxylin stains, and most of the thrombi were partially positive for fibrin.

Cortisone therapy was started, with initially 25 mg. of cortisone acetate twice daily by mouth. The improvement was dramatic; his temperature subsided in 10 hours and although occasionally elevated in the next two weeks this was never above 100° F. When the dose was increased to 50 mg. b.d. the temperature remained completely normal. Equally dramatic was the clinical improvement; his personality completely changed, he became co-operative, his appetite returned and he immediately wanted to get out of his cot. Before this he was quite miserable and inconsolable. With 50 mg. b.d. he developed features of Cushing's syndrome and prednisolone 5 mg. t.d.s. and later 5 mg. b.d. was substituted for cortisone acetate. Since that time he has required between 5 and 10 mg. of prednisolone daily; the mother has now learnt from his general demeanour and from his temperature chart (which she has kept assiduously) how much cortisone is required. The constant aim is to stop cortisone therapy but at this stage a remission has not been obtained. Clinically, however, he is very well indeed and physical examination reveals no abnormality.

Discussion

The first example of this syndrome was described by Moschcowitz (1924, 1925). Probably no more than 40 proven cases have been reported since. According to Symmers and Barrowcliff (1951) this syndrome occurs in both sexes at any age. The youngest case recorded so far was a child, aged 22 months, reported by Craig and Gitlin (1957). All cases to date have died, two-thirds of them in six weeks or less. Examples of a prolonged course are few, the longest being that of a young man reported by Brown and Norman (1946). Another case running a course of three and a quarter years was reported by Meacham, Orbison, Steele and Schaefer (1951).

The onset of the syndrome is usually sudden. Typically it is characterized by fever, purpura and haemolytic anaemia. Multifarious, fluctuating neurological disturbances often occur terminally and are of little diagnostic consequence, and death results, usually in two to four weeks.

Abnormal laboratory findings include thrombocytopenia and anaemia often associated with a raised reticulocyte count. Leucocytosis is usual and may be leukaemoid in type. The bleeding time is prolonged and clot retraction defective but the coagulation time is usually normal.

The case is of interest for several reasons: it is the youngest one on record, the mode of presentation although acute was by no means fulminating and the illness has been protracted. Frank neurological signs have been absent from the start, although there was a marked personality change consisting of extreme misery and complete lack of co-operation even after months in hospital. With a fall in the temperature the patient became quite quickly a happy and co-operative child. On one day only was the platelet count down to 100,000 per c.mm., but this was normal the next day and subsequently. Anaemia was never at any time severe, the lowest haemoglobin level recorded being 9 g. % (60%).

The clinical presentation with fever, leucocytosis, marked joint symptoms, an urticarial rash and a mild purpura, has been recorded before.

Evidence of hypersensitivity, as illustrated here, to pertussis-diphtheria-tetanus antigen and sulphonamides is not infrequent in this syndrome and reactions to iodine compounds, sulphonamides, and penicillin have been reported. Many consider this syndrome to be related to the so-called collagen diseases. We felt that the symptomatology was consistent with that of disseminated lupus erythematosus, but L.E. cells were not demonstrated. There is a good deal of pathological evidence to support this view. Verrucous endocarditis and disseminated lupus erythematosus have been reported in association with thrombotic microangiopathy. Symmers and Gillett (1951) have also reported a case of polyarteritis nodosa in which widely disseminated lesions of thrombotic microangiopathy were also present. Beigelman's (1951) concept of the aetiology of disseminated lupus erythematosus, polyarteritis nodosa, and thrombotic microangiopathy is that of a hyperergic response occurring at different sites in the vessel wall; a maximal response in the perivascular mesenchyme produces disseminated lupus erythematosus, a maximal response in the media produces polyarteritis nodosa, and a maximal response in the intima produces thrombotic microangiopathy. Similar lesions can be reproduced in animals by the Schwartzman phenomenon.

The thrombotic lesions, which are confined to the smallest calibre vessels, occur more frequently and are more numerous in the myocardium, the capsular zones of the adrenals and in the renal cortex. The hepatic and adrenal sinusoids are not involved. There has been, in the past, much speculation as to the exact nature of the occlusive thrombi. Although it was generally accepted that these thrombi were composed of agglutinated platelets, there was no definite proof. Craig and Gitlin (1957) reviewed the literature at length and discussed the inadequacy of the standard staining procedures for fibrin. Using fluorescein-labelled rabbit anti-human fibrin serum, they showed that the thrombi were composed of fibrin. Also with this fluorescent antibody technique, they failed to demonstrate platelets in the thrombi.

The names given to this syndrome in the past have been unsatisfactory. While some have stressed the thrombocytic nature of the thrombi and others the thrombocytopenia, they all lose sight of the characteristic haemolytic anaemia. Moschcowitz's syndrome was suggested as a title, but being eponymous it is not entirely satisfactory. Symmers (1952) suggested the name of thrombotic microangiopathic haemolytic anaemia or, for short, thrombotic microangiopathy, which is descriptively accurate and wisely omits controversial and inconstant features. It is to be hoped that this title finds general acceptance.

The prognosis in the present case must obviously be guarded. Cases living longer than this one have been reported but have invariably terminated fatally. However, the response to steroid therapy is the encouraging feature of this case. The recorded cases have almost always been so acute that therapy has not been successful. A.C.T.H. and cortisone have been used and splenectomy has been performed but without benefit. We feel that in this case cortisone proved of decided value in inducing the second remission. Reduction of prednisolone below 5 mg. b.d. results in elevation of the temperature, malaise and joint soreness within three days. We have persistently tried to discontinue therapy but the reappearance of pyrexia and symptoms has been prompt.

Summary

The youngest case (21 months) of thrombotic microangiopathic haemolytic anaemia is recorded. The child is alive and well after two years.

The clinical and pathological findings are given in detail. The nature of the occlusive thrombi is discussed.

The names accorded this syndrome are discussed and the title, thrombotic microangiopathic haemolytic anaemia, or for short, thrombotic microangiopathy, is supported.

Steroid therapy has been of inestimable benefit and no doubt has been life-saving. As yet it has not been possible to discontinue the maintenance dose of prednisolone. The prognosis must obviously remain guarded.

References

Beigelman, P. M. (1951). *A.M.A. Arch. Path.*, **51**, 213.
Brown, E. B. and Norman, J. W. (1946). *N.Y. St. J. Med.*, **46**, 2167
Craig, J. M. and Gitlin, D. (1957). *Amer. J. Path.*, **33**, 251.
Meacham, G. C., Orbison, J. L., Steele, H. J. and Schaefer, J. A. (1951). *Blood*, **6**, 706.
Moschcowitz, E. (1924). *Proc. N.Y. path. Soc.*, **24**, 21
—— (1925). *Arch. intern. Med.*, **36**, 89.
Symmers, W. St. C. (1952). *Brit. med. J.*, **2**, 897.
—— and Barrowcliff, D. F (1951). *J. Path. Bact.*, **63**, 552.
—— and Gillett, R. (1951). *A.M.A. Arch. Path.*, **52**, 489.

ACUTE ACQUIRED HAEMOLYTIC ANAEMIA ASSOCIATED WITH HERPES SIMPLEX INFECTION

BY

R. McLAREN TODD and N. V. O'DONOHOE

From Alder Hey Children's Hospital, Liverpool

(RECEIVED FOR PUBLICATION JUNE 13, 1958)

Acquired haemolytic anaemia in childhood is a relatively uncommon condition. Lederer (1925) described three patients with acute haemolytic anaemia and in the literature up to 1938 Atkinson (1940) found 59 cases of 'Lederer's anaemia', 30 of which were in children. Millichap (1952) reviewed the papers published between 1940 and 1951 and found reports of a further 32 children with this disorder, the youngest patient affected being 6 weeks of age.

Acquired haemolytic anaemia may develop after treatment with drugs such as quinine, sulphonamides, para-amino-salicylic acid, or after chemical poisons, for example naphthalene, benzene; it may be associated with general diseases such as leukaemia, lymphadenoma, liver diseases, lupus erythematosus; it may follow or be associated with infections either caused by bacteria (*Streptococcus*; *Cl. welchii*; *Cl. tetanis*) or by viruses (virus pneumonia, *influenza A*, *coxsackie A*, infectious mononucleosis, Newcastle disease, measles); but it is frequently unassociated with any obvious disease although investigations may point to the presence of auto-agglutinins or auto-haemolysins. Boorman, Dodd and Loutit (1946) considered that congenital and acquired haemolytic anaemias could be distinguished by the antiglobulin (Coombs) test which was thought to be positive only in acquired haemolytic anaemias; but Wright, Dodd, Bouroncle, Doan and Zollinger (1951) have shown that the Coombs test may be negative in acquired haemolytic anaemia and positive in the congenital type. The stimulus to production of the antibodies in this disorder remains a mystery in many cases but the most likely explanation is that the antigen is derived from infective agents such as bacteria or viruses. The clinical features and results of investigations in a patient recently under our care are now described.

Case Report

Ann O'D., aged 6 years 3 months, was admitted to Alder Hey Children's Hospital on February 2, 1957. Two months before admission she had a clinically mild attack of measles and no complications developed. She returned to school and remained well until five days before admission when she was off colour and did not want to eat. Her family doctor found clinical evidence of a throat infection and prescribed oral penicillin. Her condition did not improve with this therapy and her parents noticed increasing pallor. On the day before admission she vomited once and gradually became semi-comatose. No bleeding was observed from the gastro-intestinal tract or elsewhere.

Her mother, father, sister and three brothers were healthy and there was no family history of allergy, tuberculosis or other disease. When admitted to hospital she was in a semi-comatose condition, extremely pale and with a slight icteric tinge. Oral temperature was 99·8 F., pulse rate 160 per minute, respirations 25 per minute, and sighing in character. No petechiae were present in the skin or mucous membranes, but a few bruises ('normal') were present on both shins. Oral examination showed that the gums were healthy but a few herpetic lesions were present on the inside of the cheeks. There were no signs of infection in the throat, ears, or lungs and no lymphatic glandular enlargement in the neck, axillae or groins. The heart was not enlarged but generalized haemic murmurs were heard, and the systolic blood pressure was 80 mm. Hg. The liver was palpable one finger breadth below the costal margin and the spleen was enlarged to two finger breadths below the costal margin. The optic fundi and general neurological examination did not reveal any abnormal signs.

The haemoglobin was 14% (2·1 g. %); white cells 2,600 per c.mm (neutrophils 58%, lymphocytes 18%, monocytes 15%); the red cells showed spherocytosis and the platelets were present in normal numbers. Direct Coombs test was strongly positive. Total serum protein level was 5·9 g. %, albumin 2·49 g. (42·3%), globulin 3·41 g. (57·7%), A/G ratio 0·73 to 1; γ globulin 1·50 g.% (25·5%), β_2 0·21 g.% (3·6%), β_1 0·39 g. (6·6%), α_2 0·75 g. % (12·6 %) and α_1 0·56 g. % (9·4%). These results show a γ globulin level twice the normal, a slightly raised α_1, and a lowered β_1. Paul Bunnell reaction was negative. Blood transfusion was started on admission, and a total of two pints of packed red cells and one pint of blood was given over a period of 26 hours.

A.C.T.H. was given intramuscularly in a dosage of 80 units twice daily for five days, followed by prednisolone 15 mg. three times daily for five days, reducing by 5 mg. every two days and discontinued four weeks after admission. Progress has been satisfactory and hepatosplenomegaly gradually subsided over a period of 10 months. Table 1 shows the results of serial blood investigations.

TABLE 1
SERIAL BLOOD INVESTIGATIONS

Date	Hb (g. %)	Hb (%)	W.B.C. (per c.mm.)	Reticulocytes (%)	Direct Coombs
2.2.57	2·1	14	2,600		Strongly positive
6	9·2	62			Positive
12	8·9	60	11,000		Positive
20					Positive
25	11·8	80		12	
6.3.57	13·3	90		2·3	Negative
14	13·3	90			
28	10·4	70			
11.4.57	11·8	80			Positive
16	12·3	83		1·3	
9.5.57	12·3	83	9,000	7·1	Positive
23	11·5	78	7,000		Positive
20.6.57	10·4	70			Positive
25.7.57	10·9	74			Negative
5.9.57	11·7	79			Negative
29.11.57	11·4	77			Positive
11.3.58					Positive

Virus studies gave the following results:

Complement fixation tests negative for mumps and L.C.M.
positive for recent herpes simplex infection.
Day 4 1 in 20
,, 20 1 in 320
Neutralization tests herpes simplex
Day 4 positive 1 in 16
negative 1 in 32
,, 20 positive 1 in 256
(only taken to this dilution)

We failed to isolate any agent from this child's blood by inoculation of chorio-allantoic membrane of fertile hen's eggs and passage of these membranes after three days' incubation of primary eggs at 36° C. Serum still had a titre of greater than 1 in 256 in the egg neutralization test.

During the past five years, four other patients with acute acquired haemolytic anaemia have been admitted to Alder Hey Children's Hospital, and Table 2 summarizes the relevant features.

Discussion

The onset of acute acquired haemolytic anaemia is often dramatic and treatment by blood transfusion to restore the haemoglobin level to a more normal value is an urgent matter. In our patient, the initial haemoglobin reading was 14% and in the four other patients seen in this hospital the haemoglobin levels reached 17%, 22%, 31% and 40% (Table 2); in Millichap's (1952) five patients haemoglobin levels varied from 18% to 48%, and in the four patients reported by Rose and Nabarro (1953) haemoglobin levels varied from 12% to 28%. A satisfactory response to blood transfusion is usually as dramatic as the onset of the illness but sometimes transfusion makes the situation worse because the transfused blood is haemolyzed rapidly. In these circumstances a replacement transfusion has proved of considerable value (Bowman, 1955), for this procedure removes antibody attached to the red cells and free in the plasma, and the fresh blood dilutes any free antibody that might remain in the circulating blood. Among the 21 children suffering from acute haemolytic anaemia reported between 1940 and 1950 (Millichap, 1952) 18 (85%) responded to blood transfusions alone. Steroid therapy is a useful adjunct to blood transfusion and probably acts by interrupting the antigen-antibody reaction, thus leading to a fall of antibody and hence to a lessening of the haemolytic process. In idiopathic acquired haemolytic anaemia, the basic disorder appears to be the patient's ability to form antibodies which have an affinity for the red blood cells. It is thought that antibodies are contained in the γ globulin fraction of the plasma and it is of interest that in our patient the γ globulin level was twice the normal value. These antibodies are usually pan-antibodies, i.e. they attack all human red cells, irrespective of blood group but elution of the red cells of our patient yielded anti-e. Weiner, Battey, Cleghorn, Marson and Meynell (1953) have described a man of 32 years with acute haemolytic anaemia in whom the antibody was also anti-e. Dacie (1954) has found that auto-antibodies in idiopathic haemolytic anaemia are of two main kinds, warm and cold. He reported the presence of warm antibodies in 30 patients and cold antibodies in eight patients with acute haemolytic anaemia; in seven of these

TABLE 2
FEATURES OF FOUR PATIENTS WITH ACUTE ACQUIRED HAEMOLYTIC ANAEMIA

Case	Age	Duration of Symptoms Before Admission	Hb (%) On Admission	Hb (%) Lowest Level	Plasma Methaemalbumin	Direct Coombs	Coombs Test Negative After:
J.W. ..	6 m.	6 d.	22	22	+	—	*
H.W. ..	1 yr. 7 m.	6 w.	40	40	+	+	18 m.
K. McD.	2 yr. 2 m.	3 w.	48	31	+	+	8 w.
E.R. ..	12 yr.	2 w.	52	17	—	+	6 w.

* Died after 5 days. Post mortem examination showed renal cortical necrosis.

the illness followed virus pneumonia and in one measles preceded the anaemia.

Infections often precede the development of these acute anaemias and it is reasonable to suppose that the blood in its circulation through virus-infected tissue becomes contaminated with virus particles which are adsorbed on to the red cell surfaces; these virus-contaminated red blood cells may stimulate the reticulo-endothelial system to produce antibodies which destroy the red blood cells and also lead to a rising blood antibody titre. In eight patients with idiopathic haemolytic anaemia reported by Morgan (1955), tests for Newcastle disease virus, influenza, mumps, psittacosis, herpes and pox virus were negative; in the four children reported by Rose and Nabarro (1953) tests for influenza, glandular fever and psittacosis were negative. Moolten and Clark (1952) isolated Newcastle disease virus from the blood of a baby of 11 months and a patient of 37 years suffering from acute idiopathic haemolytic anaemia, and they also found an unidentified virus in the blood of 10 patients with acute haemolytic anaemia associated with general diseases such as leukaemia, Hodgkin's disease, lupus erythematosus, and infective hepatitis. Although we were unable to isolate a virus from the blood of our patient, the results of complement fixation and neutralization tests confirmed that a recent primary infection with herpes simplex virus had occurred. McNair Scott (personal communication) does not know of a report of a similar case, and we have been unable to find a similar example of the development of haemolytic anaemia following herpes simplex infection in the British or American literature.

Summary

The clinical features and results of haematological investigations of a girl of 6 years suffering from acute acquired haemolytic anaemia are recorded. Investigations suggest that the anaemia was the result of a recent primary infection with herpes simplex virus.

References

Atkinson, F. R. B. (1940). *Brit. J. Child. Dis.*, **37**, 35.
Boorman, K. E., Dodd, B. E. and Loutit, J. F. (1946). *Lancet*, **1**, 812.
Bowman, J. M. (1955). *A.M.A. Amer J. Dis. Child.*, **89**, 226.
Dacie, J. V. (1954). *Sang*, **25**, 675.
Lederer, M. (1925). *Amer. J. med. Sci.*, **170**, 500.
McNair Scott, T. F. (1958). Personal communication.
Millichap, J. G. (1952). *Arch. Dis. Childh.*, **27**, 222.
Moolten S. E. and Clark, E. (1952). *Trans. N.Y. Acad. Sci.*, **14**, 232.
Morgan, H. R. (1955). *J. Lab. clin. Med.*, **46**, 580
Rose, B. S. and Nabarro, S. N. (1953). *Arch. Dis. Childh.*, **28**, 87.
Wright, C. S., Dodd, M. C., Bouroncle, B E., Doan, C. A. and Zollinger, R. M. (1951). *J. Lab. clin. Med.*, **37**, 165.
Weiner, W., Battey, D. A., Cleghorn, T. E., Marson, F. G. W. and Meynell, M. J. (1953). *Brit. med. J.* , **2**, 125.

HAEMOLYTIC ANAEMIA IN A CHILD RECEIVING NITROFURANTOIN

BY

DAVID LEVY and ALICE PORGESS
From the Paediatric Department, Poriah Government Hospital, Tiberias, Israel

(RECEIVED FOR PUBLICATION MAY 28, 1958)

In 1956, West and Zimmerman reported a 'first case' of haemolytic anaemia, apparently caused by the use of nitrofurantoin (Furadantin). Since then, no further reports of this untoward effect of the drug have appeared in the literature.

Recently a case of acute pyelonephritis treated with Furadantin, observed in the Paediatric Department of the Poriah Government Hospital in Tiberias, developed severe haemolytic anaemia when given this drug.

Case Report

S.I., a male baby of Iraqui origin, was admitted to this department at the age of 10 months. He was born normally, after a normal full-term pregnancy, the eighth child in the family. He had been breast fed all his life. No haemolytic disease was reported among the other children or the parents of the baby.

A week before admission the infant was seen by a local physician on account of watery stools and vomiting. The treatment given was, reportedly, not effective.

On admission, the baby was severely ill. He was semi-conscious; breathing was deep and rapid, giving the impression of severe metabolic acidosis. Skin turgor was practically non-existent. The liver edge was felt 3 cm. below the costal margin. The temperature was 39° C., and weight 7·3 kg.

Laboratory examinations on admission showed the following results: Hb. 11·0 g. per 100 ml.; R.B.C. 3,900,000 per c.mm.; W.B.C. 41,000 per c.mm. (stab 7%, neutrophils 68%, lymphocytes 18%, monocytes 1%, eosinophils 1%, plasma cells 2%); reticulocytes 3%. Repeated urine examinations showed albumin +, white blood cells in large clumps and many granular casts. Stool examination was negative; stool culture was sterile for *Shigella* and *Salmonella*. Old tuberculin (5 TU) intracutaneously caused no local reaction 48 hours after injection.

It was apparent that this baby was suffering from dehydration and electrolyte imbalance; he was therefore given intravenously physiological solutions with added base. During the 24 hours after admission 600 ml. of standard solution, saline and glucose 5% aa, 400 ml. of 5% glucose solution and 50 ml. of 1/6 molar sodium lactate were administered. The baby was also given Neomycin 400 mg. daily, in four equal doses.

On the day after admission the baby's condition was markedly improved; body weight reached 8·1 kg.; the number of stools was reduced and no clinical signs of acidosis were apparent. On the fourth day of hospitalization stools were normal in appearance and number.

On the third day of his hospital stay, because of the urinary tract infection, a course of nitrofurantoin, 50 mg., three times a day, was started. On the fourth day of this treatment he passed red dark-coloured urine. Administration of nitrofurantoin was discontinued, after a total dose of 700 mg. had been given, a total of 90 mg. per kg. of body weight.

On this day the red blood cell count was 980,000 c.mm. with a haemoglobin level of 3 g. per 100 ml. The reticulocyte count was 8%, platelets 140,000 per c.mm.; haematocrit 17%. The total serum bilirubin level was 2·82 mg. per 100 ml.; urea 38·5 mg. per 100 ml. The total plasma protein was 5·8 g. per 100 ml. (3·08 albumen and 2·72 globulin). A Coombs test, direct and indirect, was completely negative. Auto-antibodies at 36° C. and at 6° C. were not found. No autohaemolysins and isohaemolysins were discovered after adding complement. Bone-marrow examination showed increased erythropoiesis with an M:E ratio of 1·7:1. Paper electrophoresis of haemoglobin showed haemoglobin A only. By alkali denaturation 3·1% foetal haemoglobin was found (normal for the patient's age). There was no bile in the urine, but haemoglobin was present.

The baby was given 450 ml. of blood over a six-hour period. Haemoglobin went up to 7·4 g. per 100 ml., the red blood cell count to 2,810,000 per c.mm. A week later further regeneration brought the red blood cell count to 3,200,000 per c.mm. and the haemoglobin rose to 9·8 g. per 100 ml. The total serum bilirubin level fell to 1 mg. per 100 ml. with a direct fraction of 0·6 mg.

Treatment was continued with Achromycin 300 mg. per day. The baby made an unhampered recovery from the urinary tract infection and was discharged after 28 days of hospitalization.

Comment

The minor side effects of nitrofurantoin are well known and the clinical picture is generally familiar to physicians. Nausea, vomiting, skin rashes, headache, diarrhoea and dizziness have been described occasionally. These effects are purported to subside rapidly when the drug is withdrawn or the dosage reduced.

Rare cases of more severe toxic effects have also been reported. Thus Hasen and Moore (1954) have reported a reduced white blood cell count of 2,900 per c.mm. with a normal differential count in one of 68 patients treated with Furadantin. West and Zimmerman (1956) described the appearance in a negro male of haemolytic anaemia following the administration of nitrofurantoin. Whereas haematological and blood chemistry examinations seemed to provide good grounds for concluding that the haemolytic anaemia was related to the administration of nitrofurantoin in this patient, the authors properly reserved judgment as proof was not unequivocal and no other reports of this untoward reaction have been published.

Therefore the appearance of haemoglobinuria, reticulocytosis, a drastic fall in the circulating red blood cells and haemoglobin and a rise in serum bilirubin in a patient with pyelonephritis when treated with Furadantin caused profound interest and every effort was made to exclude other possible causes for haemolytic anaemia at our patient's age. On the other hand no trial was made to prove experimentally *in vivo* the haemolytic influence of nitrofurantoin because of the rapid haemolysis which necessitated an immediate transfusion of blood.

The mechanism of haemolysis due to nitrofurantoin is conjectural. The similarity of the nitrofurantoin-induced haemolysis to that induced by other drugs, such as the sulphonamides, is apparent. Szeinberg, Sheba, Hirshorn and Bodonyi (1957) have postulated that a constitutional congenital anomaly, namely glutathione deficiency of the red blood cells, is essential for the pathogenesis of this reaction. Their study indicates that this abnormality is fairly frequent among Jews originating from the Arab countries in Asia (Eastern Jews). No examination of the glutathione content of the red blood cells of this patient was made, as the deficiency appears with the ageing of the red blood cells, the young ones being normal.

Summary

A case of acute haemolytic anaemia occurred in an infant receiving nitrofurantoin (Furadantin) for acute pyelonephritis. No other cause for this haemolysis could be found. Haemolysis subsided after stopping the drug. Although no experimental proof is available, it seems reasonably proved that the haemolytic anaemia was caused by the action of Furadantin on the red blood cells.

References

Hasen, H. B. and Moore, T. D. (1954). *J. Amer. med. Ass* , **155**, 1470.

Szeinberg, A., Sheba, C., Hirshorn, N. and Bodonyi, E. (1957). *Blood*, **12**, 603.

West, M. and Zimmerman, H. J. (1956). *J. Amer. med. Ass.*, **162**, 637.

ERYTHROCYTE SEDIMENTATION RATE, C-REACTIVE PROTEIN DETERMINATION, SERUM PROTEIN FRACTIONS, FIBRINOGEN LEVEL AND ANTI-STREPTOLYSIN REACTION IN 52 RHEUMATIC CHILDREN

BY

N. POPOV and S. STANISHEVA

From the Department of Rheumatism, Second City Children's Hospital, Sofia

(RECEIVED FOR PUBLICATION JUNE 16, 1958)

This paper reports the results of our investigations into the clinical significance of laboratory tests in 52 cases of rheumatic fever treated in the Rheumatic Department of the Second City Children's Hospital, Sofia. The diagnosis of active rheumatic infection is based on the history, presence of carditis (in 48 cases), changes in the electrocardiograms, and by the supporting evidence of five laboratory tests: namely the erythrocyte sedimentation rate, C-reactive protein determinations, serum protein fractions, the blood fibrinogen level and the antistreptolysin-O reaction.

Eighteen of the children were in their first attack, and 34 had had one or more attacks of rheumatic fever. Thirteen cases in first attacks and 19 cases in subsequent attacks received steroid therapy.

Five children were 6 years old or under, 36 were between 7 and 11 years, and 11 were 12 or 13 years of age.

Methods

The laboratory tests were carried out by the following methods:

1. **Erythrocyte Sedimentation Rate** (E.S.R.). By Westergren's method (1921, 1957), estimations up to 10 mm. in the first hour being accepted as normal.

2. **C-reactive Protein** (C.R.P.). Determined by the method of Anderson and McCarty (1950), using C.R.P. anti-serum produced by Schiffelin and Co., New York, and assessed as −, +, ++ or +++, in accordance with the criteria suggested by Wurhmann and Wunderly (1957).

3. **Serum Protein Fractions** (S.P.F.). By paper electrophoresis following Flynn and de Mayo (1951). Figures for each fraction expressed as percentage of the total protein, and the following figures accepted as pathological: albumen under 47%, α_1 globulin over 5%, α_2 globulin over 12%, β globulin over 14%, and γ globulin over 20% (Popov, 1956a, b). In the present paper the determinations for total protein are not discussed since deviations from the normal were slight and indeterminate.

4. **Plasma Fibrinogen Level.** By kjeldahlometric determination, normal range was 180-350 mg. per 100 ml. in accordance with our own findings (Popov and Stanisheva, 1958).

5. **Antistreptolysin Reaction** (A.S.O.). By the method described by Kalbak (1947). Standard serum from the State Serum Institute, Copenhagen, was used. Though a titre of over 200 was accepted as pathologically increased, we have previously shown (Popov and Bojadzieva, 1957) that serial estimations have a very much greater value than a single initial estimation.

In all a total of 1,743 estimations were carried out on the 52 children as follows:

E.S.R.	527 estimations
C.R.P., S.P.F. and A.S.O. ..	304 estimations each
Plasma fibrinogen	304 estimations

Results

Table 2 presents the results obtained for the five investigations on the 52 children, divided firstly into those in a first attack and those in subsequent attacks, and also divided according to whether hormone therapy was given or withheld. With each estimation the highest figure obtained during the active phase of the infection is given. Consequently for the E.S.R., C.R.P. and the fibrinogen levels, the results are obtained mainly at the beginning of the illness. For the A.S.O. the results obtained are usually in the middle of an attack, whilst the figures for the S.P.F. were obtained at various times throughout the attack.

Consideration of these results reveals the following points:

1. **Erythrocyte Sedimentation Rate.** The E.S.R. remained normal in seven children, of whom only one was in a first attack. Very high figures were obtained in 18 children, 10 in their first attack.

TABLE 2

	No.	E.S.R. (mm./1st hr.)				C.R.P.				S.P.F.				Fibrinogen Level (mg.%)			A.S.O. (units)		
										Normal	Increased								
		>10	11 to 30	31 to 60	Over 60	—	+	++	+++		α_1 α_2 γ	α_2 γ	γ only	180 to 350	360 to 550	over 550	under 200	300 to 600	800 and over
I. First attack (18) (*a*) with steroid therapy ..	13	—	2	2	9	1	—	4	8	1	8	4	—	5	3	5	1	5	7
(*b*) without steroid therapy	5	1	1	2	1	—	2	—	3	—	4	1	—	2	3	—	—	2	3
II. Subsequent Attacks (34) (*a*) with steroid therapy ..	19	2	5	6	6	—	2	10	7	—	9	7	3	10	6	3	3	7	9
(*b*) without steroid therapy	15	4	4	5	2	4	7	1	3	4	1	5	5	12	2	1	8	5	2
Totals ..	52	7	12	15	18	5	11	15	21	5	22	17	8	29	14	9	12	19	21

The follow up of the E.S.R. showed that in the children in their first attack and receiving steroids it remained raised for an average of 25 days, whilst in three of these the E.S.R. was not normal until the thirtieth day, and in another not until the forty-fifth day. Of the five children in their first attack not given steroid therapy, in one the E.S.R. was normal, in two it became normal in about 20 days, whilst in the remaining two, both of whom suffered from tonsillitis during their rheumatic infection, the E.S.R. remained raised for 60 days.

Of the children in a subsequent attack and receiving steroid therapy, 11 showed a raised E.S.R. for an average of 50 days (in two children for 65 days, in one child for about three months); of the children in a subsequent attack and not receiving steroid therapy the E.S.R. became normal also on an average in about 50 days (in two children after two months and in one after three months).

2. C.R.P. In general the C.R.P. tests showed positive or negative results much in accordance with the data quoted in the literature (Müller, 1956), but in many cases variations in the intensity of the reaction were obtained especially from + to ++ during the course of the disease. Of 18 children in the first attack 11 showed a raised C.R.P., usually ++. In one child the estimation was persistently negative in spite of clinical evidence of active infection, whilst in six children estimations varied from + to ++ from time to time.

Of 35 children with subsequent attacks, in 10 the C.R.P. was +++ steadily over a long period, in four it was constantly negative. Of the eight children in the first attack and being treated with hormones, C.R.P. tests in seven steadily improved from the onset of the disease, and in one (a protracted case with several previous attacks) the C.R.P. remained positive for about three months as did the E.S.R. and S.P.F. In general this test was usually the first to appear positive and the first to become negative with the exception of the fibrinogen level which was often the first to become negative in children with a first attack receiving steroid therapy.

3. S.P.F. Protein fractions are related to the humeral changes in the connective tissue during the different phases in rheumatic progress (Chaptal, Jean, Campo, Alram and Fraisse, 1954). In the present series also the dysproteinaemia was present at the beginning of the attack and its intensity appeared to correspond to the degree of the exudative and productive tissue changes. Moreover, the dysproteinaemia remained raised for a long time after the E.S.R. and S.R.P. had become negative. These findings are in accordance with those of Jacox (1956).

In the present series, five children showed repeatedly normal values in spite of other evidence of activity, four of whom were in subsequent attacks and not receiving steroid therapy. In the remaining 47 dysproteinaemia was marked at the beginning of the attack. In 22, there was at the beginning of the attack an increased α_1 and α_2 globulin with a moderately increased γ globulin. As the process evolved the α globulin fractions decreased and the γ globulin fraction increased up to a figure of 30%. In this group the dysproteinaemia lasted for an average of 55 days. By contrast, of the 17 children in their first attack, though there was a similar pattern for the α_2 and the γ fractions, the dysproteinaemia lasted on an average about 40 days. In two children who had an intercurrent infection of measles γ globulin dropped to 10 and 12% respectively.

We agree with the data of Payne and Forsyth (1958) that children over the age of six years have approximately adult protein fraction levels. We also agree with Klaishevitsch (1958) regarding the behaviour of the globulin fractions in the cardiac forms of rheumatism and that in a first attack great deviations from the normal are observed, also a more rapid return to normal compared with children in subsequent attacks.

4. Fibrinogen Levels. We previously studied these in 70 children (Popov and Stanisheva, 1958). It was there concluded that during the first attack without complications and also in many repeated attacks the fibrinogen level may become normal during the first week of the disease, but that if the condition becomes protracted, and particularly in repeated attacks, the fibrinogen level remains high for a long time. In the present series, in 29 children fibrinogen levels were normal, between 180 and 350 mg. %; of 23 children with high fibrinogen levels, and in three cases with previous attacks and receiving hormone treatment the fibrinogen levels remained high for 30, 40 and 60 days respectively. In the remaining cases there was a greatly raised fibrinogen level, from 360 to 850 mg. %, which became normal during the first 10 days.

5. A.S.O. Twelve of our children had a titre constantly under 200 units, i.e. within the upper limit of normal, and 11 of these had had previous attacks. In 19 the A.S.O. titre was between 300 and 600 units; seven of these were in their first attack, and 12 had had previous attacks. In 21 patients the A.S.O. titre was between 800 and 1,600 and 10 of these were in their first attack. In children with a raised A.S.O. titre the height of the curve was reached about the end of the second week, whilst in those treated with cortisone the high level was sustained for from 30 to 75 days. Two children were exceptional in that the A.S.O. fell before the twentieth day. Chaptal *et al.* (1954) and Harris, Needleman, Harris and Friedman (1956) and Lanza, Morbidelli and Papotti (1956) reported that a quick fall of the A.S.O. was brought about by steroid therapy. There were three such cases in our series receiving steroids. In general, in children with previous attacks and treated with steroids the A.S.O. level remained high for 40 days.

In eight patients there was a very high level of A.S.O. titre at the beginning of their admission to hospital. In these children there was a history suggesting that they had been admitted during the second or third week of their illness.

In nine children receiving steroid therapy, three of whom were in their first attack, when steroid therapy was discontinued or diminished there was a simultaneous increase of the E.S.R., C.R.P., S.P.F., and some tendency to elevation of the A.S.O., as also clinical deterioration of the cardiac condition. This rebound phenomenon is in accordance with the findings of Holt (1956).

An effort was made to correlate the laboratory findings of the cases given steroids with the following results: 23 cases showed a correlation between the five tests, in nine cases, a correlation between the E.S.R., C.R.P., S.P.F. and the A.S.O.; in 10 cases between the E.S.R., the C.R.P., and the S.P.F.; in four cases between the C.R.P., the S.P.F. and the A.S.O., and in three cases between the C.R.P. and the A.S.O. Completely normal laboratory findings in the presence of clinical evidence of activity was observed in three cases.

Summary

At intervals of seven to 10 days 1,743 investigations for E.S.R., C.R.P., S.P.F. and fibrinogen levels and A.S.O. titre were performed in 52 rheumatic children with active infection. Eighteen of these children were in their first attack, of whom 13 were being treated with steroid therapy, and 34 had had previous attacks, 19 of whom were receiving steroids.

In 23 cases there was good correlation between the positive findings in the five tests when related to clinical activity. In three cases the laboratory tests were normal in the face of evidence of clinical activity. In the remaining cases there was correlation between four tests in nine cases, between three tests in 14 cases, between two tests in three cases. There was a rebound phenomenon in nine cases.

References

Anderson, H. C. and McCarty, M. (1950). *Amer. J. Med.*, **8**, 445.
Chaptal, J., Jean, R., Campo, C., Alram, D. and Fraisse, J. (1954). *Arch. franç. Pédiat.*, **11**, 1055.
Flynn, F. V. and Mayo, P. de (1951). *Lancet*, **2**, 235.
Harris, T. N., Needleman, H. L., Harris, S. and Friedman, S. (1956). *Pediatrics*, **17**, 29.
Holt, K. S. (1956). *Arch. Dis. Childh.*, **31**, 444.
Jacox, R. F. (1956). *N.Y. St. J. Med.*, **56**, 672: (cf. *Abstr. Wld Med.* (1956). **20**, 215.)
Kalbak, K. (1947). *The Antistreptolysin Reaction.* State Serum Institute, Copenhagen.
Klaishevitsch, G. I. (1958). *Pediatrija*, no. 1, p. 68.
Lanza, I., Morbidelli, R. and Papotti, G. (1956). *Minerva med. (Torino)*, (*parte Sci*), **47 (1)**, 553.
Müller, W. (1956). *Z. Rheumaforsch.*, **15**, 31.
Payne, W. W. and Forsyth, C. C. (1958). *Arch Dis. Childh.*, **33**, 61.
Popov, N. (1956a). *Sovr. Med.*, **7**, 116.
—— (1956b). Scientific Works of the State Institute for Haematology and Blood Transfusion in Sofia, **3**, 64.
—— and Bojadzieva, M. (1957). *Sovr. Med.*, **8**, 33.
—— and Stanisheva, S. (1958). *Pediat. Akuš. Ginec.*, **2**, 29.
Westergren, A. (1921). *Acta med. scand.*, **54**, 247.
—— (1957). *Triangle*, **3**, 20.
Wuhrmann, F. and Wunderly, C. (1957). *Die Bluteiweisskörper des Menschen*, 3rd ed. Basel.

THE PROGNOSIS OF IDIOPATHIC RENAL ACIDOSIS IN INFANCY WITH OBSERVATIONS ON URINE ACIDIFICATION AND AMMONIA PRODUCTION IN CHILDREN

BY

ELIZABETH U. BUCHANAN and G. M. KOMROWER

From the Royal Manchester Children's Hospital and the Department of Paediatrics and Child Health, University of Manchester

(RECEIVED FOR PUBLICATION APRIL 30, 1958)

Idiopathic renal acidosis of infancy has been recognized for over 20 years since the descriptions of the morbid anatomy by Lightwood (1935) and of the clinical condition by Butler, Wilson and Farber (1936). The incidence of the condition appeared to reach a peak between 1946 and 1952 during which time 35 cases were described in The Hospital for Sick Children, London (Lightwood, Payne and Black, 1953), while 17 cases were seen in the Birmingham Children's Hospital between 1948 and 1953 (Carré, Wood and Smallwood, 1954). The prognosis has been stated to be good in infants surviving the acute phase of the illness (Hartmann, 1939; Stapleton, 1949; Lightwood *et al.*, 1953) but only isolated cases have been followed for any number of years after recovery (Kelsey, Reinhart and Fishel, 1950; Doxiadis, 1952). Our colleagues, seeing cases of renal tubular acidosis in adults, have been interested to know whether there is any relationship between this condition and that seen in infancy. It was, therefore, felt worth while to make a detailed survey of the eight children who had been in the Royal Manchester Children's Hospital with infantile renal acidosis between 1948 and 1953 and who, by the time of the review, were between 5 and 10 years of age and had been off all treatment for periods ranging from three and a half to nine years.

The review which was carried out in 1957 included recent history, physical examination, a radiograph of the abdomen to detect renal calcification, and examination of blood and urine. Distal renal tubular function was examined by a test designed to assess powers of concentration and dilution at the same time as the ability to secrete an acid urine and to form ammonia following the administration of ammonium chloride. We could find no data on normal values in children for urine acidification and ammonia production following oral ammonium chloride, so it was necessary to carry out observations on a control series.

Methods

Twenty-two normal children formed the control series. In selecting cases for this series the following criteria were observed: the child was considered to have recovered from the condition for which he had been admitted to hospital and was about to be discharged (the majority being surgical cases on the day before discharge); secondly, there was no history of renal disease, no abnormality was detected in the urine and the concentration and dilution test was normal.

The technique used for the combined concentration and dilution and acidification test was as follows. Fluids were restricted from 8.30 p.m. on the evening preceding the test until 12.30 p.m. next day, but solid foods were allowed. The child emptied his bladder at 8.30 p.m., 12.30 a.m. and 6.30 a.m.; the specific gravity was measured and the urine discarded. At 8.30 a.m. and 9.30 a.m. the child again emptied his bladder; the volume and specific gravity of the urine were measured and a specimen preserved with thymol for estimation of pH and ammonium content. Between 9.30 a.m. and 10.30 a.m. the child was given ammonium chloride in a dose of 0·1 g. per Kg. body weight (the salt being given in gelatine capsules in every instance except one where difficulty was encountered with swallowing, and a mixture was given instead). During that hour the child was also given 20 ml. water per Kg. body weight. The ammonium chloride was given over an hour to avoid nausea, and difficulty in this respect arose in only one instance. The child having the test emptied his bladder at 11.30 a.m. and this specimen was discarded. This procedure was followed to eliminate the fluctuations in ammonia production during this period resulting from the variable initial urine pH. In this way it was possible to assess more accurately the effect of the ammonium chloride. The bladder was emptied at 12.30 p.m., 2.30 p.m. and 4.30 p.m.; urine passed between these times was mixed with the next timed specimen; all collections of urine were preserved with thymol. The volume and specific gravity of each specimen was measured and pH and ammonium content estimated. The pH was measured by means of the B.D.H. capillator. Ammonium was estimated using Conway's micro-diffusion units, the rate of excretion in micro-equivalents per minute being calculated in each period and also over the two to seven-hour period following the administration of the drug.

In every case the urine pH fell below 5·3 within five hours of the administration of ammonium chloride, the range being from 4·8 to 5·2 on the B.D.H. capillator. The values obtained by this means are only accurate to within 0·2 in either direction. This has been determined by comparison with values obtained on a glass electrode pH meter. It has been found, however, that when the pH is below 5·7 the figures obtained with the B.D.H. capillator is consistently higher than that obtained with the glass electrode pH meter. It seems likely, therefore, that the ability of these children to acidify urine is even greater than that shown by our results.

The rate of ammonium excretion in the five-hour period under investigation varied considerably from one child to another but was found to bear a close relationship to the child's weight. The results obtained in the 22 normal children are shown on the accompanying graph which also includes figures for normal adult controls obtained during a similar investigation in adults. In this investigation ammonium excretion was estimated over the two to eight-hour period after ammonium chloride (Wrong and Davies, 1959, in press).

Cases Under Review

The eight children who had been in the Royal Manchester Children's Hospital with infantile renal acidosis between 1948 and 1953 had all been under the care of one of us (G.M.K.): five were boys and three girls. All had been admitted to hospital between the ages of 5 and 11 months, their symptoms having begun at between 3½ and 8 months of age. With one exception they had presented three or more of the recognized features of constipation, vomiting, anorexia, failure to gain weight and polyuria. In the exception the only presenting feature was failure to gain weight. Physical examination on admission had shown two or more of the recognized signs of hypotonia, wasting, dehydration, malar flush and palpable faeces in the abdomen. In every case except one (R.M., see Appendix) the diagnosis was confirmed shortly after admission by the finding of a systemic acidosis with serum bicarbonate of less than 35 vol. % (16 mEq./l.) associated with alkaline or faintly acid urine, the pH ranging from 6·9 to 7·9. The serum chloride was raised above 640 mg. % as sodium chloride (110 mEq./l.) in the five cases in which the estimation was carried out before treatment was begun. With one exception (R.M.) the blood urea did not rise above 50 mg. % and returned rapidly to normal when treatment was begun. Radiographs of the abdomen showed no evidence of renal calcification in any patient. In seven cases (excluding R.M.) treatment with alkalis was given, sodium citrate and citric acid being used initially and potassium citrate added later if necessary. Hartmann's solution and M/6 lactate were used in the early stages of treatment especially in the four cases where parenteral fluids were required. Treatment was continued until the biochemistry remained normal after a trial period without alkali. The length of treatment varied from five to 23 months. All the children except one were able to stop treatment between the age of 15 and 21 months. The one exception was an infant who had been very difficult to control when treatment was initiated. In her case treatment had to be continued until she was 2 years 4 months old. All the children attended the out-patient department at intervals until 1954 and their progress was considered to be satisfactory.

The review carried out in 1957 comprised two stages. In the first the children were seen as out-patients and the object of the review explained to the parents. The recent history was obtained, a physical examination carried out and a radiograph of the abdomen taken. In the second stage the child was admitted to hospital for 36 hours for examination of blood and urine, followed by the combined concentration, dilution and acidification test already described.

In every case the parents were well pleased with the child's progress and no abnormality was found on physical examination which included blood pressure estimation. Heights were close to the 50 percentile for the corresponding age, but weights were rather below it with two girls close to the 10 percentile. The percentiles used were those calculated by Tanner (1958) from data provided by Scott (1955). It is interesting, though probably not significant, that the two underweight girls were the patients whom it had been most difficult to control at the onset of treatment. A radiograph of the abdomen revealed no evidence of renal calcification in any of the children. Urine examination, including microscopy, showed no abnormality. Blood chemistry comprised serum calcium, phosphorus, chloride and bicarbonate and blood urea. The values obtained were normal in every case with the exception of the blood urea in R.M. (see Appendix).

The test designed to assess distal renal tubular function showed very satisfactory results. After 13 hours' deprivation of fluid the urine specific gravity rose to between 1,018 and 1,025, while after

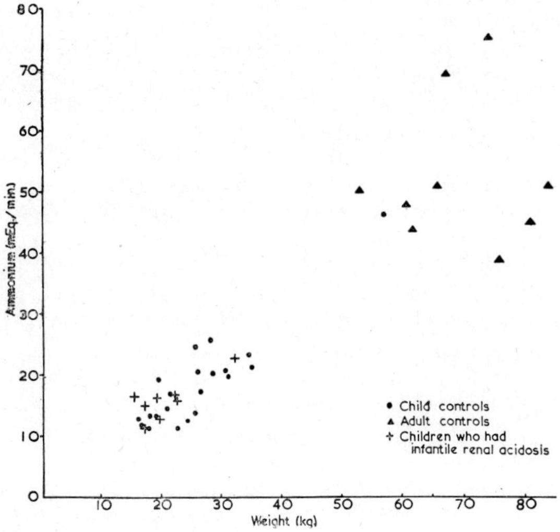

FIG. 1.—Ammonium excretion in 2-7 hours following the administration of ammonium chloride.

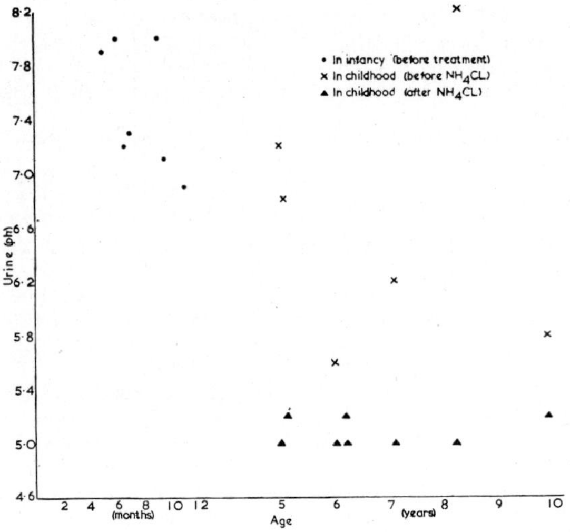

FIG. 2.—Urine pH in relation to age.

taking water (20 ml. per kg.) it fell to 1,001 or 1,000. Following ammonium chloride the urine pH fell to between 5·0 and 5·2 in every case and, bearing in mind the remarks made in connexion with the control series, the actual acidity of the urine may well have been greater. Ammonium excretion is plotted against weight in Fig. 1 and shows that these children fall within the range determined for the control series.

Conclusion

The results of the investigation confirm the clinical impression that idiopathic renal acidosis of infancy is a self-limiting disease if the affected children are brought safely through the acute phase. In particular it shows complete recovery of the ability to secrete an acid urine (Fig. 2) and to form ammonia (the latter ability being present but impaired during the acute illness) (Latner and Burnard, 1950). From these results it appears that renal acidosis associated with nephrocalcinosis in older children and adults is a different condition from infantile renal acidosis and that the one does not lead to the other.

This work was done while one of us (E.U.B.) was holding the Ashby Memorial Research Scholarship of the University of Manchester.

We should like to thank Dr. O. Wrong for permission to include his figures for adults in the graph and for his co-operation, and Miss V. K. Wilson for advice and assistance on biochemistry.

REFERENCES

Butler, A. M., Wilson, J. L. and Farber, S. (1936). *J. Pediat.*, **8**, 489.
Carré, I. J., Wood, B. S. B. and Smallwood, W. C. (1954). *Arch. Dis. Childh.*, **29**, 326.
Davies, H. E. F. and Wrong, O. (1957). *Lancet*, **2**, 625.
Doxiadis, S. A. (1952). *Arch. Dis. Childh.*, **27**, 409.
Hartmann, A. F. (1939). *Ann. intern. Med.*, **13**, 940.
Kelsey, W. M., Reinhart, J. B. and Fishel, J. (1950). *Pediatrics*, **5**, 689.
Latner, A. L. and Burnard, E. D. (1950). *Quart. J. Med.*, **19**, 285.
Lightwood, R. (1935). *Arch. Dis. Childh.*, **10**, 205.
——, Payne, W. W. and Black, J. A. (1953). *Pediatrics*, **12**, 628.
Scott, J. A. (1955). *Report on the Heights and Weights of School Pupils in the County of London in* 1954. London County Council.
Tanner, J. M. (1958). In *Modern Trends in Paediatrics*, (Second Series) ed. A. Holzel and J. P. M. Tizard. p. 325, Butterworth, London.
Wrong, O. and Davies, H. E. F. (1959). *Quart. J. Med.* In the press.

APPENDIX

Case History

R.M., a first-born male child, was born on September 15, 1947, and was admitted to the Royal Manchester Children's Hospital at the age of 7 months on account of a two-month history of anorexia, loss of weight, fretfulness, constipation and intermittent vomiting. The pregnancy and delivery had been uneventful, and birth weight was $8\frac{3}{4}$ lb. He had been breast fed for only 2 weeks, and was then changed to National Dried Milk on which he continued to thrive until he was 5 months of age. Thereafter he lost 1 lb. 10 oz. in weight in five weeks. When seen at 7 months he weighed only 14 lb. 6 oz. Apart from obvious loss of weight and dehydration, the only abnormal feature was a flush over the malar bones unassociated with pyrexia. Following admission he developed an irregular pyrexia and his weight remained stationary. Investigations included a Mantoux test, 1 in 1,000, which was negative, radiographs of chest and wrist which were both normal, haemoglobin 78% (11·5 g.%) with colour index 0·93, white cell count 12,000 with normal differential. Throughout his stay in hospital there was constant slight albuminuria and the urine specific gravity never rose above 1,010. He had intermittent pyrexia, and urine culture twice yielded *Strep. faecalis* which cleared following courses of sulphadimidine and penicillin. The urine was usually neutral or alkaline but on one occasion was acid to litmus. Blood urea was 57 mg. % on admission and rose to 105 mg. %. Intravenous pyelogram showed poor excretion of dye but no obvious renal abnormality. In the last week in hospital his weight gain improved and when discharged on June 17, 1948, he weighed 15 lb. 4 oz. From July 6 to July 28, 1948, he was an in-patient at Birmingham Children's Hospital. There he was found to have hyperchloraemia (698 mg. % as sodium chloride), a low alkali reserve (25·5 vol. %) and a serum calcium of 11·2 mg. % and a diagnosis of infantile renal acidosis was made. The urine still contained a trace of albumin and some pus cells, and the ammonia content of a 24-hour specimen was only 0·11 g. By this time there was a marked improvement in his clinical condition and his blood urea had fallen to 50 mg. %. Treatment with alkalis was therefore not considered necessary. He took his feeds well and gained weight steadily and when discharged at the age of 10½ months he weighed 17 lb.

R.M. was seen as an out-patient in Manchester at regular intervals during the next 5½ years. His progress was rather slow until he reached 2 years of age but thereafter his height and weight were well up to the average for his age and no abnormality was found on physical examination, which included blood pressure estimation. His blood urea, however, remained above normal except on one occasion in 1954 when it was 29 mg. %. When reviewed in 1957 at the age of 9 years, 10 months, his height and weight were close to the 90 percentile for his age and he appeared to be very well. Blood pressure was 95/60 and a radiograph of the abdomen revealed no renal calcification. Urine examination, including microscopy, showed no abnormality and the concentration and dilution test gave a specific gravity range of 1,022 to 1,002 after 13 hours' deprivation of fluid. In the acidification test his performance was well up to the average, the urine pH falling to 5·2 after three hours and the rate of ammonium excretion being well within the normal range for that weight (see Fig. 1). Serum electrolytes were within normal limits but blood urea was still 43 mg. %; six months later this had fallen to 38 mg. % while the urea clearance was 72% of average normal function. In this boy, therefore, renal tubular function now appears to be restored to normal but there is still some doubt about glomerular function. The height to which the blood urea rose in the acute phase of the illness suggests that there may have been some glomerular damage at that time, and that this illness may not have been a pure idiopathic renal acidosis of infancy.

DIASTEMATOMYELIA

BY

C. C. MICHAEL JAMES and L. P. LASSMAN

From the Departments of Orthopaedic Surgery and Neurological Surgery, Newcastle upon Tyne General Hospital

(RECEIVED FOR PUBLICATION MAY 12, 1958)

Diastematomyelia is a rare condition and in our opinion is tending to be recognized more frequently by the radiologist, but its clinical significance does not appear to have been stressed. The purpose of this communication is to describe a case of this syndrome and to emphasize the importance of surgical treatment.

The term diastematomyelia is used to designate a congenital condition in which the spinal cord is divided longitudinally into two portions over some part of its extent. According to Cameron (1957) the term diastematomyelia was originally used by Hertwig in 1892 to describe a split in the spinal cord which occurred as a result of experimental interference with frogs' ova. Diastematomyelia becomes of clinical importance when there is a septum across the neural canal passing antero-posteriorly between the two portions of the spinal cord. The septum may be of bone, fibrous tissue, fibro-cartilage, or a mixture of these; it transfixes the spinal cord and divides partially or completely the neural canal antero-posteriorly in the midline. It most commonly affects the lower thoracic and lumbar regions but it has been described in the thoracic region as high as T.V.2 (Cowie, 1951). A similar septum may be found, in the absence of diastematomyelia between the nerves of the cauda equina, some of which may be adherent to the septum and diverted from their normal course. It has been found to be associated with other congenital anomalies of the vertebral column, particularly spina bifida, often of the spinal cord as in myelocele and occasionally with dermoid cysts (Matson, Woods, Campbell and Ingraham, 1950).

Some authors prefer the term diplomyelia for this condition because they regard it as the result of an attempt at twinning (Herren and Edwards, 1940; Benstead, 1953) but Cameron (1957) suggests that it is a failure of development associated with the delayed closure of the human equivalent of the blastopore. Cameron also, with Kapsenberg and Lookeren (1949), regards the presence of a septum as being due to the inductive influence of the split spinal cord upon the closely associated mutual development of dura and bone column, the septum being an abortive attempt at the formation of a midline neural arch by inversion of the laminae.

A septum is liable to fix the spinal cord so that traction is exerted on it as the vertebral column grows in length relatively faster than the cord, a process usually described as 'ascent' or 'migration' of the cord. The effect of transfixion becomes more marked with growth and, if it is severe and unrelieved, paralysis is likely to ensue owing to tension upon the cord itself, upon the nerve roots, and possibly owing to reduction of blood supply by traction on the blood vessels. A septum, therefore, is likely to be the cause of a progressive neurological deficit in the lower limbs, disparity of size of the lower limbs, incontinence, paresis, trophic changes and even paralysis.

The condition is usually recognized in childhood but has also been reported in adults in their twenties. The presenting symptoms are usually progressive weakening or failure to develop strength in a lower limb, or deterioration of gait. Occasionally the parents have brought the child because they were anxious about the presence of a hairy patch or naevus on the back and a radiograph has demonstrated diastematomyelia (Matson *et al.*, 1950).

Case Report

A girl, aged 10 years, attended an orthopaedic clinic complaining of discomfort in the right fourth toe in relation to the plantar aspect of the metatarso-phalangeal joint. No obvious cause for this was found but the appearance of the lower limbs attracted attention. The legs were of equal size and the feet normal except that the right foot was slightly smaller than the left. The skin of the legs and feet was livid and the circulation poor although it was a warm day. The whole appearance resembled that commonly seen in children with a myelomeningocele. Her mother said the girl frequently suffered from chilblains and that she always had 'very poor circulation in her legs', which went blue and mottled very easily; they never went 'dead' or painful. There was no history of bladder disturbance.

On examination of the back there was no abnormality evident except an excess of sparse hair over the lumbo-sacral area. The right plantar reflex was equivocal on that day but on the next examination four weeks later was found to be definitely flexor. There was no weakness in the lower limbs. She was small for her age; her three sibs, all younger, were of normal height. On admission to hospital two months later her condition on examination was unchanged but it was not possible to elicit her right plantar reflex: there was no demonstrable loss of sensation. Diagnosis was confirmed by radiological appearance and by myelography.

Plain radiographs showed spina bifida of L.V. 3, 4 and 5, and S.1. There was also a dense bony opacity situated in the midline and apparently extending from the spinous process of L.V.2 to the posterior aspect of the body of L.V.3 (Figs. 1 and 2), which was confirmed by tomography as being a midline bone spur. On myelography, the myodil column divided about 1 cm. below the bony spur and united again above the spur. A narrow, negative midline shadow was present for about 1·5 cm. above the spur (Figs. 3 and 4).

Operation. The spinous processes were removed, starting two segments lower than the expected site of the lesion. On removal of the spine of L.V.2 a bone pillar was displayed transfixing the cord. The pillar was extradural and closely invested by the dura; it was firmly attached posteriorly at the peak of the neural arch. The pillar at its narrowest was oval in section, 4 mm. in length (cranial-caudal) and 3 mm. wide. Its anterior attachment to the body of L.V.3 was not firm and was presumably fibrous.

The dura was opened, showing a division of the spinal cord into two equal parts, the split extending cranially from the pillar for 1·5 cm. All the roots were lateral to the cord. The split did not extend caudally from the pillar. There was a thin fibrous band ascending to a higher level within the dura and above the bony pillar; the band was divided and the bone removed, piecemeal and with difficulty, through the very small hiatus in the cord since it was not possible to rotate the cord without dividing the nerve roots.

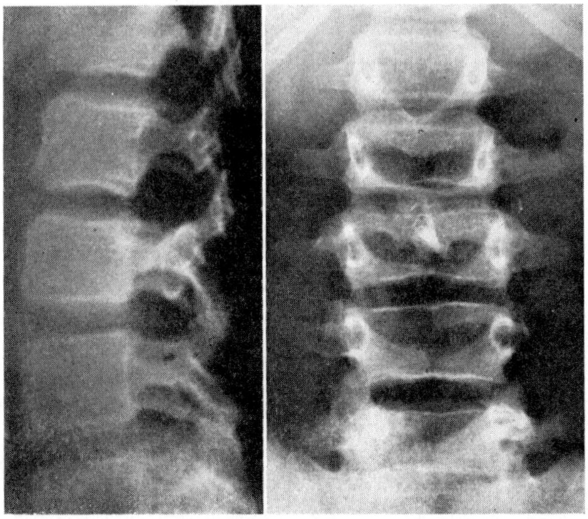

Figs. 1 and 2.—Survey views of the lumbar spine showing the bone spur lying in the sagittal plane.

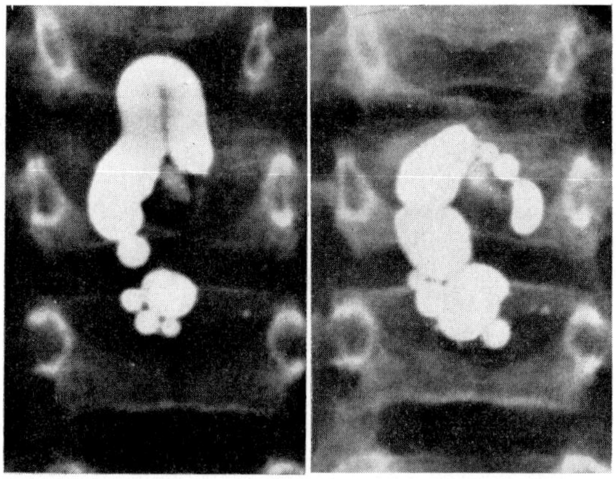

Figs. 3 and 4.—Myelography demonstrates the separation of the myodil above the spur by the fibrous membrane (Fig. 3) and below the spur by its base. (The spur is ringed in Fig. 3.)

The cord was free at the end of operation; it had not ascended when released. The conus medullaris was situated 1½ cm. below the pillar. Closure was normal.

The post-operative course was uneventful; for a few hours the patient had pain in the left buttock. About three months later she complained of pain in her left great toe, but this rapidly subsided.

Five months after operation, her legs were of normal appearance as far as her circulation was concerned; she had no pain but clinically there was slight weakness of the left flexor hallucis longus.

Nine months after operation, there was no abnormality to be found. The circulation was improved, but was still not completely normal, and she had had no chilblains.

Discussion

The preliminary radiographical examinations had quite clearly demonstrated what was actually found at operation. The curious 'narrow, negative midline shadow' seen in the myelogram was found to be due to the thin fibrous band within the dura lying in the midline cleft in the spinal cord. It was attached to the dura internally, both at the cranial edge of the bone pillar and posteriorly. It was not possible at operation to determine clearly if the fibrous band was also attached to the dura overlying the posterior aspect of the vertebral body. The myodil column divided about 1 cm. below the bony spur because of the obliquity of the spur whose anterior attachment was more caudal than its posterior attachment.

As Matson *et al.* (1950) have pointed out, the septum passing antero-posteriorly across the spinal canal may not be sufficiently calcified in young children to show on a radiograph. If the presence of a septum is suspected, repeat examinations will be necessary later on, or, as our findings showed, the condition can be demonstrated by myelography and unnecessary delay in making a diagnosis thereby avoided. Also there are two other radiographical pointers which can indicate the possibility of diastematomyelia: increased inter-pedicular distance and spina bifida. Herren and Edwards (1940) found that the spinal canal is widened where there is congenital abnormality of the cord, and both Neuhauser, Wittenborg and Dehlinger (1950) and Cowie (1951) have pointed out that increased inter-pedicular distance without pedicular erosion is a sign of congenital spinal cord abnormality and is present in cases of diastematomyelia. If the views of Kapsenberg and Lookeren (1949) and Cameron (1957) on developmental anomalies of the spinal cord are accepted, it seems to be impossible for diastematomyelia, with or without a septum, to occur without a very close relationship to spina bifida.

The decision to operate was based on the knowledge that the effects of traction on the cord were likely to be progressive. There was no reason to delay by watching to find out if indeed there would be progressive deterioration of circulation and muscle tone in the lower limbs, particularly since these effects may not appear until the age of 23 years; they may be rapid and irreversible. It is these facts which make it important to make the diagnosis early and to act to correct the anomaly. In this patient, the conus medullaris of the spinal cord was lying at a lower level (lower border of L.V.4) than is normally found at the time of birth, a state which was not demonstrated pre-operatively, and its retention at this level had so far produced remarkably little neurological result.

It is not possible to explain satisfactorily the mildness of the neurological effects of the lesion. They were not in themselves causing any disability but were noticed quite by chance during a clinical examination for another complaint. The circulatory deficiency had been present for many years. There are, however, various factors to be considered, the age at which there is the greatest differential rate of growth of bone column and spinal cord, the point of fixation of the cord and the firmness with which the cord is tethered.

There does not appear to be any information about the levels of the conus in the years between birth and completion of growth, and it is not known whether the bone column and spinal cord maintain the same rate of growth relative to each other throughout the growing period or whether, for example, they grow equally for a period and then the bone column grows much faster. Since the bone column and spinal cord are developed in close association with each other in embryo it is likely that they are closely associated throughout the post-natal growing period and it is reasonable to argue from what is known about the growth of the skeleton. The period of greatest increase in height is around puberty and it is likely to be at this time that the 'ascent' of the cord is most rapid. The dura and arachnoid normally grow at almost the same rate as the bone but keep a definite relationship with the spinal cord in that the nerve roots in the adult have only a short course within the main dural sheath before acquiring their own individual sheaths. The dura therefore is itself not normally under any great traction force and actively lengthens as the bone column grows, just as do the spinal nerves (Streeter, 1919). The spinal cord also grows, but more slowly than the bone; its length at the end of the growth period is greater than at birth. If for any reason the bone age of the individual is less than normal, the ascent of the cord will be equally delayed. In the present case the bone age was normal and the child had not attained puberty. Since there is relatively less ascent of the spinal cord at the cranial end than at the caudal end of the vertebral canal, as shown by the obliquity of the nerve roots in their course to the neural foramina, fixation caudally is more likely to produce neurological signs. In the present case the point of fixation of the cord was relatively low in the bone column and relatively high in the spinal cord but the cord was not immobilized. The bone septum was situated in a division of the spinal cord of about 1·5 cm. length and was at the caudal end of the division; when the septum was removed, the cord did not alter its position. This suggests that the spinal cord had already been able to ascend to a small extent but would in a short time have been prevented from ascending further except at the expense of the elasticity of the cord tissues with resultant pressure effects and increased neurological signs.

As already mentioned, this child was small for her age. Using the crown-rump measurement, but not as accurately as Provis and Ellis (1955), our case was 64·9 cm. long in the stem which corresponds with the average of 64·5 cm. and 66·9 cm. found in Edinburgh girls at mean ages of 6·54 and 7·49 years respectively. Her bone age as estimated by radiographs of her elbows and wrists was the same as her true age so that the delay in development of neurological signs cannot be ascribed to late bone growth.

Summary

Diastematomyelia is a congenital division of the spinal cord in its length. A case is described where there was an associated bone spur passing across the spinal canal in the lumbar region between the two halves of the cord.

The operation findings are described and discussed in relation to the clinical signs and to the radiological appearances. Preliminary tomography and myelography clearly demonstrated the anatomical state but the clinical signs bore no relation to the abnormal position of the spinal cord, fixed as it was in the vertebral canal by a bone septum, with the conus medullaris at a level below that normally found at birth. The various factors associated with this abnormality are discussed in detail in an attempt to explain the paucity of neurological signs in this case.

The need for early diagnosis and preventive surgery in cases of diastematomyelia transfixed by a septum is stressed.

Our grateful thanks are due to Dr. Sheila Cameron, radiologist, and Dr. Gordon Gryspeerdt, neuro-radiologist, Newcastle General Hospital, for their assistance in the diagnosis of this case.

REFERENCES

Benstead, J. G. (1953). *J. Path. Bact.*, **66**, 553.
Cameron, A. H. (1957). *Ibid.*, **73**, 195 and 213.
Cowie, T. N. (1951). *Brit. J. Radiol.*, **24**, 156.
Herren, R. Y. and Edwards, J. E. (1940). *Arch. Path. (Chicago)*, **30**, 1203
Kapsenberg, J. G. and Lookeren, J. A. van (1949). *Acta Anat. (Basel)*, **7**, 366.
Matson, D. D., Woods, R. P., Campbell, J. B. and Ingraham, F. D. (1950). *Pediatrics*, **6**, 98.
Neuhauser, E. B. D., Wittenborg, M. H. and Dehlinger, K. (1950). *Radiology*, **54**, 659.
Provis, H. S. and Ellis, R. W. B. (1955). *Arch. Dis. Childh.*, **30**, 328.
Streeter, G. L. (1919). *Amer. J. Anat.*, **25**, 1.

A CASE OF CUSHING'S SYNDROME IN AN INFANT

BY

E. GOLDBLATT and A. H. SNAITH

From The Hospital for Sick Children, Great Ormond Street, London

(RECEIVED FOR PUBLICATION JUNE 2, 1958)

Cushing's syndrome is rare in infancy. The present case is reported because of the unusual pathology and because to our knowledge this is the first case in which bilateral adrenalectomy has been carried out in an infant.

Case History

The patient, a girl, was born after a normal full-term pregnancy. Her birth weight was 8 lb. 4 oz. (75th percentile) and at 12 months, when she was apparently normal, her weight was 24 lb (75th percentile). Two months later she was brought to hospital because of her rapid gain in weight and increasing irritability. During this period she had gained 4 lb. 14 oz. and weighed 28 lb. 14 oz. (97th percentile). Thus the onset of her condition was short and dramatic (Figs. 1 and 2).

On examination (Fig. 2) she was obese, with a buffalo hump, her face was plethoric and she had an acneiform rash. There was slight hirsutes of the face and back. No striae were present. She had a small umbilical hernia. The height was 30 in. and the span 30¼ in. (50th percentile). The blood pressure was 140/90 mm. Hg (normal average 96/66 mm. Hg). On radiographic examination the bone age was normal and there was no osteoporosis of the spine, skull or long bones. An intravenous pyelogram suggested that there might be enlargement of the right adrenal. Glucose tolerance test: fasting blood sugar, 89 mg. %; sugar readings were 111, 111, 117, 137 and 125 mg. %. The serum sodium was 147 mEq./1, the serum potassium 4·4 mEq./1, the blood cholesterol 154 mg. %; serum proteins were 7·0 g. % and the α and γ globulins were slightly raised. The haemoglobin was 110% (16·3 g. %), and the white count normal except that no eosinophils were present. R.B.C. were 4,720,000/c.mm. Details of steroid excretion are given in Table 1.

In the expectation that an adrenal tumour would be found an exploratory laparotomy was undertaken by Mr. D. Innes Williams. Cortisone 25 mg. per day was given orally in divided doses for two days prior to the operation. Both adrenal glands were found to be slightly enlarged and nodular. The left adrenal was

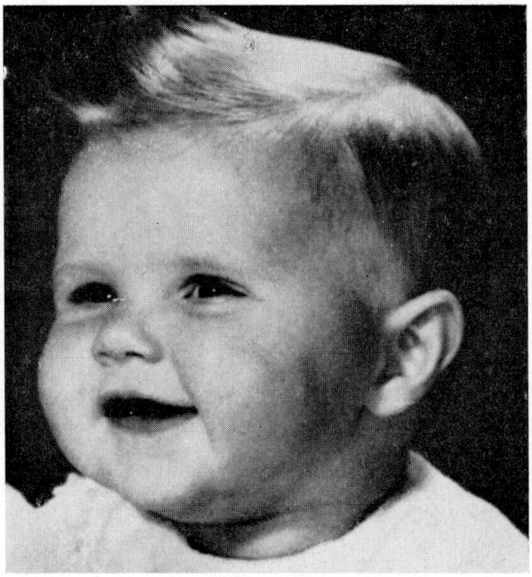

FIG. 1.—Apparently normal at 8 months old.

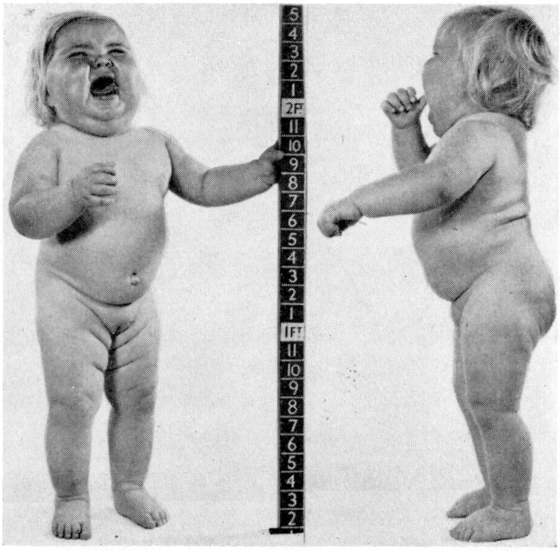

FIG. 2.—On admission aged 14 months.

TABLE 1

STEROID EXCRETION IN GIRL AGED 14 MONTHS WITH CUSHING'S SYNDROME DUE TO BILATERAL MULTIPLE ADRENOCORTICAL ADENOMATA

Stage and Treatment	17-Keto-steroids (mg./24 h.)	17-Hydroxy-steroids (mg./24 hr.)	17-Ketogenic-steroids (mg./24 hr.)
Normal for age ..	0·5	1·2	2·0
Before first operation ..	2·9	9·7	21·3
Following removal of left adrenal ..	2·4	4·2	6·0
After 5 days of:			
ACTH 25 mg./day ..	2·9	9·9	15·8
9-*a*-fluorohydrocortisone 500 µg. b.d. ..	1·6	10·4	7·5
Methyl testosterone 10 mg./day ..	3·4	3·4	8·8
Stilboestrol 1 mg. per day	2·4	3·8	6·0

Before operation aldosterone excretion was <2 µg./24 hours, total oestrogen excretion $<1\cdot0$ µg./24 hours and urinary gonadotrophins <5 m.µ./24 hours (within normal limits).

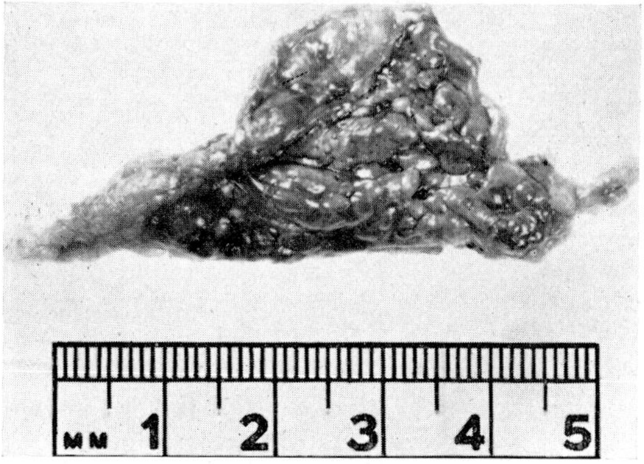

FIG. 3.—Left adrenal. Note multiple nodules.

removed (Figs. 3, 4a and 4b). The liver was large and fatty. There was a moderate hypokalaemic alkalosis for the first week after operation, during which time 1 g. of potassium chloride per day was given and cortisone was continued in the same dosage as before. Otherwise, the post-operative course was uneventful. After further investigation it was decided to remove the right adrenal. The day before the second operation 50 mg. of cortisone were given by mouth and on the day of the operation 50 mg. b.d. of cortisone were given intramuscularly. The post-operative course was uneventful, cortisone was gradually reduced and the patient was discharged two months later, by which time her appearance had become much more normal. At present she is being maintained on 20 mg. of cortisone acetate and 1 g. of salt a day. Three months after discharge from hospital she was again admitted, suffering from avulsion of two finger tips which she had caught in a train door. She withstood this trauma without any evidence of metabolic upset.

Further Investigations. After removal of the left adrenal there was a decline in steroid excretion but the clinical condition remained unchanged. The influence of ACTH, fluorohydrocortisone, methyl testosterone and of stilboestrol on steroid excretion was then studied (Table 1) and it was concluded that none of these hormones, in the dose given, strikingly influenced secretion by the remaining gland. The great increase in

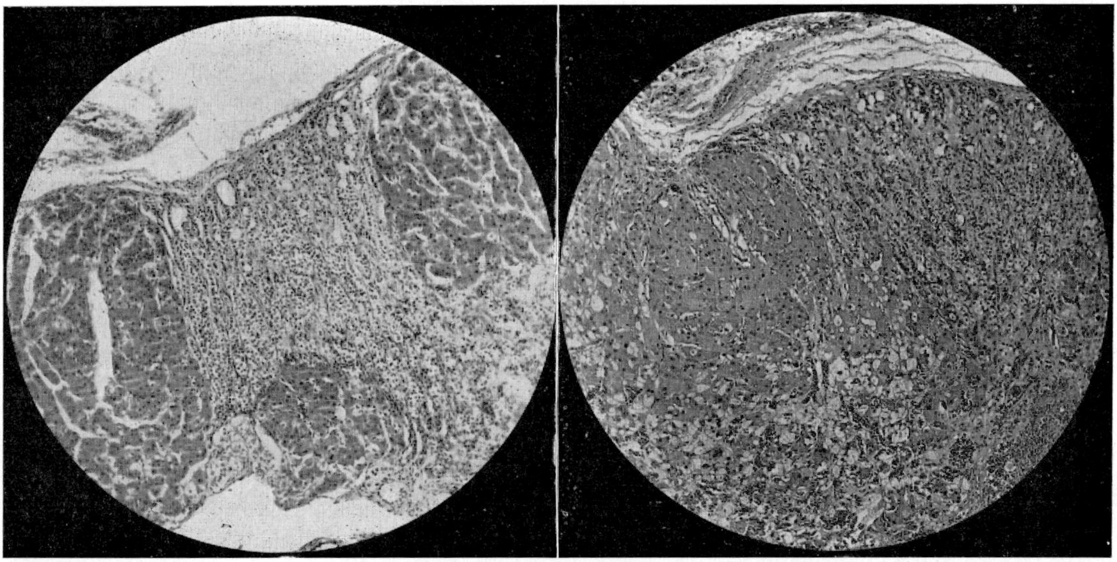

(*a*) (*b*)

FIGS. 4a and 4b.—Photomicrographs of adrenal glands × 60, illustrating multiple adenomatous nodules and intervening areas of atrophic cortical tissue.

17-hydroxysteroid excretion which might have been expected in a case of adrenal hyperplasia did not occur after the administration of A.C.T.H.

Discussion

In children Cushing's syndrome is usually due to tumour (Guin and Gilbert, 1956); a case of adrenal hyperplasia has recently been described in a child aged 8½ by Hubble and Illingworth (1957) and in a case of the same age reported by Chute, Robinson and Donohue (1949) multiple bilateral adenomatous nodules of the type present in this case were found at autopsy. The aetiology of adrenal hyperplasia with Cushing's syndrome remains obscure. Elevated blood ACTH levels have not been demonstrated and it is possible that the adrenal glands are unduly sensitive to ACTH. Jailer, Longson and Christy (1956) have suggested that the pituitary secretes in excess a hypothetical corticotrophin-potentiating substance. The response to ACTH administration in the present case was moderate, and the histological appearance of normal adrenocortical cells adjacent to nodules of abnormal cells could be compatible with the view that secretion by the abnormal cells was in fact to a large extent autonomous.

In view of the age of the patient the possibility that the hyperplastic glands were the result of abnormal development of the foetal cortices was considered. It has been suggested that the human foetal cortex may be dependent upon pituitary gonadotrophins, as is the 'X' zone in the mouse (Chester Jones, 1957). No change in steroid excretion was observed to follow the administration of stilboestrol or methyl testosterone, which might have been expected to suppress gonadotrophin secretion. No gonadotrophins could be detected in the urine.

Irradiation of the pituitary gland was not considered appropriate treatment in view of the age of the patient, since to be effective such treatment might interfere with the secretion of other trophic hormones; moreover the response to ACTH did not indicate that a diminution of ACTH secretion would necessarily be of great benefit.

Adrenal enucleation is a procedure which may be successfully carried out in the rat, a new cortex regenerating from solitary cortical cells which adhere to the capsule (Chester Jones, 1957). Such a procedure, if practicable, would have been of interest in this patient since it might have been observed whether normal or abnormal cells regenerated, and thus, perhaps, some light might have been thrown on the fundamental aetiological problem in adrenal hyperplasia. However, it does not seem surgically possible to remove the cortex so as to leave the capsule behind as an intact bag, as in the rat. Furthermore, there is some doubt whether adrenal regeneration occurs after enucleation in the human subject (Dempster, 1955). Consequently, total adrenalectomy, which is the treatment of choice in the older patient was undertaken here with the intention of maintaining the patient on cortisone for the rest of her life. The long-term prognosis remains to be seen (Fig. 5).

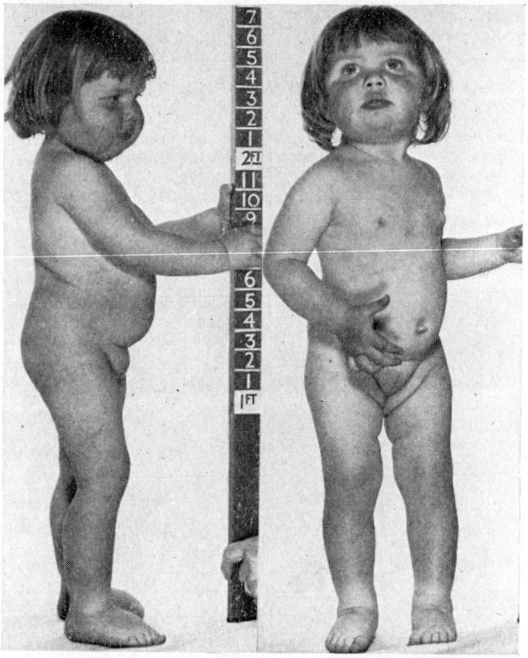

FIG. 5.—Five months after total bilateral adrenalectomy.

We wish to thank Dr. A. P. Norman for permission to publish this case, Dr. I. Chester Jones with whom we discussed the possibility of adrenal enucleation for his advice, and Mr. Derek Martin, of the Department of Medical Illustration, for the photographs.

REFERENCES

Chute, A. L., Robinson, G. C. and Donohue, W. L. (1949). *J. Pediat.*, **34**, 20.
Dempster, W. J. (1955). *Brit. J. Surg.*, **42**, 540.
Guin, G. H and Gilbert, E. F. (1956). *A.M.A. J. Dis. Child.*, **92**, 297.
Hubble, D. V. and Illingworth, R. S. (1957). *Arch. Dis. Childh.*, **32**, 285.
Jailer, J. W., Longson, D. and Christy, N. R. (1956). *J. Clin. Endocr.*, **16**, 1276.
Jones, I. Chester (1957). *The Adrenal Cortex*, p. 112 Cambridge.

EPIDEMICS OF GASTRO-ENTERITIS ASSOCIATED WITH *ESCH. COLI* O119 INFECTION

BY

K. HUGH-JONES* and G. I. M. ROSS†

From the Westminster Children's Hospital and Westminster Medical School

(RECEIVED FOR PUBLICATION JUNE 23, 1958)

Introduction

Three outbreaks of gastro-enteritis associated with the presence of *Esch. coli* O119 in the stools occurred among the infants in a baby ward between September, 1954, and February, 1956. In these epidemics altogether 45 infants were found to be infected. During the whole period the organism was also isolated from 13 out-patients and three children in other wards. This paper describes the frequency with which the organism was found in the stools of those at risk, the association between this finding and symptoms, some biochemical and antigenic characteristics of the *Esch. coli* O119, together with the results of antibiotic and sulphonamide sensitivity tests and a note of comparison with the clinical response.

Bacteriological Methods

Swabs of faeces were taken from each infant on admission and thereafter on every Monday and Thursday while in the ward.

Cultures. The routine swabs were plated on MacConkey agar and desoxycholate citrate agar. Swabs from those known to have diarrhoea were inoculated also into selenite F broth from which subcultures were made on to desoxycholate citrate agar after 24 hours' incubation. All the *Esch. coli* O119 strains isolated were stored on Dorset egg slopes for further tests.

Antigenic Identification. (*a*) O ANTIGENS. During the first year of this investigation all faecal specimens were examined for the presence of 10 different O types of *Esch. coli.* These types were O25, O26, O55, O86, O111, O114, O119, O125, O126 and O128. The antisera initially used for this purpose were most kindly supplied by Dr. J. Smith of Aberdeen. Later, sera prepared in this laboratory and polyvalent and individual O antisera supplied by the Standards Laboratory of the Central Public Health Laboratory were also used.

Mixtures of lactose-fermenting colonies of gram negative bacilli on MacConkey agar were tested for agglutination on Murray slides with these sera. Pure colonies of the various types of *Esch. coli* were then selected by slide agglutination, if necessary after further subculture. Their identity was finally determined by tube agglutination tests showing that, after boiling for one hour to destroy K antigen, they were agglutinated to the titre of the O antiserum. One of the earliest strains of O119 isolated in the first epidemic was kindly confirmed as such by Dr. Joan Taylor.

After the first year of this study tests were made routinely only for *Esch. coli* types O26, O55, O111, O119 and O128 as the numbers of the other types encountered did not justify the considerable extra work involved in searching for them. In all cases of gastro-enteritis, however, when tests were negative for these five types of *Esch. coli* and for salmonellae and shigellae, the additional antisera against the other five *Esch. coli* types were used to try and identify a possible pathogen in the stools.

(*b*) H ANTIGENS. One strain of O119 isolated in the first epidemic was found by Dr. Joan Taylor to be type H6. Then, using antiserum kindly provided by Dr. Taylor, other strains were typed by tube agglutination. Motility was readily obtained with only one or two passages through Craigie tubes.

Biochemical Tests. The fermentative ability of all the strains of typable *Esch. coli* isolated during the period of the study was tested in 1% peptone water sugars. Sugars were incubated up to 21 days if acid had not been produced before that time. Tests such as indole, Voges-Proskauer and methyl red were carried out by the standard procedures described in Topley and Wilson (1946).

Sensitivity Tests. Antibiotic sensitivity tests were performed immediately after the isolation of each strain of typable *Esch. coli* using tablets (Evans Medical Supplies Limited) containing penicillin, streptomycin, aureomycin, terramycin and chloramphenicol. Subsequently the exact bacteriostatic concentrations of these antibiotics, and of neomycin, polymyxin, tetracycline and sulphathiazole were determined by plating each organism on agar containing doubling concentrations of these agents. The sulphonamide sensitivity tests were made

* St. Bartholomew's Hospital, London, E.C.1.
† Ashford Hospital, Ashford, Middlesex.

using the medium recommended by Jewell and Pearmain (1954) but with 2% horse blood added.

General Background

These epidemics occurred in the baby ward of Westminster Children's Hospital. The ward consisted of 11 separate cubicles, one of which sometimes took two infants and seven of which were nursing-mother flats. All these cubicles were entirely separate rooms, each with a wash basin. Individual nurse's and doctor's gowns were provided for each baby and the usual barrier nursing techniques were used whenever attending to the children. Every effort was made to avoid admitting cases of gastro-enteritis to the ward, but during the period under review four infants were finally diagnosed as such and a pathogenic *Esch. coli* other than O119 demonstrated in their faeces. Two were infected with an O55, one with an O111 and one with an O128.

Clinical Findings During the Survey

First Epidemic. PRELIMINARY SURVEY. During July and August, 1954, several babies in the ward developed gastro-enteritis and in September testing for pathogenic *Esch. coli* was first begun. Four children (Cases 1-4), who had or had had gastro-enteritis recently, were found to be excreting *Esch. coli* O119. Because of this the ward was shut and this investigation begun.

MAIN SURVEY. The ward was closed for four days in Week 2 (Fig. 1) when each cubicle was scrubbed, fumigated with formaldehyde and then aired for 24 hours. On opening the ward entirely new patients were admitted. From this point onwards the routine swabbing on admission, and thereafter twice weekly, was begun and daily enquiry made regarding each infant's stools. In all, some 370 swabs were examined from 51 infants. During the first week that the ward was open (Week 3) all the children had negative swab results.

Within 12 days of reopening the ward (Week 4) *Esch. coli* O119 was demonstrated in the stools of a breast fed baby (Case 5) and the steady spread of the infection can be followed from case to case in Fig. 1. A further 22 babies were infected. Case 3 was readmitted in the ninth and reinfected in the eleventh week (Fig. 1) bringing the total to the

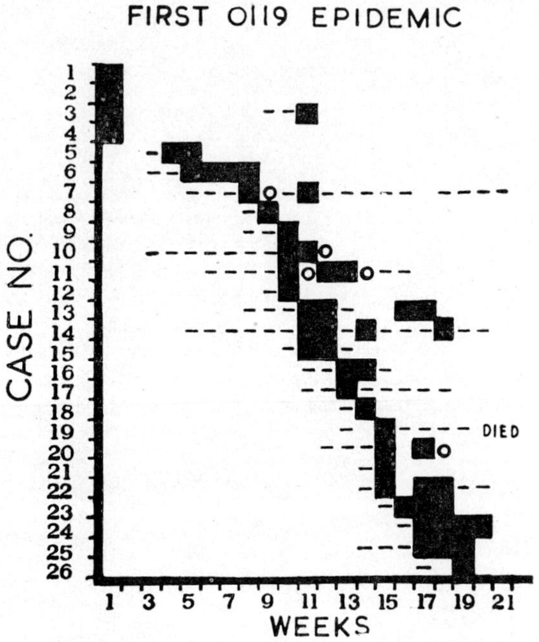

FIG. 1.—The results of culture of the faeces in each case in each week of the epidemic: ■ *Esch. coli* O119; — No typable *Esch. coli*; O No *Esch. coli*.

23 cases shown in Table 1. Fig. 2 shows the number of babies in the ward during each week, the number with positive cultures and the number with definite gastro-enteritis.

Once the organism had been demonstrated again after reopening the ward it will be seen that at least

TABLE 1

Group	Criteria			Number of Infants			
	Admission Swab	Further Swabs	Clinical Evidence of Gastro-enteritis	First Epidemic	Second Epidemic	Third Epidemic	Total
I	Negative	Negative	None	28	33	14	75
II	Negative	Positive	None	8	4	2	14
III	Negative	Positive	Mild	5	2	0	7
IV	Negative	Positive	Definite	10	8	2	20
Total infants at risk in each epidemic				51	47	18	116

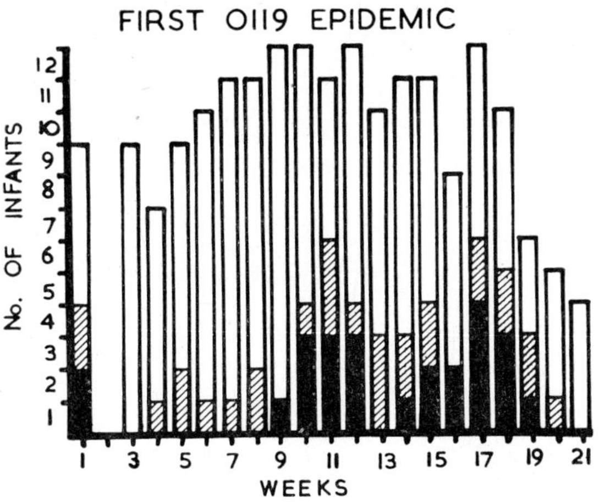

FIG. 2.—The total number of infants, those with *Esch. coli* O119 in faeces and those with gastro-enteritis, in each week of the epidemic: ■ Number with definite gastro-enteritis; ▨ Number with *Esch. coli* O119 in faeces; □ Total number of infants in ward.

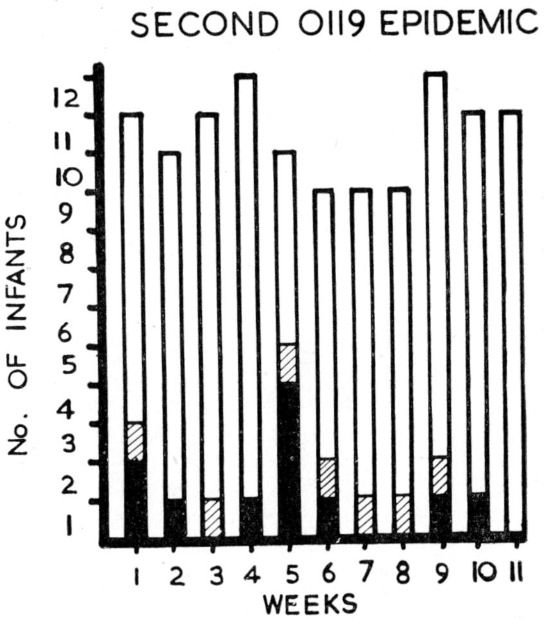

FIG. 4.—The total number of infants, those with *Esch. coli* O119 in faeces and those with gastro-enteritis, in each week of the epidemic: ■ Number with definite gastro-enteritis; ▨ Number with *Esch. coli* O119 in faeces; □ Total number of infants in ward.

one child was excreting it in each of the remaining weeks of the epidemic. There were two peaks (Weeks 11 and 17) during which 50% of the children had positive cultures. Because of the second peak of cross-infection no further babies were admitted to the ward, and so the epidemic died out at the end of January, 1955, after more than 20 weeks and the ward was then closed. During this epidemic one child attending Out-patients with gastro-enteritis was found to be infected with *Esch. coli* O119.

Interim Period between First and Second Epidemics. The ward was shut for two weeks for thorough cleaning and repainting; during this time there was a vigorous overhauling of nursing procedures and structural improvements were planned. Although no serious deficiencies in the methods of preventing cross-infections were brought to light, the discussion and general awareness no doubt improved individual techniques. It was also decided for the future that even the mildest case of gastro-enteritis due to pathogenic *Esch. coli* in that ward should be treated energetically with antibiotics.

The ward was reopened in February, 1955, and no case of *Esch. coli* O119 infection was detected for 15 weeks. During this period some 300 faecal samples from 48 infants were examined.

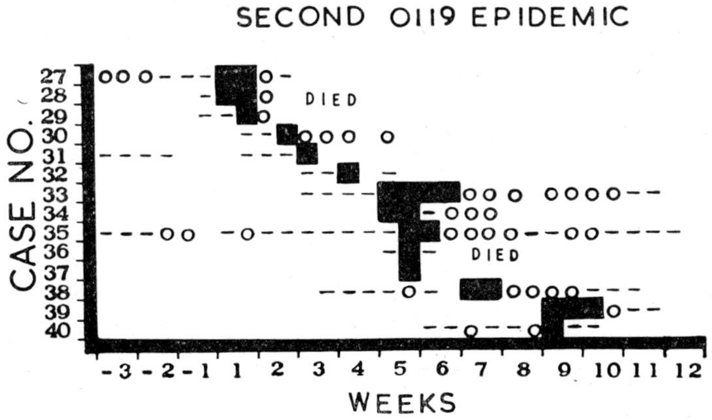

FIG. 3.—The results of culture of the faeces in each case in each week of the epidemic: ■ *Esch. coli* O119; — No typable *Esch. coli*; O No *Esch. coli*.

Second Epidemic. On June 6, 1955, two babies (Cases 27 and 28) developed gastro-enteritis and were found to have *Esch. coli* O119 in their stools on the same day (Week 1, Fig. 3). Fig. 3 shows the spread of the in-infection from case to case during the 10 weeks that the epidemic lasted. The organism was demonstrated in the faeces of at least one infant during each week except Week 8. During this week Case 38 continued to have diarrhoea though no *Esch. coli* was grown from his faeces; terramycin was being given at that time. Fig. 4

shows the number of babies in the ward, the number with positive cultures for *Esch. coli* O119 and the number with definite gastro-enteritis each week. The peak incidence of infection was in Week 5 when 50% of the children had positive cultures. In all, 14 infants were found to be infected.

The source of this infection was not known. It was unlikely that the organism had remained alive in the ward during the 18 weeks since the previous epidemic. The most likely origin was Case 27 who was admitted with whooping cough and treated with terramycin for the first three weeks. Towards the end of this course of treatment the child had some diarrhoea but this then stopped. Two weeks later, however, it recurred and *Esch. coli* O119 was first demonstrated in the faeces. Alternatively the organism may have been carried by a member of the staff from the first epidemic; or it may have been introduced into the ward, directly by the admission of an unidentified carrier, or indirectly by a member of the staff from a child with diarrhoea attending Out-patients. However, as no *Esch. coli* O119 was demonstrated either in the ward or from Out-patients before June 6 the source of infection must remain uncertain. During the epidemic the organism was found in the faeces of one infant in another ward and of five children, two in one family, attending Out-patients. It seems possible that the epidemic was part of a more widespread infection in the locality. The epidemic died out in the tenth week and thereafter till the ward was closed in Week 12 for structural alterations, *Esch. coli* O119 was not again demonstrated. During this epidemic some 180 faecal specimens from 47 infants in the ward were examined.

Interim Period between Second and Third Epidemics. This period was of 26 weeks during which over 800 faecal samples were examined. Eight infants were found to be infected with *Esch. coli* O119. One was admitted to a different ward from that in which the epidemics occurred and the others were out-patients. Seven had attended because of gastro-enteritis, the eighth was a 4-year-old symptom-free contact. Six of these cases occurred during November, 1955.

Third Epidemic. This epidemic began in February, 1956, and continued for 10 days. Four infants only in the baby ward were infected out of 18 at risk. One of these had been in the ward 10 days previously and presented with diarrhoea as an out-patient five days after the end of the epidemic. He was found to be excreting *Esch. coli* O119. It seems likely that he was infected while in hospital and only developed symptoms and positive stools after discharge. The infection appeared to have been introduced by an infant who was admitted with otitis externa. The first swab taken on admission showed the presence of the organism. This child was discharged home after five days in hospital. She was still excreting the organism in her stools but was always without any symptoms of infection. The other three infants had negative stools on admission and were presumably infected from the first child. Two of them had definite gastro-enteritis.

General Features

Incidence of Gastro-enteritis and Mortality in the Infected Infants. It can be seen from Table 1 that during the three epidemics in the ward 41 infants were found to be infected out of 116 at risk, and of those infected seven had mild symptoms and 20 definite gastro-enteritis. In this analysis Cases 1 to 4 are not included as they occurred during the preliminary survey.

In the first epidemic one child died of gastro-enteritis. In the second two died, both with severe congenital abnormalities. One had a myelomeningocoele and hydrocephalus and his death was accelerated by gastro-enteritis. The other had congenital heart disease and died aged 12 days in congestive heart failure.

Carrier State. The second group in Table 1 of 14 children who were excreting the organism but remained symptom-free supports the suggestion that a carrier state exists as it does in other intestinal infections. The finding of the two older symptom-free children aged 4 and 6 in Out-patients also supports this. Although these children are well in themselves they are a danger to others. This is especially so because the organism can often be demonstrated in almost pure culture from their stools. Such a child seemed to be the origin of the third epidemic.

Incubation Period. To try and estimate the incubation period the time relationship between the first positive culture and the development of symptoms was studied, and also the length of time at risk was calculated, i.e. in the ward before the first positive culture developed. Out of the 20 infants with definite gastro-enteritis, five developed symptoms on the day of the first positive culture, four one day after, two two days after and one three, four, nine, 10 and 11 days after. Four developed symptoms before their first positive culture, one on the day before and the others on the fifth, sixth and seventh days before.

Remembering that cultures were made only twice weekly, the fact that 13 out of the 20 developed symptoms within four days of the organism being demonstrated suggests a short incubation period. This is supported by the fact that 60% of those that did become infected were found to be excreting the organism within a fortnight, and 20% within five days, of exposure to infection in the ward.

Age. The age incidence in the epidemics can be seen in Fig. 5. Because this ward was for babies there were more children in the youngest age group; nearly 80% of the admissions were under 6 months. Most of those that became infected did so during their second to fifth months of life—a time when infants are particularly susceptible to infection, which may be related to the low level of gamma globulin in their blood. The oldest child whom we found to be infected with an O119 was aged 6 years; he was symptom free. The oldest with symptoms was aged 2½ years. Both were out-patients.

Feeding. About one-fifth of the 116 infants at risk were entirely breast fed while in hospital but of the 41 infected infants only one was breast fed and that child was symptom-free (Case 5). Although the mothers were nearly always admitted with their babies, the routine nursing procedures were still carried out by the staff.

Treatment. First Epidemic. Systematic treatment with sulphonamides or antibiotics of every infant found to be infected with O119 was not given, as the policy of treating all cases however mild, or all carriers, had not yet been accepted. Several infants received more than one course of treatment with one or more drugs while in hospital. These courses were given as treatment either for the original cause of admission or for gastro-enteritis.

Nine infants received sulphonamide orally, two streptomycin orally and seven penicillin systemically; all continued to excrete the organism while on treatment. One infant received chloramphenicol orally; he had negative swabs during treatment but was found to be excreting the organism again within seven days of stopping the drug.

Second Epidemic. Four infants were discharged from hospital within a day or so of the organism being discovered in their stools and a fifth died; these were all untreated.

Seven infants with *Esch. coli* O119 infection were treated with terramycin and two with aureomycin followed by terramycin. The dosage of terramycin ranged from 10-16 mg./lb./day (mean 12 mg./lb./day) for four to 27 days (mean 12 days). In the nine treated patients all types of *Esch. coli* disappeared completely from the stools (Fig. 3). Once the stools

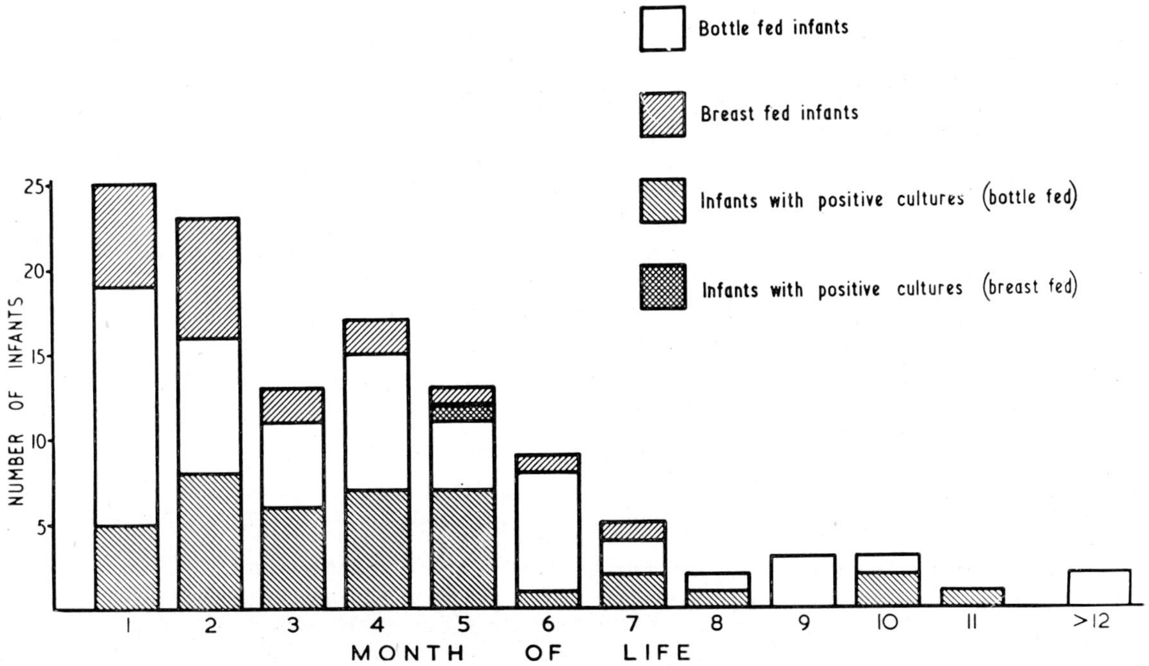

Fig. 5—The age incidence of all the infants in the three epidemics, those with positive cultures and those breast or bottle fed.

had become negative for O119 they remained so during the time the infants were in hospital.

THIRD EPIDEMIC. The two children with symptoms were given terramycin, one receiving 50 mg./lb./day, the other 120 mg./lb./day. In both the cultures became negative. One had previously been treated with sulphonamide (125 mg./lb./day) for nine days with no effect.

Sensitivity of the *Esch. coli* O119 Strains to Antibiotics and Sulphonamides. The sensitivity of the *Esch. coli* O119 strains isolated from 53 of the 61 infected infants were tested. All 53 strains had similar sensitivities. The bacteriostatic concentrations of the different drugs are shown in Table 2.

TABLE 2

SENSITIVITY OF 53 STRAINS OF *ESCH. COLI* O119

Drug	Number of Strains Completely Inhibited by Lowest Concentration of Drug (µg. per ml. or units* per ml.)							(mg. per 100 ml.)	
	1	2	4	8	16	50	100	512	1024
Polymyxin*	22	31							
Terramycin		9	41	3					
Tetracycline		19	30	4					
Chloramphenicol			24	29					
Aureomycin			11	31	11				
Streptomycin			1	27	25				
Neomycin			12	41					
Penicillin*						28	25		
Sulphathiazole								11	42

All were sensitive to therapeutic concentrations of polymyxin, terramycin, aureomycin, tetracycline, chloramphenicol, streptomycin and neomycin and all were resistant to penicillin and sulphathiazole.

In view of the resistance to the sulphonamide it is not surprising that drugs of this group proved so ineffective during the first epidemic. Terramycin given during the second and third epidemics proved effective in eradicating the organisms from the stools. Yet in spite of this the second epidemic continued for 10 weeks.

Biochemical Characteristics of the *Esch. coli* O119 Strains Isolated. Strains isolated from 53 infants were tested. These were the same strains as those on which the sensitivity tests were made. All gave identical reactions. Glucose, maltose, mannitol, lactose, sucrose, arabinose and xylose were fermented with acid and gas production within usually three days. Dulcitol was fermented with acid and gas production after two to 10 days. Variable times in the fermentation of dulcitol were found with even the same strains in several different batches of dulcitol peptone waters. Sorbitol was fermented after one day. Adonitol, inositol, inulin and rhamnose were not fermented in 21 days. All strains were indole positive, urease negative, methyl red positive, Voges-Proskauer negative and failed to liquefy gelatin. Tests for mucus production and haemolysis were negative.

H Antigen Type of the *Esch. coli* O119. One of the earliest strains isolated in the first epidemic was found to be type H6 by Dr. Joan Taylor. We subsequently typed 57 strains isolated from different infants during the period of the investigation and found all to be type H6.

Bacteriological Findings in the Whole Period of the Investigation. The findings in 1,044 specimens from 400 children studied during the three epidemic periods are summarized in Table 3. During these periods a total of 127 specimens from 53 children were found to contain O119 while about 15% contained no *Esch. coli* of any type, usually because of antibiotic or sulphonamide therapy. In the intervals between the three epidemics another 1,224 specimens from 418 children were examined. Of these specimens 260 contained no *Esch. coli* and eight out of 72 specimens with pathogenic types of *Esch. coli* contained O119. In addition 782 faecal swabs from 76 newly born infants in three different maternity units, kindly provided by Dr. I. M. Anderson, were examined. These swabs were taken daily from birth till discharge from hospital. In only one of these swabs, taken from a baby without symptoms on the tenth day after birth, was a typable *Esch. coli* found and this was an O128.

TABLE 3

FINDINGS IN 1044 FAECAL SPECIMENS FROM 400 INFANTS EXAMINED DURING THE THREE *ESCH. COLI* O119 EPIDEMICS

	Baby Ward		Other Wards	Out-patients
	O119+ve	O119−ve		
Infants (No.):				
studied	45	75	66	214
with *Esch. coli* O119	45	0	2	6
with other pathogenic types of *Esch. coli*	5	6	8	15
Specimens (No.):				
total examined	412	186	116	330
with *Esch. coli* O119	105	0	13	9
with no *Esch. coli*	80	30	14	61
with other pathogenic types of *Esch. coli*	15	11	9	18

Incidence of Other Types of *Esch. coli*. The incidence of other types of *Esch. coli* at Westminster Children's Hospital during the whole period of the study is shown in Table 4. In all, 60 infants were found to be infected, of whom 18 were in the baby ward. During the first epidemic five of the 26 infants with O119 infection in the baby ward were found to be infected with another of the 10 types of *Esch. coli* for which tests were being made. At some stage during their stay in hospital three (Cases 17, 20 and 24) were infected with O111 and two with O128 (Cases 5 and 14). One patient (Case 20) was found to be excreting O111 on admission and subsequently infected the other two; one of these was found to be excreting both O111 and O119 at the same time. The O128 was introduced by another infant who at no time excreted O119.

Other types of *Esch. coli* known to be associated with gastro-enteritis in infants were isolated from 12 other infants in the baby ward who were at no time found to be infected with O119. *Esch. coli* O128 was most common.

During the first interim period three of the five in-patients with O128 infection were in the baby ward and the organism appeared to have spread from one to another.

In the second epidemic none of the infants who were infected with O119 were found to have any other typable *Esch. coli* in their faeces. Three other infants in the baby ward and 11 others were found to be excreting one or other of the 10 types as shown in Table 4. The O26 which infected two infants in the baby ward appeared to have spread from one infant to the other.

In the second interim period the three in-patients infected with O55 were in the baby ward and again the infection appeared to spread from one to the other. This organism persisted in the ward into the third epidemic period and infected two of those who later excreted O119.

Evidence of Cross-infection. There were 23 infants infected with O119 during the main part of the first epidemic. Therefore the organism must have passed from one child to another at least 22 times; there was also evidence of cross-infection twice with O111 and once with O128. That is at least 25 incidents of cross-infection among 51 infants in 16 weeks. During the second epidemic there were 13 cross-infections due to O119 and one due to O26 among 47 infants in 11 weeks. In the three weeks of the third epidemic there were 18 at risk and three incidents of cross-infection. In the first interim period there were two examples due to O128 and in the second two due to O55. However, one other pathogenic type of *Esch. coli* was found in the ward during the second epidemic and three others during the second interim period without any spread.

Totalling up the number of days each child was at risk in the ward, there were 1,175 child-days in the first epidemic, 818 in the second and 231 in the third. Therefore there was one incident of cross-infection for every 47, 58 and 77 child-days in the three epidemics respectively.

These facts show a decreasing incidence of cross-infection. This could be due either to preventive measures or to decreasing virulence and infectivity of the organism. Table 1 does not show any decline in the incidence of symptoms in the later epidemics nor do the mortality figures suggest any decrease in the virulence of the organism as the type of infants at risk were very similar throughout the whole period. Therefore it was felt that the improved control of the infections was due to the measures taken to cut down cross-infection.

Improvements to Reduce Cross-infection. The general precautions against infectious diseases in force at the time of the first epidemic have been described earlier. During the first interim period the following improvements were made: (1) ample paper hand towels were provided; (2) taps were adjusted to be easily operated by elbow; (3) cello-

TABLE 4

NUMBERS OF INFANTS INFECTED WITH VARIOUS *ESCH. COLI* TYPES

Esch. coli Type	1st O119 Epidemic Sept. 1954-Jan. 1955		Interval		2nd O119 Epidemic June-Aug. 1955		Interval		3rd O119 Epidemic Feb. 1956	
	I.P.*	O.P.†	I.P.	O.P.	I.P.	O.P.	I.P.	O.P.	I.P.	O.P.
O119	28	1	0	0	15	5	1	7	4	0
O128	3	3	5	2	0	2	1	2	0	0
O55	1	2	2	1	2	0	3	2	2	0
O26	3	0	0	1	2	1	1	1	0	0
O111	3	0	0	0	0	1	2	2	0	0
O126	0	1	0	0	0	4	0	0	0	0
O86	0	1	0	0	2	0	0	0	0	0
O125	1	0	0	0	0	0	0	0	0	0
O114	0	0	0	0	0	0	1	0	0	0

* I.P.=In-patient in any ward of the hospital.
† O.P.=Out-patient.

phane was incorporated in face masks; (4) nurses responsible for making feeds no longer had nursing duties in the ward, leaving one sister, two staff nurses and eight student nurses to look after 12 babies. This staff was no longer called upon to help at night in Out-patients or in emergencies in other wards, but worked only in the baby ward.

The major structural improvements could not be carried out till August and September, 1955, after the second epidemic. Then the sluice room was redesigned and unnecessary equipment removed. A large bucket sterilizer and an electric incinerator were installed. Once the former was working, a special bucket and lid for soiled clothes, linens and napkins was provided for each baby. In the sluice room the nurses, using large forceps, put the napkins into one large container and the soiled laundry into another, spraying Domitol into the containers before replacing the lids. The napkins went in the inner bags of the container direct to the laundry. The soiled linen container was emptied down a shute four times a day by the porters. All the linen was then sorted and dispatched to the laundry by separate external staff from a special room in the basement.

A modern stainless steel kitchen sink unit was installed and each baby was given an individual feed tray on which was put his own feed box and lid for bottle and individual teat bowl and lid. All were sterilized before each feed and kept on a separate shelf in a cupboard.

Special precautions against infection were instituted whenever a baby passed suspicious motions. These consisted in using soluble napkins which were burnt in the electric incinerator, soaking all linen in Domitol in a separate container kept on the balcony outside the sluice, providing separate examination trays containing an auriscope, stethoscope, spatulae and torch, and keeping feeds in a separate kitchen. In addition all infants with symptoms of gastro-enteritis were treated with antibiotics, terramycin being usually chosen.

The effectiveness of these precautions has been further tested since the end of the period of this study when babies with gastro-enteritis due to *Esch. coli* O127 were admitted from the Maternity Unit. Although several babies became cross-infected, control was easy and no persistent epidemic occurred.

Discussion

Bacteriology. The association of certain types of *Esch. coli* with gastro-enteritis in infants is now well established. The subject has been thoroughly reviewed by Smith (1955). While some cases of gastro-enteritis may be caused by viruses or some yet unidentified agent there is no doubt in our minds that other cases are not only associated with the presence of certain *Esch. coli* types in the intestine but are actually caused by these organisms.

The first attempts to classify *Esch. coli* isolated from cases of gastro-enteritis used biochemical criteria but this method was insufficiently precise to definitely distinguish pathogenic from non-pathogenic strains. The serological classification of *Esch. coli* by Kauffmann (1947) based on O, K and H antigens allowed a much more exact identification. By the end of 1953 there were already 126 O groups, 62 K antigens and 34 H antigens recognized (Kauffmann, 1954). In *Esch. coli* isolated in gastro-enteritis the K antigens are of the B type, except in O25 strains in which they are of L type, and a constant B antigen appears to be associated with each O group. Each OB type may have variable H (flagellar) antigens or none at all. Variation in H antigen, then, allows subdivision of OB types which is useful in epidemiological studies.

Numerous papers incriminating at least 12 different O types of *Esch. coli* as causes of gastro-enteritis have been published. Kauffmann (1947) showed that strains collected from gastro-enteritis cases by Adam as early as 1923 and 1927 were type O111:B4 while those isolated by Bray (1945) were type O55:B5. Types O26:B6, O86:B7, O125:B15, O126:B16 and O128:B12 were found later by Taylor and Charter (1952) in infants with gastro-enteritis. More recently cases due to type O127:B8 have been described by Cooper, Walters, Keller, Sutherland and Wiseman (1955) and due to O114 by Rogers and Cracknell (1956) and Charter (1956).

Esch. coli later shown to be type O119:B14 were first isolated from calves with 'scours' (Wramby, 1948). Scours is a disease of calves in which fever, diarrhoea and pneumonia occur in the first few days after birth. Smith (1953) reported the association of this organism with diarrhoea in 21 infants in Aberdeen during 1952. Thomas and Charter (1956) record the isolation of O119 from one infant but no other paper describing this organism as a cause of epidemics of gastro-enteritis is known to us though a number of outbreaks have occurred (Smith, 1955).

The biochemical reactions of the Aberdeen strains, where tested, were similar to those of the strains isolated by us in Westminster and the strains in both epidemics were type H6 which is the most commonly found flagellar antigen in O119 strains. The virulence of the Aberdeen O119 organisms was comparatively like that of our strains. No deaths occurred in the 21 Aberdeen cases while three deaths occurred in our series of 61 cases and two of those who died had other severe disabilities. In both series the infectivity rate was high. Smith (1953) states that 10 out of 25 contacts became infected. In our first epidemic 45%, in our second 30% and in our third 22% of the infants in the ward exposed to infection were found to be excreting the organism.

The reasons for incriminating *Esch. coli* O119 as the cause of gastro-enteritis in our cases were as follows: (*a*) out of the 20 cases of definite gastro-enteritis in the three epidemics, 12 developed symptoms within two days of the first demonstration of *Bact. coli* O119; (*b*) all had almost pure cultures of the organism from their faeces at the time that they were ill. In convalescence, however, the organism usually became gradually less predominant; (*c*) there was a parallelism in the ward between the incidence of positive swabs and cases of gastro-enteritis (Figs. 2 and 4); (*d*) *Esch. coli* O119 was cultured from all cases of gastro-enteritis in the ward during the epidemics and no other causal organism was found.

In contrast was our finding of negative faecal swabs not only in hundreds of babies without diarrhoea at this hospital, but also in more than 800 swabs from infants in the maternity units mentioned earlier.

Prevention of Cross-infection. The improvements in construction, nursing care and drug treatment in the baby ward, already described, undoubtedly reduced cross-infection but did not at once prevent fresh cases, even though stools were rapidly cleared of all *Esch. coli* (Figs. 1 and 3). This indicates the extreme infectivity of the pathogenic *Esch. coli* which together with the short incubation period allows epidemics to occur even in carefully managed baby wards and leaves no time for delay in taking extra precautions. This great infectivity has been commented on by many authors including Rogers (1951) and Jameson, Mann and Rothfield (1954).

A child excreting the organism, whether with or without symptoms, is a danger to others and should be sought out and isolated. Ideally this requires an isolation-admission ward where children who have been in contact with gastro-enteritis or recently in other hospitals or day nurseries can be swabbed and observed for at least two days. Jameson *et al.* (1954) not only recommended this but did not allow infants who had been previously in a gastro-enteritis ward to be admitted for any condition to a ward other than a gastro-enteritis unit. This was because such infants may be continuous or intermittent carriers of pathogenic *Esch. coli*. For the same reason they did not allow infants who had been in a gastro-enteritis unit to be transferred to nurseries or convalescent homes. Several of our infants continued to excrete O119 for about eight weeks and one infant with O111 infection was still excreting this organism after more than four months. We certainly agree that these infants should be nursed in isolation and we consider that excretors of pathogenic types of *Esch. coli* should be at once treated with larger than normal oral doses of antibiotics, such as terramycin, 50 mg./lb./day, or neomycin, 50 mg./lb./day. Sensitivity tests should be made on all strains isolated as there is considerable variation in sensitivity of these organisms to antibiotics and sulphonamides.

Summary

Three epidemics of gastro-enteritis due to *Esch. coli* O119 involved 45 babies in one ward. Twenty-seven had symptoms and three died.

The short incubation period and high infectivity rate allowed the occurrence of these epidemics in spite of usual barrier nursing techniques and individual cubicles. Cross-infection was reduced by improved precautions and prompt administration of terramycin to all babies excreting the organism. Sensitivity tests proved useful in the choice of antibiotic. All the O119 strains were resistant to sulphonamide and sensitive to chloramphenicol, aureomycin, streptomycin, neomycin and polymyxin.

In the 18 months' study 3,048 faecal specimens from 894 infants were examined. Apart from the 45 infants in the three *Esch. coli* O119 epidemics another 16 were found to be infected with O119 and 61 with other pathogenic types of *Esch. coli*, including 18 with O128, 15 with O55, nine with O26 and eight with O111.

We wish to thank Dr. I. M. Anderson, Dr. C. F. Harris, the Hon. Mrs. N. O. Richards, Mr. D. Levi and Mr. G. H. Macnab for their help and encouragement and their permission to report on their cases; Dr. Joan Taylor and Dr. J. Smith for much valuable advice and the supply of various typing antisera, and Miss Geraldine Coats for much hard work in performing the biochemical and sensitivity tests.

References

Bray, J. (1945). *J. Path. Bact.*, **57**, 239.
Charter, R. E. (1956). *Ibid.*, **72**, 33.
Cooper, M. L., Walters, E. W., Keller, H. M., Sutherland, J. M. and Wiseman, H. J. (1955). *Pediatrics*, **16**, 215.
Jameson, J. E., Mann, T. P. and Rothfield, N. J. (1954). *Lancet*, **2**, 459.
Jewell, P. and Pearmain, G. E. G. (1954). *J. clin. Path.*, **7**, 308.
Kauffmann, F. (1947). *J. Immunol.*, **57**, 71.
—— (1954). *Enterobacteriaceae*, 2nd ed. Ejnar Munksgaard, Copenhagen.
Rogers, K. B. (1951). *Proc. roy. Soc. Med.*, **44**, 519.
—— and Cracknell, V. M. (1956). *J. Path. Bact.*, **72**, 27.
Smith, J. (1953). *Ibid.*, **66**, 503.
—— (1955). *The Aetiology of Epidemic Infantile Gastro-enteritis.* Royal College of Physicians, Edinburgh.
Taylor, J. and Charter, R. E. (1952). *J. Path. Bact.*, **64**, 715.
Thomas, M. E. M. and Charter, R. E. (1956). *Brit med. J.*, **2**, 339.
Topley, W. W. C. and Wilson, G. S. (1946). *Principles of Bacteriology and Immunity*, 3rd ed. Edward Arnold, London.
Wramby, G. (1948). *Acta path. microbiol. scand.*, Suppl. 76.

BOOK REVIEWS

The Medical Annual. Edited by SIR HENRY TIDY and Prof. R. MILNES WALKER. (Pp. xi +580; 42 plates.) Bristol: John Wright. 1958.

The seventy-sixth issue of the *Medical Annual* will be the last to bear the name of Sir Henry Tidy as medical editor, and the publisher's note rightly deplores his departure and promises an appraisal of his work for the Annual next year.

Two major changes have been made. The alphabetical arrangement according to the title of the article had become clumsy and confusing, and a certain degree of grouping into sections has been introduced, which, the publishers maintain and the reviewer agrees, will make for ease of reference. The second innovation is a series of four special articles before the "Review of the year's work" namely, Intersexuality; Wound infection in operating theatres; Dangers arising from the medical use of x-rays; and Changing emphasis in paediatrics.

These articles are presumably intended as general reviews on chosen subjects of very particular interest and should they be greatly appreciated, and as a result increase in number, it will, to some extent, change the nature of the Annual. They are, as they should be, of a high standard though the last, dealing largely with the changes that have come over the practice of paediatrics as a result of the rapid decline of mortality and morbidity in children, the growth of psychiatry and the infiltration of a more psychological outlook in hospitals, is light-weight stuff compared at least with the first two.

The section on paediatrics seems, to a paediatrician, disproportionately short; nine medical and five surgical pages in a 570-page book leaves little enough room to review even the 14 subjects discussed though these have been usefully chosen. However, subjects of paediatric interest are scattered throughout the Annual ('paediatrics' we are constantly saying, 'is only general medicine for a special age group') and one can read about polio vaccination, the treatment of obesity with a high fat diet, metabolic hypothyroidism, coarctation of the aorta, Hirschsprung's disease and, in a particularly valuable article, rheumatoid arthritis. Here the discussion is of the relation of this condition to others such as disseminated lupus erythematosus and diffuse necrotizing polyarthritis, and of the dangers of hypercortinism, which may induce mesenchymal changes closely resembling either of these two conditions.

Finally, for light reading, there is an account ('instructive', says the Annual) in the section on the urogenital tract on the size of the male urethral meatus in the circumcised and uncircumcised. Apparently this is, on an average, smaller in circumcised adults, and the earlier circumcision is performed the smaller it is! Perhaps this stupendous bit of statistical research will initiate a swing against circumcision in the States similar to that which occurred in this country when the bottom dropped out of circumcision with the advent of the National Health Service.

The Annual ends with the Practitioner's Index and Book of the Year.

Enuresis: A Clinical and Genetic Study. By B. HALLGREN. (Pp. 159.) Copenhagen: E. Munksgaard. 1957.

This monograph contains a tremendous amount of factual material derived from a retrospective study of 111 enuretics treated at a psychiatric clinic in 1945 and a current study of 119 cases in 1952. On the clinical side the aspects studied included the history (85% primary, 15% acquired), sex differences, frequency, age of cessation, depth of sleep and association with emotional disturbances, speech disorders, masturbation, etc. Environmental factors reviewed included social grading, size of family and broken homes. The genetic/statistical section reveals how much work has been put into the study and how disappointingly indefinite have been the results. Many of the conclusions, which paediatricians experienced in the handling of such cases would accept without question, have not been statistically proven partly because of the ever present difficulty of separating heredity and environment and partly because enuretics form a heterogeneous group. Nevertheless, the author concludes that there is a group of genetically determined primary enuretics in whom the symptom may be suppressed by environmental harmony, and that the acquired cases may follow an environmental stimulus. He is on less sure ground when calculating the mode of inheritance but some evidence is given to show that the mechanism is one of simple dominance with incomplete penetrance, the latter probably being mainly influenced by external factors.

This monograph makes no claim to study treatment but a passing reference reveals that only 4·4% of the cases ceased to wet within six months after treatment, i.e. a therapeutic failure rate of 95·6%! It will be invaluable for anyone writing a paper on enuresis but almost valueless to anyone endeavouring to treat the individual case.

Kinderärztliche Notfallfibel, 4th ed. By B. de RUDDER. (Pp. viii+205; 34 figures. DM 18.60.) Stuttgart: Georg Thieme. 1958.

The fourth edition of Professor de Rudder's by now well-known 'aide' to the diagnosis and treatment of medical and surgical emergencies in children has been somewhat expanded. While this increased covering of the subject must improve its value it is to be regretted that, from the point of view of the foreigner to German medicine, the table of drugs and their dosage is composed almost entirely of proprietary names which mean nothing to the reviewer.

INDEX TO VOLUME XXXIII

Abdominal pains, recurrent: field survey of 1,000 school children, 165
ABO incompatibility and haemolytic disease of newborn, 185
Abscess, acute spinal epidural, in infant with recovery, 261
Accra, intraperitoneal blood transfusion in treatment of kwashiorkor in children in, 202
Acidosis, renal, idiopathic, in infancy, prognosis of, 532
Acromegaly in a girl of 8 years, 49
Adenoma, parathyroid, in child presenting as rickets, 46
African children, phlyctenular conjunctivitis in, 292
ALLAN, J. H.: Mineralization of enamel in developing teeth, 182
Allergy to cow's milk in infancy, 265
Amino acids, plasma, in malnutrition, 499
Ammonia production in children, 532
Anaemia, haemolytic, acute acquired, associated with herpes simplex infection, 524
——, ——, associated with acute renal damage in infancy, 181
——, ——, in a child receiving nitrofurantoin, 527
——, ——, thrombotic microangiopathic, 520
Anorexia and severe inanition associated with tumour involving hypothalamus, 257
Antibodies which may be transferred to newborn baby, colostrum and milk as source of, 24
Antistreptolysin reaction in rheumatic children, 529
Aortic arch, congenital interruption of, 131
APLEY, J., and NAISH, N.: Recurrent abdominal pains; a field survey of 1,000 school children, 165
Arch, first, syndrome, 477
Archives of Disease in Childhood, on editing the, 383
ARMATA, J., *see* GIZA, T., and ARMATA, J.
Ataxia, Friedrich's, unusual findings in family with, 217
ATTA, S. B. G. O., *see* OFORI ATTA, S. B. G.
Autism, infantile, 382

B

Basophilic leucocytes in children in health and disease, 193
BENEŠ, V., *see* ELEFANT, E., VOJTA, V., and BENEŠ, V.
Beriberi in 4-month-old infant, 269
BEVERLEY, J.: Stress and pathogenicity of toxoplasma, 182
Bile ducts, intrahepatic, congenital absence of, 396
BISHTON, R. L., SAMES, C.P., and WALLIS, H. R. E.: Calcified mesenteric lymphangioma, 176
Blood transfusion, exchange, clinical and biochemical changes during, 142
—— ——, intraperitoneal, in children in Accra with special reference to treatment of kwashiorkor, 202
BOOK REVIEWS: BREMER, J. L.: Congenital anomalies of the viscera, 1957, 96; CHARNY, C. W., and WOLGIN, W.: Cryptorchism, 1957, 273; DANOWSKI, T. S.: Diabetes mellitus, 1957, 183; DAVISON, W. C., and LEVINTHAL, J. D.: The compleat pediatrician, 1958, 487; DELTHIL, P.: Les regimes du nourrisson bien portant ou malade, 1957, 274; DOUGLAS, J. W. B., and BLOMFIELD, J. M.: Children under five, 1958, 488; DUHAMEL, B., and SEGAUX, S.: Technique chirurgicale infantile, 1957, 487; DUHAMEL, J.: Affections non congénitales de l'anus et du rectum chez l'enfant, 1958, 384; EVANS, P., and MAC KEITH, R.: Infant feeding and feeding difficulties, 3rd edit., 1958, 274; FERGUSON, A. B., *et al.*: Orthopedic surgery in infancy and childhood, 1957, 272; GETZ, S. B., and REES, E. L.: The mentally ill child, 1957, 96; GUILLEMINET, M., and RICARD, R.: Pseudarthrose congénitale du tibia et son traitement, 1958, 384; HALLGREN, B.: Enuresis, 1957, 552; HINDEN, E.: A primer of paediatrics, 1957, 183; KAUFMANN, R.: Chirurgie préventive de la tuberculose ostéo-articulaire, 1958, 273; KJELLBERG, S. R., ERICSSON, N. O., and RUDHE, U.: The lower urinary tract in childhood, 1958, 274; KLEIN, M. R.: Hydrocéphalie du nourrison, 1958, 384; LIPPMAN, H. S.: Treatment of the child in emotional conflict, 1956, 275; LORAINE, J. A.: Clinical application of hormone assay, 1958, 274; Medical Annual, 1958, 552; MICHAUD, L., and DUCHÉ, D. J.: L'enfant inadapté, 1957, 276; MINSKI, L.: Deafness, mutism and mental deficiency in children, 1957, 275; MORLEY, M. E.: Cleft palate and speech, 4th edit., 1958, 276; New Zealand Commission of Inquiry. Fluoridation of public water supplies, 1957, 276; Paediatrics. Supplement, 1957, 272; ROBERTS, G. F.: Comparative aspects of haemolytic disease of the newborn, 1957, 384; RUDDER, B. de: Kinderärztliche Notfallfibel, 1958, 552; SCHAUFFLER, G. C.: Pediatric gynecology, 4th edit., 1958, 487; SPEER, F.: The management of childhood asthma, 1958, 487; VEEDER, B. S., *ed.*: Pediatric profiles, 1957, 272; WILKINS, L.: The diagnosis and treatment of endocrine disorders in childhood and adolescence, 2nd edit., 1957, 184; WISSLER, H.: Aktuelle Problem der Kindertuberkulose, 1958, 488; Year book of pediatrics, 1957-58, 272
BOORMAN, K. E., DODD, B. E., and GUNTHER, M.: A consideration of colostrum and milk as sources of antibodies which may be transferred to the newborn baby, 24
BOTHA, G. S. M.: The gastro-oesophageal region in infants, 78
Bowel negativism, implications of, in psychogenic megacolon in children, 371
BRETTELL, R. O., *see* GAIRDNER, D., MARKS, J., ROSCOE, J. D., and BRETTELL, R. O.
British Paediatric Association, 29th Annual General Meeting, 381
Bromide partition test in diagnosis of non-purulent meningitis, 440
Bronchiectasis in childhood, prognosis of, 19
BROWN, G. A., *see* WEEKS, M. M., and BROWN, G. A.
BUCHANAN, E. U., and KOMROWER, G. M.: The prognosis of idiopathic renal acidosis in infancy with observations on urine acidification and ammonia production in children, 532
BUCHANAN, M. F. G., *see* CRAIG, W. S., and BUCHANAN, M. F. G.
BULBROOK, R. D., GREENWOOD, F. C., and SNAITH, A. H.: Hormone excretion in precocious puberty in girls, 295
Burma, Upper, physical development of school girls in, 452
BURMAN, D.: Congenital spherocytosis in infancy, 335
BYWATERS, E. G. L., *see* HALLIDIE-SMITH, K. A., and BYWATERS, E. G. L.

C

Cardiovascular disease, congenital, during first year of life, electrocardiographic recognition of ventricular hypertrophy in, 346
Caries, dental, prevalence of, in relation to maturity, 455
CATHIE, I. A. B.: On editing the *Archives*, 383
CHEEK, D. B., and PERRY, J. W.: A salt wasting syndrome in infancy, 252
Chinese children, pneumatosis intestinalis, 445
CLAIREAUX, A. E., and FERREIRA, H. P.: Bilateral pulmonary agenesis, 364
COATES, S., *see* WOOLF, L. I., *et al.*
Coeliac disease, test for, 413
COGHLAN, M. K., and JOSEPH, M. C.: The disappearance of foetal haemoglobin in congenital cyanotic heart disease, 191
COLLINS, J.: Pancreatitis in young children, 432
Colon, neonatal perforation of, 362
Colostrum as source of antibodies which may be transferred to newborn baby, 24
Conjunctivitis, phlyctenular, in African children, 292
COOPER, C. E., and GRIFFIN, S.: Oesophageal stricture secondary to hiatus hernia, 383
CRAIG, W. S., and BUCHANAN, M. F. G.: Hypocalcaemic tetany developing within 36 hours of birth, 505
CRAVIOTO, J., *see* WESTALL, R. G., *et al.*
C-reactive protein determination in rheumatic children, 529
CROME, L., and SYLVESTER, P. E.: Hydranencephaly, 235
CROMPTON, C. W., *see* MAXWELL, G. M., ROWE, G. G., and CRUMPTON, C. W.
CROSSE, V. M., WALLIS, P. G., and WALSH, A. M.: Replacement transfusion as a means of preventing kernikterus of prematurity, 403
Cushing's syndrome in infant, 540

D

DAVIES, W.: Cow's milk allergy in infancy, 265
Deafness following maternal rubella; results of a prospective survey, 383
Dental caries, prevalence of, in relation to maturity, 455
Dermoid cyst, intracranial, associated with Klippel-Feil deformity and recurrent meningitis, 222
Development, assessment of, dissociation as guide to, 118
—— in children of very low birth weight, 10
Diabetes insipidus following tuberculous meningitis, 315
—— mellitus in child showing features of Refsum's syndrome, 320
Diabetic and non-diabetic women, postnatal weight loss of babies born to, 323
Diarrhoea, infantile, jaundice and, 330
Diastematomyelia, 536
DILLISTONE, F., *see* WOOLF, L. I., *et al.*
Dissociation as guide to developmental assessment, 118
DOBBS, R. H., *see* HAAS, L., and DOBBS, R. H.
DODD, B. E., *see* BOORMAN, K. E., DODD, B. E., and GUNTHER, M.
DRILLIEN, C. M.: Growth and development in a group of children of very low birth weight, 10
——: A longitudinal study of the growth and development of prematurely and maturely born children, 417, 423
Dwarfism, pituitary, autopsy findings in case of, 469
Dysautonomia, familial, 465
Dysmaturity, 123

E

EDEN, A. R., *see* ROBINSON, M. J., ORCHARD, N.P., and EDEN, A. R.
EDWARDS, M. S., GRIFFITHS, L. L., and SWIFT, P. N.: Cellular immunity at birth, 512
Electrophoresis, paper, of serum proteins in children, 61
ELEFANT, E., VOJTA, V., and BENEŠ, V.: Intraspinal neuroblastoma in a newborn baby, 212
EMERY, J. L., JOWETT, G. H., and MACDONALD, M. S.: Postnatal changes in glomeruli in the kidney, 182
Emphysema, regional obstructive, in infancy, 97
Enamel, mineralization of, in developing teeth, 182
ENGLESON, G., *see* SJÖSTEDT, S., ENGLESON, G., and ROOTH, G.
Enuresis, persistent, treatment with the electric buzzer, 160
ERICSSON, N. O., and IVEMARK, B. I.: Renal dysplasia and pyelonephritis in infants and children, 181
Erythema nodosum in children, changing aetiology of, 137
Erythrocyte sedimentation rate in rheumatic children, 529
Esch. coli O119 infection, epidemic of gastro-enteritis associated with, 543

F

FALKNER, F.: Some physical measurements in the first three years of life, 1
FARQUHAR, J. W., and SKLAROFF, S. A.: The postnatal weight loss of babies born to diabetic and non-diabetic women, 323
——, and SMITH, H.: Clinical and biochemical changes during exchange transfusion, 142
FAWNS, H. T., *see* NICOLS, V. S., and FAWNS, H. T.
Femur, traumatic subperiosteal haematoma of, in newborn, 205
FERREIRA, H. P., *see* CLAIREAUX, A. E., and FERREIRA, H. P.
Fibrinogen level in rheumatic children, 529
Fibrocystic disease, sweat analysis in, 74
FINDLAY, M., *see* GRIFFITHS, S. B., and FINDLAY, M.
First arch syndrome, 477
FISCH, L., *see* JACKSON, A. D. M., and FISCH, L.
Fluid shift from vascular compartment immediately after birth, 489
FOLEY, B. V.: Congenital interruption of aortic arch, 131
FOLL, C. V.: Physical development of schoolgirls in Upper Burma, 452
FORFAR, J. O., *see* THOMSON, J., and FORFAR, J. O.
FORSYTH, C. C., *see* PAYNE, W. W., and FORSYTH, C. C.
FRANKLIN, A. W.: The prognosis of bronchiectasis in childhood, 19
FREIMAN, I., *see* STEIN, H., and FREIMAN, I.
Friedrich's ataxia, unusual findings in family with, 217

G

GAIRDNER, D., MARKS, J., ROSCOE, J. D., and BRETTELL, R. O.: The fluid shift from the vascular compartment immediately after birth, 489
GAISFORD, W.: Poliomyelitis vaccination of newborn infants, 383
GARDNER, R., and SNAITH, A. H.: The urinary excretion of 17-hydroxysteroids in children, 305
Gargoylism; clinical, radiological and haematological features in two siblings, 229
Gastro-enteritis associated with *Esch. coli* O119 infection, epidemic of, 543
Gastro-oesophageal region in infants, anatomy of, with special reference to closing mechanism and partial thoracic stomach, 78
GEORGE, W. H., *see* WOOD, B. S. B., GEORGE, W. H., and ROBINSON, A. W.
GIZA, T., and ARMATA, J.: Frank beriberi in a 4-month-old infant, 269

Glucuronide formation, insufficient, in newborn and its relationship to pathogenesis of icterus neonatorum, 473
GOLDBLATT, E., and SNAITH, A. H.: Case of Cushing's syndrome in an infant, 540
GOMEZ, F., *see* WESTALL, R. G., *et al.*
GREENWOOD, F. C., *see* BULBROOK, R. D., GREENWOOD, F. C., and SNAITH, A. H.
GRIFFIN, S., *see* COOPER, C. E., and GRIFFIN, S.
GRIFFITHS, L. L., *see* EDWARDS, M. S., GRIFFITHS, L. L., and SWIFT, P. N.
GRIFFITHS, R., *see* WOOLF, L. I., *et al.*
GRIFFITHS, S. B., and FINDLAY, M.: Gargoylism: clinical, radiological and haematological features in two siblings, 229
Growth and development of prematurely and maturely born children, longitudinal study of, 417, 423
—— in children of very low birth weight, 10
Gumma of liver in congenital syphilis, 58
GUNTHER, M., *see* BOORMAN, K. E., DODD, B. E., and GUNTHER, M.
——, *see also* HASSAN, F., and GUNTHER, M.

H

HAAS, L.: Neonatal perforation of colon, 362
——, and DOBBS, R. H.: Congenital absence of the intrahepatic bile ducts, 396
Haemangioma, subglottic: two infants with laryngeal stridor, 210
Haematoma, traumatic subperiosteal, of femur in newborn, 205
Haemoglobin, foetal, disappearance of, in congenital cyanotic heart disease, 191
Haemolytic disease of newborn, ABO incompatibility and, 185
HALLIDIE-SMITH, K. A., and BYWATERS, E. G. L.: The differential diagnosis of rheumatic fever, 350
Hartnup disease, case of, 114
HASSAN, F. and GUNTHER, M. The serum proteins at 6 months of age in infants fed on human or cow's milk or on both, 30
Head, first arch syndrome, 477
Heart, auricular-ventricular dissociation, and Wenckebach phenomenon in children, 236
—— disease, congenital cyanotic, disappearance of foetal haemoglobin in, 191
——, ——, ——, in one of identical twins, 342
——, normal diameter of, in radiographs of preschool children, 134
——, ventricular hypertrophy in congenital cardiovascular disease during first year of life, electrocardiographic recognition of, 346
——, —— septal defect in infants, clinical and haemodynamic study of, 67
Heberden's cases of anaphylactoid purpura, 271
HENDERSON, W.: A case of Hartnup disease, 114
Hernia, hiatus, oesophageal stricture secondary to, 383
Herpes simplex infection, acute acquired haemolytic anaemia associated with, 524
—— zoster ophthalmicus in children, 437
HEWITT, D.: Normal diameter of the heart in radiographs of pre-school children, 134
HEYCOCK, J. B., and WILSON, J.: Diabetes mellitus in a child showing features of Refsum's syndrome, 320
Hiatus in infants, 82
HOLBOROW, C. A.: Subglottic haemangioma, 210
HOLDEN, H. M., *see* MISCH, K. A., and HOLDEN, H. M.
HOLT, L. E., jun., *see* WESTALL, R. G., *et al.*
Hormone excretion in precocious puberty in girls, 295
HUGH-JONES, K., and ROSS, G. I. M.: Epidemics of gastro-enteritis associated with *Esch. coli* O119 infection, 543
HUSAIN, O. A. N., *see* WELCH, R. G., and HUSAIN, O. A. N.
Hydranencephaly, 235
Hydrocephalus, natural history of, 383
α-hydroxy-butyric acid and phenylpyruvic acid, inborn error of metabolism with urinary excretion of, 109
Hypercalcaemia, infantile, severe, with special reference to the facies, 385
Hypertension, essential, changes in placenta, in, 182
Hypocalcaemic tetany developing within 36 hours of birth, 505
Hypothalamus, tumour involving, anorexia and severe inanition associated with, 257

I

Icterus neonatorum, insufficient glucuronide formation in newborn and its relationship to pathogenesis of, 473
ILLINGWORTH, R. S.: Dissociation as guide to developmental assessment, 118
Immunity, cellular, at birth, 512
Inanition, severe, and anorexia associated with tumour involving hypothalamus, 257
Infants, newborn, colostrum and milk as source of antibodies which may be transferred to, 24
——, ——, haemolytic disease of, ABO incompatibility and, 185
——, ——, hypocalcaemic tetany in, 505
——, ——, insufficient glucuronide formation in, and its relationship to pathogenesis of icterus neonatorum, 473
——, ——, intraspinal neuroblastoma in, 212
——, ——, meningitis in, small outbreak in maternity unit, 358
——, ——, perforation of colon in, 362
——, ——, poliomyelitis vaccination of, 383
——, ——, traumatic subperiosteal haematoma of femur in, 205
——, ——, urinary infection in, diagnosis of, 382
IVEMARK, B. I., *see* ERICSSON, N. C., and IVEMARK, B. I.

J

JACKSON, A. D. M., and FISCH, L.: Deafness following maternal rubella, 383
JAMES, C. C. M., and LASSMANN, L. P.: Diastematomyelia, 536
JAMES, U.: The diagnosis of urinary infection in the newborn, 382
Jaundice and infantile diarrhoea, 330
JENKINSON, V., *see* PAYNE, W. W., and JENKINSON, V.
JOLLY, H., and LAMONT, E. M.: Sirenomelia, 226
JONES, H. E.: Congenital heart disease in one of identical twins, 342
JOSEPH, M. C., and PARROTT, D.: Severe infantile hypercalcaemia with special reference to the facies, 385
——, *see also* COGHLAN, M. K., and JOSEPH, M. C.
JOWETT, G. H., *see* EMERY, J. L., JOWETT, G. H., and MACDONALD, M. S.

K

KAGAN, H.: Anorexia and severe inanition associated with a tumour involving the hypothalamus, 257
Kanner's syndrome, 328
Kernikterus of prematurity, replacement transfusion as means of preventing, 403
17-ketosteroids, urinary excretion of, in children, 301
Kidneys, acidosis, idiopathic, in infancy, prognosis of, and urine acidification and ammonia production, 532
——, acute damage of, in infancy, haemolytic anaemia associated with, 181
——, dysplasia of, and pyelonephritis in infants and children, 181
——, glomeruli of, postnatal changes in, 182

Klippel-Feil deformity and recurrent meningitis, intracranial dermoid cyst associated with, 222
KOMROWER, G. M., *see* BUCHANAN, E. U., and KOMROWER, G. M.
Kwashiorkor, intraperitoneal blood transfusion in treatment of, in children in Accra, 202

L

LA PEÑA, C. DE, *see* WESTALL, R. G., *et al.*
LAMONT, E. M., *see* JOLLY, H., and LAMONT, E. M.
LASSMAN, L. P., *see* JAMES, C. C. M., and LASSMAN, L. P.
LAURENCE, K. M.: The natural history of hydrocephalus, 383
Leucocytes, basophilic, in children in health and disease, 193
LEVY, D., and PORGESS, A.: Haemolytic anaemia in child receiving nitrofurantoin, 527
Liver, gumma of, in congenital syphilis, 58
LORBER, J.: Changing aetiology of erythema nodosum in children, 137
——: Diabetes insipidus following tuberculous meningitis, 315
Lungs, agenesis, bilateral, 365
——, chronic disease of, sweat analysis in, 74
Lymphangioma, mesenteric, calcified, 176

M

MACDONALD, M. S., *see* EMERY, J. L., JOWETT, G. H., and MACDONALD, M. S.
MACFARLANE, A., and MACGREGOR, A. R.: Malignant non-chromaffin paraganglioma of thigh, 55
MACFARLANE, P. S.: Haemolytic anaemia associated with acute renal damage in infancy, 181
MACFARLANE, W. V., *see* WHITEHOUSE, D., and MACFARLANE, W. V.
MACGREGOR, A. R., *see* MACFARLANE, A., and MACGREGOR, A. R.
MACGREGOR, M.: Osteomyelitis variolosa, 383
——: Paediatrics in Western Nigeria, 277
MCKAY, E., and SMITH, J.: A small outbreak of neonatal meningitis in a maternity unit, 358
MCKENDRICK, T.: Familial dysautonomia, 465
MCKENZIE, J.: The first arch syndrome, 477
Malnutrition, plasma amino acids in, 499
MANSBRIDGE, J. N.: The prevalence of dental caries in relation to maturity, 455
MARKS, J., *see* GAIRDNER, D., MARKS, J., ROSCOE, J. D., and BRETTELL, R. O.
MARTIN, P. B., *see* RUSHWORTH, R. G., and MARTIN, P.B.
MAXWELL, G. M., ROWE, G. G., and CRUMPTON, C. W.: A clinical and haemodynamic study of ventricular septal defect in infants, 67
Measurements, physical, in first three years of life, 1
Megacolon, psychogenic, in children: implications of bowel negativism, 371
Meningitis, neonatal, small outbreak of, in a maternity unit, 358
——, non-purulent, bromide partition test in diagnosis of, 440
——, recurrent, and Klippel-Feil deformity, intracranial dermoid cyst associated with, 222
——, Salmonella, 171
——, tuberculous, diabetes insipidus following, 315
"Mermaid", 226
Mesenteric lymphangioma, calcified, 176
Metabolism, inborn error of, with urinary excretion of α-hydroxy-butyric acid and phenylpyruvic acid, 109
Milk as source of antibodies which may be transferred to newborn baby, 24
——, cow's, allergy in infancy, 265
——, human or cow's, or on both, serum proteins at 6 months of age in infants fed on, 30
MISCH, K. A., and HOLDEN, H. M.: Sweat test for the diagnosis of fibrocystic disease of pancreas, 179
MITCHELL, R. G.: Basophilic leucocytes in children in health and disease, 193
——, and RHANEY, K.: Traumatic subperiosteal haematoma of the femur in the newborn, 205
MONCRIEFF, A., *see* WOOLF, L. I., *et al.*
MUIR, C. S.: Pneumatosis intestinalis in Chinese children, 445
MULLINS, A. G.: The prognosis in juvenile obesity, 307

N

NAISH, N., *see* APLEY, J., and NAISH, N.
Neuroblastoma, intraspinal, in newborn baby, 212
Newborn infants, haemolytic disease of, ABO incompatibility and, 185
—— ——, hypocalcaemic tetany in, 505
—— ——, insufficient glucuronide formation in, and its relationship to pathogenesis of icterus neonatorum, 473
—— ——, intraspinal neuroblastoma in, 212
—— ——, meningitis in, small outbreak in maternity unit, 358
—— ——, milk and colostrum as source of antibodies which may be transferred to, 24
—— ——, perforation of colon in, 362
—— ——, poliomyelitis vaccination of, 383
—— ——, traumatic subperiosteal haematoma of femur in, 205
—— ——, urinary infection in, diagnosis of, 382
NICOL, V. S., and FAWNS, H. T.: Observations on the bromide partition test in the diagnosis of non-purulent meningitis, 440
Nigeria, Western, paediatrics in, 277
Nitrofurantoin, haemolytic anaemia in child receiving, 527

O

Obesity, juvenile, prognosis in, 307
O'DONOHOE, N. V., *see* TODD, R. MCL., and O'DONOHOE, N. V.
Oesophagus and stomach, closing mechanism between infants, 78
——, atresia of, with common tracheo-oesophageal tube, 367
——, congenital short, 89
——, stricture of, secondary to hiatus hernia, 383
OFORI ATTA, S. B. G.: Intraperitoneal blood transfusion in children in Accra with special reference to the treatment of kwashiorkor, 202
OLDHAM, J. S.: The electrocardiographic recognition of ventricular hypertrophy in congenital cardiovascular disease during the first year of life, 346
ORCHARD, N. P., *see* ROBINSON, M. J., ORCHARD, N. P., and EDEN, A. R.
Osteomyelitis variolosa, 383

P

Paediatric Pathology Club, Proceedings of 3rd Annual Meeting, 181
—— societies in British Isles, 95
Paediatrics in Western Nigeria, 277
PAINE, C. G.: Changes in the placenta with particular reference to essential hypertension and pre-eclamptic toxaemia, 182
Pancreas, fibrocystic disease of, sweat test for diagnosis of, 179
Pancreatitis in young children, 432
Paraganglioma, malignant non-chromaffin, of thigh, 55
Parathyroid adenoma in child presenting as rickets, 46
PARKER, R. G. F.: Jaundice and infantile diarrhoea, 330

PARROTT, D., *see* JOSEPH, M. C., and PARROTT, D.
PAYNE, W. W., and FORSYTH, C. C.: Paper electrophoresis of serum proteins in children, 61
——, and JENKINSON, V.: A test for coeliac disease, 413
PERRY, J. W., *see* CHEEK, D. B., and PERRY, J. W.
Phagocytic response, mechanism and nature of, 512
Phenylketonuria, dietary treatment of, 31
Phenylpyruvic acid and α-hydroxy-butyric acid, inborn error of metabolism with urinary excretion of, 109
Phreno-oesophageal membrane in infants, 83
PINKERTON, P.: Psychogenic megacolon in children: the implications of bowel negativism, 371
Pituitary dwarfism, autopsy findings in, 469
Placenta, changes in, with particular reference to essential hypertension and pre-eclamptic toxaemia, 182
Plasma amino acids in malnutrition, 499
Pneumatosis intestinalis in Chinese children, 445
Poliomyelitis vaccination of newborn infants, 383
POPOV, N., and STANISHEVA, S.: Erythrocyte sedimentation rate, C-reactive protein determination, serum protein fractions, fibrinogen level and antistreptolysin reaction in 52 rheumatic children, 529
PORGESS, A., *see* LEVY, D., and PORGESS, A.
Prematurely born children, growth and development of, 417, 423
Prematurity, kernikterus of, replacement transfusion as means of preventing, 403
Proteins, serum, at 6 months of age in infants fed on human or cow's milk or both, 30
——, ——, in children, paper electrophoresis of, 61
PROUT, M., and SNAITH, A. H.: Urinary excretion of 17-ketosteroids in children, 301
Puberty, precocious, in girls, hormone excretion in, 295
PUGH, R. C. B.: Pyelonephritis, 181
Purpura, anaphylactoid, William Heberden's cases of, 271
Pyelonephritis, 181
——, renal dysplasia and, in infants and children, 181

R

RASMUSSEN, H., *see* WESTALL, R. G., *et al.*
Refsum's syndrome, diabetes mellitus in child showing features of, 320
RHANEY, K., *see* MITCHELL, R. G., and RHANEY, K.
Rheumatic children, erythrocyte sedimentation rate, C-reactive protein determination, serum protein fractions, fibrinogen level and anti-streptolysin reaction in, 529
—— fever, differential diagnosis, 350
Rickets, parathyroid adenoma in child presenting as, 46
ROBERTS, A. P.: Case of intracranial dermoid cyst associated with the Klippel-Feil deformity and recurrent meningitis, 222
ROBINSON, A. W., *see* WOOD, B. S. B., GEORGE, W. H., and ROBINSON, A. W.
ROBINSON, M. J., ORCHARD, N. P., and EDEN, A. R.: Thrombotic microangiopathic haemolytic anaemia, 520
ROITMAN, E., *see* WESTALL, R. G., *et al.*
ROOK, A.: William Heberden's cases of anaphylactoid purpura, 271
ROOTH, G., *see* SJÖSTEDT, S., ENGLESON, G., and ROOTH, G.
ROSCOE, J. D., *see* GAIRDNER, D., MARKS, J., ROSCOE, J. D., and BRETTELL, R. O.
ROSS, G. I. M., *see* HUGH-JONES, K., and ROSS, G. I. M.
ROSSI, M., *see* TOLENTINO, P., and ROSSI, M.
ROWE, G. G., *see* MAXWELL, G. M., ROWE, G. G., and CRUMPTON, C. W.
Rubella, maternal, deafness following: results of prospective survey, 383
RUSHWORTH, R. G., and MARTIN, P. B.: Acute spinal epidural abscess, 261

S

Salmonella meningitis, 171
Salt wasting syndrome in infancy, 252
SAMES, C. P., *see* BISHTON, R. L., SAMES, C. P., and WALLIS, H. R. E.
SANDISON, A. T.: Autopsy findings in a case of pituitary dwarfism, 469
Schoolgirls, physical development of, in Upper Burma, 452
Serum protein fractions in rheumatic children, 529
—— proteins at 6 months of age in infants fed on human or cow's milk or on both, 30
—— —— in children, paper electrophoresis of, 61
—— transaminase variations in childhood, 409
SHNIER, M. H.: The Wenckebach phenomenon and auricular-ventricular dissociation in children, 236
Sirenomelia, 226
SJÖSTEDT, S., ENGLESON, G., and ROOTH, G.: Dysmaturity, 123
SKLAROFF, S. A., *see* FARQUHAR, J. W., and SKLAROFF, S. A.
SMELLIE, J.: The effect on the infant of large therapeutic doses of vitamin D given to the mother throughout pregnancy, 383
SMITH, A. J., and STRANG, L. B.: An inborn error of metabolism with the urinary excretion of α-hydroxy-butyric acid and phenylpyruvic acid, 109
SMITH, H., *see* FARQUHAR, J. W., and SMITH, H.
SMITH, J., *see* MCKAY, E., and SMITH, J.
SNAITH, A. H., *see* BULBROOK, R. D., GREENWOOD, F. C., and SNAITH, A. H.
——, *see also* GARDNER, R., and SNAITH, A. H.
——, *see also* GOLDBLATT, E., and SNAITH, A. H.
——, *see also* PROUT, M., and SNAITH, A. H.
Spherocytosis, congenital, in infancy, 335
Spine, acute epidural abscess; case in infant with recovery, 261
——, neuroblastoma in, in newborn baby, 212
STANISHEVA, S., *see* POPOV, N., and STANISHEVA, S.
STEIN, H., and FREIMAN, I.: Phlyctenular conjunctivitis in African Children, 292
Stomach and oesophagus, closing mechanism between, in infants, 78
——, partial thoracic, in infants, 78
STONE, F. H.: Infantile autism, 328
STRANG, L. B., *see* SMITH, A. J., and STRANG, L. B.
Stridor, laryngeal, subglottic haemangioma in two infants, 210
Sweat analysis in fibrocystic disease, chronic pulmonary disease, and controls, 74
SWIFT, P. N., *see* EDWARDS, M. S., GRIFFITHS, L. L., and SWIFT, P. N.
SYLVESTER, P. E.: Some unusual findings in a family with Friedrich's ataxia, 217
——, *see also* CROME, L., and SYLVESTER, P. E.
Sympus dipus, 226
Syphilis, congenital, gumma of liver in, 58

T

Teeth, developing, mineralization of enamel in, 182
Tetany, hypocalcaemic, developing within 36 hours of birth, 505
Thigh, malignant non-chromaffin paraganglioma of, 55
THOMSON, J., and FORFAR, J. O.: Regional obstructive emphysema in infancy, 97
TODD, R. MCL.: Acromegaly in a girl of 8 years, 49
——, and O'DONOHOE, N. V.: Acute acquired haemolytic anaemia associated with herpes simplex infection, 524
TOLENTINO, P., and ROSSI, M.: Serum transaminase variations in childhood, 409

Toxaemia, pre-eclamptic, changes in placenta in, 182
Toxoplasma, stress and pathogenicity of, 182
Tracheo-oesophageal tube, common, in atresia of the oesophagus, 367
Transaminase, serum, variations in childhood, 409
Transfusion, exchange, clinical and biochemical changes during, 142
Tuberculous meningitis, diabetes insipidus following, 315
TUCKER, S. M.: Herpes zoster ophthalmicus in children, 437
Twins, identical, congenital heart disease in one of, 342

U

Urinary infection in newborn, diagnosis of, 382
Urine acidification in children, 532

V

VALENTINE, G. H.: ABO incompatibility and haemolytic disease of newborn, 185
Vascular compartment, fluid shift from, immediately after birth, 489
VEST, M.: Insufficient glucuronide formation in the newborn and its relationship to the pathogenesis of icterus neonatorum, 473
Vitamin D, large therapeutic doses of, given to mother during pregnancy, effect on infant, 383
VOJTA, V., *see* ELEFANT, E., VOJTA, V., and BENEŠ, V.

W

WALLIS, H. R. E., *see* BISHTON, R. L., SAMES, C. P., and WALLIS, H. R. E.
WALLIS, P. G., *see* CROSSE, V. M., WALLIS, P. G., and WALSH, A. M.
WALSH, A. M., *see* CROSSE, V. M., WALLIS, P. G., and WALSH, A. M.
WATSON, K. C.: Salmonella meningitis, 171
WEEKS, M. M., and BROWN, G. A.: Sweat analysis in fibrocystic disease, chronic pulmonary disease and controls, 74
Weight loss, postnatal, of babies born to diabetic and non-diabetic women, 323
WELCH, R. G., and HUSAIN, O. A. N.: Atresia of the oesophagus with common tracheo-oesophageal tube, 367
Wenckebach phenomenon and auricular-ventricular dissociation in children, 236
WESTALL, R. G., *et al.*: The plasma amino acids in malnutrition: preliminary observations, 499
WHITEHOUSE, D., and MACFARLANE, W. V.: Gumma of the liver in congenital syphilis, 58
WICKES, I. G.: Treatment of persistent enuresis with the electric buzzer, 160
WILSON, J., *see* HEYCOCK, J. B., and WILSON, J.
WOOD, B. S. B., GEORGE, W. H., and ROBINSON, A. W.: Parathyroid adenoma in a child presenting as rickets, 46
WOOLF, L. I., *et al.*: The dietary treatment of phenylketonuria, 31

PRINTED IN GREAT BRITAIN BY HEADLEY BROTHERS LTD
109 KINGSWAY LONDON WC2 AND ASHFORD KENT